FUNDAMENTALS OF VETERINARY CLINICAL NEUROLOGY

FUNDAMENTALS OF VETERINARY CLINICAL NEUROLOGY

Rodney S. Bagley, DVM

WILEY Blackwell

Fundamentals of Veterinary Clinical Neurology

Authorized reprint by Wiley India Pvt. Ltd., 4435-36/7, Ansari Road, Daryaganj, New Delhi – 110002.

Reprint: 2014

Printed at: Beekam Print & Pack, Delhi.

ISBN: 978-81-265-5251-1

To my wife Lynn and children Joshua, Jessica, and Jordan

Contents

Disclaimer

As with all clinical medicine, the recommendations in this text may not be valid in individual patient situations, as no written text can predict all the individual nuances of clinical medicine. Additionally, as information regarding disease processes develops, evolves, and improves, treatment options may change. Depending upon when current information is available, the recommendations in this text may not be valid. Similarly, drug doses may be different from those stated here.

It is the responsibility of the primary care veterinarian to use the information contained in this text as a guide only, because any patient's unique abnormalities may require a diagnostic and treatment strategy that is individualized for that patient and may be necessarily different from the recommendations described in this book.

Preface

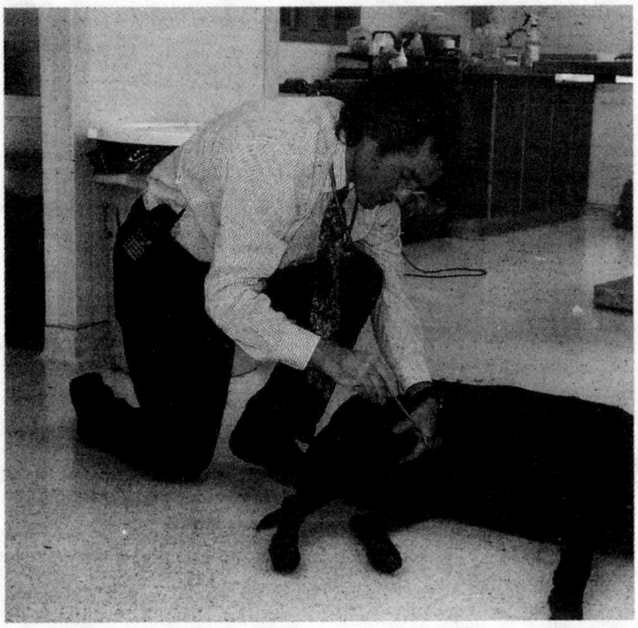

Veterinary neurology is one of the most dynamic subspecialties within the veterinary profession. No longer is neurology a "localize and euthanize" specialty. Owners now demand to have their animals made better. The advent of advanced imaging studies such as magnetic resonance (MR) imaging has revolutionized the antemortem diagnosis of animals and allows us to "see" what is going on inside the animal's nervous system. Innovative treatments, specifically in neurosurgery, can now be logically expanded and developed. All of these aspects of clinical neurology lead to an encouraging future in evaluation of animals with neurologic disease.

Animals with neurologic disease present some of the most daunting challenges in clinical practice. Teaching and learning the skills necessary to perform appropriate clinical neurologic judgments requires a basic understanding of pathophysiology of neurologic disease. Factual knowledge of disease processes and characteristics is a prerequisite for clinical integration and disease diagnosis. *Fundamentals of Veterinary Clinical Neurology* is envisioned to be used as a guide for veterinary students and veterinarians in general clinical practice in the learning (or relearning) about clinical diagnosis and management of small animals with diseases involving the nervous system. For the teacher of veterinary neurology, this book can be used as a framework for educating veterinary students in the clinical thought processing necessary for clinical evaluation of animals with neurologic disease.

The book is organized in a manner similar to how a veterinary clinician would approach evaluation of an animal with suspected neurologic disease. The initial chapters review fundamental aspects of neuroanatomy and physiology that are helpful when attempting clinical neurologic evaluation. These initial chapters are followed by discussion of the neurologic examination, neuroanatomical diagnosis, differential diagnosis, diagnostic testing, and treatment of animals with neurologic disease. For day-to-day clinical neurologic evaluations, important general aspects of disease types and presentations are often necessary. The disease chapters are designed to provide an overview of scope and clinical signs of disease processes that affect the nervous system. References are provided in the bibliographies that can be consulted when the specific information is needed and to allow the interested reader to find both historical and more in-depth information on diseases and their diagnosis and treatment.

This book was specifically written as an educational resource for veterinary students and clinical veterinarians and has grown out of my educational experiences teaching veterinary neurology to veterinary students, interns, and residents. Remember that the best clinicians are always skeptical of the "truth," and that you are only as good as your differential list.

Acknowledgments

This book is a humble summary of countless contributions, and while I may be credited with the effort, my role is more of an observer, scribe, and educator. First, this book could not have been possible without the numerous individuals who have made observations of neurologic disease and then had the courage to write about these experiences in manuscript articles, books, proceedings, and abstracts. Also, many of these same individuals had the courage to speak and lecture in continuing education forums so that we all could learn from what they knew or thought. All of these experiences and communications allow for us all to have more knowledge so that we can serve our patients better. I have endeavored to include as many of these contributions as references as possible, but I realize that some of these contributions may have been missed or inadvertently left out. This should be viewed only as my error and omission, and not a reflection of the quality of the contribution.

Second, there are many individuals who helped with the physical processing of this book. These individuals may have read or typed parts of the chapters, which helped immensely in the physical labor of putting a book such as this together. Specifically, Theresa Pfaff, Robyn Fry, Lynn Bagley, and Drs. Chad West and Annie Chen. Thanks to Charles Leathers for the anatomical spinal sections, and Henry Moore and the others at the biomedical communications unit at Washington State University for photographic artistry and processing. Included in the editors are the hundreds of veterinary students at Washington State who used a prototype of this book and have given feedback and advice on how to make it better. In addition, copy editor Carol Kromminga and all of the individuals at Blackwell Publishing including Antonia Seymour, Lynne Bishop, and Jamie Johnson have spent an incredible amount of time and effort to product this book.

Professionally, there are a number of individuals who have either encouraged me or provided me with opportunities to grow in veterinary medicine. Robert (Bob) Martin at Virginia Tech helped me get my foot in the door of Cornell for my internship. Sharon Center taught me that veterinary medicine was limitless. John Randolph taught me about precision and dedication to patient evaluation. William Hornbuckle taught me the practical realities of getting the job done. Joe Kornegay and Simon Wheeler taught me the nuts and bolts of veterinary neurology and, specifically, neurosurgery. Pat Gavin at WSU has been a great colleague and friend who allowed my academic career to flourish. We have learned a lot together. And, finally, thanks to Dr. Alexander de Lahunta, the ultimate veterinary educator and role model.

I have been lucky to be associated with the neurologic education of a number of residents: in neurology, Drs. Mike Harrington, Gena Silver, and Sean Sanders, as well as my residents Chad West and Annie Chen. They are my driving force in veterinary neurologic education, and they have advanced my learning in new and different ways. Finally, I have been lucky to have had the support, throughout my career, of my wife, Lynn, and our three wonderful children, Joshua, Jessica, and Jordan. As my friend Ron Sande once told me, the three most important letters after your name aren't "DVM," they're "DAD." Thank you to all of you.

I Fundamentals of Clinical Evaluation

1. Fundamental Concepts of Clinical Neuroanatomy
2. Pathophysiology of Nervous System Disease
3. Clinical Examination of the Animal with Suspected Neurologic Disease
4. Neuroanatomical Diagnosis
5. Clinical Features of Important and Common Diseases Involving the Intracranial Nervous System of Dogs and Cats
6. Clinical Features of Important and Common Diseases Involving the Spinal Cord of Dogs and Cats
7. Clinical Features of Important and Common Diseases Involving the Peripheral Nervous System, Neuromuscular Junction, and Muscle of Dogs and Cats
8. Formulation of the Differential Diagnosis of Animals with Neurologic Disease
9. Options for Diagnostic Testing in Animals with Neurologic Disease
10. Diagnostic Testing in Animals with Intracranial Neurologic Disease
11. Diagnostic Testing in Animals with Spinal Disease
12. Diagnosis of Important and Common Diseases Involving the Peripheral Nervous System, Neuromuscular Junction, and Muscles of Dogs and Cats
13. Treatment of Important and Common Diseases Involving the Intracranial Nervous System of Dogs and Cats
14. Basics of Treatment of Important Spinal Cord Diseases of Dogs and Cats
15. Treatment of Diseases Involving the Peripheral Nervous System, Neuromuscular Junction, and Muscle of Dogs and Cats

1 Fundamental Concepts of Clinical Neuroanatomy

The nervous system is one of the most vital and complex of all body systems. The nervous system is responsible for such important functions of life as recognition of multiple sensations and stimulations, integration of such information, and subsequent responses and reactions of the body. These activities are important to bring about what we consider to be "normal" function. Disease involving the nervous system alters these complex anatomical and physiologic relationships and creates clinical abnormalities.

The practicing clinician who deals with clinical patients needs to have a working understanding of how the nervous system is organized and functionally integrated to understand how disease, which alters these complex anatomical and physiologic relationships, results in clinical dysfunction. Remembering the location and function of specific structures such as amygdala, however, tends to be lost in the day-to-day clinical evaluations of affected patients. Contributing to this problem is the fact that there is a great deal of specific nervous system terminology to learn and understand. In addition, some terms used to describe nervous system structures and functions are ambiguous, and there is inconsistent agreement among neuroanatomists, physiologists, pathologists, and clinical neurologists as to the definition and day-to-day use of certain terms. For example, an axon may sometimes be referred to as a "fiber" or even a "nerve." A single muscle cell may also be referred to as a "fiber." The term "nerve" may be used in describing a single neuron, nerve cell body and its axon, or group of axons such as in a peripheral nerve. The term "tract" is often used to describe a group of axons, as are "pathway" or "projection." When information moves from one area to another, it is often described as being "transported," "transmitted," or "projected." Information that travels in a cranial direction, such as from the spinal cord to the brain, "ascends." Information that travels in a caudal direction, such as from the brain to the spinal cord, "descends." Neurons may affect or "influence" other neurons and organs. This effect may be through "stimulating," "exciting," "activating," or "depolarizing" another nerve or organ. The neuronal effect may also "inhibit" another nerve or organ. Due to the complexity of the nervous system and its functions, along with the sometimes confusing terminology, the practicing clinician can easily feel overwhelmed with a sense of ignorance about the components and functions of the nervous system.

While it is often important to have knowledge of how discrete neuroanatomical elements of the nervous system function as isolated entities, it is most important for the practicing clinician to have an overall understanding of how separate neuroanatomical entities within the nervous system are integrated, interrelated, and interacted, as these interactions are what are ultimately responsible for the animal to perform various normal functions or, in the case of disease, to not perform these functions normally. This is, in essence, an understanding of how information is transmitted or "flows" back and forth between structures within the nervous system. These interconnections and relationships are what are responsible for clinically important body functions. To acquire this global understanding, a conceptual understanding of how the nervous system is arranged is helpful.

Although it is complex, there is a relatively consistent pattern to the anatomical arrangements of nerves and their connections. Like many relationships in biology (e.g., DNA), simple building blocks are placed in increasingly sophisticated relationships to ultimately build increasingly complex relationships (fig. 1.1). It is sometimes easier to conceptualize the structure and the function of the nervous system through an analogous situation. Thus, the interrelationships are often thought about as a system of roadways, railways, or waterways for transporting information from point A to point B, with some resultant effect. These entities provide the concept of flow or movement of substance (information). The nervous system is often equated to an electrical system or circuit, and the brain is often compared to a "computer." Both electrical systems and the nervous system share common themes, with basic connections becoming additive to perform increasingly complex functions. As an electrical system begins with a flip of a switch, the nervous system is stimulated through activation of a receptor. Receptors are located throughout the body. The role of the receptor is to "sense" events that occur either on or within the body. A process that stimulates may then be referred to as a "sensation." An effect is defined as "a feeling evoked by a stimulus."

This sensing activity of the nervous system gives rise to

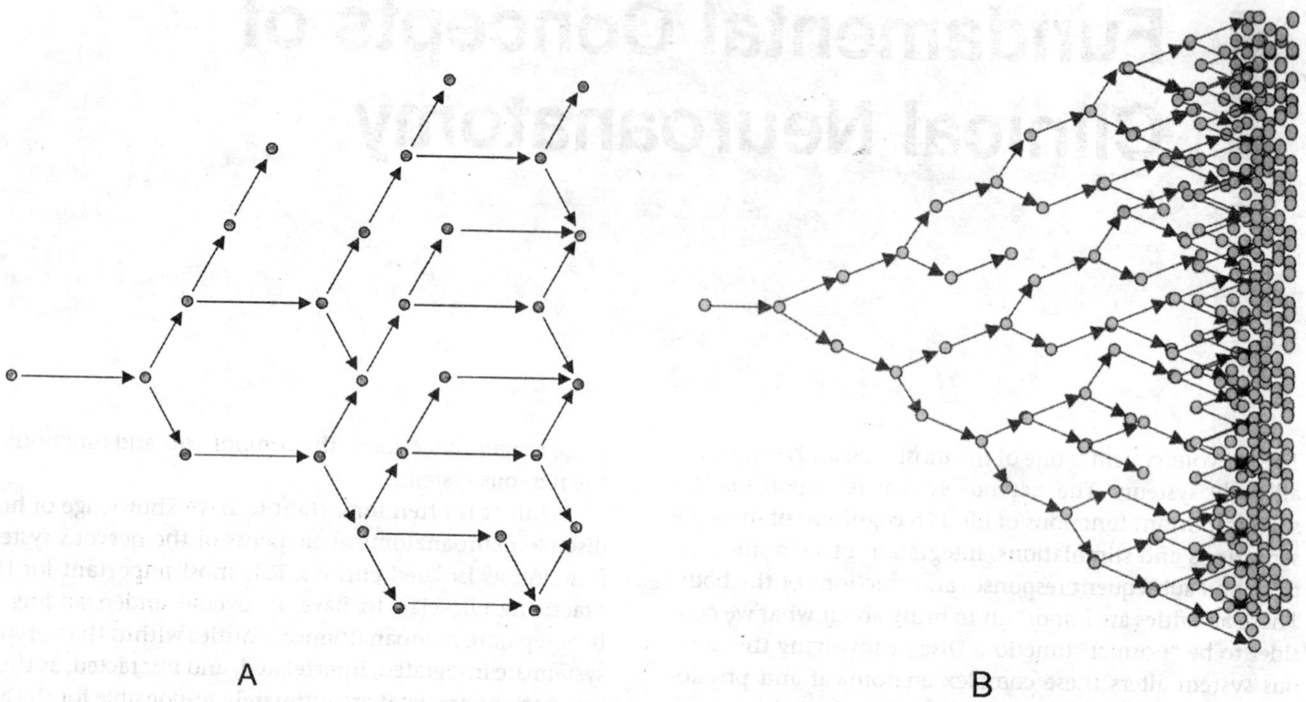

Fig. 1.1. Conceptualization of the nervous system. Single nerve elements are additive to form complex interrelationships. (A) Schematic representation of duplication of single nerve elements, and (B) schematic representation of the potential relationship of one nerve element to many others.

the terms "sensory," "feeling," or "afferent portion" of the nervous system. The term "afferent" implies "conveying toward the center," which includes both sensing information and transporting information. For a single nerve, the receptors and the mechanics for relaying this information to a nerve cell are the function of the dendrite or similar structures.

In a simple electrical circuit, information may travel from the switch along a wire to a light fixture. Once the current reaches the light fixture, the fixture "understands" that the current from the switch is ultimately attempting to bring about a change in the light (e.g., to turn the light on or off). (This analogy is obviously an artificial one, as electrical circuits, being inanimate structures, cannot think or feel.) Recognizing that the current is attempting to turn the light on or off is a reflection of integration or assimilation capacity of the system. The integration of the numerous sensations found within or on the body is one of the most important roles served by the nervous system. Integration most likely involves the summated effect of excitatory or inhibitory stimuli to the nerve cell or cells. It is rare for single nerve cells to result in significant alterations in bodily functions independently; it is more common that cells are grouped together that perform similar functions. This arrangement also adds redundancy to the nervous system, allowing for some loss or dysfunction of individual cells without affecting the overall function of the unit. The relationship of multiple elements being necessary to result in an end result also allows for a more "graded" effect, rather than a pure "all or nothing" response.

The information from the sensory receptors is transmitted to multiple areas within the nervous system, such as the spinal cord, brain stem, cerebellum, thalamus, and areas in the cerebral cortex (somesthetic areas). Processing of information is one of the major functions of the nervous system. It has been suggested that up to 99% of the incoming sensory information is discarded as irrelevant. After processing, information may be projected to areas of the nervous system that cause the desired responses (integrative function).

Considering again an electrical circuit, once the light fixture receives and "understands" the current resulting from the flip of the switch, a response is initiated that results in a current flow to the lightbulb and, finally, the production of light. In a similar fashion, once the nervous system has recognized and understood the stimulus (afferent or sensory information), a response to this stimulus can be generated. This brings about an effect (the result produced by an action). This response function is performed through the efferent portions of the nervous system. Efferent implies conveying away from the center. Once again, both terms "afferent" and "efferent" suggest a flow or movement of information in a specific direction (fig. 1.2). Flow of information in the form of electrical alterations (depolarization) in the nerve cell elements is transported to elicit an effect.

Just as flow of electricity can be directed through numerous interconnected circuits, individual nerves can be arranged in complex anatomical arrangements and relationships to allow for increasingly sophisticated functions

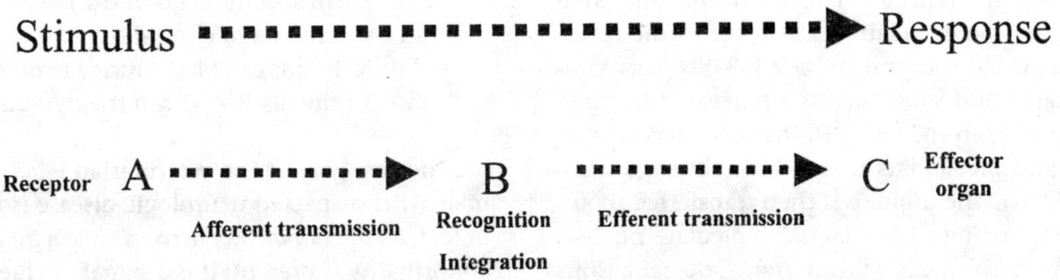

Fig. 1.2. Schematic representation of the basic flow of information within the nervous system.

(fig. 1.1). These arrangements often have intricate and extensive patterns of connections. While seemingly chaotic, the arrangement of connections within the nervous system follows patterns referred to as *somatotopic organization* (deLahunta 1983; Jenkins 1978; King 1987). This concept implies that certain specific nerves, which are associated with specific body functions or regions, are anatomically localized in discrete regions of the nervous system. Neurons may be connected in a sequence. The first neuron in the sequence is referred to as a first-order neuron, the second neuron being referred to as a second-order neuron, and so forth.

The nervous system includes a number of different structural elements. Nerves and their processes, synapses, and connections are obviously important components. Additionally, there are supporting elements (glial cells such as astroctyes and oligodendroglia cells), blood vessels, and covering membranes (meninges). As these structures are often intimately connected anatomically to neural elements, dysfunction of one of these nonneural structures may easily result in dysfunction of neural structures.

The general description of neuroanatomy that follows is not meant to suggest that the nervous system is simple in organization and structure. It is, rather, an introduction to fundamental concepts of how the nervous system is interconnected and functionally integrated. If more specific neuroanatomical information is required, multiple resources are available for consultation (Beitz and Fletcher 1993; deLahunta 1983; Evans 1993; Fletcher 1993; King 1987; Kitchell 1993; Murphy and Pollock 1993). These resources also serve as the basis for anatomical information discussed in this chapter.

ANATOMY OF AN INDIVIDUAL NERVE

A prototypical single nerve consists of sensors (*receptors, dendrites*), a cell body, an *axon* (an extension of the cell body), and a *connection* (*synapse* or *neuromuscular junction*) with another nerve, muscle, or organ (Kitchell 1993). Information from both the internal and external environment of the body is collected via receptors. Receptors are of differing types for recognition of varying stimuli. Receptors associated with nervous functions include mechanoreceptors, pressure receptors, touch receptors, proprioceptive receptors, and stretch receptors. Free nerve endings may also act as receptors, especially for functions such as recognition of painful stimuli. An individual receptor is often stimulated by a single stimulus. A receptor-specific stimulus results in a change (activation) in the receptor altering the receptor cell membrane potential and initiating an action potential. This action potential is transmitted in the dendrites in the direction of the cell body. The axon, which is an extension of the cell body, is responsible for carrying the impulse away from the cell body toward either a muscle, nerve-cell element, or another organ to affect the function of this structure. Connections with other nerves or organs are referred to as *synapses*. The specialized nerve/muscle synapse is termed the *neuromuscular junction*. This fundamental nerve structure is the basic foundation of the nervous system.

An individual nerve cell body may be found, for example, in the cerebral cortex and be responsible for receiving information from stimuli in other parts of the body regarding the basic sensations of touch, vision, smell, taste, hearing, or pain. This information is then relayed to other nerve cell groups in the brain that may affect the function of structures in the head, thorax, abdomen, trunk, or skin through the peripheral components of the nervous system. Nerve cell elements that are present primarily in the brain and spinal cord are commonly referred to as the *central nervous system* (CNS). Nerve cells or their elements that reside primarily outside the brain and spinal cord are referred to as the *peripheral nervous system* (PNS). These distinctions are somewhat arbitrary, as the interconnections of these systems may overlap in various anatomical areas. As an example, motor nerve cell bodies that are associated with peripheral nerves to the limb muscles are anatomically present within the spinal cord. The clinical effect of an abnormality in either the cell body or its elements (i.e., axonal projections) may be indistinguishable.

Nerve cell bodies with similar functions are often grouped in discrete anatomical areas. A grouping of nerve cell bodies within brain and spinal cord is referred to as a *nucleus* of cells. Nerve cell bodies can also be grouped together and located outside the central nervous system in *ganglia*, such as in the dorsal nerve root.

CONNECTIONS WITHIN THE NERVOUS SYSTEM

It is important when dealing with diseases affecting the nervous system that the "flow" of information through the interconnection of anatomical components of the nervous system be understood. For example, for the function of sight, light is initially reflected (collected) from the environment into the eye stimulating a receptor in the retina (deLahunta 1983; Murphy and Pollock 1993). A nerve impulse is generated and subsequently propagated through nerves that travel from the retina in the optic nerve, optic chiasm, and optic tract and terminate in the lateral geniculate nucleus (LGN). The impulse is then transferred to another nerve originating in the lateral geniculate nucleus that travels from the LGN within the optic radiations (nerve axons in the cerebral cortex) to terminate on nerves in the occipital region of the cerebral cortex. The nerve cells that reside in the occipital lobe and their associated connections in additional areas of the cerebral hemispheres are responsible for integrating or understanding the significance of the information generated in the retina (i.e., the visual image). While relatively simple in concept, the complexity of the visual image that is ultimately relayed to the cortex requires a variety of receptors and corresponding transport nerves. Information stimulating the visual system may also affect the parasympathetic system found in the oculomotor nerve (cranial nerve III) resulting in reflex constriction of the pupil. Still further interneuronal connections may send light information to regions of the hypothalamus that may affect the circadian rhythm or reproductive function. Via numerous interconnections and interrelationships between various nerves within the central and peripheral nervous system, multiple body functions may be affected by a single stimulus.

For some effects, there is a more direct connection from the afferent systems to the efferent system. These functions are referred to as *reflexes,* implying that there is a cause and effect relationship without an interposed integration (deLahunta 1983; Kitchell 1993). The term "reflex" also implies that conscious integration, initiation, or recognition is not necessary for the performance of the reflex activity. The *patellar reflex* is an example of a simple reflex with minimal interconnections requiring no cerebrocortical input for performance. Other reflexes, such as pupil constriction with a light stimulus or the withdrawal or flexion reflex of a limb, require extensive neuronal interconnections. In addition to their anatomical relationships, discrete areas of the nervous system that have similar functions can be grouped into more "functional" areas or relationships.

FUNCTIONAL ORGANIZATION OF THE NERVOUS SYSTEM

Components of the nervous system, functioning together, are necessary for certain "normal" body functions, such as walking, eating, and drinking. When the functions of these areas are disrupted by disease, this dysfunction is referred to as a *clinical sign.* This sign is a clue to the clinician that an area of the nervous system is abnormal.

Clinical evaluation of animals with nervous system disease is founded on certain premises:

- Disease is often isolated to specific areas of the nervous system, such as the brain or spinal cord.
- Disease of specific areas of the nervous system results in a specific set of clinical signs.
- Clinical signs can be identified to determine the location of the disease within the nervous system.

The first goal of the veterinarian when evaluating animals with suspected neurologic disease is to determine if, in fact, *an abnormality of nervous system function exists.* If an abnormality is present, it is a signal or clue to the location of the problem. After assimilating clinical clues, a determination as to where the nervous system is abnormal can be made. This determination is commonly referred to as the *neuroanatomical diagnosis.*

When identifying the numerous locations where disease can affect the nervous system, it is convenient to divide the nervous system into various anatomical and functionally related regions. Disease in these functionally related regions of the nervous system is often associated with a specific group of clinical signs (see chapter 4, Neuroanatomical Diagnosis). An important landmark for dividing the nervous system both anatomically and functionally is the foramen magnum. Structures found rostral to the foramen magnum primarily are the *intracranial* nervous system elements, and structures found caudal to this landmark are the *spinal cord* and *peripheral nerves.* The ***brain*** is the term commonly used to indicate the nervous system structures found within the intracranial region. Neuronal extensions and connections of these intracranial structures important for functions in and around the head are found in the associated *cranial nerves.* Cranial nerves are analogous to the spinal nerves, the latter of which have cell bodies within the spinal cord or associated spinal ganglia and connect to peripheral receptors or end organs. Cranial nerves have cell bodies that reside within the intracranial nervous structures (nuclei) or ganglia and connect to peripheral receptors or end organs in or around the head and, in some instances, with other parts of the body. There are 2 pairs of cranial nerves, and these are designated by name or with Roman numerals I through XII.

Within the intracranial nervous system, regions that have similar anatomical locations and physiologic functions may be further delineated. A convenient landmark to divide the intracranial nervous system structurally and functionally is the *tentorium cerebelli.* This structure resides caudal to the occipital lobes of the cerebral hemispheres and rostral to the cerebellum. If an imaginary line is extended along the axis of the tentorium cerebelli ventrally, the intracranial nervous system is divided into those structures *rostral* to this level (i.e., *supratentorial* region) and those structures found *caudal* to this level (i.e., *infratentorial* region) (fig. 1.3).

The *supratentorial* (also referred to as the *prosencephalon* or *forebrain)* region anatomically includes the cerebral hemispheres, basal nuclei, diencephalon, and rostral portion of the mesencephalon (Beitz and Fletcher 1993; deLahunta 1983; Jenkins 1978; King 1987). These structures reside *rostral* to the *tentorium cerebelli* and are responsible for many functions requiring or associated with conscious-

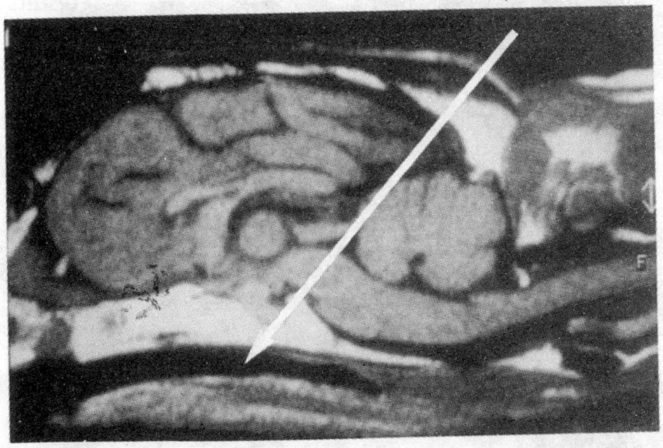

Fig. 1.3. Sagittal, magnetic resonance image of the intracranial space in a dog. The division between the supratentorial and infratentorial structures is represented by the arrow.

ness, cognition, awareness, recognition, and coordinated responses of the body. "Voluntary" or "conscious" functions are often initiated in these regions, including the initiation of movement, urination, eating, drinking, and other common motivations of life. Because of the importance of these essential functions of life and to the relatively sophisticated functions generated from these regions, supratentorial structures are often referred to as "higher centers" of the brain or nervous system.

The cerebral hemispheres (also referred to as the telencephalon) are made up of neuronal cell bodies and supporting cells (*grey matter*) as well as *white matter* (axonal processes of neurons). The cerebral cortex is located between the white matter and the pia mater (the innermost layer of the meninges). The grey matter of the cerebral cortex has been divided into approximately six cellular layers (table 1.1), however, these layers are not always discrete and identifiable in dogs and cats.

Nerves of the cerebral hemispheres may have interactions with other nerves of the body through their axonal connections. Axons of the cells in layers 1, 2, and 4 remain confined to the cortex and often within the same hemisphere (deLahunta 1983). These axons are referred to as association axons or fibers. Other cerebral cortical neuronal axons may project to the opposite hemisphere and are referred to as commissural axons or fibers. Axons in the corpus callosum are examples of commissural axons. Some axons of cerebrocortical neurons send projections from the cortex to the brain stem and spinal cord and are referred to as projection axons or fibers. The axons of layers 3, 5, and 6 tend to form association, commissural, or projection fibers. In this way, axons of the cerebral hemispheres can influence multiple regions of the nervous system.

The surface of the cerebral hemispheres resembles collections of interwoven tubes. The convex portions of the cerebral hemispheres are referred to as gyri, and the depressions between the convex portions are referred to as sulci (fig. 1.4) (Beitz and Fletcher 1993; deLahunta 1983).

Table 1.1. Layers of the grey matter of the cerebral cortex

Outer
1. Molecular (plexiform) layer
2. External granular layer
3. Pyramidal (external pyramidal) layer
4. Internal granular layer
5. Ganglionic (internal pyramidal) layer
6. Multiform (fusiform) layer
Inner

Source: deLahunta 1983.

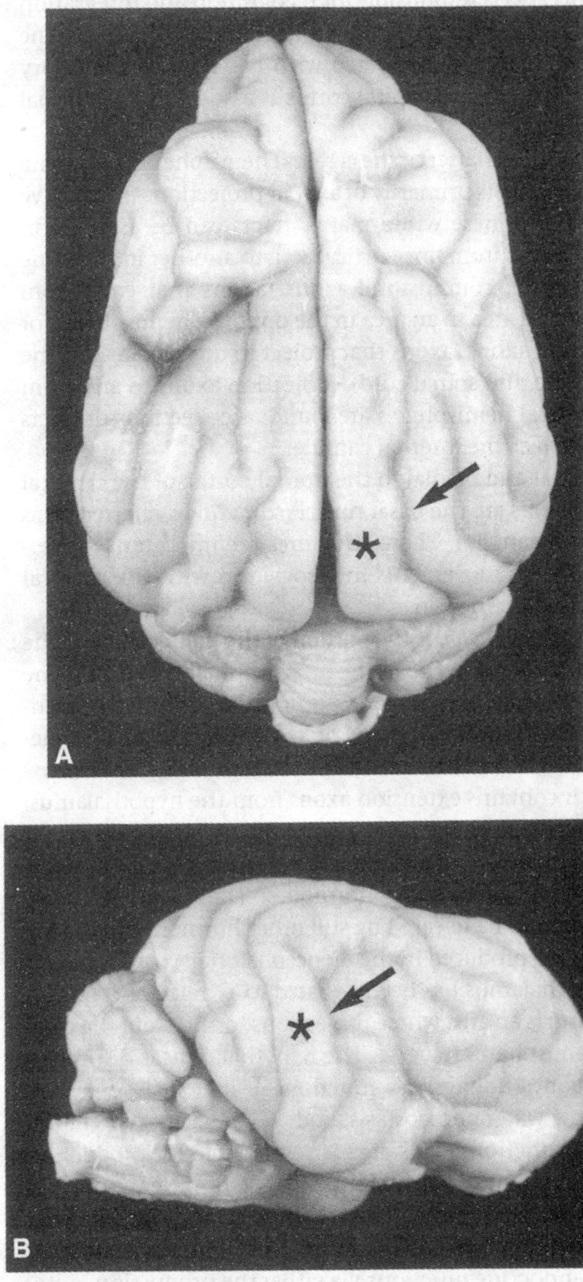

Fig. 1.4. (A) Dorsal and (B)sagittal views of the canine brain. Note the numerous gyri (*) and sulci (*arrow*).

The numerous gyri and sulci of the cerebral hemisphere are associated with differing functional systems. The gyri and sulci have various names and are associated with a variety of functions. Although somewhat similar, the gyral and sulcul pattern of the cerebral hemisphere may differ between individuals as well as between breeds of dogs.

The cerebral cortex is associated with numerous functions relating to consciousness, intellect, emotions, behavior, perception, and control of motor function. Each cerebral hemisphere is divided into four areas based on associated function. These are the *frontal, parietal, temporal,* and *occipital* cortex (fig. 1.5). General body functions are associated with individual cortices. The frontal cortex is predominantly associated with motor activity. The parietal cortex is also referred to as the somesthetic or sensory cortex. This area is responsible for recognition and integration of the multitude of sensations and stimuli of the body. The temporal cortex is associated with behavior and auditory function, and the occipital cortex is associated with visual functions.

The white matter of the cerebral hemispheres, or corona radiata, consists primarily of axonal projections from nerve cell bodies. These white matter tracts can be association axons (axons from one cortical area to another in the same hemisphere), commissural axons (axons that cross from one cortical area to an area in the opposite hemisphere), or projection axons (axons that project to nuclear areas in the brain stem and spinal cord). Projection axons to and from the cerebral hemispheres are found as collections of tracts referred to as the internal capsule.

Ventral and medial to the frontal cortex of the cerebral hemispheres are the basal nuclei (sometimes referred to as the basal ganglia). These structures are important for certain types of movements in association with the cerebral cortex and brain stem.

The *diencephalon* is the portion of the brain caudal to the basal nuclei and rostral to the mesencephalon (fig. 1.6). The *thalamus* and *hypothalamus* are located within the diencephalon. The *pituitary gland* or *hypophysis* is located immediately ventral to this area. The caudal pituitary or *neurohypophysis* contains extension axons from the hypothalamus. The rostral pituitary (adenohypophysis) is responsible for the production of many endocrine hormones such as ACTH and thyroid stimulating hormones. These hormones are stimulated to be released by still other hormones (releasing hormones) produced in the diencephalon.

The thalamus has been equated to a "relay or train station" and is an area where projections to and from the cerebral hemispheres traverse. The hypothalamus is associated with many rudimentary functions of life, such as eating, drinking, water homeostasis, body temperature, and reproductive functions. This area is responsible for production hormones that can initiate the release of other endocrine hormones that have global body effects. The pituitary gland functions in association with the hypothalamus in many endocrine functions via either the production (anterior pituitary) or release (posterior pituitary or neurohypophysis) of hormones and metabolically active elements.

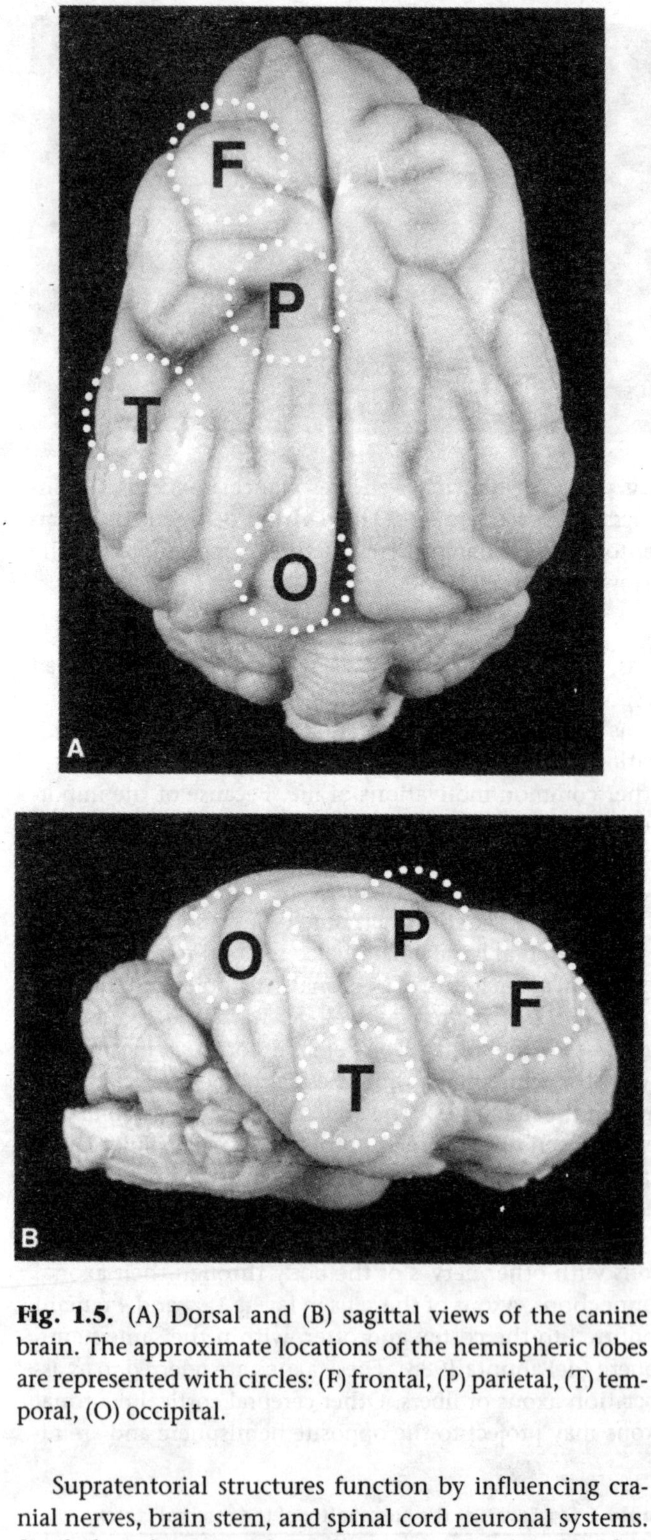

Fig. 1.5. (A) Dorsal and (B) sagittal views of the canine brain. The approximate locations of the hemispheric lobes are represented with circles: (F) frontal, (P) parietal, (T) temporal, (O) occipital.

Supratentorial structures function by influencing cranial nerves, brain stem, and spinal cord neuronal systems. Similarly, information from these structures is projected to the supratentorial structures for conscious integration and recognition. When considering the function of consciousness and awareness, the cerebral hemispheres are stimulated by brain stem elements of the *ascending reticular activating system* (ARAS) (deLahunta 1983; Jenkins 1978; King 1987). The ARAS lies in the central portion of the brain stem from the medulla to the diencephalon. Afferent projections to this area are from pathways that contain ascending sensory information from the body. The ARAS sends

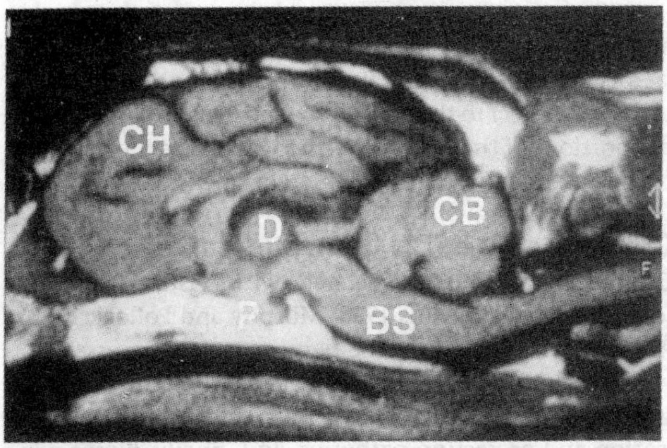

Fig. 1.6. Sagittal, magnetic resonance image of the intracranial space in a dog showing the cerebral hemisphere (CH), cerebellum (CB), brain stem (BS), diencephalon (D), and pituitary (P).

projections to the thalamus to ultimately reach the cerebral hemispheres for maintaining wakefulness.

Many structures within the supratentorial region are important for complex body functions that influence the *behavior* of the animal. The *limbic system* is the name given to portions of the brain that are commonly associated with behavior (Beitz and Fletcher 1993; deLahunta 1983; Jenkins 1978; King 1987). The name limbic (edge or border) is used because the nuclei that are primarily responsible for these functions lie in two incomplete rings on the medial aspect of the telencephalon at its border with the diencephalon. The limbic system includes these as well as other anatomically distant but functionally related nuclei such as those in the brain stem.

The limbic system influences visceral motor activity, primarily through its influence of the hypothalamus. Projections from the olfactory, optic, auditory, external, and internal sensory systems influence components of the limbic system. The limbic system functions in basic drives, sexual activity, emotional experiences, memories, fears, and pleasures.

INFRATENTORIAL NERVOUS SYSTEM

The *infratentorial structures* include much of what is commonly referred to as the *brain stem* (Beitz and Fletcher 1993; Jenkins 1978; King 1987; Selcer 1990; Shell 1990). The *cerebellum* also resides in this region dorsal to the brain stem (fig. 1.6). For this functionally related discussion, the brain stem includes part of the mesencephalon (midbrain), the metencephalon (pons), and the myelencephalon (medulla oblongata). Many of the *cranial nerve nuclei* (cranial nerves III through XII) and neurons responsible for important vital functions, such as wakefulness and respiration, reside in the brain stem.

Information flowing to and from the cerebral cortex, thalamus, and other components of the supratentorial structures travels through the brain stem to and from the spinal cord. The brain stem contains functional systems such as the vestibular system and the reticular systems that have important roles in extensor tone and maintenance of body position relative to the influence of gravity. Brain stem structures also have significant roles in gaiting and walking.

The *cerebellum* is present dorsal to the brain stem and fourth ventricle (an area normally containing cerebrospinal fluid) and has the unique function of modifying movements to keep these movements smooth and coordinated (deLahunta 1983; Holliday 1979). This control may occur by regulation of muscle tone, posture, and skilled movement.

The *vestibular system* (cranial nerve VIII and its connections) works in close association with the cerebellum influencing posture. A portion of the cerebellum (flocculonodular lobe) is primarily responsible for vestibular-associated functions such as balance in the equilibrium. The vestibular system has an important influence over body, head, and eye posture.

The *cranial nerves* are nerve projections to and from neurons in brain stem nuclei and structures in the head and neck (deLahunta 1983; Evans 1993; Evans and Kitchell 1993; Jenkins 1978; King 1987; Shell 1990). The vagus nerve (cranial nerve X) also projects to and from the viscera and other body organs including those in the thoracic and abdominal cavities. There are twelve pairs of cranial nerves ordered I through XII (table 1.2). Cranial nerves I (olfactory nerve important for smell) and II (optic nerve important for vision) are functionally associated with the supratentorial structures. Cranial nerves III through XII have cell bodies that reside within or adjacent to the brain stem. Afferent or sensory information from some cranial nerves is projected to the supratentorial structures for conscious recognition.

Cranial nerves play an important role in reflex functions of the head, but may also provide information to, and receive influences from, the cerebral cortex. Blinking, for example, may occur as a reflex function through local stimulation from the eye or periocular structures. An animal may also voluntarily or consciously blink via activation of the supratentorial motor systems which then influence the function of the facial nerve. Cranial nerve VII, the facial nerve, is composed of motor nerve cell bodies in the brain stem nuclei (CN VII or facial nucleus) and their associated axons that project from the brain stem nucleus through the skull to form the peripheral facial nerve. For initiation of blinking, this nerve synapses on the orbicularis oculi muscle surrounding the palpebral fissure. Regardless of whether the facial nerve is stimulated via a reflex synapse or by a synapse from a nerve in the cerebral motor cortex, however, this nerve is the final common pathway that results in the clinical manifestation of a blink.

Cranial Nerve (CN) I—Olfactory Nerves

Cranial nerve I is, in reality, a constellation of multiple nerve fibers and synapses (deLahunta 1983; Evans 1993). The first-order neuron is a bipolar neuron in the caudodorsal olfactory epithelium in the nose. These neurons func-

Table 1.2. Cranial nerve (CN) names and important functions

Name	Function
CN I olfactory	Smelling
CN II optic	Vision and pupillary light reflexes
CN III oculomotor	1. Primarily, medial movement of the eye through innervation of the extraocular muscles 2. Pupillary constriction through parasympathetic innervation of the iris
CN IV trochlear	Intorsion of the eye through innervation of the dorsal oblique extraocular muscle
CN V trigeminal	1. Sensation to the eye and cornea 2. Sensation to the maxillary/mandibular area 3. Motor innervation to the muscle of mastication
CN VI abducents	Innervation to the lateral rectus and retractor bulbi extraocular muscles
CN VII facial	1. Motor to the muscles of facial expression 2. Taste 3. Salivation/lacrimation 4. Skin sensation (ear)
CN VIII vestibular cochlear	1. Balance and posture 2. Hearing
CN IX glossopharyngeal	1. Motor and sensation to pharynx 2. Taste 3. Salivation
CN X vagus	1. Motor and sensation to larynx 2. Taste 3. Salivation 4. Parasympathetic innervation to viscera
CN XI accessory	Motor innervation to trapezius muscle, parts of the sternocephalicus, cleidomastoideus, and cleidocervicalis portions of the brachiocephalicus
CN XII hypoglossal	Motor to the tongue

tionally act as chemoreceptors. The distal (toward the nose) portion of these cells consists of ciliated processes (numbering 6 to 8) that penetrate the olfactory mucous membranes. Unmyelinated axons from these cells project caudally to penetrate the cribiform plate and synapse on neurons (brush or mitral cells) in the olfactory bulbs.

Axons from the mitral cells project caudally in the olfactory tract and lateral olfactory stria to the ipsilateral olfactory cortex within the (pyriform) cortex. Brush neurons project through the olfactory tract and medial olfactory stria, the rostral commissure, the contralateral medial olfactory stria, and the olfactory tract to the contralateral olfactory bulb. The two pyriform cortices are connected by commissural fibers, which allows for information to be passed between these regions. Smell, therefore, is a bilaterally integrated sensation in the brain.

Reflex pathways for smell involve projections into the nuclear areas of the limbic system. Axons in the medial olfactory stria enter the septal area. Axons in the lateral olfactory stria project to the amygdaloid nucleus and hippocampus portions of the limbic system to influence the behavior of the animal in response to different smells.

Cranial Nerve II (CN II)—Optic Nerve

Cranial nerve II is associated with visual functions (deLahunta 1983; Evans 1993; Murphy and Pollock 1993). Anatomical areas within the nervous system necessary for vision include the eye, the optic nerve, the central projection pathways to the visual (occipital) cortex, cortical association and projection pathways, and, finally, motor neurons necessary to complete motor responses to visual stimuli (fig. 1.7). Visual functions during a clinical exami-

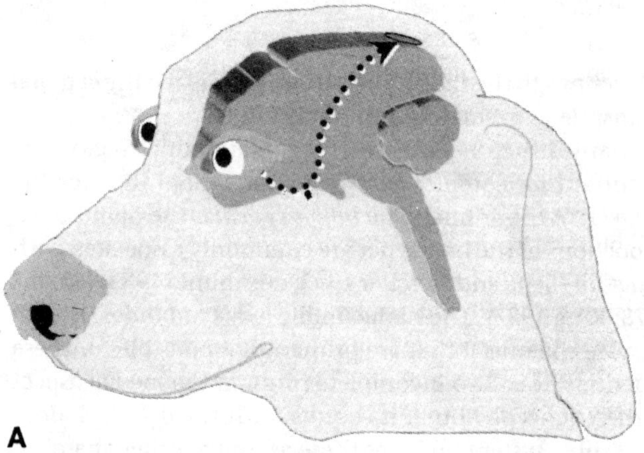

A

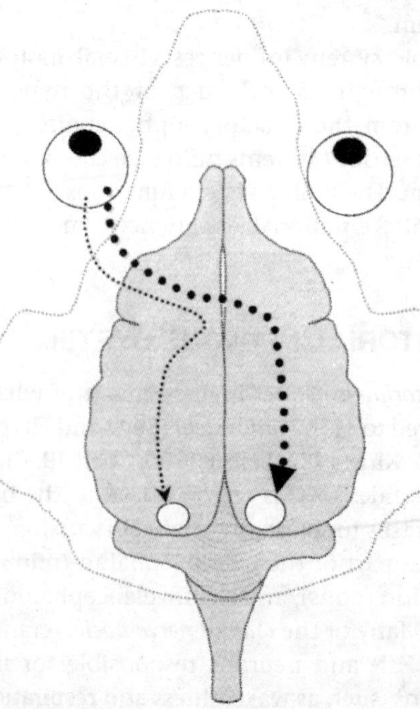

B

Fig. 1.7. (A) Lateral and (B) dorsal views, schematic representation of the flow of afferent visual information from the eye to the contralateral occipital lobe.

nation can be assessed by testing for the menace response, by observing whether the animal bumps into objects in the examination area, or by having the animal walk through an unfamiliar area with obstacles placed in its path (obstacle course).

It is important when assessing abnormalities of the visual system to perform a complete visual ophthalmic examination including a critical examination of the retina (e.g., a fundic examination). This examination will most often require a good light source, such as a Finoff transilluminator, and some form of magnification (direct or indirect ophthalmoscopy). In addition to viewing abnormalities of the retina, one can visually evaluate the rostral portion of the optic nerve. Clues to diffuse systemic disease, such as hypertension, coagulopathies, and inflammation/infection, that could also be affecting the nervous system can be assessed during a retinal examination.

Neuroanatomy for Menace Response. The menace response is used as an assessment of visual function (Braund 1994; Chrisman 1991; deLahunta 1983; Oliver et al. 1987; Oliver et al. 1997). This response is tested independently in each eye while the opposite eye is covered, usually by the examiner's hand. The menace response assesses the function of two cranial nerves, CN II (afferent) and CN VII (efferent—blinking). Other interposed components of the nervous system, such as the supratentorial structures for visual integration and the cerebellum, are also necessary for a normal menace response to be generated (also see chapter 3).

A menacing object such as the rapidly approaching hand is presented to the animal. Light reflected from the hand is first projected through the ocular structures passing through the clear structures of the globe (cornea, anterior chamber, lens, vitreous) to excite electromechanical receptors in the retina.

The retina contains 10 layers (from outer to inner: pigment epithelium, photosensitive layer, external limiting membrane, external nuclear layer, external plexiform layer, internal nuclear layer, internal plexiform layer, ganglion layer, nerve fiber layer, and internal limiting membrane). Light travels through the retina to its outer regions.

The photosensitive layer represents the dendritic zone of the photoreceptor cells (rods and cones) (Scagliotti 1990). This dendritic zone consists of modifications of cell processes arranged in orderly double-membraned stacks forming disks. Within the rods, these membranes contain rhodopsin. Rod receptors are sensitive to low levels of light. In the cones, these membranes contain iodopsin. Cone receptors are sensitive to greater levels of light and are responsible for color vision. Both of these receptor types are electromechanical receptors and convert the light stimuli into an electrical impulse through depolarization of neural elements. A three-neuron system is present in the retina. Axons from the third neuron in this series travel toward the center of the eye and form the optic nerve.

Diverse areas of the retina receive information from differing environmental areas. The visual fields in space are separated into temporal (lateral) and nasal (medial) fields. Objects in the temporal visual field are projected onto the nasal retina. Objects in the nasal visual field are projected onto the temporal retina.

Axons in the optic nerve project caudally toward the optic chiasm. In dogs, 75% of the optic nerve fibers cross over or decussate at the chiasm to enter the contralateral optic tract (deLahunta 1983). In cats, 65% of these fibers decussate to the contralateral side. This crossing of fibers allows for projection of information from one visual field to both cerebral hemispheres simultaneously (a degree of binocular vision). Axons from the nasal retinal region (lateral visual field) contribute the majority of the fibers that cross in the chiasm, and the temporal retinal axons contribute the majority of fibers that remain ipsilateral in the visual pathways.

After decussating at the chiasm, axons are projected within the *optic* tract (fig. 1.7). Via the optic tract, fibers associated with vision reach the lateral geniculate body or nucleus, which is found in the thalamus. From the lateral geniculate nucleus, axons project in the optic radiations to terminate in the visual cortex of the occipital lobe. The visual image is integrated in the visual cortex and association areas. Appropriate responses to recognition of the image are then mediated by additional cortical (motor) areas.

The afferent pathway for the menace response travel form the eye to the occipital cortex. The efferent portion of this response is mediated through CN VII (facial nerve) resulting in closure of the eyelid.

How the information actually projects from the visual cortex to the contralateral nucleus of CN VII is not well understood. It is known, however, that this pathway either projects through, or is positively influenced by, the cerebellum, as animals with cerebellar disease can lack a menace response. However, animals with cerebellar disease will have normal vision and normal CN VII function. Some animals with an absent menace response due to cerebellar disease may still blink in response to a bright light shown in the eyes. Blinking in response to light stimulation is known as the dazzle reflex (Oliver et al. 1997). With unilateral cerebellar disease, for example, an animal may have a menace deficit in the eye that is ipsilateral to the cerebellar lesion.

Visual fibers also project to the rostral colliculus in the dorsal midbrain for orientation of the head and body toward the visual stimulus. Still other axons project to the hypothalamus and other components of the limbic system for behavior responses, such as light's ability to affect reproductive function.

Neuroanatomy of Pupil Function. The pupil is innervated by both the parasympathetic and sympathetic divisions of the nervous system (Collins and O'Brien 1990). These divisions are, in turn, influenced by many diverse areas within the nervous system. When stimulated, the parasympathetic system constricts the pupil; the sympathetic system dilates the pupil. Parasympathetic innervation to the eye travels through CN III (oculomotor nerve).

The afferent pathway for pupillary constriction during light stimulation, or the pupillary light reflex (PLR), is within similar anatomical structures as those pathways that influence visual functions from the eye. Axons for the PLR travel from retinal nerves in the optic nerve, optic chiasm, and optic tract. Prior to synapse in the lateral geniculate nucleus, fibers associated with the PLR diverge from those within the visual pathways and travel to the pretectal nucleus in the midbrain (fig. 1.8). From the pretectal nucleus, fibers project bilaterally to the parasympathetic nucleus of CN III (PSN CN III) (Edinger Westfall nucleus in human beings). This nucleus is located rostral to the motor nucleus of CN III at the level of the rostral portion of the rostral colliculus and the pretectal area. Prior to the parasympathetic nucleus, information stimulating the pupillary light reflex travels primarily from the contralateral eye as a result of the predominant decussation of these fibers in the optic chiasm. Axons from the contralateral eye are projected back toward the parasympathetic nucleus, which is ipsilateral to the stimulated eye. A portion of these fibers, however, is also projected to the parasympathetic nucleus contralateral to the stimulated eye. In essence, then, light information is projected from one eye to both parasympathetic nuclei simultaneously. This bilateral projection provides for the bilateral reflex pupillary constriction seen clinically resulting from unilateral ocular light stimulation. The contralateral projection is functionally greater than the ipsilateral projection for this reflex, making the direct (in the eye receiving the light stimulation) PLR slightly stronger than the indirect (in the eye opposite to the eye receiving the light stimulation) PLR.

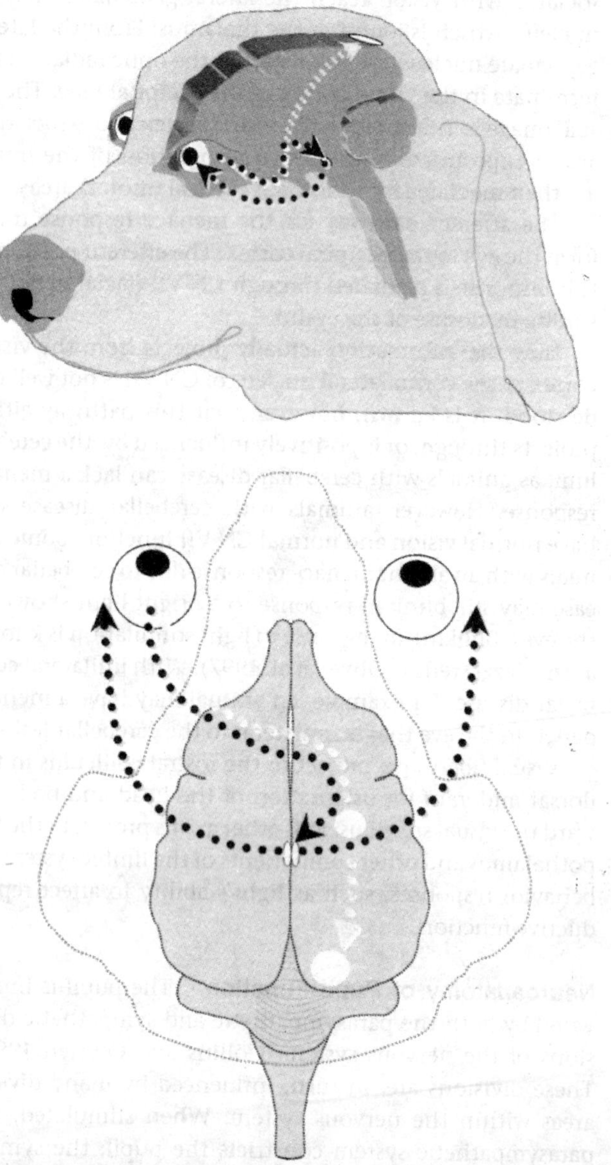

A

B

Fig. 1.8. (A) Lateral and (B) dorsal views, schematic representation of the flow of information for the pupillary light reflex (black dots).

Efferent axons from the parasympathetic nucleus (preganglionic parasympathetic axons) course ventrally through the brain stem and exit the brain stem with the motor component of CN III medial to the crus cerebri in the lateral part of the intercrural fossa (mesencephalon level). The parasympathetic portion of this nerve can usually be seen grossly on the medial side of CN III. At this level this portion of CN III is susceptible to compression during brain *herniation* (see chapter 2) (Kornegay et al. 1983). The nerve next courses in the area of the cavernous sinus (venous structure surrounding the pituitary gland or hypophysis) and exits the skull in the orbital fissure. Caudal to the globe and ventral to the optic nerve, the preganglionic parasympathetic fibers synapse in the ciliary ganglion. The postganglionic parasympathetic fibers pass by way of the short ciliary nerves along the optic nerve to innervate the ciliary muscle and constrictor of the pupil. In dogs, there are five to eight short ciliary nerves. In cats, there are only two, a nasal (medial) and malar (lateral) nerve. Stimulation of these nerves results in constriction of the iris.

Sympathetic innervation to the pupil is responsible for pupillary dilation and innervation to the vessels of the iris (fig. 1.9). Sympathetic control may be initiated in the hypothalamus of the diencephalon.

Sympathetic stimulation descends through the brain stem and cervical spinal cord in the lateral tectotegmental spinal pathway (deLahunta 1983; Jenkins 1978; King 1987). This pathway synapses on the cell bodies of the preganglionic sympathetic nerves that influence the eye structures. Cell bodies of these nerves are located in the intermediolateral grey matter in the thoracic (T)1–3 spinal cord segments. Preganglionic sympathetic nerves responsible for pupil dilation exit the spinal cord and vertebral canal and course cranially in the cervical sympathetic trunk within the cranial thorax. This pathway continues through the cervical area with the vagus nerve forming the vagosympathetic trunk. Preganglionic nerves synapse in the cranial cervical ganglion located just caudal to the ear. Postganglionic nerves travel through the middle ear, course with CN IX and then with the carotid artery to enter the skull. These axons course close to the cavernous sinus with the carotid artery, and exit the skull through the orbital fissure. Postganglionic sympathetic fibers run with the ophthalmic branch of CN V to the eye, and, via the short ciliary nerve, synapse on the dilator muscle of the pupil.

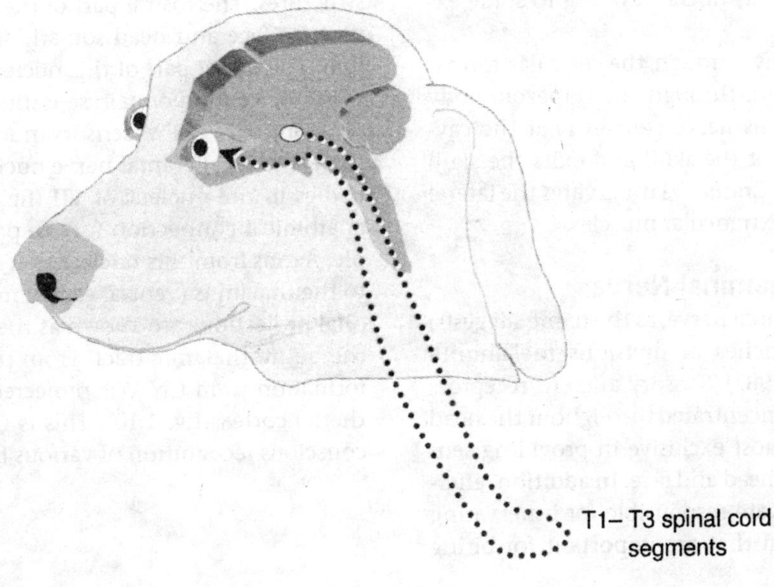

Fig. 1.9. Lateral view, schematic representation of the sympathetic innervation to the pupil. Preganglionic cell bodies are found in the T1–T3 spinal cord segments.

Sympathetic axons may also influence vascular structures surrounding the eye. Vasomotor sympathetic fibers have a similar preganglionic course. Postganglionic fibers travel along the common carotid and internal carotid arteries as part of the carotid plexus, are in close approximation with the cavernous sinus, exit the skull in the orbital fissure, enter the orbit via the superior orbital fissure traveling with various blood vessels such as the ophthalmic artery. These fibers disperse from blood vessels and pass through the ciliary ganglion without synapsing to continue toward the globe as short ciliary nerves. These nerves supply the blood vessels and branched chromatophores of the uveal tract.

Some postganglionic fibers will also innervate the smooth muscle fibers in the orbital sheath (musculus orbitalis). The sympathetic system, then, innervates the muscles of the periorbita, eyelids (Muller's muscle), the third eyelid, the dilator muscle of the iris, and the vasomotor fibers to the blood vessels and chromatophores of the uveal tract.

Pupil size is influenced by the relative activity of the parasympathetic portion of CN III and the sympathetic nerves. The concept of double reciprocal innervation suggests that both the pupil dilator muscle and sphincter are under dual innervation, and the degree of pupil change is due to the balance between these two systems (Yoshitomi 1986). A relative excess of parasympathetic stimulation or a relative decrease in sympathetic stimulation will result in a constricted pupil. Conversely, a relative increase in sympathetic stimulation or a relative decrease in parasympathetic stimulation will result in a relatively dilated pupil.

Cranial Nerve III—Oculomotor Nerve

In addition to the parasympathetic function of CN III, the oculomotor nerve also influences *movement of the eye* (deLahunta 1983; Jenkins 1978; King 1987). These differing functions (motor versus autonomic) are controlled by differing nuclear groups of CN III.

The motor nucleus of CN III is located in the rostral mesencephalon at the level of the rostral colliculus. Axons pass ventrally through the tegmentum, exit the brain stem on the lateral side, course rostrally lateral to the hypophysis near the cavernous sinus to exit the skull in the orbital fissure. The motor component of cranial nerve III is responsible for the innervation of the dorsal, ventral, and medial rectus; the ventral oblique (extorts the globe); and the levator palpebrae muscles.

Cranial Nerve IV—Trochlear Nerve

The trochlear nerve is unique of the cranial nerves in that it is the only cranial nerve in which 100% of its axons *decussates*, or *crosses*, and this nerve is the only cranial nerve that exits the dorsal aspect of the brain stem (deLahunta 1983; Jenkins 1978; King 1987). The cell bodies of the trochlear nucleus are located in the caudal mesencephalon at the level of the caudal colliculi. The axons course dorsally and caudally to exit the brain stem just caudal to the caudal colliculus. The nerve crosses midline and travels near the cavernous sinus. Axons exit the skull in the orbital fissure to innervate the dorsal oblique muscle of the eye. When activated, the dorsal oblique normally intorts or rotates the dorsal portion of the eye medioventrally toward the medial canthus and nose.

Cranial Nerve VI—Abducent

The abducent nucleus is located in the rostral medulla oblongata adjacent to midline ventral to the floor of the fourth ventricle at the level where the caudal cerebellar peduncles merge with the cerebellum (deLahunta 1983; Jenkins 1978; King 1987). The abducent nerve contains only motor (somatic efferent) fibers traveling to some extraocular muscles.

The axons pass ventrally through the reticular formation and exit the brain stem through the trapezoid body lateral to the pyramids. This nerve courses near the cavernous sinus on the floor of the skull and exits the skull through the orbital fissure. Cranial VI innervates the lateral rectus and retractor bulbi extraocular muscles.

Cranial Nerve V—Trigeminal Nerve

Cranial nerve V, the trigeminal nerve, as the name suggests, contains three main branches or divisions (deLahunta 1983; Jenkins 1978; King 1987). Sensory afferent receptors of this nerve are densely concentrated throughout the head and face. This nerve is almost exclusive in providing sensory information from the head and face. In addition, efferent axons from this nerve are responsible for innervating the muscles of mastication that are important for biting and chewing.

The three major branches of this nerve are the *ophthalmic*, the *maxillary*, and the *mandibular* nerves. The ophthalmic and maxillary branches provide *sensory afferent* information to the brain, and the mandibular nerve is responsible for *both* sensory and motor functions.

Sensory receptors of the head and the roof of the mouth send afferent information centrally through afferent fibers of all the three nerve branches. Afferent cell bodies are located in the trigeminal ganglion (Gasserian) similar to other afferent sensory cell bodies throughout the body. This ganglion resides in the trigeminal canal within the petrous temporal bone of the skull. Axons from these sensory cell bodies enter the brain stem (pons) at the level of the middle cerebellar peduncle through the trigeminal nerve. Within the brain stem, the majority of these fibers course caudally on the lateral side of the medulla oblongata to form the spinal tract of CN V. This is a relatively large structure that extends throughout much of the brain stem from the pons through the medulla oblongata. The spinal tract of CN V continues caudally into the first cervical spinal cord segment as the dorsolateral fasciculus (Lisauers's tract).

A nuclear column is located just medial to this spinal tract. In the pons, this column is referred to as the pontine sensory nucleus. In the medulla oblongata and into the first spinal cord segment, this column is the nucleus of the spinal tract of CN V that becomes continuous with the substantia gelatinosa of the spinal cord. The substantia gelatinosa of the spinal cord is found in the dorsal (sensory) grey matter and is primarily responsible for integration of sensory (painful) information projected in spinal nerves. The relationship of this portion of the spinal cord grey matter and CN V anatomically suggests similar physiologic function associated with pain recognition.

This sensory nucleus of CN V is anatomically extensive in the brain stem. In this sensory trigeminal nuclear column, afferent sensory fibers of CN V terminate. The pontine portion of this sensory nucleus is thought to be primarily associated with mechanoreception of the head structures. The rostral part of the spinal nucleus primarily projects face and head somatic sensations to the cerebellum. The major part of this nucleus, however, is associated with nociception or pain sensations.

From this CN V sensory nuclear column, axons can project to local cranial nerve nuclei such as the motor cell bodies in the nucleus of VII (fig. 1.10). This provides the anatomical connection for the palpebral reflex, for example. Axons from this nuclear area cross midline and project to the thalamus (ventral caudal medial nucleus). These axonal projections are known as the trigeminal lemniscus or the quintothalamic tract. From the thalamus, sensory information from CN V is projected to the parietal (somesthetic) cortex (fig. 1.10). This is the pathway allowing for conscious recognition of various facial sensations.

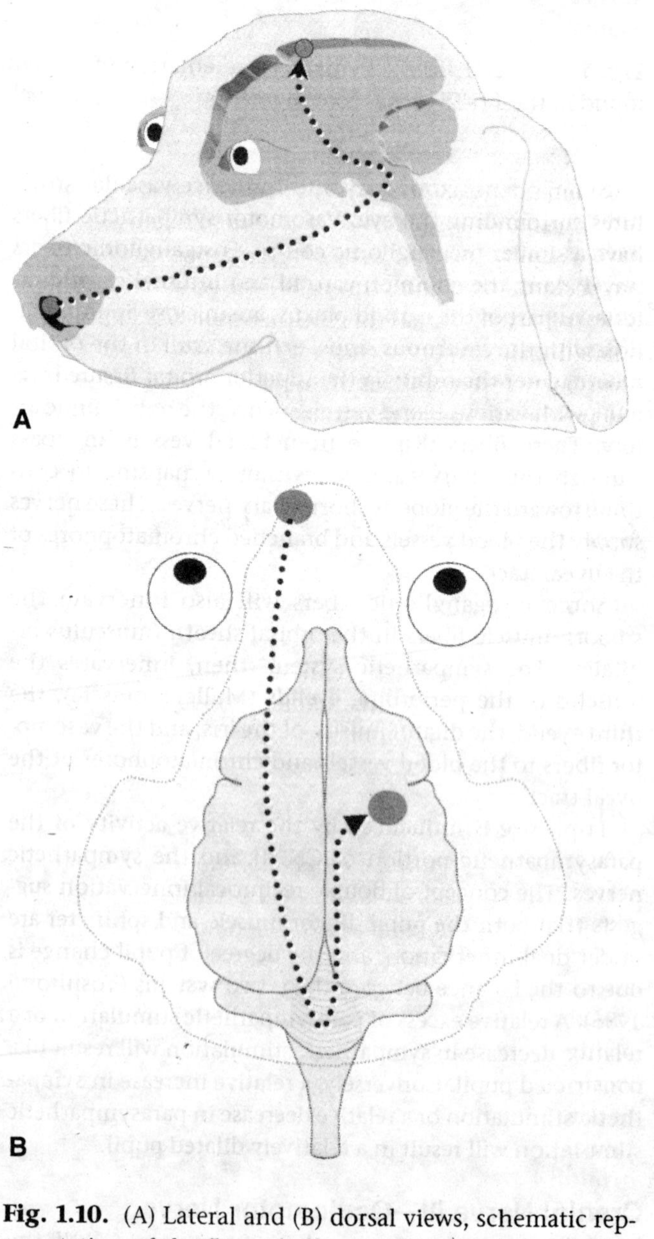

A

B

Fig. 1.10. (A) Lateral and (B) dorsal views, schematic representation of the flow of afferent sensory information in the trigeminal nerve to the contralateral parietal cortex.

Afferent projections in cranial nerve V also transmit general proprioception (position sense) information from structures of the head. Proprioceptive receptors are present in the muscles of mastication, facial and extraocular muscles, and the temporomandibular joint. Proprioceptive fibers are found in all branches of the trigeminal nerve. These fibers apparently pass through the trigeminal ganglion and enter the pons with the trigeminal nerve. These axons continue rostrally along the lateral border of the central grey substance of the fourth ventricle and the mesencephalic aqueduct in the mesencephalic tract of the trigeminal nerve. Cell bodies of these afferent fibers are located in the nucleus of the mesencephalic tract of CN V in a narrow band on the lateral border of the central grey substance throughout the mesencephalon.

Efferent functions of cranial nerve V are important for motor innervation to the muscles of mastication. Cell bodies of these motor fibers are located in the motor nucleus of cranial nerve V within the pons. This nucleus is found at the level of the rostral cerebellar peduncle in the lateral reticular formation, medial to the pontine sensory nucleus of cranial nerve V and dorsal to the dorsal nucleus of the trapezoid body. Axons pass laterally and slightly ventrally through the middle cerebellar peduncle. From the pons to the trigeminal canal, these motor neurons often can be seen as a separate nerve on the medial aspect of the primary nerve. Motor fibers pass through the trigeminal ganglion in the trigeminal canal of the petrosal bone, join the mandibular nerve, pass through the oval foramen, and are distributed to the muscles of mastication (masseter, temporal, pterygoids, rostral digastricus, mylohyoid) as well as the tensor tympani and the tensor veli palantini.

The trigeminal nerve itself emerges from the brain stem at the level of the pons and travels through the petrosal bone in the trigeminal canal before branching. The three branches of CN V traverse the skull via different foramina. In dogs, the ophthalmic branch of the trigeminal nerve enters in the orbital fissure, the maxillary branch enters through the round foramen (internally) and the rostral alar canal (externally). The mandibular branch exits through the oval foramen.

CRANIAL NERVE VII—FACIAL NERVE

Cranial nerve VII supplies innervation to the muscles associated with facial expression, to the lacrimal and salivary glands, to the middle ear and the blood vessels of the head, and to the palate and the rostral two-thirds of the tongue associated with branches of the trigeminal nerve (fig. 1.11) (deLahunta 1983; Jenkins 1978; King 1987). Neurons supplying innervation to the muscles of facial expression are located in the facial nucleus in the brain stem. This nucleus lies caudal to the trapezoid body and the attachment of the caudal cerebellar peduncle. The axons pass dorsomedially to midline near the floor of the fourth ventricle, where they pass rostrally over the nucleus of CN VI in the genu (knee) of the facial nerve. These fibers then course ventrolaterally through the medulla and emerge from the brain stem

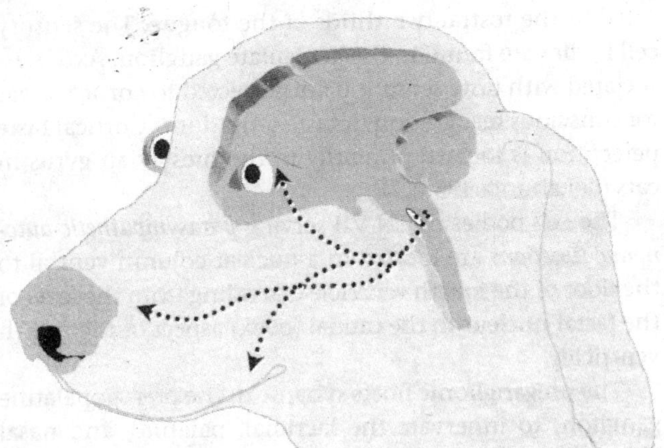

Fig. 1.11. Lateral view, schematic representation of the distribution of the facial nerve.

through the trapezoid body next to CN VIII. The facial nerve courses through the facial canal in the petrosal bone, and exits the skull through the stylomastoid foramen. The facial nerve runs through the middle ear before branching in the petrosal bone.

In the petrosal bone, the major petrosal nerve exits initially, prior to the geniculate ganglion, to innervate the lacrimal glands (Oliver et al. 1987; Oliver et al. 1997). The chorda tympani branch next exits and projects to the tongue, salivary glands, and stapedius muscle. The facial nerve proper then exits the stylomastoid foramen, courses ventral to the external ear canal, and gives rise to three branches: (1) the auricolopalpebral branch, which innervates the eye and ear muscles; (2) the dorsal buccal branch to the muscles of the maxilla; and (3) the ventral buccal branch to the muscles of the maxilla and mandibular areas. These branches of the facial nerve innervate the muscles of the ear, eyelids, nose, cheeks, lips, and caudal portion of the digastricus muscle.

Receptors for pain sensation in the middle ear and blood vessels of the head are also found at CN VII. Afferent axons course toward the central nervous system toward cell bodies located in the geniculate ganglion of the facial nerve. Axons course from these cell bodies to enter the ventrolateral aspect of the medulla oblongata into the solitary tract and nucleus (cell bodies of CNs VII, IX, X) of the solitary tract. This nucleus is predominantly responsible for reflex function of the head through synapses with the nuclei of other cranial nerves or their projection, or by way of interneurons to metabolic centers of visceral function (respiration, cardiovascular, swallowing, urination) in the reticular formation of the brain stem.

Some axons from these cell bodies may course rostrally and serve a conscious proprioceptive function. These axons travel via the contralateral brain stem in the ill-defined solitariothalamic pathway to terminate in the thalamus (ventral caudal medial) and finally the somesthetic (parietal) cortex.

The facial nerve receptors responsible for taste are located in the rostral two-thirds of the tongue. The sensory cell bodies are found in the geniculate ganglion. Axons associated with taste sensation are projected to cortical areas for conscious recognition of taste sensations. Cortical taste perception is located primarily in the presylvian gyrus in cats (deLahunta 1983).

The cell bodies of CN VII serving *parasympathetic autonomic functions* are located in a nuclear column ventral to the floor of the fourth ventricle extending from the level of the facial nucleus to the caudal (obex) aspect of the fourth ventricle.

The preganglionic fibers synapse in the pterygopalatine ganglion, to innervate the lacrimal, palatine, and nasal glands. Additional preganglionic fibers synapse in the mandibular and sublingual salivary glands. These neurons are responsible for lacrimation and salivation.

Cranial Nerve VIII—Vestibulocochlear Nerve

Cranial nerve VIII has two main divisions: vestibular and cochlear. These serve to maintain the position of the head in space (vestibular) and function in hearing (cochlear) (deLahunta 1983; Jenkins 1978; King 1987).

Vestibular Division. The *vestibular division* of CN VII is responsible for providing information of the head and other structures relative to gravity. The receptors for both the vestibular and cochlear portions of cranial nerve VIII are contained within the inner ear structures. Vestibular receptors are present within the membranous labyrinth. Within this area are three semicircular ducts containing a fluid substance called endolymph, each with a dilated portion at one end known as the ampulla. The three semicircular canals are at right angles to each other. Within each ampulla is a receptor, the crista ampullaris. This is a transverse ridge of connective tissue lined by neuroepithelium. On the surface of these cells is a gelatinous structure, the cupula. The neuroepithelium is composed of two cell types, hair cells and supporting cells. The hair cells have 40 to 80 luminal hairs and a single modified cilium (kinocilium). During movement of the head, the endolymph flows in the semicircular ducts to stimulate the hair cells.

The semicircular ducts attach to the utricle. This contains the macula utriculi, which also houses the neuroepithelium (hair cells) (deLahunta 1983; Jenkins 1978; King 1987). The utricle communicates with the endolymphatic duct and sac, which in turn communicate with the saccule. A similar macula is found in the saccule, the macula sacculi. Covering these cells is a gelatinous material known as the otolithic membrane. On the surface of this material are small calcareous crystalline bodies known as statconia (otoliths). The macula in the utriculus is located in a horizontal plane, and the macula of the saccule is in a sagittal plane. The maculae are important in sensing gravitational forces. In essence the force of gravity affects the statconia. The saccule also communicates with the auditory (cochlear) portion of this nerve via the ductus reuniens.

The dendritic zone of the vestibular division of CN VIII is in synaptic relationship with the hair cells. The axons

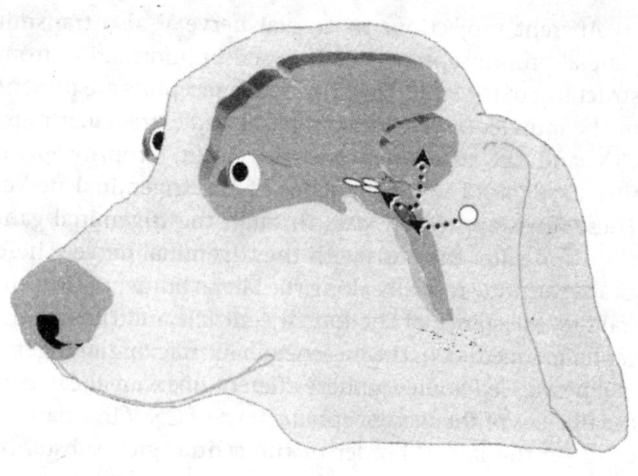

Fig. 1.12. Lateral view, schematic representation of the distribution of the vestibular nerve.

from these cells course through the internal acoustic meatus with those of the cochlear division. The cell bodies are located in the vestibular ganglion. The axons enter the brain stem at the cerebellomedullary angle at the level of the trapezoid body and the attachment of the caudal cerebellar peduncle. After entering the brain stem, the majority of these axons terminates in the vestibular nuclei (fig. 1.12). Some enter the cerebellum directly through the caudal cerebellar peduncle and terminate in the fastigial nucleus and flocculonodular lobe of the cerebellum. While there are central and peripheral vestibular components, it should be remembered that CN VIII never actually projects beyond the limits of the skull.

There are four vestibular nuclei on each side of the brain stem (rostral, medial, lateral, caudal). These nuclei send axons to many diverse areas within the nervous system. Through the vestibulospinal tract, the vestibular system sends descending axons to the spinal cord to positively affect the limb extensor muscles and negatively affect limb flexor systems. In cats, much of this input comes from the lateral vestibular nucleus (deLahunta 1983).

The medial vestibular nucleus projects into the medial longitudinal fasciculus, which descends the spinal cord to the cervical and cranial thoracic regions (deLahunta 1983; Jenkins 1978). Axons also course rostrally in the medial longitudinal fasciculus to influence the nuclei of cranial nerves III, IV, and VI, providing for some normal reflex (oculovestibular) eye movements.

Axons of CN VIII project into the reticular formation to the vomiting center. There may also be a vestibular projection pathway for conscious proprioception, traveling in similar regions as the pathways for the auditory functions of this nerve. Axons from the vestibular nuclei also project to the cerebellum via the caudal cerebellar peduncle to terminate in the flocculus of the cerebellar hemisphere and the nodulus of the caudal vermis (flocculonodular lobe) as well as the fastigial nucleus.

Cochlear Division. The *cochlear division* of CN VIII is important for auditory stimulus recognition (deLahunta

1983; Jenkins 1978; King 1987). Receptors of the cochlear division of CN VIII are located in the cochlear duct within the ear. The spiral organ (organ of Corti) contains the sensory epithelium that is present on the basilar membrane. This structure is made up of hair and supporting cells. The hair cells send processes that extend into a proteinaceous membrane, the tectorial membrane. The dendritic zone of the cochlear portion of CN VIII is in synaptic relationship with the base of the hair cells. The cell bodies are located in the modiolus at the origin of the spiral lamina, forming the spiral ganglion. The axons course through the internal acoustic meatus where they join the vestibular division of CN VIII. These axons terminate on cell bodies in the cochlear nucleus that bulges on the lateral side of the medulla.

The axons of the cochlear nuclei project in two main pathways: ventrally through the trapezoid body and dorsally as the acoustic stria. Reflex hearing functions are mediated by direct synapse with brain stem nuclei. Reflex control of sound wave frequency is sensed (afferent) by the cochlear division of CN VIII, and the efferent nerve is found in CN V, projecting to the tensor tympani muscle, and CN VII, projecting to the stapedius muscle. When a loud sound enters the ear, these muscles contract and result in increased impedance to sound in the middle ear (stapedius) and tympanic membrane (tensor tympani).

The projection pathways for sound ascend toward the cerebral cortex through the trapezoid body, lateral lemniscus, caudal colliculus, brachium of the caudal colliculus, and medial geniculate body of the thalamus. From the thalamus, axons project through the internal capsule to the temporal (auditory) cortex. The ascending auditory pathway is diffusely located in the brain stem with bilateral central projections. The predominant projection is, however, contralateral. Decussation of these pathways occurs at the trapezoid body, between the nuclei of the lateral lemniscus, and at the commissure of the caudal colliculus.

Cranial Nerve IX—Glossopharyngeal Nerve

The glossopharyngeal nerve provides motor and sensory innervation to the pharynx, as well as parasympathetic functions for salivation and taste sensation (fig. 1.13) (deLahunta 1983; Jenkins 1978; King 1987). The cell bodies of the motor (visceral efferent) fibers are located with CN X and CN XI in the nucleus ambiguus, an ill-defined column of neurons in the ventrolateral medulla oblongata. Cranial nerve IX emerges from the medulla lateral and caudal to CN VIII. The nerve courses through the jugular foramen and the tympanooccipital fissure to innervate the stylopharyngeus and other pharyngeal muscles.

Receptors for sensory (visceral afferent) fibers of CN IX are located in the caudal tongue, pharynx, and carotid body and sinus. Cell bodies of these nerves are located in the distal ganglion. The axons enter the brain stem through CN IX, and enter the solitary tract and nucleus of the solitary tract similar to CN VII. These axons function in pain recognition in the tongue and pharynx and baroreception of the great vessels.

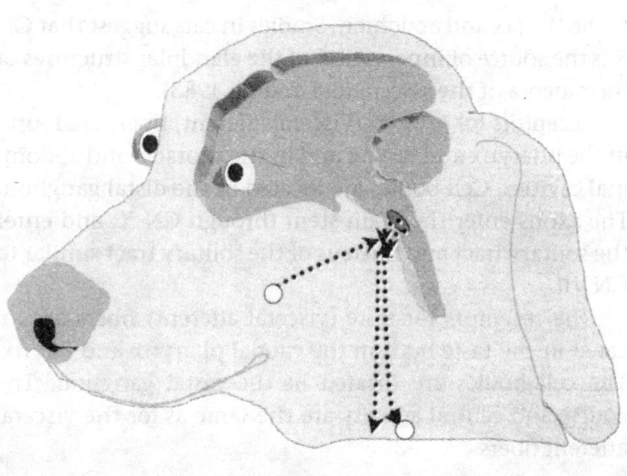

Fig. 1.13. Lateral view, schematic representation of the location of cranial nerves IX and X.

For salivation, cell bodies of the parasympathetic fibers are located in the same nuclear column as CN VII. Preganglionic fibers synapse in the otic ganglion. Post ganglionic fibers innervate the zygomatic and parotid salivary glands.

Receptors for taste (visceral afferent) are present in the caudal one-third of the tongue and the rostral pharynx. Cell bodies are located in the distal ganglion. The course and central activity is the same as for visceral afferent functions.

Cranial Nerve X—Vagus Nerve

The vagus nerve is important for motor and sensory innervation of the pharynx and provides a major component of the parasympathetic innervation to the esophagus and the gastrointestinal tract (fig. 1.13) (deLahunta 1983; Jenkins 1978; King 1987). Other functions of the vagus include taste sensation and salivation. Motor cell bodies (visceral efferent) of this nerve are similarly located in the nucleus ambiguus as are those for CN IX. The axons of CN X traverse the skull through the jugular foramen and tympanooccipital fissure. Some fibers join the pharyngeal plexus and innervate the muscles of the palate, pharynx, and cervical esophagus. Some leave the vagus nerve in the cranial laryngeal muscle to innervate the cricothyroid muscle, with the recurrent laryngeal nerve and its caudal laryngeal branch innervating all the other muscles of the larynx, cervical and cranial esophagus. In cats, these latter axons have been noted to arise from the caudal nucleus ambiguus and course to the vagus by the internal branch of the accessory nerve. Cell bodies from the nucleus ambiguus innervate the entire length of the esophagus.

Cell bodies of the parasympathetic (visceral efferent) nerves of CN X are located in the same nuclear column as for CN VII and IX. Neurons of CN X make up the majority of this column. These axons exit the lateral aspect of the medulla oblongata, course through the jugular foramen and tympanooccipital fissure, and descend in the neck, being eventually distributed to the esophagus and organs of the thorax and abdomen. Studies in cats suggest that CN X is the source of innervation of the glandular structures of the mucosa of the viscera (deLahunta 1983).

Receptors for sensory (visceral afferent) fibers are found in the pharynx and larynx and in the thoracic and abdominal cavities. Cell bodies are located in the distal ganglion. The axons enter the brain stem through CN X, and enter the solitary tract and nucleus of the solitary tract similar to CN VII.

The receptors for taste (visceral afferent) fibers are located in the taste buds in the caudal pharynx and larynx. The cell bodies are located in the distal ganglion. The course and central activity are the same as for the visceral afferent fibers.

Cranial Nerve XI—Spinal Accessory Nerve

The spinal accessory nerve provides motor innervation to the trapezius as well as portions of the sternocephalicus and brachiocephalicus muscles (fig. 1.14) (deLahunta 1983; Jenkins 1978; King 1987). Spinal accessory nerve (visceral efferent) axons project from the caudal nucleus ambiguus and emerge from the ventrolateral aspect of the medulla with the visceral efferent fibers of CN X. The cranial roots join to form the internal branch. The internal branch passes laterally and joins the external branch to form the accessory nerve. Other visceral efferent cell bodies of the external branch are located in the motor nucleus of the accessory nerve in the lateral portion of the ventral spinal cord grey matter from the first (C1) to possibly the seventh (C7) cervical spinal cord segments. The axons exit the spinal cord laterally as roots of the accessory nerve. The external branch passes through the foramen magnum. This nerve enters the jugular foramen and leaves the tympanooccipital fissure. Here the internal branch leaves the accessory nerve and joins the vagus nerve. The external branch then forms the accessory nerve to innervate the trapezius as well as portions of the sternocephalicus and brachiocephalicus muscles.

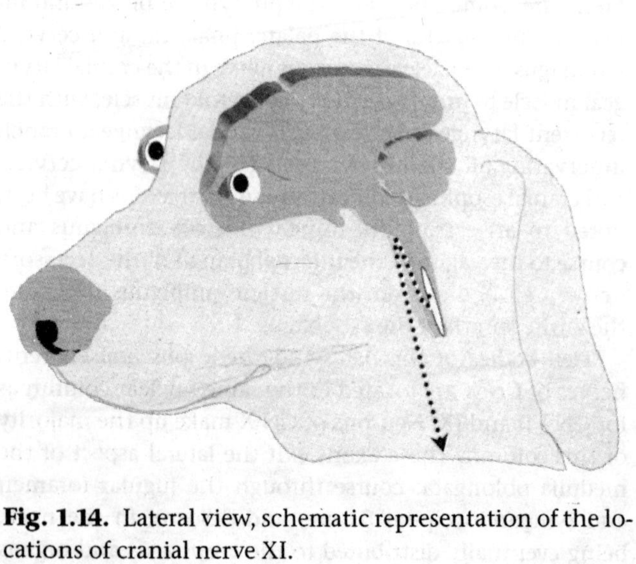

Fig. 1.14. Lateral view, schematic representation of the locations of cranial nerve XI.

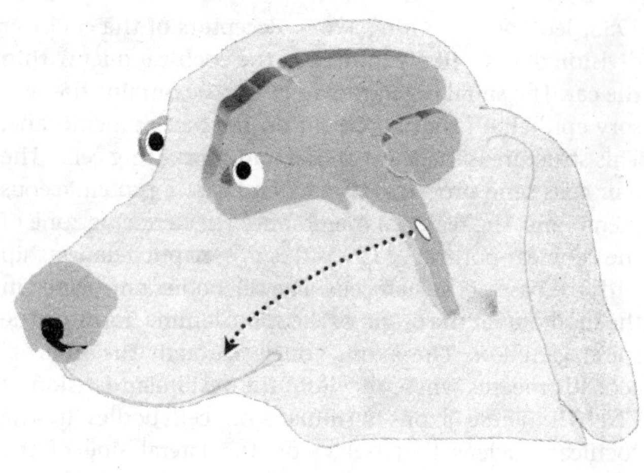

Fig. 1.15. Lateral view, schematic representation of the locations of cranial nerve XII.

Cranial Nerve XII—Hypoglossal Nerve

The hypoglossal nerve provides motor innervation to the muscles of the tongue (fig. 1.15) (deLahunta 1983). Cell bodies of these motor (somatic efferent) axons are located in the hypoglossal nucleus in the medulla oblongata, adjacent to midline on floor of the fourth ventricle. Axons of this nerve cross the lateral aspect of the olivary nucleus in the brain stem, and emerge as numerous longitudinal small roots lateral to the pyramids. These roots merge at the small hypoglossal canal to form CN XII proper. This nerve innervates the extrinsic muscles of the tongue (styloglossus, hyoglossus, and genioglossus), the intrinsic muscles of the tongue, and the geniohyoideus. A few cell bodies of neurons to the intrinsic lingual muscles are located in the caudal area of the facial nucleus. Each genioglossus muscle is innervated by neurons from both hypoglossal nuclei.

THE MENINGES

The meninges are the peripheral covering tissues of the central nervous system (figs. 1.16 and 1.17) (deLahunta 1983; Jenkins 1978; King 1987). There are three layers of the meninges: the dura mater, arachnoid, and pia mater extending from outer to inner surfaces. The dura mater is the most external and is a fibrous tissue of collagen matrix. The arachnoid is usually intimate in ventral contact with the dura. A space is present ventral to the arachnoid (subarachnoid space) where CSF is present. The pia is a thin tissue layer that is intimate with the outer surface of the nervous tissue. The pachymeninx refers to the dura mater. The leptomeninx, or meninges, refers to the arachnoid and pia mater as a unit. All of these meningeal structures are also found surrounding the spinal cord.

An invagination of the meninges is located between the dorsal cerebral hemispheres. This is the falx cerebri. Portions of the meninges may also be found more centrally around or within the ventricular system (tela choroidea).

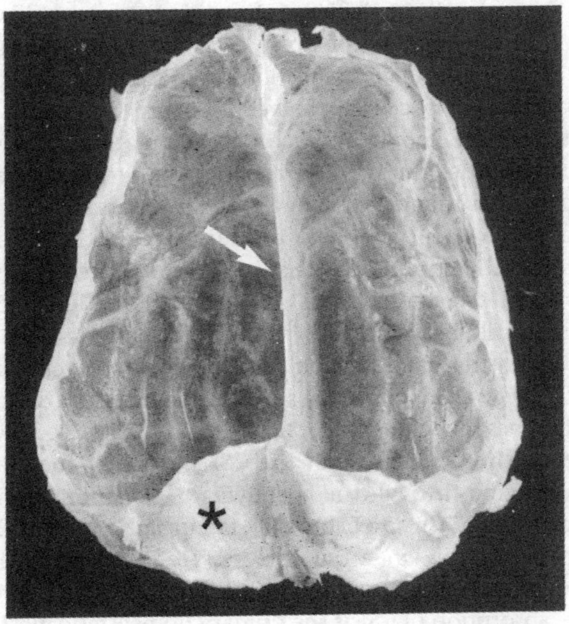

Fig. 1.16. Meningeal coverings of the brain (viewed from inside looking dorsally). Note the tentorium cerebelli (*) and the falx cerebri (*arrow*).

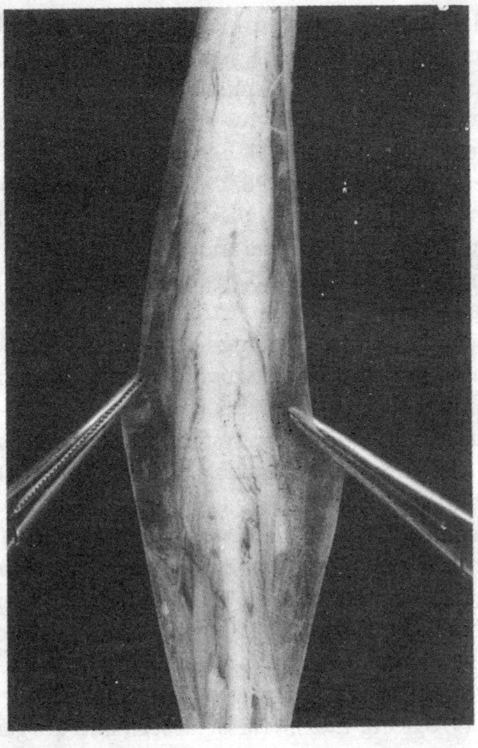

Fig. 1. 17. Meningeal coverings of the spinal cord (incised on midline and retracted by hemostats).

VENTRICULAR SYSTEM AND CSF

The brain normally contains areas that are devoid of cells but filled with cerebrospinal fluid (CSF) (fig. 1.18) (Beitz and Fletcher 1993; deLahunta 1983; Jenkins 1978; King 1987). These areas are collectively known as the ventricular system.

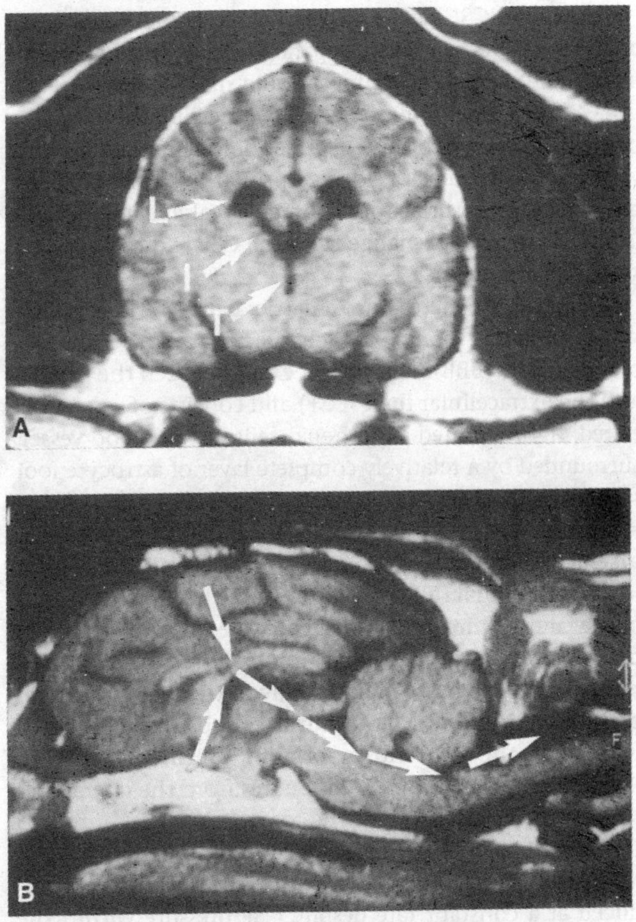

Fig. 1.18. (A) Transverse and (B) sagittal views of the brain of a dog. In (A), note the ventricular system as the blacker structures: (L) lateral ventricle, (I) interventricular foramen, (T) third ventricle. In (B), arrows represent the flow of CSF in the ventricular system.

From rostral to caudal, beginning in the cerebral hemispheres, the components of this system include the lateral ventricles, the third ventricle, the mesencephalic aqueduct, and the fourth ventricle. Extensions of the lateral ventricle may extend into the olfactory regions of the brain. The third ventricle is present in a circular pattern around the innerthalamic adhesion. The mesencephalic aqueduct is the smaller tubular connection between the third and fourth ventricle in the mesencephalon. The fourth ventricle is present between the brain stem (ventrally) and the cerebellum (dorsally). The fourth ventricle is continued into the spinal cord via the central canal. The ventricular system is lined by specialized columnar cells with microvilli known as ependymal cells. These cells are important as a partial barrier between the CSF and the brain parenchyma, and also play an important role in production of CSF. In some areas of the ventricular system, there are concentrations of a vascular structure and an associated ependymal lining known as the choroid plexus. This tissue also has an important role in CSF production, and pulsations in these structures may result in movement of CSF.

The blood-CSF barrier exists at the choroid plexus and consists of two cell layers separated by a thin basement membrane. This is a semipermeable membrane between the CSF and the plasma. The CSF-extracellular fluid (ECF) barrier occurs over the outer surface of the brain and in the ventricles. This barrier is formed primarily by the ependymal cells. On the surface of the brain, a pial-glial membrane is present to limit exchange from the CSF and the nervous system parenchyma.

Importantly, there is also a barrier between the vascular system and the brain parenchyma, termed the "blood-brain barrier" (BBB). This barrier exists between the plasma and the extracellular fluid (ECF) and consists of nonfenestrated, tightly joined endothelial cells of the blood vessel, surrounded by a relatively complete layer of astrocyte foot processes. The BBB plays an important role in preventing the free exchange of various substances within the vascular system and brain cells.

Cerebrospinal fluid originates from the choroid plexus of the lateral, third, and fourth ventricles, directly from the brain by way of the ependymal lining of the ventricular system, directly from the brain by way of the pial-glial membrane covering the external surface, and from the blood vessels of the pia and arachnoid (deLahunta 1983). Approximately 35% of CSF originates from the lateral and third ventricles, 23% from the fourth ventricle, and 42% from the subarachnoid space (deLahunta 1983).

Cerebrospinal fluid is an ultrafiltrate of plasma. It is produced at a constant rate despite CSF pressure within the ventricular system (deLahunta 1983). The rate of CSF production is independent of the hydrostatic pressure of the blood, but dependent on the osmotic pressure of the intravascular space. Hyperosmolality of blood, for example, decreases CSF production. Cerebrospinal fluid circulates from the sites of production and exits the ventricular system at the lateral apertures of the fourth ventricle, then passes dorsally over the cerebral hemispheres to the dorsal sagittal sinus. It penetrates the brain with the larger blood vessels of the perivascular space (extensions of the subarachnoid space to where the pia reflects back on these vessels). In some animals, CSF may also exit at the conus medullaris in the caudal portion of the spinal cord.

Compared to plasma, CSF has less potassium and calcium, and more chloride, sodium, and magnesium, and approximately 75–80% as much glucose (deLahunta 1983). The protein content in dogs and cats is less than 25 mg/dl from the cerebellomedullary cistern (<35 mg/dl from lumbar area). Dogs produce approximately 0.047 ml of CSF/min, whereas cats produce CSF at approximately 0.017 ml/min (deLahunta 1983).

Flow of CSF is dependent on the pulsation of the blood (systole and diastole) in the choroid plexus. With each pulsation, CSF pressure increases with flow aided by the cilia of the ependymal cells. Cerebrospinal fluid flow occurs in both directions (cranial and caudal), but primarily flows caudally in dogs. The pressure exhibited by the CSF contributes to *intracranial pressure,* the importance of which will be discussed in chapter 2.

The major site of CSF absorption is in the arachnoid villus within a venous sinus or a cerebral vein (deLahunta 1983). The villus is a prolongation of the arachnoid and the subarachnoid space into the venous sinus. Collections of these villi are known as arachnoid granulations. The venous endothelium acts like a ball valve (from transient transcellular channels that develop for the passage of fluid) so as to be open when CSF pressure exceeds the venous pressure (the normal relationship). If venous pressure rises above CSF pressure, the villi will collapse. Directional flow, therefore, is always from CSF to blood (deLahunta 1983).

Other sites of absorption of CSF include the veins and lymphatics surrounding the spinal nerve roots and the cranial nerves (olfactory and optic nerves) where these nerves traverse the skull. Some of the CSF may enter the brain parenchyma through the ependyma to be absorbed into blood vessels. This probably is an important means of CSF absorption only when the CSF pressure is elevated. With production being mostly independent of intracranial pressure, absorption of CSF is the primary homeostatic mechanism to prevent increases in CSF pressure.

STRUCTURES CAUDAL TO THE FORAMEN MAGNUM

At the level of the foramen magnum, the brain stem becomes contiguous with the spinal cord. The spinal cord serves as a conduit for transmission of information to and from the intracranial structures (Burke and Colter 1990; deLahunta 1983; Dyce et al 1996a; Dyce 1996b; Fletcher 1993; Jenkins 1978; King 1987). Also, the spinal cord contains the neuronal cell bodies that are responsible for motor functions in the limbs and trunk.

Both the spinal cord and the overlying vertebral structures are divided into segments (fig. 1.19). It is important to define whether one is referring to spinal cord segments or vertebral segments when discussing pertinent spinal neuroanatomy. During clinical neuroanatomical localization of lesions within the nervous system, for example, it is most common to refer to the particular *spinal segments* that are involved (figs. 1.19 and 1.20).

The spinal cord is divided into spinal segments (approximately 36) with some variability between individual animals as to the actual number. The cervical spinal cord normally contains 8 of these spinal segments, the thoracic area has 13 segments, and the lumbar region has 7 segment structures (Chrisman 1991; deLahunta 1983; Fletcher 1993; Jenkins 1978; King 1987). The sacral segments are generally divided into 3 segments, with the caudal segments being somewhat variable, but often 5 segments. The spinal cord segmental arrangement is variable, both between species and even within individuals within the species. Spinal segments are encased within the vertebrae throughout its length.

In the cervical area, there are 7 cervical vertebrae (vertebral segments) and 8 associated spinal cord segment structures (deLahunta 1983; Fletcher 1993; Jenkins 1978; King 1987). Therefore, there is a slight discontinuity between the

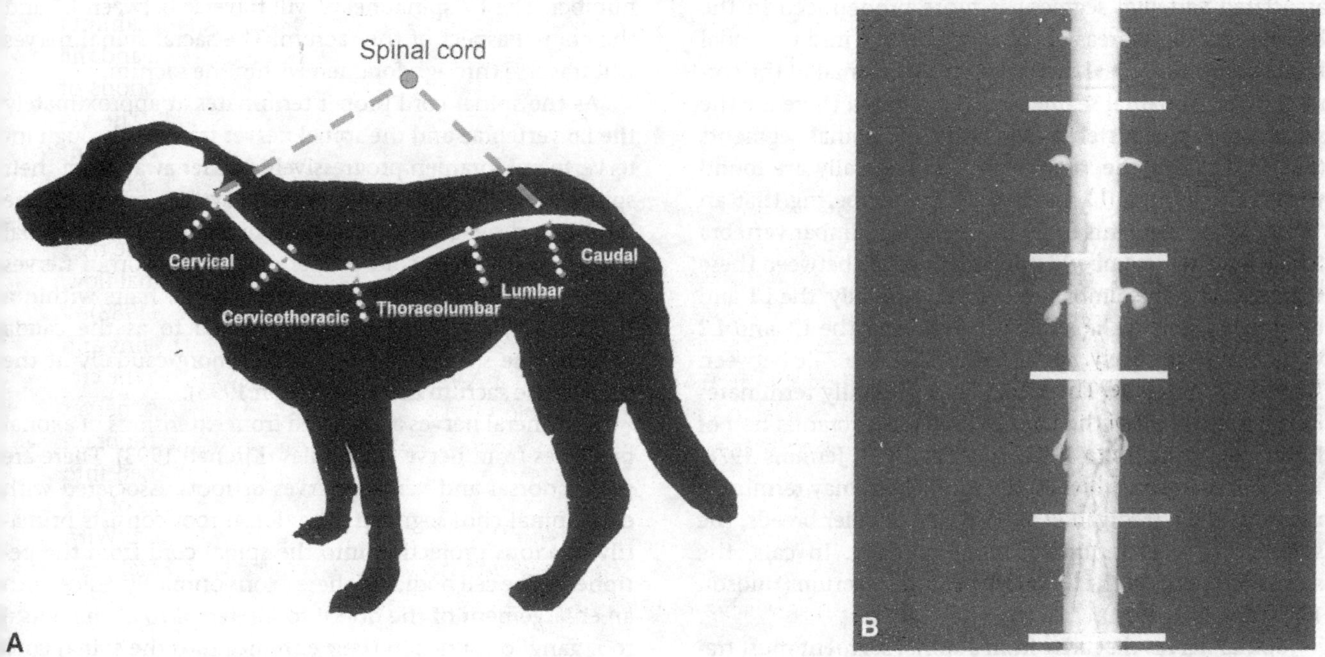

ig. 1.19. (A) Schematic view of a dog spinal cord with various regions. (B) Gross anatomical specimen of the dog thoracolumbar spinal cord showing the approximate divisions of the spinal segments.

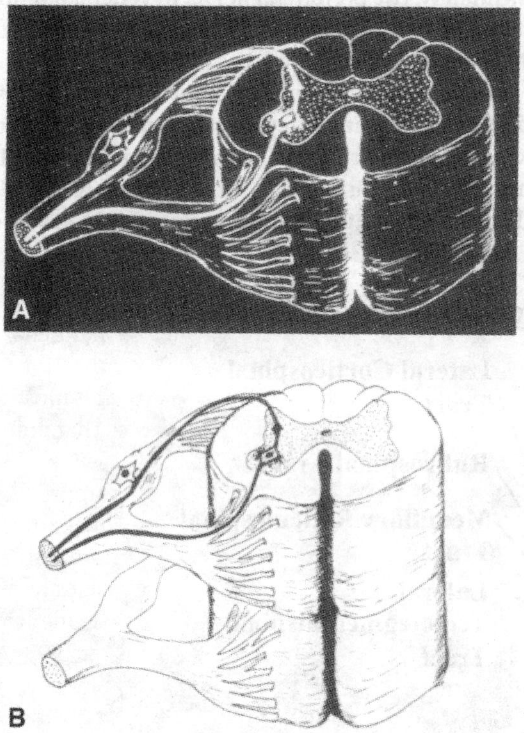

ig. 1.20. Schematic view of (A) a single spinal cord segment and (B) adjacent spinal segments.

ocation of the cervical spinal cord segments and the cervial vertebral segments, with the spinal cord segments lying ithin or slightly cranial to the vertebrae of the same numer. A single spinal cord segment will give rise to a paired set f associated spinal nerves numbered similarly as the spinal segment. For example, the first cervical, or C1, spinal cord segment will produce the first cervical, or C1, nerve. (There is also a first cervical vertebrae, the C1 vertebrae.) To reiterate, it is important to not confuse the spinal cord segments, associated spinal nerves, and cervical vertebrae during clinical communication even though each of these structures is commonly referred to as "C1." Obviously there is an extra cervical spinal segment and associated nerves (C8 segment and nerves) compared to only 7 cervical vertebrae. Spinal nerves that arise from a spinal segment must traverse the vertebral canal to terminate peripherally on a muscle or organ or to provide conduit for projection of afferent information from the periphery into the spinal cord. Spinal nerves traverse between vertebrae in the intervertebral foramen just ventral to the articular facets of the adjacent vertebrae. In the cervical area, the first cervical nerve will traverse from the vertebral canal peripherally through the lateral vertebral foramen located within the dorsal arch of C1 vertebrae. The C2 spinal nerve will traverse between C1 and C2 vertebrae. The additional cervical spinal nerves will traverse the vertebral foramen cranial to the vertebrae of the same number. The C7 spinal nerves will traverse the intervertebral foramen between the C6 and C7 vertebrae and the C8 spinal nerves will traverse the intervertebral foramen between the C8 and T1 vertebrae.

The thoracic spinal cord contains 13 thoracic spinal cord segments and 13 associated pairs of spinal nerves. Generally, the spinal segments overlie the vertebrae of the same number. The spinal nerves traverse the foramen caudal to the vertebrae of the same spinal cord segment. For example, the T7 spinal nerves will traverse the foramen between the T6 and T7 vertebrae.

The discontinuity between spinal segment location and

associated vertebral segment is more pronounced in the lumbar and sacral areas of the spine. In the mid to caudal lumbar area, the spinal cord segments lie cranial to the corresponding vertebral segments, even though there are the same number of vertebral segments and spinal segments (i.e., 7). In dogs, the sacral segments generally are found within the lumbar (L) 5 vertebrae. Remembering that an "S" for sacral segments looks like a "5" for lumbar vertebra 5 may help in remembering the relationship between these segments and the lumbar vertebrae. Generally, the L1 and L2 spinal segments lie approximately over the L1 and L2 vertebrae, respectively. Spinal segments L3 to 7 lie between L3 and L5 vertebrae. The spinal cord generally terminates in the caudal half of the L6 vertebrae to the cranial half of L7 in dog (deLahunta 1983; Fletcher 1993; Jenkins 1978; King 1987). In larger breeds, the spinal cord may terminate more cranially (Morgan et al. 1987). In smaller breeds, the spinal cord may terminate more caudally. In cats, the spinal cord ends at the L7 vertebrae or the sacrum (Hudson 1993; Kot et al. 1994).

Spinal nerves that arise from a spinal segment must traverse through the intervertebral foramen to terminate peripherally on a muscle or organ or to provide afferent information from the limb and body structures into the spinal cord (Fletcher 1993; Kitchell 1993; Kitchell and Evans 1993). Spinal nerves traverse between vertebrae in the intervertebral foramen just ventral to the articular facets of the adjacent vertebrae. In the lumbar area, as in the thoracic area, the first lumbar nerve will traverse from the vertebral canal peripherally through the foramen between L1 and L2 vertebrae or caudal to the vertebrae of the same number. The additional lumbar spinal nerves will traverse the vertebral foramen caudal to the vertebrae of the same number. The L7 spinal nerve will traverse between L7 and the cranial aspect of the sacrum. The sacral spinal nerves will traverse through foramen within the sacrum.

As the spinal cord proper terminates at approximately the L6 vertebrae and the spinal nerves traverse through intervertebral foramen progressively farther away from their spinal segment origin, the nervous system overlying the L6, L7, and sacral vertebrae is more a collection of spinal nerves than spinal cord proper. This collection of nerves viewed grossly gives off the appearance of hairs within a horse's tail, and thus is often referred to as the cauda equina. The spinal cord terminates more caudally at the level of the sacrum in cats (Hudson 1993).

Peripheral nerves are formed from extensions of axonal processes from nerve cell bodies (Kitchell 1993). There are paired dorsal and ventral nerves or roots associated with each spinal cord segment. The dorsal root consists primarily of axons projecting into the spinal cord from the periphery. The cell bodies of these axons primarily reside with an enlargement of the dorsal root referred to as the dorsal root ganglion. Prior to their entrance into the spinal cord proper, the nerve roots form multiple rootlets. The ventral root is formed primarily from axons of efferent or exiting nerves to the periphery. At the origin of these nerve roots are nerve rootlets, which coalesce to form the nerve root and, ultimately, the peripheral nerve. In general but not exclusively, the dorsal root usually contains sensory axons and the ventral root contains motor axons.

A cross section of a spinal segment reveals the relationship between the central grey matter and the more peripheral white matter structures (fig. 1.21) (deLahunta 1983; Fletcher 1993; Jenkins 1978; King 1987; Kitchell 1993). Spinal cord white matter contains groups of axons or tracts

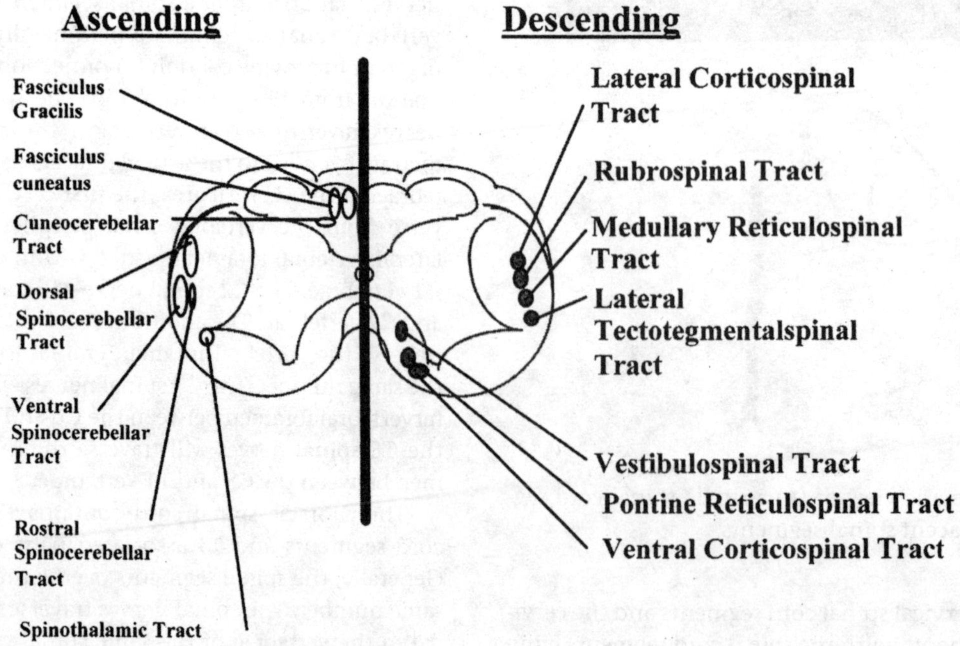

Fig. 1.21. Transverse schematic view of a single spinal cord segment showing the approximate location of the ascending and descending spinal tracts.

traversing through the spinal cord from peripheral sensory receptors and their projections to the intracranial structures. In addition, within the white matter, there are tracts descending from the intracranial structures that traverse through the spinal cord to synapse on the neuronal cells that form nerves that exit the spinal cord and project to the peripheral axial or appendicular structures.

The central grey matter of the spinal cord tends to have the appearance of an "H," but has also been described as a "butterfly" or "animal horns." The dorsal and ventral arms of the H are contiguous with the nerve rootlets either entering (dorsal) or exiting (ventral). The white matter is isolated more peripherally by the H-shaped grey matter and associated nerve rootlets into discrete regions. These regions of white matter are referred to as funiculi. Between the parallel sides of the H and the cross bar dorsally is the dorsal funiculus (or bilateral funiculi). Lateral to the parallel sides of the H is the lateral funiculus (funiculi). Ventral to the parallel sides of the H and the cross bar is the ventral funiculus (funiculi).

The dorsal funiculus contains the fasciculus gracilis and cuneatus, which are the primarily ascending sensory or afferent tracts (fig. 1.21). These tracts are the cranial projection of proprioceptive neurons from peripheral receptors in the pelvic and thoracic limbs. As a general rule, projections or tracts of similarly functioning axons are named first by their anatomical origin and last by their termination. For example, the spinocerebellar tracts project information from the spinal cord (initially from the limbs) to the cerebellum providing afferent information to the cerebellum. The spinothalamic tracts originate in neurons in the spinal cord and ascend the spinal cord to terminate in the thalamus of the supratentorial region. The corticospinal tracts originate in the motor cortex of the cerebral hemisphere and descend through the brain stem to terminate on nerves of the spinal cord. The rubrospinal tract originates in the red nucleus of the mesencephalon and descends through the brain stem to terminate in the spinal cord.

The lateral funiculus contains both ascending and descending tracts. These tracts include the dorsal and ventral spinocerebellar tracts and the rostral spinocerebellar tract, which send afferent projections to the cerebellum from the pelvic limb. The lateral corticospinal and rubrospinal are descending motor tracts primarily responsible for limb flexion. Additional tracts include the medullary reticulospinal tract (descending inhibitory motor function), the lateral tectotegmental spinal tract (descending sympathetic system), and the spinothalamic tract (ascending pain fibers).

The ventral funiculus contains the vestibulospinal and pontine reticulospinal tracts. These projections tend to have a descending facilitatory influence to limb extensor muscles. The ventral corticospinal tracts, if present, are composed of descending motor tracts.

As in other parts of the nervous system, spinal cord tracts are somatotopically organized. In the ascending tracts of the dorsal funiculus (fasciculus gracilis and cuneatus), tracts from the pelvic limbs reside more medially compared to projections from the thoracic limbs. Originating caudally, successively more cranially located projections are added more laterally (deLahunta 1983; Fletcher 1993; Jenkins 1978; King 1987). Conversely, ascending projections in the spinocerebellar tracts and the majority of the descending motor tracts projecting to the spinal cord and associated limbs tend to lie more laterally in relation to the tracts to and from the more cranial (thoracic) segments (deLahunta 1983; Fletcher 1993; Jenkins 1978; King 1987). Disease that involves specific spinal tracts may be reflected in the type of clinical signs present. For example, abnormalities affecting predominantly the tracts to and from the thoracic limbs may result in clinical signs more obvious in the thoracic limbs.

GREY MATTER

The *grey matter* is centrally positioned in the spinal segment. This area is predominantly made up of the *neuronal cell bodies,* their processes, terminations of descending axons, and interneurons (connections between neurons). The grey matter is divided into various areas based on anatomical arrangements of the cells (Rexed's laminae) (fig. 1.22) (deLahunta 1983; Fletcher 1993; Jenkins 1978; King 1987).

As a general rule, the dorsal grey matter (also referred to as dorsal horn) is involved or associated with sensory (afferent) functions. Nerve cells in the middle section, or the intermediate horn, are associated with autonomic functions. Finally, the ventral grey matter (ventral horn) is the location of the majority of nerve cells that produce nerves that ultimately terminate on limb and trunk muscles for production of movement. The grey matter is again somatotopically divided in the ventral horn, with the cell bodies of neurons projecting to the axial musculature located more medially in this area and cell bodies of neurons projecting to the appendicular musculature located more laterally (deLahunta 1983). The cell bodies of neurons to the more proximal limb musculature are located more ventrally and the neurons to the more distal limb muscles are located more dorsally in the ventral grey matter.

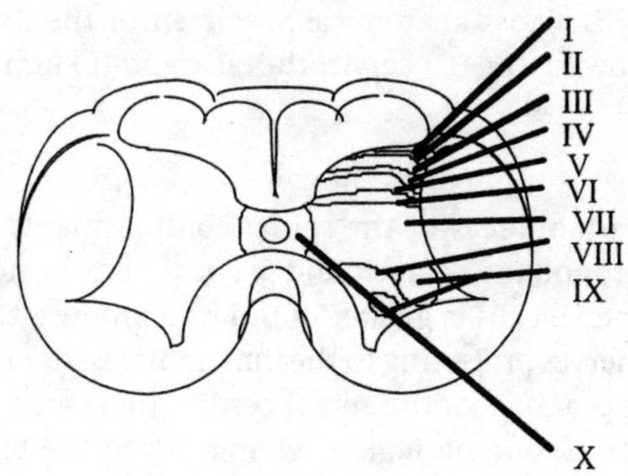

Fig. 1.22. Transverse schematic view of a single spinal cord segment showing the differing regions of the grey matter. The grey matter is divided in the ten Rexed's lamina.

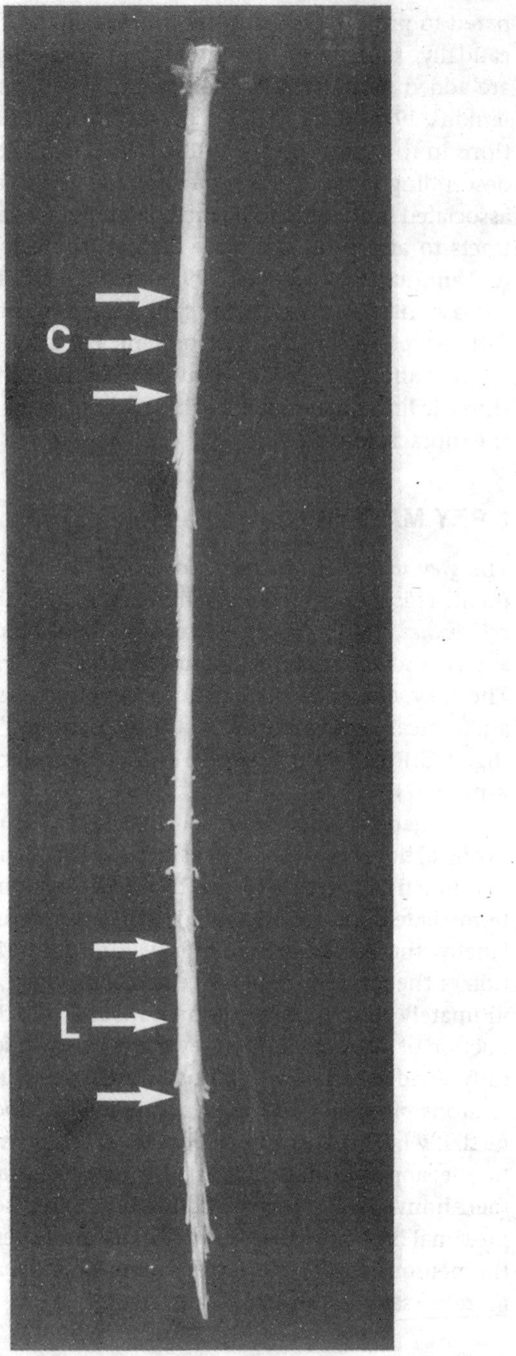

Fig. 1.23. Gross anatomical specimen of the dog spinal cord showing the (C) cervicothoracic and (L) lumbar intumescences.

In certain areas of the spinal cord, primarily concentrated around the thoracic and pelvic limbs, the number of motor nerve cells is greater in order to produce the major motor nerves projecting to the limb muscles (fig. 1.23). The gross appearance of the spinal cord in these areas is larger than corresponding regions giving rise to the term intumescence (swelling). The nerve cell bodies in the ventral grey matter of the spinal cord in these areas produce axons that form the spinal and peripheral nerves projecting from the spinal cord and peripheral muscle or organ, hence giving rise to the peripheral nerves or peripheral nervous system. The regions of the spinal cord where this concentration of nerve cells and nerve fibers arise are generally between the C6 to T2 spinal segments for the thoracic limb and the L4 through the sacral spinal segments for the pelvic limb. Considering the regions of the spinal cord that produce spinal nerves that terminate in limb muscles, the spinal cord can be divided into five major regions (table 1.3; fig. 1.19).The spinal cord can be functionally divided based upon the spinal segments and associated clinical signs of disease affecting the various segments. This division is also based upon whether the associated spinal segments contain cell bodies that give rise to peripheral nerves projecting to the limbs or not.

Table 1.3. Functional areas of the spinal cord

C1—C5
C6—T2
T3—L3
L4—S3
Caudal

Some peripheral nerves may coalesce distal to their traversing the intervertebral foramen. This coalescence of nerves is commonly referred to as a plexus. In the thoracic limb axillary area, these nerves are referred to as the brachial plexus. In the medial pelvic limb area, these peripheral nerves form the pelvic plexus.

The innervation of regional nerves, as well as the corresponding origin of these nerves from spinal segments forming the plexus, may vary between individual animals. When regional nerves forming the brachial plexus arise from more cranial spinal rootlets compared to the normal distribution, the plexus is said to be prefixed. When the nerves originate from more caudal spinal cord segments than normal, the plexus is said to be postfixed. Allam studied the nerves that form the brachial plexus in dogs and found the following percentages of dogs had the brachial plexus derived from the associated spinal segments: 58.6% were formed by C6, C7, C8, and T1; 20.7% were formed by C5, C6, C7, C8, and T1; 17.24% were formed by C6, C7, C8, T1, and T2; and 3.4% were formed by C5, C6, C7, C8, T1, and T2 (Allam et al. 1952). The ratio of dogs with prefixed, median, and postfixed plexus types is approximately 1:3:1.

THE PERIPHERAL NERVOUS SYSTEM

The peripheral nervous system includes any nerve myelinated by a Schwann cell (fig. 1.24) (deLahunta 1983; Jenkins 1978; King 1987; Kitchell 1993). Schwann cells begin myelinating peripheral nerves to the limbs at the intervertebral foramen of the vertebral column. Using this strict definition, other components of the peripheral nerve, such as the cell body of the motor neuron in the ventral grey matter of the spinal cord, the synapse, or the effector organ, would not be included in the peripheral nervous system. Functionally, however, a lesion of the peripheral nerve or cell body would result in identical clinical signs.

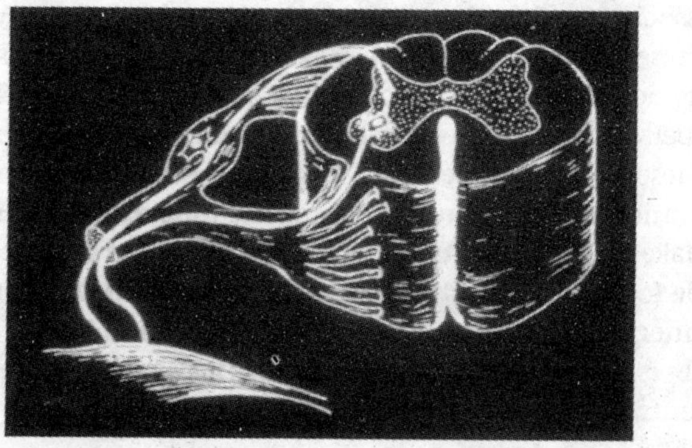

Fig. 1.24. Transverse schematic view of a single spinal cord segment showing the association with the peripheral nervous system connecting to a limb muscle.

Therefore, the term "peripheral nervous system" is sometimes used as a functional definition to includes all components from the cell body to the effector organ.

In essence, the peripheral nervous system forms the ultimate link between the central integrating pathways of the nervous system and the body structures necessary for performance of a specific function. Without this connection, regardless of what initiating events occur in the central nervous system, the function within the body will not be completed. These structures are sometimes referred to as the final common pathway for ultimate expression of nervous system function.

Sensory Receptors of the Peripheral Nervous System

There are five basic types of peripherally located sensory receptors (Guyton and Hall 1996): (1)mechanoreceptors, (2)thermoreceptors, (3)nociceptors, (4)electromagnetic receptors, and (5)chemoreceptors.

Numerous sensations perceived by the body are initiated in many anatomically different types of receptors (table 1.4). For example with the sensation of touching, Meissner's corpuscles are important for recognition as to exactly what part of the body is being touched and the texture. Expanded tip tactile receptors (e.g., Merkel's discs) provide steady state signals that allow one to determine continuous touch of objects against the skin. Ruffini's end organs are multibranched, encapsulated receptors important for continual signaling. Paccinian corpuscles are stimulated only by rapid movement, thus being important for detecting tissue vibration or other rapid changes in the mechanical state of tissue.

Each type of receptor is highly sensitive to one type of stimulus for which it is designed (also referred to as the labeled-line principle). In essence, there is specificity of nerve fibers for only one modality of sensation. A modality is a form of energy converted by the receptor organ into a neuronal impulse. Some receptors can be stimulated by various modalities with the type of sensation determined by the area in the nervous system where that nerve fiber terminates.

Table 1.4. Stimulus sensation and the associated nervous system receptor type

Sensation perceived	Receptor type
Pain, cold, warmth	Free nerve endings
Pressure	Paccinian corpuscles
	Expanded tip receptor
Touch	Meissner's corpuscles
Muscle spindle stretch	Intrafusal fiber (annulospiral organ)
	Extrafusal fibers
Tendon stretch	Golgi tendon organ

Source: Guyton and Hall 1996.

In all instances, the basic change is in the receptor membrane permeability, which allows ions to diffuse more or less readily through the membrane and change the transmembrane potential (Guyton and Hall 1996). This results in a receptor potential. If this receptor potential is of an appropriate magnitude (threshold), an action potential is elicited. The greater the receptor potential is above a threshold level, the greater the frequency of action potential generation becomes.

Once a receptor is stimulated, receptors have the ability to adapt to continual stimulation (Guyton and Hall 1996). Some receptors adapt quickly to extinction (fast adapting, e.g., Paccinian corpuscle); others adapt more slowly (non-adapting:tonic, e.g., muscle and joint receptors). The longest adaptation time of a mechanoreceptor is approximately 2 days by the carotid and aortic baroreceptors. The adaptive mechanism depends on the individual receptor. This accommodation may occur, for example, because of the inactivation of the Na channel.

Rapidly adapting receptors fire while a change is taking place, that is, the number of impulses produced is directly related to the rate at which the change takes place (rate or phasic receptors). These rate receptors are important because they allow the organism to predict the state of the body over the next few seconds.

The peripheral nerve fibers may be categorized in a number of different ways based upon anatomic or physiologic properties, or in some instances, a combination of both properties (table 1.5). In some schemes, classification depends upon the amount of myelin (i.e., nerve fiber diameter) present. A simple classification scheme divides these into afferent and efferent peripheral nerves. Afferents project information to, and efferents project information from the CNS in most instances. Afferent nerves usually serve a sensory function, and efferents serve a motor function.

Considering the structure of a sensory nerve, the cell body is often found in a ganglion outside the central nervous system. Receptors recognize stimuli and project this information in dendritic processes toward the cell body. Depending upon the stimulus and receptor, various-sized nerve fibers may be involved. The diameter of the axon will determine the velocity of conduction of the nervous impulse. In general, the size of the axon is determined by the degree of myelin present. Myelin is formed by Schwann cells (for the peripheral nervous system) and oligoden-

Table 1.5. Categories of neurons

A All myelinated fibers except the preganglionic autonomic efferents
- Afferent fibers
  - I From annulospiral organ and Golgi tendon organs
  - II Mainly from cutaneous mechanoreceptors
  - III From pinprick pain receptors and sensory ending from blood vessel walls and hair follicles.(* Also called A delta fibers)
- Efferent fibers
- Subgroups
  - Alpha—Supply extrafusal muscle fibers only
  - Beta—Similar size to alpha: give a branch to muscle spindle fibers; then innervate "slow twitch" extrafusal fibers.
  - Gamma—Supply intrafusal fibers only

B Preganglionic autonomic efferents

C Unmyelinated fibers

Sources: Guyton 1996; Jenkins 1978.

drogliocytes (for central nervous system axons). Myelin has been equated to an "insulator," which will increase the speed of conduction of a neural impulse. Larger fibers have more myelination and therefore conduct impulses relatively more rapidly. Small fibers may have little or no myelin and conduct impulses relatively slower. It is important to understand that speeds of nerve impulse conduction are relative, as even unmyelinated fibers conduct impulses at a comparatively rapid rate.

Sensations such as touch are often associated with relatively rapid conduction of impulses. These receptor types are associated with relatively larger A beta nerve fibers or axons (Guyton and Hall 1996). These A beta fibers conduct at velocities of between 30 and 70 m/sec. Conversely, free nerve endings that sense certain painful stimuli are associated with A delta fibers or axons that conduct impulses at between 5 and 30 m/sec. Tickle and itch sensations are carried in C fibers, which are small unmyelinated axons and conduct impulses relatively slowest (Guyton and Hall 1996).

Once information is projected toward the cell body, axons from the cell body enter the spinal cord through the dorsal nerve root. Sensory axons may then be projected in the central nervous system pathways in the spinal cord, or may terminate on additional neuronal elements within the spinal cord (i.e., interneurons or motor neurons).

Neuronal cell bodies responsible for movement are found primarily in the ventral grey matter of the spinal cord. These neurons tend to be relatively larger cells with larger, myelinated axons such as alpha fibers. These motor neuron cell elements may be stimulated by local neurons in the spinal cord or from the terminations of axons descending from more cranial sites in the central nervous system, such as the brain and brain stem. In this way, the components of the central nervous system may signal movement in the muscles of the limb, for example. Local axons from the dorsal root ganglion cells may also terminate on these motor neurons allowing for local spinal reflex functions.

Muscle fibers are categorized as either intrafusal or extrafusal. Intrafusal fibers are a small subset of fibers that are associated with the afferent elements from the muscle. These fibers are modified, small striated muscle cells that are positioned parallel to the larger extrafusal fibers. These fibers may act as receptors for stretch or proprioception. These fibers are innervated by gamma efferent neurons, activation of which provide for muscle tone. Extrafusal fibers make up the majority of the muscle fibers and are responsible for the overall strength of the muscle. These fibers are innervated by alpha neurons. When stimulated, these fibers are primarily responsible for the majority of muscle contraction.

Neuronal Excitation

The normal negativity of the resting membrane is maintained by the sodium-potassium pump, which extrudes three sodium (Na) ions out of the cell and at the same time allows two potassium (K) ions to enter the cell. These are negatively charged ions (proteins, phosphates) that cannot diffuse out of the cell. With the Na-K pump extruding more positive ions than it brings in, the inside of the cell becomes negative compared to the outside. Any charge difference that occurs in the cell is distributed equally.

An excitatory neuron will increase the cell membrane's permeability to Na and K. Because of the large electrochemical gradient, Na rushes into the cell. This increase in intracellular Na causes the resting membrane potential to become less negative, an excitatory postsynaptic potential. The result is that an action potential is formed in the cell. This occurs where the axon leaves the cell, a region referred to as the axon hillock. The action potential is initiated here because there is an increase in the concentration of voltage-gated Na channels in this area.

Inhibitory synapses, by contrast, open K and chloride (Cl) channels. This allows K to leave the cell and Cl to enter, making the center of the cell more negative (hyperpolarized). This is called an inhibitory postsynaptic potential. Inhibition of nerve impulses can also occur at the presynaptic terminal referred to as presynaptic inhibition. The end result of which is to decrease the amount of Ca ions that enter the terminal, and therefore decrease the amount of transmitter released.

Conduction that occurs in the normal direction along the afferent or efferent nerves is called orthodromic conduction. Conduction of impulses in the direction opposite to the way these impulses normally travel is referred to as antidromic conduction.

Synapses and the Neuromuscular Junction

A synapse is the junction between one neuron and another (deLahunta 1983; Guyton and Hall 1996; Jenkins 1978; King 1987). If a neuron terminates on a muscle, this synapse is called a neuromuscular junction.

There are two different types of synapses, one chemical and the other electrical. Almost all synapses in the CNS are chemical, and the chemical secreted is a neurotransmitter (e.g., acetylcholine, norepinephrine, epinephrine, etc.). Conduction across the synapse occurs in one direction, from the presynaptic neuron to the postsynaptic neuron.

The synapse is one way that the direction the impulse will travel is controlled. The impulse can either be facilitated or inhibited in this area.

The presynaptic terminals are frequently called boutons. The presynaptic terminal is separated from the postsynaptic receptor by a synaptic cleft (200 to 300 Angstroms) (Guyton and Hall 1996). These presynaptic terminals have synaptic vesicles (which contain the neurotransmitter substance) and mitochondria (which provide ATP to produce more transmitter). The substance released will be either excitatory or inhibitory, depending on the receptor (either excitatory or inhibitory), on the postsynaptic terminal. There are numerous substances now known to be neurotransmitters. Examples include glutamine, aspartate, taurine, GABA, and glycine.

When an action potential reaches the presynaptic terminal, the membrane depolarization causes release of the neurotransmitters from the presynaptic vesicles. This release is dependent on calcium ions that enter the terminal. Some disease processes such as botulism result in an abnormality of presynaptic release of ACH that prevents normal synaptic function.

The neurotransmitter substance is synthesized and degraded or reabsorbed in this area. For example, ACH is synthesized from acetyl CoA and choline in the presence of choline acetyltransferase. When ACH is released into the synaptic cleft, it is rapidly degraded to acetate and choline by acetylcholinesterase.

At the postsynaptic receptor, there exists a large number of receptor proteins. These receptor proteins have two important components, a binding protein and an ionophore. The ionophore is either a chemically activated ion channel or an enzyme that activates the internal metabolic system of the cell. The chemically activated channels are either Na, K, or Cl channels. Depending on which of these channels is opened, the impulse can be excitatory (if Na channels are opened) or inhibitory (if K or Cl channels are opened).

After the neurotransmitter binds, the transmitter is rapidly removed from the synaptic cleft by either diffusion or enzymatic destruction, or is actively transported back into the presynaptic terminal (especially with norepinephrine).

ANATOMY OF SPINAL REFLEX FUNCTION

Spinal reflex function requires a local reflex arc for initiation and completion of this function (Braund 1994; Chrisman 1991; deLahunta 1983; Fletcher 1993; Jenkins 1978; King 1987; Oliver et al. 1987; Oliver et al. 1997; Pearson and Gordon 2000). While voluntary functions are ultimately performed through the reflex system, reflex functions do not require voluntary initiation or input. The reflex arc includes the stretch or touch receptor (sensory receptor), the afferent peripheral nerve, the associated spinal segments, the efferent nerve, neuromuscular junction, and muscle. Reflexes can contain only one nerve-to-nerve connection (i.e., monosynaptic) or have numerous nerve-to-nerve connections (i.e., polysynaptic). The patellar reflex is an example of a relatively simple, monosynaptic reflex (deLahunta 1983).

When performing the patellar reflex, for example, the straight patellar tendon is struck with a reflex hammer or similar instrument. The deformation of the tendon results in a small elongation or stretching of the muscle fibers. Subsequently, an afferent impulse is generated and projected proximally in the afferent peripheral nerve, through the dorsal root, to synapse on the cell body of the motor neuron in the ventral grey matter of the spinal cord. This motor cell is stimulated, an impulse is generated through the ventral root, distally in the peripheral nerve (alpha motor nerve), across the neuromuscular junction to depolarize the muscle and result in movement.

With other reflexes such as the withdrawal or flexion reflex, synapse from the dorsal root occurs on an intermediate neuron (interneuron) that in turn synapses on the cell body of the motor neuron. These intermediate neurons are the referred to as interneurons. These interneurons may also be connected to neurons innervating muscles of the opposite limb. This, for example, allows for the extension of one limb concurrent with flexion of the opposite limb (i.e., crossed extensor reflex) (deLahunta 1983; Jenkins 1978, King 1987).

For the majority of spinal reflexes, the cell body for the afferent (sensory) nerve is present in a dorsal root ganglion. This is a bipolar or pseudounipolar neuron that has its dendrites or receptors coming from the distal parts of the body, and whose axon synapses on a cell body in either the CNS or PNS. Considering the patellar reflex, the receptor is in the annulospiral organ of the intrafusal fibers of the muscles of the quadriceps. The intrafusal fibers are modified, small striated muscle cells that are positioned parallel to the larger extrafusal fibers. There are two types of intrafusal fibers, a nuclear bag type and a nuclear chain type (deLahunta 1983; Jenkins 1978; King 1987). The nuclear bag type is interrupted near the center by a dilation containing many cell nuclei. The nuclear chain type has centrally placed nuclei but no central dilation.

When a muscle is stretched, sensory information ascends from the nuclear bag region of the intrafusal fiber in the Ia afferent fibers, whose cell bodies are in the dorsal root ganglion type (deLahunta 1983; Jenkins 1978; King 1987). The axons from these fibers synapse directly on the cell bodies of the alpha motor neuron innervating the extrafusal fibers of the muscle (Tonic loop mechanism) type (deLahunta 1983). Efferent innervation to the intrafusal fibers results from the gamma fibers and is responsible primarily for maintenance of muscle tone. This can be equated to a continual but low-grade muscle contraction. When an intense muscle contraction is necessary, the alpha motor neuron excites the more numerous extrafusal fibers.

Collaterals of the Ia fibers synapse on interneurons in the ventral grey matter of the spinal cord, which are inhibitory to alpha motor neurons innervating muscles whose contraction is in opposition (antagonistic) to the muscle contraction necessary for the reflex function.

Information from the nuclear chain region ascends in the Group II sensory neurons. These terminate upon interneurons that are inhibitory to the extensor muscles and facilitatory to the alpha neurons to flexors (the phasic gamma loop). Renshaw cells are an example of inhibitory interneurons primarily influencing alpha motor neurons affecting antigravity muscles. These inhibitory neurons are themselves inhibited, for example, by tetanus toxin, and this disinhibition results in rigid extension of the limbs (tetany) (deLahunta 1983; Jenkins 1978; King 1987).

The nuclear bag and nuclear chain regions of the intrafusal fibers receive efferent information through the gamma plate and gamma trail neurons, respectively (deLahunta 1983). Via these gamma neurons, muscle is tonically influenced, maintaining muscle tone.

Additional receptors are present in the tendons of muscles referred to as Golgi tendon organs. Information from these receptors is projected in Ib afferent nerves. These receptors have a higher threshold for stimulus than the receptors in the annulospiral organ. The Ib afferents project to interneurons, which in turn synapse on inhibitory neurons to alpha nerves innervating the contracting muscle, and synapse on facilitatory neurons to alpha nerves to muscle with opposing or antagonistic functions. This provides for smooth coordination of skeletal muscle activity and protects against overstretching of tendons.

DERMATOMES (CUTANEOUS) AND AUTONOMOUS ZONES

The skin on the surface of the body is innervated by sensory nerves. The entire area of the skin innervated by a single nerve is termed a dermatome (fig. 1.25) (Bailey and Kitchell 1987; deLahunta 1983; Jenkins 1978; King 1987; Kitchell et al. 1980; Oliver et al. 1997). An area of skin innervated by only one nerve is termed the autonomous zone (Bailey and Kitchell 1987; deLahunta 1983; Jenkins 1978; King 1987; Kitchell et al. 1980; Oliver et al. 1997). Autonomous zones have been determined for dogs based upon fixed anatomical points (Bailey and Kitchell 1987; deLahunta 1983; Jenkins 1978; King 1987; Kitchell et al. 1980). Individual variation of innervation patterns and movement of the skin overlying these points can lead to false assessments (Bailey and Kitchell 1987). It is sometimes important when determining the number and distribution of peripheral nerves involved in a disease to stimulate only the autonomous zone of the peripheral nerve to identify dysfunction of the sensory component of individual peripheral nerves.

THE FUNCTIONAL CONCEPTS OF UPPER VERSUS LOWER MOTOR NEURON

As has been emphasized, many functions of the nervous system cannot be explained by the contribution of its discrete elements, nor are these functions the result of single or groups of neuronal elements. In general, the nervous system can be conceptualized into two parts: a more centralized controlling system, and a local reflex system. The central controlling system is analogous to the brain, brain stem, cerebellum, and portions of the spinal cord that contain or are important for descending controlling information usually to local spinal or cranial nerves. These controlling functions are performed by numerous neuronal systems and pathways within the central nervous system, depending upon the type of activity to be performed. This functional concept of a central controlling system is often referred to as the upper motor neuron (UMN) system as many of the controlling and coordinating functions are associated with control of muscle movement. The UMN is a neuron or group of neurons that does not exit the central nervous system and influences, either positively or negatively, the local reflex system (fig. 1.26).

Conversely, as the central nervous system does not directly connect to the organs or muscles, a second functional nervous system is necessary for ultimate stimulation

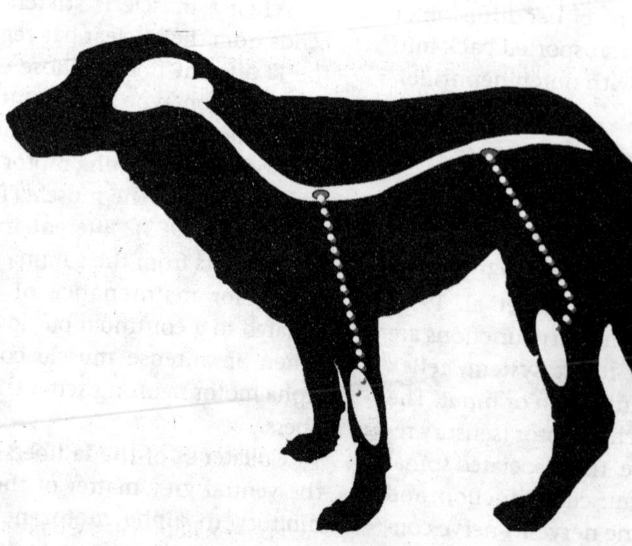

Fig. 1.25. Schematic view of a dog showing concept of dermatomal distribution.

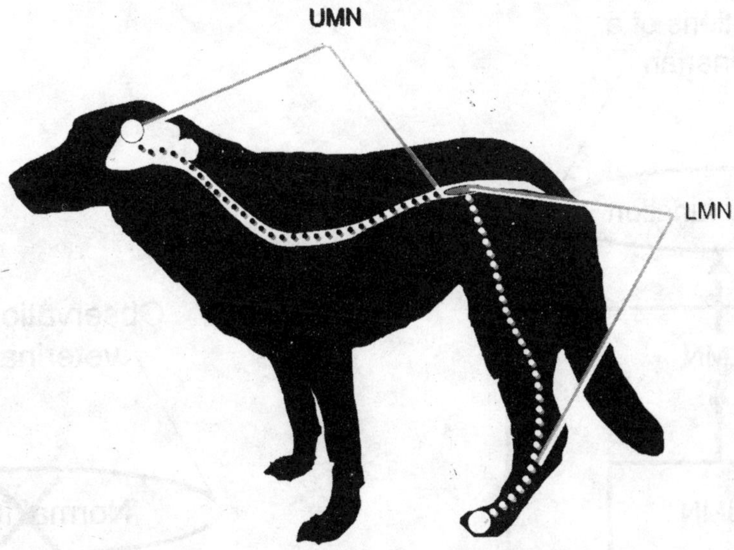

Fig. 1.26. Schematic view of a dog showing concept of UMNs compared to LMNs.

of a muscle or organ. This system is conceptualized as more rudimentary, or reflex in function, with these reflex functions being primarily performed by components of the peripheral nervous system and cranial nerves. This component of neural control is referred to as the lower motor neuron (LMN) system. The LMN is analogous to the efferent (motor) peripheral nervous system and the effector organs (primarily muscles). The peripheral nervous system includes any nerve myelinated by a Schwann cell. Schwann cells begin myelinating peripheral nerves to the limbs at the intervertebral foramen. Using this strict definition, other functional components of the LMN, such as the cell body of the motor neuron in the ventral grey matter of the spinal cord, would not be included in the peripheral nervous system. Functionally, however, a lesion of the peripheral nerve or cell body would result in identical clinical signs. Therefore, the terms "peripheral nervous system" and "LMN" are used interchangeably in some descriptions.

An important evaluation of LMN function in the clinical setting is the determination of local reflex functions. As many reflex functions also require peripheral sensory input (see Anatomy of Spinal Reflex Function above), diseases of the afferent peripheral sensory systems may result in decreased or absent spinal reflexes, and diseases of the peripheral sensory nervous system are often grouped under diseases affecting the LMN.

As veterinarians, we clinically evaluate animals based on our observational and physical evaluations. Conceptually, a two-box system can be used to represent clinical neurologic assessments (fig. 1.27). We, as veterinarians, are "outside the box," and cannot directly see the nervous system function. We evaluate body functions such as walking, barking, eating, drinking, urinating, and blinking through observation of an animal to determine if the nervous system is functioning properly. These functions are performed via the central controlling systems' (UMNs) influence on the local reflex system (LMNs), or in some instances (i.e., spinal reflex function) by the independent function of the local reflex system.

If a clinical function is normal, then we, as evaluators, assume that both the UMNs and LMNs are functionally normally. If, however, we determine that a function is abnormal, then we are uncertain if the abnormality resides in the UMN, the LMN, or both. We then evaluate the function of the LMN, for example, by assessing local spinal reflex function. If the local spinal reflex function is normal, and the animal is dysfunctional, then we assume that the problem lies within the UMN. If, however, the LMN is dysfunctional, we have lost some of our ability to assess for a concurrent UMN problem. Obviously, the UMN is a complex functional system, and potentially influences a vast array of clinical functions, such as behavior or consciousness. By evaluation of these other functions of the UMN, we may still be able to determine the integrity of the UMN.

Much of the basis of appropriate clinical medicine depends upon the accurate assessment of "normal" functions, compared to "abnormal" functions. The knowledge of function comes with experienced observation of both normal and abnormal function. Knowledge of neuroanatomy becomes important in determining the location of the abnormal function within the nervous system (neuroanatomical diagnosis), which leads to the consideration of appropriate differential diagnoses, application of appropriate diagnostic testing, and, finally, an accurate diagnosis of the cause of the neurologic dysfunction. An accurate diagnosis is the cornerstone of the formulation of an accurate treatment plan and prognosis. The remaining portions of this book will be helpful in that pursuit.

EXAMPLES OF FUNCTIONAL SYSTEMS IN THE NERVOUS SYSTEM

The anatomical components of the nervous system are interconnected to form various *functional systems*. A func-

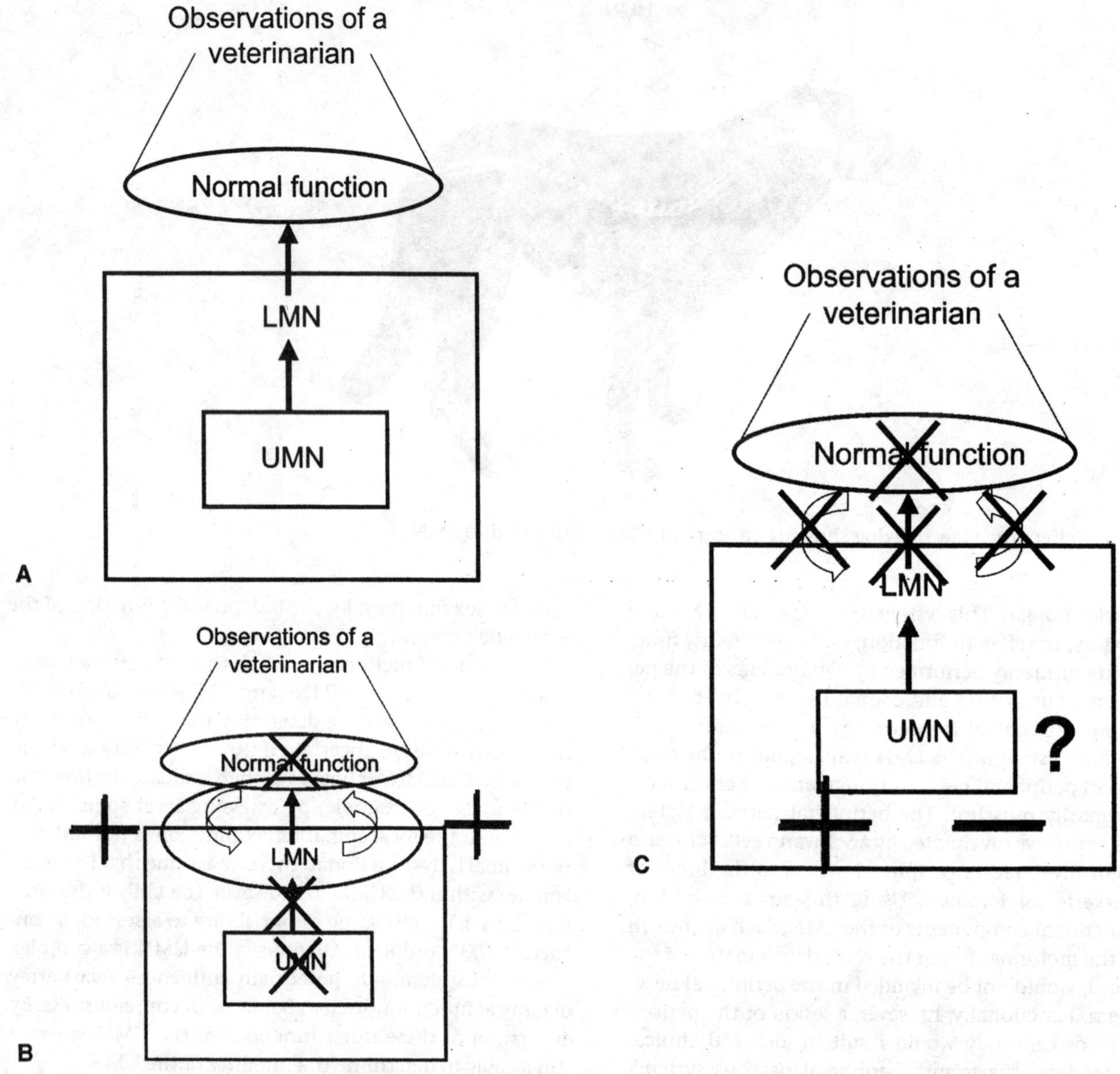

Fig. 1.27. (A) Schematic conceptualization of the veterinarian's observations of UMN and LMN signs. (B) If both the UMN and LMN are normal, normal function will be observed. If the animal is dysfunctional, and the LMN is normal, the abnormality is assumed to be in the UMN systems. (C) If the animal is dysfunctional and the LMN is abnormal, function of the UMN may not always be observed.

tional system may be defined as a constellation of neuronal elements or groups that function in some particular pattern that results in a body reaction such as movement. Selected functional systems will be discussed below as an introduction to show the anatomical complexity of some apparently "simple" body functions. Additional functional systems will be discussed in other chapters dealing with the clinical neurologic abnormalities.

Proprioception and Movement

Proprioception is the knowledge of one's position in space and is an important body function under neurologic control (fig. 1.28). Kinesthesia is an awareness of the precise position and movement of the parts of the body and especially the limbs. Kinesthesia information is initially identified via muscle and joint receptors. Projections from these receptors are present to both the cerebral cortex for conscious recognition and the cerebellum for unconscious proprioception.

Proprioceptive functions are initiated through activation of mechanoreceptors, stretch, or touch receptors. When excited, the impulse is projected from these receptors (dendrites of sensory system) proximally in the limb toward the spinal cord (orthodromic conduction). The impulse will be projected to synapse on the cell body which is usually located in the dorsal root ganglion of the dorsal spinal nerve (deLahunta 1983; Jenkins 1978; King 1987). From this cell body, an impulse will ascend in through the

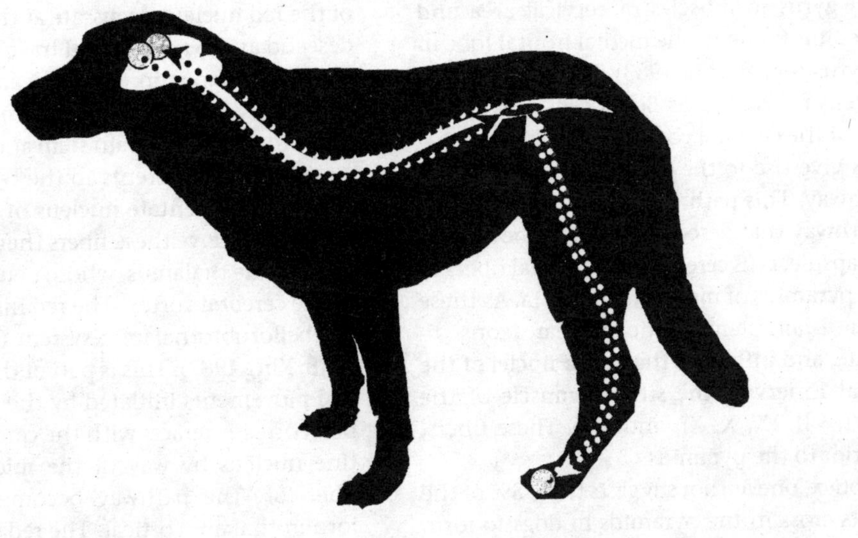

Fig. 1.28. Schematic view of a dog showing pathways for conscious proprioception.

spinal cord on the same (ipsilateral) side and enter the fasciculus gracilis (for information from pelvic limb proprioception receptors) in the dorsal funiculus of the spinal cord. Axons from receptors in the thoracic limbs are found in the fasciculus cuneatus. The dorsal funiculus is organized in a somatotopic orientation. The axons from the most caudal levels of the spinal cord are most medial in location. Axons that enter at more cranial levels are added successively laterally. Therefore, the fasciculus gracilis is more medially located in the dorsal funiculus than the fasciculus cuneatus (deLahunta 1983; Jenkins 1978; King 1987).

Axons in these pathways project cranially and ipsilaterally in the spinal cord to the level of the caudal aspect of the brain stem medulla oblongata. In the medulla oblongata, axons in the fasciculus gracilis and cuneatus synapse on neurons in the corresponding nuclear areas, the nucleus gracilis and medial cuneatus nucleus, respectively (deLahunta 1983; Jenkins 1978; King 1987). Considering that elements of a single neuron essentially extend from the peripheral receptor to the caudal brain stem termination, axons in this projection system are comparatively sizeable in length. As neuronal functional systems are often connected in series, this initial neuron is often referred to as the first-order neuron. These first-order neurons will synapse on the next neuron in the system or the second-order neuron. The cell bodies of these second-order neurons are present in the brain stem nuclear areas of the gracilis and cuneatus.

Second-order axons from these nuclei course ventrally through the medulla oblongata as the deep arcuate fibers to the opposite side (contralateral) of midline. Axons continue rostrally (ascend) in the medial lemniscus to the ventral caudal lateral nucleus of the thalamus. From the thalamus, axons ascend in the internal capsule and corona radiata of the cerebral hemispheres to the somesthetic cortex. The somesthetic cortex is part of the parietal lobe caudal to the cruciate sulcus (caudal part of the postcruciate gyrus and rostral suprasylvian gyrus). The cruciate sulcus is orientated perpendicular to midline on the dorsal and more rostral cerebral hemispheres. This sulcus is often the division between the parietal and frontal cerebral hemispheres.

Additionally, general proprioceptive pathways project from the first three cervical spinal cord segments through cells found within the lateral cervical nucleus (deLahunta 1983; Jenkins 1978; King 1987). This nucleus receives afferent information from the spinocervical tract. The cell bodies of the axons in this tract are located predominantly in lamina IV of the dorsal grey matter of the spinal cord. The axons from the lateral cervical nucleus ascend cranially and cross to the contralateral side of the caudal medulla to join the medial lemniscus pathways.

Once proprioceptive information reaches the level of the parietal cortex, the position of the limbs is "consciously" recognized. Once the limb is determined to be malpositioned, neuronal systems are activated to return the limb to its normal resting or standing position. To reposition the limbs, descending motor pathways must be recruited. In general, the two motor systems that are recruited are referred to as the pyramidal and extrapyramidal systems. The pyramidal system is essentially made up of motor pathways from the cerebral motor cortex that project caudally to the spinal cord (corticospinal pathways). Additionally, some of these projections from the cortex terminate on the brain stem nuclei of the cranial nerves for movements of the facial muscles (corticobulbar fibers or tracts) (deLahunta 1983; Jenkins 1978; King 1987). The pyramidal system is an important system in humans for controlling finely skilled movements such as of the fingers and hands. Subsequently, as animals are deficient of fingers, the significance of this system in domestic species is debatable.

Pyramidal tracts are poorly developed in most domestic animals (deLahunta 1983; Jenkins 1978; King 1987). The cell body is located somatotopically in the motor cortex. In carnivores, this is found in the postcruciate and rostral suprasylvian gyrus (postcruciate to appendicular musculature; suprasylvian gyrus to muscles of cervical area and head); in ungulates it is found in the medial frontal lobe in the precruciate gyrus (deLahunta 1983). Many of the cell bodies are large cells referred to as Betz's cells and are located in lamina V of the cerebral cortex.

These neurons give rise to the axons contained in the corticospinal pathway. This pathway is an uninterrupted, monosynaptic pathway that descends through the corona radiata, internal capsule, crus cerebri, longitudinal fibers of pons, and ventral pyramids of medulla oblongata. As these axons descend the brain stem, corticonuclear axons diverge and decussate, and influence the motor nuclei of the cranial nerves that innervate the striated muscle of the head (III, IV, V, VI, VII, IX, X, XI, and XII). These fibers, thus, terminate prior to the pyramids.

Caudal to the obex, one author suggests that 75% of the corticospinal tracts cross in the pyramids in dogs to form the lateral corticospinal tract (lateral funiculus) in the spinal cord (deLahunta 1983). Fifty percent of these axons terminate on cell bodies in the cervical gray matter, 20% in the thoracic area, and 30% in the lumbosacral grey matter. The remaining 25% continue ipsilaterally in the ventral funiculus adjacent to the ventral medial fissure as the ventral corticospinal tract. This tract descends only as far as the midthoracic level, and decussates at termination.

Another author suggests that the decussation of these tracts at the pyramid is 100% in dogs, and almost 100% in cats, so that there is only a small ventral tract in cats that reaches only the upper segments of the cervical area (King 1987). The corticospinal tracts form approximately 10% of the total spinal cord white matter in dogs, 20% in monkeys, and 30% in human beings (deLahunta 1983). These axons synapse on the cell bodies of the lower motor neurons in the spinal cord grey matter.

The extrapyramidal system is somewhat less discretely defined, but it is the term commonly used to describe all other motor systems besides the pyramidal (corticospinal) system (deLahunta 1983; Jenkins 1978; King 1987). The extrapyramidal system is a multisynaptic motor pathway. The cell bodies are located in all divisions of the brain. In the supratentorial regions, extrapyramidal elements are found in the frontal and parietal lobes of the cerebral cortex and the basal nuclei (septal nuclei, amygdala, claustrum, caudate nucleus, putamen, pallidum). The basal nuclei are part of a feedback mechanism from cortical extrapyramidal nuclei involving the caudate to pallidum to the thalamus, and back to the cerebral cortex. At the time of cortical initiation of voluntary movement, these pathways modify the intended movement. Extrapyramidal elements are also found in the diencephalon and the mesencephalon (substantia nigra, tegmental nucleus, red nucleus). Only the cells located in the mesencephalon caudally have axons that descend the spinal cord.

Some of the neurons in the substantia nigra project to the caudate nucleus. (nigrostriatal pathway) (deLahunta 1983; Jenkins 1978; King 1987). The red nucleus receives afferents from the ipsilateral motor cortex by way of the internal capsule and crus cerebri. Axons from the cell bodies of the red nucleus decussate at the level of the nucleus and descend as the rubrospinal tract (lateral funiculus of spinal cord). The axons in this tract are primarily facilitatory to flexor muscles. Rubrobulbar neurons descend to the cranial nerve nuclei in the brain stem and influence their function.

Additional afferents to the red nucleus come from the contralateral dentate nucleus of the cerebellum. The neurons that receive these fibers then project to the rostral nucleus of the thalamus, whose neurons subsequently project to the cerebral cortex. The red nucleus becomes part of the cerebellorubrothalamic system (deLahunta 1983; Jenkins 1978; King 1987). This is part of the feedback system to control movements initiated by the cerebral cortex. The cerebral cortex interacts with the cerebellum through the pontine nucleus by way of the middle cerebellar peduncle. Therefore the pathway becomes corticopontinocerebellorubrothalamocortical. The red nucleus is also connected by both afferents and efferents to the basal nuclei.

In the more caudal brain stem, the reticular formation in the pons has a facilitatory influence on the motor neurons of the extensor muscles (deLahunta 1983; Jenkins 1978; King 1987). This pontine reticulospinal tract descends mostly in the ipsilateral ventral funiculus. An area in the medulla has an inhibitory influence over motor neurons to extensor muscles and descends the spinal cord in the medullary reticulospinal tract in the lateral funiculus in a medial intermediate position mostly on the ipsilateral side.

The olivary nucleus receives afferents from many of the extrapyramidal nucleus. It projects to the contralateral portion of the cerebellum through the caudal cerebellar peduncle and is a primary source for extrapyramidal projection to the cerebellum. A feedback circuit also exists through this nucleus to the cerebral cortex.

Following the integration of proprioceptive information, multiple motor systems may be recruited to result in return of the limb to a normal position. The major motor response pathways include the corticospinal tracts (pyramidal functions), and the rubrospinal, medullary, and pontine reticulospinal (extrapyramidal) tracts. Other descending tracts, such as the vestibulospinal, medial longitudinal fasciculus, and tectospinal tracts, also influence motor tone and activity.

Unconscious Proprioception and the Role of the Cerebellum

Occurring concurrently with the conscious knowledge of where a limb or body part is in the environment is the additional input from proprioceptive systems that are not consciously recognized. Of these unconscious proprioceptive systems, the cerebellum system plays a significant role in determining proprioceptive information for integration into motor functions.

The cerebellum is a unique nervous system structure that is located dorsal to the brain stem and fourth ventricle in the infratentorial region (see fig. 1.6) (Chrisman 1990; deLahunta 1980; deLahunta 1983; Holliday 1979; Jenkins 1978; King 1987). It consists of a more rounded center region with bilateral conical projections. The surface appearance contains numerous undulations. The cerebellum consists of a central median region, the vermis (wormlike), and a lateral hemisphere on each side. The uvulonodular fissure separates the large body of the cerebellum from the smaller flocculonodular lobe (ventral aspect of cerebellum near the center). The nodulus is the most rostral part of the caudal vermis and is adjacent to the fourth ventricle. The flocculus is on the ventral aspect of the cerebellar hemisphere.

The vermis is divided into rostral and caudal lobes by the primary fissure (deLahunta 1983; Jenkins 1978; King 1987). On cut section, there is an extensive area of white matter in the cerebellum called the cerebellar medulla. The branching of this white matter into the folia is referred to as the arbor vitae.

The folia are small folds seen in the cerebellum and consist of white matter tracts and the associated three layers of the cerebellar cortex. The outer portion of the folium is covered by leptomeninges (pia and arachnoid). Similar to the cerebral hemispheres, the cerebellum has a cortical region and a more central nuclear and projection pathway region.

The cerebellum cortex consists of three layers (deLahunta 1983; Jenkins 1978; King 1987). The outermost layer of the cerebellar cortex is the molecular layer. It is composed mostly of axons (unmyelinated) and telodendria (synapses) of granular neurons and the dendritic zone of Purkinje cells. The cells of the molecular layer include the basket and stellate cells, which are inhibitory to the Purkinje cells. The middle layer is the Purkinje cell layer. These are large, easily recognized flask-shaped cells in a single layer. Their dendritic zone is in the molecular layer of the cerebellum, where their dendrites are located transversely to the longitudinal axis of the cerebellum. The Purkinje cells are the important source of inhibitory input that travels from the cerebellum and also projects to the deep cerebellar nuclei. The inner layer is the granule layer. This contains mostly granule cells, but also some Golgi cells. The granule cell is the only cell of the cerebellar cortex that is facilitatory. The Golgi cells are inhibitory to the granule cells. This layer varies from 5 to 6 cells in thickness at the bottom of a folium to 15 to 20 cells thick at the top of a folium. The axons of the granule cells project up the molecular layer, bifurcate, and run parallel with the long axis of the folium, intersecting at right angles to the dendritic areas of the Purkinje cells.

The deep cerebellar nuclei are mirrored on each side of the median plane and include, from lateral to medial, the dentate, interpositus, and fastigial nucleus. These cells are influenced by the Purkinje cells (inhibitory) or from afferents (mossy and climbing fibers) to the cerebellum (excitatory). Therefore, depending on the strength of each impulse, the output from these nuclei to the command centers of the motor system can either be nil or excitatory.

The cerebellum is connected to other central nervous structures via three groups of white matter tracts on each side of the brain stem. These structures are named the rostral, middle, and caudal cerebellar peduncles.

AFFERENT PROJECTIONS TO THE CEREBELLUM

There are two main collections of afferent fibers to the cerebellum: the mossy fibers, which carry fibers from the pontine nuclei, tectum, red nucleus, reticular formation, vestibular nuclei, and the spinocerebellar tracts, and the climbing fibers, incoming fibers from the olivary nuclei (table 1.6 ; fig. 1.29) (deLahunta 1983; Jenkins 1978; King 1987). The spinal projections to the cerebellum come primarily from four spinocerebellar pathways. These pathways transmit proprioceptive (unconscious) information from the muscle spindles and Golgi tendon organs to the cerebellum. The spinocerebellar pathways from the pelvic limb include the dorsal and ventral spinocerebellar tracts (deLahunta 1983; Jenkins 1978; King 1987). The first-order neuron of the dorsal spinocerebellar tract has its cell body located in the dorsal root ganglion of the spinal nerve serving the pelvic limbs. The dendrite region of these cells is located in the muscle spindle. From the cell body, axons project to synapse in the base of the dorsal (horns) grey matter of the spinal cord (thoracic nucleus, Clarke's nucleus). Axons from these second-order neurons project cranially in the superficial dorsolateral funiculus ipsilaterally to enter the cerebellum via the caudal cerebellar peduncle.

The cell body of the first-order neuron of the ventral spinocerebellar tract is located in the dorsal root ganglion. The receptor is the Golgi tendon organ. These axons synapse in the base of the dorsal horn, decussate immediately, and project cranially in the ventral spinocerebellar tract located in the superficial, ventrolateral funiculus. This pathway enters the cerebellum via the rostral cerebellar peduncle, and decussates a second time to end on the same side of the cerebellum from which the impulse originated.

The cerebellar projections from the thoracic limbs include the spinocuneocerebellar pathway and the cranial spinocerebellar tract (deLahunta 1983; Jenkins 1978; King 1987). The first-order neuron receptor of the spinocuneocerebellar pathway is in the muscle spindle (some Golgi tendons may be involved). The cell body is located in the dorsal root ganglion of the spinal nerves serving the thoracic limb. The axons enter the ipsilateral fasciculus cuneatus of the dorsal fasciculus and projects cranially to the lateral cuneate nucleus.

The lateral cuneate nucleus is located in the medulla oblongata. Axons from here travel in the cuneocerebellar tract to enter the cerebellum via the caudal cerebellar peduncle to end in the ipsilateral cerebellum.

The cranial spinocerebellar tract has its receptor in the Golgi tendon organ (deLahunta 1983; Jenkins 1978; King 1987). The cell body is again located in the dorsal root ganglion. The second-order neuron cell body is located in the base of the dorsal horn from C1 to T1. The axon enters the ipsilateral cranial spinocerebellar tract, which lies medial to the ventral spinocerebellar tract, and enters the cerebellum via both the rostral and caudal cerebellar peduncles to end in the ipsilateral cerebellar cortex.

Some of the kinesthesia information carried in the

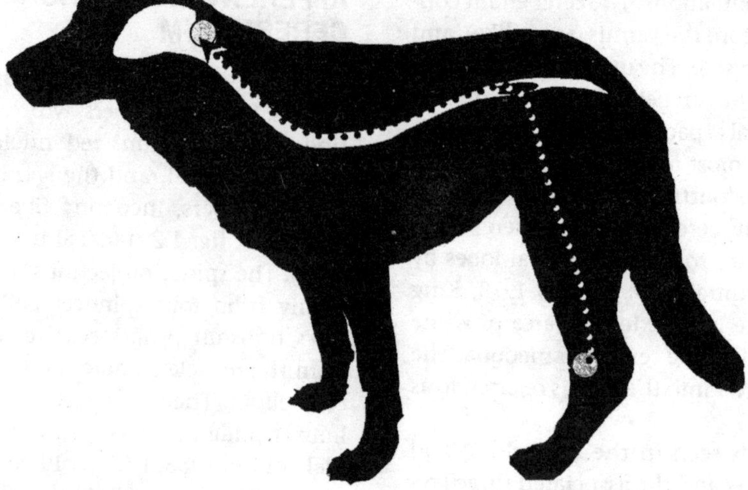
A

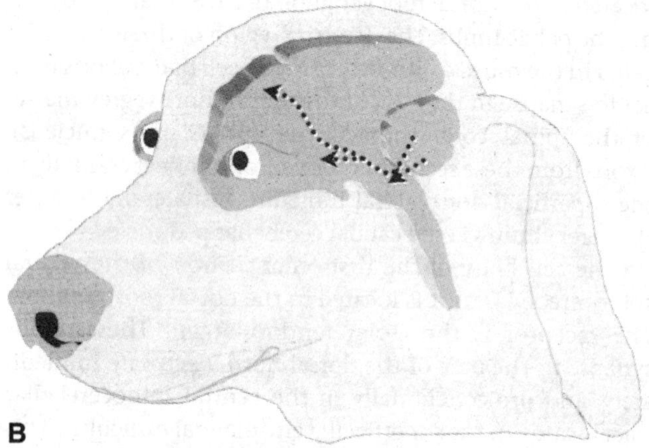
B

Fig. 1.29. (A) Schematic view of a dog showing afferent pathways from joint receptors in the pelvic limb to the cerebellum. (B) Schematic view of dog showing efferent projections from the cerebellum to the central area responsible for movement (cortex, basal nuclei, brain stem).

spinocerebellar tracts is not projected to the cerebellum, but to the cerebral cortex. Muscle proprioception from the pelvic limb is projected in the dorsal spinocerebellar tracts. At the medulla, these fibers form collaterals, and these synapse in a displaced fragment of the nucleus gracilis known as the nucleus Z (King 1987). From here, axons project in the medial lemniscus to the ventral thalamic nuclei, and then to the sensory cortex.

A similar pathway from the thoracic limbs is probably present, coming from the muscle proprioception of the thoracic limb and running in the spinocuneocerebellar tract to synapse in the nucleus X, which lies next to the lateral cuneate nucleus (King 1987). From here, the pathway to the cerebral cortex is the same as from the nucleus Z.

The pontine projections to the cerebellum come from the cerebral cortex (deLahunta 1983; Jenkins 1978; King 1987). These fibers then travel in the internal capsule, the crus cerebri, and the longitudinal fibers of the pons. Axons leave these fibers and synapse on ipsilateral pontine neurons. These axons cross midline (forming the transverse fibers of the pons) and enter the cerebellum via the contralateral middle cerebellar peduncle. This pathway is important for skilled motor function.

The fibers from the red nucleus project through the rostral cerebellar peduncle via the rubrocerebellar pathways. Fibers from the reticular formation project via the reticulocerebellar processes to enter the caudal cerebellar pathway.

Axons of the cell bodies in the vestibular nuclei project to the cerebellum via the ipsilateral caudal cerebellar peduncle. These terminate mostly in the flocculus of the hemisphere and the nodulus of the caudal vermis (the flocculonodular lobe) and the fastigial nucleus.

The mossy axonal fibers enter the cerebellum and synapse in two places: either on the deep cerebellar nuclei or on the granule cells (deLahunta 1983; Jenkins 1978; King 1987). These fibers are facilitatory at these synapses. The extrapyramidal fibers of the telencephalon and brain stem project information to the cerebellum via the olivary neurons. This nucleus is located in the ventrolateral portion of the caudal medulla, extending rostrally to the facial nucleus and caudally to the obex. The axons from the olivary nuclei cross midline and enter the cerebellum via the caudal cerebellar peduncle.

The climbing axonal fibers are of olivary nerve cell origin and enter the cerebellum via the caudal cerebellar peduncle. Their axons synapse in the deep cerebellar nuclei and in a one-to-one relationship with the Purkinje cells. The impulses from these axons are facilitatory.

EFFERENT PROJECTIONS FROM THE CEREBELLUM

The efferent fibers for the cerebellum include fibers originating in the Purkinje cells and the cells of the deep cerebellar nuclei. Efferents influence motor activity by modifying activity initiated by other nervous system areas. Because of this, no substantial cerebellar efferents descend the spinal cord.

The Purkinje cells, derived mostly from the flocculonodular lobe, project directly to the vestibular nuclei via the caudal cerebellar peduncle (table 1.6). Axons from the fastigial nucleus project to the vestibular nuclei and the reticular formation via the caudal cerebellar peduncle. The interpositus nuclei neurons project to the red nucleus and reticular formation via the rostral cerebellar peduncle. The neurons from the dentate nucleus project to the red nucleus, reticular formation, pallidum, and ventral lateral nucleus of the thalamus through the rostral cerebellar peduncle. The lateral cuneate nucleus receives axons from the cuneocerebellar tracts.

This cerebellar system of connections is important in determining, primarily at a subconscious level, the position of the limbs and other body parts, and relaying that information to the appropriate areas that will ultimately affect movement. By providing appropriate "input data" to the motor systems, the cerebellar system allows for a coordination of this activity so that movement is more "smooth."

PAIN AND SENSATION

Pinprick pain can be elicited by stimulation of the skin with a fine needle. This information is transmitted initially in thin, myelinated fibers (A III or A delta fibers) (Guyton and Hall 1996). The sensations are conducted relatively quickly, are accurately localized, and do not outlast the stimulus. Pinprick axons form collaterals, which project and excite short inhibitory interneurons that are enkephalinergic. These inhibit neurons that project true pain from the substantia gelatinosa to the reticular formation. Pinprick information is transmitted centrally in the spinothalamic tract.

Table 1.6. Summary of afferents to and efferents from the cerebellum

Afferent projections to the cerebellum
Spinal cord
Spinocerebellar (dorsal and ventral)
Spinocuneocerebellar
Cranial spinocerebellar
Vestibular system
Tectocerebellar
Brain stem
Olivary nucleus
Pontine nucleus
Red nucleus
Reticular formation
Efferent projections from the cerebellum
From flocculonodular lobe to the vestibular nucleus
From the fastigial nucleus to the vestibular nucleus and reticular formation
From interpositał nucleus to red nucleus and reticular formation
From the dentate nucleus to the red nucleus, reticular formation, pallidum, ventral lateral nucleus of the thalamus

Sources: deLahunta 1983; Jenkins 1978; King 1987.

Pain receptors in the skin are more numerous than pressure receptors. True pain is initially carried in thin, unmyelinated (C) fibers, which enter into the substantia gelatinosa (dorsolateral tract or Lissauers's tract; Rexed's lamina II). A delta fibers are responsible for initial pain sensations and C fibers are responsible for delayed pain sensations. A pain stimulus results in an inhibition of inhibitory pain fibers resulting in projection of pain information. The substantia gelatinosa receives collaterals from the large-diameter cutaneous mechanoreceptor axons that form the gracile and cuneate fascicles and can cause presynaptic inhibition of pain information (i.e., rubbing a painful area may make it feel better). This sensation is projected centrally through nonspecific pathways of the ascending reticular formation. This information is eventually projected in the medial lemniscal system.

In human beings, pain information pathways decussate and ascend in the spinothalamic tract on the opposite side of the spinal cord (Guyton and Hall 1996). Therefore, a unilateral lesion in the spinal cord of humans will cause an ipsilateral motor deficit and a contralateral sensory deficit. This is referred to as Brown-Sequard syndrome (deLahunta 1983). This is rarely seen in animals because the ascending pain pathways are more diffuse in nonprimate species (deLahunta 1983).

Ascending pain information from the ascending reticular formation (possibly also through the spinothalamic tracts) projects to the periaqueductal grey of the brain stem to excite enkephalinergic neurons in the nucleus raphe magnus possibly through serotonergic mechanisms. Inhibitory synapses on pain responses are projected down the spinal cord in the raphe spinal tract.

Pain can have numerous qualities. Initial pain is sharp and localizable (Guyton and Hall 1996). Delayed pain is dull and has a latency of 0.5–1.0 second. Deep pain is dull and poorly localizable. Visceral pain is dull, diffuse, and poorly localized. This may be because, in comparison to the general somatic afferent fibers, there are fewer general visceral afferent fibers, and these are infrequently recognized by conscious perception.

Endogenous Modulation of Pain

The body itself may inhibit pain conduction recognition through central and peripheral antinociceptive mechanisms. Stimulation of many central nervous system areas, such as periaqueductal grey, nucleus reticularis paragigantocellularis, nucleus gigantocellularis pars alpha, prefrontal cortex, septal nuclei, caudate, amygdala, or lateral hypothalamus may result in pain relief. This is likely mediated through the release or alteration in concentrations of neurotransmitters such as endorphins, enkephalins, serotonin, norepinephrine, and others.

Additionally, pain transmission may be blocked locally at the spinal cord level in the substantia gelatinosa (gating). These endogenous antinociception mechanisms may be a physiological explanation for why acupuncture and acupressure may be beneficial.

THE AUTONOMIC NERVOUS SYSTEMS

The autonomic system components of the nervous system subserve many of the homeostatic functions of the body (deLahunta 1983; Jenkins 1978; King 1987; Kitchell 1993). These systems are often thought of as more primitive and basic to the body, often associated with internal organ or visceral functions. As with most neuronal systems, the autonomic systems are as much functional conceptualizations as discrete anatomical elements. These systems are based on a two neuron concept of a preganglionic and a postganglionic nerve. These nerves may be influenced by other neuronal systems from the intracranial structures or spinal cord. The hypothalamus is an influential controlling center with regard to autonomic functions (Jenkins 1978; King 1987).

The neuronal functions of the autonomic systems are usually categorized as either parasympathetic or sympathetic (fig. 1.30). The parasympathetic systems are important for functions such as pupillary constriction, salivation, urination, and defecation. Neurons functioning in the parasympathetic system are concentrated in some cranial nerves and in the pelvic areas of the body. Cranial nerves III (oculomotor), VII (facial), IX (glossopharyngeal), and X (vagus) have parasympathetic functions associated with them. Cranial nerves III and VII tend to be contained in and around the head, whereas CN IX, and especially CN X, innervate visceral structures of the pharynx, larynx, and thoracic and abdominal cavities.

Autonomic nervous systems tend to consist of 2 interconnected neurons. In the two-neuron concept, the parasympathetic system tends to have relatively longer preganglionic neurons. The postganglionic neurons tend to be short and reside intimately with the effector organ. For ex-

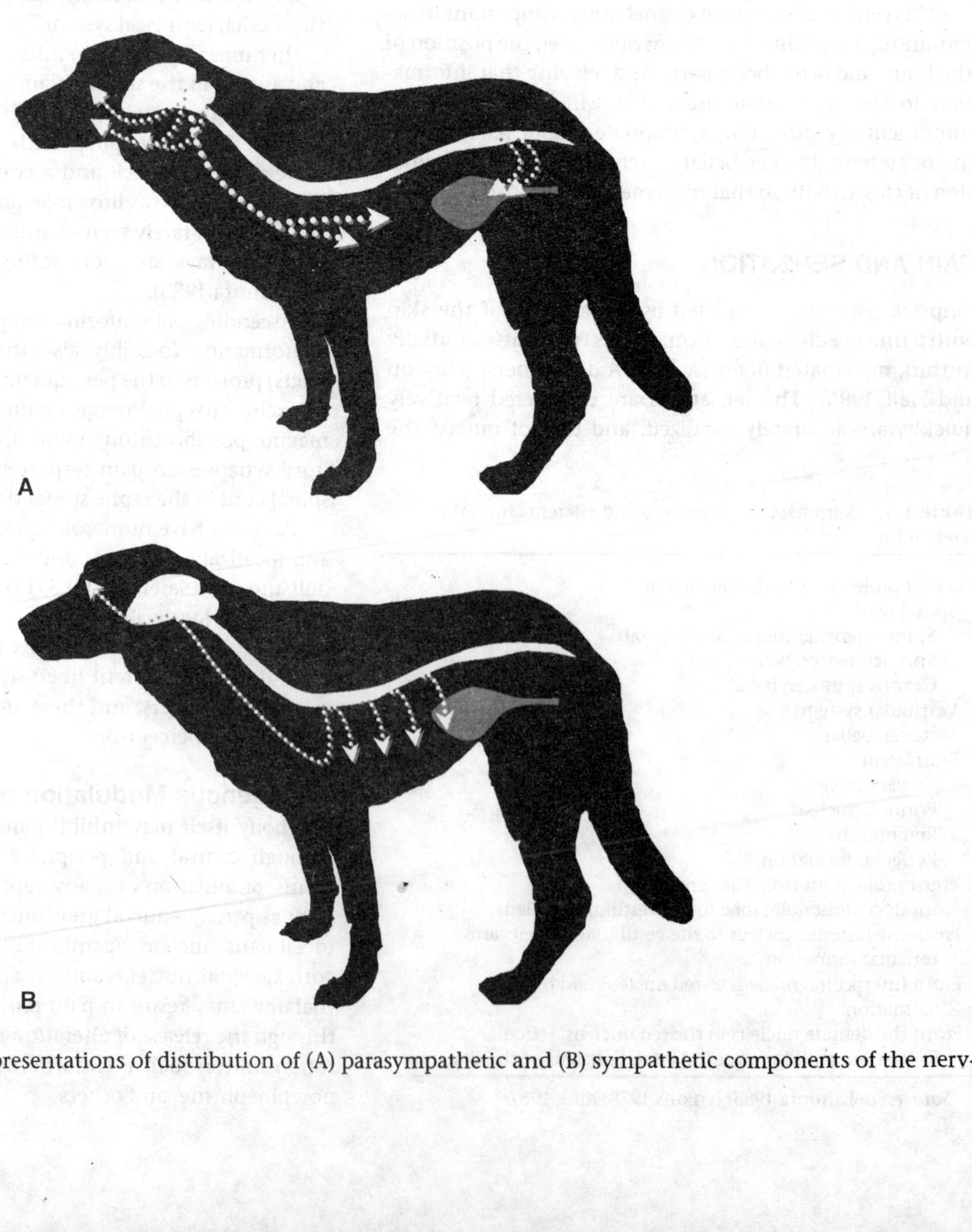

Fig. 1.30. Schematic representations of distribution of (A) parasympathetic and (B) sympathetic components of the nervous system.

ample, the parasympathetic preganglionic cell bodies that are responsible for pupillary constriction are present in the parasympathetic nucleus of the oculomotor nerve in the brain stem. The preganglionic axons exit the brain stem as a component of the oculomotor nerve and project to the iris. Within the iris, the preganglionic fibers terminate on the postganglionic fibers, which being already in the iris are relatively shorter in length.

The preganglionic cell bodies of the sympathetic neuronal system are concentrated primarily in the thoracolumbar region of the spinal cord. Cell bodies of preganglionic axons are found in the grey matter between the dorsal and ventral horns (intermediolateral grey matter). The preganglionic cell bodies are influenced by descending neurons from the intracranial nervous system via projections through the cervical spinal cord. As an example, a stimulus such as a loud sound may be transmitted into the intracranial structures via the cochlear nerve. Subsequently, axons of the central sympathetic pathways are excited, which transmits information caudally through the brain stem and cervical spinal cord (the lateral tectotegmental spinal pathway) to terminate on the preganglionic cell bodies in the cranial thoracic spinal cord segments T1–3. The preganglionic cell body is excited, which sends its axons out through the intervertebral foramen, through the thoracic cavity and thoracic inlet, cranially in the cervical area in the vagosympathetic trunk to terminate on the postganglionic sympathetic cell bodies in the cranial cervical ganglion just caudal to the ear. The postganglionic nerves send axons in through, along the floor, and then out of the skull to eventually terminate in the iris and periocular structures. The sound stimulus that initially excites the sympathetic system ultimately results in dilation of the pupil. In this example, both the preganglionic and postganglionic sympathetic nerve systems travel relatively longer distances to reach the effector organ.

Urinary Function

Urination is an important function of the nervous system (fig. 1.31). It involves both conscious and unconscious (reflex) modalities (deLahunta 1983; Oliver et al. 1987; Oliver et al. 1997). Conscious urination involves the cerebral cortex. Unconscious urination involves the brain stem and the parasympathetic and sympathetic systems within the spinal cord and peripheral nerves. Simplistically, the sympathetic system prevents while the parasympathetic system allows for urination.

Urination is a complex reflex function with central control, the purpose of which is to void urine from the body. This reflex most likely involves brain stem structures as well as local spinal cord segments, and therefore may be termed a suprasegmental reflex. Normal urination requires the coordinated function of both the peripheral and central nervous systems. The peripheral nerves that innervate the bladder are the pelvic, pudendal, and hypogastric nerve groups.

The cell bodies of the pelvic nerve which provide parasympathetic innervation to the detrusor and bladder neck (internal urethral sphincter) are located in the intermediate grey matter of the S1–3 spinal cord segments. The pudendal nerve provides somatic innervation to the striated muscle of the external urethral sphincter. Cell bodies of this nerve are located in the same area as for the pelvic nerve. The hypogastric nerve provides sympathetic innervation to the bladder. Cell bodies of this nerve are located in the L1 to L4 spinal cord segments.

Sensory receptors are located in the wall of the bladder and are responsive to stretch and/or pressure. Information from these receptors travels in the afferent pelvic nerve entering the sacral spinal cord. Afferent cell bodies of the pelvic nerve are present in the spinal ganglia of the S1–3 segments. Axons of the pelvic nerve terminate either on interneurons in the grey matter of the sacral spinal cord, or ascend in projection pathways to the brain.

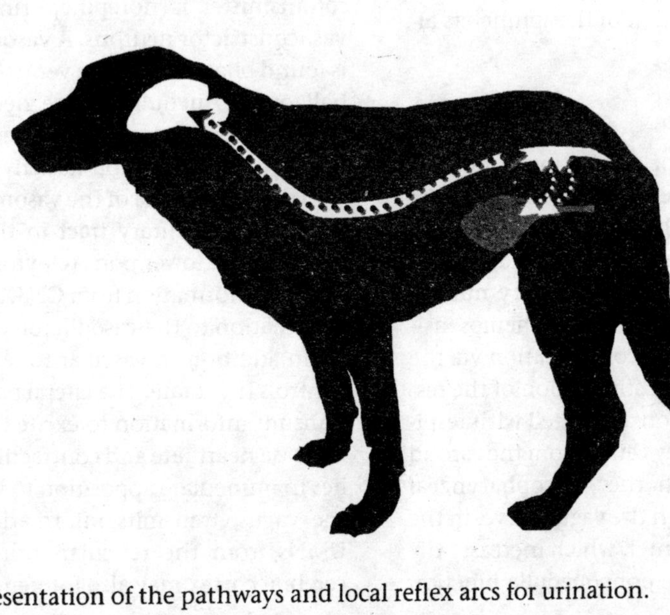

Fig. 1.31. Schematic representation of the pathways and local reflex arcs for urination.

Pelvic nerve axons terminate on interneurons that then terminate on the cell bodies of the preganglionic pelvic nerve of the parasympathetic system, which results in contraction of the detrusor muscle (smooth muscle of the bladder). Additional interneurons synapse on pudendal efferent nerves innervating the striated muscle of the urethra to inhibit its activity. Of unknown importance, interneurons also ascend to the sympathetic centers of the hypogastric nerve to inhibit its normally inhibitory influence on urination. The preganglionic cell bodies of the hypogastric nerve are located at the L1–4 spinal segments and terminate in the caudal mesenteric ganglion. From here, the second-order neurons project to the bladder wall. While both alpha and beta receptors are found in the bladder wall, the beta activity predominates, and, therefore, the normal function of the stimulated hypogastric nerve is to allow bladder wall relaxation.

Sensory information that ascends in the spinal cord from the pelvic nerve does so in the spinothalamic tract and fasciculus gracilis and eventually reaches the somesthetic cortex (deLahunta 1983; Oliver et al. 1987; Oliver et al. 1997). Some ascending information reaches the reticular formation of the pons, midbrain, and medulla oblongata. These areas modulate normal storage and evacuation of urine. Descending information from these areas travels through the tectospinal and reticulospinal pathways. Voluntary urination is initiated in the cerebral cortex, with descending impulses going to the pudendal nerve to either excite or inhibit the external urethral sphincter. The cerebellum apparently has an inhibitory influence on urination.

Defecation

Defecation is controlled like urination, locally at the spinal cord level as well as having descending conscious input. The sacral spinal segments and the pelvic and pudendal nerves will innervate the colon and rectal sphincter, respectively. When the colon is distended with feces, afferent signals in these nerves may set up reflex stimulation of the colonic smooth muscle and relaxation of the sphincters allowing for stool to be passed.

Respiration

Animals can have impairment of respiration functions with nervous system disease (Bagley et al. 1993). The UMN respiratory centers are located in the pons and medulla oblongata of the brain stem (Guyton and Hall 1996). In the medulla, there are dorsal and ventral respiratory nuclear groups, which control respiration, as well as a chemosensitive area that senses changes in CO_2 concentration via the formation of H+ ions. Besides direct stimulation of the respiratory center, afferent information associated with respiration is projected to the respiratory center from the carotid bodies (chemoreceptors) through the glossopharyngeal nerve and the aortic bodies through the vagus nerve. In the pons, there is the pneumotaxic center, which increases the number of breaths/minute. At the pons/medulla junction is the apneustic center, which prevents the switch off of respiration.

From these brain stem centers, the signal for respiration travels caudally through the cervical and cranial thoracic spinal cord to the LMNs for respiration. These LMNs are the phrenic nerve (spinal segments C4–C7), which innervates the diaphragm and the intercostal nerves (from the corresponding segmental spinal cord segments in the thoracic area) to the intercostal muscles.

There are numerous nonneurological influences upon respiration. For example, an increase in body temperature increases respiration both directly by effects on the respiratory center and indirectly by increasing metabolism with subsequent CO_2 production. In dogs and cats, panting may be used as a heat-dissipating mechanism. When the temperature of the blood increases, the hypothalamus signals a panting center to increase respirations. The panting center is closely related to the pneumotaxic center.

Cardiovascular Functions

Vasomotor tone is maintained through interaction between the peripheral receptors and the vasomotor center in the brain stem (Guyton and Hall 1996). The peripheral receptors are baroreceptors. These are spray-type nerve endings located in the walls of arteries being extremely abundant in (1) the wall of the internal carotid artery slightly above the carotid bifurcation in the carotid sinus, and (2) the wall of the aortic arch. Information is transmitted from the carotid sinus through the glossopharyngeal nerve to the solitary tract in the medulla oblongata. Information from the arch of the aorta is transmitted through the vagus nerve. This information eventually reaches the vasomotor center in the reticular substance of the medulla oblongata and the lower pons. This area transmits information caudally in the spinal cord through sympathetic vasoconstrictor fibers to the blood vessels of the body.

Within the vasomotor center, there is a vasoconstrictor area (also called C1) that is found bilaterally in the upper medulla and lower pons (Guyton and Hall 1996). The neurotransmitter is norepinephrine and these fibers excite vasoconstrictor neurons. A vasodilator area (also called A1) is found bilaterally in the ventrolateral portion of the lower half of the medulla. These neurons also secrete norepinephrine, but these fibers project rostrally to the vasoconstrictor area and inhibit its activity.

The sensory area of the vasomotor center is located bilaterally in the solitary tract in the dorsolateral part of the medulla and lower pons (Guyton and Hall 1996). This area receives information from CN IX and CN X and projects this information to the vasodilator and vasoconstrictor centers.

In addition to vascular tone the vasomotor center also controls heart rate. The lateral parts of the vasomotor center transmit information to excite the sympathetic nerves and increase heart rate and contractility. The medial part, which lies in immediate apposition to the dorsal motor nucleus of the vagus, transmits information to decrease heart rate. UMNs from the reticular formation, diencephalon, and cerebral cortex may also influence the vasomotor center.

Coughing

The cough reflex occurs when the bronchi and trachea are irritated by a foreign substance (Guyton and Hall 1996). The larynx and carina are especially sensitive. Afferent impulses pass from the respiratory passages through the vagus nerve to the medulla oblongata. This results when a large volume of air is inspired and the vocal cords shut tightly to entrap the air in the lungs. The abdominal muscles forcefully contract, pushing against the diaphragm while the intercostal muscles also forcefully contract. The vocal cords and epiglottis are suddenly opened wide and the air is forcefully ejected from the lungs.

Sneezing

The sneeze reflex is similar to the cough reflex (Guyton and Hall 1996). Irritative stimuli to the nasal passages excite CN V to the medulla. Reflex events are similar to that of a cough except that the uvula is depressed to allow a large amount of air to pass through the nasal passages.

Eating

Hunger may be elicited by a number of stimuli (Guyton and Hall 1996; Jenkins 1978). Mechanoreceptors detecting stretch of the stomach wall may play a minor role. Glucoreceptors appear to be present in the diencephalon, liver, stomach, and small intestine, signaling a reduced availability of glucose and stimulating hunger. Other long-term regulators of hunger include thermoreceptors (which sense body heat, directly proportionally to energy utilization) and liporeceptors (sensing amounts of body fat). The role of these stimuli for appetite is suggested, however, not proven.

Satiety is the process that stops feeding. There is both a preabsorptive and postabsorptive satiety. The preabsorptive phase results from the feeding behavior itself before absorption of nutrients. Postabsorptive satiety is most likely dependent upon adequacy of nutrient intake.

Preabsorptive satiety is the result of stimulation of a variety of receptors, including olfactory; gustatory; mechanoreceptors of the mouth, throat, and esophagus; and, most importantly, stretch receptors of the stomach. Chemoreceptors in the stomach, for assessment of glucose and amino acid content of food, may also be important. Postabsorption satiety is dependent upon the availability of glucose, increased heat production, and changes in fat metabolism induced with feeding.

Central recognition of hunger occurs in the hypothalamus. Bilateral destruction of certain ventromedial regions of the hypothalamus results in overeating (loss of satiety) (Jenkins 1978). Destruction of the more lateral areas results in lack of eating. The cortex and limbic system have influences over these centers, and to complete the eating process, complex motor integration is necessary to perform the motor acts required.

Drinking

Thirst is a sensation indicating the need to replace lost body water (Bagley 1994; Guyton and Hall 1996). Body water is constantly in a state of flux, with noticeable losses occurring in the urine. These obvious losses of body water are referred to as sensible losses. Nonrenal losses, such as through the respiratory or gastrointestinal tract, are normally not perceivable and are, therefore, referred to as insensible losses.

Body water depletion results in hypovolemia, hyperosmolality of the extracellular fluid (ECF), or both. These water aberrations signal for numerous physiologic adaptations to counterbalance the effects of the water loss. Important physiologic adaptations include release of antidiuretic hormone (ADH) and stimulation of thirst. Both of these adaptations tend to increase body water, the latter through stimulation of drinking. Antidiuretic hormone increases water reabsorption and conservation by the kidney.

Body water is replaced primarily through drinking, but also through the intake of nondipsetic sources of water. An example of a nondipsetic source of water is the water contained in food. While these nondipsetic sources of water may be adequate to maintain hydration and osmolality under normal conditions, the intake of nondipsetic water is not physiologically controlled. During periods of excessive water loss, nondipsetic water intake will not necessarily compensate for that loss. Thirst, in contrast, is signaled by a physiologic need for body water, and is the ultimate physiologic safeguard against dehydration.

Experimental studies suggested that thirst is recognized primarily within the hypothalamus of the diencephalons (Anderson and McCann 1956). The role of the central nervous system in the generation of thirst was shown in dogs, wherein electrocoagulative destruction of an area in the rostral hypothalamus resulted in adipsia (Bagley 1994).

The importance of these hypothalamic areas for thirst and drinking was shown in dogs, wherein electrocoagulative destruction of an area in the rostral hypothalamus resulted in adipsia (Anderson and McCann 1956). This area of the hypothalamus responsible for thirst is close to, but different from, the areas associated with ADH production. Extrahypothalamic areas of the brain such as the amygdala and subcommissural organ may also play a role in thirst and drinking. Additional sensory receptors for thirst may occur in the mouth, pharynx, and vascular system such as the portal system. The combination of receptors signal thirst to replace the body water deficit prior to significant ECF osmolality alterations.

The hypothalamic receptor cell necessary for thirst recognition is referred to as an osmoreceptor. When the ECF is hyperosmolar relative to intracellular fluid, these cells lose water and shrink. This shrinkage signals the need for drinking. The composition of the osmole resulting in ECF hyperosmolality appears to influence the degree of stimulation of thirst. Sodium is the most potent osmole stimulating thirst. Experimentally in dogs, ECF hyperosmolality induced by infusion of hypertonic sodium chloride stimulates thirst. When hypertonic solutions of glucose or urea were infused, however, thirst was not stimulated. Sodium is relatively impermeable to the cell membrane, whereas, glucose and urea are more permeable.

Thirst stimulation seems to relate inversely to the rate at which a particular solute crosses the osmoreceptor cell membrane, and the more freely the solute moves across the cell membrane, the less effective that solute is at stimulating thirst.

While ECF hyperosmolality is an important stimulus for thirst, other effects of body water depletion can also signal thirst. For example, hypovolemia can be a potent stimulator of thirst, with a decrease in vascular volume of between 5 and 10% being necessary to result in drinking (Guyton and Hall 1996). Stretch receptors or humoral factors such as those of the renin/angiotensin system may stimulate thirst. Additional receptors in the mouth detecting dryness of the mucous membrane may elicit or alter thirst. In comparison, plasma osmolality only need increase as little as 5% above normal to stimulate thirst equally. Therefore, hyperosmolality and hypovolemia/hypotension can occur concurrently or independently to stimulate thirst. These two factors appear synergistic in their effects on thirst. When an animal is hypotensive, the osmoreceptor threshold is altered so that a smaller degree of osmolality increase is required to result in thirst. Similarly, in a hypervolemic or hypertensive animal, a greater increase in osmolality is required to stimulate thirst equally.

If the ECF is hypo-osmolar to the intracellular fluid (ICF), then the cell imbibes water and swells, thus eliminating the signal for thirst. How thirst ultimately results in drinking is less clear, but presumably this sensation involves cerebral cortical structures and conscious control.

2 Pathophysiology of Nervous System Disease

Neuronal cells, like most cells of the body, require essential structural elements and metabolic processes to function effectively (Guyton and Hall 1996). Disease can affect the nervous system in a number of ways. Some disease processes directly alter the structural integrity of nervous system elements, while others result in cellular metabolic derangements. Similar to other body systems, normal physiology or function of the nervous system is dependent upon healthy cellular activity. The basic nervous system physiology is primarily dependent upon normal cell membrane physiology. Transmembrane electrical charge is generated and altered through energy-dependent movement of charged particles such as sodium, potassium, and chloride. Alterations in cellular membrane potentials give rise to depolarization and action potential generation, which terminate in synaptic activity. Synaptic activity results in alterations in neuronal and effector organ function.

The normal brain cell maintains an unevenly distributed electrical charge across the cell membrane. The interior of the cell is negative with respect to the exterior, and this charge difference is maintained in the resting state primarily via the Na^{+2}-K^{+} ATPase pump that extrudes three Na^{+2} molecules in exchange for moving two K^{+} molecules into the cell. This pump requires energy to maintain the interior of the cell approximately negative 70 to 85 mv with respect to the exterior.

When the cell is excited, this resting membrane potential moves toward positive until threshold is reached (depolarization), and an action potential is generated. This occurs primarily via Na^{+2} entering the interior of the cell. After threshold is reached and the action potential is generated, Na^{+2} will then be extruded, the molecular charge at the cell membrane will become more negative, and the cell will repolarize to its resting membrane potential.

Pathophysiologic processes that alter the ability of a nervous system cell to generate an action potential ultimately result in clinical dysfunction. Energy is utilized to generate and maintain normal axon potential generation. Cellular energy is heavily dependent upon the availability of oxygen as well as the appropriate metabolism of oxygen. Oxygen becomes available to the nervous system primarily through its transport in the vascular system. When many of the acquired nervous system disease processes are assessed at a fundamental pathophysiologic basis, dysfunction and destruction of the nervous system most commonly result from a lack of oxygen permeating the cells or from the cell's inability to extract or utilize oxygen available. Glucose, electrolytes, neurotransmitters, and other elements are also important for neuronal function in many instances. Without oxygen, however, most central neuronal functions cease rapidly.

A neuronal element and its metabolic dependence on oxygen become a simple supply and demand relationship. A nervous system cell has a fundamental requirement for oxygen to support its metabolic processes. Oxygen is delivered to neuronal cells primarily through the arterial side of the vascular system. Delivery of oxygen is dependent on the flow characteristics of blood, including the integrity and size of the vascular system, the component of blood and plasma, and the pressure required to move a fluid (blood) through the system.

PATHOPHYSIOLOGIC SEQUELAE OF INTRACRANIAL DISEASE

The intracranial nervous system resides in a unique physiologic environment. Protected by, but also confined within, the bony limits of the cranium, nervous tissue exists with cerebrospinal fluid (CSF) and blood (fig. 2.1). Disease of the brain parenchyma or other intracranial tissues commonly alters this existing physiologic equilibrium (fig. 2.2). Many of these processes increase the relative volume within the intracranial cavity, ultimately affecting intracranial pressure (ICP) (fig. 2.3). Individual and unique disease processes involving the intracranial structures are discussed in chapter 5.

Intracranial disease can alter normal physiological relationships in numerous ways. These include, but are not limited to, physical invasion and/or destruction of neurons, metabolic alterations in neuronal or glial cells, impairment of vascular supply to normal tissue (ischemia or hypoxia), impairment of autoregulation, hemorrhage (intratumoral or intraventricular), irritation (seizure generation), obstruction of the ventricular system, edema formation, production of physiologically active substances, and increased intracranial pressure (ICP) (Bagley 1996a, 1996c; Kornegay 1993; Olby and Jeffery 2003). These processes

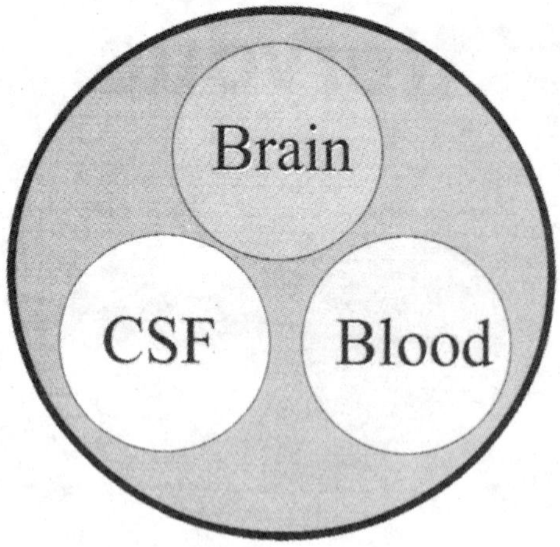

Fig. 2.1. Schematic relationship of important intracranial volume components within the skull.

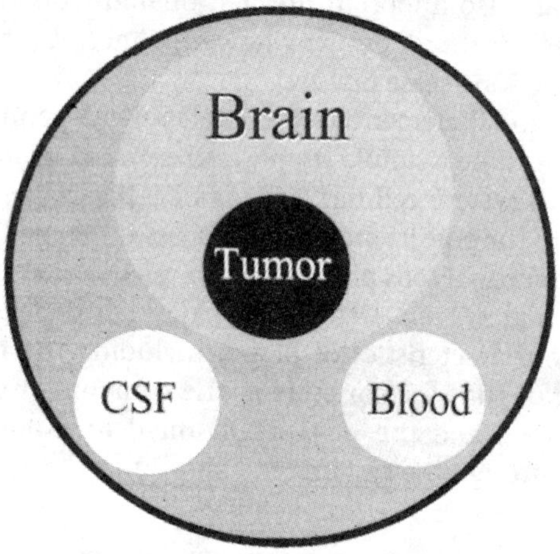

Fig. 2.2. Schematic relationship of important intracranial volume components within the skull associated with a brain tumor.

may initiate and perpetuate each other. Some of the more common aforementioned pathophysiologic disturbances are described further.

Ischemia

One of the most important consequences of structural intracranial disease is the effect of these diseases on cerebral blood flow. Blood normally flows to the brain from the heart, aorta, brachiocephalic trunk, and carotid arteries (Beitz and Fletcher 1993) (fig. 2.4). There are apparent species differences in the anatomical arrangement of vessels responsible for cerebral perfusion from the carotid level. In dogs, blood flows into the circle of Willis from the internal carotid artery (deLahunta 1983; King 1987). In cats, the internal carotid artery is apparently often nonpatent shortly following birth, and blood is directed from

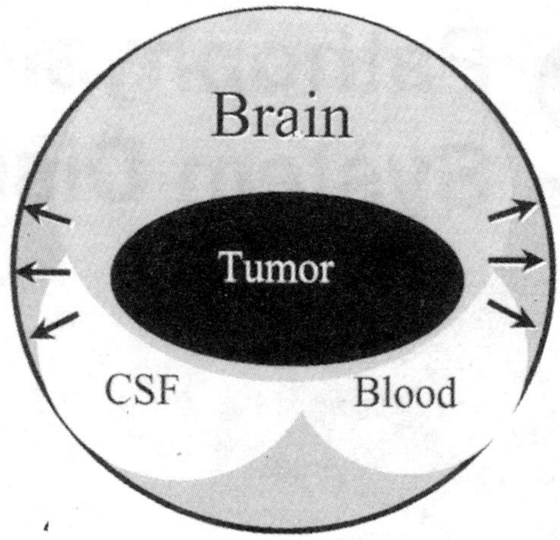

Fig. 2.3. Schematic relationship of important intracranial volume components within the skull associated with a brain tumor increasing the intracranial pressure (ICP).

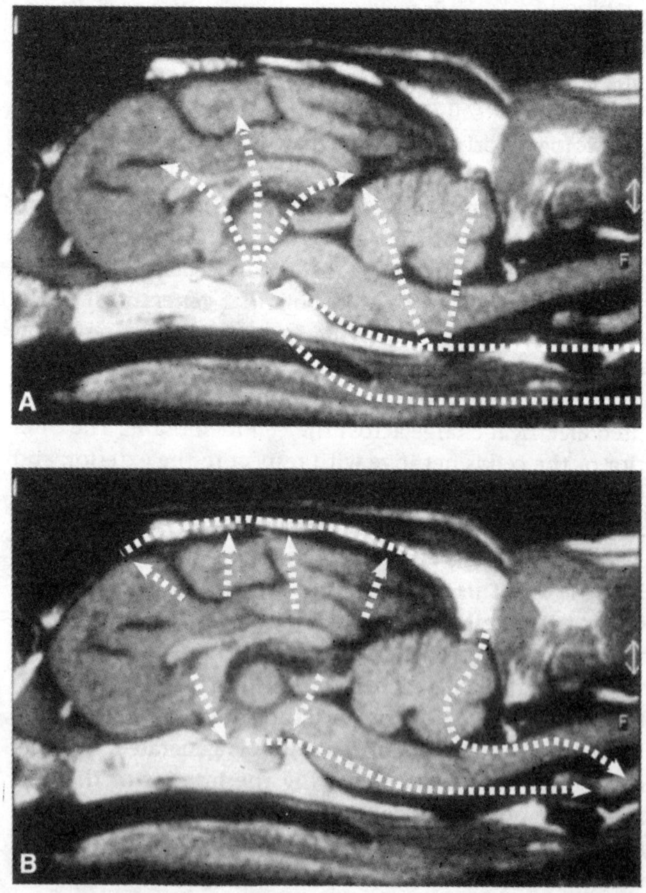

Fig. 2.4. Sagittal, magnetic resonance view of the dog brain. The important (A) arterial and (B) venous vascular systems are shown (*lines with arrows*).

the external carotid artery through the maxillary artery to the ventral arterial system (King 1987).

The circle of Willis supplies the majority of arterial blood flow to the cerebral cortex. Blood also reaches the

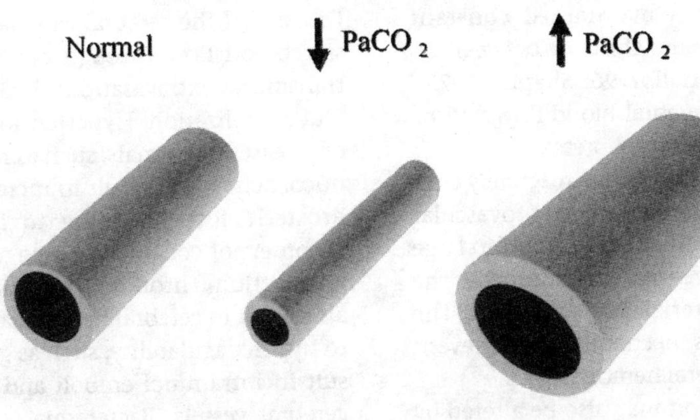

Fig. 2.5. Schematic relationship of the cerebral vessels to alterations in $PaCO_2$ concentrations.

caudal brain stem from the subclavian arteries via the vertebral arteries and, ultimately, the basilar artery. In cats, blood flow has been suggested to be reversed in the basilar artery and the majority of the blood supply to the intracranial nervous system results from blood flow from the maxillary artery (King 1987). This reversed blood flow in the basilar artery in cats, however, is debatable.

Because normal function of neurons depends on an adequate supply of oxygen, abnormalities of blood flow can significantly impair normal brain function. Also, the metabolic rate of brain/mass is high compared to most tissues. For normal function, the brain cells require an almost constant supply of oxygen. Continuous oxygen delivery is necessary as the brain is very inefficient at anaerobic metabolism. Additionally, neurons have minimal storage of glycogen to support anaerobic metabolism.

Cerebral blood flow is influenced by at least three factors: CO_2 concentrations, H+ concentrations, and oxygen concentrations (Shapiro 1975). Cerebral vessels are directly responsive to local $PaCO_2$ concentrations, with cerebral blood flow coupled to cerebral metabolic rate. As $PaCO_2$ concentrations increase, cerebral vessels dilate to increase blood flow to the brain (fig. 2.5). The opposite effect is seen with decreased $PaCO_2$. This $PaCO_2$-dependent cerebrovascular alteration is a component of what is termed *autoregulation.* The cerebral vessels have the ability to change diameter in response to $PaCO_2$ (chemical autoregulation) concentrations as well as alterations in blood pressure (pressure autoregulation) in order to maintain a relatively constant cerebral blood flow during minor fluctuations in cerebral blood flow. The diameter of cerebral vessels is primarily dependent upon local pH in the perivascular environment. Alterations in local pH are a direct result of $PaCO_2$ concentrations, similar to mechanisms in the chemosensitive area of the medulla oblongata for stimulation of respiration. If chemical autoregulation is intact, hyperventilation to decrease $PaCO_2$ will cause cerebral vasoconstriction, decreased cerebral blood volume, and, subsequently, decreased intracranial pressure (ICP). The opposite may result from hypoventilation.

Unfortunately, cerebrovascular autoregulatory capability is affected by a variety of intracranial processes (Shapiro 1975). For example, local acidosis, common in many hypoxic and ischemic events, will disrupt local autoregulatory functions. Cerebral vessels may lose vasoconstrictive mechanisms and become inappropriately dilated. In this situation, hyperventilation will not alter the vascular diameter in the affected area. In this instance, at least two consequences are possible, both dependent upon the premise that cerebrovascular autoregulatory capacity is absent due to local disease.

As $PaCO_2$ is decreased by hyperventilation, vessels in the surrounding normal brain will vasoconstrict. Vessels in the damaged or abnormal area of the brain are already maximally dilated and, as such, unable to constrict. Because of the vasoconstriction in the surrounding normal brain, vascular resistance increases in this area, shunting blood into the abnormal area (inverse steal or Robin Hood phenomenon) (Shapiro 1975). This has the positive effect of increasing cerebral blood flow to the abnormal and potentially hypoxic areas of the brain. The negative effect, however, is potentiation of hemorrhage and cerebral edema in the abnormal area due to the increased flow.

The opposite may occur as $PaCO_2$ increases. In this instance, vessels in normal brain surrounding the diseased area will dilate. Again, vessels in the abnormal area are already maximally dilated due to loss of autoregulation. Vascular resistance will be decreased in surrounding normal brain, blood will be shunted away from abnormal areas, potentially decreasing hemorrhage and edema but resulting in further hypoxia (steal phenomenon) (Bagley 1996b, 1996c; Shapiro 1975).

Autoregulation of cerebral blood flow also can occur in response to systemic blood pressure changes in order to maintain cerebral blood flow relatively constant during times of both hypo- and hypertension. This cerebrovascular autoregulatory mechanism prevents underperfusion and subsequent ischemia during times of hypotension and hemorrhage and edema at times of hypertension. In most instances, cerebral blood flow is maintained constant throughout systemic blood pressure shifts of between 60 and 150 mm Hg (Guyton and Hall 1996; Shapiro 1975). Above and below these limits, cerebral blood flow will be directly dependent upon systemic blood pressure.

The sympathetic system may play a role in actively constricting cerebral vessels in the presence of cerebrovascular hypertension. In this situation, constriction occurs in large and intermediate-sized cerebral vessels, which impedes the further distribution of the arterial pressures into the smaller arteries of the brain. This mechanism may prevent small vessel disruption and cerebral hemorrhage.

Normal pressure autoregulation may also be altered by intracranial disease. An assessment of whether pressure autoregulation remains intact in brain disease is difficult to predict clinically. Global pressure autoregulatory function has been assessed in human patients with head injury and found to be intact in approximately 70% of head trauma patients (Bouma et al. 1992). It has been suggested that a crude clinical estimate of intact autoregulatory function is the level of consciousness, with conscious patients having more intact autoregulatory capacity. Local loss of autoregulation, however, is almost impossible to predict in the clinical setting without sophisticated testing that is not practically available.

Additionally, at least in the instance of exogenous head trauma, discrepancies can occur between the intact function of pressure versus chemical ($PaCO_2$-responsive) autoregulatory capacities (Enevoldsen and Jensen 1979). With head trauma, pressure autoregulation is often abnormal; however, $PaCO_2$-responsive autoregulation remains intact. This is termed *dissociative vasoparalysis* and has important ramifications during treatment. As the cerebrovascular response to blood pressure changes are abnormal, a more intimate control of systemic blood pressure and central venous pressure is required to prevent large shifts of blood pressure and subsequent cerebral blood flow. If pressure autoregulation is defective, significant increases in mean arterial blood pressure will increase cerebral blood flow and, ultimately, ICP. If pressure autoregulation is intact, decreased blood pressure will cause cerebrovascular vasodilation, increasing cerebral blood flow and, ultimately, increasing ICP.

Pressure autoregulation may also falsely appear intact (false autoregulation) even when vasomotor paralysis is present. In this situation, cerebral blood flow is found to not increase when systemic blood pressure is increased, suggesting intact pressure autoregulation. Because of associated cerebral swelling, however, further dilation of cerebral vessels is prevented. Therefore, no additional increase in cerebral blood flow is possible, regardless of blood pressure. All of these factors contribute to a myriad of intracranial blood flow alterations that can affect intracranial pressure.

Cerebrovascular Disease

Primary cerebrovascular disease is reportedly less common in dogs compared to humans, however, clinically apparent cerebrovascular diseases have been recognized in animals. Diseases of the cerebral vasculature may result from excessive blood flow through cerebral vessels (hypertension), transmural extravasation of blood, ischemia, thrombosis, and embolization. Hypertension, associated with a variety of diseases in animals, such as renal disease and hyperadrenocorticism, can result in increases in cerebrovascular hydrostatic forces leading to intracranial hemorrhages. Disorders of coagulation (coagulopathies, DIC) and platelet function (thrombocytopenia and thrombopathies) can also result in cerebral hemorrhage. Diseases that predispose to hypercoagulability, such as glomerulonephritis, may result in intramural emboli and subsequent thrombosis of cerebral vessels. Bacteremia (endocarditis) may result in septic embolization of intracranial vessels. Vessel wall integrity can be disrupted by neoplastic infiltration or inflammatory diseases, including vasculitis syndromes, and can result in thrombosis and hemorrhage. Less commonly, arteriovenous malformations and aneurysms have been reported in dogs. All of these intracranial vascular abnormalities may predispose to cerebral hypoxia and ischemia, as well as intracranial hemorrhage.

Cerebrovascular disease results primarily in ischemia and hemorrhage. Other secondary consequences include edema formation, mass effect, and increases in intracranial pressure. Ischemic damage, regardless of cause, results in endothelial cell damage predisposing to thrombosis, necrosis, and hemorrhage. One of the most devastating effects of severe intracranial vascular disease is intracranial hemorrhage. Hemorrhage into and around the brain can result in an associated inflammatory reaction, increases in overall intracranial volume, and increases in intracranial pressure (Brinker et al. 1992; Foley et al. 1994; Regan and Panter 1993). Intraventricular bleeding and bleeding into the cerebrospinal fluid are irritating to local nervous tissue and may result in inflammation (meningitis, myelitis, or encephalitis). Hemorrhage into the third ventricle is often associated with fever, most likely due to local alterations in the thermoregulatory center. If bleeding is substantial enough, hematomas may subsequently form, altering CNS volume/pressure relationships and potentially increasing intracranial pressure and decreasing cerebral blood flow.

Hypertension is an underrecognized cause of cerebrovascular disease in animals. Autoregulation of cerebral blood flow occurs in response to systemic blood pressure changes in order to maintain cerebral blood flow relatively constant during both hypo- and hypertension. This prevents underperfusion and subsequent ischemia during times of hypotension and hemorrhage and edema at times of hypertension. In most instances, cerebral blood flow is maintained constant throughout systemic blood pressure shifts of between 50 and 150 mm Hg (Shapiro 1975). Above these limits, cerebral blood flow will be directly dependent upon systemic blood pressure, and the risk of hypertensive encephalopathy and cerebrovascular damage increases.

More commonly, however, complications of systemic hemostatic diseases can affect the CNS (Bagley 2000). Examples include thrombocytopenias and coagulopathies.

Animals being given anticoagulant drugs (heparin, coumadin) may have apparent spontaneous hemorrhagic episodes in or around the nervous system. Disseminated intravascular coagulopathy, anticoagulant rodenticide intoxication, and hemophilia and other congenital hemostatic diseases may also be associated with CNS bleeding.

Hemorrhage into and around the brain and spinal cord can adversely affect nervous tissue. Intraventricular bleeding and bleeding into the cerebrospinal fluid are irritating to local nervous tissue and may result in inflammation (meningitis, myelitis, or encephalitis). Hemorrhage into the third ventricle is often associated with fever, most likely due to local alterations in the thermoregulatory center. Hemorrhage into the spinal cord usually results in severe paresis or plegia.

Most devastating, however, is when the bleeding is substantial enough to form excessive additional volume within the CNS (Hopkins and Wheeler 1991). Hematomas may subsequently form. These alter CNS volume/pressure relationships with the possibility of increasing intracranial pressure and decreasing cerebral blood flow. Similar events probably occur in the spinal cord, however, they are less well defined. While the initial hematoma will create a certain degree of pressure, clinical signs may worsen as the hematoma is resorbed ("ages"). This was originally thought to result from the hyperosmolar environment of the resolving hematoma increasing the movement of fluid (water) into the hematoma, actually increasing its volume, however, this is not always found. Increasing hematoma volume may ultimately cause worsening clinical signs compared to those associated with the initial hemorrhagic event.

Water Balance in the Brain

In disease state, cells in the brain are susceptible to alterations in intracellular and extracellular water (ECF) content (Guyton and Hall 1996). Local osmolality is an important component of brain water content. Normally, the brain cells and the extracellular environment share an equal osmolality. If the osmolality of the intravascular or extracellular fluid increases, fluid will shift from the brain cells to the extracellular environment. Brain cells will become smaller, which may affect cellular metabolic functions. If the ECF remains hyperosmolar, brain cells compensate for this persistently hyperosmolar ECF environment by the intracellular production of osmolytes (historically known as idiogenic osmoles) (Bagley 1994). The composition of these osmoles is unclear, but they may be glucose moities or amino acids such as glutamate, aspartate, and GABA.

Osmolytes are initially produced between 1 and 4 hours after persistent ECF hyperosmolality (Bagley 1994). These osmolytes serve to increase the intracellular osmotic environment, resulting in transmembrane movement of water into the cell. This is an attempt to stabilizes brain cell volume. Osmolytes are maximally effective at stabilizing brain water content by 7 days following the presence of a persistently hyperosmolar extracellular environment.

While osmolytes are produced relatively rapidly following persistent ECF hyperosmolality, these products are dismantled more slowly. If, after osmolytes are produced and a rapid decrease in the ECF osmolality occurs, osmolytes present in the brain's cells will now result in the intracellular osmotic environment to be hyperosmolar relative to the ECF. Transmembrane shifts in water will result in a significant increase in intracellular water content causing cellular edema. This may ultimately result in disruption of the cell membrane and cellular destruction.

Conversely, if a normal brain cell is exposed to ECF hypoosmolality, this cell may initially imbibe water. This can result in demyelination in specific areas of the brain and is known as central pontine myelinolysis. In human beings, the brain stem is often affected, which is reflected by the pontine portion of the name. In dogs, areas in the thalamus are more classically affected. Once intracellular water volume is again stabilized, if the ECF becomes hyperosmolar, water will be shifted from the cell to the ECF, resulting in cellular shrinkage. This will result in dehydration of brain cells, making them smaller. Shrinkage of the brain may rupture fragile bridging veins causing these vessels to rupture and resulting in intracranial hemorrhages.

Cerebral Edema

Many intracranial diseases result in or are associated with brain edema. Following an acute injury, brain edema becomes maximal between 24 and 48 hours after injury. Edema may persist for a week or more. Brain edema has been described as vasogenic, cytotoxic, or interstitial based upon cause and anatomic areas of involvement (fig. 2.6) (Fishman 1975; Reulen 1976). Any or all of these types of edema may be present in an animal with brain disease.

Types of Cerebral Edema. Cytotoxic edema (intracellular edema) results from failure of cellular energy with resultant failure to appropriately extrude sodium from within the cell. Intracellular water increases and cells swell. This edema most often results in disease processes such as toxicity, ischemia, or hypoxia.

Interstitial edema is increased water content of the periventricular white matter due to movement of CSF across the ventricular walls in instances of hydrocephalus. Periventricular white matter is reduced due to the disappearance of myelin lipids secondary to increases in white matter hydrostatic pressure or decreases in periventricular white matter blood flow (Rosenberg et al. 1983).

Vasogenic edema is the most common form of edema associated with CNS neoplasia. This type of edema results from vascular injury secondary to physical disruption of the vascular endothelium or functional alterations in endothelial tight junctions. Differences in transmural pressure gradients result in extravasation of fluid from cerebral vessels to the extracellular fluid spaces of the brain (Rosenberg et al. 1983). These abnormalities allow for fluid to move from the vascular to perivascular spaces.

Areas of the brain where ECF is normally enlarged provide a natural conduit for fluid movement. Increases in intravascular pressure due to loss of autoregulation, vascular

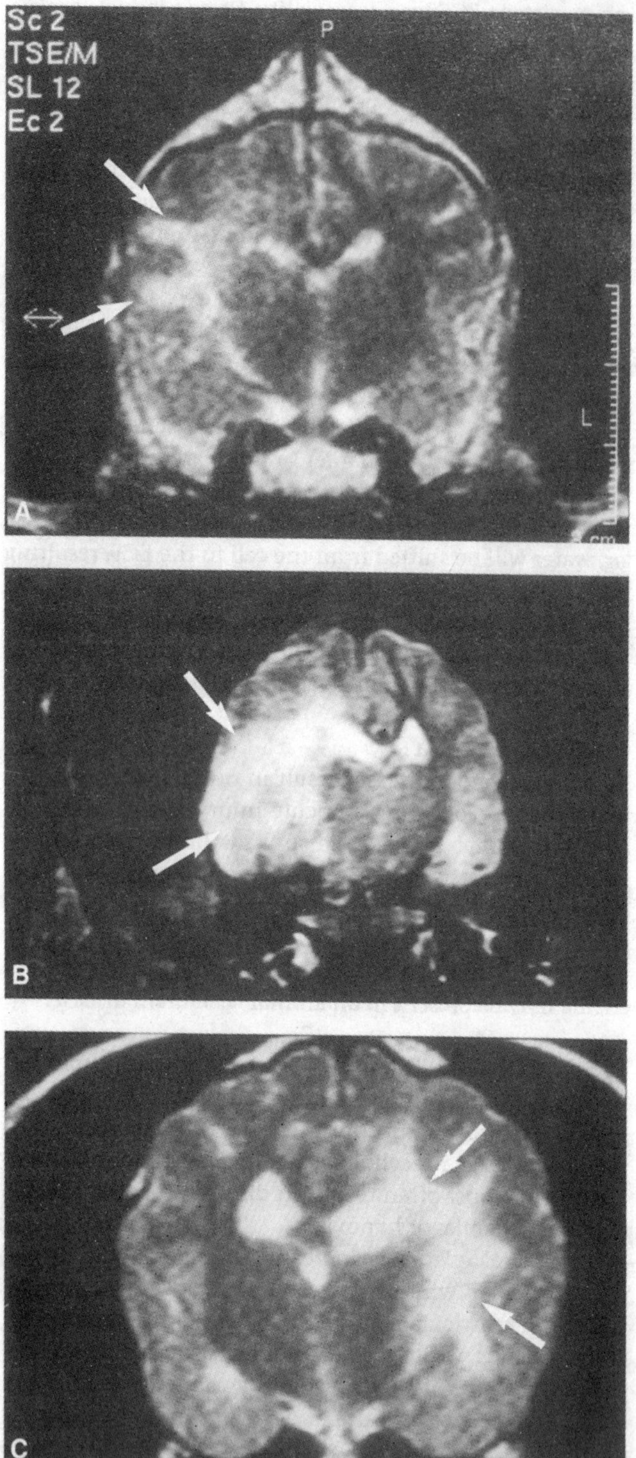

Fig. 2.6. Transverse, T 2-weighted magnetic resonance images from three (A, B, C) dogs showing cerebral edema (hyperintense or whiter in appearance). The edema of these dogs is within the white matter (*arrows*).

obstruction, or hypertension (Cushing's response, cerebral ischemic response) may perpetuate edema formation.

Vasogenic edema migrates away from areas of vascular disruption via bulk flow. Fluid movement depends upon a balance between the opposing forces of capillary hydrostatic pressure and tissue resistance pressure. Vasogenic edema usually spreads readily through the white matter, possibly because of the orderly arrangement of nerve fibers found there. Also, the movement of this type of edema may be related to low capillary density and blood flow in normal white matter. Deep white matter of the affected cerebral hemisphere is preferentially affected (fig. 2.6).

Seizures

Seizure activity is a common sequela to intracranial disease (Bagley and Gavin 1998; Bagley 1999). A seizure is defined as a paroxysmal, transitory disturbance of brain function that has a sudden onset, ceases spontaneously, and has a tendency to recur. Seizures are usually associated with autonomic disturbances such as urination, salivation, and defecation. Epilepsy is a recurrent seizure disorder irrespective of cause (Podell 1996).

Pathophysiology of Seizures. Seizures result from spontaneous depolarization of intracranial neurons (March 1998; Russo 1981). On one hand, the cell is available to be excited by excitatory postsynaptic potentials. This stimulation will result in depolarization. In opposition, the cell may be inhibited or prevented from depolarizing by stimulation from inhibitory postsynaptic potentials.

The basic pathophysiological processes that result in seizures, then, are excessive excitation or loss of inhibition (disinhibition). Hypoglycemia, for example, will cause loss of energy substrate for the Na^{+2}-K^{+} ATPase pump, failure to extrude Na^{+2}, and the cell moving toward positivity and depolarization (excessive excitation). In a disease process where inhibitory transmitters are unable to function (hepatic encephalopathy ?), the lack of inhibition will allow for unregulated depolarization.

A seizure can occur when certain proportion of brain cells spontaneously depolarize referred to as a seizure focus. For a seizure to have clinical consequences, a group of cells must depolarize, referred to as a paroxysmal depolarization shift (PDS). Normal neurons may display sporadic, low-frequency activity. The brain normally contains these minor electrical events without clinical consequence. In seizure foci, the firing pattern is one of regular recurrent high-frequency bursts of action potentials. The PDS usually remains localized to a small area if the brain is able to contain much of this activity by preventing the spread of depolarization to other cells (surround inhibition).

When a depolarization is of a sufficient magnitude, the impulse may be conducted to a more widespread area or even the entire brain. When the entire brain becomes involved a generalized seizure will be produced. This spread of depolarization most likely occurs through normal anatomic connections between neurons. Propagation of abnormal electrical activity can occur in milliseconds and a generalized seizure will be seen from the onset, or, if the spread is slower, an initial focal seizure (confined to one body part/area) may eventually be followed by a generalized seizure. If the spread of the electrical discharge is terminated prior to generalization, a focal seizure will be the extent of the disturbance.

Focal seizures may become generalized through normal

brain interconnections, or may become generalized by synchronized depolarizations controlled from the thalamus and other subcortical structures. This centrencephalic theory of seizure propagation suggests that generalized seizure activity originates in structures in the brain stem and thalamus, which is then projected to the cortex (March 1998; Russo 1981). Experimental evidence suggests that both brain stem and cortical stimulation may result in seizure activity.

Seizure activity may perpetuate the likelihood of additional seizure activity. This is referred to as kindling. Kindling may occur locally or at distance sites removed from the initial seizure focus. A mirror focus, for example, is where a seizure focus creates similar activity in a homologous area of the contralateral hemisphere. With time, both mirror foci and kindled foci may become autonomous and form a new, independent seizure focus.

Why seizures terminate as rapidly as they begin is also uncertain. Metabolic exhaustion of neurons does not appear to be an adequate exclusive explanation for such termination. Extracortical inhibitory centers, such as within the cerebellum, may play a role. Ablations of the cerebellum, for example, facilitate seizure activity (Russo 1981). Phenytoin, a commonly used anticonvulsant in human beings, dramatically increases the rate of firing of Purkinje neurons. Other areas such as the caudate and parts of the thalamus and reticular formation may also help to terminate seizure activity.

Ventricular Obstruction

Cerebrospinal fluid originates from the choroid plexus of the lateral, third, and fourth ventricles, directly from the brain by way of the ependymal lining of the ventricular system, directly from the brain by way of the pial-glial membrane covering the external surface, and from the blood vessels of the pia and arachnoid (deLahunta 1983). Cerebrospinal fluid is produced at a constant rate despite CSF pressure in the ventricular system. This rate is independent of the hydrostatic pressure of the blood, but dependent on the osmotic pressure. As an example, hyperosmolality of blood decreases CSF production and may be one of the mechanisms by which mannitol therapy decreases intracranial pressure.

Cerebrospinal fluid circulates from the sites of production and exits the ventricular system at the lateral apertures of the fourth ventricle, then passes dorsally over the cerebral hemispheres to the dorsal sagittal sinus. CSF penetrates the brain with the larger blood vessels of the perivascular space (extensions of the subarachnoid space to where the pia reflects back on these vessels). In some animals, CSF may also exit at the conus medullaris of the spinal cord.

From rostral to caudal, beginning in the cerebral hemispheres, the components of the ventricular system include the lateral ventricles, the third ventricle, the mesencephalic aqueduct, and the fourth ventricle (deLahunta 1983). The third ventricle is formed in a circular pattern around the thalamus. The mesencephalic aqueduct is a relatively smaller connection between the third and fourth ventricle. The fourth ventricle is located between the brain stem (ventrally) and the cerebellum (dorsally). The fourth ventricle is continued into the spinal cord via the central canal.

Table 2.1. Cerebrospinal fluid pressure in normal dogs (in mm Hg)

	Mean*	Range*
Schirmer (1958)	5	NA
Hoerlein (1965)	7	NA
Parker (1972)	NA	5–10
Novak (1974)	9	4–16
Simpson and Reed (1987)	6	4–10

*Pressures converted from mm CSF to mm Hg and rounded to nearest whole number.

Flow of CSF is dependent on the pulsation of the blood in the choroid plexus. Systole results in a small increase in intracranial pressure. With each pulsation, CSF pressure increases and CSF may then move toward the lateral apertures, aided by the cilia of the ependymal cells. Cerebrospinal fluid flow occurs in both directions (cranial and caudal), but there appears to be a predominant caudal flow in dogs.

The pressure exhibited by the CSF contributes to intracranial pressure and expansion of the brain. Cerebrospinal fluid pressure has been historically measured in animals as a reflection of intracranial pressure. Normal cerebrospinal fluid pressures for dogs are found in table 2.1 (Hoerlein 1965; Novak et al. 1974; Parker 1972; Schirmer 1958; Simpson and Reed 1987). Slightly lower CSF pressures have been found in cats as compared to dogs.

The major site of CSF absorption is in the arachnoid villus within a venous sinus or a cerebral vein (deLahunta 1983). The villus is a prolongation of the arachnoid and the subarachnoid space into the venous sinus. Collections of these villi are known as arachnoid granulations. The venous endothelium acts like a ball valve (from transient transcellular channels that develop for the passage of fluid) so as to be open when CSF pressure exceeds the venous pressure (the normal relationship). If venous pressure rises above CSF pressure, the villi will collapse. Flow direction, therefore, is always from CSF to blood.

Other sites of absorption include the veins and lymphatics around the spinal nerve roots, and the cranial nerves (olfactory and optic) where they leave the skull. Some of the CSF may enter the brain parenchyma through the ependyma to be absorbed into blood vessels. This apparently is only an important means of CSF absorption when the CSF pressure is elevated. With production being mostly independent of intracranial pressure, absorption is the primary homeostatic mechanism for maintenance of intracranial pressure.

Hydrocephalus can result from obstruction of the ventricular system, irritation of the ventricle (from inflammation or hemorrhage), and increased size of the ventricles due to loss of brain parenchyma (hydrocephalus ex vacuo), and it can be present without an obvious cause (congenital) or, rarely, can be the result of overproduction of CSF associated with a choroid plexus tumor (fig. 2.7). Ventricular ob-

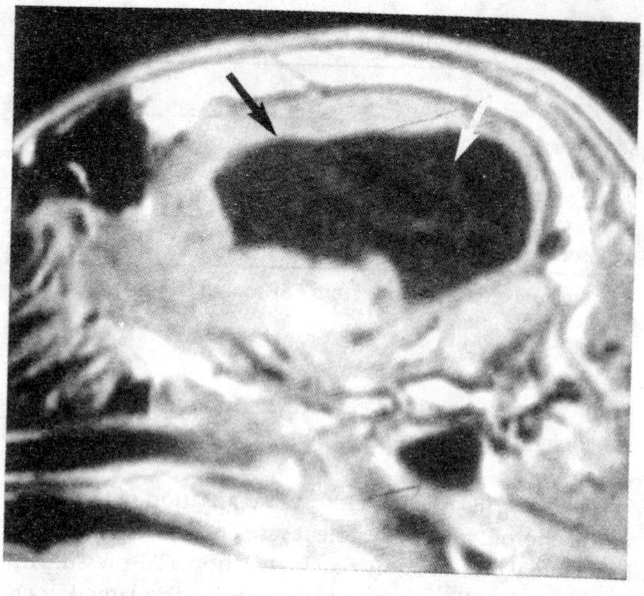

Fig. 2.7. Sagittal, T 1-weighted magnetic resonance image from a dog showing severe dilation of the lateral ventricles (*arrows*).

struction can occur both from intraventricular and extraventricular obstruction. Diffuse ventricular enlargement suggests congenital ventricular dilation or obstruction at the level of the lateral apertures or foramen magnum. Focal ventricular enlargement suggests focal obstruction or parenchymal cell loss. It is not uncommon to have bilateral lateral ventricle enlargement that is asymmetric. Animals with asymmetric appearance of the ventricles should be critically evaluated for focal obstruction of or impingement on the ventricular system due to mass effect. Hemorrhage into the ventricular system can occur with head trauma, hypertension, and bleeding disorders. Blood products are irritating to the ependyma, and result in associated inflammation (Brinker 1992; Foley 1994; Regan and Panter 1993).

If the ventricular system is obstructed, CSF will be trapped behind the level of obstruction. This may also be referred to as a noncommunicating hydrocephalus (deLahunta 1983). As some small amounts of CSF may pass the level of the obstruction, this may not always be the most appropriate description of the pathophysiological state. Anatomically smaller areas of the ventricular system are common sites of obstruction. These include the interventricular foramen and the mesencephalic aqueduct. Obstruction can result from tumor, granuloma, hemorrhage, or inflammation. Rarely, abnormalities of ependymal cilia function can result in ventricle dilation, probably due to poor or absent CSF flow. Immotile cilia syndrome and Kartagener's syndrome would be examples.

Hydrocephalus can result in clinical signs due to loss of neurons or neuronal function, alterations in intracranial pressure, and associated pathophysiological effects of intracranial disease. Interstitial edema, for example, is increased water content of the periventricular white matter due to movement of CSF across the ventricular walls in instances of hydrocephalus. Periventricular white matter is reduced due to the disappearance of myelin lipids secondary to increases in white matter hydrostatic pressure or decreases in periventricular white matter blood flow. Increased CSF pressure may contribute to intracranial disease through alterations in intracranial pressure. Consequences of increased intracranial pressure are described later in the chapter.

If formation of CSF equilibrates with absorption, a compensated hydrocephalic state may occur. In some instances, CSF production may decrease, possibly due to pressure damage to the choroid plexus or ependyma.

Increases in Intracranial Pressure

Intracranial pressure (ICP) is the pressure exerted between the skull and the intracranial tissues (Lyons and Meyer 1990). As the skull is relatively inelastic compared to the other intracranial tissues, ICP is determined primarily by changes in intracranial tissue volume and the compensatory ability of these tissues to accommodate for volume changes.

The three major volume components residing within the intracranial space are the brain tissue (intracranial cellular elements), the cerebrospinal fluid, and blood. Intracranial disease often increases the volume of one of these components. A brain tumor, for example, will increase the volume of the brain tissue component. For ICP to remain normal, an increase in volume of one of these three intracranial components must be compensated for by a decrease to an equal amount in one or both of the other components (intracranial compliance). While compliance can initially aid in stabilizing ICP, this compensatory mechanism has finite limits. When compliance is exhausted, ICP will increase (fig. 2.8) (Shapiro 1975). The limits of compliance may vary between individual patients and may be influenced by the extent and location of an intracranial mass as well as cerebral blood flow. As ICP increases, the pressure within the intracranial space decreases cerebral blood flow. With decreased cerebral perfusion, neuronal ischemia, hypoxia, dysfunction, and death ultimately result.

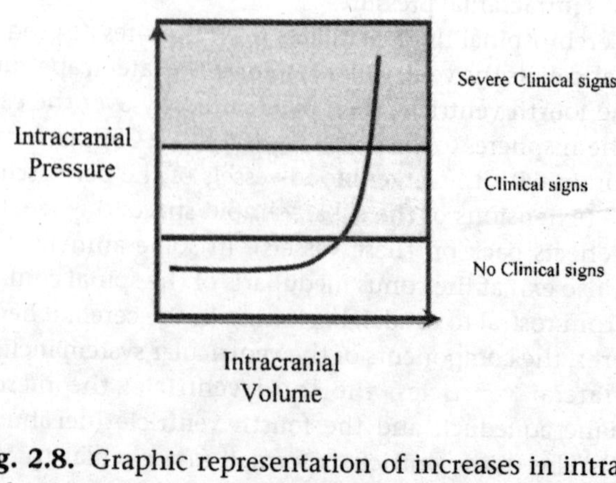

Fig. 2.8. Graphic representation of increases in intracranial pressure (ICP) subsequent to increases in intracranial volume.

Cerebral blood flow and CSF are in constant flux. Subsequently, ICP is dynamic and pulsatile, with a small pressure wave occurring almost simultaneously with each heart beat (Cardoso et al. 1983; German 1988). This wave form is referred to as the intracranial pulse pressure wave (ICPPW). The ICPPW is best visualized when ICP is measured with a pressure transducer placed within a lateral ventricle. The ICPP wave form has three separate peaks or spikes contraction (Cardoso et al. 1983; German 1988). The P1 or first spike is referred to as the percussion wave and is thought to originate from the pulsation of blood vessels within the choroid plexus associated with each heart contraction (Cardoso et al. 1983; German 1988). The origins of the second and third components of the ICPP wave are not definitively established. The amplitude of the second component, the P2 or tidal wave, however, is altered by ventilation status. With hyperventilation, the amplitude of this peak will decrease (Barlow et al. 1985). The opposite is seen with hypoventilation, as the amplitude of P2 will increase. The third component is the P3 or dicrotic wave. Its amplitude may be altered by changes in venous pressure, possibly the result of changes in intrathoracic pressure during breathing (Cardoso et al. 1983; German 1988).

Mean ICP normally remains relatively constant. Periodic, and sometimes dramatic, fluctuations may occur in response to normal body functions such as coughing or abdominal straining via increases in intrathoracic pressure and venous pressure impairing venous return from the intracranial space. With intracranial disease that alters intracranial volume, ICP may be elevated persistently or episodically, resulting in persistent or episodic clinical abnormalities, respectively. Monitoring ICP over time provides the most accurate reflection of alterations of ICP in disease states. As exemplified by Lundberg, periodic elevations in ICP (plateau waves) with ensuing return of ICP to normal levels can occur in humans with intracranial disease (Lundberg 1960). These periodic elevations are thought to originate from cerebral vasodilation secondary to decreased cerebral perfusion in patients with intact cerebrovascular autoregulatory capacity (Rosner and Becker 1984). In this situation, single time measurements of ICP may not accurately reveal these episodic elevations, and critical periods of raised ICP will be overlooked.

The configuration of the ICPPW may also change depending upon the level of ICP. With increasing ICP, the P2 component becomes progressively increased in amplitude, with the P1 amplitude changing minimally (Cardoso et al. 1983; German 1988). This ICP increase results in the normal sawtooth-shaped wave becoming rounded and the individual peaks becoming one. The change in the ICPPW may occur prior to clinically significant elevations of absolute ICP and suggests decreasing compliance within the intracranial space.

How Is ICP Measured? Intracranial pressure can be measured from numerous intracranial compartments. Cerebrospinal fluid pressure (CSFP), as a reflection of ICP, can be measured within the ventricles of the brain, at the cerebellomedullary cistern, in the subarachnoid space overlying the brain, or in the lumbar area (cistern in humans). Historically in animals, measurements of CSFP have been taken to infer ICP (Hoerlein 1965; Novak et al. 1974; Parker 1972; Schirmer 1958; Simpson and Reed 1987). Needle puncture and manometer readings have been employed to provide this information, however, this method does not lend itself easily to chronic measurement of ICP. As stated previously, ICP may be dynamic and these fluctuations are important to recognize and objectively measure. Also, to perform needle puncture safely, anesthesia is required in all but the comatose animal. If ventricular obstruction or herniation occurs, the CSF spaces may become compartmentalized. In this situation, depending upon where CSFP is measured, CSFP may also not accurately reflect global ICP. Evidence from humans with unilateral structural brain lesions suggests that the most accurate assessment of ICP occurs when measured ipsilateral to the lesion (Weaver et al. 1982).

When measuring CSFP, intraventricular measurements are the most accurate reflection of ICP. These measurements are most often taken from within the lateral ventricle. Measurements obtained in this way, however, are associated with a higher infectious complication rate in comparison to other less invasive methods (Allen 1986; Aucoin et al. 1986). Also, if the ventricle is obliterated by the disease process, accurate cannulation may be difficult. Epidural, subarachnoid, and subdural screws were developed to avoid entering the brain parenchyma during ICP monitoring, but they have yielded inconsistent and inaccurate results in comparison to intraventricular measurements (Barlow et al. 1985; Ostrup et al. 1987;). Measurement of brain tissue pressure (BTP) is a potential compromise, allowing for accurate measurements of ICP in comparison to intraventricular measurements, but avoiding ventricular catheterization (fig. 2.9) (Brock et al. 1972; Crutchfield 1990; Iannotti 1984; Shores et al. 1991).

Numerous physiological and nonphysiological vari-

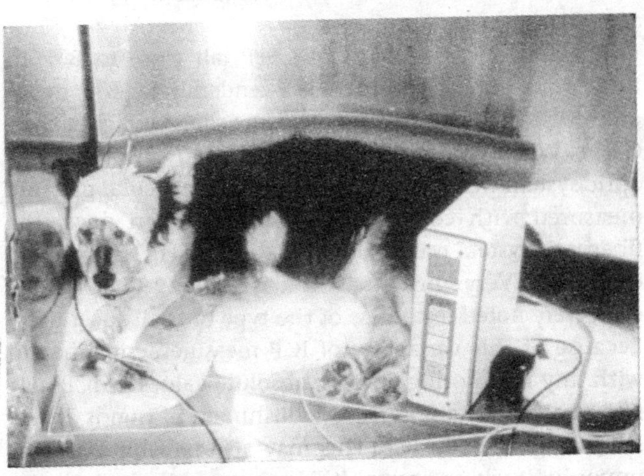

Fig. 2.9. Dog following intracranial surgery with a fiberoptic ICP pressure monitoring system implanted within the cerebral hemisphere.

ables influence ICP measurements. These include anesthetic agents (Cornick 1992; Shores 1985) and body weight (Simpson 1987; Simpson and Reed 1987). The effects of anesthetic agents on ICP are variable, and the need for anesthesia to measure ICP will potentially alter values obtained (Cardoso et al. 1983; German 1988).

Most inhalant anesthetics increase ICP due to their vasodilatory effects on cerebral vessels and resultant increase in cerebral blood flow (Cornick 1992; Shores 1985). Of the commonly used inhalant anesthetics, halothane causes the largest degree of cerebral vasodilation. Increases in cerebral blood flow can increase ICP due to the associated increase in intracranial volume. The ultimate effect on ICP of increased cerebral blood flow depends upon whether cerebral vascular autoregulation is intact.

Body size may also influence measured ICP. Larger dogs, for example, have slightly greater ICPs as compared to smaller dogs (Simpson and Reed 1987).

With these considerations and limitations in mind, ICP values have been determined for clinically normal dogs. In most instances, the ICP values were taken from cerebrospinal fluid pressures measured at the cisterna magna (Hoerlein 1965; Novak 1974; Parker 1972; Schirmer 1958; Simpson 1987; Simpson and Reed 1987). A summary of CSFPs and ICP values for clinically normal dogs is given in (table 2.2). The majority of CSFPs fall between 5 and 12 mm Hg in normal dogs.

To address the need for chronic recording of ICP, a fiberoptic ICP monitoring system (Olm Intracranial Pressure Monitoring System, Camino Laboratories, San Diego, CA; Digital Pressure Monitor, Model 420, Camino Laboratories, San Diego, CA) has been developed for use in humans. This same system has been used for ICP monitoring in dogs and cats. With this system, pressures can be measured from the CSF compartments or the brain tissue (BTP) itself. This system yields accurate measurements chronically in clinical patients and has gained widespread acceptance in clinical practice. The same system has been used by us and others to monitor ICP both experimentally and clinically in dogs and cats (Bagley 1996; Pluhar 1996; Shores et al. 1991).

Previous measurements of CSFP fall close to BTP in these groups, however, there is a tendency for BTP measured with the fiberoptic system to be slightly higher than CSFPs. When BTP measurements obtained with this fiberoptic system were compared with intraventricular pressure measured with conventional transducers in dogs, the fiberoptic system was accurate to +/- 3 mm Hg (Crutchfield et al. 1990). Very similar magnitudes of change in ICP, however, were noted regardless of the type of transducer used. Because of this variability of ICP measurement inherent with any monitoring devices, absolute values of ICP may not be as important as the establishment of trends of persistent increases in ICP. This may also be why a specific upper limit where normal ICP becomes pathologically increased is unclear.

Previous studies have reported the utility of fiberoptic intracranial pressure monitoring in dogs. This fiberoptic

Table 2.2. Brain tissue pressure in normal dogs measured under isoflurane anesthesia with a fiberoptic ICP monitoring system (in mm Hg)

	Mean*	Range
Shores et al. (1991)	9.8	8–13
Keegan et al. (1995)	10.0	8–12
Bagley et al. (1995)	11.0	8–14
Pluhar et al. (1996)	9.6	8–12

Note: Olm Intracranial Pressure Monitoring Kit—Model 110-4B. Camino Laboratories, San Diego, CA; Digital Pressure Monitor, Model 420, Camino Laboratories, San Diego, CA.
*Values rounded to nearest whole number.

ICP monitor has been used for establishing changes in ICP under anesthesia and during intracranial surgery. In animals with isoflurane as a maintenance anesthetic, mean intracranial pressure was found to be approximately 10 mm Hg (range 8–13 mm Hg) (Bagley 1996b). Mean ICP in dogs we have evaluated was slightly higher, but the range of pressures measured was similar. Again, values obtained with this method of ICP monitoring are slightly higher overall in comparison to results from previous studies measuring cerebrospinal fluid pressure via a cisterna magna puncture and manometer readings.

Proper positioning of the fiberoptic transducer can influence the absolute ICP measurements obtained. Placing the tip of the transducer just slightly (~3–5 mm) into the brain parenchyma is attempted. This can be performed by roughly judging, prior to implantation, how far the transducer extends out of the retaining bolt. Usually, prior to encountering brain tissue, recorded measurements remain <5 mm Hg. When brain parenchyma is encountered, a sharp increase in pressure above 5 mm Hg is noted. Ideally, at this time, the ICPPW is present. Black dots on the transducer cable allow for assessment of distance when advancing the cable. If the transducer cable is advanced too far into the brain parenchyma, falsely elevated measurements will be obtained and increased brain damage may occur.

In addition to proper placement of the transducer cable, we have noted in small dogs and cats that screwing the bolt into the skull too far may also falsely elevate ICP measurements. This is because approximately 3 mm of the bolt tip extends beyond the threads of the bolt on the implanted side. To prevent obtaining a falsely elevated ICP, screwing the bolt just far enough into the skull so that it is secure is most desirable.

Obviously, measuring ICP with this system is invasive with the potential for iatrogenic brain damage. When properly placed, however, associated brain damage is usually minimal (Bagley, Baszler, et al. 1995; Bagley, Keegan, et al. 1995). Besides the mechanical damage produced by the cable, focal hemorrhage and edema are seen in the cortex where the cable is implanted.

Information regarding ICP in normal awake dogs is scarce. As well, the objective influence of normal physiological alterations, such as eating, drinking, coughing, and sneezing, on ICP is not established. In our hospital, we have monitored ICP in nonanesthetized animals following brain trauma or surgery. The fiberoptic system seems well suited for this purpose, and few complications have been encountered. However, in animals that are violent, propulsive, or uncoordinated in their movements, the potential exists for the cable and/or bolt to be dislodged. The fiberoptic cable is susceptible to breakage if bent and will subsequently malfunction. The transducer cable can be disconnected from the monitor, without apparent inaccuracy in measurement, for transport of the animal from area to area within the hospital.

Newer, noninvasive techniques for measurement of the cerebral blood flow with Doppler may give an indirect measure of ICP. In humans with increasing ICP, transcranial Doppler ultrasound wave forms showed low, then zero, and finally reversed diastolic blood flow velocities correlated to increasing ICP (Hassler et al. 1988).

What Constitutes Increased ICP? An absolute level wherein ICP is elevated has not been established. This may be the result of the inherent inaccuracies of the monitoring equipment and the variation in baseline ICPs normally. Most importantly, the rapidity with which ICP increases and the subsequent compensatory mechanisms of a patient have the most effect on the clinical ramifications of any ICP increase. Most information from humans suggest that persistent ICP >15–20 mm Hg is pathologically elevated. Cerebral blood flow may not be significantly decreased until ICP reaches ~ 30 mm Hg (Hassler et ai. 1988). Experimentally, however, ICP has been raised to very high levels (>100 mm Hg) before brain death occurred (van Loon et al. 1993). We have seen ICPs as high as 30–40 mm Hg in dogs that subsequently have recovered from brain injury. A large number of similar cases needed to establish treatment and prognosis recommendations, however, is not currently available. In other instances, when ICP is rapidly increased from normal to 25 mm of Hg in experimental models of increased intracranial pressure in dogs, cerebral blood flow can be stopped and actually reversed (Bagley unpublished observations).

Intracranial pressures in dogs with intracranial abnormalities have been reported uncommonly (Bagley et al. 1995). It is noted that not all animals with space-occupying intracranial diseases have associated increases in ICP. In our hospital, dogs and cats with ICPs greater than 15–20 mm Hg are treated and pressures are monitored. In dogs that have recovered from brain injury, ICPs have decreased within the first 24–48 hours. This fact, alone, does not ensure functional recovery in all instances.

Clinical Effects of Intracranial Pressure Alterations. Acute reductions in intracranial volumes, such as may occur with ventriculoperitoneal shunting, CSF leakage, or cerebral dehydration, may result in damage to intracranial vessels and subsequent intracranial hemorrhage (Coulter and Gooch 1993). Vascular structures that traverse between the meninges and the brain are easily torn or disrupted when the brain becomes smaller and the distance between the meninges and the brain increases. This vessel disruption can result in intracranial hemorrhage.

More commonly, clinical abnormalities result from increased ICP. The major intracranial effect of increasing ICP is alteration of cerebral perfusion pressure (CPP), cerebral blood flow, and, ultimately, brain ischemia. Increases in intracranial volume and ICP may also result in shifts of brain tissue termed brain herniation (fig. 2.10, 2.11) (Shapiro 1975). Cerebral perfusion is dependent upon systemic blood flow and intracranial pressure expressed via the formula CPP = MABP - ICP (CPP—cerebral perfusion pressure; MABP—mean arterial blood pressure). For CPP to remain constant, the negative effects of increased ICP on blood

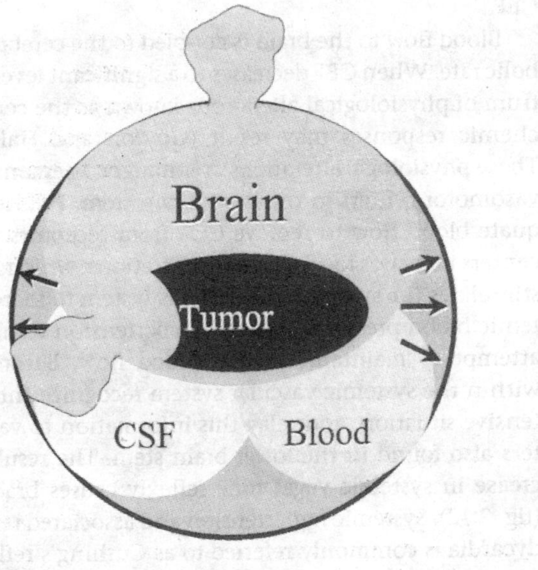

Fig. 2.10. Schematic relationship of important intracranial volume components within the skull associated with a brain herniation.

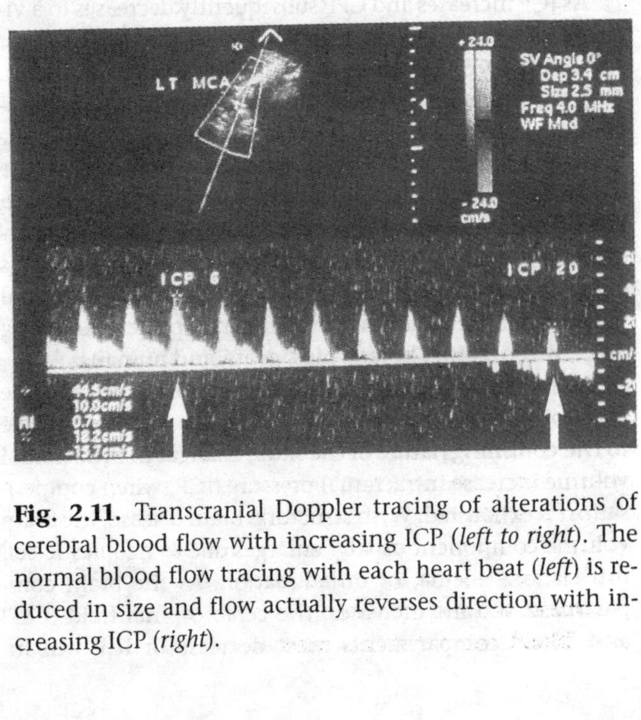

Fig. 2.11. Transcranial Doppler tracing of alterations of cerebral blood flow with increasing ICP (*left to right*). The normal blood flow tracing with each heart beat (*left*) is reduced in size and flow actually reverses direction with increasing ICP (*right*).

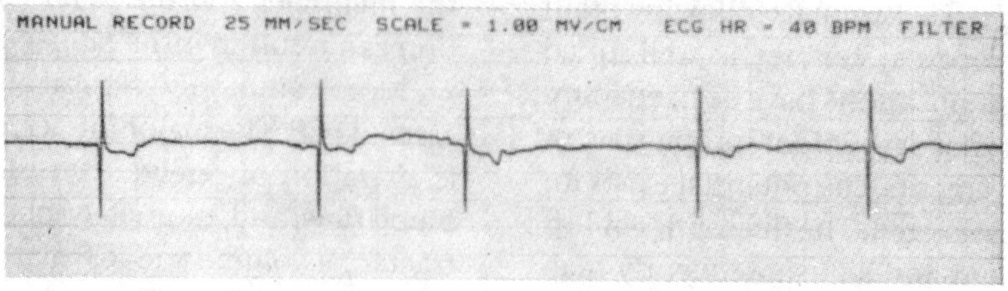

Fig. 2.12. Electrocardiogram from a dog with increased ICP, hypertension, and bradycardia.

flow to the brain must be compensated for by increases in systemic blood pressure. Cerebral perfusion pressure is a determinant of cerebral blood flow but is not always equivalent; in many instances, however, as CPP decreases so does CBF.

Blood flow to the brain is coupled to the cerebral metabolic rate. When CBF decreases to a significant level, a spectrum of physiological alterations known as the cerebral ischemic responses may result (Guyton and Hall 1996). These physiologic alterations are thought to emanate from vasomotor centers in the lower brain stem. Failure of adequate blood flow to remove CO_2 from receptors in these centers increases local CO_2 concentrations, which, in turn, stimulates the sympathetic nervous system to increase systemic blood pressure. Systemic hypertension results as an attempt to maintain cerebral blood flow. Baroreceptors within the systemic vascular system recognize this hypertensive situation, and relay this information to vagal centers also found in the lower brain stem. The resultant increase in systemic vagal tone reflexly causes bradycardia (fig. 2.12). Systemic hypertension and associated reflex bradycardia is commonly referred to as Cushing's reflex. This often explains why many animals with intracranial disease have sinus bradycardia (Guyton and Hall 1996). Increased ICP may also result in pulmonary edema (Pender and Pollack 1993).

As ICP increases and CPP subsequently decreases to a vitally low level, a large catecholamine release occurs (Graf and Rossi 1978; Salvati et al. 1992; van Loon et al. 1993). This catecholamine release may result in myocardial ischemia known as brain-heart syndrome. Clinically, arrhythmias are noted. Focal myocardial ischemia is the pathological lesion, with focal white streaks seen grossly in the myocardium (King et al. 1982). Histologically, myocardial degeneration is common. Brain-heart syndrome has been described with numerous intracranial and spinal pathological lesions and in different species including dogs, sheep, cattle, horses, pigs, goats, and humans.

Intracranial pressure alterations are often responsible for clinical decline in many animals with brain disease. Due to the confining nature of the skull, changes in intracranial volume increase intracranial pressure (ICP) when compensation is exhausted. With structural brain disease, the brain volume component usually enlarges due to neoplastic cell infiltration, edema, or inflammation. As the brain compartment volume increases, the cerebrospinal fluid (CSF) and blood compartments must decrease or ICP will increase. Compensation for increased brain tissue volume initially involves shifting of CSF out of the skull, decreased CSF production, and, eventually, decreased cerebral blood flow.

These compensatory mechanisms prevent increases in ICP for some undetermined period of time. In general, the more slowly the volume increase occurs, the more readily this volume increase is compensated for. When compensatory mechanisms are exhausted, relatively small increases in intracranial volume result in dramatic elevations of ICP. At this time clinical signs become apparent. Initial signs of increased ICP may be nonspecific and limited to alterations in mental status (progression to stupor and coma), cranial nerve dysfunction, and paresis. Unfortunately, clinical signs of increased ICP often become most obvious relatively later in the course of the disease.

Terminal Effects of Compartmentalized ICP Increases: Brain Herniation. As intracranial volume continues to increase beyond the limits of compensation, ICP may increase so precipitously that shifts of brain parenchyma, termed *brain herniation*, will occur (fig. 2.10, 2.13) (Kornegay et al. 1983). If herniation occurs rapidly, coma and severe neurological impairment result. Unfortunately, in many instances, brain herniation becomes a terminal event.

At least five major types of brain herniation have been described: rostral or caudal transtentorial, subfacial or cin-

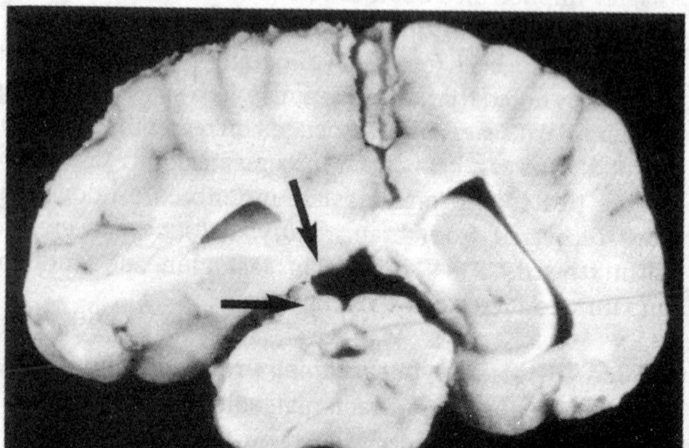

Fig. 2.13. Gross brain specimen from a dog showing unilateral caudal transtentorial brain herniation with resultant compression of the midbrain (*arrows*).

gulate gyrus, foramen magnum, and herniation through a craniotomy defect (Fishman 1975; Kornegay et al. 1983). Of these, caudal transtentorial, subfacial, and foramen magnum occur most commonly. Clinical signs of caudal transtentorial herniation are frequently the result of pressure distributed downward through the midbrain with subsequent compression of the oculomotor nerve (fig. 2.13). With unilateral herniations, an ipsilateral dilated pupil, unresponsive to light stimulation, may be seen. Monitoring for clinical signs of this type of herniation, therefore, should include frequent pupillary evaluations. If unilateral mydriasis is noted in this setting, immediate and aggressive attempts to decrease ICP should be instituted.

Foramen magnum herniation may occur quickly and results in respiratory arrest due to associated pressure on the respiratory centers in the caudal brain stem (fig. 2.14). Foramen magnum herniation is invariably fatal, and surgical attempts at decompression after this type of herniation have not been helpful in affected dogs.

SPINAL CORD PATHOPHYSIOLOGY

Similar to the intracranial structures, the spinal cord may be affected by a variety of disease processes. Degeneration of nervous system elements may result from metabolic derangements of cellular functions. Spinal cord disease may also result from mechanically damaged cellular elements due to diseases that affect spinal cord structural integrity. Most importantly, many diseases that alter spinal cord structure also alter spinal cord blood flow. This results in spinal cord ischemia as common pathophysiologic sequelae to spinal cord compression.

The spinal cord receives blood flow segmentally at multiple levels along the vertebral axis (Fletcher 1993; King 1987). In the cervical area, blood flows to the spinal cord from the heart, brachiocephalic trunk, and left subclavian arteries. From these arteries, blood flows into the vertebral arteries, as well as the dorsal scapular artery, deep cervical artery, and thoracic vertebral artery. The vertebral arteries will supply primarily the C1 to C7 spinal segments. The dorsal scapular artery gives rise to the C8 cervical spinal branch. The deep cervical artery gives rise to the first thoracic spinal branch. The thoracic vertebral artery gives rise to the spinal branches between T2 and T4.

Within the spinal canal, the spinal branch arteries divide into dorsal and ventral branches. The dorsal branch is smaller than the ventral branch. The ventral branch becomes contiguous and forms the ventral spinal artery. This artery is unpaired and is present in the ventral median fissure. The ventral spinal artery extends longitudinally along the ventral aspect of the spinal cord. The ventral spinal artery will give rise to numerous dorsally directed branches, which enter the spinal cord ventral to supply the ventral grey matter and ventral funiculi.

The dorsal branches of the spinal arterial system enter the spinal cord around and often in association with the dorsal nerve roots to supply primarily the dorsal lateral grey and white matter. On the surface of the cord in the pia, there are incomplete anatastomic connects, which may encircle the spinal cord. In some instances, the dorsal lateral arteries can also travel longitudinally along the length of the spinal cord in a dorsal lateral direction. Although this basic pattern occurs in the arterial blood supply to the spinal cord, there is often significant individual variation among these arterial channels. The ventral spinal artery system is more consistent in location and anatomy.

Within a spinal cord segment, the arteries that penetrate into the parenchyma tend to be relatively small and thin walled. While some regions of a spinal segment are supplied by one primary arterial system (ventral or dorsal), other regions of the spinal cord are in an overlapping zone, being supplied partially by both arterial systems. These areas of arterial overlap may be more susceptible to ischemic changes and subsequent spinal damage.

Experimentally induced spinal cord injury has provided a significant proportion of the data regarding basic patho-

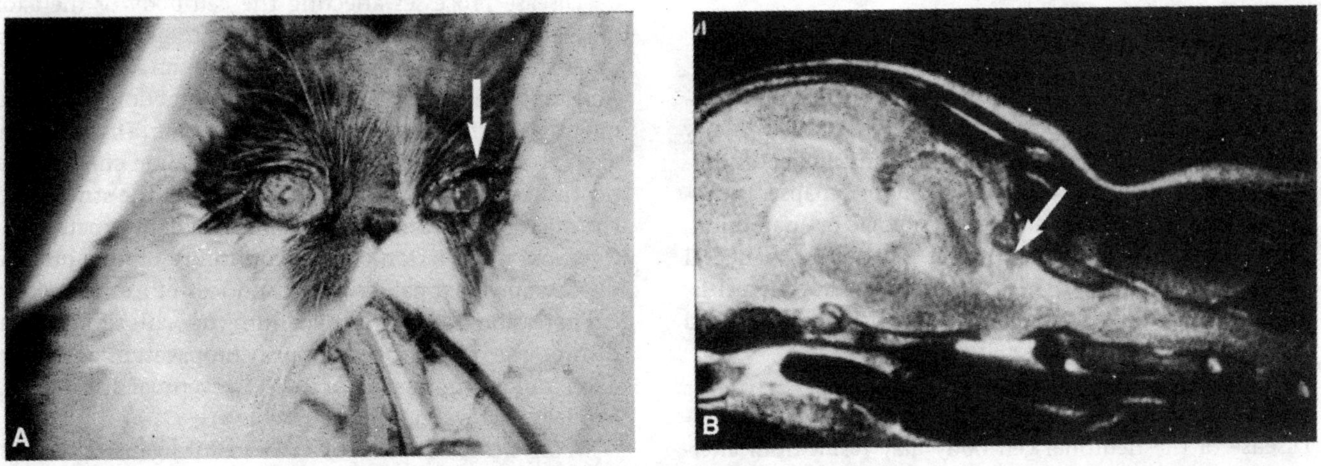

Fig. 2.14. (A) Photo of a cat with anisocoria (*arrow*). This cat had both a caudal transtentorial brain herniation and a foramen magnum herniation. (B) Sagittal, proton-density MR image from this cat showing herniation of the cerebellum into the foramen magnum (*arrow*).

physiologic alterations in the diseased spinal cord. The pathophysiologic changes that occur in the spinal cord have been extensively reviewed (Berg and Rucker 1985; Janssens 1991; Braund et al. 1990; Rucker 1990; Brown and Hall 1992; Quencer and Bunge 1996; Turner 1987). Spontaneous spinal cord injury and other forms of spinal cord disease may result in similar or slightly different pathological processes depending upon the disease present.

Briefly, when the spinal cord is injured due to an external impact, two major consequences result (i.e., the primary mechanical injury and its resultant pathophysiologic sequelae, or the "secondary injury"). The primary injury usually includes shearing and disruption of axonal processes, nerve cell bodies, and supporting structures such as glial cells and vascular elements resulting in physiologic or morphologic disruption of nervous impulses. Any change in the vertebral canal diameter may cause spinal cord displacement and compression, and increases in intraspinal pressure. Nervous impulses in this area may be disrupted due to increasing pressure applied to the axons and nerves or from ischemia due to alteration in spinal cord blood flow or hemorrhage. These pressure increases set in motion numerous pathophysiological consequences including ischemia, further hemorrhage, and edema. Because the grey matter normally receives proportionally higher blood flow compared to white matter, ischemic-related damage is often seen here first. Central hemorrhagic necrosis is the pathological consequence. All of these events lead to a self-perpetuating process of damage to the spinal cord that often is equally, if not more, detrimental to the spinal cord than the initial mechanical injury (second injury theory). Putative mediators of this self-perpetuating process include excitatory neurotransmitters, endorphins, catecholamines, lipid peroxidation, and free radicals released after the initial insult.

Other spinal cord diseases may result from primary degeneration of neural or supporting cell elements. The pathophysiology of these disease processes are discussed in chapter 6.

PERIPHERAL NERVE PATHOPHYSIOLOGY

Disease processes affecting the peripheral nerves and associated cell bodies can be varied (Summers et al. 1995). Many of these diseases, however, result in a finite number of alterations in the neuronal cell body, axon, or synapse. Pathophysiologic alterations may be physiologic or anatomical. The ultimate consequence, however, is disruption of neural impulse generation or destruction of neural elements. Specific peripheral nerve, neuromuscular junction, and muscle diseases are discussed in chapter 7.

Disease of the Neuron

Disease of the neuronal cell body may result from alterations in structural components (such as DNA and other proteins), failure of energy for metabolic processes (such as from ischemia or hypoxia), disruption of axons and synaptic connections, programmed cell death, accumulation of metabolic by-products (i.e., storage diseases), or due to "lack of a vital substance" for survival (abiotrophies) (Summers et al. 1995). Disease of the cell body is referred to as a neuronopathy. If the neuronal cell is a motor nerve cell, then these diseases are often referred to as "motor neuron" diseases. These same basic pathophysiologic processes may also affect neurons within the brain or spinal cord.

Disease of the Axon

The axon is an extension of the cell body that serves to form a connection with other nerve elements or muscle cells. Along the axon a neural impulse is propagated to eventually depolarize the synapse. Many axons are surrounded by a myelin sheath. The myelin sheath serves to increase the speed of propagation of a neuronal impulse. Disease affecting the axon or the myelin sheath may alter or delay the conduction of a neural impulse along these structures leading to inappropriate synaptic depolarization and subsequent ineffectual neurologic function.

The axon contains structural elements known as neurofilaments and microtubules. These elements serve as a scaffolding along the axon. They are produced in the cytoplasm of the neuronal cell from proteins and other molecules. These structures are also important in the transport of neurotransmitters and other vital substances from the cell body to the terminal axon (bouton) at the synapse or neuromuscular junction. Even within the axon there is a "flow" of structural elements, referred to as axonal transport. This transport can occur toward (anterograde) or away (retrograde) from the synapse. This system of axonal structure and transport is conceptually similar to wooden logs being transported by floating in a river. The logs (tubules and filaments) are cut in the forest (the cell body), placed in the river (the axon), and transported down river to the sawmill (the synapse). A person may jump on one of the logs and ride on the log down river. Similarly, a neurotransmitter can be produced in the cell body, attached to a filament, and transported to the terminal bouton for storage or release during depolarization of the terminal axon.

Disease processes affecting the cell body or the axon may affect the production and structure of the microtubules and neurofilaments necessary for the axon function. Abnormalities of axon structure and function can subsequently affect action potential propagation. Disease of the axon is referred to as an axonopathy. Some chemotherapeutic agents (e.g., vincristine) may affect the structure of the microtubules and therefore affect axonal structure and function. A laceration of the axon can result in a physical disruption of axonal structure and loss of axon function. Compression of the axon, depending upon its severity, may disrupt the physiologic impulse propagation along the axon (mild compression) or result in eventual disruption of axonal structure (severe compression).

A physical disruption of an axon during disruption will result in morphologic alterations in the axon as well as the neuronal cell body. This alteration is referred to as Wallerian degeneration. In essence, these alterations are a result of the physical disruption of the axon and the attempt of the neuron to regenerate its axon. Following transection of the axon, the axon distal to the laceration will degenerate. The axon slightly proximal to the laceration will also degenerate. This axon proximal to this damaged region may enlarge. Dilated axons proximal to an area of axonal damage when viewed microscopically in cross section are referred to as spheroids. Eventually multiple sprouts (collaterals of the axon) will develop from the distal axonal area in an attempt at axonal regeneration. These axonal collaterals elongate in an attempt to find the outer layers (basal lamina) of the distal degenerated axon.

Concurrent with these changes in the axon, there are alterations in the neuronal cell body, also as a reflection of the cell's attempts at regeneration of the axon (Summers et al. 1995). The nucleus may become eccentrically placed within the cytoplasm, often away from the axon. The ribosomal structures in the cytoplasm (Nissl substance) can be condensed and become located in specific areas of the cytoplasm. Often, the Nissl substance will be displaced toward the periphery of the cytoplasm. As Nissl substance has a more dark-staining appearance compared to the cell cytoplasm when viewed under a light microscope, the condensation of the Nissl substance results in a "clearing" of the more central regions of the cytoplasm. This appearance is referred to as central chromatolysis. In rarer instances the Nissl substance becomes condensed centrally, resulting in peripheral chromatolysis. The constellation of morphologic alterations in the cell body and axon may also be referred to as the "axon reaction."

Similar changes can occur in an axon and associated cell body when the axon is damaged by disease. If the axonal disease is severe enough, the axonal structure may be disrupted. Again, as a component of regeneration, alterations can occur in cell body and axon as described previously with Wallerian degeneration. As the term "Wallerian degeneration" is often reserved to describe only those changes induced by a physical cutting of the axon, the term "Wallerian-type or Wallerian-like" degeneration is used.

Independently, or concurrently, disease or damage to the myelin may affect the speed of neural impulse propagation along the axon. As myelin encircles the axon, damage to the axon resulting in disintegration of the axon structure will also result in disruption of myelin. Myelin can also be damaged independently of the axon. This is referred to as demyelination and can result from acquired diseases that affect myelin or result from compression of the axon. In some diseases, myelin is not produced adequately or effectively (i.e., hypomyelination and dysmyelination).

Trauma (and by extension, disease) of a nerve can also be categorized in a combination of anatomical disruption and functional consequences. A *neuropraxia* is a physiologic interruption in function and conduction in the nerve, usually associated with a lesion of the myelin without severe axonal involvement or a functional axonal alteration. Neuropraxia is the least severe of the types of nerve damage or dysfunction, which also usually equates to the greatest likelihood of reversal and clinical improvement. *Axonotmesis* suggests separation and damage of some axons. Again, this usually occurs through mechanical disruption, but may also result from diseases of the axon. Some regeneration of axons may occur, so this type of injury may be somewhat reversible. Improvement in function will depend upon the magnitude of the axon loss (i.e., percentage of axonal damage) and the degree and extent of regeneration. *Neurotmesis* is complete severance of all structures of the nerve and is the most severe form of injury. The likelihood of regeneration is less with neurotmesis as compared to neuropraxia or axonotmesis.

Unfortunately, it is not always possible to determine the morphologic extent of the damage to neuronal elements, and therefore, the likelihood of axonal regeneration. Additionally, axonal regeneration is more likely with peripheral nerve injury compared to central axonal injury.

Disease of the Synapse or Neuromuscular Junction

The synaptic connection may also be primarily affected with disease. If the synapse is of an axon on a muscle cell, this is referred to as the *neuromuscular junction.*

The presynaptic terminals are frequently called *boutons.* Presynaptic terminals have synaptic vesicles (which contain the neurotransmitter substance) and mitochondria (which provide ATP to produce more transmitters). When an action potential reaches the presynaptic terminal, the membrane depolarization causes release of the neurotransmitters from the presynaptic vesicles. This release is dependent on calcium ions that enter the terminal. Obviously, if the terminal axon disintegrates, the synapse will as well. Disease may also affect the presynaptic release of neurotransmitters, and consequently prevent activation of the synapse, preventing activation of the effector organ or muscle.

At the postsynaptic receptor, there exists a large number of receptor proteins. These receptor proteins have two important components, a binding protein and an ionophore. The ionophore is either a chemically activated ion channel or an enzyme that activates the internal metabolic system of the cell. The chemically activated channels are either Na, K, or Cl channels. Depending on which of these channels is opened, the impulse can be excitatory (if Na channels are opened) or inhibitory (if K or Cl channels are opened).

If disease alters or prevents neurotransmitter binding, affects neurotransmitter production, release, or degradation, or alters the structure or function of the postsynaptic receptors, the effector organ will not be activated. Clinical dysfunction will result. Some disease processes such as botulism and tick paralysis prevent the release of neurotransmitter from the presynaptic region of the neuromuscular junction. Other diseases such as myasthenia gravis affect the postsynaptic structures and receptors, preventing neurotransmitter binding, and subsequent lack of postsynaptic depolarization. Still other processes such as organophosphate intoxication alter the breakdown and metabolism of neurotransmitters within the synaptic cleft.

Disease of Functional Systems

On a grander scale, these basic pathophysiologic alterations occurring in single neuronal elements can be mirrored in multiple neurons and axons. As with most systems, there is a degree of disease or injury that will not result in clinical dysfunction. This is most likely a reflection of the redundancy of functional elements in a neuronal system. Damage or disease to a single axon is clinically inconsequential. Damage or disease to a certain proportion of neural elements (a threshold) results in clinically recognizable dysfunction. Intuitively, the degree of neuronal element dysfunction will correlate with the degree of clinical dysfunction.

3 Clinical Examination of the Animal with Suspected Neurologic Disease

Insufficient examination and inaccurate observations are more common causes of incorrect diagnoses than false conclusions from correct and sufficient facts.

—R. N. DeJong (paraphrase)

Clinical examination is the foundation of good medical practice. A thorough clinical evaluation is most likely to yield accurate and appropriate clinical information. Clinical clues are the foundation of clinical intuition and diagnostic acumen. Adopting a stereotypic approach to clinical assessment ensures that critical observations are not missed during the evaluation process.

The neurologic examination process is arguably the epitome of clinical examination. The process of clinical neurologic assessment involves collection of data regarding normal as well as abnormal function. In general, the steps followed during evaluation of animals with neurologic disease include:

- Determination and clarification of the presenting problem (the *chief complaint*). Why is the animal here?
- Determination of the temporal course of the problem (*historical perspective*). When did the problem start? Is the problem getting better, worse, or staying the same?
- Performance of a physical (*neurological examination*) and assessment of physical clues
- Determination of which portion of the nervous system is involved with the disease. This is arguably the most important aspect of clinical neurologic evaluation and is often referred to as the *neuroanatomical diagnosis.*
- Establishment of a list of diseases that can affect or cause disease in the particular area of the nervous system in question. This is often referred to as the *differential diagnosis.*
- Determination of which diagnostic test will establish if the disease is present and its extent. This is the *diagnostic testing* portion of clinical evaluation.
- Establishment of a *treatment* plan for this disease
- Providing the owner a realistic idea as to what to expect in the future (the *prognosis*)

THE PURPOSE OF THE NEUROLOGIC EXAMINATION

Information collected during the neurologic examination is used for two main purposes:

1. To determine if abnormalities exist in neurologic function
2. To determine the location of the abnormalities within the nervous system

Through examination and assessment of functions controlled by the nervous system, clues to the presence and location of disease within the nervous system are found. As the nervous system is a part of the entire body, the neurologic examination is an extension of a complete physical examination. It is important to perform a complete physical examination in addition to any specialty assessment to avoid overlooking important abnormalities that might ultimately lead to the clarification of the disease process.

NEUROLOGICAL EXAMINATION

Observing, touching, and manipulating the animal are paramount in determining the presence, location, and extent of any disease process. Patient examination identifies functional and anatomical abnormalities associated with disease. The significance of abnormalities identified by subsequent diagnostic testing can be determined only by an understanding of the associated clinical signs found in the animal. Many clinically detectable neurologic abnormalities are indicative of dysfunction of specific functional components within the nervous system. Clinical signs resulting from dysfunction of the nervous system, however, are rarely pathognomonic for a specific disease process. Instead, clinical neurologic abnormalities reflect the location of involvement of the nervous system with disease.

The neurologic examination process should be used to assess important functional components or subdivisions of the nervous system. The various components of the examination are used to determine the functional capabilities of specific components of the nervous system. The complete neurological examination commonly contains an evaluation of the following main assessments:

- Consciousness and awareness
- Involuntary movements
- Posture
- Gait
- Conscious proprioception (knowledge of where the limbs are in the environment)
- Spinal and other reflexes
- Cranial nerve assessment
- Special functions such as urination, eating, drinking, and respiration
- Pain and sensation

Some neurologic assessments are determined through owner questioning, some are observational assessments, and still others require a "hands-on" approach, wherein the animal is palpated and manipulated. Surprisingly, a significant amount of information can be collected relatively quickly by simply observing how the animal is postured, reacts in the environment, moves, and walks. In some instances, observation of specific movements or postures is extremely helpful in determining where abnormalities exist within the nervous system.

Astute clinicians will mentally prepare for clinical evaluation by anticipating abnormalities that may be found during the examination process. If, for example, an animal is presented with a specific abnormality, a mental review prior to the physical examination of pathophysiologic processes that can result in the particular presenting abnormality may help in focusing the clinician's attention on necessary physical assessments to determine the degree and extent of the abnormality. As an example, an animal is being presented for inability to stand in the pelvic limbs. A mental review of general body systems that, when affected with disease, could result in pelvic limb movement abnormalities might include the musculoskeletal, neurologic, cardiovascular, and metabolic systems of the body. This preevaluation mental assessment might help to focus physical evaluations on critical assessment of these body systems. Obvious clinical findings, such as the lack of a pulse in a limb, are less likely, therefore, to be overlooked.

Signalment, History, and Chief Complaint

Basic patient characteristics (age, breed, gender) are usually gathered prior to physical assessments, except in some emergency situations. As many diseases are breed associated, the signalment may provide a fundamental clue to the etiology of the disease (Braund 1994; Kornegay 1986; Oliver et al. 1997; Wheeler 1989) (appendix 2). The age of the animal at the onset of clinical signs is helpful, as some diseases, such as inherited or congenital defects, affect younger animals whereas others, such as brain neoplasms, generally affect older animals. A few diseases occur specifically in one gender of animal.

Chief Complaint and History

Historical information is obtained through communication with the owner and review of historical records of the patient. An appropriate historical review is adapted to the particular clinical situation. Commonly, historical information includes a general history of systemic health and prophylactic care (vaccination). With regard to the nervous system, questions should be asked to assess the *owner's concern* or *chief complaint,* the *duration,* and the clinical *course* (progressive, unchanged, improving) of the problem.

It is always important to determine why the owner has presented the animal for evaluation. Initially, the owners are asked to describe what abnormality they are concerned about. Unfortunately, owners' descriptions of clinical problems can be misleading. The accuracy of an owner's observation is dependent upon how knowledgeable the owner is regarding medical abnormalities, how familiar the owner is with normal animal behavior and movement, and how astute he or she is in previous observation of the animal. In some instances, the clinical abnormalities found by the clinician may be different from those that the owner has concerns about. Addressing the reason that caused the owners to present the animal for evaluation is important for client relations and overall client satisfaction, however, assessment for all clinically significant problems is important for successful clinical outcomes.

Clarification of the *temporal course* of the presenting complaint is invaluable, but is also sometimes difficult due to inaccuracies of owner interpretation of signs. It is a common trait of human beings, once a clinical problem is identified, to go back and mentally search the past for causes, factors, or events that may have contributed to the abnormality. For example, many animals are presented for evaluation of abnormalities in walking. In some cases, the animal may have historically fallen, which focused the owner's attention toward the walking problem. However, it is also plausible that the animal had dysfunctional limbs prior to falling, but that this dysfunction was unrecognized. Possibly the clinical problem was the cause of or was exacerbated by the falling episode. It is important for the clinician to keep an open mind and guard against being too trusting of historical accounts as nonscientific observations may be subject to inaccuracies. Some of the best clinicians are *always skeptical* of apparently obvious facts.

When verbally communicating with owners, it is important to ask questions that are not inherently biased, leading, ambiguous, or intimidating. Open-ended questions such as "what did you see" or "what did your animal do" are helpful, as they allow the owner the opportunity to describe abnormalities and events in their own words. For example, evaluation of seizure disorders often requires an accurate historical record of the activity of the animal. Many owners have heard the word "seizure" at some point in their lives, and have a preconceived idea of what a seizure is. Unfortunately, owners' understanding of a seizure may be vastly different from an educated medical professional's definition. For many, a "seizure" is taken to mean any event wherein an animal acts strangely episodically or intermittently. Falling down from a heart problem (e.g., syncope), a behavior abnormality, painful episodes, and even getting stung by a bee might fit into the owner's determination of a "seizure." Asking the owner to describe what the animal did before during, and after the seizure might allow the clinician to more accurately determine if the event was, in fact, a true seizure or some other episodic disturbance.

Historical questions will need to be adapted for each individual animal's situation to clarify the presenting problem (table 3.1). Specific questions (i.e., was the animal exposed to toxic substances or has similar disease been observed in genetically associated animals, siblings, offspring, or housemates) are asked depending upon the presenting complaint.

Table 3.1. Common historical questions

General history questions:
Coughing? Sneezing? Vomiting? Diarrhea?
PU/PD/PP? Water consumption? Food Consumption?
Vaccinations? When and What?
Heartworm tested (Dog)? FeLV/FIV tested (Cat)?
Travel history?
Current medications? History of drug reaction?
Disease in parents, siblings, offspring, others in the environment?
Toxin exposure?
Specific historical questions directed toward the nervous dysfunction:
Chief complaint?
Clinical signs getting better, worse, or staying the same?
Behavior or personality change?
Any relation of clinical signs to eating?
Worse with exercise?
Crying or vocalizing as if in pain?

Physical Examination

As the nervous system is integrated with virtually all other systems within the body, disease of multiple body systems may adversely affect the nervous system. Therefore, a complete physical examination is a must prior to the neurological assessment. Body system abnormalities that are commonly confused for neurologic abnormalities include abnormalities of the visual, cardiovascular, pulmonary, musculoskeletal, and metabolic systems.

Information Gathered Through Observation of the Animal

What does the examiner observe about the animal when viewing the animal from a distance? Astute and accurate observation is one of the most important of all clinical skills during physical and neurologic assessments. The way an animal moves, acts, or looks often provides important clues to the location and type of clinical dysfunction.

Subjective Assessments

A subjective evaluation (what does the examiner observe about the animal when viewing the animal from a distance?) can be made concurrently with collection of the history as well as throughout all phases of the clinical examination. As nervous system dysfunction is often reflected in abnormalities of movement, it is helpful to allow the animal to move freely around the examination room while watching for movement traits and characteristics. An obvious exception to allowing the animal to move freely would apply to the animal that may have a traumatic vertebral fracture or subluxation or is dangerous to itself, the owner, or the health care team such as by being unduly aggressive. In the former instance, the animal should be physically immobilized (i.e., taping to a rigid surface such as a spinal backboard) as soon as possible, as acutely traumatized animals may have an unstable vertebral segment that could worsen and result in further deterioration of clinical signs with manipulation. Neurological examination will have to be altered to accommodate immobilization in traumatized animals (see chapter 22).

As the veterinary hospital often contains many new and different sights and smells, most animals presented for clinical examination are at least somewhat apprehensive in this environment. These animals should remain alert and orient themselves to obvious environmental visual, sound, smell, or touch stimuli. Owner questioning is often necessary to clarify the personality of the individual animal and obtain information concerning how the animal has acted in similar environments in the past. Owner comments such as, "He's much more quiet (depressed) than he usually is" or "He's always this scared when he comes to the veterinarian" are often very helpful for making a subjective assessment of the animal's overall awareness of various environmental stimuli.

Abnormal postures and movement disorders are usually observed during this portion of the examination. Examples of these types of abnormalities include head tilting, head turning, falling, wandering, circling, limping, or vocalizing as if painful.

As an example, a tendency to propulsively walk in a circular direction (i.e., circling) may be seen in animals with disease involving either the supratentorial or vestibular areas of the nervous system. Usually, but not always, the animal circles toward the side of a unilateral supratentorial lesion or vestibular disease lesion. Animals with vestibular disease tend to circle in tighter, smaller circles as compared to the wider circling seen with supratentorial lesions. Circling, in this latter instance, may be a component of the adversive syndrome (deLahunta 1983). Some animals with behavior disorders or pain may also circle in an attempt to constantly orient themselves to a particular body area such as the tail. Subjective observations help in the determination of whether an abnormality exists of nervous system function. Correlation of the specific functional abnormality with the neuroanatomical structures responsible for the particular function aids in determination of the location of the dysfunction within the nervous system. Specific abnormalities and their significance are discussed later in this chapter.

ABNORMALITIES OF MENTAL AWARENESS, CONSCIOUSNESS, AND BEHAVIOR

Clinical signs of alterations in consciousness and behavior range from subtle (e.g., an animal that is just less active than normal) to severe (e.g., comatose and unable to respond to any external stimuli) (Chrisman 1991; deLahunta 1983; Oliver et al. 1987; Oliver et al. 1997). The "normal" state of an animal's consciousness is dynamic and is dependent on a complex interaction between stimuli and response, which varies from individual to individual and, in some cases, from moment to moment. Most importantly, it is virtually impossible for a clinician to determine what an animal "thinks." Clinical assessments of consciousness, therefore, are often crudely categorized into general groups of responses (table 3.2).

An animal is assessed as alert if it responds to a given stimulus as would the majority of other normal animals interacting with the same stimulus in the same environment. Normal animals are alert and acutely aware of changes in their environment. They orient themselves to alterations in activity, sound, and light. Unless the clinician is very familiar with the animal's normal personality and response to a range of environmental stimuli, subtle abnormalities of consciousness are more difficult to determine. It is often only through owner questioning to establish the "normal" personality of the animal that subtle alterations of consciousness are elucidated.

Terms used for the state of inappropriate mental function between alert (normal) and severe impairment (stupor or coma) are not well agreed upon in veterinary medicine. Terms such as "depressed" (lowering or decrease of functional activity), "obtund(ed)" (dull or blunt), "dementia" (organic loss of intellectual function), and "delirium" (mental disturbance marked by illusions, hallucinations, cerebral excitement, physical restlessness, and incoherence) have been used to describe the condition of being mentally abnormal, yet at least partially aware and responsive.

Animals with severe abnormalities of consciousness may not be as physically mobile, tend to stay in one location, may sleep more than normal, and may be less responsive to external stimuli such as light, touch, and sound. These animals may not eat and drink normally. Stuporous animals tend to remain in a sternal or lateral recumbent position and are relatively unresponsive to environmental stimulation. These animals still react to painful stimuli. Comatose animals are similarly unresponsive to environmental stimuli, however, these animals do not react even to painful stimuli. Abnormalities of cranial nerve functions and pupil reactivity, posture, and proprioception may also be present with intracranial derangements. Decerebrate rigidity, wherein the animal has opisthotonus, extensor rigidity of all limbs, and either stupor or coma is present with severe midbrain lesions.

Some animals with alterations of consciousness and awareness may *head press.* Head pressing is the term used to describe a situation where animals stand and push the dorsal aspects of their head or nose against a wall or other stationary object (fig. 3.1). This behavior suggests a deficiency of awareness and cognition.

Episodic or short-term loss of consciousness with periods of normal consciousness in between may be found with *narcolepsy, syncope,* and *seizure.* Narcolepsy (excessive daytime sleepiness) is an episodic disorder that results in rapid progression to deep sleep, usually following some triggering stimulus such as eating. Syncope is a short, episodic loss of consciousness that results from transient cerebral hypoxia or anoxia. Syncopal episodes may mimic a seizure or narcoleptic/cataplexic event. If hypoxia is prolonged, actual seizure may result and confound the clinical interpretation. Syncope is most often the result of a cardiopulmonary disorder (usually a bradyarrhythmia) and, therefore, attention should be given to the cardiopulmonary systems during the routine physical examination (Adams and Victor 1993).

Diseases that affect a variety of nonneural body systems resulting in systemic metabolic derangements can secondarily alter the function of the intracranial nervous system and result in impairment of consciousness. With metabolic diseases, overt neurologic examination deficits other than alterations in awareness may not be present. If clinical ex-

Table 3.2. Mental status categories of animals

Alert	Normal
Inappropriate	• Quiet, unwilling to perform normally but responsive to environmental stimuli • Responsive to environmental stimuli, but responses are not normal
Stuporous	• Remains unresponsive to environmental stimulation but responsive to painful sensation
Comatose	• Nonresponsive to either environmental or painful stimulation

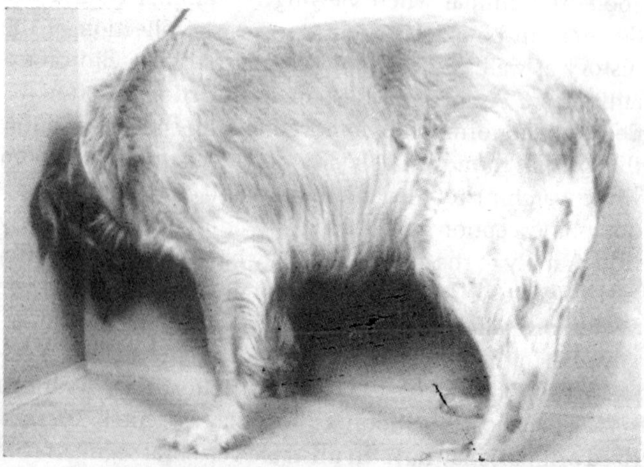

Fig. 3.1. Dog shown head pressing in a corner.

amination abnormalities do result from metabolic dysfunction, the neurologic deficits present in the animal are often symmetrical. It is also possible that a metabolic process can secondarily result in edema or hemorrhage in the brain, which results in anatomical alteration of brain structure and subsequent focal neurologic examination abnormalities. Increases in intracranial pressure or poor cerebrovascular perfusion may result in decreases in consciousness and awareness (see chapter 2).

Severely altered consciousness usually indicates significant central nervous system dysfunction and constitutes an emergency evaluation. As metabolic derangements from numerous nonneurologic causes may alter consciousness to this degree, a complete systemic as well as neurological evaluation is imperative in these instances.

BEHAVIOR

Not only the presence of consciousness, but also the quality of the consciousness is important. The quality of consciousness is essentially the ability to behave normally (Parker 1990). Normal behavior is commonly determined for a population of animals, but is also dependent on individual patient characteristics. Alterations in behavior may include aggression; vocalization; excessive or abnormal sexual activity; changes in eating, chewing, drinking, urinating, defecating; as well as changes in personality. Frenzied activity (excessive compulsive?) and repeated unusual behavior such as tail chasing or fly biting might also occur. Changes in behavior in relation to stimulating events, such as increases in abnormal behavior after eating in animals with hepatic encephalopathy, may also be important clues to an underlying metabolic disease process.

Primary behavioral abnormalities can be difficult to differentiate from those alterations in behavior associated with abnormalities of cognition. In general, clues to an underlying behavior problem may be suggested by whether the abnormality occurs when the owner (audience) is not present, if the animal's movements can be interrupted, and whether the abnormality occurs at a consistent time during the day or in response to a consistent stimulus or context (i.e., the owner's leaving or coming home). Animals whose episodic behavioral abnormality occurs only in the presence of the owner or an audience, who can be interrupted from the activity, who have the abnormality only in response to a specific stimulus, and who are otherwise normal when the behavior is interrupted are more likely to have a primary behavioral problem.

Narcolepsy/Cataplexy

Narcolepsy (excessive daytime sleepiness) and cataplexy (periods of acute muscular hypotonia) are episodic disorders that may mimic syncope and seizure. An abnormal sleep/awake cycle is operant. Normal sleep appears to be controlled by areas within the reticular formation of the brain stem. There are two phases of sleep. Initial sleep is non-REM (rapid eye movement) sleep. Rapid eye movement sleep begins approximately 20 minutes after initiation of non-REM sleep. This is characterized by relaxation of the neck and back muscles and irregular respiration. Flurries of movement occur phasically. During REM sleep, the brain is highly active, however, most motor activity associated with this period is inhibited from dorsal pontine tegmental areas. Other areas within the CNS such as the cortex, cerebellum, and spinal cord may also contribute to this inhibition. REM sleep lasts approximately 10 minutes. Dogs, but usually not cats, may have paddling movements of the limbs, possibly mimicking seizure activity.

Acute onset of REM sleep, usually occurring with stimulation such as eating, is characteristic of narcolepsy. Disordered neurotransmitter metabolism or abnormalities of the reticular activating system are thought to be responsible, however, a true cause is not known. The actual anatomic or physiologic abnormality may lie within the brain stem ascending reticular activating system (ARAS), however, clinical signs usually reflect a diffuse cerebral disturbance.

Some breeds of dogs are predisposed to narcolepsy including Doberman pinschers, Labrador retrievers, miniature poodles, dachshunds, beagles and Saint Bernards. Clinical signs usually begin at a young age, however, dogs as old as 7 years have been diagnosed with this disorder.

Other types of sleep disorders are rarely seen (Hendricks and Morrison 1981). Violent movements that occur during sleep disorders may be mistaken for seizure activity.

Syncope

Syncope is a short, episodic loss of consciousness that results from transient cerebral hypoxia or anoxia. Usually animals will collapse sternally and be unable to stand for relatively short periods of time. Syncopal episodes may mimic a seizure or narcoleptic/cataplexic event. If cerebral hypoxia is prolonged, actual seizure may result and confound the clinical interpretation. Syncope is most often the result of a cardiopulmonary disorder (usually a bradyarrhythmia) and, therefore, attention should be paid to the cardiopulmonary systems during the routine physical examination.

ABNORMALITIES OF POSTURE AND BODY POSITION AT REST

Posture is evaluated at rest and as the animal is placed in abnormal positions throughout the examination. Postural abnormalities offer important clues to neurologic dysfunction.

Abnormalities of Head Posture

A *head tilt* is an abnormal posture wherein one ear is deviated more ventrally than the opposite (figs. 3.2, 3.3). For reference, when the animal is viewed from the front, an imaginary line can be drawn from one side of the head to the other along the horizon. A second imaginary line can be drawn perpendicular to this horizontal line that transects through the philtrum of the nose. In normal animals, these imaginary lines will form a 90° angle. In animals with a head tilt, the imaginary line drawn through the philtrum will form an acute angle less than 90° (fig. 3.3).

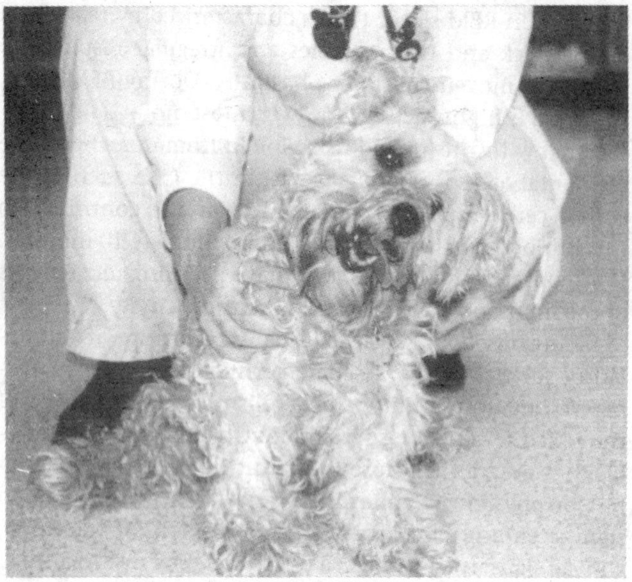

Fig. 3.2. Dog with a head tilt to the left side.

When severe, the animal may be rolled on the dorsal aspect of its body. In some cases, the animal may continually fall and roll.

Head tilting is most often associated with disease of the vestibular or cerebellar systems. The head tilt is usually directed toward the side of the lesion in the nervous system especially if the lesion involves the peripheral vestibular apparatus. Occasionally, with lesions involving the caudal cerebellar peduncle between the brain stem and cerebellum or flocculonodular lobe of the cerebellum, the head tilt is directed away from the side of the lesion, the so-called paradoxical vestibular syndrome (Holliday 1979/1980; deLahunta 1983).

The cerebellum will send inhibitory efferent connections through the caudal cerebellar peduncle to the ipsilateral vestibular nuclei. If there is a lack of inhibition to the vestibular nuclei on the same side as the cerebellar lesion, then the vestibular nuclei will be disinhibited and, through a similar mechanism discussed above, result in facilitation of the extensors on the ipsilateral side and facilitation of the contralateral flexors (Thomas 2000). Therefore, the body will lead away from the side of the lesion and the head tilt will be in the opposite direction, as well.

A *head turn* is where the nose remains parallel to the horizon, however, the nose is directed toward the flank or caudal aspect of the body (fig. 3.4). This has sometimes been referred to as a "yaw" (Oliver et al. 1997). This posture may be a component of the adversive syndrome, which consists of a head turn (sagittal axis of head perpendicular to the ground) and circling (deLahunta 1983). The animal may also intermittently orient the head laterally or toward the caudal aspect of the body.

A head turn occurs most often with supratentorial lesions. The head turn and circling are usually toward the side of the lesion. A similar abnormality, termed "hemi-inattention" or "hemi-neglect," may be seen wherein the animal will only eat from one side of its food bowl (Holliday 1991; O'Brien 1993). In some situations of lesions of the (caudal) brain stem or cervical region, the head may be turned to be positioned tightly against the neck or trunk.

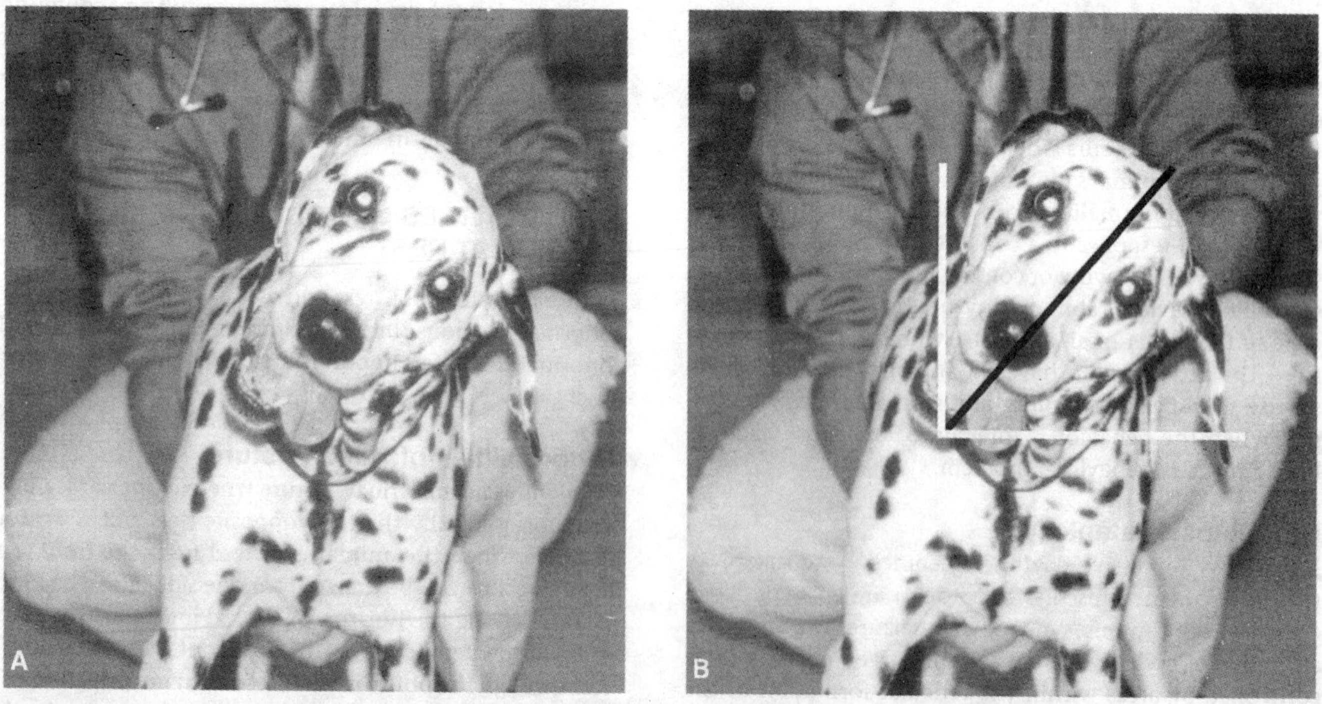

Fig. 3.3. (A) Dog with a head tilt to the left side showing the angulation of the head. (B) The same dog is shown with imaginary lines drawn to represent the degree of tilt from midline.

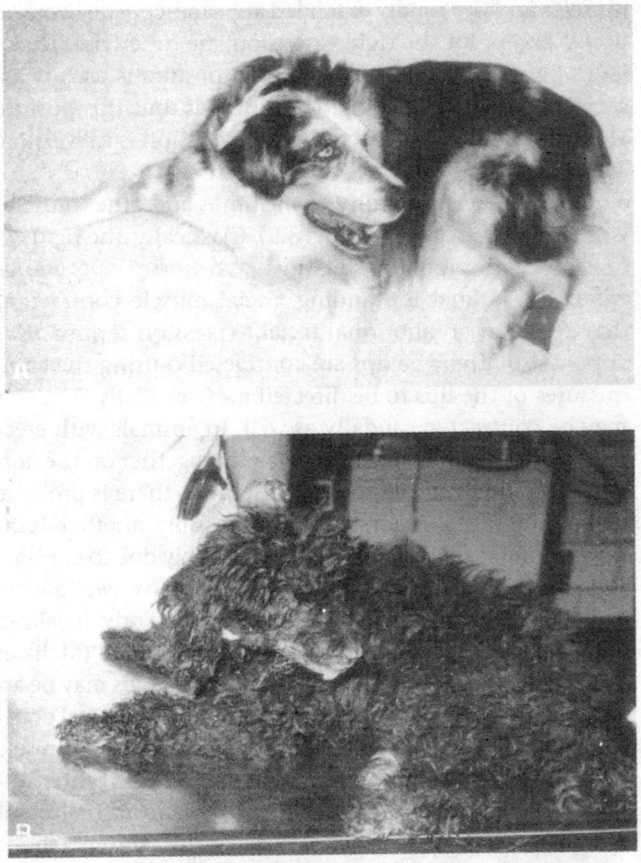

Fig. 3.4. (A, B) Two dogs with a head turn to the left.

Abnormalities of Limb Posture

Animals with neurologic dysfunction may stand with their limbs more laterally positioned than normal. This is often referred to as a *wide-based stance* (fig. 3.5). This appearance is most often associated with an abnormality of proprioceptive function. Lesions of the nervous system commonly associated with a wide-based stance include the vestibular system, cerebellum, and spinal cord. This posture may be an attempt by the animal to prevent itself from falling to one side. Conversely, animals that stand with the limbs very close together and directly under the trunk may have abnormalities of muscle strength, such as with disease of the peripheral nerves, neuromuscular junction, or muscles themselves.

Spasticity is increased tone of the muscles of the limbs (fig. 3.6). Opisthotonus is a body posture where the neck is held in extension with the top of the head directed toward the midback region. In a recumbent animal, spasticity and/or opisthotonus can be seen in numerous situations. These include decerebrate rigidity, decerebellate rigidity, and Schiff-Sherrington syndrome.

Decerebrate rigidity is characterized by opisthotonus and extension of all limbs. Usually the animal is stuporous or comatose (fig. 3.7). This is due to loss of descending input (from the supratentorial structures) to the brain stem structure responsible for flexion and extension of the limbs. The medullary reticulospinal system normally responsible for

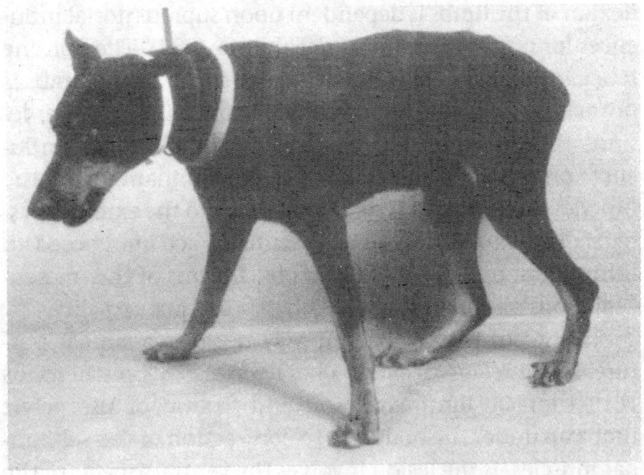

Fig. 3.5. Dog showing a wide-based stance. (From R. Bagley and I. Mayhew, Clinical examination of the nervous system, in Veterinary Clinical Examination and Diagnosis, eds. O. M. Radostits, I. G. J. May, and D. M. Houston [Harcourt Publishers Ltd., London, W. B. Saunders, 2000], fig. 19.6.)

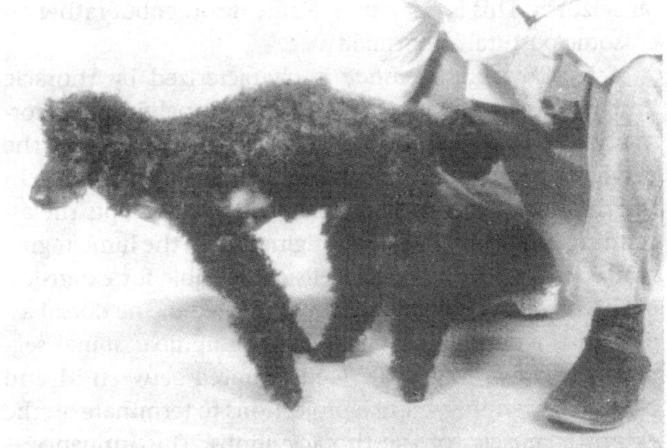

Fig. 3.6. Dog with increased extensor tone (spasticity) of the thoracic limbs from cervical lesion.

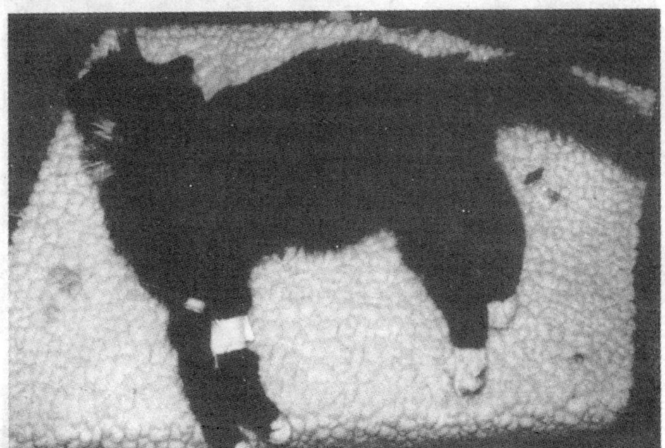

flexion of the limbs is dependent upon supratentorial influences for normal functions (deLahunta 1983). The pontine reticulospinal system influencing extension of the limbs is normally not under supratentorial control. Therefore, lesions that interrupt the descending supratentorial influences on the brain stem will more predominantly alter the function of the flexor systems compared to the extensor systems. The extensor systems essentially act unopposed to bring about extension of the limbs. Lesions of the (mesencephalon) midbrain result in this postural abnormality.

Lesions of the cerebellum may result in a similar posture. *Decerebellate rigidity* is characterized by opisthotonus with thoracic limb extension and flexion of the pelvic limbs up under the body due to contraction of the sublumbar muscles. If the lesion involves the ventral aspects of the cerebellum, extensor rigidity of all limbs is seen (Holliday 1979/1980). Importantly, as the lesion associated with this posture does not affect consciousness, the animal with decerebellate rigidity has normal mental awareness and consciousness. This clinical feature serves to differentiate decerebellate from decerebrate rigidity.

Affected animals can assume decerebellate posture episodically resulting in some referring to this as a "cerebellar seizure." This is not a true seizure disorder but rather an episodic postural abnormality.

Schiff-Sherrington posture is characterized by thoracic limb extension and inability to move the pelvic limbs normally (fig. 3.8) (deLahunta 1983). Spinal reflexes in the pelvic limb are usually normal. This results from a lesion in the thoracolumbar spinal segments that interrupts the ascending inhibitory impulses originating in the lumbar grey matter and terminating on cells responsible for extension of the thoracic limbs. Border cells located in the dorsal aspect of the ventral grey matter in the lumbar spinal segments between L1 and L7 (concentrated between L1 and L4) send ascending, cranial projections to terminate on the extensor muscles of the thoracic limbs. This influence is normally inhibitory to these extensor muscles. Spinal lesions that interrupt this ascending inhibitory influence result in unopposed function of the thoracic limb extensor muscles and the rigidly extended appearance. The thoracic limbs, except for the rigid extension, are otherwise neurologically normal. Schiff-Sherrington posture is usually associated with severe spinal cord injuries, but this posture alone does not indicate that the spinal lesion is irreversible as has been suggested.

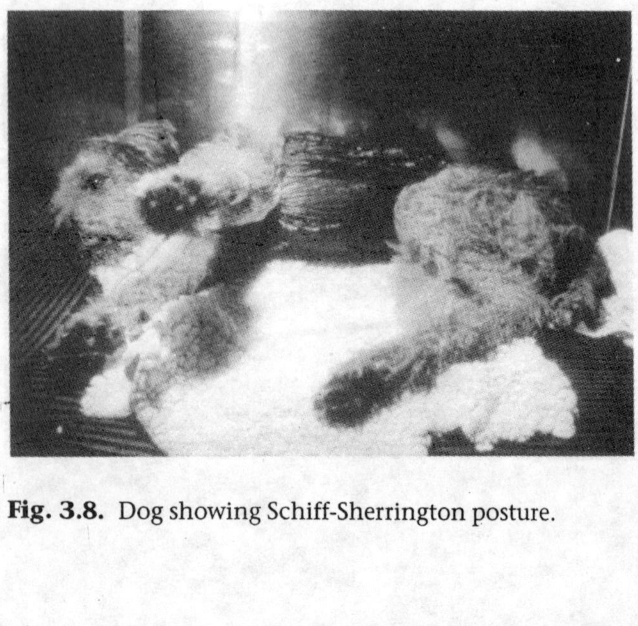

Fig. 3.8. Dog showing Schiff-Sherrington posture.

Severe extensor rigidity of the limbs and other muscles is characteristic of *tetanus* (fig. 3.9). Classically, the rigid extension of the limbs results in a "sawhorse" appearance when the animal is standing. Facial muscle contraction may result in an abnormal facial expression termed *risus sardonicus.* Often the lips are contracted causing the commissures of the lips to be directed more caudally. The ears may be contracted caudally as well. In animals with erect ears, the ears may be positioned closer together on the dorsal aspect of the head. In other instances, there is prolapse of the nictitating membranes and possibly miotic pupils. Affected animals may also salivate, possibly due to contraction of the pharyngeal muscles and ineffective swallowing.

While tetanus usually affects the entire body, localized tetanus involving one limb is occasionally noted (Malik et al. 1989). Episodic extensor rigidity of the limbs may be associated with a variety of abnormalities of the central or peripheral nervous systems and muscles. Episodic muscle contraction resulting in a stiff appearance, albeit intermittently, can result in disorders such as *myotonia* (failure of muscle relaxation), *reflex myoclonus, seizure,* and metabolic abnormalities such as *hypoglycemia, electrolyte abnormalities,* and muscle *cramping* syndromes ("Scotty cramp") (Myers et al. 1969).

In some instances of chronic lower motor neuron disease with muscle atrophy and fibrosis, one or both pelvic limbs may be held in *chronic rigid extension.* This posture is often seen with toxoplasmosis or neosporosis infection in young dogs (fig. 3.10). Spasticity can be seen at rest or at gait and is usually associated with upper motor neuron (UMN) disease.

A consistent flexion of a limb may be associated with soft tissue injury of the limb, muscle fibrosis, and skeletal and joint abnormalities. When walking, this is commonly referred to as a (non-weight bearing) *lameness.* If the limb is not anatomically fused in this position, this posture most often is the result of pain somewhere around the limb. If the pain originates from a spinal or peripheral nerve abnormality, this is termed a *nerve root signature* (fig. 3.11). Nerve root signature may involve either the thoracic or pelvic limbs (Palmer 1970; Prata and Stoll 1973; Bagley et al. 1997).

Abnormalities of Body Trunk Posture

Scoliosis is an abnormal lateral deviation of the vertebral column. This may be due to a problem of the vertebrae, ribs, or associated muscles and ligaments. Abnormal muscle support due to denervation of the paraspinal musculature contributes to asymmetric lateral muscle tension and subsequent vertebral deviation. In dogs, scoliosis often occurs secondary to intramedullary spinal cord lesions such as syringomyelia or hydromyelia (Child et al. 1986; Bagley et al. 1997; Bagley et al. 2000). Associated damage to spinal

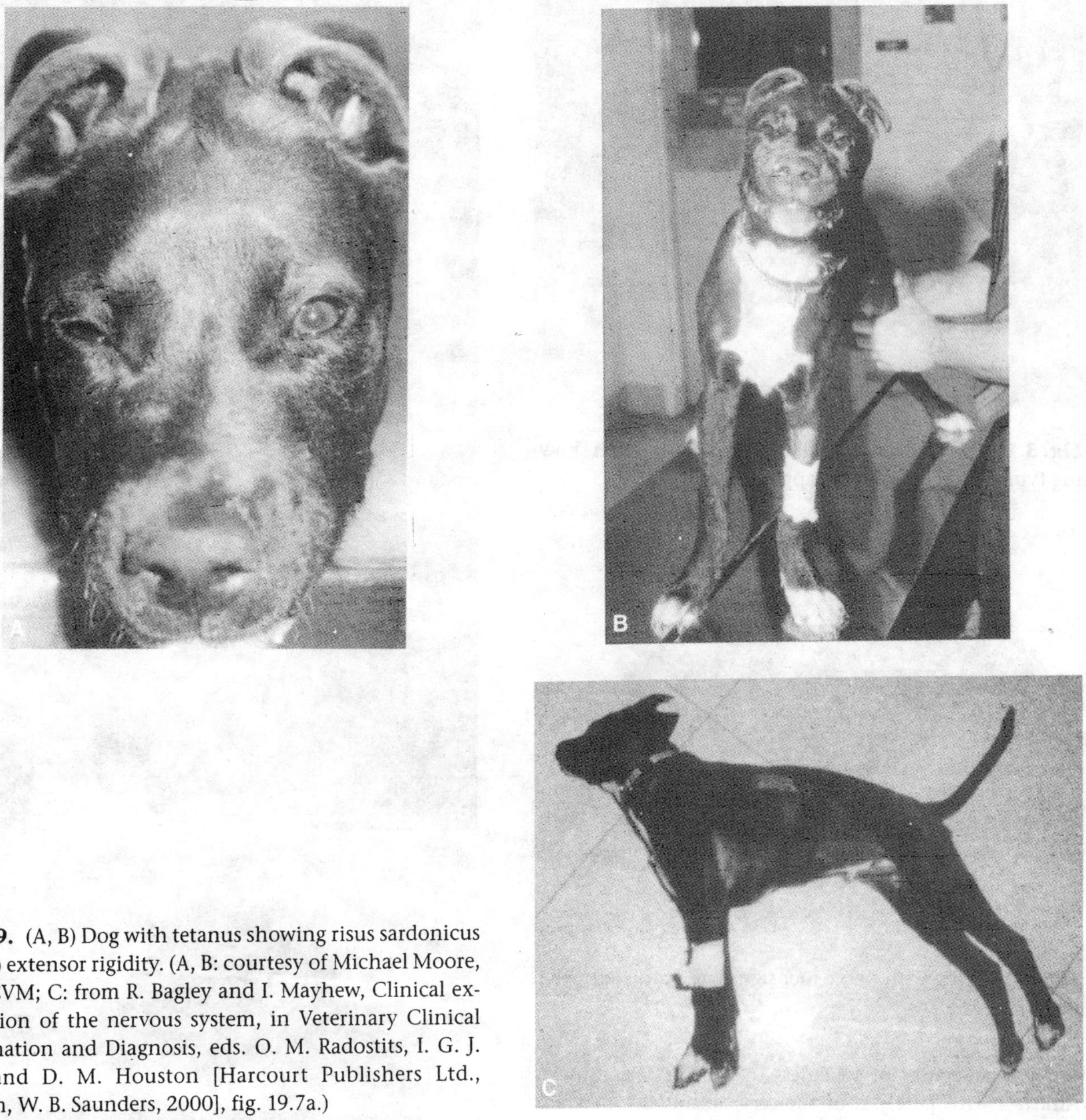

Fig. 3.9. (A, B) Dog with tetanus showing risus sardonicus and (C) extensor rigidity. (A, B: courtesy of Michael Moore, WSU-CVM; C: from R. Bagley and I. Mayhew, Clinical examination of the nervous system, in Veterinary Clinical Examination and Diagnosis, eds. O. M. Radostits, I. G. J. May, and D. M. Houston [Harcourt Publishers Ltd., London, W. B. Saunders, 2000], fig. 19.7a.)

cord LMN cells that are responsible for paraspinal muscle innervation may result in abnormal paraspinal muscle function.

Kyphosis, an abnormal flexion primarily of the thoracolumbar spine, may be a postural abnormality associated with pain, or may result from abnormalities of the vertebrae, ligaments, ribs, paraspinal muscles, and spinal and other peripheral nerves. Often, a kyphotic posture is the result of pain originating in the cervical area, thoracolumbar spine, or abdomen (fig. 3.12). Dogs with cervical pain also will often keep their neck muscles rigid with their heads held in the same horizontal plane as their spine, or lower to the ground. Doberman pinschers with cervical vertebral malformation/malarticulation will often keep their cervical area straight in relation to their thoracolumbar area presumably as a result of pain or possibly to relieve some of the associated spinal compression (see chapter 6). Lack of muscle tone dorsally may allow for overpulling of the ventral spinal muscles.

Lordosis is a ventral deviation of the spine and is uncommon in small animals. This may be a reflection of weakness or impairment of the paraspinal muscles. Occasionally, animals with thoracic vertebral or thoracic cavity disease will tend to flex the thoracic spine ventrally compared to the cervical and lumbar regions. In some instances, the neck and head may secondarily be positioned in a more extended position.

Ventral flexion of the neck (ventral neck flexion) is most commonly seen in cats and immature dogs (fig. 3.13). The animal's head will be directed ventrally toward the ground and usually caudally toward the ventral thoracic region. While this posture may result from cervical pain, it is more

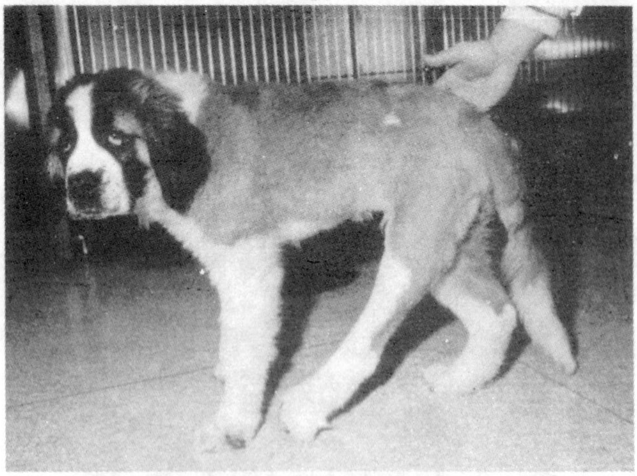

Fig. 3.10. Dog with muscle fibrosis and contraction showing typically straight-legged appearance.

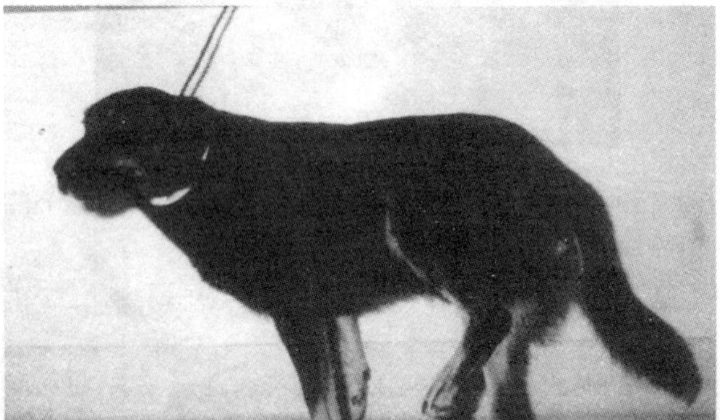

Fig. 3.11. Dog with nerve root signature of the left pelvic limb.

often a reflection of weakness of the cervical muscles. Animals with paralysis of the cervical muscles may also have a head and neck that appear to "flop" in a dependent (compared to gravity) direction.

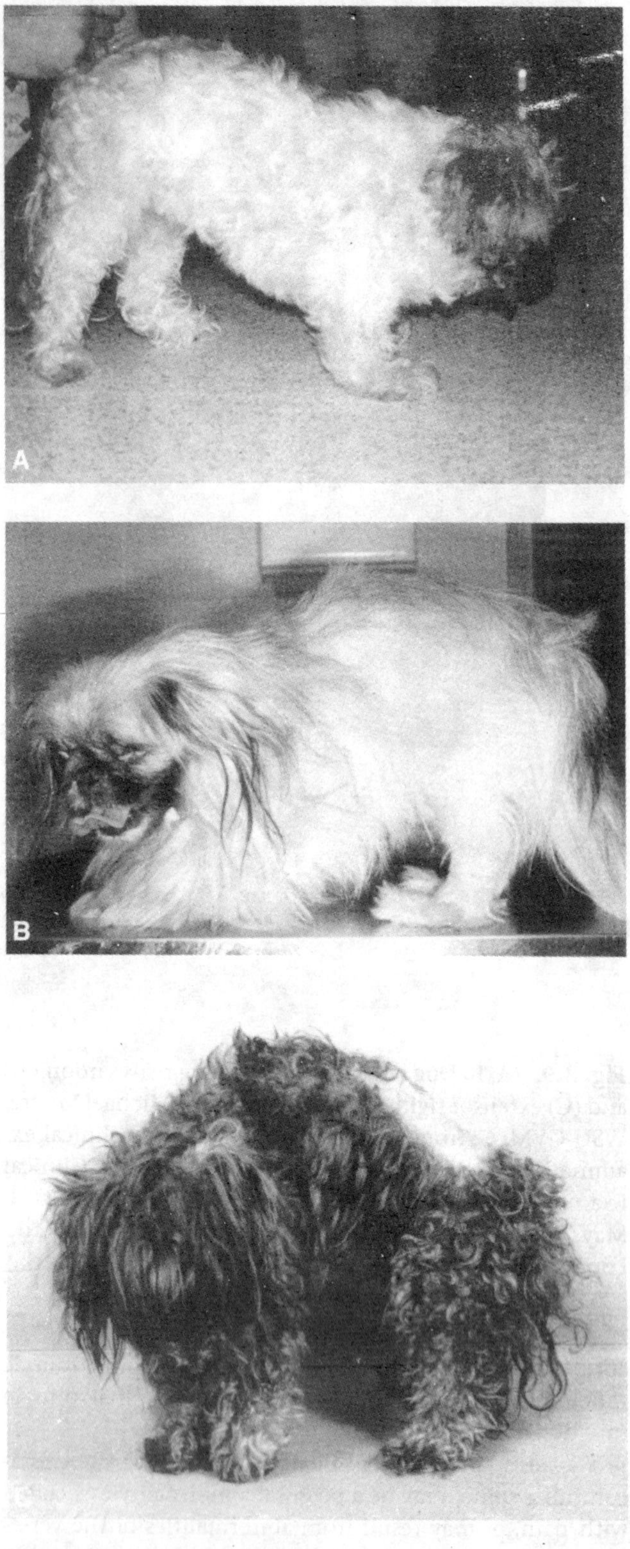

Fig. 3.12. (A, B, C) Kyphotic appearance of three dogs with cervical pain.

ABNORMAL SPONTANEOUS AND INVOLUNTARY MOVEMENTS

Abnormal movements commonly result from dysfunction of the nervous system due to the significant influence of the nervous system on muscular functions. Movement can be voluntary or involuntary. Abnormalities of voluntary movement are discussed below under Assessment and Abnormalities of Gait in this chapter.

Involuntary movement disorders are less well classified in animals compared to humans. Terms such as tics, twitches, shivering, shuddering, and fasciculation are often used to describe episodic, irregular muscle movements or depolarizations associated with muscle contraction. Some movement disorders are classified as "hyperkinetic" or *dyskinesias* or *myokymias* (Nakahata et al. 1992; Penderis and Franklin 2001; Ramsey et al. 1999; Reading and McKerrell 1993). Dyskinesias are defined as impairment of the power of voluntary movements resulting in fragmented or incomplete movements. Involuntary movements are usually manifested through abnormal motion of

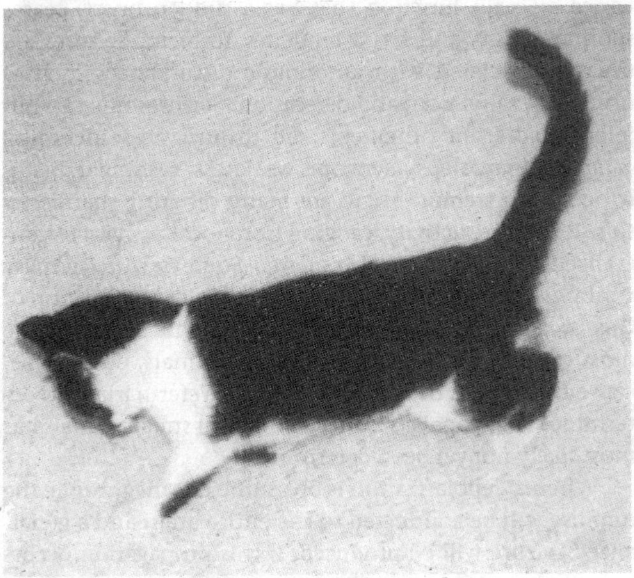

Fig. 3.13. Cat with ventral neck flexion.

the limbs, trunk, or head. Flexing movements of the limbs may occur. These types of episodes need to be differentiated from partial seizure activity and muscle disorders.

Tremor is a rhythmic, oscillatory, involuntary disorder of movement resulting from alternate or synchronous contraction of reciprocally innervated, antagonistic muscles (Bagley 1992). Electromyographically, tremor is characterized by rhythmic bursts of motor neuron activity occurring in opposing muscle groups. The contraction of muscles with opposing function gives tremor a biphasic nature. This biphasic character differentiates tremor from other abnormalities of movement. While seen during the awake state, true tremor should cease with sleep.

Tremor can be localized to one body area or be generalized (whole body). Localized tremor usually involves the head or pelvic limbs.

Tremor is ultimately a disorder of movement. Therefore, regions of the nervous system primarily responsible for normal movement, when abnormal, may generate a tremor. In humans these areas include the basal nuclei and other components of the extrapyramidal system, cerebellum, diffuse neuronal cell bodies involved in segmental and supraspinal reflex mechanisms, components of the lower motor neuron, and the interconnecting pathways. Additionally, abnormalities of mechanical apparatus of the limbs (e.g., bones, joints, and tendons) may also result in tremor. Species differences exist as to which anatomical areas within the nervous system, when abnormal, result in tremor. For example, lesions involving the basal nuclei and substantia nigra commonly result in tremor in human beings but this is not clear for dogs.

The cerebellum functions in control of movement once that movement is initiated. Tremor seen with cerebellar disease is most obvious when the animal intends to move in a goal-oriented effort and it is therefore referred to as an *intention tremor.* This type of tremor often becomes more obvious when an animal attempts to lower its head to eat or drink from a bowl or dish. Intention tremors may involve the head or the entire body, and may be accompanied by other signs of cerebellar dysfunction such as ataxia and hypermetria.

Tremor in human beings can either be normal (physiological) or abnormal (pathological) (Adams and Victor 1993). Physiological tremor is present in all muscle groups in the waking state. This tremor may partially result from passive vibration of body tissues produced by mechanical activity of the heart, however, its true origin is not yet known. Normally, this tremor is at a low enough amplitude that it is almost imperceptible.

Tremor is considered pathological when it impairs normal function. Pathological tremor is thought to result from imbalances of neurotransmitters, such as dopamine, acetylcholine, and gamma-aminobutyric acid. Various pathological tremor syndromes exist in human beings including resting (Parkinsonian) tremor, intention or ataxic tremor, action tremor, hysterical tremor, and a mixed tremor having components of various types of tremor (Adams and Victor 1993; Cooper and Rodnitzky 2000).

Myoclonus is a shocklike contraction of a muscle or muscles that tends to occur repeatedly in a rhythmic pattern (deLahunta 1983). It is akin to the rhythmic depolarization and contraction that occurs in the heart with each beat. Myoclonus, if present, often involves the thoracic limb, however, a pelvic limb or the facial muscles including the tongue may also be involved (Silver et al. 1997). Myoclonus in dogs is usually the result of distemper infection that establishes a pacemaker-like depolarization of local motor neurons, however, it has been associated with lead toxicity and other forms of nervous system inflammation (Breazile et al. 1966).

Reflex myoclonus is characterized by episodic, stimulation-evoked extensor rigidity of the body and is most commonly seen in Labrador retrievers (Fox et al. 1984; March et al. 1993). Affected animals become stiff, usually when excited or stimulated. Other breeds (Dalmatian) are occasionally affected. As this is a congenital disorder, young (weeks to months of age) animals are affected.

Dancing Doberman syndrome is a disease characterized by alternating pelvic limb flexion when the animal is standing. A peripheral neuropathy or myopathy of the pelvic limb nerves is suspected (Chrisman 1990). Some animals with tendon, muscle, and other musculoskeletal injuries may stand with a similar appearance. In instances of gastrocnemius tendon avulsion, for example, the flexed toe stance may be clue to this abnormality (fig. 3.14). Other dogs with apparent dyskinesias or limb pain may stand with the limb in a flexed position.

Myotonia occurs as a congenital problem in various breeds including the Chow-Chow and cats. Animals with myotonia have sustained muscle contraction, which is initiated voluntarily or with stimulation, and sustained involuntarily. The excessive muscle contraction is thought to be due to an abnormal muscle cell membrane that supports persistent depolarization. Animals with myotonia may

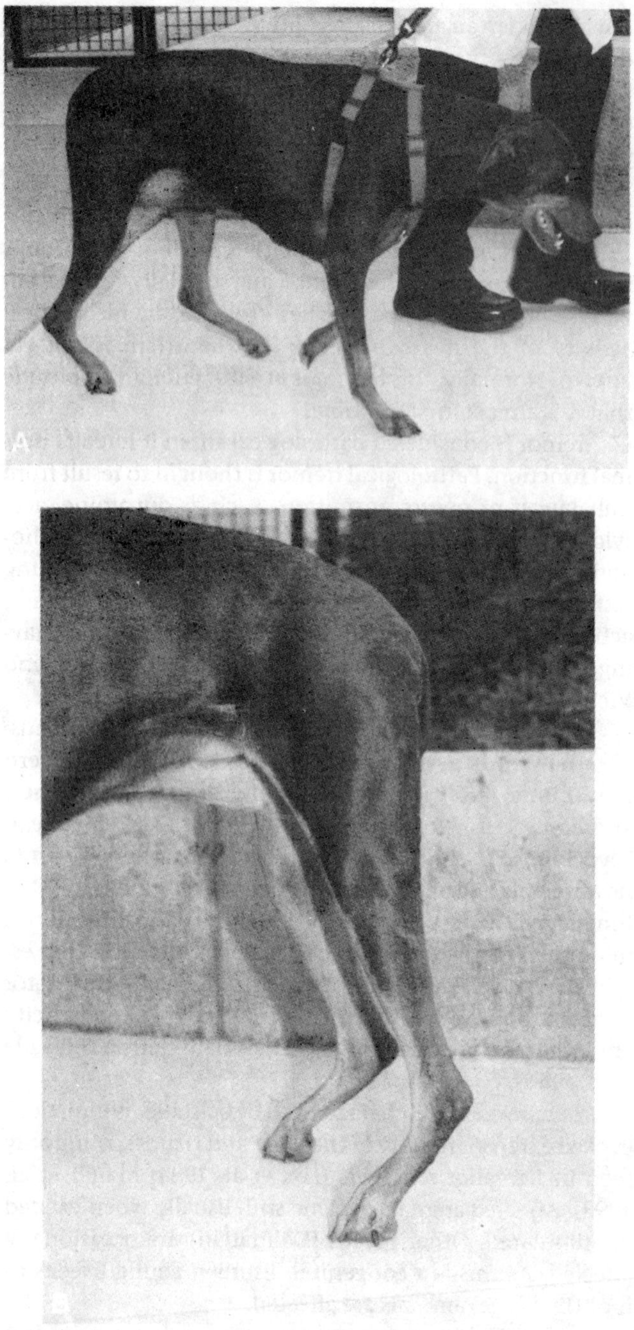

Fig. 3.14. (A, B) Doberman with rupture of the gastrocnemius tendon showing typical flexed toe posture.

have a short-stilted gait and apparent stiffness or extensor rigidity of the limbs. Affected animals also may have large, bulky muscles on palpation. Muscle dimpling may occur with direct muscle percussion.

Scotty cramp is characterized by paroxysms of muscular hypertonicity, usually precipitated by excitement or exercise (Myers et al. 1969). Animals appear stiff and stilted at gait. Some animals (Cavalier King Charles spaniel) may fall over and become laterally recumbent (Herritage and Palmer 1983). This disease has also been seen in Dalmatians and Norwich terriers.

Seizures are an important and common sign of neurological disease. A seizure is a paroxysmal, transitory disturbance of brain function that has a sudden onset, ceases spontaneously, and has a tendency to recur. Seizures are usually associated with autonomic disturbances such as urination, salivation, and defecation. Seizures must be differentiated from other episodic disturbances including cataplexy/narcolepsy, syncope, weakness, vestibular disturbances, and tremor. There are many differing manifestations of seizure activity, ranging from focal activity to generalized tonic clonic movements. Some seizure activity contains characteristic features that help in clarification of this problem. The generalized tonic, clonic seizure is the most common seizure recognized in animals, possibly because this type is the most obvious for veterinarians to determine. The scope of seizure disorders of small animals has most likely not yet been determined.

When a depolarization is of a sufficient magnitude, the impulse will be conducted to the entire brain and a generalized seizure will be produced. If this propagation occurs in milliseconds, a generalized seizure will be seen from the onset. If the spread is slower, an initial focal seizure (confined to one body part/area) can eventually become generalized. If the spread of the electrical discharge stops, a focal seizure will be the extent of the disturbance.

Focal seizures remain localized to one body region such as a limb or facial muscles. They are of value in localization of the seizure focus to a side of the brain as they often occur in the side of the body opposite to a supratentorial lesion. Additionally, focal seizures are more often associated with structural brain disease.

Bizarre behaviors may be manifestations of seizure disorders, possibly initiated in components of the limbic system (temporal lobe epilepsy). Fly biting would be one example and may be more common in breeds such as the Cavalier King Charles spaniel. At one extreme, even some gastrointestinal abnormalities such as vomiting have been suggested to be the result of seizure activity (Breitschwerdt et al. 1979). Other behavior disorders, such as flank sucking or tail biting, may result from a seizure focus, but definitive proof is lacking. These disorders are usually a primary behavior abnormality.

Seizures can occur as the result of a structural brain abnormality, a metabolic abnormality within the body that secondarily affects the brain, or without apparent cause (idiopathic epilepsy) (see chapter 17). Clinical evaluation initially depends upon two important features: the age of onset of the first seizure and the presence of interictal neurological deficits. Certain breeds of dogs such as beagles, Belgian Tervurens, German shepherds, keeshonds, and collies have an increased incidence of idiopathic epilepsy. Other high incidence breeds include the Saint Bernard, golden retriever, Irish setter, American cocker spaniel, wirehaired fox terriers, Alaskan malamutes, Siberian huskies, and miniature poodles.

Idiopathic seizures are not associated with interictal neurological deficits. Obvious deficits found upon neurological examination in animals with seizures suggest a structural cause. Some animals, however, may have reversible neurological deficits during the postictal period.

These deficits usually resolve within 48 hours; occasionally deficits may last for days after the seizure. Knowledge of when the seizure(s) occurred in relationship to the examination is important for this determination.

Metabolic causes of seizure usually do not result in persistent neurological deficits. Deficits are possible, especially when mental status is also abnormal. Metabolic disease-associated deficits are usually symmetric if present unless associated structural abnormalities such as edema or hemorrhage are concurrently present.

ASSESSMENT AND ABNORMALITIES OF GAIT

Gait is commonly defined as a regularly repeating series of leg movements during walking or running (also see chapter 20). The nervous system controls the actions of the muscles, bones, joints, and associated connective tissue important for this function (table 3.3). Disease of any or all of these components can result in a gait abnormality. Normal walking is produced by the recruitment of stepping reflexes, which alternate between the extensor and flexor muscles. There is, however, a complex of actions involving multiple nervous system pathways associated with voluntary movement. As an example, the vestibulospinal and reticulospinal tracts are facilitatory to the extensor muscles, important for maintenance of body tone against gravity (the stance or propulsive phase). The corticospinal and the rubrospinal tracts are facilitatory to the flexor muscles, important for the protraction (flight) phase of limb movement. The upper motor neuron control for locomotion is thought to be located in the brain stem, however, a discrete anatomic gait center (nucleus) has not been identified. Supratentorial (forebrain) structures are likely important for voluntary control, especially of intricate movements. The cerebellum contributes to the coordination of movement.

Table 3.3. Structures necessary for movement

Requirements for movement
- Nerves to signal muscle and sense joint position
- The muscles contract and provide the force for limb movement.
- Bones, tendon, and ligaments for support
- Oxygen, via blood flow, to support muscle metabolism
- Nutrients and other metabolic building blocks of muscles

Components of the nervous system required for movement
- Supratentorial (forebrain) structures are important for voluntary control, especially of intricate movements.
- Brain stem structures are important for gait generation.
- The cerebellum , while not necessary for the initiation of movement, is important for coordination of movement. Cerebellar influences coordinate and smooth body movements by controlling rate, range, and force of limb motion. The cerebellum most likely is responsible for inhibition of the flexor component of gait.
- The spinal cord allows for information to be transferred from the intracranial structures to the limbs. The grey matter of the spinal cord is where the nerve cell bodies that give rise to the efferent peripheral nerves are found.
- The peripheral nerves carry efferent and afferent information to and from the muscles, respectively.
- The neuromuscular junction provides a means for transfer of nervous information to the muscles.

Clinical Gait Assessment

Animals have varying normal gait characteristics depending upon such factors as their body size, limb conformation, and shape (also see chapter 20). The degree of diversity even among a single species such as dogs is great, and can result in characteristic stepping movements and body movements for that breed. While seemingly simple, one of the first questions to be addressed when evaluating animals for abnormalities of movement is, "Does this animal have a gait abnormality or is this movement normal for the breed?"

As abnormalities of numerous body components can affect gait, it is important to determine which of these components is the cause of the dysfunction. Some gait abnormalities are more characteristic of nervous system disease, while other abnormalities are more characteristic of musculoskeletal or other system abnormalities.

Gait Abnormalities Characteristic of Nervous System Disease

Ataxia is a failure of muscular coordination or an irregularity of muscle action. In some situations, it is defined as lack of an axis, implying an inability to travel along a straight line. Ataxia is usually associated with a "falling" or "swaying" of the body from side to side. It is also commonly present in association with other forms of abnormal limb movements such as dysmetria.

Ataxia results from a variety of anatomic lesions within the nervous system, most commonly of the cerebellum, vestibular system, and spinal cord sensory pathways. Ataxia, without motor involvement (paresis), usually implies cerebellar or cerebellar pathway disease. Sensory ataxia due to loss of joint position sense is often made worse by blindfolding the animal, effectively preventing visual compensatory mechanisms.

Dysmetria is improper estimation of distance during muscular activity. Dysmetria includes both *hypo-* and *hypermetria.* With hypermetria, voluntary muscular movement overreaches the intended goal and is essentially a failure to limit the degree of flexion (fig. 3.15). With hypometria, voluntary movement falls short of the intended goal. Hypermetria is more commonly recognized than hypometria. Both of these abnormalities are most often associated with lesions of the cerebellum or cerebellar pathways. In the instance of hypermetria, for example, the loss of cerebellar input, which normally limits the flexion phase of gait, results in the exaggerated movement.

Spasticity is a state of increased muscle tone (fig. 3.6). This is reflected as a stiff appearance of the limbs, a lack of normal flexion, or limbs that are maintained more extended during the flight phase of gait. This is occasionally referred to as "floating." Spasticity commonly results from upper motor neuron (UMN) lesions.

Paresis is derived from the Greek word for relaxation and

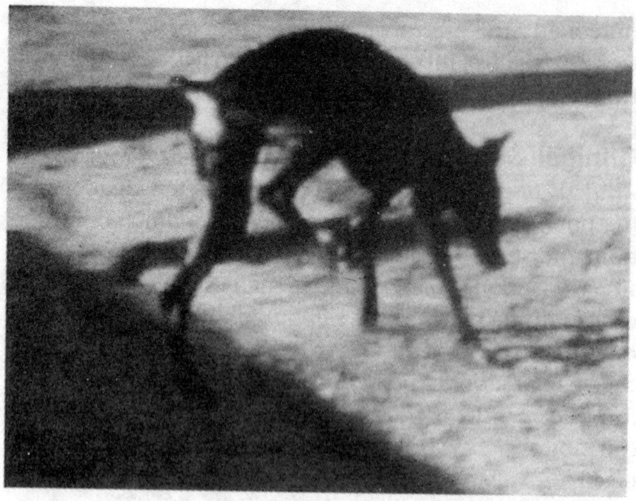

Fig. 3.15. Dog with hypermetria of the right pelvic limb. (From R. Bagley and I. Mayhew, Clinical examination of the nervous system, in Veterinary Clinical Examination and Diagnosis, eds. O. M. Radostits, I. G. J. May, and D. M. Houston [Harcourt Publishers Ltd., London, W. B. Saunders, 2000], fig. 19.9.)

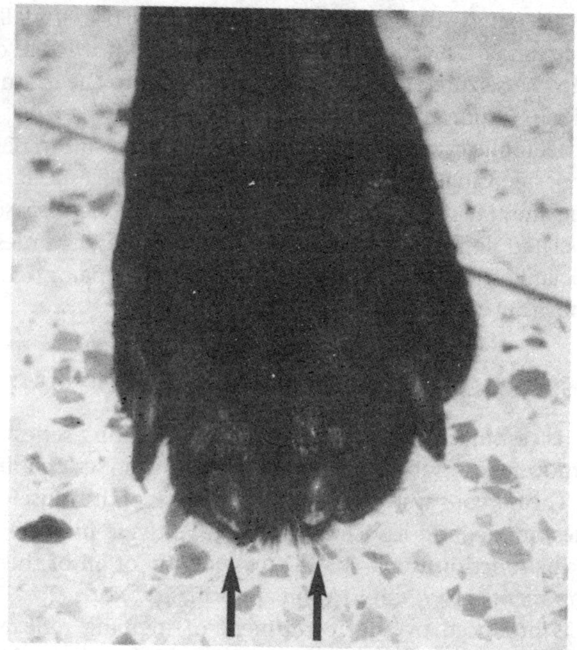

Fig. 3.16. Dog with paresis showing abnormal toenail wear (*arrows*).

implies weakness of motor function without complete paralysis (some voluntary motion remains). *Paralysis* implies loss of motor function from either a neurologic or muscular abnormality. The term "paresis," however, has different connotations including limb dysfunction from various causes. In many clinical descriptions, paresis and conscious proprioceptive abnormalities are used interchangeably, with the term "paresis" implying a conscious proprioceptive abnormality.

Varying degrees of paresis exist; some animals retain the ability to walk while others are unable to support weight. During gait, paresis may be manifested in a number of ways. This is most obvious when the animal contacts the dorsum of the paws (drags) along the ground. Abnormal toenail wear, especially when the toenails of the two longest toes (P3 and P4) are worn to a greater extent than the shorter (P2 and P5) toes, may suggest underlying paresis (fig. 3.16). In some animals, when the limb contacts the ground or when the animal's body weight is placed on limb, the paw rotates or twists. In other instances, the limb may overflex when the animal contacts the ground. This is often followed by an overflexion during the subsequent flight phase of the gait. In still other instances, the animal impacts the ground with greater force than normal. This may be a reflection of poor proprioceptive knowledge of where the limb is in space and subsequently when this limb should impact the ground.

Animals that are paretic often will have irregular step distances (see The Importance of Step Distance below). These same animals tend to have greater impact with their limbs and the ground. This may reflect an abnormality of proprioception wherein the animal is uncertain when and where the limb will touch the ground. When the foot does impact the ground the animals may swivel or twist, usually with the caudal aspect of the limb moving more laterally and the toes becoming more medially placed (i.e., the front of the foot ends up pointing more medially).

Supratentorial disease will not dramatically affect gait. Paresis at gait is usually evident with lesions in the midbrain caudal to the level of the red nucleus (deLahunta 1983). The severity of the gait impairment increases as the lesion occurs progressively more caudally in the central nervous system. For example, supratentorial lesions may result in significant hemiparesis when postural reactions are tested, however, gait remains relatively normal. With brain stem or spinal cord lesions, the associated paresis usually results in obvious gait impairment. Depending upon where within the nervous system the lesion occurs, gait may be altered differently. Wide circling toward the side of a unilateral supratentorial lesion is common. Occasionally, spasticity may be noticed, with the limb (primarily a thoracic limb) appearing stiff, floating, and overreaching.

Lesions of the brain stem and cervical spinal cord will often have dramatic effects on gait, frequently impairing the ability to stand and generate a gait. If the lesion occurs unilaterally, ipsilateral hemiparesis is noted. If pathways are affected bilaterally, tetraparesis will be present. Spinal reflexes should reflect the UMN nature of the lesion.

Circling is propulsive walking in circles (fig. 3.17). This is usually found in animals with disease involving either the supratentorial or vestibular areas. Usually, but not always, the animal circles toward the side of a unilateral supratentorial lesion or vestibular disease lesion. Animals with supratentorial disease will also tend to overstep with the thoracic limb contralateral to the direction of the circling. The paw appears to be "thrown" cranially, wherein the paw is quickly overextended prior to impacting the ground and

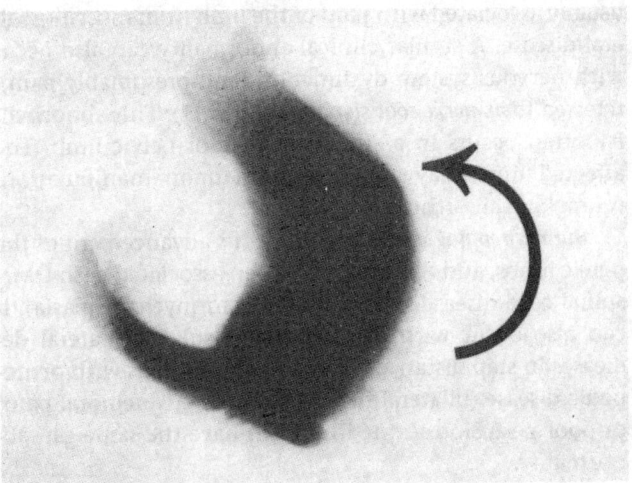

Fig. 3.17. Cat shown circling to right. (From R. Bagley, Recognition and localization of intracranial disease, Vet Clinic N Am (Small Anim Pract) [1996], 667–709, fig. 1.)

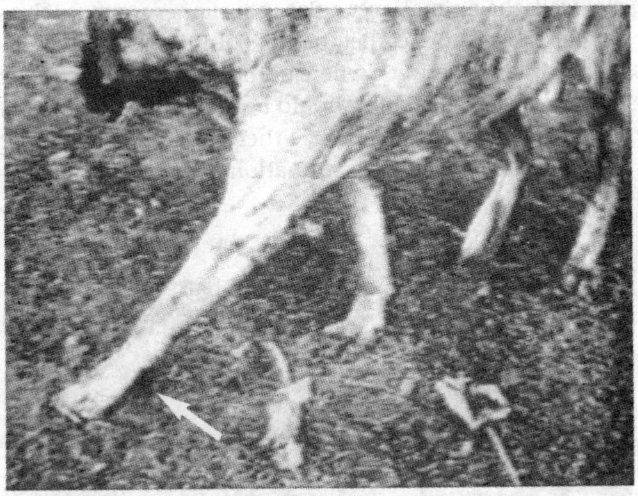

Fig. 3.18. Dog with a right supratentorial lesion, which oversteps with the contralateral thoracic limb.

may result in a "flipping" movement of the paw (fig. 3.18). Animals may propulsively direct their attention toward the caudal aspects and exhibit a circling behavior. This phenomenon may be a reflection of a compulsive obsession (behavior disorder) or a directed attention toward a particular stimulus such as pain or itching.

Gait Abnormalities and Lesions of Selective Peripheral Nerves

Lesions of the *femoral nerve* result in an inability to extend the stifle and support weight. The animal may have difficulty bringing the limbs forward and may "bunny-hop" or have shorter step distance in the affected limb. Bunny-hopping is the simultaneous advancement of the pelvic limbs, and has classically been associated with UMN spinal cord disease (spinal dysraphism/myelodysplasia). Animals with orthopedic disease (bilateral hip dysplasia or coxofemoral pain) may have the same gait abnormality.

Lesions of the *obturator nerve* often do not affect gait in dogs and cats. If an animal is placed on a slippery surface, however, the affected pelvic limb(s) may slide laterally with weight bearing.

Lesions of the *sciatic nerve* result in a characteristic gait wherein the distal foot is almost "thrown" forward by the movements of the more proximal muscles of the limb. When the animal is weight bearing, the hock joint may overflex resulting in the dropped-hock appearance. Atrophy of the muscles of the limb is common with LMN disease. Atrophy associated with sciatic disease is often obvious in the cranial tibial muscle group. With lesions of the *cranial gluteal nerve,* the stifle may become abducted during the stance phase of gait.

Lesions of the *radial nerve* affect the animal's ability to extend the carpus. If the lesion occurs proximally in the radial nerve, the elbow may be positioned more ventrally than normal. The limb may be carried off of the ground with the elbow flexed if the musculocutaneous nerve is intact.

With lesions of the *medial, ulnar, musculocutaneous,* and *suprascapular nerves,* gait is usually unaffected. The carpal joint may be overextended with medial and ulnar lesions. With musculocutaneous nerve paralysis, elbow flexion is poor and this joint may be held overextended.

Gait Abnormalities and Musculoskeletal Problems

Certain gait abnormalities are more characteristic of a problem in the musculoskeletal system. *Fibrotic myopathy* of the semimembranous and semitendinous muscles results in one such characteristic gait abnormality (Lewis 2000). At faster speeds, there is an awkward jerking in a medial direction of the affected limb during the flight phase of limb movement. If the animal is observed from behind, as the affected pelvic limb begins to be lowered following the zenith of the flight phase of gait, the distal foot (from the hock level) is rapidly pulled in a medial direction due to the decreased elasticity of the fibrotic muscle.

With fibrosis of the *infraspinatous* and *supraspinatous muscle,* the thoracic limb at the shoulder lever may be more outwardly rotated, with the foot contacting the ground in a more sideways position (fig. 3.19).

Animals with *rupture of the gastrocnemius tendon* may sink at the hock joint when weight bearing. A similar phenomenon may occur with abnormal sciatic innervation to the gastrocnemius muscle. If, however, the gastrocnemius tendon ruptures and the superficial digital flexor tendon remains intact, as weight is placed on the limb and the hock sinks, the toes will be held in a more flexed position (fig. 3.14). This characteristic toe position does not occur with neurologic weakness of the gastrocnemius muscle. Affected animals may have a leg-carrying lameness, and stand straight in the stifles when weight bearing. Animals often have associated muscle atrophy of the limb including the semimembranous, semitendinous, and gastrocnemius muscles. This may sometimes be confused with dancing Doberman syndrome.

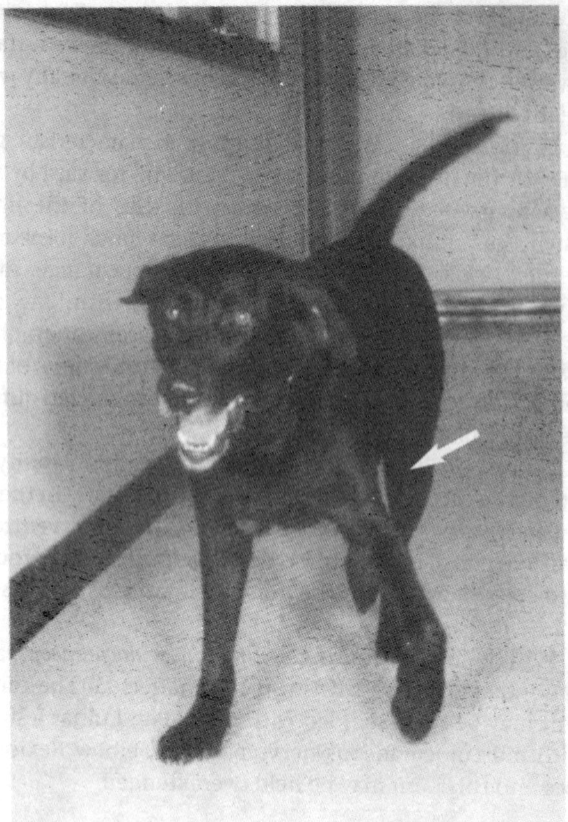

Fig. 3.19. Dog with infraspinatous contraction and an outwardly rotated shoulder (*arrow*). (Courtesy of James D. Lincoln, WSU-CVM)

Iliopsoas muscle disease may result in pelvic limb lameness. Animals may position the hocks in a more adducted way (cow-hocked).

Gait Abnormalities and Various System Diseases

Stiffness associated with *decreased step length* is commonly seen with diseases of the peripheral neuromuscular apparatus (LMN cell body, nerve roots, peripheral nerve, neuromuscular junction, and muscle), musculoskeletal disease, metabolic weakness, or poor perfusion of the limb.

Dogs with neuromuscular disease may also have a stiff, stilted, choppy gait due primarily to muscle weakness. These abnormalities may be episodic and worsen, as in the case of myasthenia gravis, as the level of exercise increases. A similar appearance may occur in dogs with pain, primarily from orthopedic disease.

Poor perfusion to the limb, as associated with a cardiovascular or local vascular problem, results in decreased limb oxygenation, increased anaerobic metabolism, and subsequent muscle weakness. Systemic metabolic disease may also result in abnormalities of muscle metabolism and subsequent muscle weakness. Differential cyanosis may be presence with some shunting of limb perfusion such as in the instance of a right-to-left PDA.

Lameness (decreased or non-weight bearing on a limb) is usually associated with pain of the limb from musculoskeletal disease. A similar clinical abnormality can also occur with nervous system dysfunction (and presumably pain), referred to as *nerve root signature* (fig. 3.11). This abnormality often occurs in a single thoracic or pelvic limb. The affected limb may appear painful upon manipulation, mimicking an orthopedic problem.

Bunny-hopping is the simultaneous advancement of the pelvic limbs, and has classically been associated with UMN spinal cord disease (spinal dysraphism/myelodysplasia). It can also occur with diseases that result in bilateral decreases in step distance. Occasionally, animals with orthopedic disease (bilateral hip dysplasia or coxofemoral pain) or poor perfusion to the limbs can have the same gait abnormality.

The Importance of the Step Distance

Clinical evaluation of gait usually involves observation of the animal's movements during walking and, when indicated, running. This is best accomplished by having a handler walk the animal over a flat, nonslippery area (such as concrete, black top, carpet, or grass). Initially, the step distance (distance between where both thoracic limbs contact the ground, for example) should be determined (fig. 3.20). The step length is assessed as either normal, increased, or decreased. Step length determination will help in establish-

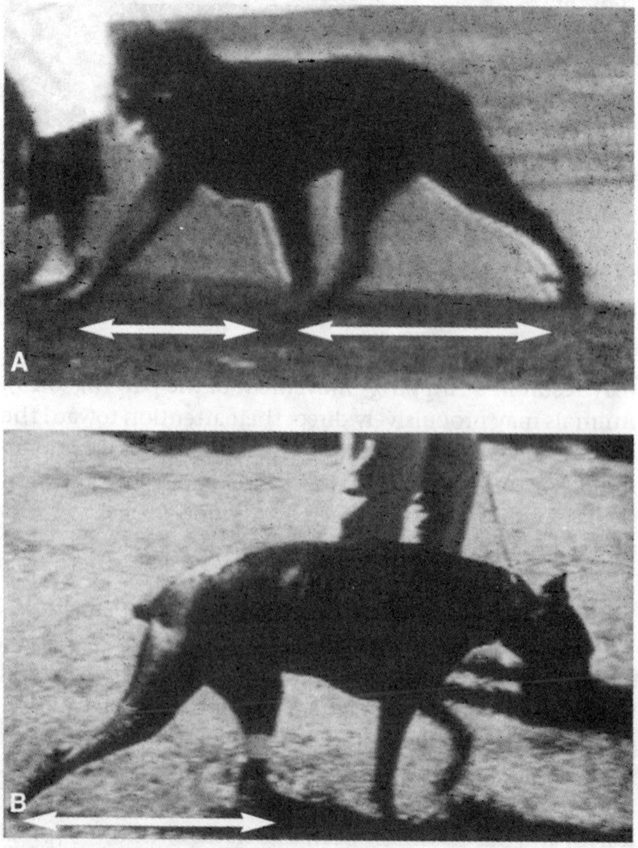

Fig. 3.20. (A, B) Two dogs with UMN disease showing increased step distance (*arrow*).

ing whether a gait abnormality is associated with disease of the nervous system.

Generally, animals with UMN neurological disease have normal or increased step and stride lengths, where dogs with orthopedic or neuromuscular disease have shortened step and stride lengths. Animals with UMN disease may appear irregular and uncoordinated, having a tendency to sway from side to side; some may fall to the side. Their feet may contact the ground with increased force. Doberman pinschers with cervical vertebral malformation/malarticulation, for example, may overflex or "sink" in the hock joints during weight bearing, presumably the result of motor or sensory weakness. These animals may rebound from this sinking resulting in hypermetria during the flight phase of the subsequent step. Also, many dogs with neurologic disease vary the step distance with subsequent steps, giving the gait an irregular temporal pattern. This results in some steps being longer and some steps being shorter. Irregular step distances is often a clue to an underlying neurologic disease compared to, for example, a musculoskeletal disease where the step distance, while being abnormal, tends to be consistently abnormal in the same way. These same animals tend have greater impact with their limbs and the ground. This may reflect an abnormality of proprioception wherein the animal is uncertain when and where the limb will touch the ground.

Dogs with LMN disease may hold the head low (possibly because of neck muscle weakness) and take short, choppy steps. Some have a kyphotic posture (figs. 3.21, 3.22). They may tire easily and appear unwilling to perform. Animals with orthopedic disease may have a similar gait abnormality. Bilateral cruciate ligament rupture is one such example wherein the pelvic limb step length is short. Normal conscious proprioception should suggest the possibility of an underlying orthopedic or musculoskeletal disease. Poor limb perfusion, such as from a partial bilateral iliac arterial thrombus or from a right-to-left PDA, may also result in a short, choppy pelvic limb gait. The clinical signs

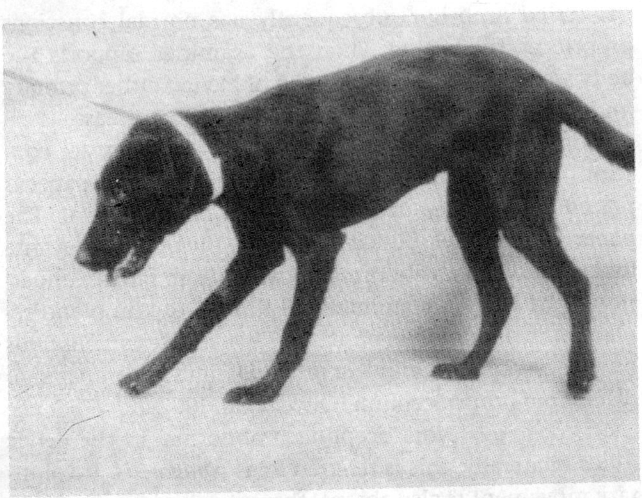

Fig. 3.21. Dog with a myopathy showing a kyphotic posture when walking.

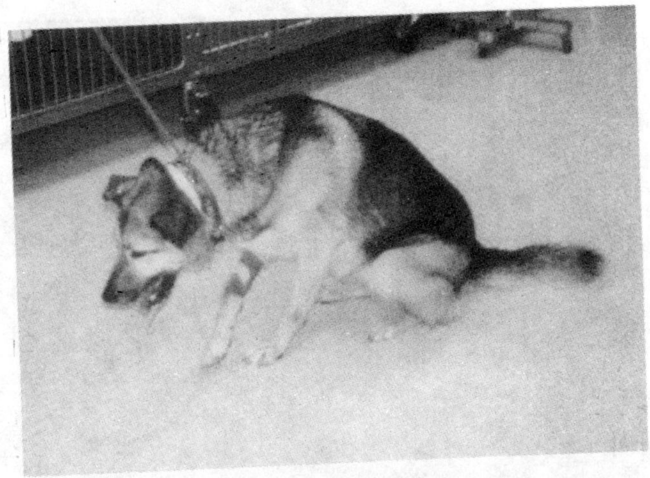

Fig. 3.22. Dog with a neuromuscular junction disease and muscle weakness showing a kyphotic posture when walking.

may worsen with exercise (similar to myasthenia gravis) and differential cyanosis (caudal aspects of the body) may be seen with the latter disease. Dogs with vertebral pain may also have short steps or be reluctant to move.

ASSESSMENT AND ABNORMALITIES OF PROPRIOCEPTION

Proprioception is the inherent knowledge of where the limbs and other body components are in relation to the environment and each other. Conscious proprioception is often assessed clinically by observing how the animal moves in space and by physically testing postural reactions. Information obtained in this component of the neurological examination is often extremely important in separating animals with neurological causes of limb dysfunction from those with disease of other systems.

Conscious Proprioception

Proprioceptive abilities are assessed subjectively during evaluation of body posture, limb position, and gait and movement. When physically testing conscious proprioception, the paw is placed in an abnormal position and the animal's response to this new limb position is observed. Conscious proprioceptive testing is usually accomplished with the animal standing, and the body weight equally distributed on the limbs. Animals with a variety of painful limb conditions may shift their weight from the affected limb to the contralateral limb making proprioceptive assessments more difficult. If testing conscious proprioception in the pelvic limbs, the examiner can place a hand between the legs in the groin area to determine if the body weight is equally supported by both limbs. If testing the thoracic limbs, a hand can be placed ventral to the chest. Animals may also shift their weight from both pelvic limbs to both thoracic limbs, or vice versa.

When the animal is positioned correctly, the paw to be tested is placed in an abnormal position. Usually this is accomplished by placing the paw on its dorsum. An under-

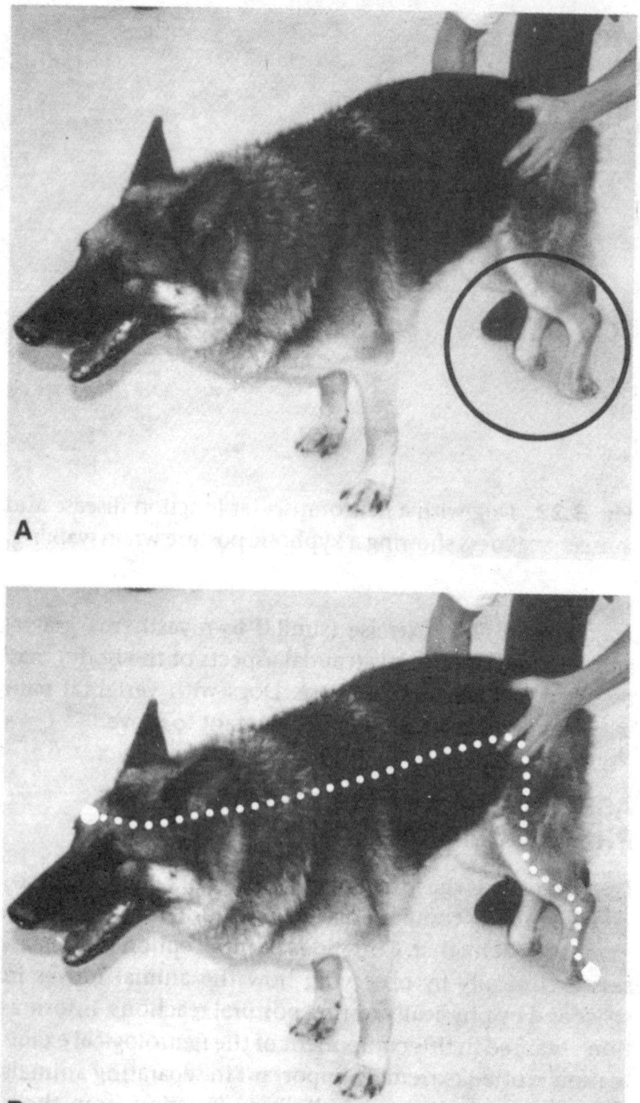

A

B

Fig. 3.23. Dog (A) with conscious proprioceptive deficits of the pelvic limbs and (B) showing the basic pathways.

standing of the flow of proprioceptive information to and from the limbs within the nervous system is important for accurate interpretation of conscious proprioceptive testing. Initially, the mechanoreceptors (touch and pressure) are excited to fire. This impulse is projected from these receptors proximally in peripheral nerves of the limb toward the spinal cord. The impulse ascends the spinal cord through the brain stem and thalamus to finally reach the sensory (parietal) cortex of the supratentorial region (fig. 3.23). The animal then *consciously* recognizes that the paw is in an abnormal position.

Subsequently, a motor response is generated, most likely in the motor portions of the supratentorial structures. An impulse is then caudally propagated through the brain stem, spinal cord, efferent (motor) peripheral nerve, and neuromuscular junction to excite the muscles necessary for correction of the paw. A normal animal should correct the paw immediately (less than 1 sec). This correction normally requires milliseconds. The smoothness of the muscle activity during correction of the paw is influenced by the cerebellum. In general, however, it is stated that with disease exclusively of the cerebellum, there is no delay in the initiation or performance of conscious proprioception.

A delay in correction of the paw is almost exclusively indicative of neurological or muscular disease. As can be seen from the extensiveness of the pathways involved, abnormal conscious proprioceptive function is not localizing to a specific area of the nervous system (see chapter 1). Importantly, a conscious proprioceptive deficit in a limb may be the result of either a UMN or LMN abnormality.

Conscious proprioceptive testing in this way provides important information in assessing the integrity of the nervous system. Contrary to popular belief, conscious proprioceptive testing, if performed properly, will not be abnormal in well-trained dogs.

Although relatively simple to perform, conscious proprioceptive testing can easily be misinterpreted. If, for example, an animal shifts its body weight to the nontested limb, when the tested paw is placed in the abnormal position, there is less impetus for the animal to react by replacing the paw. This is especially true if the animal is painful in the limb. In instances were pain of the limb may be confusing the results of the testing, the examiner may try to pull the lower limb slightly more caudally when turning the paw on its dorsum. This may excite other proprioceptive receptors in other regions of the limb (such as more proximately), and subsequently provide the animal with an additional stimulus to replace the limb.

In an animal with exclusive muscle weakness, conscious proprioception may be abnormal when the animal's full body weight is placed on the limb (fig. 3.24). This animal "understands" that the limb is abnormally positioned, but lacks adequate muscle strength to replace the limb. If this is suspected, the examiner should support the majority of the animal's body weight for the retest. In these animals, when their weight is supported by the examiner, they can often replace the paw normally. An animal that has conscious proprioceptive deficits when its body weight is placed on the tested limb but subsequently has normal conscious proprioceptive testing when the examiner supports the body weight should be suspected of having either primary muscle weakness or neuromuscular junction disease.

Some recommend the use of a paper slide test for conscious proprioceptive testing, wherein a piece of paper is placed below the weight-bearing foot of the animal. The paper is then slowly pulled laterally by the examiner. As the limb slides into an abnormal location from farther underneath the body, the animal will flex up the limb and replace it in its original position. This also tests conscious proprioception but may test proximal limb as compared to distal limb proprioception (Oliver et al. 1997).

If conscious proprioception is abnormal in the pelvic limbs bilaterally, this is referred to as *paraparesis*. If voluntary movement is also absent, this is referred to as *paraplegia* (fig. 3.25). If conscious proprioception is abnormal in only one limb, this is *monoparesis*. If all four limbs are ab-

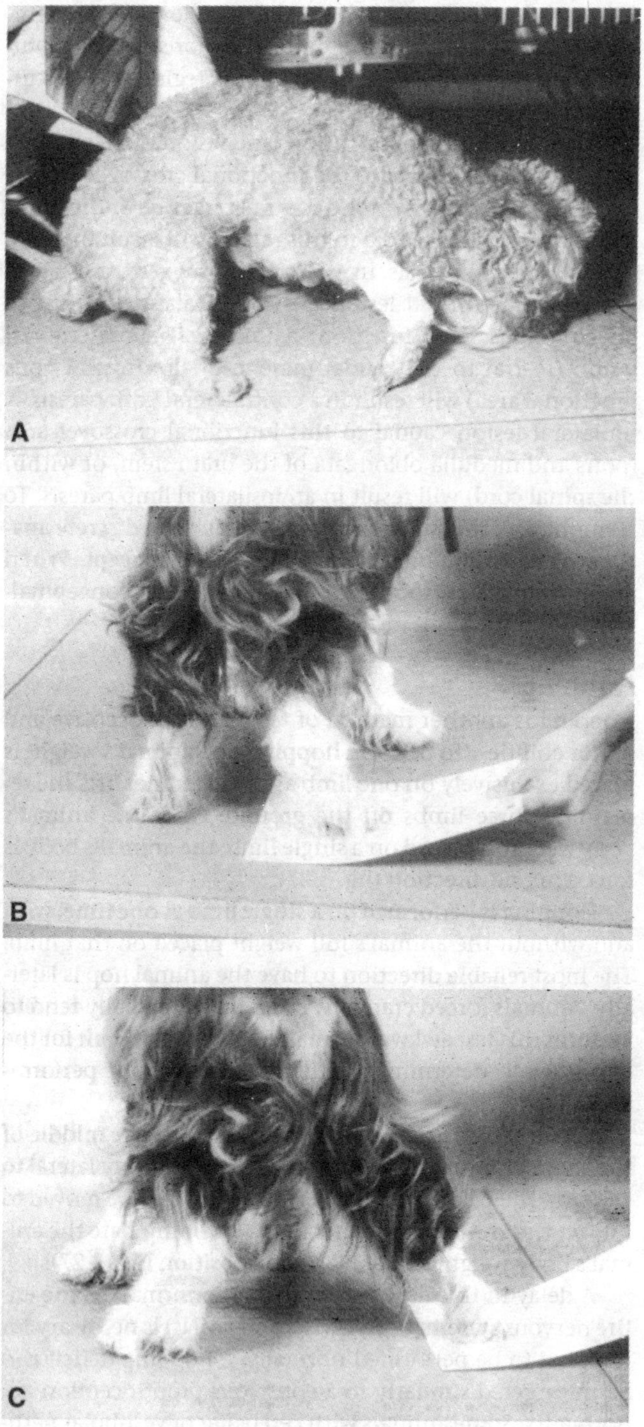

Fig. 3.24. (A) Dog with muscle weakness that is unable to support its own body weight. Paper slide test: (B) A piece of paper is placed under the foot; (C) the paper is then pulled laterally.

normal, the animal has *tetraparesis.* If the thoracic and pelvic limbs are affected on one side and on the same side, this is a *hemiparesis.*

In some animals with cervical or, occasionally, more rostral lesions, paresis is dissimilar in the thoracic compared to the pelvic limbs. More commonly in this situation, paresis is more obvious in the pelvic as compared to

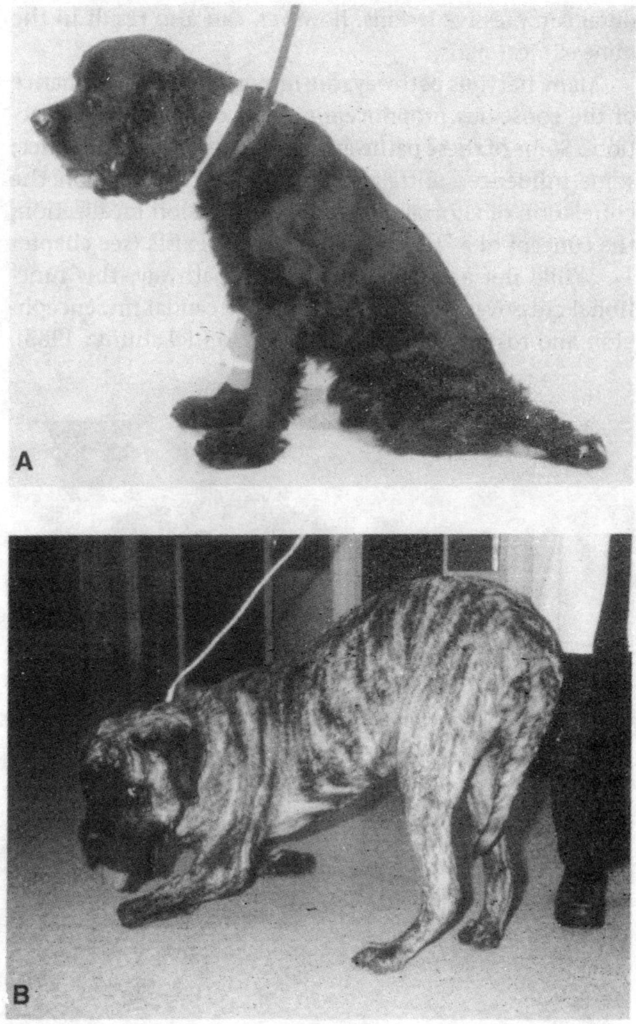

Fig. 3.25. (A) A dog with paraplegia and (B) a dog with conscious proprioceptive deficits in both thoracic limbs.

the thoracic limbs. Explanations for this include (1) there are quantitatively more UMN tracts influencing thoracic than pelvic limb function, (2) the pelvic limbs are farther from the center of gravity, and (3) tracts descending to the pelvic limbs are located more superficially in the spinal cord than those traveling to the thoracic limbs (deLahunta 1983; King 1987). This final explanation is based upon the somatotopic orientation of spinal cord tracts wherein tracts influencing specific body areas lie in specific anatomically discrete areas of the brain and spinal cord.

This somatotopic organization may be the same reason that some animals with a cervical spinal cord lesions present with paresis that is worse, or exclusively present, in the thoracic limbs as compared to the pelvic limbs (fig. 3.25). This presentation, termed *central cord syndrome,* implies that the more centrally (medially) located tracts influencing thoracic limb function are involved with the disease process preferentially as compared to the more laterally placed tracts traveling to the pelvic limbs. Often when these clinical signs are seen, intramedullary spinal lesions, such as syringomyelia or hydromyelia, are present. Extradural compressive lesions, however, can also result in the same clinical signs.

Many nervous pathways are important for performance of the conscious proprioception and other postural reactions. Some of these pathways have an ipsilateral influence; some influence contralateral structures. Based upon the correlation of clinical observation and lesion localization, the concept of a "functional crossover" exists (see chapter 1). While not a discrete anatomical pathway, this functional crossover is in the region of the caudal mesencephalon and rostral pons (figs. 3.22, 3.26) (deLahunta 1983).

A

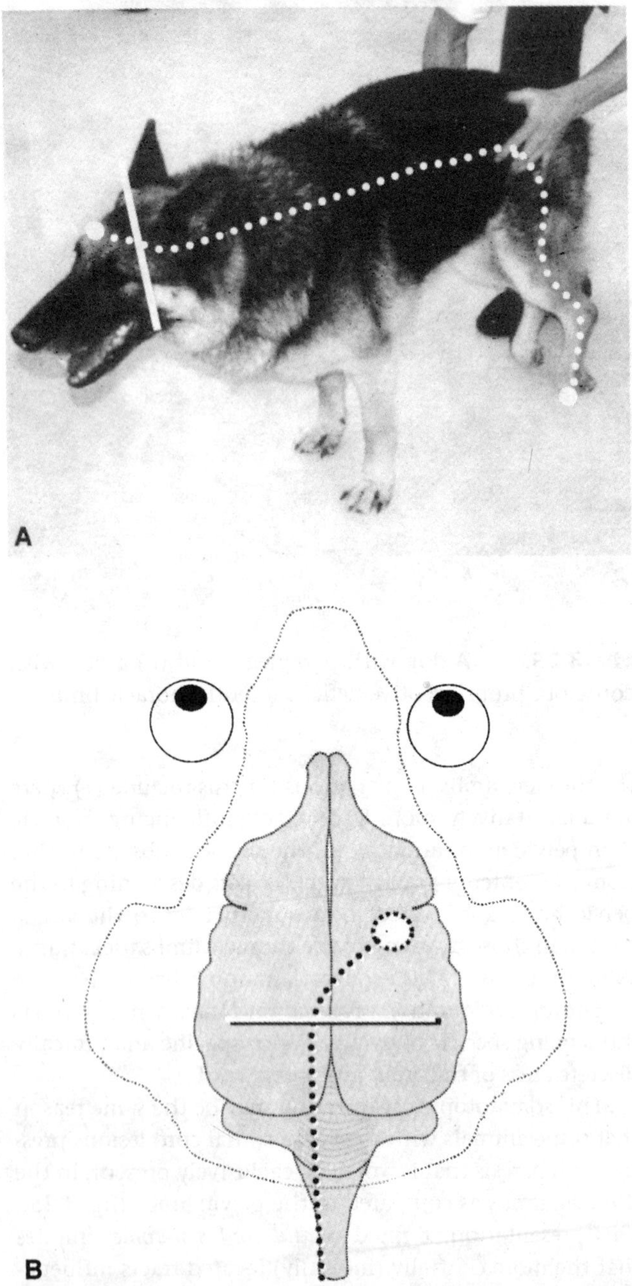

B

Fig. 3.26. (A) Dog with conscious proprioceptive deficits of the pelvic limbs showing the approximate level of the "functional cross-over." (B) Schematic dorsal view of the functional cross-over.

Somewhat conveniently, this is the same level of the nervous system where the supratentorial regions are conceptually separated from the infratentorial regions of the intracranial nervous system.

Based on clinical observations and lesion correlations, a unilateral lesion rostral to the functional crossover will result in (hemi-) paresis on the contralateral side of the body. A unilateral lesion caudal to this region will result in an ipsilateral (hemi-) paresis. In essence, this suggests that a unilateral supratentorial lesion has a contralateral influence on conscious limb function; a unilateral supratentorial lesion (rostral to the caudal mesencephalon/rostral pons junctional area) will result in a contralateral limb paresis. A unilateral lesion caudal to this functional crossover area (pons and medulla oblongata of the brain stem, or within the spinal cord) will result in an ipsilateral limb paresis. To reemphasize, the functional crossover is not a discrete anatomical structure, but rather a functional concept. When attempting lesion localization, however, this conceptualization is important.

Hopping

Hopping is another method of testing proprioceptive and motor abilities. To perform hopping, the animal's weight is placed exclusively on one limb as the examiner lifts the remaining three limbs off the ground. Once the animal's body weight is placed on a single limb, the animal's body is forced in one direction (fig. 3.27).

Hopping is performed on a single limb at one time, with and without the animal's full weight placed on that limb. The most reliable direction to have the animal hop is laterally. Animals forced cranially, caudally, or medially tend to perform this test awkwardly making it more difficult for the examiner to determine subtle abnormalities of performance.

When the animal's center of gravity (i.e., the middle of the thorax for the thoracic limb) is forced slightly lateral to the paw, the paw should be flexed and quickly be moved to impact the ground more laterally to accommodate the animal's body weight in the new body position (fig. 3.27).

A delay in this limb movement is abnormal. As the entire nervous system (both UMNs and LMNs) is necessary for hopping to be performed normally, a hopping deficit can be interpreted similarly to a conscious proprioception abnormality. Some animals with cerebellar or vestibular pathway lesions may have exaggerated limb movement when hopping (fig. 3.27).

Animals with neuromuscular weakness such as myasthenia gravis will not be able to hop normally when their full weight is placed on the limb, however, they will hop normally if the examiner supports the majority of the animal's weight. An animal that has a hopping deficit when full weight bearing, but not when its weight is supported by the examiner is, therefore, suspected of having neuromuscular disease.

In larger dogs, hopping becomes more difficult for the average examiner to perform. Also, animals with painful limbs, such as from musculoskeletal disease, may be unwill-

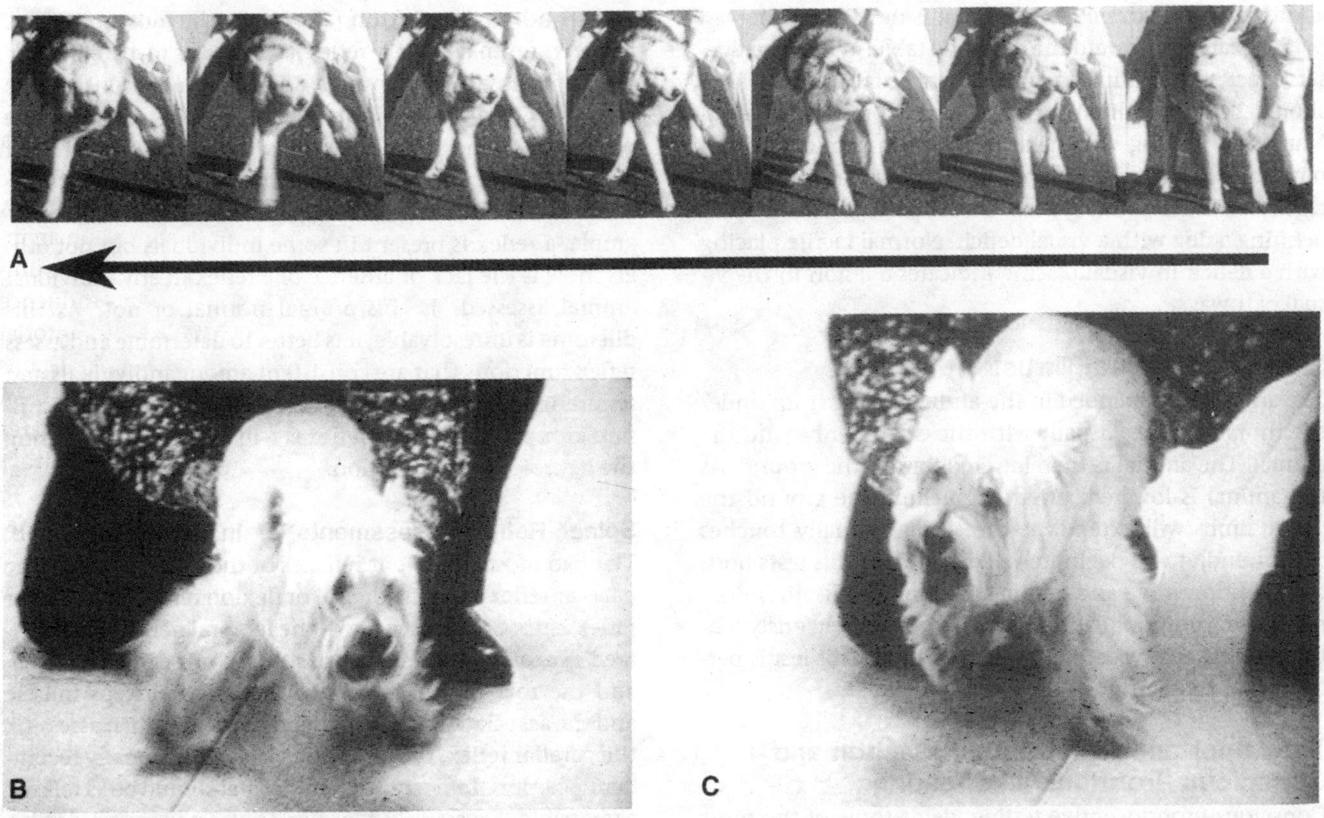

Fig. 3.27. (A) Dog showing hopping from right to left. Second dog shown hopping to (B) the right and (C) the left. Notice the exaggerated limb movement when hopping to the right. (A: from R. Bagley and I. Mayhew, Clinical examination of the nervous system, in Veterinary Clinical Examination and Diagnosis, eds. O. M. Radostits, I. G. J. May, and D. M. Houston [Harcourt Publishers Ltd., London, W. B. Saunders, 2000], fig. 19.14a.)

ing to perform due to the pain of moving and impacting the limb. A condition that limits limb mobility or contributes to the awkwardness of the animal's movement increases the difficulty of test interpretation. Hopping is, therefore, often reserved for use in smaller dogs and cats that are free of musculoskeletal or other painful conditions of the limbs.

Wheelbarrowing and Hemiwalking

These tests can be performed if conscious proprioception and hopping testing yields equivocal results or in large dogs where single-limb hopping is physically difficult for the examiner. For wheelbarrowing, the thoracic or pelvic limbs of the animal are lifted by the examiner so that the animal's weight is placed either on both pelvic or both thoracic limbs exclusively. The animal is then forced by the examiner to move its body. When testing the thoracic limbs, the animal is usually forced cranially or forward. When testing the pelvic limbs, the animal is usually forced backward or caudally. The animal should make normal walking movements in the limbs touching the ground. Wheelbarrowing of the thoracic limbs, especially if the head is concurrently held dorsally extended by the examiner, may be very helpful in assessing for subtle thoracic limb paresis not revealed by other tests. This test can be negatively influenced by similar factors that negatively influence hopping.

For hemistanding and hemiwalking, the thoracic and pelvic limbs on the same side of the animal are lifted by the examiner so that the animal's weight is placed either on one side of the limbs (thoracic and pelvic) or on the other exclusively. For assessment of hemistanding, a determination of how well the animal can stand and support weight is made. For hemiwalking, the animal is then forced by the examiner to move its body, usually in a lateral direction, as with hopping. With hemiwalking, however, the combination of movements of the thoracic limb and ipsilateral pelvic limb is assessed. As the animal is forced laterally, the animal should move the limbs, usually one at a time, to a more lateral location as when hopping.

If an animal has obvious abnormalities on conscious proprioceptive testing and hopping, it is not necessary to perform these tests as no additional clinical information will be obtained. This test also can be negatively influenced by similar factors that negatively influence hopping.

Placing

Placing is performed by supporting the animal's weight and moving the animal toward a table edge, for example. Placing can be performed when the animal is able to see the table edge, or nonvisually by covering one or both of the animal's eyes. The nonvisual reactions are assessed first. The animal is suspended off the ground by the examiner and its eyes are covered. The animal is next slowly moved by the examiner toward the edge of a table. When the dorsal aspect of the animal's paw touches the table, the animal should bring the limb forward to rest on the tabletop. Nonvisual placing will yield information similar to hopping and conscious proprioception tests concerning the integrity of the nervous system. Visual placing may help in defining a dog with a visual deficit. Normal tactile placing with a deficit in visual placing indicates a lesion in the visual pathways.

Extensor Postural Thrust

The animal is suspended in the air by picking it up under the thoracic limbs, usually with the examiner behind the animal. The animal is then lowered toward the ground. As the animal is lowered, prior to touching the ground the pelvic limbs will extend. As the animal actually touches the ground, it will begin to walk backward. This tests both the proprioceptive and vestibular systems and often does not yield additional information to that previously obtained with other postural reaction testing. This test is performed infrequently.

The Importance of Postural Reaction and Conscious Proprioceptive Testing

Conscious proprioceptive testing yields some of the most important information concerning the integrity of the central and peripheral nervous systems. Conscious proprioceptive testing is commonly abnormal with lesions of the peripheral nerves, spinal cord, and intracranial nervous structures. The muscular system is necessary to perform movements initiated and controlled by the nervous system. Conscious proprioceptive testing is often used to distinguish neurologic from nonneurologic causes of limb dysfunction.

ASSESSMENT AND ABNORMALITIES OF SPINAL REFLEXES

Spinal reflex function does not require conscious or voluntary input for performance. Reflex function is more of a localized nervous system function. The reflex arc includes the stretch or touch receptor (sensory), the afferent peripheral nerve, the associated neuron elements of specific spinal segments, the efferent nerve, neuromuscular junction, and muscle. Reflexes can be fairly simplistic, such as when having a monosynaptic connection, or involve more complex associations of regional nerve connections or polysynaptic. Reflex functions can be performed through the spinal nerve and associated peripheral nerves, the cranial nerves, or through autonomic nerves. Cranial nerve reflex function is discussed under Cranial Nerve Assessment below.

Assessment of Spinal Reflexes

Spinal reflexes are primarily evaluated in the limbs of the thoracic and pelvic limbs. Reflexes classically assessed in the pelvic limb include the patellar, cranial tibial, gastrocnemius, and flexion or withdrawal, however, the patellar and withdrawal or flexion reflexes are the most consistent between animals. For a reflex assessment to be clinically useful, it must be present in a way that can be consistently assessed. Certain historically described reflex functions are present in some normal animals but are not present in other normal animals. These inconsistencies create difficulties for the clinician during patient evaluation. If, for example, a reflex is present in some individuals but not others, how is the lack or absence of a reflex in any individual animal assessed? Is this animal normal or not? As this dilemma is unresolvable, it is better to determine and assess reflex functions that are consistent among individuals and ignore inconsistently present reflexes. Assessment of a finite group of consistent reflexes will also save time during the neurologic examination.

Spinal Reflex Assessments of in the Pelvic Limb. The two most consistent reflexes of the pelvic limb are the patellar reflex and withdrawal or flexion reflex. The patellar reflex assesses the integrity of the femoral nerve, the associated neuronal elements of the spinal cord segments L4–L6, and the mechanical apparatus of the quadriceps muscle and the associated straight patellar tendon. When assessing the patellar reflex, the animal is placed in a laterally recumbent position. Importantly, the animal should be as relaxed as possible. Excessively tense or contracted muscles in an animal that is apprehensive or constantly trying to stand up can override the reflex contraction of the quadriceps muscle.

The upside limb reflex is most accurately assessed. The straight patellar tendon is palpated and assessed for disease. The straight patellar tendon should feel like a taut band of tissue between the distal end of the femoral and the proximal tibia. In rare instances, this tendon will be ruptured and will feel slack. In other situations where there is severe, usually chronic disease of the stifle joint, the dimensions and the definition of the tendon may be inconspicuous. Sometimes it is helpful for the examiner to place a hand on the inside of the limb in the groin area to elevate the limb slightly. Ideally, the limb will be suspended freely to avoid any mechanical hindrance to reflex performance.

The straight patellar tendon is lightly tapped with a reflex hammer or similar instrument (fig. 3.28). As assessment of reflex functions is based on the subjective opinion of the examiner, it is important to maintain consistency in examination technique between patients. Therefore, it is ideal to use the same instrument for percussion on all patients similarly tested. The straight patellar tendon does not need to be struck aggressively, therefore the percussion hammer should be held relatively lightly between the fingers and hand of the examiner. In many instances, the hammer is used more as a pendulum to strike the tendon.

Almost instantaneously as the straight patella ligament is tapped, there is a quick extension of the stifle and an associated leg-kicking action. Lack of this reaction indicates either that the animal is tense, the reflex was performed incorrectly, there is a mechanical problem with the tendon or stifle joint, or the reflex is absent due to neurologic disease.

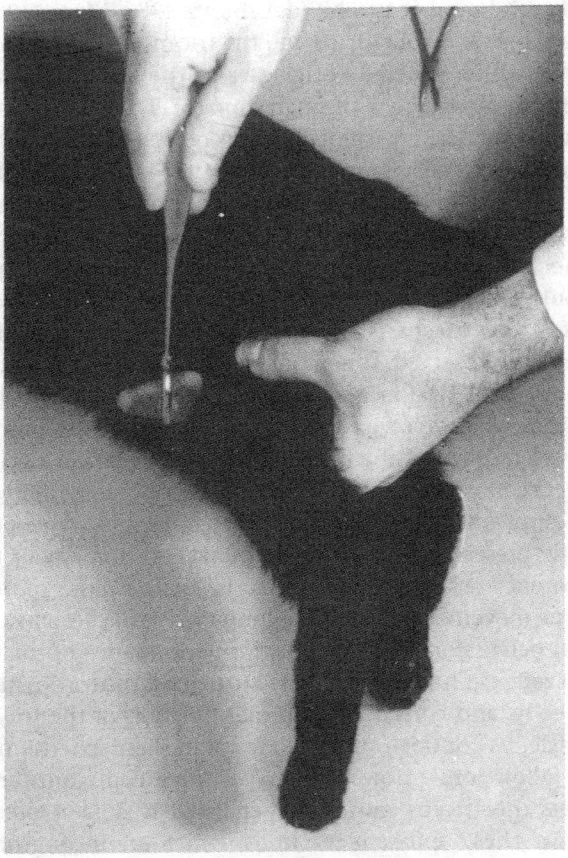

Fig. 3.28. Position of the limb for performance of the patellar reflex.

If no reaction is initiated, the examiner should repeat the test as many times as necessary to determine the integrity of the reflex arc. The degree and extent of the extension of the stifle is used as a measure of the strength of the reflex. Again, assessment of reflex functions is directly dependent on the knowledge and experience of the examiner, as all reflex assessments require subjective interpretation. The most accurate assessments will be made by those examiners experienced in the spectrum of reactions possible in both normal and abnormal animals. Assessment of numerous normal dogs with regard to reflex functions ensures accurate assessment of abnormal reflex functions.

If the animal is tense, or if there is conformation change in the stifle, no reflex may be present in otherwise neurologically normal animals. Sometimes, although it is not ideal, assessing the reflex in the down limb may help in the determination of whether the animal is overriding the reflex by being tense in the upside limb. As the animal is lying on the down limb, it is less likely to feel compelled to tense or move that limb, and therefore a reflex is more likely to be obvious. If when the limb is in an upward position, no patellar reflex is encountered, however, when the limb is assessed in the downward position a reflex is present in the same limb, the examiner should be suspicious that lack of reflex in the upward position is misleading. It may not be possible to accurately assess the quality of the reflex in the down limb, as the contact with the floor and other parts of the body may inhibit the full extension of the stifle.

Table 3.4. Assessment of spinal reflexes

Functional score	Assessment
0	Absent
1	Decreased
2	Normal
3	Exaggerated
4	Clonus (persistently contracted muscle)

In some animals that are tense, the degree of muscle reaction may appear excessive relative to the stimulus. This is more common in younger animals and in apprehensive or excited animals. The reflex in these individuals is also falsely exaggerated.

When evaluating spinal reflex function, the presence or absence as well as the magnitude of response are important. Spinal reflexes are usually graded on a scale ranging from absent to decreased to excessive or exaggerated (table 3.4). Obviously, a normal reflex would be found in the middle of these extremes.

It is important to remember that the functional score given to a reflex is a subjective evaluation based upon examiner experience. The clinician should examine as many normal animals as possible to gain this experience. It is most important for the examiner to determine if the reflexes are at least normal versus decreased or absent. In the presence of signs of neurologic dysfunction, as in an animal with conscious proprioceptive deficits, reflex assessments are used to determine the integrity of the LMN. If the animal has conscious proprioceptive deficits in a limb and the spinal reflexes are intact, the lesion in the nervous system most likely is in the UMN. Animals with UMN lesions most commonly have normal but sometimes exaggerated spinal reflexes.

Conversely, if the lesion resulting in the deficit of conscious proprioception involves the LMN, the reflex function of LMN will usually be affected. Therefore, the spinal reflexes tend to be decreased to absent. An animal is determined to have an LMN abnormality based on the decreased to absent character of the spinal reflexes.

The withdrawal or flexion reflexes in the pelvic limb are used primarily to assess the integrity of the sciatic nerve and its associated spinal segments (L6 to sacral [S] 1). This reflex is elicited by pinching the toes and looking for appropriate flexion of the hock and stifle joints to move the paw away from this stimulus. If, however, the toe is pinched more aggressively, pain pathways projected to the brain may also be elicited. In this situation, the animal may enhance the reflex withdrawing with added voluntary withdrawing of the limb. The amount of toe pressure that elicits an added voluntary withdrawal of the limb varies in individual dogs. Some dogs are extremely sensitive to palpation of the paws and toes and, therefore, have excessive voluntary reactions. This variability adds to the subjective interpretation of the reflex on the part of the examiner.

Also important to remember is that a reflex withdraw-

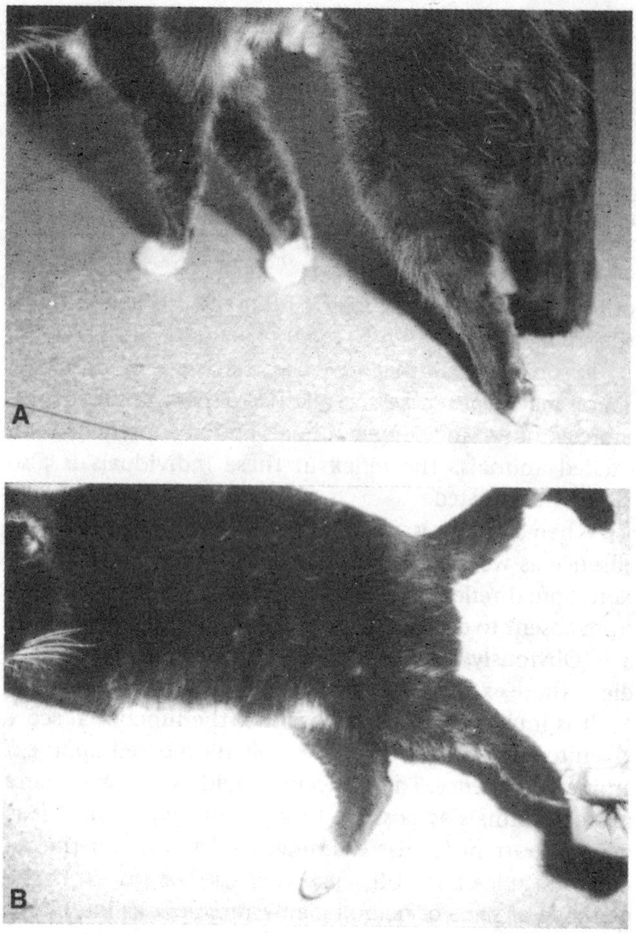

Fig. 3.29. Cat showing (A) decreased conscious proprioception and (B) poor withdrawal reflex with poor hock flexion.

ing of the limb should not be interpreted as a conscious activity of the animal. For example, animals with spinal cord transactions cranial to the lumbar spinal cord may not consciously recognize their pelvic limbs, however, they can often still withdraw the limb as a result of local reflex mechanisms.

The withdrawal reflex is similarly assessed as being absent, decreased, normal, or exaggerated. Decreased ability to adequately flex the hock is usually the most notable spinal reflex abnormality when sciatic disease is present (fig. 3.29).

The cranial tibial and gastrocnemius reflexes are sometimes suggested as assessments of the sciatic nerve (L6–S1). The cranial tibial reflex assesses the peroneal branch, and the gastrocnemius reflex assesses the tibial branch. As with the thoracic limb muscles, the muscle bellies or tendon of insertion are percussed and an appropriate response is seen. When the cranial tibial muscle is percussed, slight hock flexion should be seen. Percussion of the gastrocnemius muscle should result in hock extension. Unfortunately, these apparent reflexes are less consistent in normal animals and, therefore, less clinically useful.

Spinal reflexes classically assessed in the thoracic limb include the extensor carpi radialis, the biceps, the triceps, and withdrawal or flexion (deLahunta 1983; Moore 1992). The extensor carpi radialis and the triceps assess the radial nerve, which generally originates in the spinal cord segments of cervical (C)7 through thoracic (T)1. The biceps reflex assesses the musculocutaneous nerve (spinal cord segments C6–C8). These reflexes are elicited by percussing the muscle belly to tendon of insertion of the individual muscles and observing for the appropriate muscle response. When the extensor carpi radialis is percussed, the carpus should extend slightly due to contraction of this muscle. When the triceps is percussed, slight elbow extension should be observed. When the biceps muscle is stimulated, slight elbow flexion may be seen. With the latter reflex, movement may be slight and not visualized. The examiner, however, may feel the muscle contract by placing a finger over the muscle during percussion. Unfortunately, many of the apparent reflexes of the thoracic limb are inconsistently present among normal animals. Also, many of the apparent "reflex" reactions may in fact be more spontaneous movement of multiple limb muscles in response to local percussion. For example, for performance of the triceps reflex, it has been suggested to percuss the triceps muscle belly, and considering normal function of the triceps muscle, its contraction should result in slight extension of the elbow joint. However, what is more commonly seen when the triceps muscle is percussed is flexion of the elbow. These apparent reactions, which are incongruous with normal anatomical functions of a muscle group, make these reactions questionable at best.

The flexion or withdrawal reflex of the thoracic limb is elicited by pinching the toes and looking for flexion of the carpal and elbow joints in order to move the paw away from this stimulus. This reflex assesses all major nerves of the thoracic limb including the radial, ulnar, median, musculocutaneous, and axillary. This reflex is dependent upon examiner interpretation, as there is probably a component of voluntary withdrawal that may be present concurrently with any reflex withdrawal. The degree to which the animal voluntarily pulls its limb away from the stimulus primarily depends upon the degree of stimulus intensity (i.e., how hard the toes are pinched).

The Importance of Clinical Assessment of Spinal Reflex Function. In essence, the nervous system works through the influence of central controlling systems or UMNs and their interaction with nerves that exit the central nervous system to terminate on effector organs such as muscles. As the central nervous system does not directly connect to the organs or muscles, a second functional nervous system is necessary for stimulation of a muscle or organ. This system is conceptualized as more rudimentary, or reflex in function, with these reflex functions being primarily performed by components of the peripheral nervous system and cranial nerves. This system is referred to as the lower motor neuron (LMN). The LMN is analogous to the efferent (motor) peripheral nervous system and the effector organs (primarily muscles). The peripheral nervous system includes any nerve myelinated by a Schwann cell.

Schwann cells begin myelinating peripheral nerves to the limbs at the intervertebral foramen. Using this strict definition, other functional components of the LMN, such as the cell body of the motor neuron in the ventral grey of the spinal cord, would not be included in the peripheral nervous system. Functionally, however, a lesion of the peripheral nerve or cell body would result in identical clinical signs as a lesion in the peripheral nerve. Therefore, the terms "peripheral nervous system" and "LMN" are used interchangeably in some publications.

An important assessment of LMN function in animals occurs through assessment of spinal reflex function. As many reflex functions also require peripheral sensory input (see Spinal Reflex Function, chapter 1), and disease of the afferent peripheral sensory systems may result in decreased or absent spinal reflexes, diseases of the peripheral sensory nervous system are often grouped under diseases affecting the LMN.

Abnormalities of Reflex Function

Upper motor neuron lesions do not diminish local spinal reflex functions. Therefore, spinal reflexes in the presence of disease of the UMN are at least normal. In some instances, the UMN systems have a "dampening" effect on spinal reflexes. When this dampening effect is removed with UMN lesions, spinal reflexes may become exaggerated.

Conversely, disease of the LMN usually affects the reflex arc at some level, and therefore results in decreased to absent reflexes. Hypo- or areflexia can signify either peripheral nervous system, neuromuscular, or muscle disease. With spinal cord disease, depending upon which reflexes are affected, the level of spinal segment involvement can be identified. For example, a decreased patellar reflex might result from a lesion of the L4 to L6 spinal segments. A decreased withdrawal reflex might result from a lesion of the L6 to S1 spinal segments (see chapter 1).

With most reflexes, some muscle or muscle group is stimulated. Muscles that counterbalance the activity of the stimulated muscle may be concurrently inhibited. As an example, when the quadriceps muscle contracts during performance of the patellar reflex, antagonistic muscles such as the semimembranous and semitendinosis, innervated primarily by the sciatic nerve, prevent excessive movements of the stifle. With sciatic disease, when the patellar reflex is initiated, loss of innervation to the antagonistic muscles for this result may result in unopposed contraction of the quadriceps and apparently exaggerated stifle extension. This apparent increase in reflex performance resulting from the loss of sciatic nerve innervation to the antagonistic muscles of this reflex is termed *pseudohyperreflexia*.

Lower motor neuron innervation to muscles is also important for muscle tone. Tone is the low-intensity state of resting muscle activity and provides some resistance to passive range of motion of the limb. Muscles may also be actively depolarized resulting in muscle contraction, therefore causing active muscle tone. Resting muscle tone is likely mediated through the gamma efferent innervation to the intrafusal muscle fibers. Resting tone is partially regulated by the UMN influence on the gamma efferent system. In an activated state, UMN influences may result in contraction of muscles and hence increase muscle active tone. Resting tone in the limbs may be increased with lesions of the UMN systems. This is commonly referred to as spasticity and results in a stiff or rigidly extended limb.

With LMN lesions, resting muscle tone is often decreased. In this instance, when the limb is passively manipulated, the muscle appears flaccid or like a "wet noodle." This decrease in resting muscle tone is often an important clue to the presence of LMN disease.

When the withdrawal reflex is tested, some animals with UMN lesions may extend the opposite limb, termed the *crossed extensor reflex* (deLahunta 1983). The description is somewhat confusing, as the term "crossed extensor reflex" is actually the normal reflex when the animal is standing. However, the term has been applied in the veterinary literature to describe an abnormal reaction of this reflex.

The crossed extensor reflex is actually more a reaction to flexion of a limb in a standing animal. In a normal animal standing on both limbs, the body's weight is usually equally distributed on these limbs. As one limb is flexed, the contralateral limb reflexly extends in preparation to support more of the animal's weight that is not supported by the flexed limb. When an animal is placed in a laterally recumbent position, descending UMN systems normally inhibit this reflex as the crossed extensor phenomenon is unnecessary (i.e., no body weight being supported by the limbs). Therefore, when assessing the up limb withdrawal reflex, there is no contralateral limb extension. If the withdrawal reflex is tested in the down limb, the animal may sense the need to roll away from the down limb in preparation for standing and, therefore, reflexly extend the up limb. This is a normal reaction when the down limb withdraw reflex is tested.

With some UMN abnormalities, when the animal is placed in the laterally recumbent position and the up limb is tested for the withdrawal reflex, the down limb may reflex extend. This is an abnormal reflex when the animal is lying on its side. Damage to the descending UMN pathways that normally inhibit this reflex allow this reflex to resurface inappropriately. With UMN abnormalities, then, when the up limb is flexed, the down limb may reflexly extend. Even though it is a normal reflex in a standing animal, this phenomenon in a laterally recumbent animal is still termed a crossed extensor reflex. A more accurate description of this clinical phenomenon may be an *abnormal crossed extensor reflex*.

An abnormal crossed extensor reflex is more apt to be present when the UMN lesion has been present a longer time (i.e., chronically). It is rare to observe an abnormal crossed extensor reflex with acute UMN abnormalities. This abnormal reflex can occur in either the pelvic or thoracic limbs, but is more commonly identified in the pelvic limbs. If this abnormal reflex occurs in the pelvic limbs, the UMN lesion is cranial to the L3 spinal segments; if this reflex occurs in the thoracic limb, the UMN lesion is cranial to C6 spinal segments.

Because the connection between the peripheral nerve and the muscle is required to maintain muscle mass, atrophy that occurs after a complete peripheral nerve injury is severe (neurogenic atrophy) and evolves over a shorter period of time (may be present within 5 days of a severe peripheral nerve injury). This is discussed further under Muscle Atrophy below.

In summary, in an animal with neurologic impairment (i.e., conscious proprioceptive deficits), decreased to absent spinal reflexes, decreased to absent resting muscle tone, and acute, relatively severe muscle atrophy are hallmarks of a lesion involving the LMN. Conversely, normal to exaggerated spinal reflexes, normal to increased resting muscle tone, and disuse muscle atrophy (more slowly evolving, and less severe in degree) are hallmarks of a lesion involving the UMN systems. This distinction becomes extremely important when considering the location of lesions involving the nervous system.

ASSESSMENT OF OTHER REFLEX FUNCTIONS

Reflex functions can be performed by other nerves originating in the spinal cord, cranial nerves, or autonomic nerves. *Anal reflex* function, for example, is assessed by stimulating the perianal area and observing for the contraction of the external anal sphincter muscles. The tail will often be flexed concurrently. An anal contraction can usually also be elicited by squeezing the penis of a male or the clitoris of a female dog. Stimulation during direct rectal palpation should also result in anal sphincter contraction. This reflex is mediated through the pelvic and pudendal nerves to the internal and external anal sphincter, respectively. Both the pelvic and pudendal nerves arise from the S1–S3 spinal cord segments. Decreased anal sphincter reflex function and decreased anal tone may result in a dilated anus and poor to absent anal contraction with local stimulation. In most instances, however, direct rectal palpation to assess the tone of the anal sphincter region is more sensitive to detect decrease in tone and local reflex function.

The *Babinski reflex* is another abnormal reflex commonly observed in human beings with UMN disease (Chrisman 1991). When the ventral foot or paw is stroked, such as with the handle end of a percussion hammer, the toes normally should curl (flex) toward the sole of the foot. With UMN lesions in adult human beings, when the sole of the foot is stroked, the toes may extend and flair outward. This is referred to as a positive Babinski reflex. This abnormality may be seen in some dogs with UMN lesions but is inconsistently present (Chrisman 1991).

The *cutaneous trunci reflex* or *panniculus reflex* tests superficial pain receptors, the spinal cord, and the lateral thoracic nerves. This reflex is elicited by pinching the skin over the dermatomal areas associated with the dorsal thoracolumbar area. The efferent response is contraction of the cutaneous trunci muscles bilaterally (fig. 3.30).

The receptor in the dermatomal distribution over the dorsal trunk is excited by the pinching stimulus, which sends an impulse through the dorsal sensory afferent nerve to the spinal cord. Within the spinal cord, prior to where the lateral thoracic nerves exit, this pathway becomes bilateral in function. The impulse travels cranially in the spinal cord to reach the cell bodies of the lateral thoracic nerves. These cell bodies are located at the C8–T1 spinal cord segments. The lateral thoracic nerves exit the spinal cord and course to the cutaneous trunci muscles.

The cutaneous trunci reflex is most helpful when evaluating lesions in the T2–L3 area and the brachial plexus. With lesions in the T2–L3 area, the cutaneous trunci reflex may be absent caudal to the spinal segment involved. Since the dermatomal distribution of the cutaneous nerves in the thoracolumbar area is caudal to the corresponding spinal cord segments, the lesion is approximately one vertebral segment cranial to where the cutaneous trunci reflex is lost.

While there is some debate as to the exact dermatomal distribution in the flank area, it appears clinically that the T12 through L1–L2 dermatomes are distributed from the last rib to the cranial border of the wings of the ilium (Griffiths 1989). Therefore, a dog with a normal cutaneous trunci reflex and UMN signs to the pelvic limbs should have a lesion in the L2–L3 spinal cord segments.

With a unilateral lesion of the lateral thoracic nerve (or its associated cell bodies) such as might occur with a brachial plexus injury, contraction of the cutaneous trunci muscle occurs only on the side opposite the lesion, without regard to which side of the body the dermatomes are excited. Because the normal side contracts no matter which side of the body is stimulated, the spinal pathways for this reflex are assumed to be intact.

Muscle Atrophy

The muscles should be assessed for loss of muscle mass or atrophy. Muscle size is most readily assessed by palpating both sides of the animal simultaneously in the standing animal. Muscle atrophy may be evidenced by decreases in muscle size or more prominence underlying bony structures. Muscle mass may be altered depending upon the degree of previous activity of the animal. Muscle mass may also vary between individuals and individual breeds. When muscle atrophy is present, this may be due to three general processes.

As the connection between the peripheral nerve and the muscle is required to maintain muscle mass, atrophy can occur following peripheral nerve disease that interrupts the muscle nerve connection. This type of atrophy is relatively severe and evolves over a shorter period of time (may be present within 5 days of a severe peripheral nerve injury). It is not uncommon that underlying bony structures are very prominent. This type of muscle atrophy is referred to as neurogenic atrophy.

Muscles may also atrophy when they are not used normally. The hallmark of this atrophy is the muscle atrophy that occurs when a limb is immobilized as in a cast. Disuse atrophy may occur with UMN lesions as the inappropriate coordination of muscle activity leads to improper normal

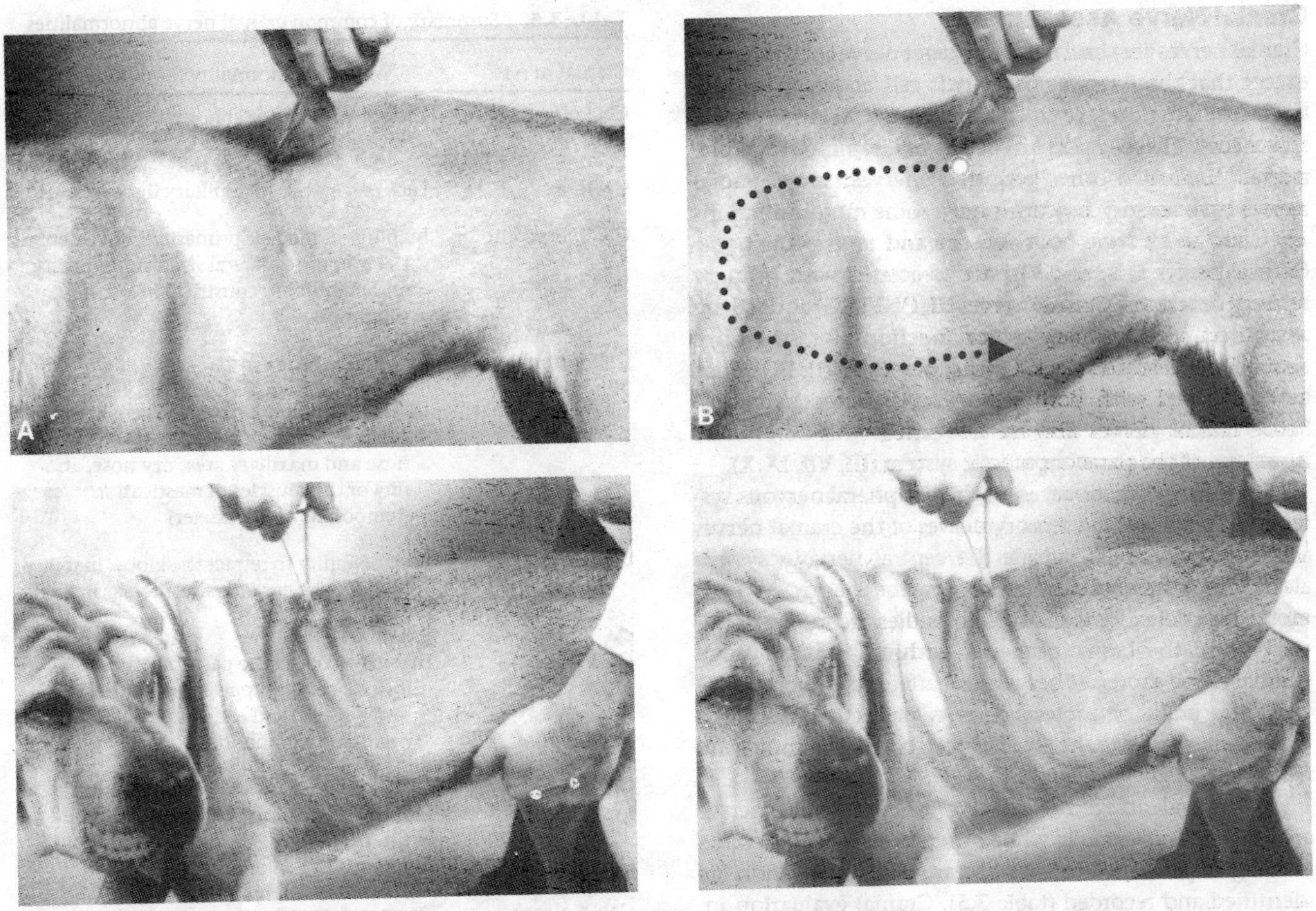

Fig. 3.30. (A) Dog before (*top*) and after (*bottom*) stimulation of the cutaneous trunci reflex and subsequent contraction of the cutaneous trunci muscle. (B) Dog before (*top*) and after (*bottom*) stimulation of the cutaneous trunci reflex with schematic representation of the pathway.

use. Disuse atrophy tends to evolve more slowly (i.e., over weeks to months) and is usually less severe than LMN atrophy unless the atrophy is very chronic in duration.

Finally, muscle atrophy may occur due an inherent abnormality of the muscle itself. Primary muscle diseases are referred to as myopathies.

Within these guidelines, the types of muscle atrophy may be difficult to separate in the clinical patient. Localized atrophy within a single muscle group suggests a neurogenic cause, however, in some instances such as infraspinatous contracture, a primary myopathic cause is present. With sciatic disease, muscle atrophy of the cranial tibial muscles is often easily assessed. Significant paraspinal muscle atrophy is often associated with diskospondylitis (fig. 3.31).

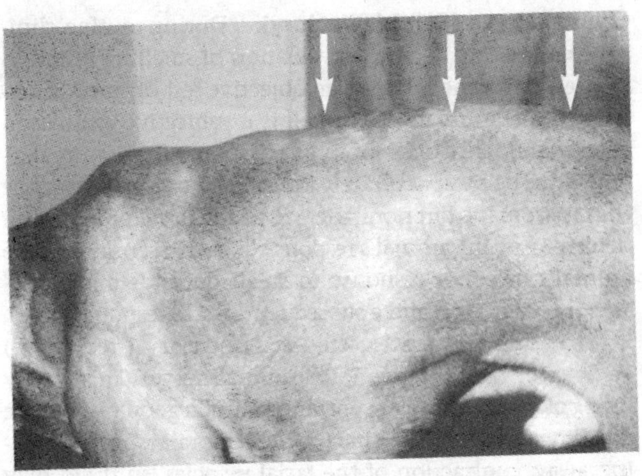

Fig. 3.31. Dog with diskospondylitis and paraspinal muscle atrophy (*arrows*).

Palpation

At the time the muscles are palpated for atrophy, the rest of the body can be palpated for abnormalities. In the head region, an incomplete fusion of the skull bones, or "soft spot," is termed a *fontanel*. While not pathognomic, this clinical finding in animals older than a few weeks of age may indicate an associated hydrocephalus (Spaulding and Sharp 1990). A fontanel is most often present over the dorsal aspect of the skull over the frontal and parietal areas.

Enlargements or swellings of the limbs may be present. Vertebral incongruities may also be palpated. Most importantly, focally painful regions can be identified (see Hyperesthesia below).

Cranial Nerve Assessment

Cranial nerves are similar to peripheral nerves of the limbs, except that these nerves have their cell bodies in the intracranial structures, or in the case of CN XI, the cervical spinal cord. There are 12 pairs of bilateral symmetric cranial nerves. Similar to other peripheral nerves, some cranial nerves have sensory functions only, some motor functions only, and some have both sensory and motor functions. Cranial nerves I, II, and VIII are associated with primary sensory functions. Cranial nerves III, IV, VI, XI, and XII are associated with primary motor functions for structures around the head and neck. Cranial nerves V, VII, IX, and X are associated with both sensory and motor functions. Some cranial nerves also are associated with autonomic functions of the parasympathetic system (III, VII, IX,X).

For sensory functions, as for the peripheral nervous system, cell bodies of the sensory nerves of the cranial nerves are found in ganglia outside the central nervous system along the course of the nerve. For cranial nerves with motor functions, motor nerve cell bodies are found in nuclei within the brain, primarily within the brain stem. Cranial nerve axons, either sensory afferents projecting toward the brain or motor efferents projecting from the brain, enter or exit the skull through the foramina and fissures.

When evaluating cranial nerve function, some nerves are assessed individually while others are assessed as functional groups. Abnormalities of cranial nerve function are identified and recorded (table 3.5). Cranial evaluation includes both observation and active testing of conscious reactions and local reflexes. Usually, a systematic evaluation is followed so that all important cranial nerve functions are assessed during the clinical examination.

Table 3.5. Summary of common cranial nerve abnormalities

Cranial nerve	Abnormality
CN I olfactory	Lack of smelling or abnormalities of smelling
CN II optic	Lack of vision and pupillary light reflexes
CN III oculomotor	Inability of medial (primarily) movement of the eye, ventrolateral strabismus, ptosis, and inability to constrict the pupil (mydriasis)
CN IV trochlear	Extorsion of the eye
CN V trigeminal	Lack of sensation to the eye and cornea, corneal ulcers, lack of sensation to the nose and maxillary area, dry nose, atrophy of the muscles of mastication (temporalis and masseter)
CN VI abducents	Lack of ability to retract the globe, inability to move the eye laterally, medial strabismus
CN VII facial	Inability to close the palpebral fissure (blink); droopy appearance of the lips, lower eyelid, and ear; abnormal taste; decreased lacrimation
CN VIII	
Vestibular portion	Loss of balance and posture, ataxia, head tilt, nystagmus, falling or rolling
Cochlear portion	Abnormal or loss of hearing
CN IX glosso-pharyngeal	Decreased gagging or swallowing
CN X vagus	Decreased gagging or swallowing, alterations in esophageal and gastrointestinal motility, megaesophagus
CN XI accessory	Atrophy of the trapezius muscle, turning the neck
CN XII hypoglossal	Lack of movement of the tongue, atrophy of the tongue, deviation of the tongue laterally from the mouth

Cranial Nerve (CN) I (Olfactory). During routine clinical examination, a critical evaluation of smelling function is rarely performed. Unless an objective test of smell is performed, determination of smell is a subjective evaluation (the examiner's) of a subjective response (the animal's). Smell can be most accurately assessed by using a substance that is aromatic but nonirritating to the nasal mucosa and determining the animal's response to such a sensation. The animal's behavior response to smell depends upon conscious recognition and a subsequent motor response.

Irritating substances will excite sensory (free nerve) endings of cranial nerve V (trigeminal nerve). This is why using alcohol or similar substance is not a good test of true smelling function. The olfactory behavioral response (turning away, contraction of the facial muscles, sniffing) may be used to test for the presence or absence of olfaction. If a more objective assessment of smelling function is necessary, electroencephalographic (brain electrical activity) monitoring may provide it (Myers 1990). Odors used include eugenol, a pure olfactory nerve stimulant, and benzaldehyde, which stimulates both olfactory and trigmenial receptors.

Anosmia (loss of smell) is most often recognized secondary to bilateral nasal passage disease. Unilateral lesions in the supratentorial structure will not cause anosmia as the integration of smell is a bilateral function. Bilateral olfactory lobe disease can result in anosmia. Viral infections such as distemper and parainfluenza may also cause anosmia. Clinically, dysosmia (abnormal smell) is almost impossible to determine unless further objective testing with various smells is performed.

Assessment of Vision and Pupils. Disease of the ocular structure or nervous system can result in visual or pupillary abnormalities. For assessment of ocular health, an ophthalmic examination is important. Vision is a function of cranial nerve II and other portions of the central nervous system. Pupillary functions are controlled by a reciprocal relationship between the sympathetic and parasympathetic nervous systems. Parasympathetic function to the pupil is the result of activation of CN III.

Cranial Nerve (CN) II (Optic Nerve). Cranial nerve II is associated with visual functions. Anatomical areas within the nervous system necessary for vision include the eye, the optic nerve, the central projection pathways to the visual cortex (occipital), cortical association and projection pathways, and finally, motor neurons necessary to complete motor responses to visual stimuli. Visual functions during a clinical examination can be assessed by performing the menace response testing, by observing whether the animal bumps into objectives in the examination area, or by having the animal walk through an unfamiliar area with obstacles placed in its path.

It is important when assessing for abnormalities of the visual system to perform a complete visual ophthalmic examination including a critical examination of the retina (e.g., a fundic examination). This will most often require a good light source such as a Finoff transilluminator and some form of magnification (direct or indirect ophthalmoscopy). In additional to the abnormalities of the retina, portions of the optic nerve can be visually evaluated. Clues to diffuse systemic disease, such as hypertension, coagulopathies, and inflammation/infection, that could also be affecting the nervous system can be helpful in the clinical evaluation process.

The Menace Response. The menace response is used as a clinical assessment of visual function. This response is performed independently in each eye while the opposite eye is covered (figs. 3.32–3.34). The menace response tests the function of two cranial nerves, CN II (afferent) and CN VII (efferent, blinking). Other components of the nervous system, such as the supratentorial structures for visual integration and the cerebellum, are also necessary for a normal menace response (McCormick and Thompson 1984).

With cerebellar disease, however, animals will have normal vision and normal CN VII function. Some animals with an absent menace response due to cerebellar disease may still blink in response to a bright light shown in the eyes (dazzle reflex) (Oliver et al. 1987). With unilateral cerebellar disease, an animal will have a menace deficit in the eye ipsilateral to the cerebellar lesion.

Other tests of vision are more subjective. Rolling a roll of tape in front of an animal is not a good test of vision, as other senses such as hearing may be elicited simultaneously. It is important to realize that even though we may not perceive these objects moving, dogs, because of their superior sense of hearing, may hear these objects moving and subsequently orient to this stimulus. Dropping cotton balls may get around this problem, but some animals will not respond to these objects consistently. Having the animal navigate through an unfamiliar obstacle course may be the best test of vision. Using soft structures as obstacles will be less traumatic to the animal if it does have a visual deficit and contacts these obstacles during testing. If vision is thought to be absent in only a single eye, blindfolding the normal eye will help in determining vision in the questionable eye.

In some animals, it may be possible to establish a visual

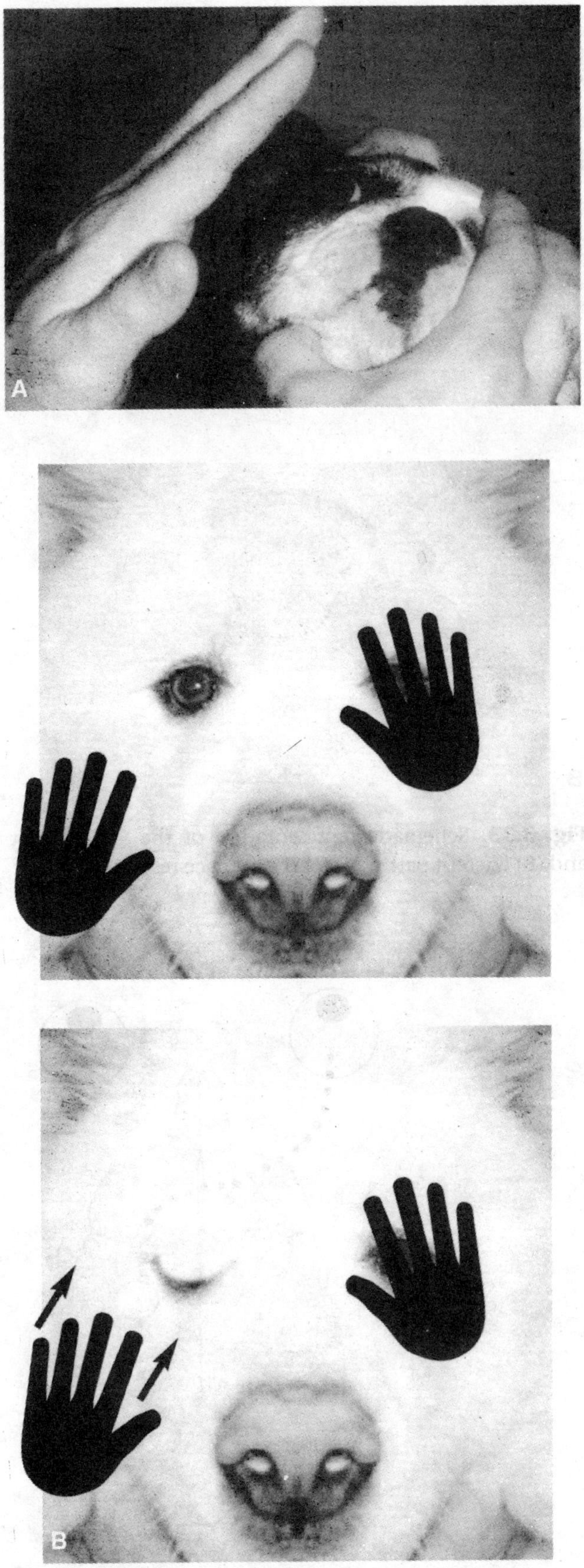

Fig. 3.32. (A) Performing the menace response. (B) Schematic representation of the menace response.

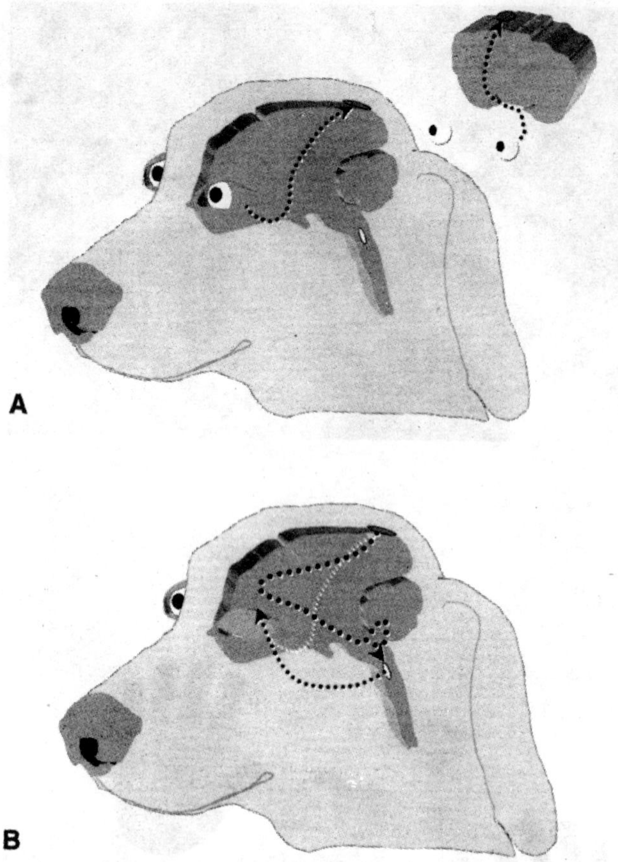

Fig. 3.33. Schematic representation of the (A) afferent and (B) efferent pathways for the menace response.

deficit in a single visual field or more commonly, in one-half of the visual fields. This requires menacing the animal from both the lateral and medial directions in each eye, while covering other visual fields. A visual deficit in one-half of the visual fields is referred to as a hemianopia.

Visual information from a single visual field is directed to the contralateral portion of the eye. The lateral (temporal) visual field of the eye, therefore, is projected to the medial (nasal) retinal receptors (fig. 3.35). Deficits in a visual field are described relative to the visual field, not the retinal field. A visual deficit in corresponding visual fields, for example the nasal visual field in one eye and the temporal visual field of the opposite eye, is referred to as a homonymous hemianopia. This may seem incongruous. However, another way to consider this problem is to consider that in each eye there is a left and right visual field. If viewing the animal from behind the head, in the left eye, for example, the lateral (temporal) visual field is on the left side, and the medial (nasal) visual field is on the right side. In the right eye, the lateral (temporal) visual field is on the right side, and the medial (nasal) visual field is on the left side of the right eye. A visual field deficit in the lateral visual field (left side) of the left eye and the nasal visual field (left side) of the right eye would be a homonymous hemianopia. Therefore, this type of hemianopia involves both left visual fields (corresponding or homonymous).

A unilateral lesion involving the supratentorial visual structures or optic tract would result in such an abnormality. A clinical clue to an optic tract lesion as compared to a supratentorial lesion is the presence of an anisocoria that

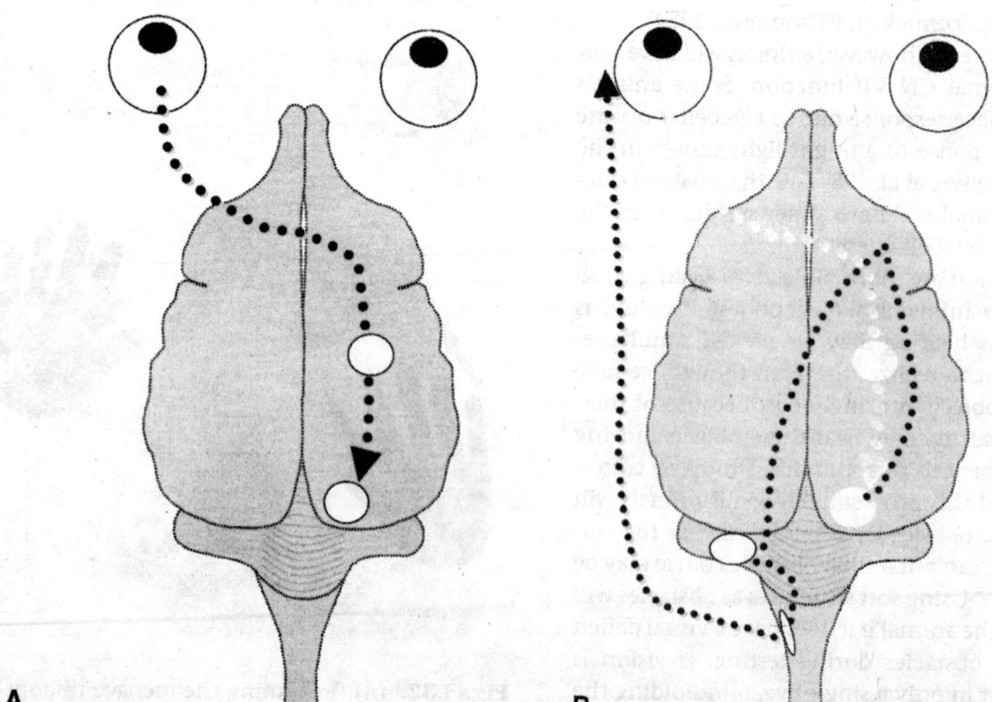

Fig. 3.34. Dorsal view, schematic representation of the (A) afferent and (B) efferent pathways for the menace response.

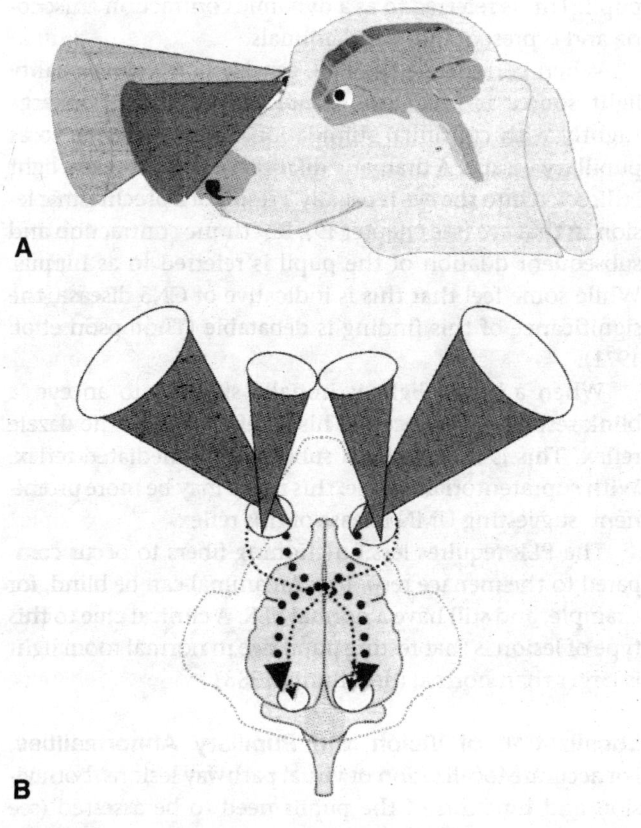

Fig. 3.35. (A) Lateral and (B) dorsal schematic views of the visual fields in the dog.

persists in all phases of light response; the dilated pupil is found in the eye contralateral to the optic tract lesion (fig. 3.36) (Antonini et al. 1979).

A hemianopia in noncorresponding visual fields (i.e., in both temporal or both nasal fields) is referred to as a heteronymous hemianopia. This type of hemianopia is very difficult to determine in animals.

Neuroanatomy of Pupil Function. The pupil is innervated by both the parasympathetic and sympathetic systems, which are, in turn, controlled by many different areas

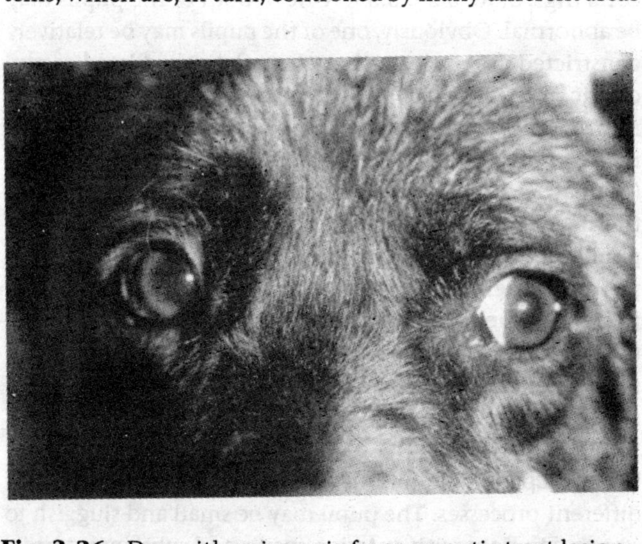

Fig. 3.36. Dog with anisocoria from an optic tract lesion.

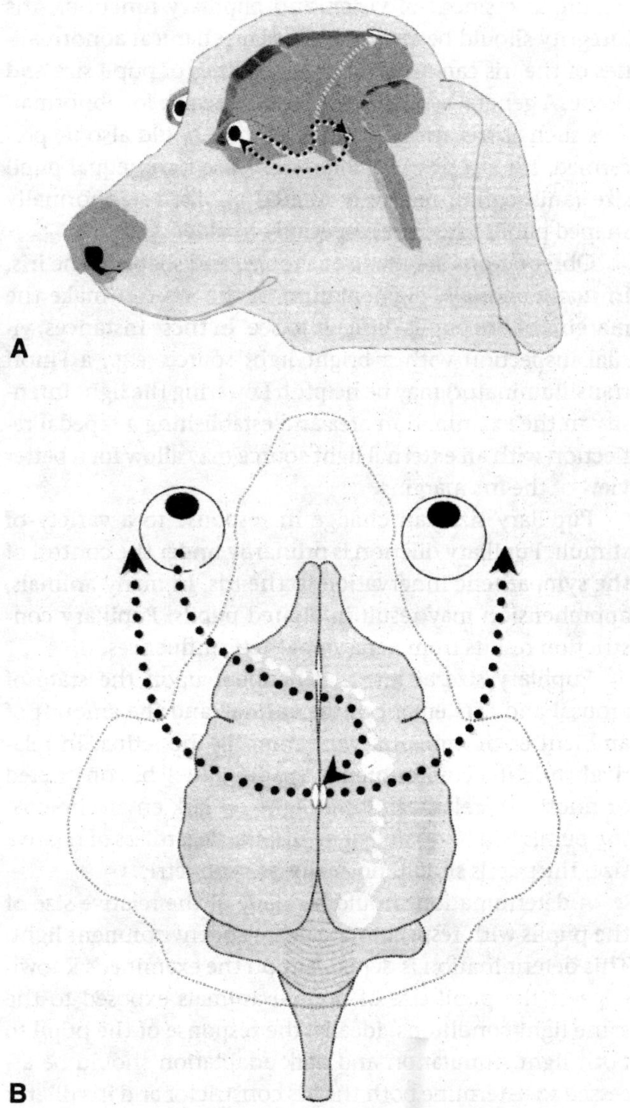

Fig. 3.37. (A) Lateral and (B) dorsal schematic representations of the pupillary light reflex (black dots).

within the nervous system (Collins and O'Brien 1990; Scagliotti 1990). When stimulated, the parasympathetic system constricts the pupil; the sympathetic system dilates the pupil. Parasympathetic innervation to the eye travels through CN III (oculomotor) (fig. 3.37).

Sympathetic innervation to the pupil is responsible for pupillary dilation and innervation to the vessels of the iris. Sympathetic control may be initiated in the hypothalamus of the diencephalon. The concept of double reciprocal innervation suggests that both the pupil dilator muscle and sphincter are under dual innervation, and the degree of pupil change is due to the balance between these two systems (Yoshitomi and Ito 1986).

Assessment of the Pupils. Pupillary assessments occur in connection with assessment of vision, ocular integrity, and iris integrity and function (Neer 1984; Neer and Carter 1987) (also see chapter 19 and appendix 4). Visual assessments have been discussed under cranial nerve II function.

During assessment of vision and pupillary functions, iris integrity should be determined, as mechanical abnormalities of the iris can result in abnormalities of pupil size and shape. A general assessment of ocular health for abnormalities such as iris atrophy and synechia should also be performed. Iris atrophy is a common cause for unequal pupil size (anisocoria), relatively dilated pupils, or abnormally shaped pupils (dyscoria) especially in older dogs.

Observations are made of the size and shape of the iris. In many animals, pigmentation of the iris can make the margins of the pupils difficult to see. In these instances, visual inspection with a bright light source (e.g., a Finoff transilluminator) may be helpful. Lowering the light intensity in the examination area and establishing a tapedal reflection with an external light source may allow for a better view of the iris margins.

Pupillary size can change in response to a variety of stimuli. Pupillary dilation is primarily under the control of the sympathetic innervation to the iris. In many animals, apprehension may result in dilated pupils. Pupillary constriction results from parasympathetic influences.

Pupillary size at rest is dependent upon the state of arousal and excitement of the animal, and the amount of ambient environmental light entering the retina. In relatively brighter environments, the pupils will be constricted or miotic. In relatively lower light or dark environments, the pupils will be dilated or mydriatic. Regardless of relative size, the pupils should normally be symmetric.

A determination should be made of the relative size of the pupils with respect to the degree of environment light. This determination is dependent on the examiner's knowledge of the pupil size of normal animals exposed to the same light conditions. Ideally, the response of the pupil to both light stimulation and dark adaptation should be assessed to determine both the iris constrictor and iris dilator functions, respectively.

Assessment of the Pupillary Light Reflex. The pupillary light reflex (PLR) is used to assess portions of the afferent visual pathway to approximately the level of the lateral geniculate body (thalamus), CN III, and the iris motor functions. The efferent portion of this reflex is performed by parasympathetic fibers of cranial nerve III (CN III) resulting in constriction of the pupil. This is a subcortical reflex and therefore requires no conscious input.

For performance of the PLR, a relatively bright light is shone into one eye at a time. If a relatively weak light source is used, poor or slow pupil response may be encountered lending confusion to the appropriateness of the reflex. When the light is shone in one eye, both pupils will constrict. The constriction of the light stimulated pupil is referred to as a direct pupillary light response. Constriction of the pupil contralateral to the stimulated eye is referred to as the consensual papillary response. Depending upon the intensity of the light stimulation, and the astuteness of the examiner, the pupil directly stimulated by the light may constrict slightly faster and to a slightly greater extent (1–2 mm smaller) compared to the consensually stimulated pupil. This is referred to as a dynamic contraction anisocoria and is present in normal animals.

When performing the PLR, especially if a poor quality light source is used, the stimulated pupil may enlarge slightly with continual stimulation. This is referred to as pupillary escape. A dramatic dilation of a pupil when light is directed into the eye is usually a result of a prechiasmic lesion in that eye (see chapter 19). Rhythmic contraction and subsequent dilation of the pupil is referred to as hippus. While some feel that this is indicative of CNS disease, the significance of this finding is debatable (Thompson et al. 1971).

When a bright light is initially shone into an eye, a blink response may occur. This is referred to as the dazzle reflex. This is most likely a subcortically mediated reflex. With supratentorial disease, this reflex may be more prominent, suggesting UMN release of this reflex.

The PLR requires less functioning fibers to occur compared to the menace response. An animal can be blind, for example, and still have a normal PLR. A clinical clue to this type of lesion is that resting pupil size in normal room light is larger than normal (deLahunta 1983).

Localization of Vision and Pupillary Abnormalities. For accurate localization of visual pathway lesions, both vision and function of the pupils need to be assessed (see chapter 19 and appendix 4). Initially the menace response is assessed. Next, the presence or absence of any resting pupillary abnormalities is recorded. Finally, direct and indirect PLRs are noted. Combined with a complete ophthalmologic examination including fundic exam and assessment of CN VII function, logical localization of lesions affecting these pathways can be made. Fundic examination is important to determine retinal integrity and to look for clues to systemic abnormalities that may secondarily affect the central nervous system. Fundic examination will also allow visualization of a portion of the optic nerve to assess for abnormalities such as papilloedema (Palmer et al. 1974).

Anisocoria. A resting inequality in pupil size is an anisocoria (figs. 3.36, 3.38, 3.39). One or both of the pupils may be abnormal. Obviously, one of the pupils may be relatively constricted or miotic, or the other relatively dilated or mydriatic. If the integrity of the visual system has been determined, this would suggest that the abnormality resulting in the pupillary change is the result of the efferent nervous (sympathetic or parasympathetic) system effects or within the iris itself. The sympathetic system is responsible for pupillary dilation. Conversely, an abnormality of the sympathetic innervation to the iris will result in a miotic pupil. Parasympathetic stimulation results in pupillary constriction. An abnormality of the parasympathetic innervation to the iris, which is provided through CN III, will result in a mydriatic pupil.

Miotic Pupil(s). Pupils may be miotic due to a number of different processes. The pupil may be small and sluggish to respond to light with anterior uveitis and subsequent iridic

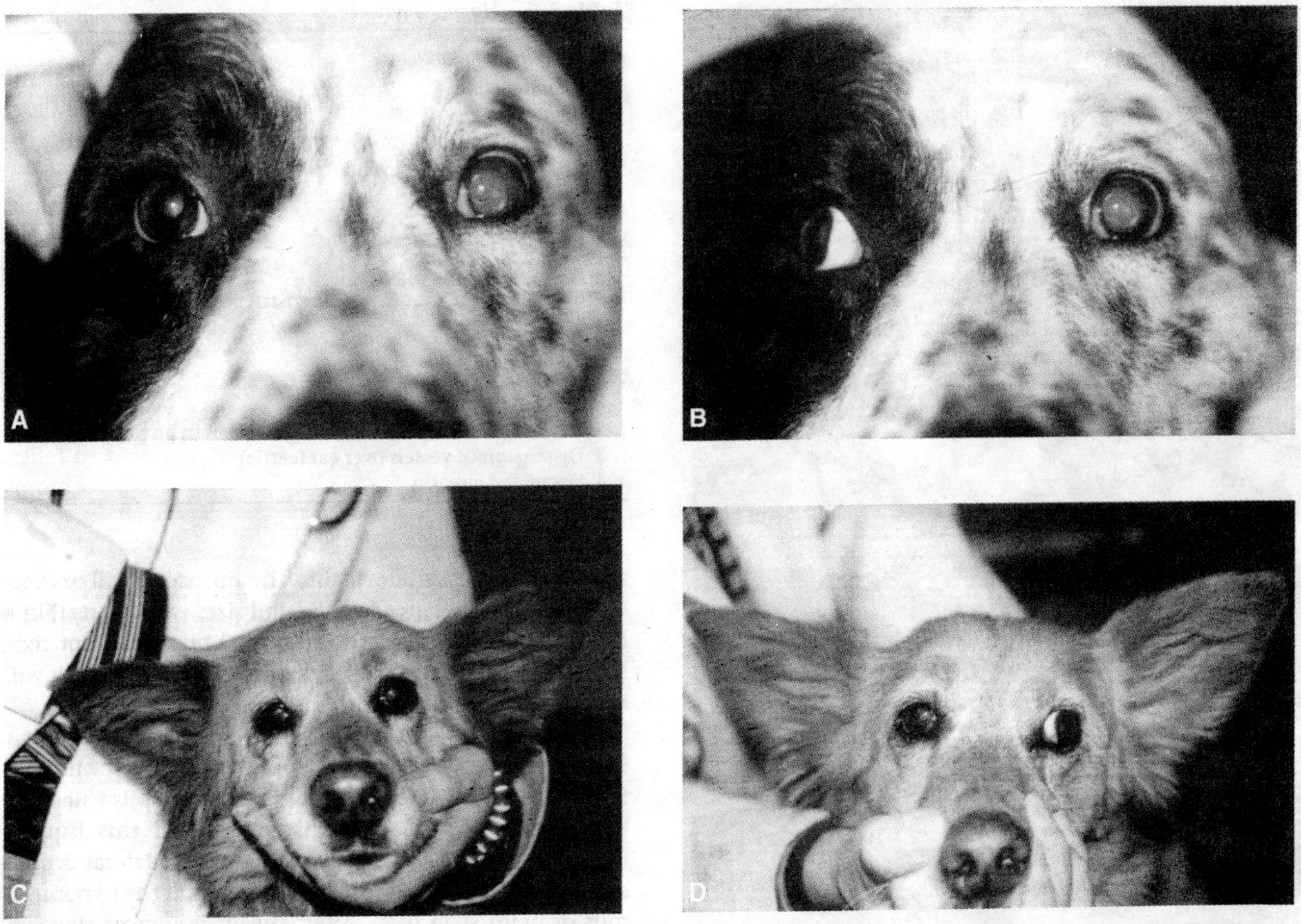

Fig. 3.38. (A, B) Dog with a cranial nerve III lesion resulting in anisocoria and inability to move the left eye medially. (C, D) Another dog with a cranial III abnormality, which is unable to move the right eye medially. (A: reprinted with permission from R. Bagley and I. Mayhew, Clinical examination of the nervous system, in Veterinary Clinical Examination and Diagnosis, eds. O. M. Radostits, I. G. J. May, and D. M. Houston [Harcourt Publishers Ltd., London, W. B. Saunders, 2000], fig. 19.21a.)

vascular congestion and edema. Painful conditions of the cornea may cause a miosis. This is a bilateral phenomenon mediated afferently through CN V (oculosensory pupillary reflex) and efferently through stimulation of the parasympathetic system of CN III. Instillation of parasympathomimetic drugs into the eye may cause miosis. The spastic pupil syndrome is a static anisocoria of cats that remains essentially unchanged during dark adaptation. Many of these cats are positive for the feline leukemia virus.

Considering the autonomic influence on the pupil, an abnormality of sympathetic innervation to the eye can result in a miotic pupil alone (Horner's pupil) or in signs of complete sympathetic denervation of the orbit (Horner's syndrome) (fig. 3.39). Clinical signs of sympathetic denervation of the eye include miotic pupil, prolapsed third eyelid, ptosis, enophthalmos, and peripheral vasodilation. All species except horses show decreased sweating.

A lesion anywhere along the sympathetic pathway can result in clinical signs of a sympathetic pupillary abnormality. Central nervous system abnormalities (brain and spinal cord) may result in only a miotic pupil and not the full constitution of clinical signs seen with Horner's syndrome. The miotic pupil alone associated with sympathetic innervation abnormalities may be referred to as Horner's pupil. Clinical signs of Horner's syndrome differ somewhat between species (table 3.6). Various causes for Horner's syndrome in dogs and cats have been described (Kern et al. 1989; Morgan and Zanotti 1989).

With sympathetic abnormalities resulting in miosis, a simple test that can aid in this determination is to place the animal in both bright light (sunlight) and darkness while assessing changes in pupil size. With a lesion of the sympathetic system, the pupil will not dilate fully in the dark. If the animal has an anisocoria and a miotic pupil from sympathetic abnormality, the anisocoria will be exacerbated (i.e., the difference in the pupil size will be great) in a darker environment. In a brighter environment, both pupils will become miotic making the anisocoria less obvious.

Mydriatic Pupil(s). A mydriatic pupil is a large, poorly responsive or unresponsive pupil. Mydriasis may be associated with parasympathetic denervation of the iris. This can result from disease of CN III or its nucleus. Parasympatholytic drugs, such as atropine, instilled in the eye that affect

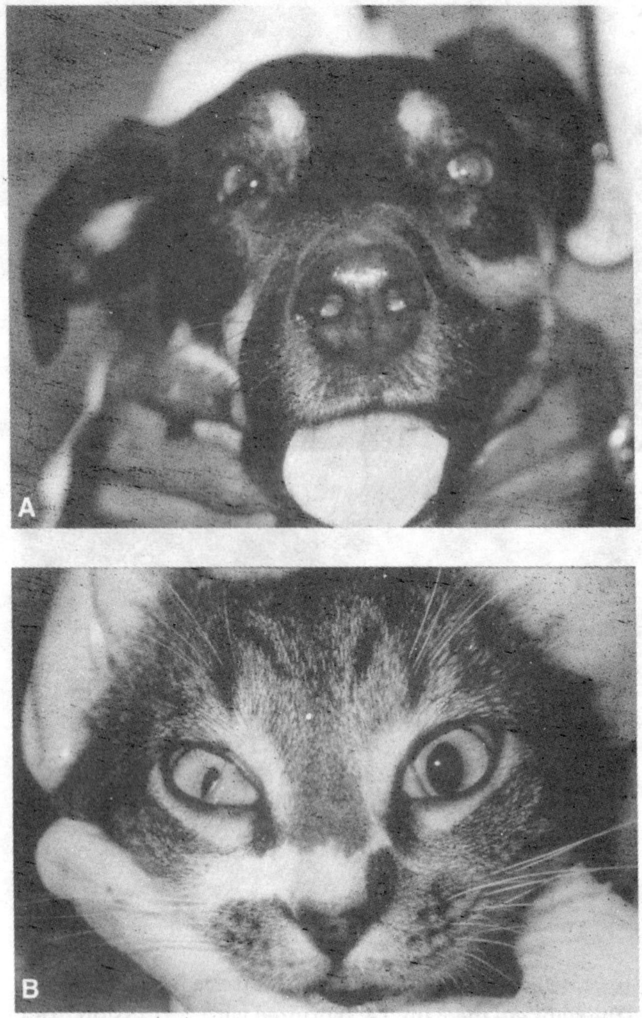

Fig. 3.39. (A) Dog and (B) cat with anisocoria and Horner's syndrome in the right eye. (B: reprinted with permission from R. Bagley, Recognition and localization of intracranial disease, Vet Clinic N Am (Small Anim Pract) [1996], 667–709, fig. 2).

Table 3.6. Horner's syndrome

Dogs and Cats
1. Miosis
2. Ptosis
3. Enophthalmos
4. Protrusion of third eyelid
5. Vasodilation
Horses
1. Ptosis most consistent
2. Miosis less obvious (greater constriction in affected eye)
3. Sweating
Cattle, Sheep, and Goats
1. Ptosis most consistent
2. Miosis less obvious (greater constriction in affected eye)
3. Distension of vessels over ear (cattle)
4. Decreased sweating

the synapse or the iris muscle itself will dilate the pupil. The affect of atropine may last for several days after one instillation. Primary disease of the iris, such as iris atrophy, is common in older dogs. A dyscoric pupil and an irregular pupillary margin may be clues. Primary disease of the eye such as synechia or glaucoma can result in a dilated pupil. An idiopathic postganglionic parasympathetic denervation of the pupil is referred to as Adie's syndrome (Goldfarb and Swann 1984). This is rare in dogs. Dysautonomia is a disease characterized by dysfunction of the autonomic system occurring in both dogs and cats (Sharp et al. 1994; Wise and Lappin 1991; O'Brien and Longshore 2000). In addition to other clinical signs, such as vomiting and constipation, dilated, poorly to unresponsive pupils may be seen.

Altering the amount of light presented to the pupils may also be helpful for diagnosis in instances of a parasympathetic system abnormality. A determination is made of the pupil size in both bright light (sunlight) and darkness. If the animal has an anisocoria and a mydriatic pupil from a parasympathetic abnormality, the anisocoria will be exacerbated (the difference in the pupil sizes will be great) in a lighter environment as the abnormal pupil will not constrict in the light. In a darker environment, both pupils will become dilated making the anisocoria less obvious.

Pupillary Changes with CNS Disease. With bilateral, usually severe cerebrocortical disease, the pupils will often be miotic. Two theories exist to explain this finding (deLahunta 1983). One is that there is a bilateral central sympathetic system abnormality, possibly at the hypothalamus or brain stem level. Alternatively, it appears that systems of the supratentorial area normally provide descending inhibitory influences on the parasympathetic nucleus of CN III. This may be useful to have the pupils relatively larger to increase the amount of information presented to the supratentorial structures. If the supratentorial systems responsible for this descending inhibitory influence are damaged, there is a release of this inhibitory influence over the parasympathetic pupillary constriction and these neurons become hyperresponsive (excessive parasympathetic tone).

If unilateral transtentorial herniation occurs, pressure from the herniated parahippocampal gyrus may be exerted ventrally onto the brain stem. As the brain stem is compressed, CN III may be trapped along the floor of the skull. Compression on this nerve may result in parasympathetic dysfunction and the ipsilateral pupil will dilate and become nonresponsive to light (Kornegay et al. 1983).

Pharmacological testing is infrequently used as an aid in localization of pupillary abnormalities resulting from autonomic disease to either the pre- or postganglionic segment. This type of testing, however, often yields inconsistent and inconclusive results (Kern et al. 1989). Pharmacological localization to the postganglionic segment is based upon the phenomenon of *denervation hypersensitivity.* When the postganglionic nerve of the autonomic system has lost its nervous innervation, the postsynaptic neuromuscular junction will become supersensitive to normally ineffective concentrations of neurotransmitter such as acetylcholine (ACH).

Drugs are administered to work locally at the postganglionic/iris synapse. A dilute concentration of phenylephrine may be used as a direct acting sympathomimetic. This drug will act to stimulate the iris directly through activation of postsynaptic sympathetic receptors. With bilateral instillation of this drug, the abnormal pupil from a postganglionic sympathetic lesion should dilate in less time than the normal pupil. This suggests denervation hypersensitivity.

An indirect acting sympathomimetic agent that has been used as a test of the integrity of the postganglionic sympathetic segment is hydroxyamphetamine or similar product. This drug will result in release of neurotransmitter from the presynaptic membrane. A positive response to this drug is dilation of the affected pupil, suggesting that the presynaptic area, and therefore the postganglionic segment of the sympathetic innervation to the pupil, is intact. With an appropriate response to this drug, the lesion should be in the preganglionic segment or central components.

Topical instillation of autonomic drugs can also be similarly used to detect parasympathetic lesions. Physostigmine is an indirect acting parasympathomimetic drug and dilute pilocarpine is a direct acting parasympathomimetic drug used when localizing parasympathetic (CN III) lesions.

Unfortunately, pharmacologic testing to determine the location of the autonomic lesion is inaccurate and is rarely performed clinically. An important caveat that influences pharmacological localization of pupillary abnormalities is that with some preganglionic lesions, *transsynaptic degeneration* may occur and secondarily cause destruction of the postganglionic segment. In this instance, pharmacological testing may falsely localize the lesion to the wrong segment (Jacobson 1990).

Cranial Nerve III (Oculomotor), Cranial Nerve IV (Trochlear), Cranial Nerve VI (Abducent). Cranial nerves III, IV, and VI are considered together as these innervate the extraocular muscles to result in ocular movement. In addition, cranial nerve III is necessary for normal constriction of the pupil.

Cranial Nerve III (Oculomotor). The oculomotor nerve has two main functions, *movement of the eye* and *pupillary constriction*. Pupillary constriction occurs via the autonomic fibers of CN III. This function is discussed under pupil assessment. The parasympathetic function of CN III is described above under Assessment of the Pupillary Light Reflex.

Clinical Assessment of Cranial Nerve III Motor Function. The motor function of CN III can be assessed by observing the eye position at rest. If CN III influence to the extraocular muscle is abnormal, the eye may be deviated from a normal position. Abnormal eye position is termed *strabismus*. Lesions of this portion of CN III produce a lateral and ventral strabismus. Ptosis (droopy upper eyelid) may result due to paralysis of the levator palpebrae muscle (fig. 3.40).

In some instances, dysfunction of the oculomotor nerve will not result in a resting strabismus, but the eye will be unable to move normally through the phases of gaze (fig. 3.38). Ocular movement can be assessed by the examiner by physically moving the head from side to side in a horizontal direction and determining if a normal physiological quick and slow movement (termed physiologic or normal nystagmus) is evoked (the oculovestibular response) (deLahunta 1983; Joseph 1992). When a normal dog's head is turned to one side in a horizontal plane, the eyes will move toward the direction of the movement. With the head moving, the eyes will attempt to maintain eye direction toward the area where the dog was initially looking (straight ahead). This will result in a slow drifting of the eyes in the direction opposite the movement of the head relative to the movement of the head. As the head continues to be moved laterally, the extraocular muscles of the eyes, as influenced by the vestibular system via the medial longitudinal fasciculus pathway in the brain stem, will result in a quick deviation of the eyes in the direction of the movement. This slow/quick

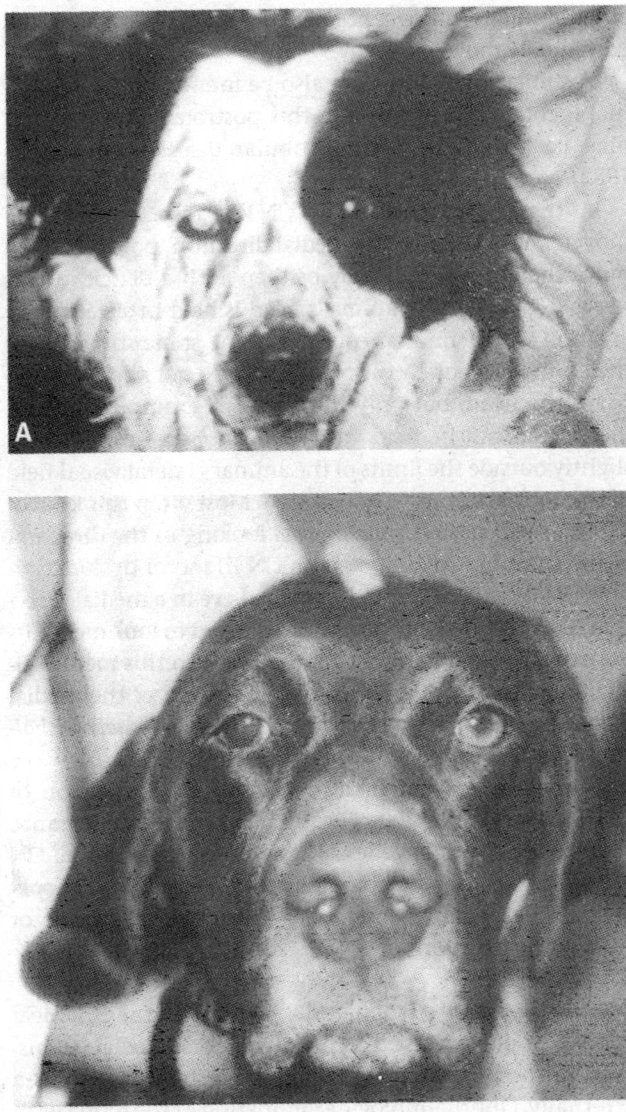

Fig. 3.40. (A, B) Dogs with right-sided ptosis from a cranial nerve III lesion.

eye movement will be continued in succession as the head is continually moved laterally.

A similar nystagmus can also be induced when an animal is rotated. A decrease in this postrotation nystagmus may be associated with vestibular disease (deLahunta 1983).

As the motor component of CN III is responsible for eye movement, primarily in a medial direction, poor ability to move the eye medially may be seen with a deficit of this nerve (fig. 3.38). The animal's head is held in a stationary position while simultaneously creating some stimulus for the animal to look in various directions, not allowing it to move the head, but only the eyes. For example, the animal's head can be held and a loud noise can be created slightly outside the limits of the animal's lateral visual field of the contralateral eye to be tested. Most often this kind of stimulus will result in the animal looking in the direction of the stimulus. An animal with CN III motor dysfunction may not be able to move the affected eye in a medial direction (fig. 3.38). When the animal is forced to look medially, the eye may not be moved appropriately in this medial direction primarily due to loss of innervation of the medial rectus muscle. This may be referred to as an *external ophthalmoplegia*.

Stimulation through the parasympathetic division of CN III results in pupillary constriction during performance of the pupillary light reflex. A lesion of this portion of CN III will result in a dilated pupil referred to as *internal ophthalmoplegia*. Animals may have abnormalities of one or both of the functions of CN III.

Cranial Nerve IV (Trochlear). Lesions of the trochlear nucleus or nerve cause a contralateral dorsomedial strabismus. In species with a round pupil, no strabismus is seen externally. Ophthalmologic examination of the retina with a direct ophthalmoscope, however, reveals the superior retinal vein to be deviated laterally. If indirect visualization is used, the superior retinal vein will be directed medially.

As cats have a vertical pupil, the dorsal aspect of the vertical pupil is deviated laterally with such a lesion. Isolated lesions of this nerve, however, are extremely rare in small animals.

Cranial Nerve VI (Abducent). Disease of CN VI results in a *ventromedial strabismus*. The eyeball cannot abduct fully and may not be retractable within the orbit. Again, isolated lesions of CN VI are extremely rare.

Abnormalities Cranial Nerves III, IV, and VI Combined. Paralysis of all muscles responsible for eye movement is termed *complete ophthalmoplegia*. Cranial nerves III, IV, VI, the sympathetic innervation, and CN V (ophthalmic branch) lie ventrally in the skull close to the *cavernous sinus* (venous system that encircles the pituitary fossa). These nerves all exit the skull through the orbital fissure. Lesions on the floor of the skull in this area may damage this combination of nerves and result in what is commonly referred to as *cavernous sinus syndrome* (Lewis et al. 1984).

Abnormalities of CNs III, IV, and VI can result in various types of strabismus. However, strabismus associated with these cranial nerve abnormalities is usually present at rest, hence the term "resting strabismus." A strabismus seen only when the head is placed in an unusual orientation is termed a *positional strabismus* (fig. 3.41). If present, a positional strabismus is most easily evoked by extending the head dorsally so that the gaze is directed dorsally toward the ceiling. As the head is moved to this new position, the vestibular receptors in the ear become activated. Vestibular information is projected cranially through the medial longitudinal fasciculus in the brain stem to influence the functions of the cranial nerves (III, IV, and VI) to the extraocular muscles (fig. 3.42). These nerves are either excited or inhibited to move the eyes to the new direction of gaze (i.e., dorsally).

As the dog's head is extended dorsally, the eyes will remain positioned in the orbit so that the gaze is directed forward (or in this position, dorsally). If one or both eyes' position deviates from this direction, this is a positional strabismus. Most commonly, the abnormal eye(s) will deviate comparatively ventrally and is most easily appreciated by observing the more prominent dorsal sclera of the affected eye (fig. 3.41). As there is no strabismus at rest, this finding implies that the vestibular input to CNs III, IV and VI is abnormal. This clinical abnormality is usually associated with an ipsilateral vestibular abnormality most commonly in the peripheral, but sometimes the central, vestibular system.

Siamese and other breeds of cats can have a strabismus (usually esotropia) due not to an abnormality of the oculomotor nerves but rather to congenitally abnormal visual projection pathways (fig. 3.43) (Johnson 1991). This eye position is an adaptation of eye position to abnormal visual information projection pathways. Siamese and similarly affected cats have increased numbers of decussating or crossed visual projections from the retina to the thalamus. The eye is deviated to result in improved visual acuity.

Cranial Nerve V (Trigeminal). Cranial nerve V—the trigeminal nerve—as the name suggests, contains three main branches or divisions. Sensory afferents of this nerve are heavily represented throughout the head and face and are almost exclusive in providing sensory information from the head and face. In addition, efferent axons from this nerve are responsible for innervating the muscles of mastication important for biting and chewing.

The three major branches of this nerve are the ophthalmic, the maxillary, and the mandibular nerves. The ophthalmic and maxillary branches provide sensory afferent information, while the mandibular nerve is responsible for both sensory and motor functions. The three branches of cranial nerve V can be evaluated independently. The ophthalmic branch can be tested by assessing for a palpebral reflex (afferent, CN V; efferent, CN VII) and by assessing corneal sensation (figs. 3.44, 3.45, 3.46).

When the medial canthus of the eye (or other skin areas directly around the eye) is touched, the animal should

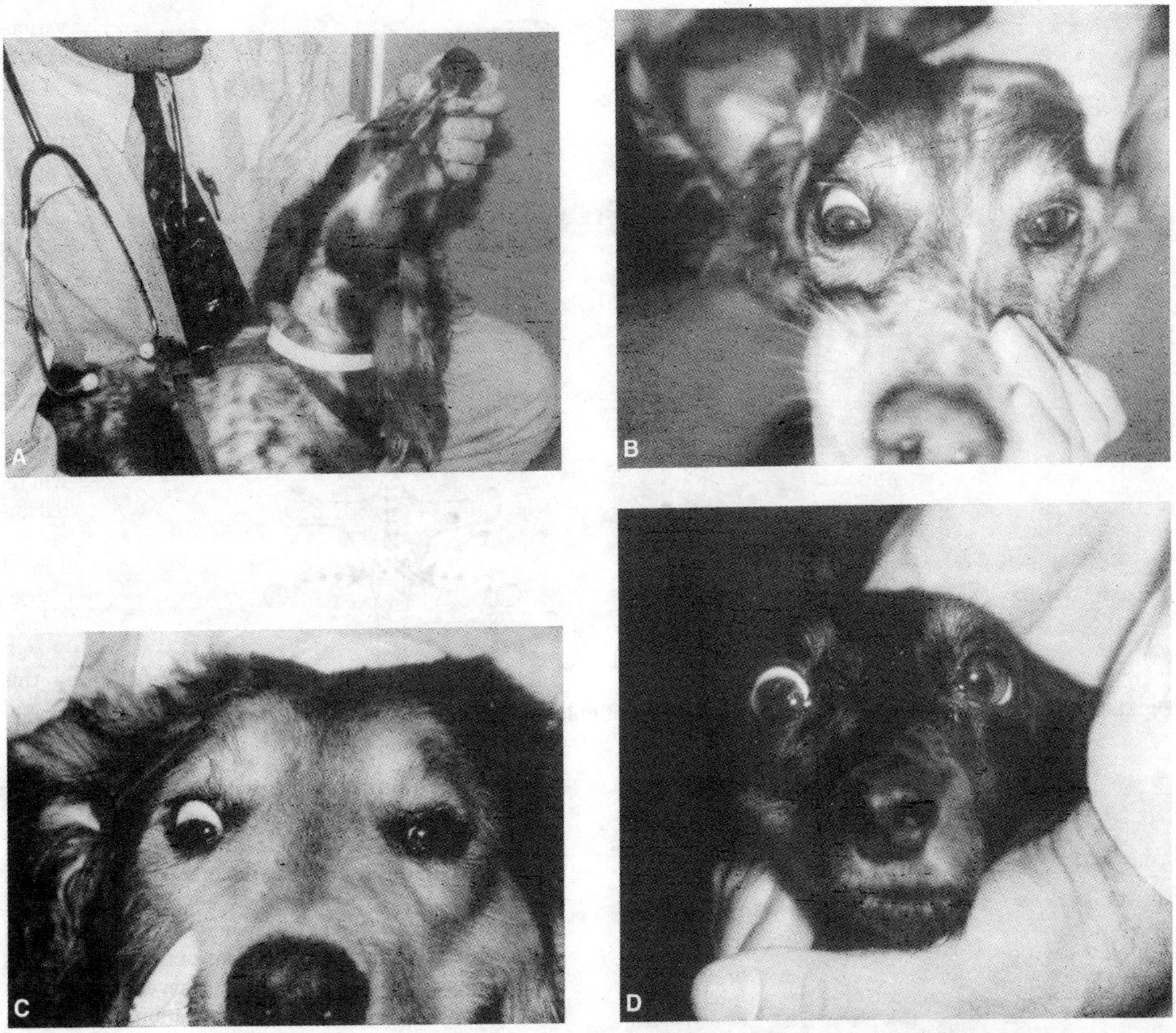

Fig. 3.41. (A) Placing a dog with vestibular disease in an extended head position. (B) View of the same dog with a positional strabismus in the right eye. (C, D) Two dogs in a head-extended position with right-sided positional strabismus when viewed from above.

blink. This is referred to as the palpebral reflex. If the cornea itself is touched, the animal usually retracts the eye in the globe as well as blinks (corneal sensation). It is important to ensure that the palpebral fissure is closed completely during performance of the palpebral reflex, as some animals with poor periocular sensation may not close the palpebral fissure completely.

The cornea can be assessed for appropriate sensory innervation by lightly touching the cornea with a nontraumatic object (e.g., a wisp of cotton) (fig. 3.45). Another method, which avoids the need for touching the cornea and potentially damaging the cornea structure, is to blow air onto the cornea. This can be accomplished by placing a 20 g flexible catheter tip on a 6 or 12 cc syringe, filling the syringe with room air, and then quickly depressing the syringe plunger to expel the air onto the cornea (fig. 3.46). Either when the cornea is touched, or when air is expelled on the cornea, the normal animal should blink immediately following the stimulus. A delayed or absent blink may indicate a deficit of corneal sensation.

Additionally, normal ophthalmic branch of CN V innervation of the cornea is needed for maintenance of the integrity of the corneal epithelium. If ophthalmic nerve function is abnormal, the corneal structure may focally be disrupted, become cloudy, and a corneal ulcer can develop. This ulcer is usually centrally positioned. This corneal alteration is known as neurotropic keratitis (figs. 3.47, 3.48). Tear production can also decrease when corneal sensation is abnormal as afferent sensory inputs through the ophthalmic branch of CN V are important for reflex tear production. With ophthalmic branch lesions, tear production is decreased but is less commonly absent. The ipsilateral nasal mucosa may also become dry and the nasal passages can become crusted.

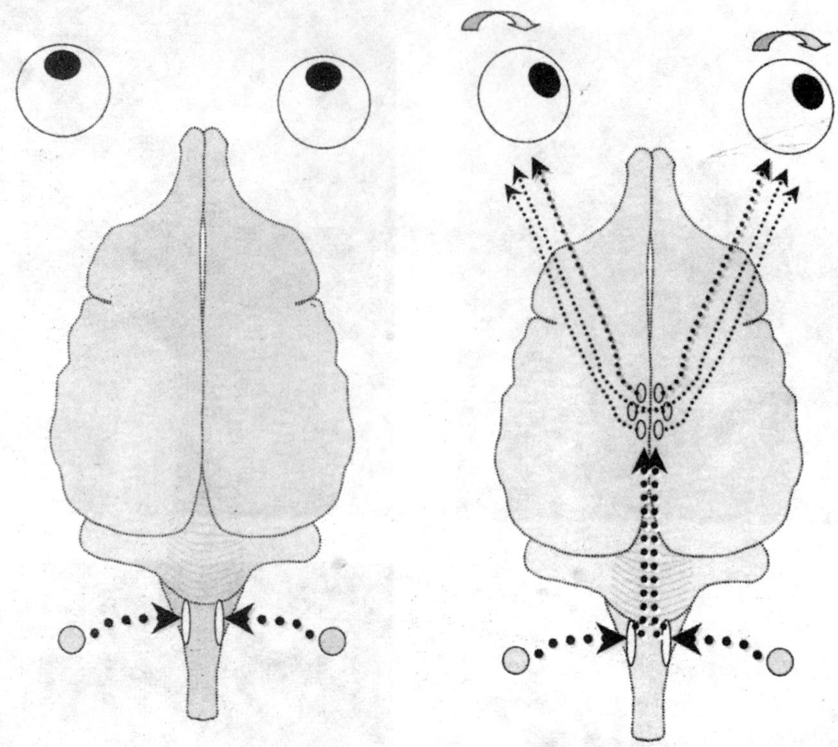

Fig. 3.42. Schematic representation of the pathway for vestibular input into ocular position.

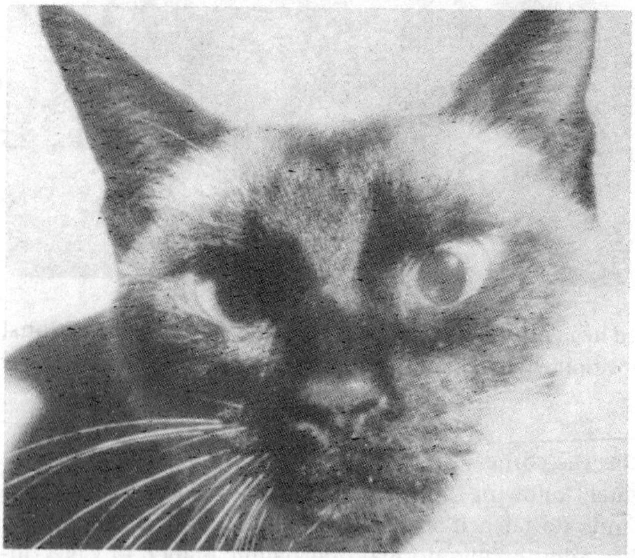

Fig. 3.43. Siamese cat with esotropia. (Reprinted with permission from R. Bagley and I. Mayhew, Clinical examination of the nervous system, in Veterinary Clinical Examination and Diagnosis, eds. O. M. Radostits, I. G. J. May, and D. M. Houston [Harcourt Publishers Ltd., London, W. B. Saunders, 2000], fig. 19.25.)

The maxillary branch of CN V is responsible for projection of sensory information from the maxillary area of the face. However, the ophthalmic branch of CN V may be responsible for some internal nasal sensation. Animals with abnormalities of the maxillary branch of CN V may lack sensation in the muzzle area. This may lead to traumatizing this area more readily, such as by biting through the anesthetic lip (fig. 3.49). Animals with abnormal sensations (paresthesia) in this region may rub or scratch the face and muzzle.

The function of the maxillary nerve is most readily assessed by stimulating the medial part of the nasal mucosa as the animal's eyes are covered (to prevent the patient from seeing you) (fig. 3.50). This stimulation is performed quickly with a slightly blunt-ended instrument such as a hemostat or cotton-tipped applicator. It is important to apply reasonably strong stimulus, however to not appear overly aggressive in performance of this test in front of the owner. It is also helpful to explain why you are performing this test to relieve the owner's fears that you are unnecessarily harming their animal.

When the nasal mucosa is stimulated, the animal is observed for two associated responses. First, the stimulation is projected centrally through the maxillary nerve to the nucleus of CN V. From this nucleus, axons are projected directly to the ipsilateral nucleus of CN VII. This reflex arc (CN V to CN VII) evokes an ipsilateral movement of the muscles of facial expression (blinking; wrinkling of the facial muscles). This is a subcortical reflex and requires no conscious input.

Concurrently, a consciously mediated, more coordinated movement (pulling) of the head away from the stimulus occurs. This response requires conscious recognition of the stimulus via pathways projecting from the nasal mucosa through the maxillary nerve to eventually reach the contralateral parietal cortex. The stimulus initiates

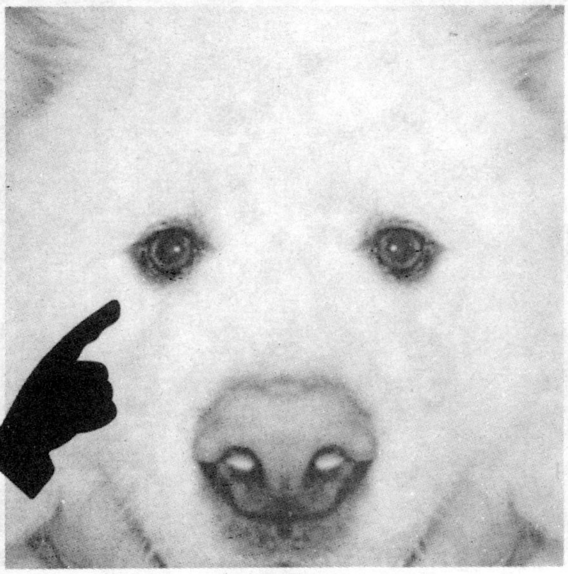

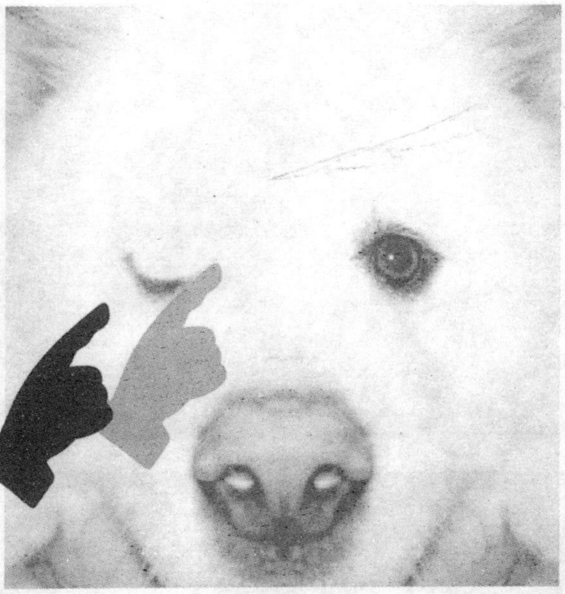

Fig. 3.44. Representation of the palpebral reflex.

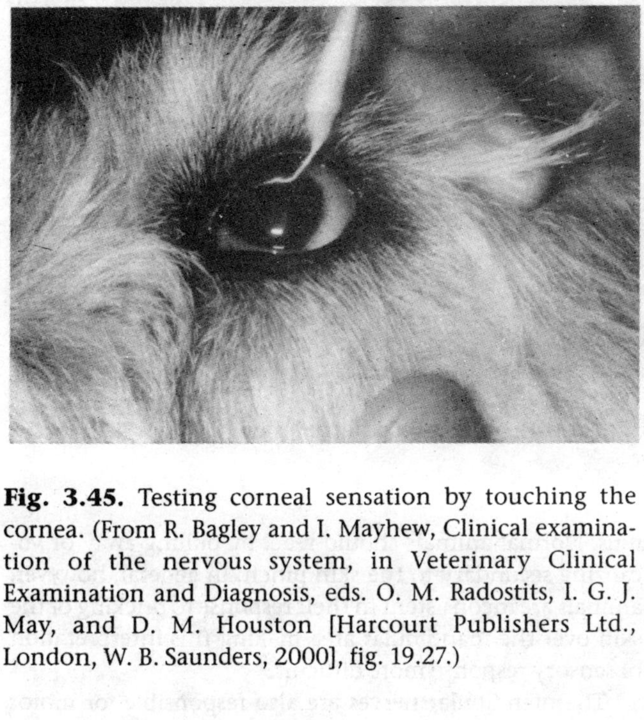

Fig. 3.45. Testing corneal sensation by touching the cornea. (From R. Bagley and I. Mayhew, Clinical examination of the nervous system, in Veterinary Clinical Examination and Diagnosis, eds. O. M. Radostits, I. G. J. May, and D. M. Houston [Harcourt Publishers Ltd., London, W. B. Saunders, 2000], fig. 19.27.)

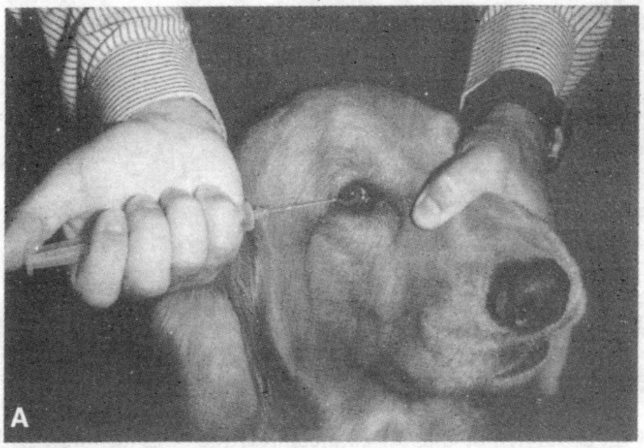

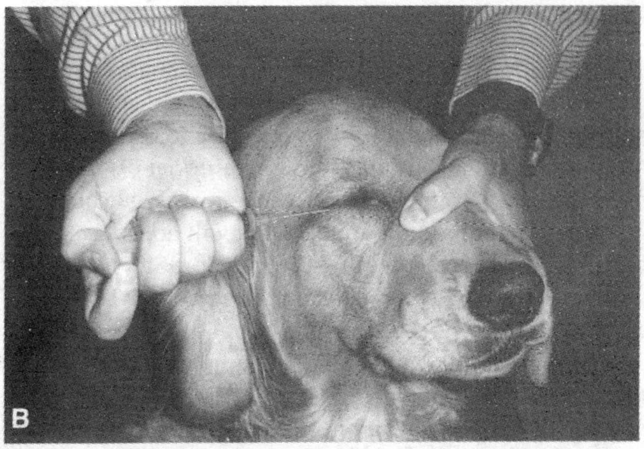

Fig. 3.46. (A) Testing corneal sensation by forcing air across the cornea. (B) The normal reflex is for the animal to blink.

projection of this sensory information afferently in the maxillary nerve to the sensory nucleus of CN V in the brain stem. This sensory information is projected across midline and rostrally to the thalamus, then subsequently to the parietal cortex. Once this sensory stimulus is recognized in the cortex, a coordinated motor response requiring primarily movement of the neck muscles is initiated. The animal rapidly moves the head and nose away from the stimulus.

Interpreting both the reflex and the conscious response

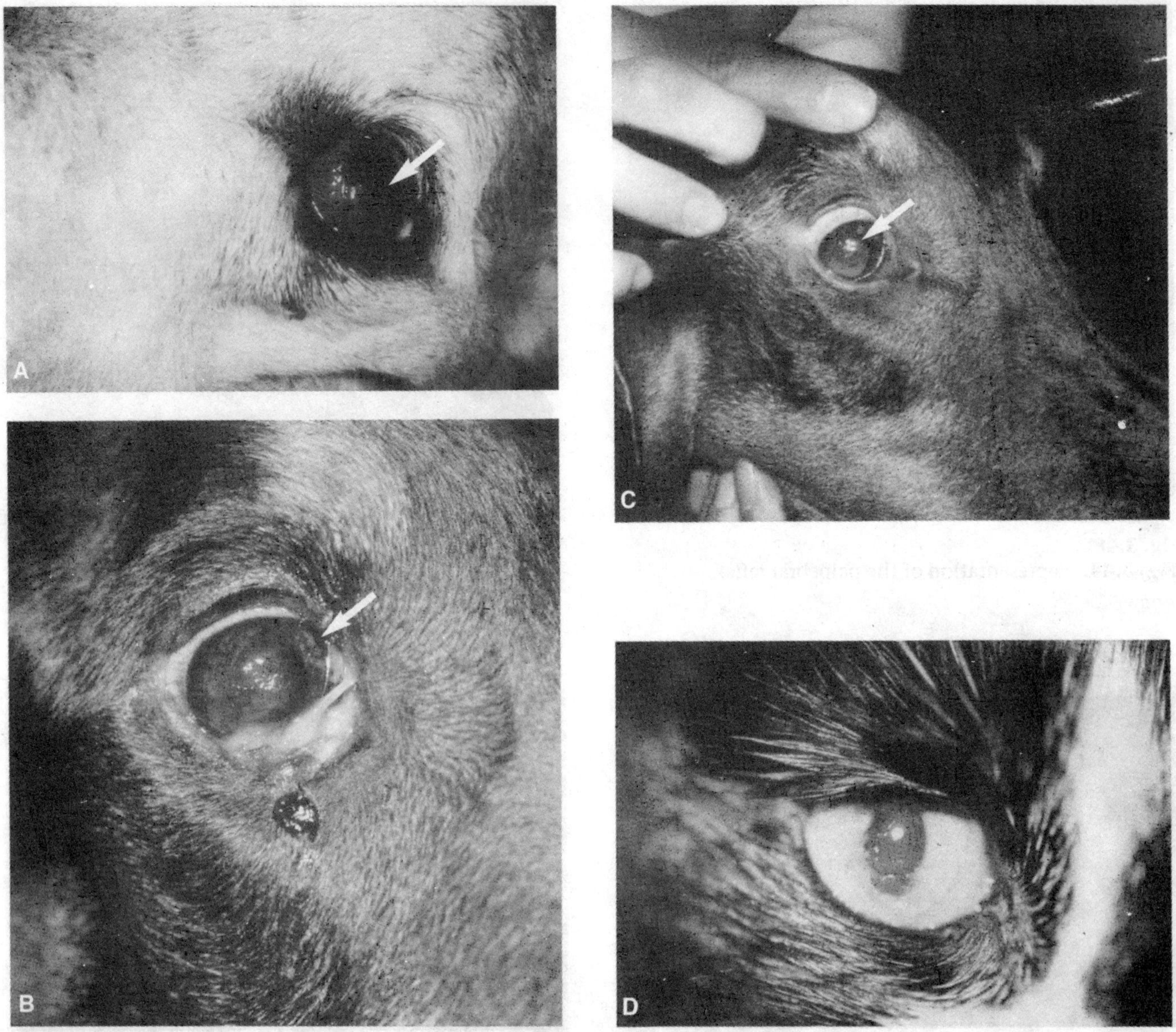

Fig. 3.47. (A, B, C) Cornea ulcer in three dogs (*arrows*); and (D) one cat with a trigeminal nerve lesion.

of the animal to this type of nasal stimulation is important for localization of an abnormality of this evaluation. An animal with a CN V maxillary branch abnormality will have neither the reflex nor conscious response to this stimulus. An animal with a contralateral supratentorial disease may have the reflex component (i.e., the animal will blink or lick when the stimulus is applied), but will not consciously move the head away from the stimulus. Some animals with cervical pain will also be reluctant to aggressively move the cervical area.

The mandibular branch of CN V supplies sensory innervation to the mandibular region of the head and face. Areas of the skin can be pinched in this region to assess sensory recognition through the mandibular nerve. A portion of the skin can be initially isolated between the jaws of a hemostat, and then that portion of skin can be squeezed tighter in the jaws to provide an increasingly painful stimulus. Normal animals should react by pulling away or vocalizing secondary to the skin pinch. In general, however, animals are inconsistent in their response to pricking of the skin over the mandibular area making this interpretation of sensory response more difficult.

The mandibular nerves are also responsible for motor innervation of the muscles of mastication, primarily the temporalis and masseter muscle (figs. 3.51, 3.52, 3.53, 3.54). Assessment of muscle tone in these muscles is performed by passively opening and closing the jaw and determining the degree of resistance. Importantly, as nervous innervation is necessary for maintenance of normal muscle mass, atrophy of the temporal and masseter muscles is common with mandibular nerve disease that results in denervation of these muscles. Bilateral atrophy of the temporalis and masseter muscles is not pathognomonic for denervation, as primary muscle diseases such as mastica-

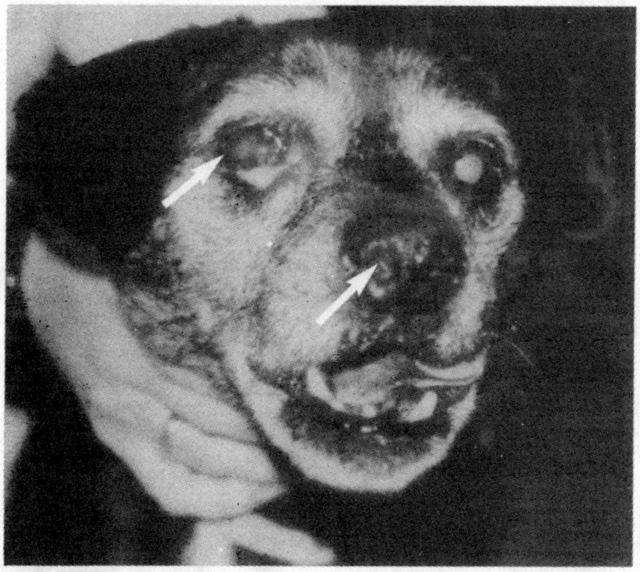

Fig. 3.48. A dog with neurotropic keratitis of the right eye (*arrow*). The dog also has a crusty nostril on the same side (*arrow*).

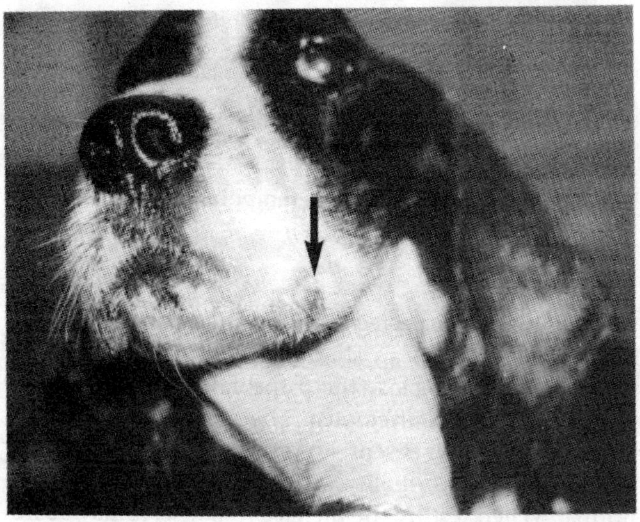

Fig. 3.49. Dog with decreased facial sensation from a trigeminal nerve lesion that is biting through its lip (*arrow*).

tory myositis may also cause atrophy of these muscles. Unilateral atrophy of the temporalis and masseter muscles is more likely to be the result of a CN V abnormality.

Animals with bilateral mandibular nerve disease may have a dropped jaw and are unable to close the mouth (fig. 3.51). The jaw area is not painful on palpation or with passive range of motion assessments. The jaw can be manipulated easily as tone of the muscles is poor. Affected animals may salivate and have difficulty prehending food as they cannot mechanically close the jaw to keep these substances in the mouth. Because of these clinical findings, affected animals are often assumed to have poor swallowing function.

An isolated unilateral dysfunction of all three branches of CN V is almost always associated with a peripheral cranial nerve (outside the brain stem), because the nuclear areas of CN are so extensive within the brain stem that destruction of all of these nuclei would usually result in other clinical signs such as proprioceptive abnormalities. It is important to remember that an intracranial lesion can affect the peripheral (outside the brain stem) aspects of CN V as the nerve travels in the trigeminal canal of petros temporal bone prior to exiting the skull.

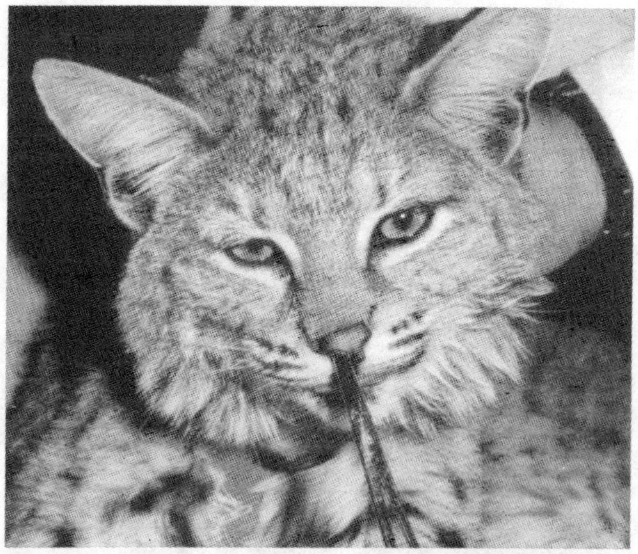

Fig. 3.50. Stimulation of the nasal mucosa in testing facial sensation. (From R. Bagley and I. Mayhew, Clinical examination of the nervous system, in Veterinary Clinical Examination and Diagnosis, eds. O. M. Radostits, I. G. J. May, and D. M. Houston [Harcourt Publishers Ltd., London, W. B. Saunders, 2000], fig. 19.29.)

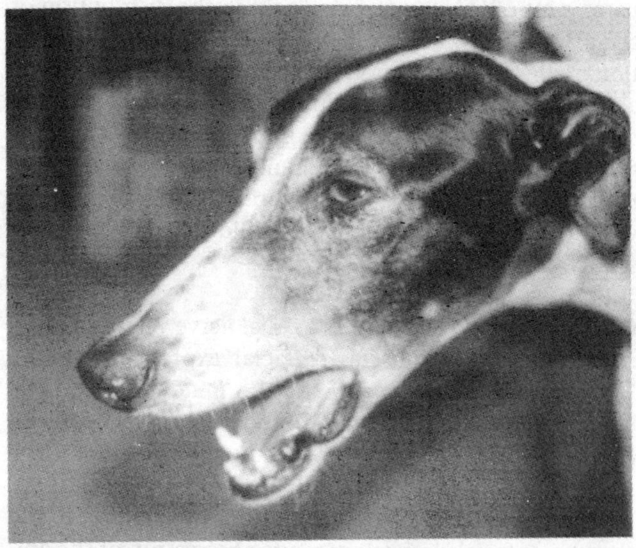

Fig. 3.51. Dog with bilateral mandibular nerve paralysis with a dropped jaw.

Painful sensations in the sensory distribution of the

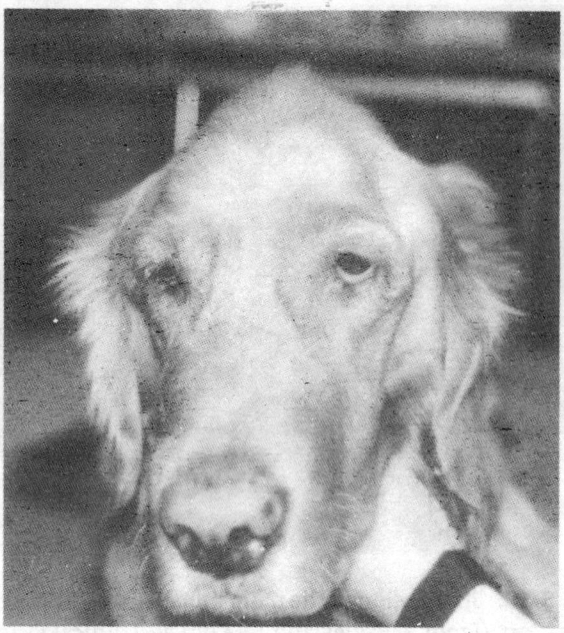

Fig. 3.52. Dog with bilateral temporalis muscle atrophy.

trigeminal nerve are referred to as trigeminal neuralgia, or Tic Douloureux in humans. These sensations are usually paroxysms of intense, stabbing pain in the distribution of the mandibular and maxillary nerves. Pain in the distribution of the trigeminal nerves is more difficult to quantify in animals. Some animals with trigeminal sensory nerve disease may rub their faces on the floor or on objects such as furniture. Animals with apparent abnormal sensations may scratch their faces and self-mutilate. Similarly, animals with dry mouths (xerostomia) or swallowing difficulty may scratch or rub their faces.

Cranial Nerve VII (Facial). Cranial nerve VII supplies innervation to the muscles of facial expression, to the lacrimal and salivary glands, to the middle ear and the blood vessels of the head, and to the palate and the rostral two-thirds of the tongue associated with branches of the trigeminal nerve.

As the facial nerve is responsible for innervation to the muscles of facial expression, astute observation of the animal's head and face may reveal abnormalities of symmetry and facial muscle movement. Animals with facial nerve disease often have abnormalities of position and movement of the lips, ears, and eyelids. Clinical signs of a lesion in the facial nerve may include paresis or paralysis of the facial muscles (figs. 3.55, 3.56. 3.57).

Facial nerve motor function is most easily assessed by testing the palpebral reflex. When the medial aspect of the palpebral fissure is touched, the animal should blink rapidly and completely. The touch is sensed through CN V, ophthalmic branch, and the muscle contraction is elicited through the motor functions of CN VII resulting in contraction of the orbicularis oculi muscle. If the more lateral aspects of the periorbital region are touched, the afferent

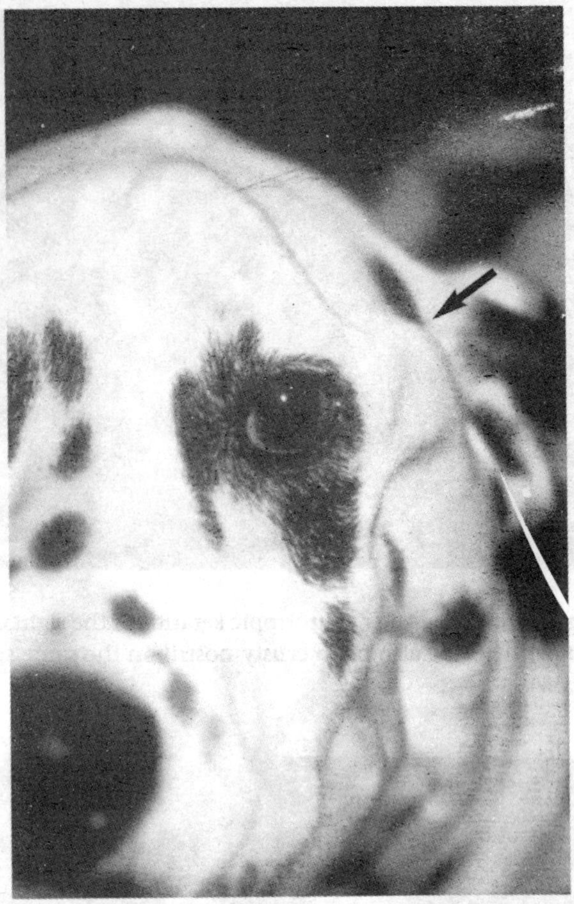

Fig. 3.53. Dog with unilateral temporalis muscle atrophy. Note the zygomatic arch (*arrow*).

stimulus may be projected in the maxillary branch of CN V fibers. Animals with an abnormality of CN VII function will not be able to close the palpebral fissure completely when this reflex is attempted. The menace response will also be decreased or absent; however, if the animal has only a facial nerve abnormality, the animal's vision should be normal. When testing the menace response, it may be noticed that the eye can be retracted in the orbit away from the menacing gesture suggesting the afferent components of this response are normal. Often, when the eye is retracted in the globe, the nictitating membrane will be prolapsed up and over the eye in a rapid movement. Similarly, when the palpebral area is touched, the animal may retract the eye but not be able to close the lids. The nictitating membrane will often be rapidly prolapsed concurrently.

Localization of the lesion within the facial nerve may be accomplished by knowledge of where this nerve branches after exiting the brain stem (Oliver et al. 1987). With lesions distal to the stylomastoid foramen, innervation to the facial muscles will be abnormal, however, taste, lacrimation, and the innervation of the stapedius muscle will be normal. With lesions in the petrosal bone, innervation to the facial muscles will be abnormal and functions of the other areas may or may not be affected. Intracranial, extramedullary lesions will result in all functions of CN VII

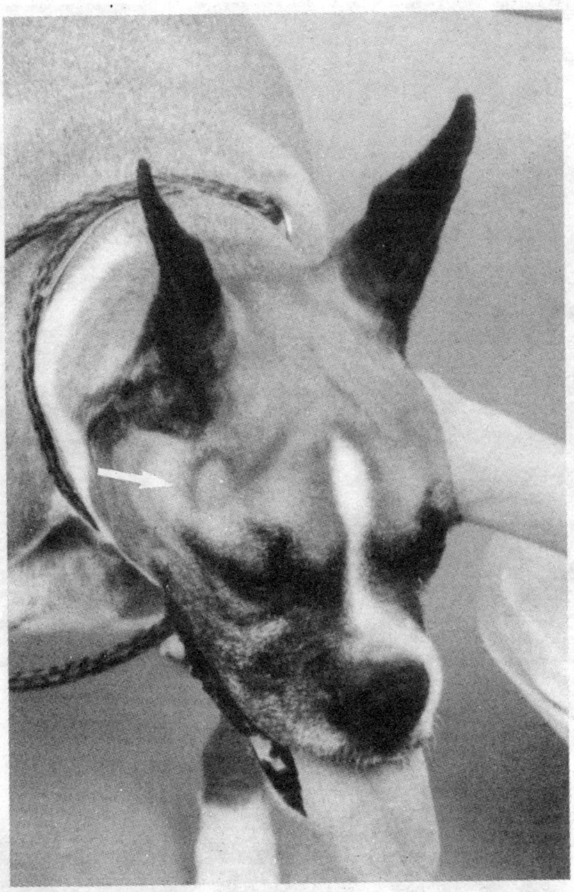

Fig. 3.54. Dog with unilateral temporalis muscle atrophy. Note "sunken head" appearance (*arrow*).

being abnormal. Brain stem nuclear lesions usually result in abnormal function of the facial muscles and stapedius muscle, with variable effects on taste and lacrimation.

With facial nerve irritation, the facial muscle may remain in a constant state of contraction or spasm referred to as a hemifacial spasm (fig. 3.58) (Roberts and Vainisi 1967). Hemifacial spasm in dogs most notably results in deviation of the philtrum of the nose toward the side of the spasm. Often the palpebral fissure is smaller on the affected side of the face, and the ear may be directed more caudally. When testing the palpebral reflex in these dogs, the animal usually can attempt movement of the eyelids, and in some cases can completely close the lid margins. This more appropriate movement of the lids coupled with the abnormal facial expression provide a clue to the underlying spasm. Similar clinical features may be seen with chronic facial nerve paralysis that has resulted in fibrosis and resultant contracture of the ipsilateral facial muscles (fig. 3.59).

Supratentorial lesions may occasionally result in facial muscle weakness (suprabulbar paralysis). Weakness of the facial muscles contralateral to a supratentorial lesion is seen. These animals often have an abnormal facial expression at rest, with a droopy lip contralateral to the supratentorial abnormality. When stimulated, the facial muscle can move appropriately, however.

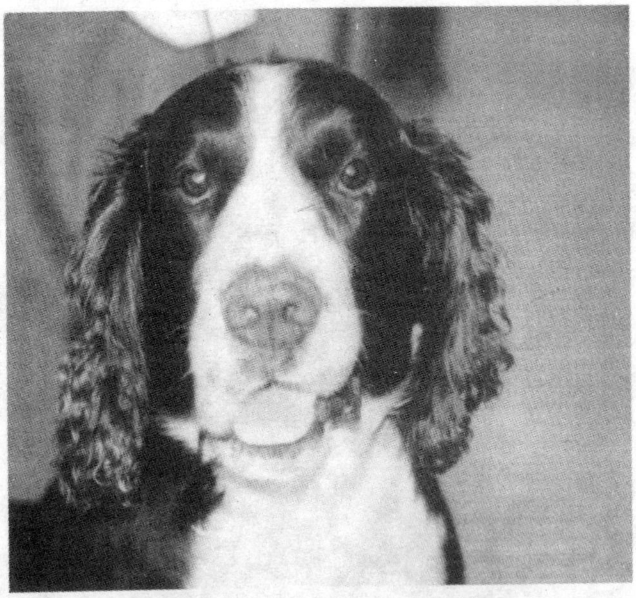

Fig. 3.55. Dog with an abnormal facial expression (droopy right lip) from a facial nerve paralysis.

The parasympathetic divisions of the facial nerve are primarily responsible for lacrimal gland secretion and salivation. Keratoconjunctivitis sicca (KCS) may be seen with involvement of this innervation. Lesions of the nerve occurring distal to the facial canal in the temporal bone, however, should not affect these fibers. Lacrimal function is most readily assessed through performance of a Schirmer tear test. Salivation can be crudely assessed by examining for moist mucosa within the mouth.

The taste functions of the facial nerve are difficult to test clinically, being a subjective sensation similar to smell. An atropine-soaked cotton-tipped applicator swab touched to the tongue may evoke a conscious response (jerking the head away from the stimulus, shaking of the head) and salivation, suggesting some normal functioning taste fibers.

Cranial Nerve VIII (Vestibulocochlear). Cranial nerve VIII has two main portions, the vestibular portion and the cochlear portion. These serve to maintain the position of the head in space (vestibular) and function in hearing (cochlear). Vestibular dysfunction can commonly be recognized by observation of the animal's head and body position and of how the animal moves. Clinical signs of the vestibular division of CN VIII include ataxia, head tilt, nystagmus, and positional strabismus. Many of these signs are present at rest and do not have to be elicited.

Ataxia results from a variety of anatomic lesions within the nervous system, most commonly of the cerebellum, vestibular system, and spinal cord sensory pathways. Ataxia, without motor involvement (paresis), usually implies cerebellar or cerebellar pathway disease, but can also result from vestibular dysfunction. Ataxia can accompany both peripheral and central vestibular dysfunction. Animals with bilateral vestibular disease may have ataxia, a wide-based stance, and tend to hold the head lower to the

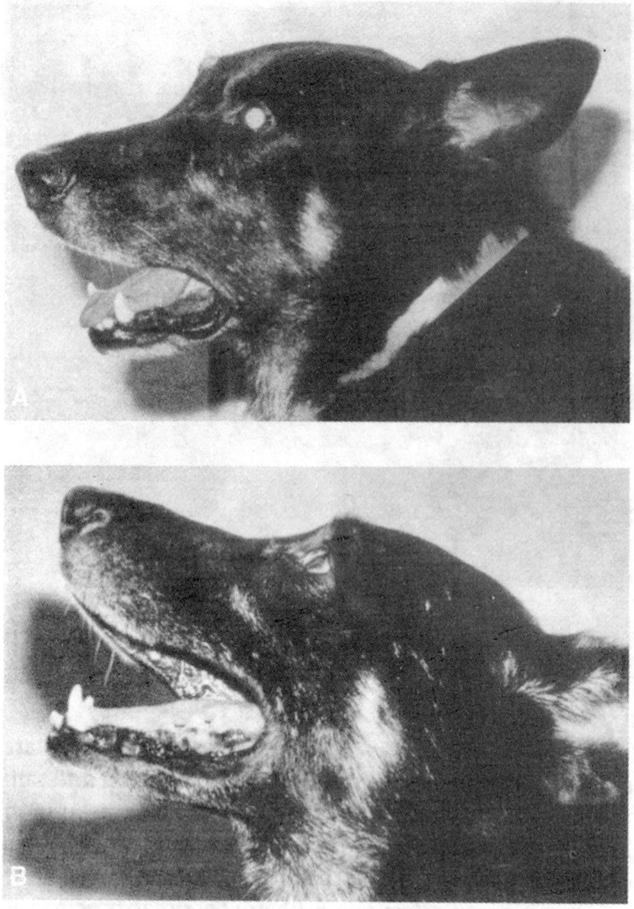

Fig. 3.56. (A) Dog with an abnormal facial expression (droopy left lip) from a facial nerve paralysis. (B) The normal side of the dog is shown for comparison. (Reprinted with permission from R. Bagley and I. Mayhew, Clinical examination of the nervous system, in Veterinary Clinical Examination and Diagnosis, eds. O. M. Radostits, I. G. J. May, and D. M. Houston [Harcourt Publishers Ltd., London, W. B. Saunders, 2000], fig. 19.31.)

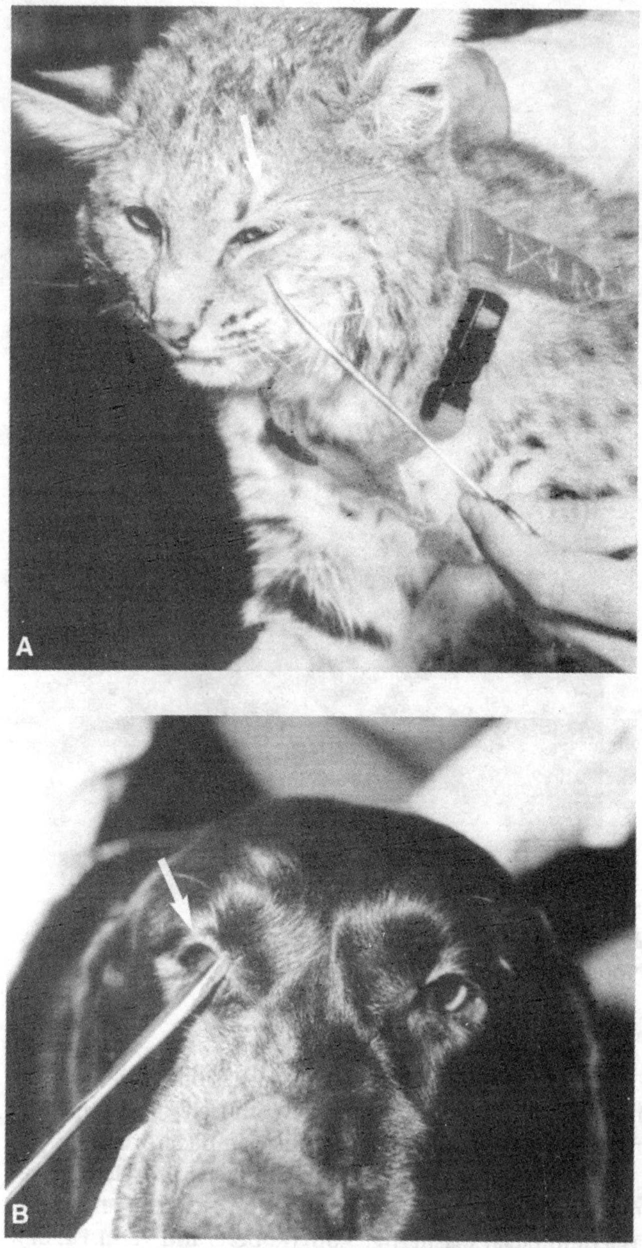

Fig. 3.57. (A) Bobcat showing closure of the left palpebral fissure following a touch stimulus of the facial region. (B) Dog showing inability to close the palpebral fissure with touch stimulation due to a facial paralysis (*arrow*). (Reprinted with permission from R. Bagley, Recognition and localization of intracranial disease, Vet Clin N Am (Small Anim Pract) [1996], 667–709, fig. 6.)

ground (fig. 3.60). The head may also be swung in wide excursions from side to side. These animals often do not have a normal physiologic nystagmus, which is a clue to the bilateral nature of this abnormality.

A *head tilt* is a common clinical sign of vestibular dysfunction. A head tilt is an abnormal posture wherein one ear is deviated more ventrally than the opposite (fig. 3.2, 3.3). For reference, when the animal is viewed from the front, an imaginary line can be drawn from one side of the head to the other along the horizon. A second imaginary line can be drawn perpendicular to this horizontal line, which transects through the philtrum of the nose. In normal animals, these imaginary lines will form a 90° angle. In animals with a head tilt, the imaginary line drawn through the philtrum will form an acute angle less than 90°.

When severe, the animal may be positioned in a laterally recumbent position or rolled on the dorsal aspect of its body. Animals with vestibular disease that are laterally recumbent tend to lie with the side of lesion in the downward position. In some cases, the animal may continually fall and roll. Head tilting is most often associated with disease of the vestibular or cerebellar systems. The head tilt is usually directed toward the side of the lesion in the nervous system, especially if the lesion involves the peripheral vestibular apparatus. Occasionally, with lesions involving the caudal cerebellar peduncle between the brain stem and cerebellum or flocculonodular lobe of the cerebellum, the head tilt is directed away from

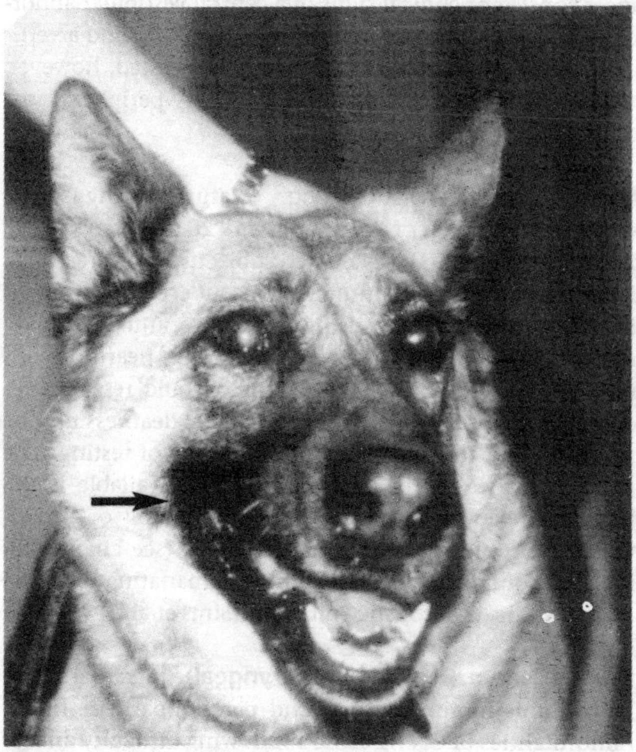

Fig. 3.58. Appearance of a dog showing hemifacial spasm (right-sided, *arrow*).

the side of the lesion, the so-called paradoxical vestibular syndrome (Holliday 1979/1980; deLahunta 1983).

Nystagmus is a spontaneous eye movement that has both a fast and slow phase. When the vestibular system is abnormal, the eyes have a tendency to drift in the direction of the lesion (slow phase), and through a brain stem mechanism the eyes are reset to their initial location (fast phase). With a peripheral lesion, the direction of the fast phase of the nystagmus is always away from the side of the lesion (slow—side). A nystagmus may be spontaneous (found as the animal is stationary) or may be present when the animal positions itself or is positioned by the examiner in an abnormal position (positional nystagmus). A positional nystagmus, if present, is most commonly elicited by rolling the animal onto its back (i.e., upside down).

Nystagmus can be in three general directions described in relation to the horizon or in the direction of the palpebral fissure. If the nystagmus is in the same direction as the palpebral fissure, this is a horizontal nystagmus. If the nystagmus is perpendicular to the palpebral fissure, this is a vertical nystagmus. In some instances, the eye will move in a rotatory direction, either clockwise or counterclockwise. This is referred to as a rotatory nystagmus. Nystagmus is most commonly seen in both eyes simultaneously; it is rare to have a single eye affected.

Dogs with vestibular dysfunction may have an associated positional strabismus. Normally, as a dog's head is extended dorsally, the eyes will remain positioned in the orbit so that the gaze is directed forward (in this instance in the direction of the ceiling). If one or both eyes' position deviates from this direction, this is a positional strabismus. Most commonly, the abnormal eye(s) will deviate ventrally and is most easily appreciated by observing the more prominent dorsal sclera of the affected eye (fig. 3.41). As there may be no strabismus at rest, this finding implies that the vestibular input to CNs III, IV, and VI is abnormal. This clinical abnormality is usually associated with an ipsilateral peripheral vestibular abnormality. Occasionally, this is seen with a brain stem disease.

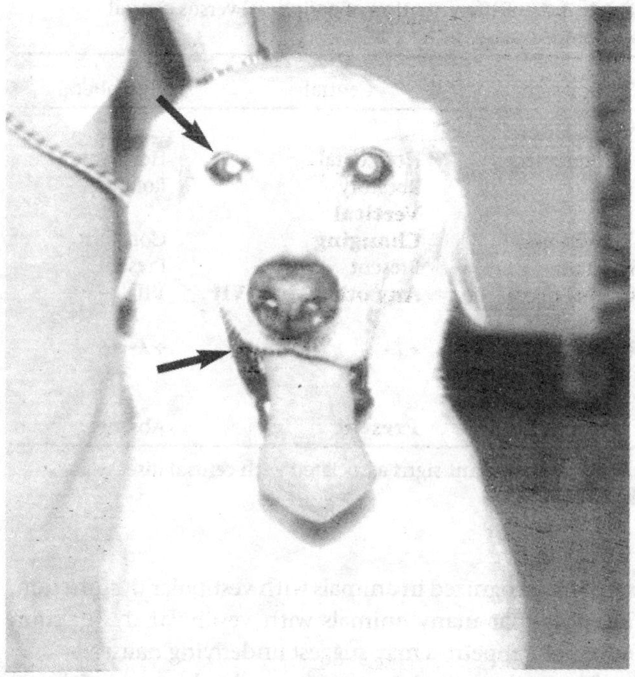

Fig. 3.59. Dog with a chronic facial nerve paralysis with fibrosis (right-sided, *arrow*). Note the smaller palpebral fissure (*arrow*).

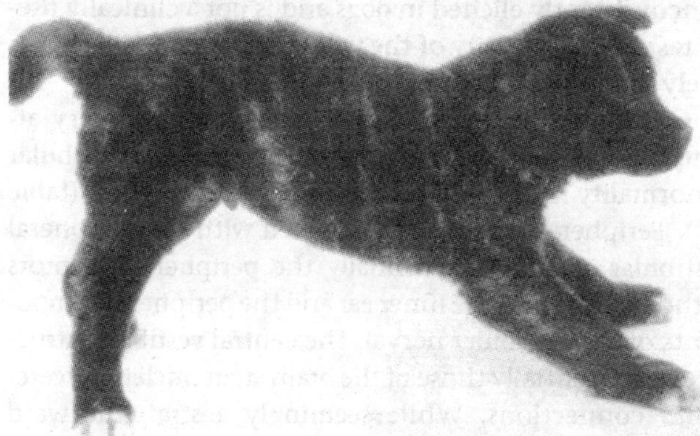

Fig. 3.60. Dog with congenital bilateral peripheral vestibular disease showing a wide-based stance and the head held lower to the ground.

Vomiting is common in humans with vestibular abnormalities, more often associated with disease of the peripheral vestibular system. Vomiting is uncommon but occa-

Table 3.7. Differentiation of peripheral versus central vestibular disease

Clinical sign	Central	Peripheral
Nystagmus		
Spontaneous	Horizontal Rotatory **Vertical**	Horizontal Rotatory
Positional	**Changing**	Constant
Head tilt	Present	Present
Cranial nerve deficits	**Any other than VII**	VII
Horner's	+ / -	+ / -
Conscious proprioceptive deficits	**Present**	Absent

Note: Important signs associated with central disease are boldfaced.

sionally recognized in animals with vestibular dysfunction. The fact that many animals with vestibular dysfunction have poor appetites may suggest underlying nausea.

The oculovestibular response may be abnormal with vestibular lesions. In dogs with bilateral vestibular abnormalities, no oculovestibular response is elicited upon head movement. When the animal moves the head, the head may be swung from side to side in wider excursions than normal.

Caloric nystagmus, the induction of a spontaneous nystagmus by irrigating cold water into the external ear canal, is inconsistently elicited in dogs and is not a clinically useful test of the integrity of the vestibular system. This test is rarely if ever performed in the modern era.

Once a vestibular abnormality is identified, every attempt should be made to determine whether the vestibular abnormality is due to a central or peripheral lesion (table 3.7). Peripheral lesions are associated with the peripheral vestibular apparatus (essentially the peripheral receptors within and around the inner ear and the peripheral components of the vestibular nerve). The central vestibular structures are essentially those of the brain stem nuclei and cerebellar connections. While seemingly a straightforward clinical distinction, clinical signs of peripheral and central vestibular dysfunction often overlap. Also, in a severely affected animal, assessments such as postural reaction testing that help to establish the presence of central disease are made difficult by the animal's posture and attempts to right itself. As with most cranial nerves, the peripheral components of the nerve travel within the skull for a distance before entering or after exiting the brain stem. Therefore, the peripheral vestibular nerve can still be affected by an intracranial disease process.

Differentiation as to whether the lesion is central (brain stem) or peripheral (CN VIII proper) is important for diagnosis, therapy, and prognosis. With unilateral central vestibular lesions, hemiparesis may be seen ipsilateral to the lesion. Occasionally, a hemiparesis is on the side of the body opposite to the direction of the head tilt (paradoxical vestibular syndrome). In this situation, the lesion is present on the side of the body ipsilateral to the hemiparesis. The most consistent clinical signs of a central vestibular abnormality are deficits of conscious proprioception and a vertically directed nystagmus. It has been suggested, however, that a vertical nystagmus may accompany peripheral vestibular lesions in rare instances.

Clinical Assessment of Hearing. Mature hearing is present by 30 to 40 days of age in dogs and 20 to 30 days of age in cats. Hearing can be evaluated subjectively by creating a loud noise in the environment (without creating other vibration currents) and assessing for ear, eye, and other body movements suggesting that the animal has heard (Pryor's reflex) (Sims 1989). Bilateral deafness would result in no clinical response to this sound. Unilateral deafness may be more difficult to determine with this type of testing. The most objective test of hearing currently available is the brain stem auditory evoked potential (BAEP or BAER), which is an electrodiagnostic evaluation (see chapter 9). Rarely, a sound can actually be heard emanating from the animal's ears (otoacoustic emission) (Sims et al. 1991).

Cranial Nerve IX (Glossopharyngeal). Cranial nerve IX contains motor, sensory, and parasympathetic fibers. Abnormalities of CN IX cause swallowing difficulty and/or laryngeal muscle abnormalities (fig. 3.61). Physically, the function of this nerve can be evaluated by eliciting a gag or swallow reflex. This is most easily elicited by the examiner placing a finger in the caudal aspect of the animal's throat. This should not be performed in aggressive animals or those suspected of having a zoonotic disease such as rabies. Also, if a zoonotic disease such as rabies is suspected, gloves should be worn during the examination process. A less-consistent way of inducing a swallow occurs when putting pressure on the laryngeal/pharyngeal area externally usually with one's finger. Dysfunction is suggested by a poor gag or swallowing reflex. Some dogs that are submissive

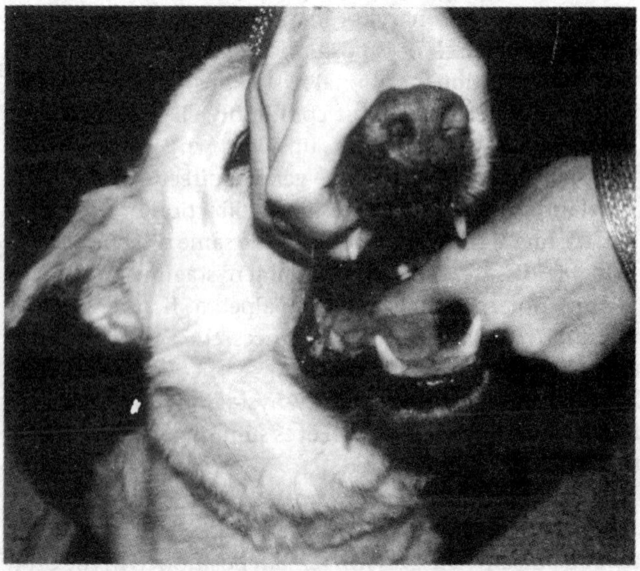

Fig. 3.61. Dog showing a decreased gag reflex.

may allow the examiner to place his or her hand in the dog's pharynx without gagging, however.

Glossopharyngeal neuralgia is paroxysmal pain in the throat or tonsilar region commonly provoked by swallowing, talking, chewing, yawning, or laughing. This may also be associated with bradycardia and syncope presumably due to triggering of cardiovascular regulatory fibers by afferent pain impulses (Shores et al. 1991). Animals may have a dry mouth (xerostomia) from a lesion of CN IX, but this has been difficult to definitively prove.

Cranial Nerve X (Vagus). While the vagus nerve is vastly important for most of the parasympathetic functions of the body, its functions are difficult to assess during a neurologic examination. As the vagus nerve is important for innervation of the esophagus and gastrointestinal systems, vagal abnormalities should be considered with abnormalities of these structures. This would include clinical signs of regurgitation, vomiting, constipation, and diarrhea. The vagal role in heart rate may be reflected in either bradycardia or tachycardia.

Abnormalities of CN X, along with the accessory branch of XI, the recurrent laryngeal or caudal laryngeal nerve, result in paralysis of the laryngeal muscles. Inspiratory dyspnea or stridor may be present in animals with laryngeal and arytenoid dysfunction. Bilateral lesions result in paralysis of the larynx, with inspiratory stridor, dyspnea and cyanosis, and abnormal esophageal function.

Cranial Nerve XI (Spinal Accessory). Abnormalities of this nerve result in trapezius muscle atrophy. Decreased resistance to lateral passive movement of the head and neck contralateral to the side of the lesion may be noted (Oliver et al. 1997). The neck may be deviated toward the affected side in chronic cases (fig. 3.62) (Moreau 1989).

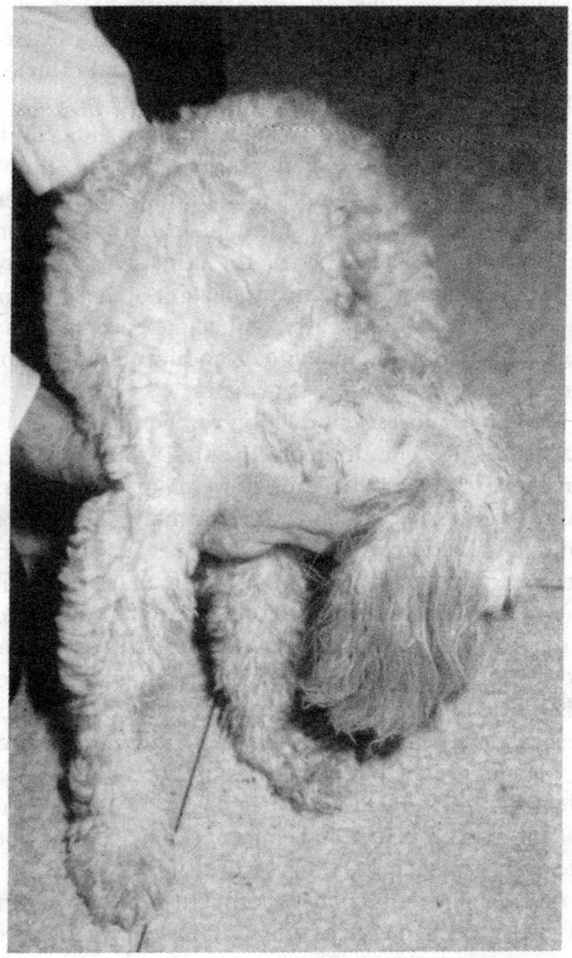

Fig. 3.62. Dog with accessory nerve lesion and associated neck deviation.

Cranial Nerve XII (Hypoglossal Nerve). Clinical signs of disease of CN XII include problems with deglutition, prehension, mastication, and speech. The tongue will be weak or paralyzed. With acute lesions, some state that the tongue will deviate toward the lesion (Braund 1994). With unilateral lesions, the tongue will be pushed toward the side of the lesion by the intact muscles on the normal side. With a chronic unilateral tongue lesion, the tongue will protrude toward the side of the lesion (ipsilateral) and there may be atrophy (ipsilateral) (fig. 3.63). Atrophy may occur on the affected side of the tongue. When this nerve was experimentally transected, however, atrophy of the tongue muscles was not found within the first 4 weeks following transection (Suter and Watrous 1980). Occasionally, UMN lesions will result in dysfunction of CN XII.

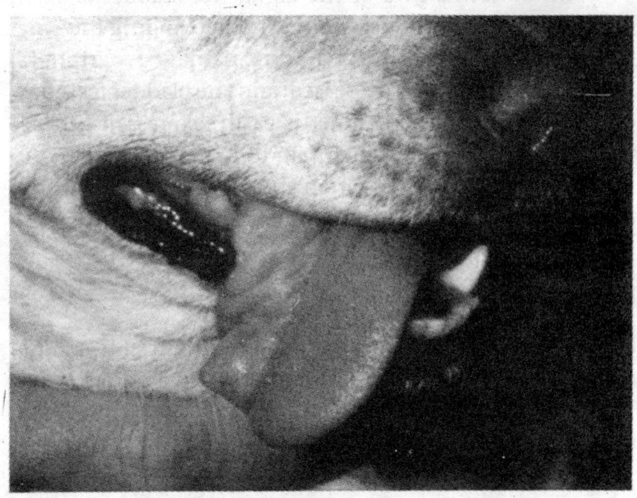

Fig. 3.63. Dog with unilateral hypoglossal nerve disease. (Reprinted with permission from R. Bagley and I. Mayhew, Clinical examination of the nervous system, in Veterinary Clinical Examination and Diagnosis, eds. O. M. Radostits, I. G. J. May, and D. M. Houston [Harcourt Publishers Ltd., London, W. B. Saunders, 2000], fig. 19.34.)

URINARY FUNCTION, SENSATION, AND OTHER SPECIAL FUNCTIONS

Urination is an important function that involves both conscious and unconscious (reflex) modalities. Urination is a coordinated body function associated with alterations in body posture. Differences in body posture exist between males and females. Males may lift one limb and urinate in a lateral direction. Females tend to lower the perineal region toward the ground by flexing the pelvic limbs. Therefore, in addition to reflex urinary system, normal abilities to move limbs and trunk are important. Alterations in urinary function can indicate a variety of problems ranging from abnormalities of the urinary systems, systemic illness that affects urine production, spinal and limb musculoskeletal abnormalities with altered posturing, and alterations in the conscious understanding of the appropriateness of when and where to urinate.

The actual process of urination can be thought of as a local spinal reflex under central control, similar to other spinal reflexes. Urinary reflexes, however, may involve anatomically distant structures within the brain stem, cerebellum, and spinal cord. Although urination is a complex function, clinically recognizable abnormalities may be present.

With abnormalities of the UMN, both ascending information to recognize that the bladder is full and descending information to result in bladder emptying is interrupted. This will result in a distended bladder (table 3.8). Because the local peripheral nerves to the bladder are not impaired, the bladder muscle has good tone, and because of hyperreflexia of the bladder outflow region, the UMN bladder is difficult to express. This is a concept similar to the hyperreflexia of a spinal reflex often seen with UMN lesions.

Additionally with UMN abnormalities, poor coordination between the phases of urination may occur (i.e., poor synchrony between detrusor contraction and urethral sphincter relaxation). Affected animals may begin to urinate normally but then stop abruptly before completely emptying the bladder. This abnormal urinary pattern is referred to as *reflex dysynergia.*

With abnormalities of the LMN, the bladder is again distended because the ascending and descending information cannot project through the damaged peripheral nerves. Bladder tone is decreased, and the bladder feels flaccid. Additionally, the bladder is easily expressed because the local tonic reflex to maintain tone in the bladder outflow tract is not present. Often animals with LMN bladder disease leak or dribble urine frequently or constantly.

DEFECATION

Defecation is controlled like urination, locally at the spinal cord level as well as having descending conscious input. The sacral spinal segments and the pelvic and pudendal nerves will innervate the colon and rectal sphincter, respectively. When the colon is distended with feces, afferent signals in these nerves may set up reflex stimulation of the colonic smooth muscle and relaxation of the sphincters allowing for stool to be passed. With lesions affecting the sacral spinal segments or associated nerve, contraction of the colon may not occur leading to constipation, obstipation, megacolon, or incontinence (Guilford et al. 1990). With UMN abnormalities, reflex defecation persists and is usually adequate for evacuating stool from the colon but may occur at inappropriate times. Also, with UMN disease, normal posturing to defecate may not occur.

Table 3.8. Clinical differentiation of UMN from LMN bladder

	Size	Ease of expression	Tone
UMN	Large	Difficult	Good
LMN	Large	Easy	Poor

CLINICAL ASSESSMENT OF RESPIRATION

There are a number of abnormal respiratory patterns that may be seen associated with alterations in the nervous system. Cheyne Stokes respiration is characterized by waxing and waning depth of respiration with regularly occurring periods of hyperpnea and apnea (Adams and Victor 1993; Guyton and Hall 1996). This is seen with bilateral cerebral or diencephalic disease. Biot's breathing is irregular periods of apnea alternating with periods of four to five breaths of identical depth. This is seen with increased intracranial pressure. Mesencephalic lesions may result in central neurogenic hyperventilation. Tachypnea to the point of panting is seen. Apneustic breathing occurs with pontine lesions and is characterized by periods of breathing and apnea that are very short, with cycles of respiration consisting of only one or two breaths interposed with periods of apnea. Caudal brain stem (medulla oblongata) lesions involving the respiratory centers may cause irregular or ataxic breathing.

Rostral cervical spinal cord lesions interrupt the pathways between the brain stem respiratory centers and the LMNs for respiration. This may result in mechanical respiratory failure. Dysphonia and abdominal respiration, where the abdomen moves out instead of in during inspiration, may be present (Bagley et al. 1993). Dysphonia in these dogs is usually characterized by a "whispering" bark. This is most likely the result of inability to create enough air flow across the arytenoids due to poor inspiratory filling of the lungs.

CLINICAL ABNORMALITIES AND ASSESSMENT OF HEART RATE AND RHYTHM

Bradycardia can occur secondary to increased intracranial pressure. As intracranial pressure increases, perfusion to the brain through the cerebral vessels decreases. The body tries to counterbalance this effect by increasing systemic blood pressure to maintain (increase) cerebral perfusion pressure. This is referred to as Cushing's response. In so doing, the increase in systemic blood pressure is sensed by the baroreceptors as hypertension. This hypertension results in a reflex bradycardia.

Arrhythmias may also be seen with central nervous system lesions. Ventricular premature contractions are seen most commonly, and this is referred to as Brain-Heart syndrome (King et al. 1982). Grossly, at necropsy, small white streaks indicative of myocardial necrosis are seen in the myocardium. This is thought to result from an imbalance in sympathetic stimulation to the heart. As cerebral perfusion drops to critical levels, there is significant release of catecholamines from the adrenal glands. This level of catecholamine results in myocardial damage.

Pulmonary edema can also result from neurogenic mechanisms. Edema occurs most commonly secondary to a seizure, and is thought to arise due to excessive sympathetic stimulation and alpha receptor-mediated vasoconstriction in the pulmonary vasculature. Pulmonary edema is most commonly seen in the caudal dorsal lung fields.

Rarely, with abnormal stimulation from CNs IX and X, syncopy can result (Shores et al. 1991). These clinical abnormalities also are associated with painful stimulation of the pharynx and larynx.

ABNORMALITIES OF EATING AND DRINKING

The diencephalon is responsible for control of many visceral functions and vital functions for life. The hypothalamic portion of the diencephalon is often referred to as the "UMN of the autonomic system."

The hypothalamus is important for eating, drinking, temperature control, sexual function, and other basic drives of life. Lesions in this area of the diencephalon can cause anorexia or hyperphagia, polydipsia (primary; diabetes insipidus) or adipsia, and hyper- or hypothermia. These systemic abnormalities may be important clues to a lesion in this area of the brain.

Abnormalities of Hunger

Central recognition of hunger occurs in the hypothalamus. Bilateral destruction of certain ventromedial regions of the hypothalamus results in overeating (loss of satiety) (Jenkins 1978). Destruction of the more lateral areas results in lack of eating. The forebrain and limbic system have influences over these centers, and to complete the eating process, complex motor integration is necessary to perform the motor acts required.

The adiposogenital syndrome (Froehlich's syndrome) is characterized by obesity and genital atrophy (deLahunta 1983). This results from lesions involving the satiety center and the medial basal nuclei of the diencephalon concerned with gonadal stimulation.

The diencephalic syndrome occurs with lesions in the diencephalon wherein eating is normal, but animals continue to lose weight (Nelson et al. 1981). This has been reported in animals with structural abnormalities of the diencephalon.

The hypothalamus is also involved with glucose metabolism, as lesions involving the ventral wall of the third ventricle have been associated with hyperglycemia, glycosuria, and abnormal glucose tolerance. Neoplasia of the pars intermedia in horses, for example, may cause this. Cats with acromegaly often have increased serum glucose (diabetes mellitus) with exogenously administered insulin resistance. These cats often have tumors of the pituitary gland that also may involve the hypothalamus.

Drinking

Thirst in animals ultimately results in drinking. Drinking is the conscious motor response to thirst that allows for water replacement. Drinking involves coordinated movements of the mouth, lips, tongue, pharynx, larynx, and other gastrointestinal structures. The sensory and motor processes of drinking may transiently relieve thirst. This preabsorptive satiety precedes postabsorptive satiety and prevents consumption of too much water. In animals, which are unable to verbalize their desires, drinking becomes the clinical hallmark of thirst.

Adipsia is lack of thirst, manifested in animals by lack of drinking (Bagley 1994). Adipsia is usually easier to recognize than hypodipsia, or partial lack of thirst. Causes of adipsia can be separated into those due to lack of thirst sensation, lack of central integration, or lack of ability to physically drink (Bagley 1994). Adipsia may occur without associated structural CNS abnormalities (osmoreceptor dysfunction) while in other animals associated structural brain disease is present (Bagley 1994).

ABNORMALITIES OF BODY TEMPERATURE REGULATION

A heat loss center appears to exist in the rostral hypothalamus and a heat conservation center exists in the caudal and lateral hypothalamic areas. The heat loss center responds to increased body temperature by initiating sweating, increased respirations, vasoconstriction, panting, and hyperhidrosis. The heat conservation center responds to decreased body temperature by initiating piloerection, shivering, vasoconstriction, and increased metabolic rate.

Lesions in the heat loss area result in hyperthermia; lesions in the heat conservation center result in hypothermia. Bilateral destruction of the descending hypothalamotegmental tracts may result in poikilothermia. Additionally, hemorrhage into the ventricular system may result in elevated body temperature.

PAIN AND SENSATION

Sensations from the skin can include touch, pressure, warmth, coolness, and pain. Superficial pain testing can be used to determine the integrity of the peripheral nerve innervation to the area. The presence of superficial or skin pain sensation, however, is inconsistent in normal animals and may be hard to elicit in stoic animals.

The entire area of the skin innervated by a single nerve is termed a *dermatome* or *cutaneous zone.* An area of skin innervated by only one nerve is termed the *autonomous zone.* Testing of sensations in the autonomous zone of the peripheral nerve may be helpful in determining the integrity of this particular nerve. Autonomous areas have been determined for dogs and are based upon fixed anatomical points. Individual variation of innervation patterns and movement of the skin overlying these points can lead to false assessments, however.

A two-step pinch technique is used to assess cutaneous

sensation (Bailey and Kitchell 1987). A small area of skin is first lightly tented between the jaws of a mosquito hemostat and subsequently squeezed further in order to elicit reactions indicating conscious recognition of this stimulus (vocalizing or quickly orienting toward the stimulus area).

The *cutaneous trunci reflex* or *panniculus reflex* tests superficial pain receptors, the spinal cord, and the lateral thoracic nerves. This reflex is elicited by pinching the skin over the dermatomal areas associated with the thoracolumbar area. The efferent response is contraction of the cutaneous trunci muscles bilaterally (fig. 3.30).

The receptor in the specific dermatomal distribution over the dorsal trunk is excited by the pinching stimulus, which sends an impulse through the dorsal sensory afferent nerve to the spinal cord. Within the spinal cord, before the lateral thoracic nerves exit, this pathway becomes bilateral in function. The impulse travels cranially in the spinal cord to reach the cell bodies of the lateral thoracic nerves. These cell bodies are located at the C8–T1 spinal cord segments. The lateral thoracic nerves exit the spinal cord and course to the cutaneous trunci muscles.

The cutaneous trunci reflex is most helpful when evaluating lesions in the T2–L3 spinal cord segments and the brachial plexus. With lesions in the T2–L3 spinal cord, the cutaneous trunci reflex may be unable to be elicited caudal to the spinal segment involved. Since the dermatomal distribution of the cutaneous nerves in the thoracolumbar area is caudal to the corresponding spinal cord segments, the lesion is approximately one vertebral segment cranial to where the cutaneous trunci reflex is lost.

While there is some debate as to the exact dermatomal distribution in the flank area, it appears clinically that the T12 through L1–L2 dermatomes are distributed from the last rib to the cranial border of the wings of the ilium (Griffiths 1989). Therefore, a dog with a normal cutaneous trunci reflex and UMN signs to the pelvic limbs should have a lesion in the L2–L3 spinal cord segments.

Clinical Assessments of Pain

Because pain is a subjective sensory experience by the one experiencing it, and because animals cannot verbally communicate their feelings to us, how do we know that they are painful? Commonly, we look for both physiological and behavioral responses that are associated with pain in human beings, and we assume that painful stimuli result in the same responses in animals (Hansen 1990). Some of these abnormalities include abnormal activity (varying from reclusive to restless and agitated, disruption of sleep/wake cycle, orienting toward the painful area, aggression), changes in body posture (tense muscles, disuse or guarding of a painful region), changes in interaction with the examiner, vocalization, and physiological alterations (increased body temperature, tachycardia, tachypnea, increased blood pressure).

Evaluation of sensation, especially with spinal cord lesions, is one of the most important evaluations to assess correctly, as prognosis is dependent on the presence or absence of conscious deep pain sensation.

Special and Abnormal Forms of Pain

In human beings there are a number of specific painful syndromes (Adams and Victor 1993). These are less well clarified in animals, however, some may have analogous examples in animals. Neuralgia occurs when a noxious stimulus acts on a nerve for a long time, then eventually results in spontaneous pains that occur in waves or sudden attacks. This pain is restricted to the region supplied by the affected nerves.

Trigeminal neuralgia (Tic Douloureux) is paroxysms of intense, stabbing pain in the distribution of the mandibular and maxillary nerves. This is impossible to determine in animals. Some animals with abnormalities of the trigeminal nerve may scratch or rub their faces. This could be speculated to be the result of an abnormal sensation (pain or paresthesia) or numbness.

Glossopharyngeal neuralgia includes paroxysmal pain in the throat or tonsilar region commonly provoked by swallowing, talking, chewing, yawning, or laughing. This may also be associated with bradycardia and syncope presumably because of triggering of cardiovascular regulatory fibers by afferent pain impulses (Shores et al. 1991).

Anesthesia dolorosa is agonizing pain in a limb when the dorsal roots are torn, even though the limb itself is analgesic. It is occasionally seen in animals with brachial plexus avulsion. Thalamic pain is spontaneous, almost unbearable pain in the contralateral half of the body associated with thalamic lesions.

Pain asymbolia occurs in humans with simultaneous defects in the frontal lobe, insula, and parietal lobe. The patient becomes indifferent to pain, probably because the brain areas responsible for the pain experience have become less active or inaccessible to normal inputs. Patients repeatedly expose themselves to injurious stimuli and often mutilate themselves.

Causalgia is agonizing pain in an area supplied by a damaged nerve with simultaneous trophic and circulatory disturbances in the affected region (sympathetic nervous system involvement). This may also occur with reflex sympathetic dystrophy (Schwartzman and McLellan 1987).

Hyperesthesia

Hyperesthesia can be very helpful in localizing lesions, especially within levels of the spinal cord. For example, a focal area of spinal hyperesthesia can often be found in dogs with intervertebral disk extrusion, which may localize to a few spinal cord segments within a given spinal level (i.e., T13–L1 pain in a dog with a T3–L3 presentation) (fig. 3.64). Diffuse spinal pain could be indicative of meningitis. Cervical pain may also be indicative of intracranial disease (Coates and Dewey 1998).

Hyperesthesia associated with minimal pressure stimulation of the paws is characteristic of polyradiculoneuritis (Coonhound paralysis) (deLahunta 1983). Animals with sensory neuropathies, conversely, may have decreased or absent skin sensation. These animals may self-mutilate themselves presumably due to this lack of sensation (Cummings et al. 1981).

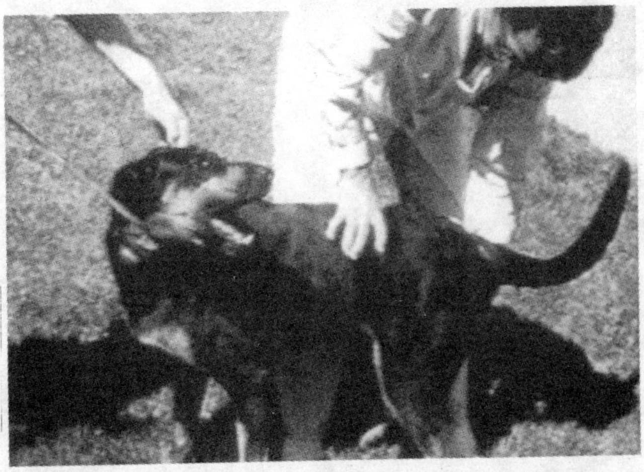

Fig. 3.64. Dog showing a painful reaction with palpation of the lumbar spine. (Reprinted with permission from R. Bagley and I. Mayhew, Clinical examination of the nervous system, in Veterinary Clinical Examination and Diagnosis, eds. O. M. Radostits, I. G. J. May, and D. M. Houston [Harcourt Publishers Ltd., London, W. B. Saunders, 2000], fig. 19.39.)

Deep Pain

The presence or absence of deep pain sensation (pain elicited by pressure on periosteum) is important for prognosis, as deep pain sensation is the final function to be lost with a severe spinal cord lesion. This is because the fibers that carry the deep pain pathways are the small myelinated or unmyelinated nerves (less susceptible to pressure), and these tracts cross and re-cross widely in the spinal cord. Therefore, a near complete functional or anatomical transection of the cord is necessary to result in loss of deep pain.

Deep pain is assessed by placing pressure with a hemostat on the periosteum of the abnormal toe and looking for either crying or attempts to bite the examiner. If neither of these occur, deep pain, for all intentional purposes, is absent. Important: Just because an animal withdraws its limb from the pressure, do not think that deep pain is present. This withdrawal function is purely a local reflex and will be present even in animals with spinal cord transactions cranial to the level of the spinal segments necessary for the spinal reflex function.

Neuroanatomical Diagnosis

Following the completion of the neurologic examination, clinical abnormalities are identified. The type and constellation of abnormalities present provide clinical clues to the location within the nervous system wherein a disease process may be present. This is referred to as neuroanatomical diagnosis and is the focus of chapter 4.

4 Neuroanatomical Diagnosis

WHERE IS THE LESION?

During performance of the neurological examination, abnormalities of nervous system function, if present, are identified and quantified. Each problem provides a clinical clue to the location of the disease or dysfunction within the nervous system. An understanding the neuroanatomic structures that are responsible for a particular neurologic examination finding are important when attempting to determine the location of the lesion resulting in the neurologic dysfunction. Some problems identified result from abnormalities of very specific regions of the nervous system. For example, decerebrate rigidity is associated with a lesion of the midbrain. A head tilt indicates an abnormality of the vestibular or cerebellar regions. In the instance of a head tilt, however, the lesion resulting in these clinical signs may be in the peripheral vestibular apparatus, in the vestibular regions of the brain stem, the cerebellum, or the connections between the vestibular nuclei and the cerebellum (cerebellar peduncles). Other abnormalities found during the neurologic examination help to determine that a lesion exists in the nervous system, but it is more difficult to determine exactly where within the nervous system the dysfunction is originating. Conscious proprioceptive deficits, for example, are a clinical sign that is an important indicator of dysfunction of the nervous system, yet the lesion resulting in the proprioceptive deficits could be found anywhere from the animal's foot to the brain. An animal that has inappropriate mentation could have a lesion in either the supratentorial regions or the brain stem, but could also have a systemic metabolic abnormality that secondarily affects the function of these areas.

The determination of where the nervous system is abnormal is referred to as the *neuroanatomical diagnosis* (Braund 1994; Chrisman 1991; deLahunta 1983; Oliver 1990; Oliver et al. 1997; Oliver et al. 1987). Determining the location of any lesions or abnormalities in the nervous system is one of the most important aspects of appropriate clinical management of animals with neurologic disease. Once the location of these abnormalities is determined, disease processes (*differential diagnosis*) that can affect that particular region of the nervous system can be more logically considered. Once a list of possible disease processes is formulated, appropriate *diagnostic tests* to establish the specific disease processes can be performed and interpreted.

Abnormalities of nervous system function are anatomically localized to as discrete a location within the nervous system as possible. If multiple clinical signs are present that cannot be explained by a single lesion within the nervous system, this could indicate either that there is a *single disease* process affecting *multiple regions* of the nervous system, or that there are *multiple disease processes* affecting different neuroanatomical areas. If subsequent diagnostic tests reveal a lesion in a region other than that suggested by the clinical examination, either the clinical findings have been identified or interpreted incorrectly, the diagnostic test has identified a subclinical abnormality, the disease process is multifocal in character, or more than one disease is present in the same dog.

Diseases involving individual anatomical areas within the nervous system tend to result in a "classic" set of corresponding clinical signs. One, some, or all of these classic clinical signs may be present in any individual animal. While being as discrete as possible with the neuroanatomic diagnosis is ideal, a practical initial goal for most clinicians is to determine if disease within the nervous system is present in either the intracranial region (and associated cranial nerves), spinal cord segments, or the peripheral/neuromuscular junction/muscle complex (fig. 4.1).

When considering where disease can affect the nervous system, it is convenient to divide the nervous system structures into anatomically and physiologically related regions. Structures rostral to the foramen magnum include the intracranial nervous system (supratentorial, infratentorial, cerebellum) and the specific cranial nerves. Structures caudal to the foramen magnum include the spinal cord segments, specific peripheral nerve, neuromuscular junction, or the muscular systems (fig. 4.1).

CLINICAL SIGNS REFLECTING INTRACRANIAL DYSFUNCTION

Clinical signs suggestive of intracranial disease include, but are not limited to, alterations in mental acuity, behavior abnormalities, cranial nerve abnormalities, seizures, and conscious proprioceptive deficits in the limbs. Once it has been

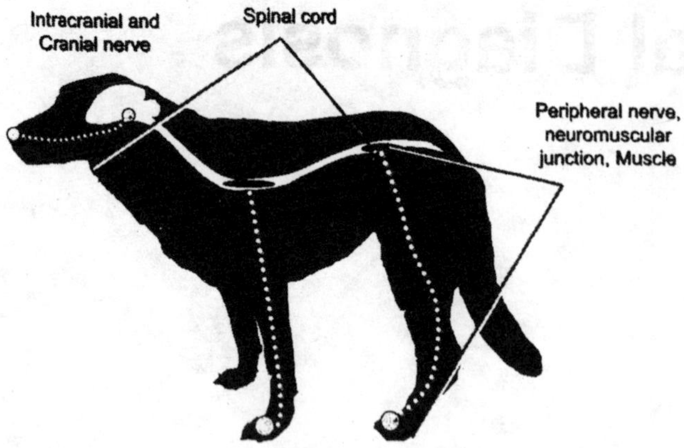

Fig. 4.1. Schematic representation of the functional divisions of the nervous system.

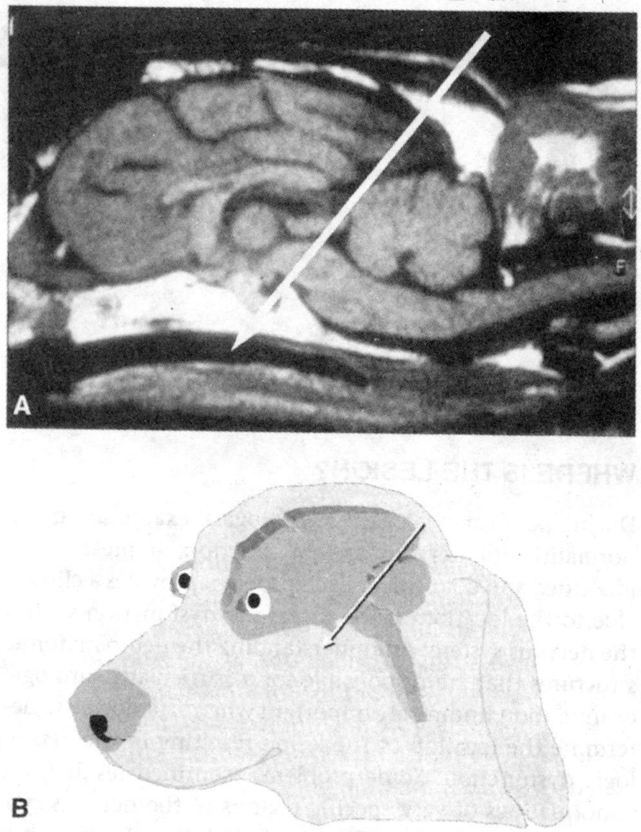

Fig. 4.2. (A) Sagittal, magnetic resonance view of the canine brain. The arrow separates the supratentorial from the infratentorial structures. (B) Schematic view of a dog's head showing division between supratentorial and infratentorial structure.

determined that an intracranial abnormality exists, further delineation of the location of the lesion may be possible based on the clinical signs present. For this discussion, an abnormality may also be referred to as a lesion (a pathologic or traumatic discontinuity of tissue or loss of function of a part) or a disease (any deviation from or interruption of the normal structure or function of a body part). These terms are not to be taken to designate any specific disease process.

Clinical Signs of Supratentorial Disease

The *supratentorial* structures include the cerebral hemispheres, basal nuclei, diencephalon, and rostral portion of the mesencephalon (fig. 4.2). These structures are located rostral to the tentorium cerebelli and are responsible for many functions requiring or associated with consciousness or awareness. For this discussion, clinical signs associated with a unilateral abnormality will be described, with the understanding that bilateral or diffuse abnormalities will potentially result in these same clinical signs, however, affecting both sides of the body. In many instances of diffuse disease, one side or region will be more predominantly affected. In general, the clinical signs will also be more severe associated with the region of predominant disease.

Unilateral lesions involving the supratentorial region predominantly result in clinical signs in parts of the body on the side opposite to the lesion (table 4.1). These are referred to as being contralateral to the abnormality. Clinical signs on the same side of the body as the disease are referred to as ipsilateral. Importantly, there is a constellation of clinical signs that may be present; however, all of these clinical signs may not be present in every affected animal. In some instances, only a single clinical sign may be present. Additionally, because of the somatotopic organization of the nervous system, very discrete abnormalities may result in localized clinical signs (for example, dysfunction of a single limb). The type and extent of any disease process ultimately will determine the specific associated clinical signs.

Classic clinical signs of an abnormality of supratentorial structure or function are discussed in the following sections.

Contralateral Menace Deficit with Normal Facial Nerve Function and Pupillary Light Reflex. A menace deficit may be associated with poor or absent vision in the eye contralateral to a supratentorial abnormality. This is the result of the predominant decussation in animals of the visual fibers at the optic chiasm. If the lesion involves the structures of lateral geniculate nucleus caudal to the occipital cortex, the visual deficit is predominantly in the lateral visual field of the eye opposite to the lesion. The medial (quantitatively smaller) visual field is also affected in the eye ipsilateral to the lesion. This combination of visual field abnormalities is referred to as a hemianopia (or hemianopsia). Clinically, because the predominant (75% in dogs) visual fields of a single eye project information to the contralateral cerebral cortex, the visual function of the eye contralateral to a supratentorial lesion appears globally *deficient*. Rarely, visual field distinctions can be recognized in clinically affected animals.

As the afferent and efferent fibers for the pupillary light reflex (PLR) should not be affected by a supratentorial le-

Table 4.1. Summary of supratentorial deficits

- Menace deficit (Contralateral to an ipsilateral lesion) with normal PLR and palpebral reflex
- Paresis (contralateral to unilateral lesion)
- Facial sensation deficit (contralateral)
- Alterations in consciousness or behavior
- Seizures
- Circling (usually toward the side of the lesion)
- Head pressing
- Head turn (usually toward the side of the lesion)
- Miotic pupils

sion, the PLR is normal in dogs with supratentorial disease. Similarly, the palpebral reflex should remain intact. Therefore, the classic constellation of clinical signs of the visual system subsequent to a supratentorial abnormality usually include an absent or decreased menace response, absent or decreased vision, a normal PLR, and a normal palpebral reflex.

Contralateral Facial Sensation Deficit. Cranial nerve (CN) V projects information from facial sensation receptors to the brain stem. This pathway then crosses to the contralateral side of the brain stem to ascend to the thalamus (supratentorial region) and, via the internal capsule, to the parietal cortex (supratentorial region) on the side opposite from the stimulation. A lesion in the supratentorial region will result in a deficit of facial and head sensation from the opposite side of the body.

Contralateral Hemiparesis. While numerous tracts associated with proprioception may have either a predominant contralateral or ipsilateral influence, unilateral abnormalities rostral to the level of the caudal mesencephalon and rostral pons predominantly affect the limbs on the contralateral side of the body. Unilateral lesions caudal to this level result in an ipsilateral hemiparesis. Therefore, this region approximately at the level of the caudal mesencephalon and rostral pons level is often referred to as the "functional crossover."

Seizures. Seizure activity is associated predominantly with abnormalities of the supratentorial structures. There is experimental evidence that seizures can also be associated with brain stem disease and possibly even spinal disease. In animals affected with spontaneous disease processes, however, seizures are most often associated with supratentorial abnormalities. In some instances, disease of the brain stem may result in secondary pathophysiologic alterations in the supratentorial structures, such as hydrocephalus, and result in seizures.

Behavior Abnormalities. Significant components of the limbic system are present in the supratentorial areas of the brain. Alteration in an animal's behavior, such as becoming somnolent or aggressive may be associated with intracranial and, specifically, supratentorial disease.

Circling, Head Pressing. These specific behavior abnormalities—circling and head pressing—are often associated with supratentorial disease. *Circling* is propulsive walking in circles. This is usually found in animals with disease involving either the supratentorial or vestibular areas. Usually, but not always, the animal circles toward or in the direction of the side of a unilateral supratentorial lesion or vestibular disease lesion. Animals with supratentorial disease will also tend to overstep with the thoracic limb contralateral to the direction of the circling. The paw appears to be "thrown" cranially, wherein the paw is quickly overextended prior to impacting the ground. This may also appear as a "flipping" motion of the distal limb just prior to placing the limb on the ground. In some instances, this contralateral limb appears more extended, stiff, or spastic. Circling, however, may also be associated with abnormalities of the vestibular system.

Head pressing occurs when animals push the dorsal aspect of their heads or noses into a wall, door, or other stationary object continually or propulsively. In some instances, animals will become stuck in a corner and won't move from that area. This abnormal behavior is assumed to reflect abnormalities of cognition and awareness. It is possible that this might indicate a response to pain in or around the head.

Head Turn. Also referred to as a ***head adversion***, a ***head turn*** occurs when the nose remains parallel to the horizon, however, the nose is directed toward the flank or caudal aspect of the body. This has sometimes been referred to as a "yaw" (Oliver et al. 1987). This posture may be a component of the adversive syndrome, which consists of a head turn (sagittal axis of head perpendicular to the ground) and circling (deLahunta 1983). The animal may also intermittently orient the head laterally or toward the caudal aspect of the body.

A head turn occurs most often with supratentorial lesions. The head turn and circling are usually toward the side of the lesion. A similar abnormality termed "hemi-inattention" or "hemineglect" may be seen where an animal will eat only from one side of its food bowl (Holliday 1991; O'Brien 1993). In essence, affected animals are unaware of portions of their external environment.

Pupillary Abnormalities. With bilateral supratentorial disease, the pupils can become miotic. This may be due to loss of descending UMN influences over the parasympathetic nuclei of CN III. Unopposed CN III function results in pupillary constriction. In other instances, this may be a reflection of an abnormality of central sympathetic input to the pupils.

Clinical Signs of Infratentorial Disease

The *infratentorial structures* include the *brain stem* and the *cerebellum*. What constitutes the brain stem varies between descriptions. Embryologically, the brain stem extends from the diencephalon to the myelencephalon. Lesions of the diencephalon and part of the mesencephalon result in clin-

Table 4.2. Summary of clinical signs of infratentorial (brain stem) disease

- Cranial nerve deficits
- Paresis (ipsilateral to unilateral lesion)
- Abnormalities of consciousness and awareness
- Vital function (cardiac and respiratory) abnormalities

ical signs that are difficult to distinguish from lesions of the cerebral cortex. These structures, therefore, are functionally placed with the supratentorial or forebrain abnormalities. For this discussion, the brain stem includes part of the mesencephalon (midbrain), the metencephalon (pons), and the myelencephalon (medulla oblongata).

Clinical signs of *brain stem disease* are listed in table 4.2.

Cranial Nerve Deficits (CNs III–XII). Neuronal cell bodies or processes of cranial nerve III through cranial nerve XII are found in the brain stem. Disease of the brain stem can result in these cranial nerve abnormalities (see table 3.5).

Coma, Stupor, and Other Abnormalities of Consciousness and Awareness. Abnormal mental status may be due to abnormalities of the *ascending reticular activating system (ARAS)* found in the reticular formation of the brain stem. This system normally sends information to the supratentorial structures to result in wakefulness. Abnormalities of this portion of the brain stem can result in stupor and coma. *Narcolepsy* may rarely result from brain stem disease.

Ipsilateral Hemiparesis. As brain stem centers responsible for movement are found caudal to the functional crossover (caudal mesencephalon/rostral pons) in the brain, conscious proprioceptive abnormalities may be present with brain stem disease. If the lesion is predominantly one-sided, hemiparesis or hemiplegia is seen. Hemiparesis, because of the caudal position of the brain stem to the functional crossover, will be ipsilateral to the lesion. In some instances with lesions at the level of functional crossover, hemiparesis may be found contralateral to the lesion. If the lesion involving the brain stem is bilateral, tetraparesis to tetraplegia can be seen. In instances where brain stem disease results in conscious proprioceptive deficits, the spinal reflexes in the limbs should be normal or exaggerated providing a clue to the UMN nature of the lesion resulting in the paresis.

If the lesion in the brain stem is bilateral but asymmetric, tetraparesis may be present, however, one side of the body may be more affected. Again, because of the relationship between the brain stem (more caudal) and the functional crossover, the limbs on the same side (ipsilateral) to a more predominant lesion will be more predominantly affected in most instances.

Respiratory Abnormalities. The respiratory centers are found primarily in the caudal brain stem (medulla oblongata). Brain stem disease can result in respiratory irregularities and failure of respiratory function.

Clinical Signs of Infratentorial Disease Involving the Cerebellum

The cerebellum is a unique structure of the central nervous system. The cerebellum receives proprioceptive information from the body (primarily through the spinocerebellar pathways) from the limbs, identifies the location of body components, then shares this information with multiple brain stem and supratentorial areas responsible for movement.

By providing input data to motor areas of the cortex and brain stem, the cerebellum serves an important role in helping to provide for smooth, coordinated movements of the body. Clinical signs of cerebellar dysfunction therefore reflect failure of smooth, coordinated movements (table 4.3). Portions of the cerebellum are intimately associated with the vestibular system. Clinical signs of vestibular function (head tilt, nystagmus) may also result from cerebellar disease or disease of the connecting pathway (caudal cerebellar peduncle) to the vestibular system. It is important to consider that the cerebellum does not work in isolation from the rest of the nervous system. If, for example, the afferent projections to the cerebellum, such as the spinocerebellar pathways, are affected with disease, the cerebellum may not receive appropriate input data in order to coordinate movement. In this way, disease of the spinal cord cerebellar pathways may also result in clinical signs of "cerebellar" disease. It may be more appropriate to refer to clinical signs of cerebellar system disease, so as to not forget about the contribution of the afferent and efferent cerebellar pathways necessary for appropriate cerebellar functions.

Because of the unique function of the cerebellum, clinical signs of cerebellar disease are often characteristic (deLahunta 1983; Holliday 1979/1980) (table 4.3). Unilateral lesions of the cerebellum result in ipsilateral clinical signs.

Ataxia and *dysmetria* are commonly seen with disease of the cerebellar systems. The animal's strength is normal with isolated cerebellar disease, however, movements may be somewhat delayed or compensations may be exaggerated. If the head is extended and dropped, it may descend farther ventrally than normal (rebound phenomenon). Dysmetria with cerebellar system disease in dogs and cats is most often reflected as *hypermetria*. Hypermetria is evident as overflexion and overstepping with the limbs during

Table 4.3. Clinical signs of cerebellar disease

- Ataxia and dysmetria
- Intention tremor
- Vestibular signs
- Menace deficits with normal vision and normal CN VII function
- Decerebellate rigidity
- Pupillary abnormalities
- Increased frequency of urination

walking or moving. This abnormality is essentially caused by the inability of the diseased cerebellum to limit flexion of the limb.

Ataxia is a failure of muscular coordination or an irregularity of muscle action. In some situations it is defined as lack of an axis, implying an inability to travel along a straight line. Ataxia is usually associated with a "falling" or "swaying" of the body from side to side. It is also commonly present in association with other forms of abnormal limb movements such as dysmetria.

Ataxia results from a variety of anatomic lesions within the nervous system, most commonly of the cerebellum, vestibular system, and spinal cord sensory pathways. Ataxia, without motor involvement (paresis), usually implies cerebellar or cerebellar pathway disease. Sensory ataxia due to loss of joint position sense is often made worse by blindfolding the animal, effectively preventing visual compensatory mechanisms.

Dysmetria is improper estimation of distance during muscular activity. Dysmetria includes both *hypo-* and *hypermetria.* With hypermetria, voluntary muscular movement overreaches the intended goal. This is essentially a failure to limit the degree of flexion. With hypometria, voluntary movement falls short of the intended goal. Hypermetria is more commonly recognized than hypometria in small animals. Both of these abnormalities are most often associated with lesions of the cerebellum or cerebellar pathways.

Intention tremors may involve the whole body but are usually most obvious in the head. A tremor is a to and fro movement of the body part. The head usually moves in an up and down ("yes") direction at a frequency of 2–4 Hz (flexions and extensions per second). This type of tremor is exaggerated by goal-oriented movement such as eating. As the animal puts its head downward toward the food or water bowl, the head appears to "bounce" or "rock" back and forth.

Involvement of the *flocculonodular lobe* or *fastigial area* of the cerebellum may result in abnormalities indistinguishable from a vestibular disturbance such as *lack of balance, head tilt, nystagmus,* and a *broad-based stance.* The nystagmus may only be seen when the head is flexed to one side, with the fast phase directed toward the side on which the head is tilted. A *pendulous eye movement,* wherein the eyes oscillate from side to side, may also be seen with cerebellar disease.

A *menace response deficit* can be seen ipsilateral to a unilateral cerebellar lesion. The cerebellum appears to influence, either anatomically or physiologically, the menace response. Importantly, animals with cerebellar causes of lack of menace response have *normal vision* and *normal CN VII* function. If tested in an obstacle course, these animals perform appropriately. Therefore, this menace deficit is not a reflection of a visual system abnormality.

Occasionally, animals with cerebellar disease may have abnormal postures. The rostral cerebellum is inhibitory to stretch in the antigravity muscles, and lesions here may result in opisthotonus with the thoracic limbs extended *(decerebellate posture*). The pelvic limbs are usually flexed forward under the body by the hypertonia of the hypaxial muscles that flex the coxofemoral joints. If the lesion also involves the ventral lobules, the pelvic limbs may be in rigid extension. Reflexes are usually exaggerated.

With unilateral lesions of the fastigial or interpositál nuclei, a *pupillary dilation* that is slowly responsive to light may be seen (Holliday 1979/1980). Occasionally, the third eyelid may protrude and the palpebral fissure may be enlarged. The pupillary dilation occurs in the eye ipsilateral to an interpositál nuclear lesion and contralateral to a fastigial nuclear lesion.

The cerebellum normally has an inhibitory influence on urination. Rarely, a cerebellar abnormality will result in frequent urination due to loss of this inhibitory input.

Paradoxical Vestibular Syndrome. Abnormalities of the caudal cerebellar peduncle or flocculonodular lobules may cause clinical signs more often associated with vestibular dysfunction (deLahunta 1983; Holliday 1979/1980). The head tilt, however, is to the side away from the lesion. The cerebellum sends inhibitory efferent connections through the caudal cerebellar peduncle to the ipsilateral vestibular nuclei. If there is a lack of inhibition to the vestibular nuclei on the same side as the cerebellar lesion, then the vestibular nuclei will be disinhibited, and through a similar mechanism discussed above, result in facilitation of the extensors on the ipsilateral side and facilitation of the contralateral flexors (Thomas 2000). Therefore, the body will lead away from the side of the lesion and the head tilt will be in the opposite direction, as well.

Diseases resulting in a paradoxical head tilt tend to affect the structure of the caudal cerebellar peduncle or flocculonodular lobe. Because of this, there is usually associated involvement of the pathways necessary for normal conscious proprioception. As this region of the nervous system is caudal to the functional crossover, the postural reaction deficits will be ipsilateral to the lesion. The conscious proprioceptive deficits establish the side of the lesion. If, for example, a dog is presented with a head tilt to the left side and has conscious proprioceptive deficits in the right thoracic and pelvic limb, the lesion is most likely on the right side in the caudal cerebellar peduncle area. The head tilt, being in the direction opposite the lesion, would then be considered paradoxical.

Clinical Signs of Infratentorial Disease Involving the Vestibular System

Clinical signs of the vestibular division of CN VIII include ataxia, head tilt, nystagmus, and positional strabismus. Many of these signs are present at rest and do not have to be elicited.

Ataxia results from a variety of anatomic lesions within the nervous system, most commonly of the cerebellum, vestibular system, and spinal cord sensory pathways. Ataxia, without motor involvement (paresis), usually implies cerebellar or cerebellar pathway disease, but can also result from vestibular dysfunction. Ataxia can accompany both peripheral and central vestibular dysfunction.

A *head tilt* is a common clinical sign of vestibular dysfunction. Head tilting is most often associated with disease of the vestibular or cerebellar systems. The head tilt is usually directed toward the side of the lesion in the nervous system especially if the lesion involves the peripheral vestibular apparatus. Occasionally, with lesions involving the caudal cerebellar peduncle between the brain stem and cerebellum or flocculonodular lobe of the cerebellum, the head tilt is directed away from the side of the lesion, the so-called paradoxical vestibular syndrome (Holliday 1979/1980; deLahunta 1983).

Nystagmus can be in all three general directions (horizontal, rotatory, or vertical) in association with vestibular dysfunction. Nystagmus is most commonly seen in both eyes simultaneously; it is rare to have a single eye affected.

Dogs with vestibular dysfunction may have an associated *positional strabismus*. Normally, as a dog's head is extended dorsally, the eyes will remain positioned in the orbit so that the gaze is directed dorsally (if the head is extended dorsally). If one or both eyes' position deviates from this direction, this is termed a positional strabismus. Most commonly, the abnormal eye(s) will deviate ventrally and is most easily appreciated by observing the more prominent dorsal sclera of the affected eye. If the strabismus is not present at rest, this implies that the function of CNs III, IV, and VI is normal. A positional strabismus is usually associated with an ipsilateral peripheral vestibular abnormality. Occasionally, this type of strabismus is seen with brain stem disease.

Vomiting is common in humans with vestibular abnormalities and is more often associated with disease of the peripheral vestibular system. Vomiting is uncommon, but it is occasionally recognized in animals with vestibular dysfunction. The fact that many animals with vestibular dysfunction have poor appetites may suggest underlying nausea. The oculovestibular response may be abnormal with vestibular lesions. In dogs with bilateral vestibular abnormalities, no oculovestibular response is elicited upon head movement. The head may be swung widely from side to side.

Diseases that involve the central vestibular components of the brain stem may result in abnormalities of conscious proprioception. If the lesion is predominantly one sided, hemiparesis or hemiplegia is seen. Hemiparesis, because of the caudal relationship of the brain stem to the functional crossover, will be ipsilateral to the lesion. In instances where brain stem disease results in conscious proprioceptive deficits, the spinal reflexes in the limbs should be normal or exaggerated providing a clue to the UMN nature of the lesion resulting in the paresis.

If the lesion in the central vestibular components of the brain stem is bilateral but asymmetric, tetraparesis may be present, however, one side of the body may be more affected. Again, because of the relationship between the brain stem (more caudal) and the functional crossover, the limbs on the same side (ipsilateral) of a more predominant lesion will be more predominantly affected in most instances. Some animals with vestibular disease may remain laterally recumbent and are unable to stand. Animals with

Table 4.4. Clinical signs of vestibular disease

Signs consistent with central vestibular disease
- Conscious proprioceptive deficits
- Vertical nystagmus
- Changing nystagmus with changing head positions
- Multiple cranial nerve deficits excluding CN VII

Signs consistent with either peripheral or central vestibular disease
- Head tilt
- Horizontal or rotatory nystagmus
- Ataxia
- Falling
- Rolling
- Positional strabismus
- Positional nystagmus (as long as the direction of the nystagmus does not change with changing head positions)

vestibular disease that are laterally recumbent seem to lie with the abnormal side of the body in the dependent or down position.

Every attempt should be made to determine whether the vestibular abnormality is due to a "central" or a "peripheral" lesion (table 4.4). Peripheral lesions are associated with the peripheral vestibular apparatus (essentially the peripheral receptors within and around the inner ear). The central vestibular structures are essentially those of the brain stem nuclei and cerebellar connections. While seemingly a straightforward clinical distinction, clinical signs of peripheral and central vestibular dysfunction often overlap. Also, in a severely affected animal, assessments such as postural reaction testing are made difficult by the animal's posture and its attempts to right itself. As with most cranial nerves, the peripheral components of the nerve travel within the skull for a distance before entering or after exiting the brain stem. Therefore, the peripheral vestibular nerve can still be affected by an intracranial disease process.

Differentiation as to whether the lesion is central (brain stem) or peripheral (CN VIII proper) is important for diagnosis, therapy, and prognosis. With unilateral central vestibular lesions, hemiparesis may be seen ipsilateral to the lesion. Occasionally, a hemiparesis is on the side of the body opposite to the direction of the head tilt (paradoxical vestibular syndrome). The lesion is found on the side of the body ipsilateral to the hemiparesis. The most consistent clinical signs of a central vestibular abnormality are deficits of conscious proprioception and a vertical directed nystagmus. It has been suggested, however, that a vertical nystagmus may accompany peripheral vestibular lesions in rare instances.

Clinical Signs and Localization of Spinal Cord Disease

Clinical signs of spinal cord disease vary with the location of the disease within the spinal cord. As pathways from the intracranial nervous system structures ascend and descend through the spinal cord to affect limb function, abnormalities of conscious proprioception are often found with spinal cord disease. Once the affected limbs are identified,

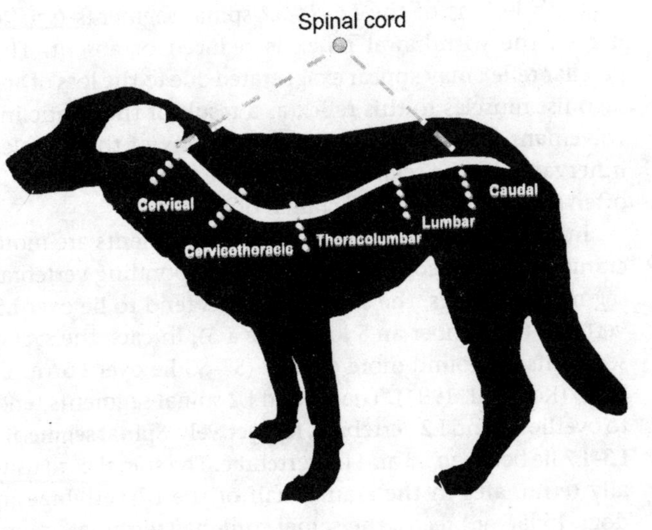

Fig. 4.3. Functional division of the spinal cord.

spinal reflex assessments are performed to determine if the lesion involves the *upper motor neuron (UMN)* or *lower motor neuron (LMN)* systems. After obtaining this information, the examiner should be able to localize the lesion into one of five spinal cord areas (fig. 4.3) (table 4.5).

The spinal cord is divided into functional areas based primarily on the presence of either *UMN* or *LMN* clinical signs to the limbs (see chapter 3) (fig. 4.4). The presence or absence of these characteristic signs is based upon the concept of local spinal reflex (does not require conscious control) functions and the normal control of these reflex functions from intracranial (higher) nervous system centers. An UMN is a neuron or group of neurons that does not exit the central nervous system, and influences, either positively or negatively, the LMN. Clinical signs of UMN include proprioceptive abnormalities, hyper- or normoreflexia, hyper- or normotonia, and disuse atrophy. Hyperreflexia is due to loss of descending UMN inhibitory influence over the gamma neurons to the intrafusal muscle spindles.

The LMN includes the peripheral nervous system and the effector organs (primarily muscles). This functional unit, however, also includes the cell bodies of the peripheral nervous system in the grey matter of the spinal cord. Clinical signs of LMN disease include proprioceptive abnormalities, hypo- to areflexia, hypo- to atonia, and neurogenic atrophy.

Both UMN and LMN abnormalities can result in proprioceptive deficits. Therefore, evaluation of spinal reflex function becomes important in separating lesions of these two functional systems.

Lesions of the *C1–C5* spinal segments can result in ataxia and tetraparesis or, if severe, tetraplegia. Descending pathways from the respiratory nuclei of the brain stem to the LMNs for respiration (phrenic nerve to the diaphragm and the intercostal nerves to the intercostal muscles) travel in the cervical spinal cord, and lesions that interrupt these pathways may compromise respiratory functions. Respiratory function is severely compromised usually only in animals that lose voluntary movement (i.e., are tetraplegic). Often, animals will have a concurrent "whispery" bark due to inadequate tidal volumes.

Table 4.5. Functional areas and associated clinical signs of the spinal cord

Functional areas	Clinical signs
C1–C5	UMN tetraparesis /plegia, neck pain
C6–T2	UMN signs to pelvic limbs; LMN signs to thoracic limbs
T3–L3	UMN signs to pelvic limbs; thoracic limbs normal
L4–S3	LMN signs to pelvic limbs and/or bladder
Caudal	Tail abnormalities

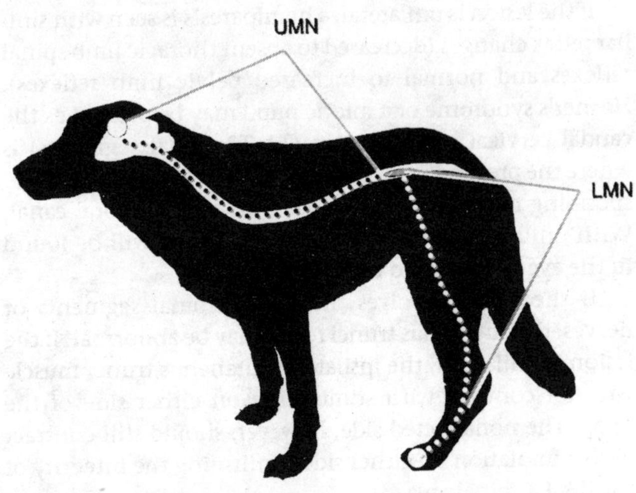

Fig. 4.4. Schematic representation of UMN compared to the LMN systems.

If the lesion occurs unilaterally within the spinal cord, a hemiparesis may be found on the side ipsilateral to the lesion (the spinal cord is caudal to the functional crossover). Cervical hyperesthesia is present with many cervical spinal cord diseases. Some animals with intracranial diseases may also have cervical hyperesthesia, however. Horner's syndrome may be present due to involvement of the descending sympathetic fibers in the lateral tectotegmental spinal tract. With unilateral lesions, Horner's syndrome will be found in the eye ipsilateral to the lesion. Spinal reflex function should be normal to exaggerated, as the LMNs in the cervical and lumbar intumescence are not affected.

In some instances of abnormalities involving the UMNs in the cervical area, the withdrawal reflexes may appear decreased. This type of clinical abnormality is more commonly found in animals with severe impairment of voluntary motor function. This apparent decreased in withdrawal reflexes may be explained by the fact that in most normal animals the strength of the withdrawal reflex determined clinically is the result of a combination of local reflex withdrawal and some associated voluntary supplementation of the muscle movements. When the supplemental voluntary component of withdrawing is affected with the UMN lesions, this leaves only the "true" local reflex component of the withdrawal, which subsequently appears weaker in comparison to the "normal" withdrawal reflex. If this apparent decreased reflex is misinterpreted, however, a diffuse LMN compared to a UMN lesion may be contemplated.

Lesions of the *C6–T2* spinal segments (cervical intumescence) may also result in tetraparesis or tetraplegia like lesions of the *C1–C5* spinal segments. Spinal reflexes in the pelvic limb will be normal or exaggerated, while those in the thoracic limbs should be decreased to absent due to involvement of the motor neuron cell bodies that make up the nerves to the thoracic limb.

If the lesion is unilateral, a hemiparesis is seen with similar reflex changes (decreased to absent thoracic limb spinal reflexes and normal to increased pelvic limb reflexes). Horner's syndrome or a miotic pupil may be present as the caudal cervical intumescence (T1–T3 spinal segments) is where the preganglionic cell bodies lie and where the corresponding nerves exit the spinal cord and vertebral canal. With unilateral lesions, Horner's syndrome will be found in the eye ipsilateral to the lesion

If the lesion involves the C8–T1 spinal segments or nerves, the cutaneous trunci reflex may be abnormal. If the lesion is unilateral, the ipsilateral cutaneous trunci muscle will not contract with stimulation on either side of the body. The nonaffected side, however, should still contract with stimulation on either side confirming the integrity of the T3–L3 spinal area.

Lesions of the *T3–L3* spinal segments may result in paraparesis or, if severe, paraplegia. Spinal reflex function in the pelvic limbs will be normal to exaggerated. The thoracic limbs and cranial nerves should function normally.

The *cutaneous trunci reflex* may be absent caudal to the location of the lesion, especially with more severe spinal lesions. The level of where the cutaneous trunci reflex stops is usually within one to three spinal segments of the lesion. With severe lesions, *Schiff-Sherrington* posture may be seen.

Focal hyperesthesia in the area of the lesion is present with many compressive and inflammatory spinal cord diseases. With unilateral lesions, a UMN monoparesis of the pelvic limb may be found.

Hyperesthesia may be present on palpation or manipulation of the vertebral segments. Focally painful regions are usually associated with local spinal diseases.

Urinary function may be abnormal with T3 to L3 spinal segment lesions. The animal often cannot urinate voluntarily. The bladder may be large, but has good tone on palpation and is difficult to manually express.

Lesion of the *L4–S3* spinal segments (lumbar intumescence) may also result in paraparesis/plegia. Pelvic limb reflexes, however, will be decreased to absent. Depending upon which area of the intumescence is involved, specific reflexes may be abnormal. With a lesion of the L4–L6 spinal segments (femoral nerve), the patellar reflex is reduced or absent. Quadriceps muscle atrophy may be present. Sensation on the distal medial side of the pelvic limb may be reduced or absent due to involvement of the saphenous nerve (sensory), which is a branch of the femoral.

With lesions of the *L6–S1–S2* spinal segments (sciatic nerve), the withdrawal reflex is reduced or absent. The patellar reflex may appear exaggerated due to the loss of antagonist muscles to this reflex as a result of the sciatic involvement (pseudohyperreflexia). Atrophy of the muscles innervated by the sciatic nerve may be present. Atrophy is often most obvious in the cranial tibial muscle.

In the lumbar area, the spinal cord segments are more cranially located compared to the corresponding vertebral segments. In dogs, the sacral segments tend to lie over L5 vertebra (remember an S looks like a 5). In cats, the sacral segments are found more distally (S2–S3 lie over L6 vertebrae) (Kot et al. 1994). The L1 and L2 spinal segments tend to overlie L1 and L2 vertebrae, respectively. Spinal segments L3–L7 lie between L3 and L5 vertebrae. The spinal cord usually terminates in the cranial half of the L7 vertebrae in dogs. In larger breeds, the spinal cord may terminate more cranially, and in smaller breeds, more caudally (Morgan et al. 1987). In cats, the spinal cord ends at the L7 or the sacral vertebrae.

With lesions of the S1–S3 spinal segments, bladder and colonic dysfunction are seen. The external anal sphincter may be dilated and have poor muscle tone for contraction. The bladder may be large, flaccid, and easily expressed. Many animals with LMN bladders will expel urine with minimal abdominal pressure.

With lesions of the *caudal* segments, tail dysfunction and reduced or absent tail sensation are seen. The tail often cannot be extended dorsally. *Hyperesthesia* may be present on palpation or manipulation of the vertebral segments. Focally painful regions are usually associated with local spinal diseases.

Clinical Signs and Localization of Peripheral Nerve, Neuromuscular Junction, and Muscle Disease

The peripheral nervous system includes any nerve myelinated by a Schwann cell. Schwann cells begin myelinating peripheral nerves to the limbs at the intervertebral foramen. Using this strict definition, other components of the LMN, such as the cell body of the motor neuron in the ventral grey of the spinal cord, would not be included in the peripheral nervous system. Functionally, however, a lesion of the peripheral nerve or cell body, the neuromuscular junction (NMJ), or the muscle could result in similar clinical signs.

In animals, LMN disease primarily results in muscle weakness. If a gait is able to be generated, the limb movements are usually short strided and "choppy". Animals are often described as "stiff" due to inability to take an appropriate step distance. The limbs may appear flaccid, and may tremor and buckle with weight bearing. Animals may stand with the limbs placed more centrally under the body. In some instances, this may result in a kyphotic or even cowhocked posture.

With some diseases, muscle weakness is exacerbated with exercise (e.g., myasthenia gravis). Animals with primary afferent or sensory neuropathies may have an awkward gait wherein they tend to "flap" the limbs and strike the ground on the more proximal palmar and plantar regions of the paw and lower limb. Dogs and cats with LMN weakness may lie down frequently. Cats particularly may rest their head on their thoracic limbs when lying down. Cats tend to have ventral neck flexion, or inability to lift their heads, presumably due to cervical muscle weakness.

Animals with LMN may also have abnormalities of limb carriage. Carpi and hocks tend to be abducted or adducted. Dogs with infraspinatous contracture tend to stand with their affected thoracic limb in an adducted position. Animals with myotonia or other muscle disorders may have hypertrophy of their muscle. Their muscle groups may be well defined anatomically. Their gaits are often stiff and short strided. Similarly, animals with muscle cramping or myotonia may have episodic bouts of stiffness and apparent extensor rigidity. Animals with peripheral nerve, NMJ, or muscle disease may be too weak to stand. When in a recumbent position, these animals often remain sternal or laterally recumbent.

Muscle weakness may be seen in visceral structures such as the esophagus resulting in megaesophagus (Shelton et al. 1990). This may result in regurgitation, excessive salivation, gagging, or aspiration pneumonia. Lower motor neuron involvement of the cranial nerves, such as the glossopharyngeal and vagus, may result in dysphagia, dysphonia, gagging, and coughing. Inspiratory stridor may be present with laryngeal paralysis seen in association with some peripheral nerve diseases. If the diaphragm and intercostal muscles are involved, decreases in effective respiration may result. Animals with respiratory muscle weakness tend to initially become tachypneic to compensate for decreased inspiratory volume. As the condition worsens, abdominal breathing, wherein the abdomen moves out during inspiration may be present.

Animals with peripheral nerve disease often have abnormalities of conscious proprioceptive testing. When evaluating conscious proprioception in animals with suspected LMN disease, it is important to evaluate the animal when full weight bearing and again when the animal's weight is supported by the examiner, as some diseases affect only the motor functions of the nerve. Diseases of the NMJ are one such example. Animals with disease of the NMJ or muscle may have proprioceptive deficits during weight bearing, but not when their weight is supported by the examiner. With many peripheral nerve and UMN lesions, animals often have both motor and sensory weakness occur concurrently. Conscious proprioceptive deficits will be present regardless of weight-bearing status in these animals.

Spinal reflexes are usually reduced or absent in animals with LMN disease. This is an important clue to the location of the lesion in the LMN. Resting muscle tone and muscle resistance to passive range of motion in the limbs will be poor or absent. In some diseases such as those of the NMJ (e.g., myasthenia gravis) and muscle, spinal reflexes are normal as relatively minimal muscle strength is necessary to perform simple reflex functions.

The atrophy of muscles that occurs is neurogenic in origin. This atrophy occurs relatively rapidly after an LMN injury (within 5 to 10 days) and is severe. Often the underlying bony structures become prominent. With single nerve disease, muscle atrophy may be in focal muscles or muscle groups corresponding to the distribution of the affected peripheral nerve innervation.

Individual peripheral nerves may be selectively involved with various pathological processes (table 4.6). Evaluation of the sensory distribution loss may be helpful in this localization. The dermatomes and autonomous zones of the limbs may have sensory deficiencies.

Table 4.6. Peripheral nerves of the limbs

Nerve	Spinal cord segments	Muscle innervated	Function of muscles
Thoracic limb			
Suprascapular	(C5) C6, C7	Supraspinatus Infraspinatus	Shoulder extension (supraspinatus) Shoulder flexion or extension
Subscapular	C6, C7	Subscapularis	Shoulder extension
Musculocutaneous	C6, C7, C8	Biceps brachi Brachialis Coracobrachialis	Elbow flexion (biceps and brachialis) Shoulder extension and abduction
Axillary	(C6) C7, C8	Deltoidies Teres major/minor (Subscapularis)	Shoulder flexion and abduction
Radial	C7, C8, T1, (2)	Triceps Extensor carpi radialis Ulnaris lateralis Common digital extensor Lateral digital extensor	Elbow, carpal, and digital extension
Median	C8, T1 (2)	Flexor carpi radialis Superficial digital flexor (Deep digital flexor)	Carpal and digital flexion

(*continued*)

Table 4.6. Peripheral nerves of the limbs (*continued*)

Nerve	Spinal cord segments	Muscle innervated	Function of muscles
Ulnar	C8, T1 (2)	Flexor carpi ulnaris Deep digital flexor	Carpal and digital flexion
Pelvic Limb			
Femoral	L4, L5, L6	Iliopsoas Quadriceps Sartorius	Stifle extension Coxofemoral flexion
Obturator	(L4) L5, L6	External obturator Pectineus	Coxofemoral adduction
Gracilis		Adductor	
Cranial gluteal	L6, L7, S1	Middle gluteal Deep gluteal Tensor fascia lata	Coxofemoral adduction
Caudal gluteal	L7, (S1, S2)	Superficial gluteal (middle gluteal)	Coxofemoral extension
Sciatic	L6,L7, S1 (S2)	Biceps femoris Semimembranosis	Stifle flexion
Semitendinosus		Coxofemoral extension	
Common peroneal	L6, L7	Peroneus longus Lateral digital extensor Deep digital extensor Cranial tibial	Hock flexion Digital extension
Tibial	L1, S1	Gastrocnemius Popliteus Superficial digital flexor Deep digital flexor	Hock extension Digital flexion
Pudendal	S1, S2, S3	External anal	Anal and external urethral
(Caudal rectal)		Sphincter	Sphincter

Source: Adapted from deLahunta 1983.

Multifocal or Diffuse Lesions of the Nervous System

Some diseases can affect multiple regions of the nervous system simultaneously. Additionally, two or more different diseases can affect the nervous system in differing areas. If the clinical signs cannot be adequately explained by a single focal abnormality, then consideration should be give to (1) a single disease with multifocal or diffuse lesions or (2) the presence of multiple disease processes.

5 Clinical Features of Important and Common Diseases Involving the Intracranial Nervous System of Dogs and Cats

Ultimately, the overriding goal of the clinical examination process is to provide physical clues for the clinician as to the specific disease process affecting the patient. Following principles of medical logic, an accurate diagnosis affords the best chance of making appropriate treatment decisions and establishing accurate prognoses. Diseases with known or established clinical features have been identified through prior observation and investigation. A specific disease process associated with an established set of clinical or pathophysiologic criteria is referred to as the *definitive diagnosis*. Once a clinical abnormality is established, a search ensues for the disease process resulting in the particular clinical abnormality present. At the time of clinical examination, however, the specific disease process is often unknown to the clinician. Primarily through deductive reasoning, clinical abnormalities (or premises) are logically formulated together to conclude what disease process is occurring in an individual patient.

After the neuroanatomical diagnosis has been established, consideration is given to diseases that affect the particular area of the nervous system in question. As it is not always possible to make accurate diagnoses via the clinical examination alone, the clinician initially often considers a number of disease processes that may result in similar clinical signs to the ones found in the patient. Using information gained through historical aspects of the abnormality, knowledge of disease pattern or clinical course, and clinical disease features, a disease process may be considered more likely or less likely depending upon the number of clinical features that are common between the known disease and the suspected or unknown disease.

Clinical practice, therefore, often revolves around a process of "playing the odds." Considering the location of the lesion and the associated clinical signs, what is the chance that a particular disease is affecting this particular individual animal? In rare instances, a disease process may have a characteristic clinical sign or group of clinical signs that are pathognomonic for a particular disease. More often, however, a number of diseases may affect the same region of the nervous system and result in the same or very similar clinical signs. As clinical signs reflect the region of the nervous system that is involved with the disease process, but not the individual disease, multiple disease processes that can result in similar clinical signs need to be considered as potential causes of the clinical signs. This is commonly referred to as the *differential diagnosis*.

The scope of neurologic diseases that have been recognized, established, and clarified through the years is sizable (Braund 1994; Chrisman 1991; deLahunta 1983; Dewey 2003; Oliver et al. 1997; Oliver et al. 1987; Summers et al. 1995). Additionally, the current knowledge and understanding of individual diseases is dynamic and constantly evolving. To add more challenges, disease processes described historically may be referred to by different names in the current era. With other diseases, there is a more complete or even entirely different understanding of the pathological process resulting in an updated or modified description of the disease pathophysiology. In clinical neurology, for example, some diseases previously classified as abiotrophies are now often referred to as "channelopathies," reflecting an improved understanding of the underlying pathological defect (Celesia 2001; Kullman 2002). New diseases, or new variants of previously described diseases, are identified sometimes daily. As new diseases are constantly being recognized and reported, and historical disease processes are better clarified, veterinary medical knowledge expands. Therefore, the current veterinary literature should be consulted for updates on specific neurologic disease processes.

The sizable number of disease processes and associated clinical signs makes it almost impossible for the clinician to command to memory each detailed set of clinical disease features. It becomes important in clinical practice, however, to understand general clinical features for groups of diseases, and mechanisms by which disease of the nervous system can occur. For example, while there are many different diseases known as *abiotrophies* (historically thought of as lack of a vital substance for life), many of these diseases affect younger animals and have progressive clinical signs. Therefore, the clinical signs or disease pattern in individual and specific diseases may be similar. These *patterns of disease* are important clues in the process of disease determination. Diseases are presented in this and the other disease chapters (see chapters 6 and 7) as representative of how the pathophysiologic processes of disease of the nervous system may be manifested. Once the important clinical features of a particular type of disease process are understood, it is more likely that the clinician will recognize these same clinical features in other animals with this same disease encountered in the future.

As stated previously, some diseases affect only specific areas of the nervous system. Conversely, other diseases affect multiple areas of the nervous system simultaneously. This chapter summarizes important nervous system disorders in dogs and cats that affect the *intracranial nervous system* and *cranial nerves*. Certain diseases (encephalomyelopathies) affect both the brain and spinal cord simultaneously. These diseases will be discussed under the predominant region (brain or spine) of the major clinical signs. Important clinical features and clues helpful for clinical diagnosis will be emphasized. Histologic and necropsy findings of these diseases have been reviewed elsewhere (Summers et al. 1995). In some cases, anatomical alterations of the nervous system are discussed, as these may be evident on advanced imaging studies, such as magnetic resonance (MR) imaging, if this imaging modality is used for diagnosis.

An important clue to a specific disease is afforded by its historical breed associations (see appendix 2). Although some of the diseases reported have been recognized in only a single animal or few related animals, there is no reason to suspect that these same diseases could not be manifested in other individuals, breeds, or even species.

The diseases are presented in a *DAMNNIITT(V)* order under each neuroanatomical heading (tables 5.1 and 5.2). This acronym stands for the subheadings of major disease categories such as degenerative (D) or anomalous (A) disease processes. Diseases are presented as examples and representatives of disease entities that may affect the intracranial nervous system structures. Bibliographic references provided at the end of the book can be consulted for a more in-depth discussion of the disease processes and a historical perspective on the disease description.

Table 5.1. Major categories of disease processes

D	Degenerative diseases
A	Anomalous and congenital diseases
M	Metabolic diseases
N	Neoplastic diseases
N	Nutritional diseases
I	Inflammatory diseases
I	Idiopathic disorders
T	Traumatic diseases
T	Toxicities
V	Vascular diseases

Table 5.2. Important disease processes involving the intracranial nervous system

Degenerative
- Primary degenerative brain diseases
  - Leukodystrophies
  - Spongiform encephalopathies
  - Neuronal cell body disorders
- Storage diseases
- Age-related dysfunction
- Cognitive dysfunction

Anomalous
- Hydrocephalus
- Hydranencephaly
- Lissencephaly

Metabolic (secondary affect brain function)
- Liver disease (hepatic encephalopathy)
- Renal encephalopathy
- Glucose abnormalities
- Thyroid abnormalities
- Hyper- and hypoadrenocorticism
- Electrolyte abnormalities

Neoplastic
- Primary brain tumor
- Metastatic tumors
- Local extension

Nutritional
- Thiamine deficiency

Inflammatory brain diseases
- Infectious
  - Viral
    - Distemper (dog)
    - Herpes virus
    - Parvovirus

Inflammatory brain diseases *(continued)*
    - Parainfluenza virus
    - Feline infectious peritonitis (cat)
  - Fungal
  - Protozoal
    - Toxoplasmosis
  - Rickettsial
    - Rocky Mountain spotted fever (Vestibular)
    - Ehrlichia
  - Bacteria
  - Parasites

Noninfectious encephalitis
- GME
- Breed-specific meningitis
- Generalized tremor syndrome
- Idiopathic noninfectious encephalitis

Trauma
- Head trauma
- Intracranial hemorrhage
- Subdural hematoma

Toxicity
- Metaldehyde
- Strychnine
- Metronidazole (vestibular)
- Lead

Vascular
- Arteriovenous malformation
- Infarction
- Primary hemorrhage (coagulopathies or platelet disorders)
- Hypertension-related cerebrovascular disease
- Feline ischemic encephalopathy

DISEASES ASSOCIATED WITH CLINICAL SIGNS OF SUPRATENTORIAL OR INFRATENTORIAL DYSFUNCTION

Degenerative Diseases of Younger Animals

While all diseases can potentially result in degeneration of nervous tissue, there are some diseases wherein the primary pathologic process is degeneration of neuronal elements (Braund 1994; Chrisman 1991; deLahunta 1993; Dewey 2003; Oliver et al. 1997; Oliver et al. 1987; Summers et al. 1995). As a broad category, degenerative diseases result from failure of the neuronal elements to survive. This is often the result of some primary intracellular pathophysiologic defect. An unidentified environmental factor, such as an infectious agent or toxin, may also result in the cellular degenerative process. In still other cases, apoptosis may be occurring in neurons. Still other degenerative diseases may be the result of abnormalities of cellular mechanisms or lack of substances necessary for the neuron or its supporting cellular elements to continue its intracellular functions or maintain its structural integrity. Some of these diseases have been referred to historically as *abiotrophies,* essentially meaning lack of the vital substance for life. With clarification, many of these diseases are associated with defects in transmembrane ion and other membrane channel function and may be referred to as "channelopathies." In some instances, a metabolic by-product may accumulate within the cell disrupting its structure or function. *Storage* or *lysosomal storage diseases* are examples of diseases in this group. In the vast majority of primary neuronal degenerative diseases, however, the actual pathophysiologic processes resulting in neuronal element death has not been determined.

There are several diseases associated with primary degeneration of neural elements. Some examples are discussed further in this chapter to emphasize the scope of these diseases in animals. Most of these diseases likely have a genetic basis, and therefore tend to result in clinical signs beginning in younger animals (Braund 1987; Coates and Mine 1995; March 1996; Summers et al. 1995). Less commonly, degenerative intracranial disease processes are found in adult or older animals (Bagley 1997).

Primary degenerative diseases may result in loss of nervous parenchymal elements (table 5.3). When examined histologically, this loss of neural elements or supporting structures results in vacuolation ("holes") of the nervous system. These vacuolations resemble the holes in a sponge and are therefore referred to as spongiform degeneration or spongiform encephalopathies (Braund 1994; Chrisman 1991; deLahunta 1993; Dewey 2003; Oliver et al. 1997; Oliver et al. 1987; Summers et al. 1995) (table 5.3). If this pathologic alteration primarily affects the white matter (axon), these diseases are referred to as *leukodystrophies.* Abnormalities of the white matter of the central nervous system have been described in both dogs and cats, including such breeds as Labrador retrievers, Dalmatians, Silky terriers, Samoyeds, Shetland sheepdogs, Scottish terriers, and miniature poodles (table 5.3).

If the pathologic process is primarily within the neuron, diseases are referred to as neuronal degenerations, neuronopathies, or polioencephalopathies (fig. 5.1) (Braund 1994; Chrisman 1991; Cummings et al. 1988; Cummings et al. 1991; deLahunta 1993; Dewey 2003; Jaggy and Vandevelde 1988; Oliver et al. 1997; Oliver et al. 1987; Palmer and Blakemore 1989; Summers et al. 1995). Primary neuronal disease often occurs in specific neurons or neuronal groups but may be widespread in distribution. Clinical signs may then be reflective of widespread neuroanatomical dysfunction.

As primary degenerative diseases usually result from inherent cellular degenerations and are not associated with neuronal inflammation or compression, affected animals are rarely painful. Clinical signs are invariably progressive. When these diseases involve intracranial structures, common associated clinical signs are behavioral abnormalities, cranial nerve dysfunction, paresis, and ataxia of the limbs. Affected animals often appear to have abnormalities of cognition and movement. Clinical suspicion for these diseases

Table 5.3. Selected breeds affected with degenerative diseases

Breeds
Spongiform degenerations or leukodystrophies
Dalmatian
Egyptian mau (cats)
Labrador retrievers
Miniature poodle
Samoyed
Scottish terrier
Shetland Sheepdog
Silky terrier
Cats—Several unclassified leukodystrophies exist
Neuronal degenerations, neuronopathies, or polioencephalopathies
Cairn terrier
Cocker spaniel
Belgian Malinois
Mastiffs
Rottweiler
Saluki

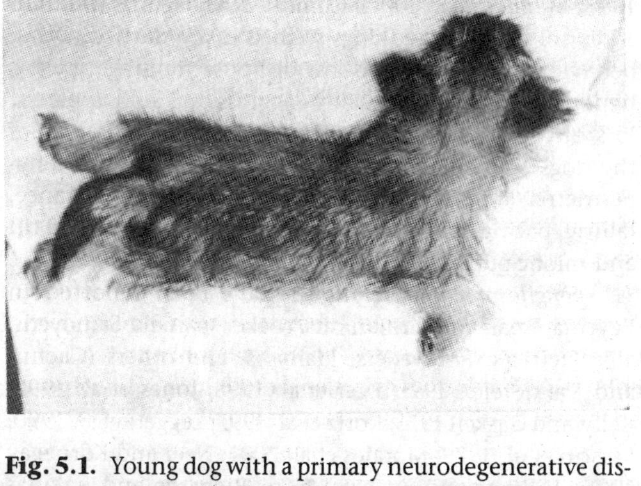

Fig. 5.1. Young dog with a primary neurodegenerative disease. The dog was blind, unable to stand, and had multiple postural abnormalities.

is increased in *young animals* with *progressive neurologic disease*, often with a diverse variety of clinical abnormalities of nervous function.

Clinical Clues to Degenerative Diseases

- Younger animals (less than 1 year of age)
- Progressive clinical signs
- Nonpainful
- Often multifocal or widespread clinical signs
- Organ enlargement (such as hepatomegaly) with some of the storage diseases

Examples of Primary Degenerative Diseases. *Primary degenerative diseases* have been described in multiple breeds of animals in association with a variety of clinical signs and disease patterns. Some specific examples are provided to illustrate the spectrum of clinical entities that can result in primary degeneration of nervous elements.

Dalmatian leukodystrophy affects both male and female dogs and is thought to be inherited in an autosomal recessive pattern (Bjerkas 1977). Histologically, there is caviation of central white matter of the cerebral hemispheres. Clinical signs begin by 3 to 6 months of age. Reported clinical signs include visual deficits, ataxia, and limb weakness.

Fibrinoid encephalomyelopathy (Alexander's disease or fibrinoid leukodystrophy) occurs in dogs including Labrador retrievers, a Scottish terrier, and a miniature poodle (Cox et al. 1986; McGrath and Batt 1975; Richardson et al. 1991). Clinical signs usually began by 3 to 6 months of age. Clinical signs included paraparesis, ataxia, generalized weakness, tremor, falling, and alterations in personality or behavior. The single Scottish terrier also had a head tilt, seizurelike activity, thoracic limb extension, and opisthotonus.

Irish setter quadriplegia and amblyopia is an autosomal recessive disease of Irish setter puppies (Palmer et al. 1973). Clinical signs were present at birth. Affected animals make paddling movements but are unable to stand.

Multisystem neuronal degeneration of cocker spaniels occurs in red-coated cocker spaniels (Jaggy and Vandevelde 1988; Morales et al. 2001). Clinical signs begin at less than 1 year of age. Affected dogs seemed easily startled. Other behavioral signs included loss of house training, apathy, hyperactivity, hypersexuality, aggression, and apparent loss of cognition. Menace responses were absent in all of the dogs evaluated. Additional clinical signs included hypermetria, intention tremors, ataxia, wide-based stance, falling, pacing, and circling. One dog had a slight head tilt and miotic pupils.

Spongiform encephalopathies have been reported in Egyptian mau and Birman cats, cocker spaniels, Samoyeds, Silky terriers, Rottweilers, Malinois, and others (Cachin and Vandevelde 1991; Eger et al. 1998; Jones et al. 1992; Kelly and Gaskell 1976; Kortz et al. 1997; Leggett et al. 1990; Mason et al. 1979; Morales et al. 2001; Neer and Kornegay 1995; O'Brien and Zachary 1985; Richards and Kakulas 1978; van den Ingh et al. 1998; Wells and McGill 1992; Wood and Patterson 2001; Wyatt et al. 1991). Some of these diseases may be forms of abnormalities of myelination, primary axonal diseases, or storage diseases. Affected animals were usually young (weeks of age) when clinical signs began. Clinical signs in the Egyptian mau cats included pelvic limb ataxia, hypermetria, depression, and frequent flicking movements of the distal pelvic limbs at full flexion. A Samoyed puppy had pelvic limb tremors from 12 days of age. Uncontrolled intermittent contractures of the spine, especially in the thoracolumbar area, in the Silky terrier were present from birth. Malinois had head tremors from 3 weeks of age, balance problems, wide-based postures, stilted, hypermetric gaits, and a fine oscillation of the eyes. The diversity in clinical signs within this category of degenerative diseases most likely reflects the diversity of pathologic changes.

Feline spongiform encephalopathy has been reported in cats in the United Kingdom (UK) between 3 and 12 years of age (Wells and McGill 1992; Wyatt et al. 1991). Clinical signs reported included muscle tremors, ataxia, dilated unresponsive pupils, jaw champing, salivation, and behavioral abnormalities such as aggression, biting, excessive grooming, hiding, and scratching. Some of these animals appeared to have periods of vacant staring and were easily startled by noise. Signs sometimes progressed to ataxia, hypermetria, and head tremor.

Hypomyelination or *dysmyelination* of the central nervous system (CNS) has been reported in a variety of breeds of dogs and some cats. These abnormalities usually result in tremor and other signs of cerebellar dysfunction and are discussed under the cerebellar diseases section of this chapter. In some instances, more diffuse clinical signs including signs of supratentorial or spinal cord dysfunction may be evident.

Storage diseases are a group of degenerative neurologic diseases associated with neuronal cell death or dysfunction due to an inborn error of metabolism and absence of a vital enzyme necessary to breakdown an endogenous body substance (see bibliography under Storage Diseases). These substances then accumulate within the neuron or other cells associated with the nervous system and eventually cause cellular dysfunction (fig. 5.2). The numerous storage diseases of small animals are listed in table 5.4. These diseases often occur in younger animals of specific breeds and, therefore, most likely have a proven or suspected genetic basis. Clinical signs of these diseases are variable depending upon the primary disease but usually begin in younger (usually less than 1 year of age) animals. Multifocal clinical signs are common. In some animals with certain storage diseases, visceral organ enlargement may be present due to accumulation of metabolic by-products in these tissues. Clinical signs associated with many of the storage diseases are invariably progressive resulting in significant clinical deterioration and dysfunction.

There are a number of storage diseases of animals. Examples are provided of disease types and associated clinical signs of this class of disease entity.

Ceroid lipofuscinosis has been reported in cats and in a number of breeds of dogs including English setters, Tibetan

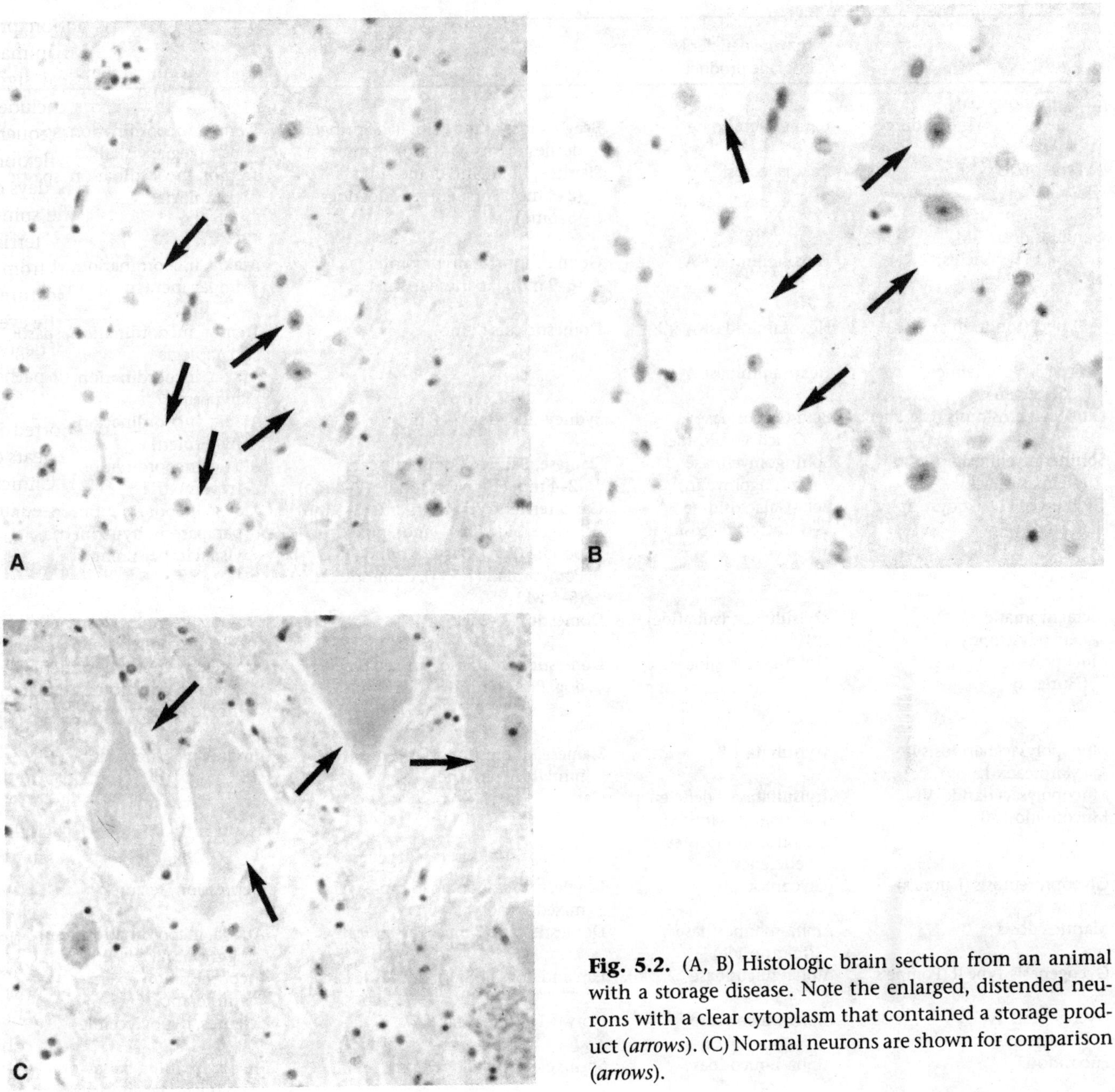

Fig. 5.2. (A, B) Histologic brain section from an animal with a storage disease. Note the enlarged, distended neurons with a clear cytoplasm that contained a storage product (*arrows*). (C) Normal neurons are shown for comparison (*arrows*).

terriers, Border collies, Chihuahuas, dachshunds, terrier-mixed breeds, Salukis, corgis, Japanese retrievers, blue heelers, Yugoslavian sheepdogs, Dalmatians, and cocker spaniels, and others (see bibliography under Ceroid Lipofuscinosis). Animals have been affected between 1 and 9 years of age. Most affected animals, however, are under 2 years old. Clinical signs are variable but include personality change, aggression, hyperactivity, loss of learned behavior, self-mutilation, visual impairment, ataxia, head tremors, seizures, and tetraparesis.

Fucosidosis has been reported primarily in male English Springer spaniels. Signs usually begin between 6 and 12 months. Clinical signs include anxiousness, apprehension, ataxia, hypermetria, and conscious proprioceptive deficits. Anatomical enlargement of many cranial and spinal nerves occurs, some of which may be palpated. By 18 to 24 months, there are visual and menace deficits and nystagmus. Death usually occurs by 3 to 4 years of age.

Gangliosidosis includes two major disease variants and separate subtypes (see bibliography under Gangliosidosis). Gangliosidosis type I occurs in Siamese, Korat, and domestic shorthair cats as well as English Springer spaniels, Portuguese water dogs, Alaskan huskies, and other dog breeds. Diffuse body organs may be involved as well as the nervous system. Skeletal lesions and widened disk spaces may occur in English springers and Portuguese water dogs. Dwarfism is also seen in English springers. Visceral body organ involvement is not reported in Siamese cats. Clinical signs of neurologic involvement include ataxia, head tremor, dysmetria, spastic paraplegia or tetraplegia, visual impairment, dementia, seizures, aggression, and death. Corneal clouding has been seen in feline gangliosidosis due

Table 5.4. Storage diseases of animals

Disease	Enzyme deficient/ storage product	Breed/Onset	Clinical signs
Gangliosidosis GM_1			
Type 1 (Norman Landing)	Beta-galactosidase	Beagle-cross (3 mo), English Springer, domestic cats (2–3 mo), Siamese	Tremor, incoordination, spastic paraplegia; visual
Type 2 (Derry's)	Beta-galactosidase	Siamese, Korat and domestic cats (2–3 mo), Portuguese water dogs (5–6mo)	Tremor, incoordination, spastic paraplegia Cerebellar
Gangliosidosis GM_2			
Type 1 (Tay-Sach's)	Hexosaminidase A	German short-haired pointer (6–9 mo), Japanese spaniel	Ataxia, incoordination, visual impairment, dementia
Type 2 (Sandhoff's)	Hexosaminidase A & B	Domestic cats (2 mo)	Tremor, incoordination, spastic paraplegia
Type 3 (Bernheimer-Seitelberger)	Hexosaminidase A		Ataxia, incoordination, hypermetria
Glucocerebrosidosis (Gaucher's)	Beta-Glucosidase (Glucocerebroside)	Sydney silky dog (6–8 mo)	Ataxia, incoordination, hypermetria
Sphingomyelinosis (Neimann-Pick)[1]	Sphingomyelinase (Sphingomyelin)	Siamese, Balinese, domestic cats (2–4 mo) (Type C); Poodle (2–4 mo)	Ataxia, incoordination, hypermetria
Globoid cell Leukodystrophy (Krabbe's)	Beta-Galactosidase (galactocerebrosidase)	Cairn terrier; West Highland (2–5 mo), beagle, blue tick (4 mo), mixed, poodle (2 yr), Basset hound (1 –2 yr), Pomeranian (1.5 yr), domestic cat (5–6 wk)	Ataxia, incoordination, tremor, paraparesis, hypermetria, visual impairment
Metachromatic Leukodystrophy	Arylsulfatase (sulfatide)	Domestic cat (2 wk)	Progressive motor dysfunction, seizures, opisthotonus
Mucopolysaccharidosis I (Hurler's)	Alpha-L-iduronidase	Domestic cat (10 mo), mixed breed dog, Plott hound	Progressive motor dysfunction, seizures, opisthotonus; high incidence of meningioma in these cats
Mucopolysaccharidosis II (Maroteaux-Lamy)	Arylsulfatase B	Siamese, domestic cat (4–7 mo), miniature pinscher	Progressive paraparesis
Mucopolysaccharide VI	Arylsulfatase B deficiency	Cats	
Mucolipidosis II	n-acetylglucosamine-1-phosphotransferase deficiency	Cats	
Glycoproteinosis (Lafora's)	(Glycoprotein?)	Beagle, basset, poodle (5 mo–9 yr), mixed breed	Depression, seizures
Mannosidosis	Alpha-mannosidase (mannoside)	Domestic cats (7 mo), Persian cat	Ataxia, incoordination, tremor, aggression
Gycogenesis Type II (Pompe's,	Alpha-glucosidase	Lapland dogs (1.5 yr), domestic cats	Incoordination, exercise intolerance
Gycogenesis Type IV (Andersen's)	Alpha-glucosidase	Norwegian forest cat	Seizures, hypoglycemia
Fucosidosis	Alpha-L-fucosidase	Springer spaniel dogs (2 yr)	Incoordination, behavioral changes, dysphonia
Ceroid lipofuscinosis (Batten's)	Unknown	English setter (1 yr), dachshund (3.5–7 yr), cocker spaniel (1.5 yr), Chihuahua, Saluki (2 yr), Australian cattle dogs, poodles, border collie, blue heeler; Tibetan terrier, Dalmatian, Yugoslavian sheepdog, Terrier mixed breed Siamese, domestic cats (2–7 yr)	Personality change, visual impairment, ataxia, incoordination, jaw champing, seizures

Note: An unclassified lysosomal storage disease also exists in Abyssinian cats.
[1]Six types of Niemann-Pick disease are recognized in human beings (A–F) based upon age of onset, degree of hepatosplenomegaly, extent of nervous system involvement, and reduction in sphingomyelinase activity; Type C in cats, sphingomyelinase activity not dramatically decreased.

to associated proteoglycan storage in the corneal epithelial fibroblasts.

Glucocerebrosidase deficiency (Gaucher's disease) is found in Australian Silky terriers with clinical signs beginning around 6 months of age (see bibliography under Glucocerebrosidosis). Clinical signs include incoordination, wide-based stance, stiff gait, generalized tremors, and hypermetria.

Globoid Cell leukodystrophy is seen in cats and a variety of dog breeds including cairn terriers, West Highland white terriers, beagles, bluetick hounds, poodles, mixed breeds, basset hounds, Pomeranians, and others (see bibliography under Globoid Cell Leukodystrophy). Clinical signs include ataxia, tremor, and paresis. Occasionally, decreased spinal reflexes are present.

Glycogenosis also is associated with various disease subtypes (see bibliography under Glycogenosis). Lapland dogs with type I glycogenosis usually show signs by 6 months of age. There is progressive muscle weakness, frequent vomiting, regurgitation, megaesophagus, dysphonia, panting, and cardiac abnormalities. Death usually occurs by 2 years of age. This disease is believed to be inherited in an autosomal recessive pattern.

Type III disease occurs in German shepherds and Akitas. Muscle weakness is seen as early as 2 weeks of age. Abdominal distention due to hepatomegaly may be found concurrently.

Type IV disease occurs in Norwegian Forest cats. Clinical signs begin around 5 months of age. Signs include fever, generalized muscle tremors, bunny hopping, weakness, severe generalized muscle atrophy with contracture of the caudal antebrachial and cranial thigh muscles, and cardiac (ventricular) hypertrophy.

Type VII disease is seen in English Springer spaniels. Clinical signs are more the result of anemia, however, a subclinical myopathy is possible. Neurologic signs are usually not present.

Mucopolysaccharidosis is also divided into differing disease subtypes (Type I: Hurler's syndrome; Type II: Maroteaux-Lamy syndrome, Type VI) (see bibliography under Mucopolysaccharidosis). These diseases are most often seen in cats, but mixed breed dogs, Plott hounds, miniature pinschers, and others have been reported with this disease. Interestingly, cats with mucopolysaccharidosis I (Hurler's) have an increased incidence of intracranial meningioma, which may contribute to any intracranial signs (Haskins and McGrath 1983).

Glycoproteinosis (Lafora's disease) occurs in beagles and basset hounds (see bibliography under Glycoproteinosis). Clinical signs are variable but include seizures. Dogs may be affected from 5 months to 7 years of age.

Mannosidosis occurs in domestic shorthair and longhair cats as well as Persians (see bibliography under Mannosidosis). Clinical signs are seen beginning between 2 and 15 months of age. Cats tend to have variable signs but often reflect cerebellar dysfunction. Bizarre behavior, dementia, corneal abnormalities, and persistent cranial suture lines may be present.

Sphingomyelinosis, or Niemann-Pick disease, occurs in miniature poodles and in domestic shorthair, Siamese, and Balinese cats (see bibliography under Sphingomyelinosis). Clinical signs include ataxia, hypermetria, head tremors, and splaying of limbs.

Degenerative Diseases: Older Animals

Many of the primary degenerative diseases of dogs and cats are inherited or congenital and, therefore, are seen primarily in young animals. Less commonly described are degenerative diseases of older animal. *Primary age-related degenerative brain diseases* of humans, such as Alzheimer's, have not been well documented in dogs and cats but are suspected to occur (Chapman 1995; Cummings et al. 1996; Hart 2001; Houpt 2001; Milgram et al. 1993, 1994; Neilson et al. 2001; Ruehl et al. 1995; Ruehl et al. 2000; Shimada et al. 1992; Yoshino et al. 1996). Deterioration of sensory integration and motor capabilities most likely occurs to some degree in older animals, but this dysfunction is rarely objectively documented. Loss of cortical parenchyma with age may contribute to the enlargement of intracranial ventricles seen with advanced imaging studies (see below, Clinical Features of Hydrocephalus). Some of these primary age-related clinical and pathologic changes are referred to as *cognitive dysfunction disorders*. Behavioral abnormalities of older animals can also be associated with many metabolic or systemic diseases.

Loss of cognitive function or awareness with age is associated with behavior abnormalities such as somnolence, alterations in sleep-wake cycles, and inappropriate urination and defecation. Aimless wandering, pacing, aggression, and apparent irritability are also possible. Recent onset of behavioral abnormalities in older animals can result from structural brain disease, such as tumor or cerebrovascular disease, and should warrant a complete evaluation of intracranial structural integrity. In some instances, bizarre behaviors may be a reflection of seizure activity.

Anomalous Disease

Anomalous conditions of the supratentorial structures are often incompatible with life, and therefore result in the animal's death either in utero or shortly after birth (Coates and Sullivan 2001; deLahunta 1983; Summers et al. 1995; see bibliography under Anomalous Disease). *Anencephaly*, for example, is developmental lack of the cerebral hemispheres often resulting in embryonic or neonatal death. *Exencephaly* is a mass of skin-covered meninges and cerebral hemispheres that project through an opening in the cranial cavity. This as well as other malformations, such as cyclopia and agenesis of the corpus callosum, have been seen in kittens exposed to griseofulvin during gestation. In many of these instances, portions of the nervous system fail to develop normally (fig. 5.3).

Meningoencephalocele, wherein neural elements are protruded into a meningocele, are usually lethal but some animals may survive past the neonatal period (fig. 5.4) (Sponenberg and Graf-Webster 1986; Zook et al. 1983). Malformations of the intracranial structures may also in-

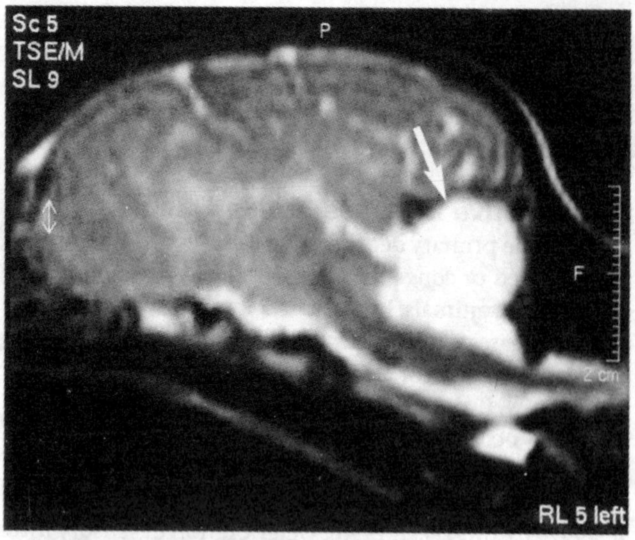

Fig. 5.3. (A) Sagittal, magnetic resonance view of the canine brain. The cerebellum is developmentally a cystic, fluid-filled structure (*arrow*).

clude hypoplasia and duplication of the prosencephalon (cerebral hemispheres and diencephalons), porencephaly, hydranencephaly, and lissencephaly. In some instances, animals with intracranial anomalies survive and are presented for clinical evaluation (fig. 5.4). The author has evaluated a dog with partial hypoplasia of prosencephalic structure that resulted in adipsia (lack of thirst). In some instances, the gross structure of the brain may appear normal, however, there are abnormalities of cellular migration or development that are noted microscopically. These abnormalities may result in seizures. Only selected portions of the nervous system structure may be affected with these malformations.

Porencephaly is essentially cavitation within the brain. In primary cases, this is thought to be due to fetal vascular maldevelopment. Cystic areas may result from abnormal development of the intracranial cellular elements or abnormalities of development of the ventricular system (see Clinical Features of Hydrocephalus below).

Hydranencephaly occurs where the cerebral hemisphere is reduced to a fluid-filled sac with the wall of the sac containing the leptomeninges, a glial membrane, and ependyma. Hydranencephaly has been described in kittens where panleukopenia virus was implicated as a cause of neural element death (fig. 5.5) (Greene et al. 1982; Sharp et al. 1999). This disease has also been described unilaterally in an 8-month-old miniature poodle (deLahunta 1983). The abnormalities were limited to the cortical area supplied by the middle cerebral artery suggesting the possibility of a vascular abnormality resulting in ischemia or hypoxia.

Lissencephaly is a smooth brain appearance with no or minimal gyri and sulci (fig. 5.6). Pachygria, where the cortical tissue is thickened, is often present concurrently. Lissencephaly is seen primarily in Lhasa Apso dogs and Korat cats and may be a cause of supratentorial signs in the postneonatal period (Greene et al. 1976; Zaki 1976; Summers et al. 1995). Often these clinical signs include seizures. Clinical signs may also include deficient or poor learning capabilities. In wirehaired terriers, Irish setters, and Samoyeds, lissencephaly has been in association with cerebellar hypoplasia (Summers et al. 1995).

Primary meningeal cystic structures, possibly the result

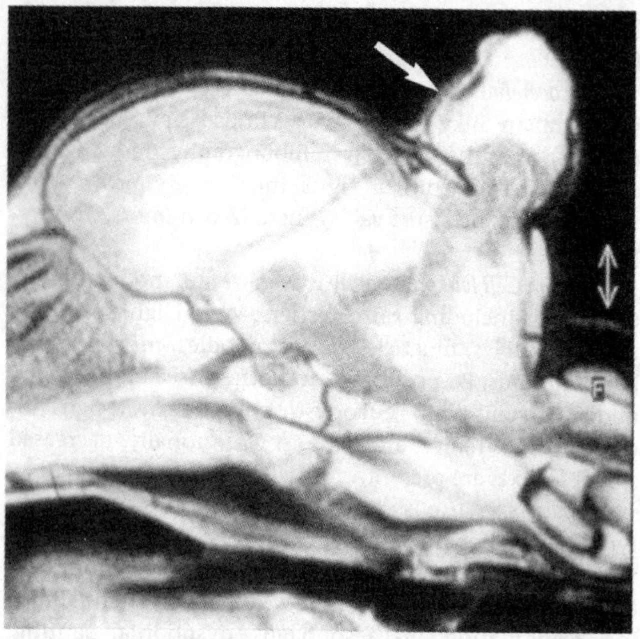

Fig. 5.4. (A) Sagittal, magnetic resonance view of an animal brain with a cerebellar meningocele (*arrow*).

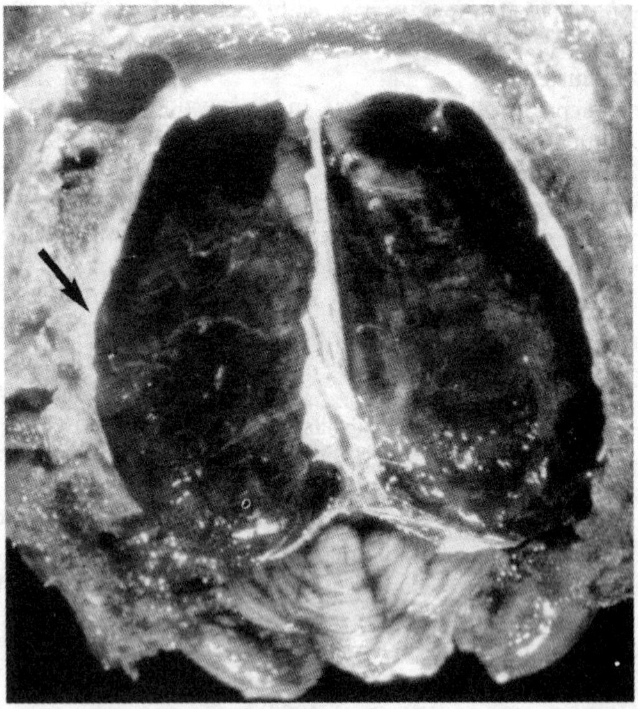

Fig. 5.5. Gross pathological view of an animal brain with hydrencephaly.

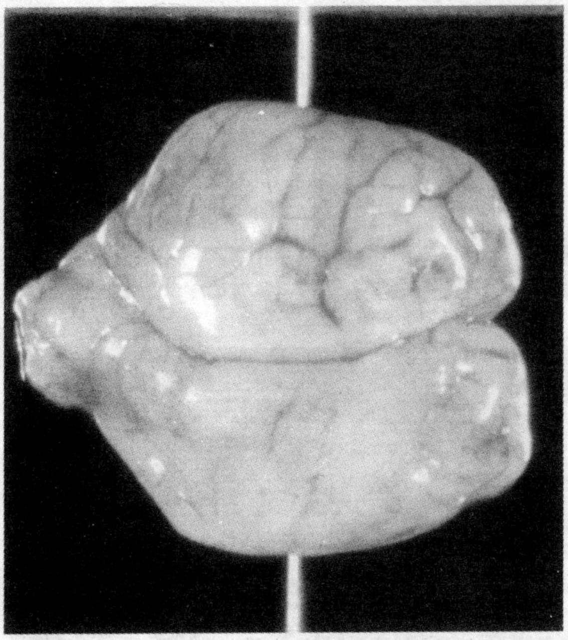

Fig. 5.6. Gross pathological view of an animal brain with lissencephaly.

of maldevelopment, may also be present in the intracranial region. These structures are different from those intraparenchyma cystic regions associated with porencephaly. Some of these cystic abnormalities may involve the ventricular system. Focal cystic structures involving the meninges are often referred to as *arachnoid* or *subarachnoid cysts* (see fig. 10.2) (Milner et al. 1996; Verneau et al. 1997). It is debatable whether these abnormalities are present at birth or are acquired during postnatal development. Extraparenchymal cysts typically are found in or around the dorsal midbrain, third ventricular region (quadrigeminal cistern), rostral and dorsal to the cerebellum, or at the cerebellopontine angle. In some animals, these abnormalities may be associated with hydrocephalus and possibly represent a rupture or outpocket of the ventricular system.

Epidermoid or *dermoid cysts,* which contain varying amounts of epidermal and dermal structures, result from congenitally displaced embryonic remnants that proliferate with age (fig. 5.7) (Howard-Martin and Howles 1988; Kornegay and Gorgacz 1982; Platt et al. 1999). During embryological invagination of neuroectoderm, portions of ectoderm destined to differentiate into skin become entrapped as the neural tube closes. Because the neural canal closes from a caudal to cranial direction beginning at the brain stem level, the fourth ventricle and cerebellomedullary and fourth ventricular region are common sites for these abnormalities to be present. Congenital epidermoid or dermoid cysts are sometimes thin walled and contain mucinous material, keratin, or desquamated epithelial cells. Abnormally displaced cells are likely present at birth, however, the onset of clinical signs usually occurs later in life. Some animals are not presented for evaluation until adulthood or middle age. Theoretically, these cysts can

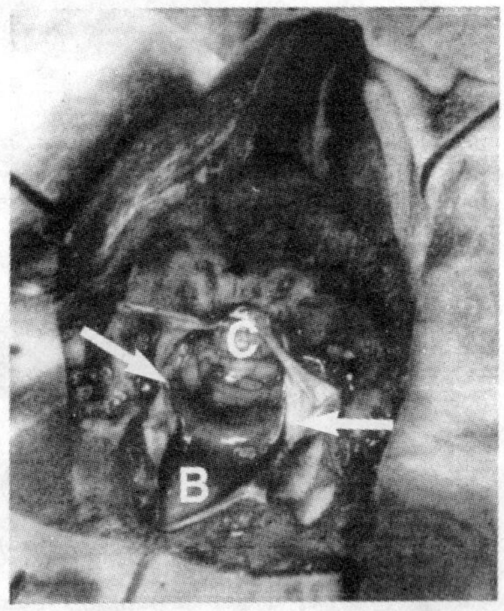

Fig. 5.7. Surgical view of the foramen magnum area of an epidermoid cyst between the cerebellum (C) and the brain stem (B) (*arrows*).

also occur iatrogenically due to laceration and inward displacement of a skin fragment during cerebrospinal fluid collection performed at the cisterna magna (see also chapter 9).

Of the clinically important intracranial anomalies, *hydrocephalus* is the most likely to result in intracranial signs in postnatal animals (fig. 5.8, 5.9, 5.10; also see figs. 10.4 and 10.5) (see bibliography under Hydrocephalus). Hydrocephalus is the term used to describe a condition of abnormal dilation of the ventricular system within the cranium. Hydrocephalus can result from obstruction of the ventricular system, irritation of the ventricle (from inflammation or hemorrhage), and increased size of the ventricles due to loss of brain parenchyma (hydrocephalus ex vacuo); it will rarely be the result of overproduction of CSF associated with a choroid plexus tumor, or be present without an obvious cause (congenital). Hydrocephalus may also be associated with cystic spinal cord abnormalities, such as syringomyelia and hydromyelia (see under Anomalous Diseases, chapter 6) (fig. 5.9).

Ventricular obstruction can occur due to intraventricular or extraventricular abnormalities. Diffuse ventricular enlargement suggests congenital ventricular dilation or obstruction at the level of the lateral apertures or foramen magnum. Focal ventricular enlargement suggests focal obstruction or parenchymal cell loss. It is not uncommon to have bilateral lateral ventricle enlargement that is asymmetric with one side larger than the other. Animals with asymmetric appearance of the ventricles should be critically evaluated for focal obstruction of, or impingement on, the ventricular system. In some instances, CSF will accumulate on the surface of the brain. This is referred to as an *external hydrocephalus* (Dewey 2002).

Hydrocephalus can result in clinical signs due to loss of neurons or neuronal function, alterations in intracranial pressure, or other associated pathophysiological effects of intracranial disease. Interstitial edema results from increased water content of the periventricular white matter

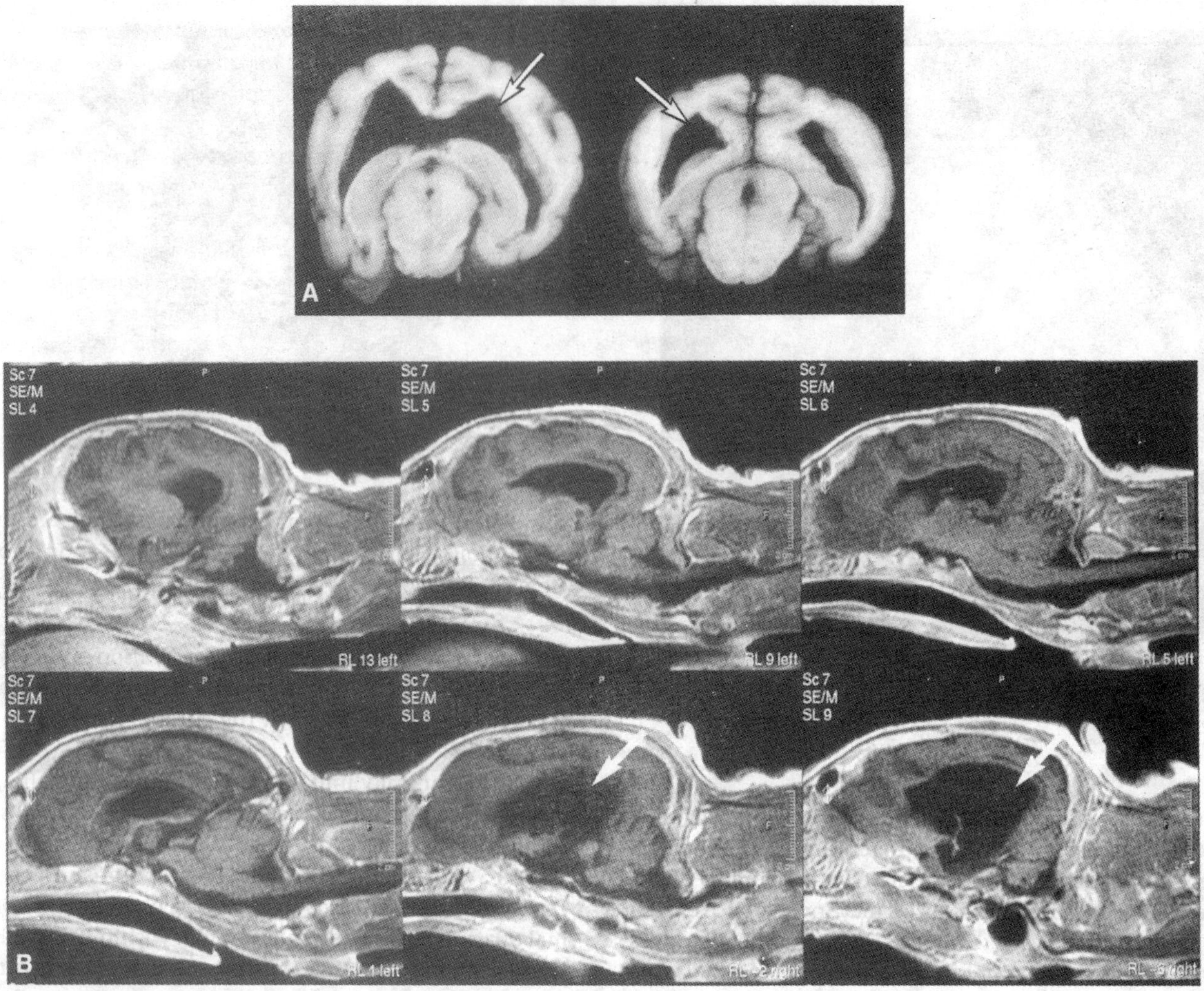

Fig. 5.8. (A) Pathologic specimen showing the gross appearance of the brain ventricles (*arrows*) of a dog with hydrocephalus. (B) Parasagittal, T1-weighted MR images from a dog with hydrocephalus. Note the ventricular dilation (*arrows*).

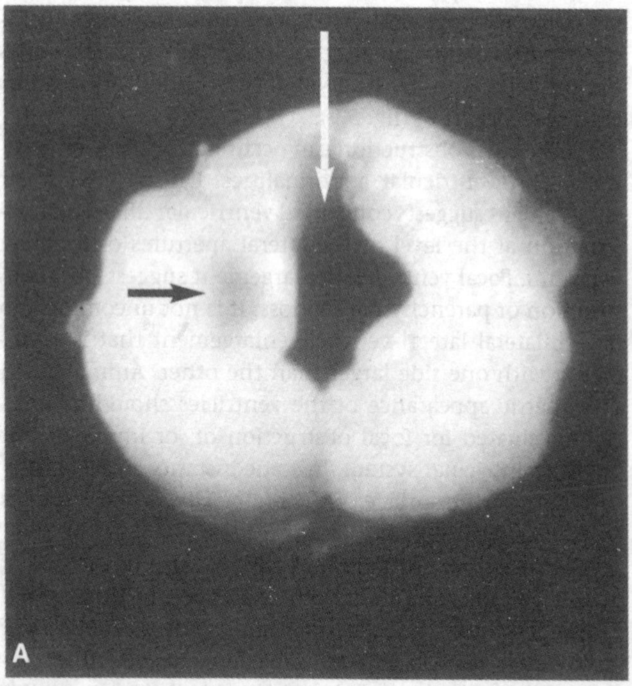

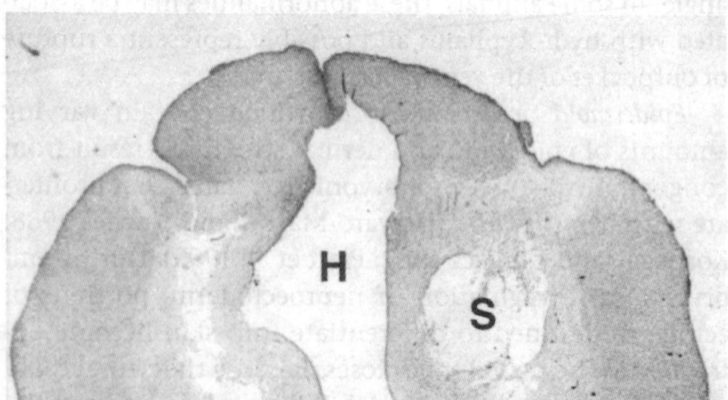

Fig. 5.9. (A) Gross pathologic spinal cord from a dog with hydromyelia and syringomyelia. Note the abnormalities within the spinal cord of a dilated central canal (*large arrow*) and a syrinx cavity (*small arrow*). (B) Histologic section of the spinal cord showing the syringomyelia (S) and the hydromyelia (H).

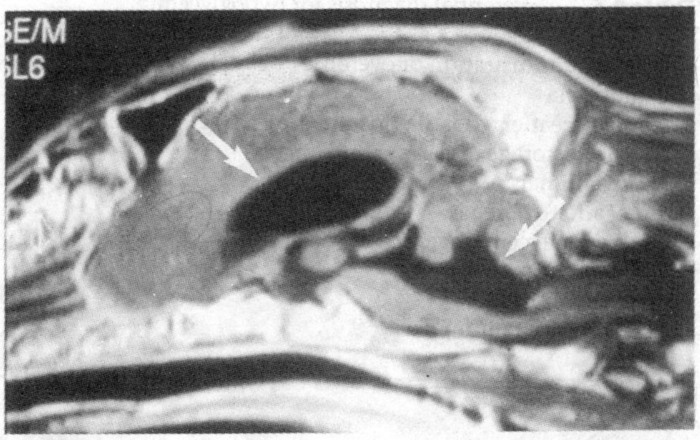

Fig. 5.10. Sagittal, T1-weighted MR images from a dog showing dilation of the lateral and fourth ventricles (*arrows*).

due to movement of CSF across the ventricular walls in instances of hydrocephalus. Periventricular white matter is reduced in size due to the disappearance of myelin lipids secondary to increases in white matter hydrostatic pressure or decreases in periventricular white matter blood flow. Increased CSF pressure may contribute to intracranial disease through alterations in intracranial pressure.

Hydrocephalus and *periventricular encephalitis* have been reported in 2- to 3-month-old puppies where a bacterial cause was suspected (Cantile et al. 1997). Clinical signs are acute and progressive including both supratentorial (behavior change, blindness, circling) and some brain stem signs (head tilt ataxia). Cerebrospinal fluid shows a mixed cell pleocytosis, with increased protein, and xanthochromia.

Clinical Features of Hydrocephalus. Breeds predisposed to congenital hydrocephalus include the Chihuahua, Pomeranian, Yorkshire terrier, English bulldog, Lhasa Apso, toy poodle, cairn terrier, Boston terrier, pug, Pekingese, and Maltese terrier. In fact, hydrocephalus for many of these animals is a genetically associated trait of the breed. In Siamese cats, hereditary hydrocephalus is transmitted as an autosomal recessive trait (Silson and Robinson 1969). In other animals, hydrocephalus may be a component of multiple intracranial abnormalities (see Dandy-Walker syndrome in the Anomalous Diseases section below). In young bullmastiffs, for example, hydrocephalus has been described in association with cerebellar ataxia (Carmichael et al. 1983). Hydrocephalus may also be associated with spinal cord abnormalities, such as syringomyelia and hydromyelia (Itoh et al. 1996; Johnson et al. 1992) (see Anomalous Diseases, chapter 6).

Clinical signs of hydrocephalus reflect the anatomical level of disease involvement. Supratentorial, brain stem, vestibular, and cerebellar signs are possible depending upon which portion of the ventricular system is affected. Severity of clinical signs is not necessarily dependent upon the degree of ventricular dilation, but rather on a host of contributing factors including any primary underlying disease process, associated intracranial pressure changes, intraventricular hemorrhage, and the acuity of ventricular obstruction (i.e., more acute ventricular obstruction is often associated with more severe clinical signs). In young dogs prior to ossification of the cranial sutures, hydrocephalus may contribute to abnormalities of skull development, such as a thinning of the bone structure, a dome-shaped or bossed appearance to the head, or persistent fontanels. A ventral and/or lateral strabismus has been noted in humans and some animals with hydrocephalus. This has been referred to as the "setting-sun sign" as the eyes in the orbit resemble the sun setting on the horizon. Confusion remains as to the underlying pathophysiologic reason for this clinical finding. It has been suggested that this appearance is associated with the skull deformity and distortion of the bony orbits. Others suggest that because this abnormality can be improved with treatment (ventricular CSF shunting) of the lateral and third ventricles that this strabismus is associated with pressure on the mesencephalic tegmentum.

Clinical Clues to Hydrocephalus

- More common in breeds with dome-shaped skulls
- Palpation for a persistent fontanel
- Intracranial signs often reflective of dysfunction of supratentorial structures

As the supratentorial structures are often involved with hydrocephalus, alterations in awareness and cognition are common. Animals with congenital hydrocephalus are often described as not as "smart" as littermates or other animals at similar points in development. Affected animals may not be able to learn housetraining or other obedience activities. Many animals affected congenitally may appear to be less intelligent than normal. In more severe cases, circling, paresis, and seizures may also be seen.

Metabolic Encephalopathies

Numerous systemic metabolic abnormalities may have secondary effects which alter intracranial functions (Cuddon 1996) (see bibliography under Metabolic Diseases). Liver disease (hepatic encephalopathy), renal disease (renal encephalopathy), pancreatic disease (pancreatic encephalopathy), glucose abnormalities (hyper- or hypoglycemia), abnormalities of thyroid and corticosteroid hormone production, electrolyte abnormalities (sodium, potassium, chloride, calcium, magnesium), and acid base abnormalities are examples.

Generally, clinical signs of metabolic encephalopathy are episodic and reflect a diffuse derangement of cerebrocortical function. If neurologic examination abnormalities are present, these abnormalities are usually symmetric within the body. Occasionally, a primary metabolic abnormality can result in focal pathology or dysfunction of intracranial neural elements. In this instance, focal clinical signs of a localized intracranial abnormality may present.

Clinical Clues to Metabolic Encephalopathies

- Clinical signs often wax and wane.
- Physical examination may reveal systemic abnormalities.
- Clinical signs of nervous system dysfunction are often symmetric.
- Ptyalism is commonly associated with hepatic encephalopathy, especially in cats.
- Hypoglycemia often occurs with episodic body or facial jerking as though the animal has been electrically shocked.

Hepatic encephalopathy (HE) results when various putative neurotoxins reach the brain unmetabolized as they pass from the portal system through an abnormally functioning liver or through a vascular diversion around the liver. Suspected toxins include GABA, aromatic amino acids, mercaptans, ammonia, and skatoles. Animals with HE usually are admitted for seizures, ptyalism (especially in cats), and mentation changes. Clinical signs may be episodic and are classically worse following eating, which may result in increased endogenous toxic substances entering the portal system.

Renal encephalopathy is associated with a number of systemic pathophysiologic derangements such as increased parathyroid hormone (PTH), production of neurotoxins, electrolyte imbalances, hyperosmolality, hypercoagulation, hypercalcemia, hypertension, uremic vasculitis, and acid-base imbalances. Clinical signs, in addition to those associated with the renal disease, include abnormal mentation, seizures, muscle tremors, generalized weakness, alterations in respiration, and coma.

Pancreatitis has been rarely associated with encephalopathy. It is unclear if these signs are the direct toxic effects of specific pancreas-related abnormalities (release of circulating enzymes or proteases) on the nervous system or the result of other associated systemic abnormalities such as fluid imbalances, hypotension, vascular abnormalities, and electrolyte disorders.

As the CNS requires a continuing supply of glucose, clinical signs of *hypoglycemia* are reflective primarily of CNS dysfunction. In addition, as a counterregulatory mechanism, sympathetic nervous system may be activated and add to clinical signs of hypoglycemia. Hypoglycemia in adult animals can result secondary to insulinoma, nonpancreatic tumors (such as of the liver, spleen, gastrointestinal elements, which may produce hypoglycemia through excess IGF-2 production), liver disease, hypoadrenocorticism, and insulin overdose (table 5.5). In younger animals and smaller (toy) breeds, inadequate stores of glycogen may predispose to hypoglycemia. Hypoglycemia is most often associated with insulin overdose in diabetic cats, but is also rarely caused by an insulinoma in older cats.

Clinical signs of hypoglycemia-related CNS dysfunction include decreased consciousness and awareness, seizures, weakness, and tremors. Clinical signs are the result of either decreased CNS glucose supply (neuroglycopenic signs) or because of sympathetic nervous system activity. Sympathetic system stimulation may result in apprehension and apparent anxiety. Clinical signs include pupillary dilation, tremors, irritability, vocalization, and a hunger response. Neuroglycopenic signs tend to include alterations in behavior, alterations in mental status, seizures, and visual deficits.

Table 5.5. Differential diagnosis for hypoglycemia

- Insulin administration or overdose
- Insulinoma
- Nonpancreatic neoplasia (insulin growth factor secretion)
- Glycogen storage diseases
- Young animals
- Small and toy breeds
- Oral hypoglycemic agents
- Hypoadrenocorticism
- Hypothyroidism
- Liver disease (failure)
- Sepsis

Affected animals may have intermittent and somewhat characteristic twitches, appearing as though they have been electrically stimulated or shocked. In dogs with extrapancreatic neoplasia, tumors are usually relatively large and may be palpable within the abdominal cavity. In dogs with insulinoma, a peripheral neuropathy has been noted concurrently with insulinoma (see also chapter 7). This may compound clinical weakness and affect prognosis for return of systemic activity.

Hyperglycemia more commonly results in clinical signs of peripheral nerve disease, most often in older cats. Dogs with diabetic ketoacidosis may have cerebral signs (depression), but whether these changes relate to the hyperglycemia or other physiologic derangements such as alterations in osmolality is not always discernible. Animals with hyperglycemia that require large doses of insulin to control blood glucose should be evaluated for acquired *acromegaly*, most often associated with a *pituitary tumor*. Enlarged facial features and body organs are usually found due to the excessive production of growth hormone. Compression on the diencephalon and other supratentorial structures resulting from the expanding pituitary tumor may also contribute to clinical signs.

Hyperthyroidism of cats has been associated with both central and peripheral nervous system abnormalities (see also chapter 7) (Joseph and Peterson 1992). Clinical signs include restlessness, hyperexcitability, irritability, aggression, wandering, pacing, circling, insomnia, and seizures. Apathy, lethargy, and depression occur infrequently. Focal neurological deficits may result from associated cerebrovascular accidents, most likely secondary to hypertension. Hyperthyroidism in cats is often also associated with clinical signs of neuromuscular disease (Joseph and Peterson 1992). Physical abnormalities include generalized weakness, neck ventroflexion, muscle tremors, gait abnormalities, and muscle atrophy. Muscle weakness often manifests as a decrease or inability to jump. Neck ventroflexion may occur with other diseases including myasthenia gravis, polymyopathy (including hyperkalemic polymyopathy), and organophosphate toxicity.

Conversely, *hypothyroidism* has been associated with intracranial and cranial nerve abnormalities in dogs. In some situations, the diagnosis of hypothyroidism was based solely on serum T4 concentrations, which may or may not have been an accurate reflection of a true hypothyroid state. Whether neurologic signs associated with hypothyroidism reflect a primary metabolic disturbance or secondary structural abnormalities associated with underlying vascular disease is not always determined. Larger breeds are more often affected with hypothyroid-associated neurologic signs. Cranial (vestibular, facial, trigeminal) and appendicular peripheral nerves may be abnormal. Head tilts and facial paralysis are commonly reported. Other neurologic signs associated with hypothyroidism include ventrolateral strabismus, nystagmus, hemiparesis, circling, and decreased corneal or facial sensation. Myxedematous coma is a severe intracranial manifestation of hypothyroidism.

Morphological changes in peripheral and cranial nerves included demyelination, remyelination, and axonal necrosis. These changes, however, are not specific for hypothyroid neuropathy. Clinical response to thyroid supplementation has been variable, suggesting a multifactorial pathophysiologic disease process.

Hyperadrenocorticism (Cushing's disease) primarily results in clinical signs of muscle and peripheral nervous system dysfunction, but also can result in signs of intracranial dysfunction. Hyperadrenocorticism is associated with multiple derangements of systemic function such as hypertension and hypercoagulability, potentially predisposing to concurrent cerebrovascular disease. Corticosteroids may also be directly toxic to selected regions of the nervous system. Some animals with hyperadrenocorticism may develop hydrocephalus, possibly the result of neuronal cell loss from corticosteroid-induced neuronal damage or hypertensive encephalopathy.

If hyperadrenocorticism results from a *pituitary tumor*, compression or infiltration of the diencephalon or other supratentorial structures as a result of local (dorsal) tumor expansion may result. Clinical signs due to compression of these intracranial structures include alterations in behavior and consciousness, seizures, and visual deficits. In some instances, abnormalities of the facial nerve function are present. While not directly compressed by these tumors, a shift of the brain stem as a result of displacement by the tumor may stretch or pull on cranial nerves resulting in dysfunction. Clinical signs of neurologic dysfunction may also result acutely following adrenolytic therapy (Nelson's syndrome). This is thought to be due to rapid expansion of a pituitary tumor in response to decreased negative feedback following loss of adrenal corticosteroid production.

Hypoadrenocorticism (Addison's disease) primarily results in clinical signs of weakness (possible muscle and peripheral nervous system dysfunction), but occasionally results in limb paresis. The classic nonspecific signs of this disease and its associated metabolic imbalances (hyperkalemia, hypoglycemia) can result in apparent alterations in mental acuity.

As cell membrane function is dependent upon a balance of electrolytes, *alterations in electrolytes* can result in neurologic abnormalities. Both hypernatremia and hyponatremia may affect the central nervous system and result in abnormalities of mentation. *Hypernatremia* is most extreme in animals with abnormalities of thirst and drinking, which may also be associated with hypothalamic disease (Bagley 1994). Too rapid correction of hypernatremia with intravenous fluid administration can result in cerebral edema and severe alterations in mentation if not death. Similarly, too rapid correction of an established *hyponatremia* can result in thalamic lesions thought to be similar to central pontine myelinolysis in humans (O'Brien et al. 1994; Laureno and Karp 1997). Alterations in potassium tend to affect muscle function more so than CNS function. However, poor cerebral blood flow secondary to cardiac arrhythmias from alterations in potassium may affect intracranial functions. Decreases of chloride may result in depolarization (excitation) of neurons, wherein increases in chloride may cause hyperpolarization of neuronal cell membranes and functional inhibition.

Hypocalcemia decreases the threshold for neuronal and muscle depolarization. Hypocalcemia most often results from iatrogenic injury to the parathyroid gland during surgical removal of thyroid tumors (primarily in cats). Primary hypoparathyroidism is possible but rare. Hypocalcemia associated with lactation (eclampsia) is also possible. Other causes include dietary calcium or vitamin D deficiency, renal disease, acute pancreatitis, ethylene glycol toxicity, and intestinal malabsorption.

Clinical signs of hypocalcemia usually reflect muscle dysfunction including weakness, tetany, and tremors. Spontaneous muscle depolarization can manifest as muscle fasciculation, cramping, rigidity, and twitching.

Hypercalcemia may result in decreased function of the nervous system. Hypercalcemia may also result in cerebral vessel vasoconstriction and subsequent alteration in cerebral blood flow. Associated alterations in cerebrovascular blood flow may also affect intracranial functions. In some instances, cerebrovascular disease, infarction, and hemorrhage may result.

Hypertriglyceridemia results primarily in seizures. This may be due to alterations in cerebral blood flow secondary to the lipid content of the blood or other metabolic derangements. This is primarily seen in schnauzers and sheltie dogs. Lipemia retinalis may be present on fundic examination.

Primary Intracellular Metabolic Defects (Mitochondrial Encephalopathy). Diseases thought to be due to a cellular metabolic defect affecting *mitochondria* and cellular metabolic functions have been described (Brenner et al. 1997; Brenner et al. 2000; Harkin et al. 1999; Wakshlag et al. 1999). A representative disease process is referred to as Leigh's syndrome in people. Affected breeds include Alaskan huskies and Australian cattle dogs. This disease is suspected in an English springer, Yorkshire terriers, and some kittens. Animals usually show signs between 6 months and 12 months of age. One Alaskan husky was 2.5 years old and another 6 years old when clinical signs were recognized. An English springer had clinical signs at 15 months old.

Clinical signs described have been diverse ranging from seizures and generalized ataxia, behavior abnormalities, difficulty prehending food, visual deficits, facial hypalgesia, head tremor, hypermetric gait, and loss of balance progressing to spastic tetraparesis. In Australian cattle dogs, signs included progressive spastic tetraparesis with weakness and extensor rigidity of the thoracic limbs, head tilt, and nystagmus. In the English springer, there was loss of menace, visual deficits, positional vertical nystagmus, excitement-induced hypermetria, and balance loss.

Neoplasia

Brain tumors primarily affect older dogs and cats (see bibliography under Brain Tumor). While some estimates exist on the frequency of brain tumors in dogs (Vandevelde 1984), the actual incidence is not known. Brain tumors may arise primarily from the brain or its surrounding tissues, extend into the brain from adjacent structures, or metastasize to the brain from another location in the body. The increased reporting of brain tumors is no doubt the result of increased diligence on the part of owners to pursue the causes of intracranial signs coupled with the increased availability and use of advanced imaging modalities such as computed tomography (CT) or magnetic resonance (MR) imaging for antemortem diagnosis of intracranial disease (fig. 5.11).

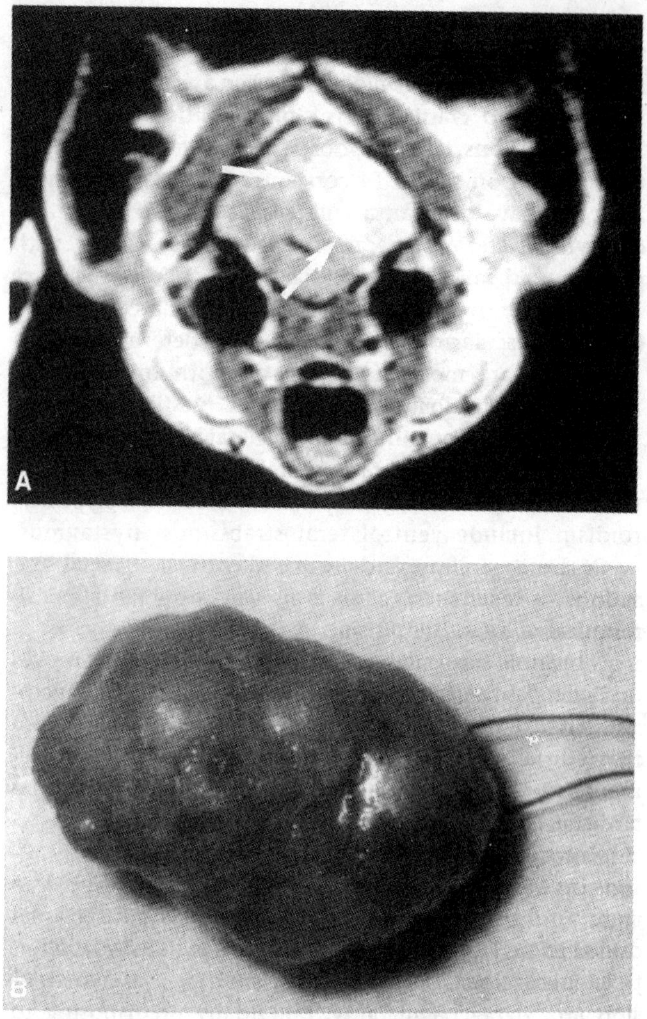

Fig. 5.11. (A) Transverse, T1-weighted MR images following intravenous contrast administration from a cat with a brain tumor (*arrows*). (B) Gross appearance of the tumor following surgical removal. Histologic diagnosis was a meningioma.

Clinical Features. Clinical signs in animals with brain tumors result not only from mechanical destruction of normal brain but also from associated pathophysiologic alterations that occur secondary to the tumor (Bagley and Kornegay et al. 1996). These sequelae include, but are not limited to, physical invasion and/or destruction of neurons, metabolic alterations in neuronal or glial cells, impairment of vascular supply to normal tissue (ischemia or hypoxia), impairment of autoregulation, hemorrhage (intratumoral or intraventricular), irritation (seizure generation), obstruction of the ventricular system, edema formation, and production of physiologically active substances. Many of these processes increase the relative volume within the intracranial cavity, ultimately affecting *intracranial pressure (ICP)*. Clinical signs are not pathognomonic for a brain tumor, but rather signal the presence of a variety of intracranial disease processes. Neurological examination findings often reflect the predominant intracranial area involved in the pathophysiologic process.

Animals with brain tumors tend to be older dogs. In a retrospective review of 97 dogs with brain tumors diagnosed at the Washington State University College of Veterinary Teaching Hospital, 95% of the affected dogs were aged 5 years or older at the time of diagnosis (Bagley et al. 1999). The median age of dogs diagnosed with brain tumor was 9 years (range 4 to 13 years). The most commonly affected breeds included golden retrievers, mixed breeds, Labrador retrievers, boxers, collies, Doberman pinschers, schnauzers, and Airedales.

Most dogs (76%) with brain tumors in our hospital had lesions of the supratentorial space. The most common presenting complaint in these dogs was seizures. While seizures are often reported to be a clinical manifestation of brain tumor in dogs, the actual incidence of seizures associated in intracranial tumors is not well established. In a series of 21 dogs with brain tumor, 8 had seizures. McGrath described the clinical features of 79 dogs with brain tumor wherein 36 dogs (46%) had seizures (McGrath 1960). In another series of 43 dogs with rostral cerebral tumors, 22 (51%) had seizures (Foster et al. 1988).

Of 44 dogs with seizures and brain tumors in our hospital, all but one dog had a tumor located in the supratentorial structures. Tumors in these dogs were located in the frontal (44%), olfactory (20%), and parietal lobes (20%).

Seizures are sometimes the only sign of a structural intracranial abnormality with the remaining neurological examination findings being normal. This is especially true with more rostral and olfactory lobe lesions (Foster et al. 1988; Palmer et al. 1974). Seizures that occur for the first time in dogs older than 5 years of age, regardless of associated neurologic examination abnormalities, should increase one's level of suspicion that a brain tumor may be present.

Clinical Clues to Brain Tumors

- More common in dogs greater than 5 years of age (median age of onset 9 years)
- Rare in dogs less than 4 years of age
- Golden retrievers commonly affected
- Seizures common

Of the dogs with tumors of the infratentorial space, the majority have vestibular or cerebellar signs as presenting complaints. Ataxia and head tilts are most common (Bagley et al. 1999).

Tumors of the intracranial space may be primary (arise from tissues in the intracranial space) or secondary (arise from tissues adjacent to intracranial space or from metastasis from far-removed tumors) (Bagley et al. 1992). Primary intracranial tumors include meningiomas; gliomas, including astrocytomas and oligodendrogliomas; ependymoma; and choroid plexus tumors. Pituitary tumors, while potentially arising from nonneural tissue, are sometimes included in this group.

Meningiomas are the most common brain tumors in dogs and cats. These tumors arise from the arachnoid layer of the meninges developing from the periphery of the brain parenchyma and expand inward. Often these tumors are calcified and contain psammoma bodies. Meningiomas may arise intraventricularly from the tela choroidea mimicking a choroid plexus tumor. Predominantly cystic meningiomas, often involving the olfactory area, have also been described (Bagley, Kornegay et al. 1996). Dogs often have a single site of meningioma. Cats, however, may have multiple intracranial meningiomas.

Meningiomas are usually histologically benign. In dogs, meningiomas tend to be more infiltrative to cortical parenchyma in comparison to cats, where meningiomas are often well encapsulated. Metastasis of meningiomas to extraneural sites is rare but possible (lung). Solitary brain masses are usually seen in dogs. These tend to be superficially whitish to dark red in color. Many contain a fine meshwork of vessels internally. On cut section, a granular or multilobular appearance is common and the tissue is often friable. A well-encapsulated, firm whitish mass is most often encountered at surgery in cats.

Gliomas arise from the supporting cells of the brain parenchyma. These include astrocytes and oligodendrogliocytes. Brachycephalic breeds of dogs such as boxers and Boston terriers may be more often affected with these tumors. Ependymal and choroid plexus tumors arise in or around the ventricle system. Choroid plexus tumors arise from areas where the choroid plexus is concentrated (the lateral, third, and fourth ventricles) (Ribas et al. 1989). Because of their association with the ventricular system, associated hydrocephalus is common (see fig. 10.8).

Pituitary tumors may result in signs of endocrine diseases (hyperadrenocorticism, acromegaly) or signs primarily related to CNS dysfunction (Davidson et al. 1991; Sarfaty et al. 1988). Macroadenomas may enlarge dorsally from the sella tursica and compress the diencephalon (see fig. 10.10). Neurologic impairment can be surprisingly minimal. The relative size of a pituitary tumor can not be predicted from endocrine testing results (Kipperman et al. 1992).

Neoplasia secondarily involves the brain via metastasis or via direct extension from extraneural sites. Primary tumors within the skull, nasal cavity, or frontal sinuses can extend directly into the brain (Moore et al. 1991; Smith et al. 1989). Often, with caudal nasal cavity tumors, signs of intracranial extension such as seizures occur prior to or without other signs of nasal disease.

Numerous tumors of animals can metastasize to the brain including hemangiosarcoma, lymphosarcoma, and mammary gland and other carcinomas (Fenner 1990; Moore and Taylor 1988; Waters et al. 1989). The incidence of intracranial metastasis is often underestimated as the brain is not always examined during a routine necropsy. Tumors that readily metastasize to the lungs may be more likely to metastasize to the brain (Waters 1989). The cortical grey/white junction is a common location of metastasis due to the increased vascularity, with brain stem and spinal cord metastasis occurring less frequently. Choroid plexus tumors and ependymomas may metastasize through the CSF to other areas in the brain or spinal cord ("drop-mets") (Adams and Victor 1989). In some instances, spinal signs from choroid plexus metastasis may be the first sign of the presence of the tumor. Diffuse intracranial tumor such as carcinomatosis is also possible.

Other tumors involving the brain are less common but may include lymphosarcoma, germ cell tumors, and craniopharyngiomas. Many of these tumors, surprisingly, are seen primarily in younger animals.

Nutritional Diseases

Thiamine deficiency is the most commonly recognized nutritional abnormality affecting the intracranial structures (see bibliography under Thiamine Deficiency). This is primarily a disease of cats. Dogs are occasionally affected. Thiamine deficiency can result due to lack of intake of thiamine, or due to a diet high in thiaminase (i.e., all fish diet). This deficiency results in polioencephalomalacia of the oculomotor and vestibular nuclei, the caudal colliculus, and the lateral geniculate body of small animals. Initial clinical signs are often nonspecific, such as lethargy and inappetence. Neurologic signs are often associated with the vestibular system including ataxia, broad-based stances, and loss of balance. Animals may be weak and unable or reluctant to walk. Cats may have ventral flexion of the neck. Other diseases such as hypokalemic myopathy, myasthenia gravis, polymyositis, and organophosphate toxicity can all cause ventral flexion of the neck.

Pupils in affected cats are often dilated and are poorly responsive or nonresponsive to light. If untreated, signs may progress to semicoma, persistent vocalization, opisthotonus, and death. Episodes of spastic opisthotonus or ventroflexion of the neck and generalized muscle spasm may occur, especially when cats are manipulated or stressed. These events may be interpreted as seizures, however, actual seizure activity is rare.

Inflammatory Diseases

Central nervous system inflammatory diseases are referred to as *encephalitis* or *meningitis* (see bibliography under Encephalitis). Encephalitis literally refers to inflammation of the brain parenchyma, and meningitis is inflammation of the meninges. In animals, both of these pathological processes often exist concurrently. *Myelitis* is the term used to describe an inflammation of the spinal cord parenchyma. A diffuse inflammation of the brain and spinal cord may be referred to as an *encephalomyelitis* or *meninigoencephalomyelitis*. The central nervous system is somewhat immunologically isolated from the rest of the body, primarily due to the blood-brain barrier (BBB). The BBB often prevents systemic infection and inflammation from reaching the nervous system. Conversely, infection and inflammation within the CNS may not be recognized by the general immunologic response systems of the body and may be less susceptible to the positive effects of the systemic immune system making treatment more difficult.

Inflammatory diseases of the central nervous system can initially be separated into those that are associated with an *infectious* organism and those that are *noninfectious* in origin. Numerous infectious agents have been incriminated as causing inflammation of the central nervous system. Incidence of infectious agents causing meningitis varies with geographic location. In general, most encephalitis and meningitis syndromes (~ 60% or greater) in small animals do not have a definable infectious cause. This can be taken to indicate that an infectious cause may have been present at some point in the course of the disease and is either no longer actively present or escapes clinical recognition.

Infectious agents causing brain disease include *viral* (distemper, parvovirus, parainfluenza, herpes, feline infectious peritonitis, pseudorabies, rabies), *bacterial*, *rickettsial* (Rocky Mountain spotted fever, *Ehrlichia*), *spirochetes* (Lyme disease, leptospirosis), *fungal* (blastomycosis, histoplasmosis, cryptococcosis, coccidioidomycosis, aspergillosis), *protozoal* (toxoplasmosis, neosporosis), and *unclassified organisms* (protothecosis). Other infectious organisms, such as *Bartonella vinsonii*, are suspected of causing CNS inflammatory disease (Breitschwerdt 2001).

Clinical signs often reflect multiple levels of neurological involvement. Systemic signs may reflect diffuse body system involvement in addition to the nervous system involvement (fig. 5.12). Joint, skin, heart, liver, kidney, and bone marrow are examples of other commonly affected

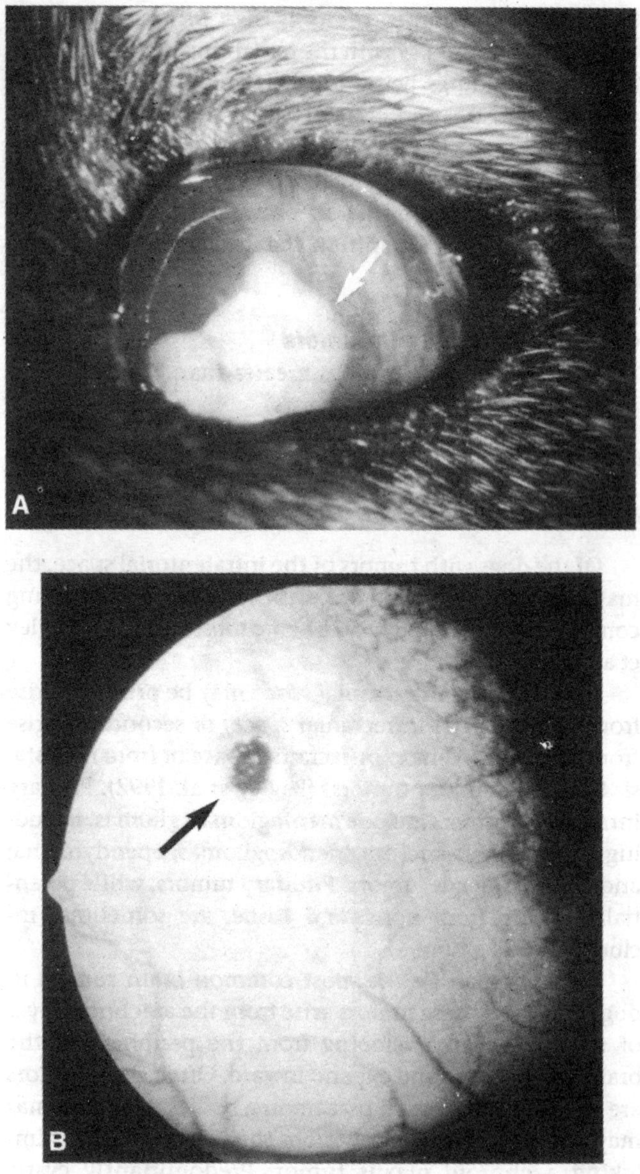

Fig. 5.12. (A) A dog with GME showing hypopyon (*arrow*). Fundic examination showing (B) an inflammatory lesion (*arrow*).

body systems. Associated organ dysfunction is often different for differing disease processes. A fundic examination may often reveal abnormalities in the retina suggestive of a systemic inflammatory process (fig. 5.12). Rarely, anterior chamber abnormalities such as hypopyon may be found in animals with inflammatory brain diseases.

Intracranial signs (behavior changes, mental status abnormalities, visual deficits) including cranial nerve dysfunction and spinal cord signs (paresis, ataxia) are common. Neck pain is often a prominent clinical feature of meningitis, but may be less obvious with pure parenchymal involvement (e.g., myelitis). A painful reaction may be observed by vocalization during direct palpation or by reluctance to move the head and neck freely or with manipulation (decreased range of motion). Diffuse spinal pain is also possible. As these diseases are often polysystemic, diffuse pain may also result from an associated polyarthritis or myositis. Some animals will react as if painful to minimal palpation anywhere on the body, especially of the limbs and face. Many animals become irritable and uncharacteristically aggressive. As chorioretinitis is often concurrently present, fundic examination may yield important clues to the polysystemic nature of the problem.

Clinical Clues to Encephalitis and Meningitis

- Often have multifocal or diffuse nervous system signs
- May have polysystemic clinical signs such as fever
- Neck pain or diffuse spinal pain common

Specific Inflammatory Diseases

Bacteria. Bacterial encephalitis and meningitis are rare in dogs and cats. Often, a concurrent disease that results in persistent bacteremia is present and bacteria can enter the nervous system through a hematogenous route. Diseases that are associated with significant bacteremia that secondary infect the CNS commonly in dogs include endocarditis and pyometra. Extension of a local bacterial disease process, most commonly from the nasal passages, middle ear, foreign body migration, or intracranial trauma is also possible. Immunosuppression, either naturally or as the result of iatrogenic steroid administration, may play a role in establishment and perpetuation of CNS infection.

Dogs and cats with bacterial meningitis usually have rapidly progressing clinical signs and the disease is often fatal. Clinical progression is due as much to the secondary inflammatory response in the CNS as to the primary infection. Multifocal signs are common including signs of systemic organ dysfunction such as chorioretinitis; polyarthritis; and kidney, liver, and respiratory abnormalities. Fever and cervical pain are common, however, they are present in less than 50% of cases. In some dogs, a cerebral abscess will form (see fig. 10.13). The associated mass effect may increase intracranial pressure rapidly to life-threatening levels.

A variety of causative bacteria may be associated with encephalitis. Most commonly, *Staphylococcus*, *Escherichia*, *Streptococcus*, and *Klebsiella* species are encountered. Other organisms include *Pasteurella multocida*, *Actinomyces*, and *Nocardia*. Anaerobic infections with *Bacteroides*, *Peptostreptococcus*, *Fusobacterium*, and *Eubacterium* occasionally have been causative. Often, multiple (mixed) bacterial species are present.

Lyme disease (*Borrelia burgdorferi*) has occasionally been associated with neurologic disease. Clinical signs primarily include alterations in mentation, paresis, and cranial nerve (VII) deficits (Azuma et al. 1993; Levy et al. 1993; Mandel et al. 1993). In some animals with CNS signs, antibodies to the organism have been present in the CSF. It is unknown whether the presence of these antibodies is evidence of primary CNS infection or nonspecific leakage of the antibodies from serum through an abnormal blood-brain barrier.

Rickettsia. Infection with rickettsial organisms associated with Rocky Mountain spotted fever (RMSF) and *Ehrlichia* commonly may involve the intracranial structures. Clinical signs most often reflect dysfunction of the brain stem, particularly the vestibular system. With RMSF there is often a history of systemic illness (usually with a thrombocytopenia) 5 to 10 days prior to development of neurological signs. As the animal's fever is decreasing, neurological signs appear. Dogs with clinical features of vestibular disease following a systemic febrile illness associated with thrombocytopenia should increase the suspicion of RMSF. Other polysystemic signs such as petechia, skin necrosis, joint inflammation, bone marrow disease, and nonneural organ dysfunction may also occur with these rickettsial diseases.

Viral. *Viral encephalitis* remains a common cause of brain inflammation. Many viral etiologies may affect the CNS. Still other viral etiologies are suspected but not yet confirmed as a cause of neurologic diseases (Quesnel et al. 1997; Rand et al. 1994). Some viral infections are more commonly reported in only very young dogs. These include herpes virus, parvovirus, and parainfluenza virus. Parvoviral encephalitis, for example, has been reported in a 7.5-week-old Dalmatian puppy. Parainfluenza virus has a propensity for causing hydrocephalus (Baumgärtner et al. 1982). Occasionally, these viruses will cause encephalitis/meningitis in adult dogs. Additionally, viral infection (herpes) has been implicated in cranial nerve abnormalities (primarily cranial nerve VII) in humans.

Canine distemper remains a common cause of neurologic dysfunction in dogs. This disease is caused by a paramyxovirus. Clinical signs can occur in any age of dog, regardless of vaccination status. Most commonly, young dogs with inadequate vaccinations are affected with the polysystemic signs (i.e., gastrointestinal, respiratory) as well as the neurologic signs of infection (fig. 5.13). Hyperkeratotic pads that sometimes accompany systemic distemper infection have been suggested to occur prior to CNS disease. However, in the modern era of prophylactic vaccination for distemper, the distemper infection may only result in clinical signs of nervous system disease without other systemic manifestations of disease. Nervous system disease associated with distemper is characterized pathologically by two main entities: neuronal and glial cell death (polioencephalomyelopathy) and demyelination (leukoencephalomyelopathy). It has been suggested that those animals with an inadequate antibody response to the virus tend to have the former pathological entity, and those with an adequate immune response to the virus tend to have the latter, immune-mediated demyelination. Any region of the nervous system can be involved. As well as persistent neurologic deficits, a chronically relapsing encephalomyelitis has been reported in a dog attributed to distemper virus infection.

Canine distemper virus may affect dogs of any age, however, there is a pattern to the destruction of nervous system tissue that is age dependent (Zurbriggen and Vandevelde 1994). Those dogs affected with the disease early in life suffer from a polioencephalomyelopathy (grey matter disease), usually have a history of seizures, and rarely survive.

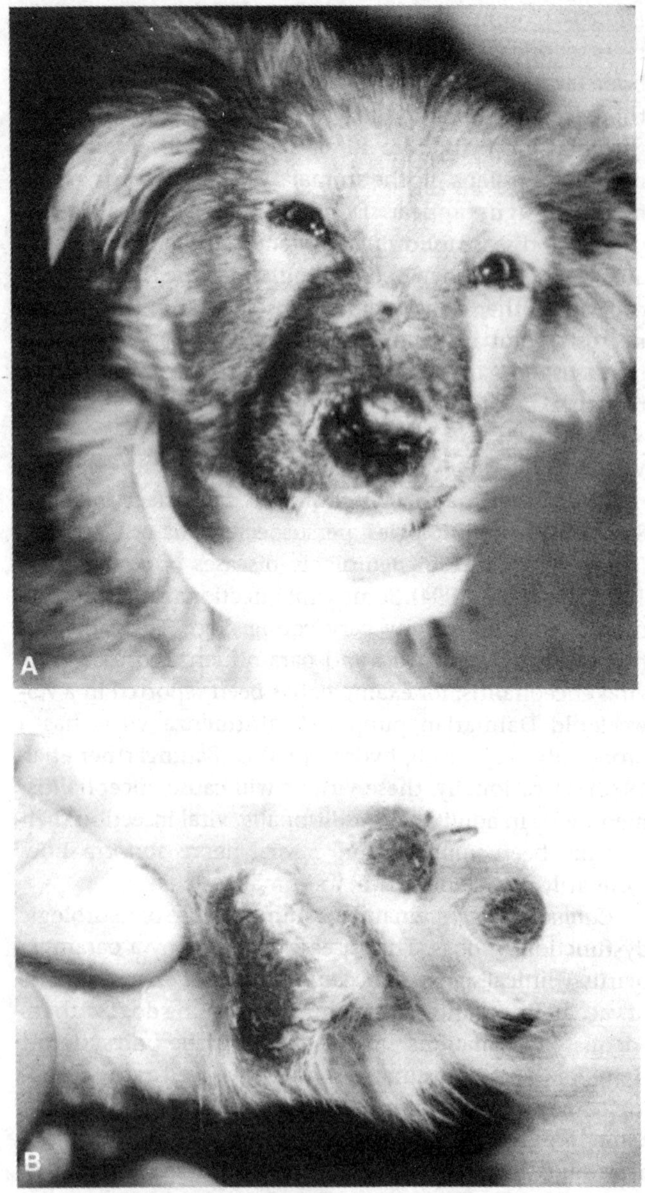

Fig. 5.13. (A) Facial appearance and (B) hyperkeratotic foot pads in a dog with systemic distemper infection.

Dogs affected by the disease later in life may have brain stem, cerebellar, and vestibular signs. They typically have a leukoencephalomyelopathy (white matter disease) or a combination of grey and white matter disease, and in most cases the disease is less severe. The type and distribution of the lesions are often reflected in widespread types of clinical dysfunction.

Myoclonus, a rhythmic, shocklike contraction of a muscle or group of muscles, is almost always the result of previous or concurrent distemper infection (Breazile et al. 1966). Rarely, myoclonus has been associated with lead toxicity and nonspecific encephalitis. Muscles of the limbs are most commonly involved, however, other muscles or muscle groups including the tongue may be affected. Clinical signs of a prior or concurrent systemic illness (respiratory, gastrointestinal) are not always found in dogs with neurologic signs associated with distemper.

Distemper virus infection has historically been associated with a variety of clinical syndromes. One of these is what is referred to as "old dog encephalitis" (deLahunta 1983). This disease is characterized histopathologically by a subacute or chronic progressive panencephalitis. This entity has also been referred to as disseminated encephalomyelitis in mature dogs, subacute diffuse sclerosing encephalitis, and chronic dementional distemper. Clinical signs in older dogs include visual impairment, increasing mental depression, compulsive circling, hyperkinesias, head pressing, and bilateral menace deficits. Overall, this is a rare diagnosis in the modern era.

Feline infectious peritonitis (FIP) results from a coronavirus-induced vasculitis in cats (see bibliography under Feline Infectious Peritonitis). This disease can involve various areas of the nervous system but primarily affects the intracranial structures and spinal cord. Very young and, conversely, very old cats seem predisposed. Of the two forms of FIP that exist in cats, the "dry" form commonly affects the nervous system. This viral infection results in an immune complex vasculitis, which is responsible for most of the pathological effects.

The pyogranulomatous (dry) form of feline infectious peritonitis virus can affect the central nervous system and may result in inflammation of the ependyma, choroid plexus, or meninges that surround the brain stem and at the junction of the cerebellum and medulla. This disease can be a challenge to diagnose, as there is no definitive antemortem test to prove a cat has the disease. It has been reported that over 45% of cats affected with the dry form of the disease will have signs of central nervous system dysfunction. This results from an inflammatory response to the virus but a lack of a protective cell-mediated immune response. Because the disease occurs as a multifocal pyogranulomatous meningoencephalomyelitis in the central nervous system, the clinical signs often reflect a diverse neuroanatomical localization. The disease is usually fatal.

Feline immunodeficiency virus has been associated with nervous system signs including behavior changes, seizures, anisocoria, and muscle twitching. As the clinical spectrum of this disease evolves, it may represent an important central nervous system pathogen of cats. Feline leukemia virus may result in lymphoma that can affect the intracranial nervous system. Direct effects of the virus on the intracranial nervous system are unclear. Feline leukemia virus, however, has been associated with a myelopathy independent of the presence of lymphoma (see spinal cord diseases discussed in chapter 6). Feline Borna disease (staggering disease) has been described in Europe and is associated with progressive pelvic limb ataxia, mental alterations, sacral hyperesthesia, fever, loss of appetite, aggressiveness, staring, seizure, hypersalivation, hypersensitivity to light and sound, inability to retract claws, and increased affection toward owners in cats. Clinical signs are progressive over the first month. This disease may have a viral cause.

Herpes virus encephalitis is mostly a clinical entity in very young puppies. Clinical signs include acute onset crying, diarrhea, dyspnea, and abdominal pain. Clinical signs usually progress to death in 1 to 3 days. Infectious canine hepatitis infection has been associated with central nervous system signs. It is unclear, however, whether these signs are the result of primary CNS infection with encephalitis, or the result of hepatic encephalopathy secondary to viral-inducted liver disease. Overall, the role of herpes virus in a variety of intracranial and cranial nerve dysfunctions in adult animals is suspected but poorly documented.

Pseudorabies is often a rapidly fatal CNS infectious disease. Affected dogs usually have some contact or exposure to swine or swine carcasses. Clinical signs include excessive salivation, fever, restlessness, anorexia, vomiting, dyspnea followed by incoordination, vocalization, anisocoria, ptosis, trimus, cervical rigidity, and muscle spasms. Animals may rub themselves or self-mutilate. Aggression is quickly followed by seizures, coma, and death.

Even though relatively uncommon, *rabies* always warrants consideration as a cause of neurologic dysfunction in dogs and cats. Unvaccinated and free-roaming animals are at greater risk of contracting this virus. Clinical signs may be initially similar to those seen with a variety of CNS diseases. Common signs include apprehension, restlessness, anorexia, and vomiting. There is often a change in temperament and excessive salivation. Approximately 25 to 30% of animals have the "furious" form of the disease with restlessness, wandering, viciousness, howling, polypnea, salivation, and seizures. Other animals have what is referred to as the "dumb" form with progressive ascending paresis or paralysis, paralysis of the lower jaw, pharyngeal and hypoglossal paralysis, facial paralysis, and possibly a change in bark due to laryngeal paralysis. Death usually results from respiratory failure. This is a fatal zoonotic disease.

Postvaccinal or *allergic encephalomyelitis* is primarily an historically described entity that followed *rabies vaccination* with phenolized brain tissue. This disease was a disseminated, demyelinating encephalitis or encephalomyelitis, which resulted as an allergic reaction to vaccine components. Clinical signs are usually of an ascending paralysis with initial signs in the pelvic limbs. This disease does suggest that reactions to a variety of antigens may result in neurologic abnormalities. Some types of noninfectious encephalitis may have an allergic or immune-mediated initiation. Other vaccines have been incriminated in immune-mediated or direct infection of the nervous system. For example, 1 week following coronavirus vaccination, a group of dogs showed seizures, tremors, and hypermetria. The role of vaccination in the genesis of many associated neurologic abnormalities, however, is often unclear.

Protozoal. *Toxoplasma gondii* and *Neospora caninum* are protozoal organisms that can affect any area of the nervous system resulting in encephalitis, myelitis, peripheral neuropathy, or myositis in cats and dogs. A classic sign of the infection in young animals is a hyperextended pelvic limb(s) (see also chapter 3). Other systemic signs such as chorioretinitis may also be present. Cats also commonly have toxoplasmosis within the nervous system, however, neosporosis has only been established experimentally in this species. A sarcocystis-associated meningoencephalomyelitis has been reported in a cat (Dubey et al. 1994).

Clinical signs depend upon the location of nervous system involvement and include intracranial, spinal cord, and lower motor neuron presentations. Intracranial signs can include supratentorial, brain stem, and cerebellar dysfunction. Clinical signs can be focal or diffuse and animals may only have signs of central or intracranial nervous system dysfunction.

Cats are more likely to have an associated systemic illness from toxoplasmosis, but may have intracranial signs exclusively. Signs are most severe in cats under 1 year of age, especially young kittens, although any age of cat can be affected. Lethargy, anorexia, and dyspnea due to pneumonia are the most frequent signs of generalized infection. Fever may be present. Gastrointestinal or hepatic signs such as icterus, vomiting and diarrhea, and abdominal effusion may occur as a result of diffuse organ involvement or from a granuloma.

These organisms damage the nerve and muscle either primarily or secondarily through the associated inflammatory reaction. Weakness may be present if the spinal cord, peripheral nerves, or muscles are involved. Hyperesthesia on muscle palpation, stiff gait, or shifting leg lameness suggests myositis.

Babesia infection rarely has been associated with neurologic signs. Signs include seizures, weakness, ataxia, and sudden death. These signs may also reflect the secondary effects on the nervous system from consequences of anemia, red cell destruction, and hypoxia.

Encephalitozoonosis is a disease caused by an obligate intracellular protozoal parasite that may be associated with neurologic abnormalities primarily in young dogs. Clinical signs are attributed to an associated vasculitis. Clinical signs may include poor growth, ataxia, tremors, blindness, seizures, aggression, abnormal vocalization, coma, and death. Cats may have severe muscles spasm, paralysis, and death.

Trypanosomiasis is rarely associated with an encephalitis. Weakness and ataxia may be seen.

Mycosis. Of the fungal diseases that can affect the nervous system, cryptococcus, blastomycosis, coccidiomycosis, candidiasis, and aspergillosis are most common. Immunodeficiency may play a role in these uncommon nervous system infections. Cryptococcosis is a common fungus involving the intracranial structures in cats. Suspicion of fungal encephalitis is increasingly based on geographic incidence of the disease and subsequent exposure of the animal. In some instances, a history of respiratory, gastrointestinal, or nasal signs accompanies signs of neurologic dysfunction.

Parasites. Involvement of the intracranial nervous system can occur with parasites such as *Cuterebra* larvae,

Toxocara, Baylisascaris procyonis, and aberrant heartworm migration. Parasite migration, and specifically *Cuterebra* larval migration, has been speculated in a number of intracranial diseases such as feline ischemic encephalopathy and feline idiopathic vestibular disease. Clinical signs will reflect the region of the nervous system mechanically damaged from the parasitic migration or damaged from the associated immunologic reaction secondary to the parasite's presence.

Other Types of Infectious Organisms. *Prototheca wickerhamii* and *Prototheca zopfii* are species of ubiquitous algae that have been reported to cause central nervous system disease. The disease is rare and it is thought that an abnormality of the animal's immune system must contribute to the pathogenesis of the disease. Animals will present with systemic signs of illness and multifocal neurological disease, the clinical signs of which will be dependent upon the area of the nervous system affected. The pyogranulomatous lesions seen in the brain of dogs with protothecosis may cause cerebellovestibular signs. In one case, an eosinophilic pleocytosis was reported. The organism has a predilection for the eyes, and ocular changes may therefore accompany signs of multifocal neurologic disease. Bloody diarrhea, visual impairment, paresis, tetraplegia, deafness, head tilt, facial hypalgesia, anosmia, and dementia are possible. The combination of acute blindness and deafness was reported in a dog with protothecosis.

A *spongiform encephalopathy* occurs in older cats in the United Kingdom and may be associated with a *prion* similar to other infectious spongiform encephalopathies. This disease occurs in older cats, and clinical signs include muscle tremors, ataxia, dilated unresponsive pupils, jaw champing, salivation, and behavior abnormalities. In one cat, tremor was most obvious in the pelvic limbs. Signs progressed to severe ataxia and hypermetria.

Noninfectious Diseases. Of the spectrum of inflammatory diseases that can affect the CNS, more often the cause of the inflammation is either undetermined or not associated with an established infectious agent. These diseases are primary inflammatory CNS diseases without a clinically identified cause. Some of these inflammatory diseases are given specific names based on common clinical features. It is rare that features are pathognomonic for a specific inflammatory CNS disease. Therefore, in clinically affected animals, the actual cause of the inflammation is always presumptive until additional testing is performed to help clarify the specific cause of the inflammation. Histologic confirmation of the actual disease process is rarely performed in animals that do not die as a result of their disease. Therefore, many encephalitic and meningitis syndromes are not classified definitively.

A noninfectious disease of the brain that is commonly overdiagnosed is *granulomatous meningoencephalitis (GME)*. Granulomatous meningoencephalitis can occur as a disseminated disease, as a focal mass-lesion, or as a primary ocular disease. The cause is not known. Some animals initially thought to have this disease have been shown, upon further study, to have lymphoma, but this is not universally true. This disease has been reported in two related Afghan hounds suggesting a genetic influence or a common environmental or infectious cause.

Young to middle-aged (6 months to 10 years, mean age slightly less than 5 years) animals are most commonly affected. Of reported cases, 80% are in small breeds of dogs, with 30% being poodles.

Clinical signs can vary. With the focal mass form, localizing CNS abnormalities may be present (fig. 5.14). With either the focal or diffuse form, both intracranial and spinal cord disease are possible. In the ocular form, animals are often presented for unilateral blindness with reduced or absent pupillary light reflexes. On fundic examination, the optic disk may be protruded into the vitreous, and may be hyperemic and edematous. Retinal vessels may be dilated and focal retinal hemorrhages may be present. In rare instances, dogs with GME may have hypopyon.

Eosinophilic meningoencephalitis occurs without apparent cause in dogs and cats. Male dogs between 4 months and 5.5 years have been affected. Half of these dogs were golden retrievers. Clinical signs included depression, somnolence, behavioral abnormalities, circling, pacing, and seizures. Systemic eosinophilia may not be present.

Spinal cord vasculitis syndromes result in signs and CSF changes of meningitis. Many of these diseases occur in specific breeds such as in beagles, German short-haired pointers, and Bernese mountain dogs. In beagles, this disease is commonly referred to as *beagle pain syndrome*. Clinical signs often include cervical pain and paresis. Intracranial signs are uncommon but possible. Aseptic meningitis and polyarthritis have been reported in Akita dogs.

There are a number of CNS inflammatory diseases that occur in specific breeds of animals, referred to as *breed-specific meningitis*. For example, *pug encephalitis* is a supratentorial inflammatory disease recognized in pug dogs (see fig. 10.16). Young pugs (6 months) are commonly affected,

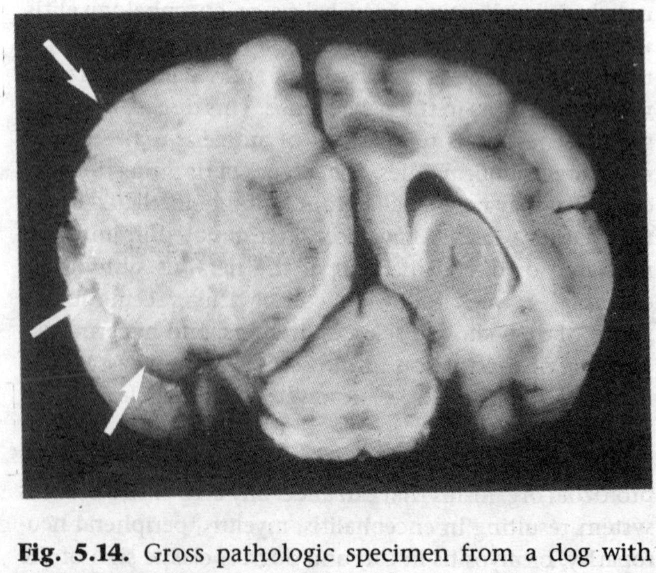

Fig. 5.14. Gross pathologic specimen from a dog with focal GME (*arrows*).

however, dogs as old as 7 years of age may have this disease. Clinical signs may include seizures, cervical pain, circling, head pressing, blindness, opisthotonus, and intermittent vocalizing. Affected dogs may have a rapidly deteriorating clinical course over a matter of hours. If cervical pain is the predominant clinical feature, initial concerns might be directed toward a cervical spinal cord lesion. This disease is essentially a necrosis of the cerebral hemispheres and other intracranial structures resulting in secondary inflammation (Cordy and Holliday 1989). In one dog, a herpes virus was incriminated as the cause, however, this has not been a consistently confirmed etiology. Similar breed-associated meningitis syndromes have been reported in Yorkshire terriers, Maltese terriers, a Pekingese dog, and others. A viral etiology has been speculated but not proven.

There is a unique clinical syndrome (generalized tremor syndrome or white shaker dog syndrome) associated with *generalized tremoring* that is usually associated with CNS inflammation. Affected dogs present with diffuse, fine, whole body tremor. Dogs with white hair coats (Maltese terrier, West Highland white terrier) are more commonly affected, however, dogs with other coat colors are also affected (Farrow 1986). Miniature pinschers are commonly affected. Additional neurological abnormalities include nystagmus, menace response abnormalities, proprioceptive deficits, and seizures. This syndrome is most often the result of a mild lymphocytic encephalitis. No etiologic agents for this disease have been established to date.

Idiopathic Diseases

Any disease that doesn't have a specific etiology is referred to as idiopathic (occurring without known cause). Having a disease without cause, however, does not provide the patient, owner, or clinician with much comfort. Some diseases, such as many of the noninfectious encephalitis and meningitis syndromes, are known to cause CNS inflammation, however, the actual cause of the inflammation is not established. These diseases might therefore be diagnosed as idiopathic inflammatory brain diseases. Also, the more exhaustive the attempts at diagnosis, the more credible it becomes to use the term "idiopathic" to describe a disease process. For example, an animal has a disease, and only a complete blood cell count (CBC) is performed to help clarify the cause of the disease. If the CBC is normal, and no further testing is done, then the cause of the disease would not be known, and a label of an idiopathic disease could be rendered. It should seem obvious, however, that this level of testing is too minimal, and therefore the confidence that the clinician has that he or she has extensively searched for the disease etiology should be low. If a diagnosis of "idiopathic" is rendered, the clinician should always feel clinically unfulfilled and remain concerned that a disease process has been overlooked or underrecognized.

With some disease processes, even with exhaustive clinical, biochemical, and histologic evaluations over years of observation, no etiology has been established for the disease process. *Idiopathic epilepsy* would be an example of a disease that would fit into this category. Idiopathic epilepsy is recurrent seizures without an underlying gross or microscopic cause (see also chapter 17). Seizures in animals with idiopathic epilepsy begin between 6 months and 4 years of age. Certain breeds of dogs may be predisposed and a hereditary basis is proven in some animals and suspected in others.

A variety of apparent behavior abnormalities may mimic signs of intracranial dysfunction or may even be suspected of seizure-associated abnormalities. Tail chasing (in bull terriers), self-mutilation, flank sucking, and fly biting are examples. *Feline hyperesthesia syndrome* is a unique and poorly understood phenomenon of cats. With stimulation such as stroking or petting over the thoracolumbar region, cats may become agitated and aggressive and show skin rippling and muscle spasms, usually localized over the lumbar area. Cats may appear as though they were startled, then exhibit frenzied behavior such as licking or biting at the flanks, back, and tail, or running. Other cats may appear as though they are hallucinating and have dilated pupils. Sudden startling, running, frantic meowing, growling, hissing, and swishing of the tail may also occur. Episodes may occur multiple times in a day and last 1/2 minute to 5 minutes.

The cause is unknown. It has been suggested that this activity is a manifestation of a focal seizure. Others suggest that it is a form of an "obsessive-compulsive" behavior. Similar clinical signs have been associated with a vacuolar myopathy in cats and toxoplasmosis. At other times, this hyperesthesia syndrome may begin with a local inflammatory stimulus such as flea or food allergy dermatitis. Focal spinal pain from a variety of diseases may predispose this region to hypersensitivity. It is also important to determine that a cat is not just exhibiting normal behavior during estrus.

Other types of movement disorders may have signs that suggest a seizure or some other central nervous disorder. Examples include dyskinesias and "Chinook (and other similar) seizures" in dogs (see D. P. O'Brien at http://www.canine-epilepsy.nect/chinook/chinook.htm).

Narcolepsy (excessive daytime sleepiness) and *cataplexy* (periods of acute muscular hypotonia) usually occur without underlying structural brain disease. The actual anatomic or physiologic abnormality may lie within the brain stem, however, clinical signs usually reflect a cerebral disturbance. Rarely, a structural brain abnormality is found. Abnormal neurotransmitter metabolism, possibly within the reticular activating system, is thought to be responsible, however, a true cause is not known.

Breeds of dogs predisposed include the Doberman, Labrador retriever, miniature poodle, dachshund, beagle, and Saint Bernard. Clinical signs usually begin at a young age, however, dogs as old as 7 years have been diagnosed with this disease. Acute onset of REM sleep, usually occurring with stimulation such as eating, is characteristic of narcolepsy. Physostigmine (0.025–0.1 mg/kg IV) potentiates the attacks for up to 45 minutes. The tricylic antidepressant imipramine, which potentiates serotonin, may be helpful as both a diagnostic test and as therapy for narcolepsy.

Trauma

Traumatic injury remains a common cause of brain dysfunction in dogs and cats (see also chapter 22). The diagnosis of trauma is usually straightforward when the trauma is witnessed. Clinical signs of intracranial trauma usually begin acutely in association with the traumatic incident. In some instances, animals are presented with an acute onset of neurological signs and an unknown history. Examining for external signs of trauma on the body, such as lacerations or skull fractures, is important. Evaluating the retinas and external ear canals for acute hemorrhage may also provide clues to the diagnosis. Clinical signs of intracranial dysfunction may be focal or diffuse depending upon the primary mechanical injury and any secondary pathophysiologic consequences.

Toxicity

Numerous toxins can affect the nervous system either primarily or secondarily. Examples of primary toxins include organophosphates, metaldehyde, lead, bromethalin, and hexachlorophene (table 5.6). When product information is examined, most chemical intoxications can result in some type of neurologic manifestations. Intoxication can result in a variety of clinical presentations depending upon the nature of the toxin involved. Polysystemic signs of toxicity such as respiratory or gastrointestinal signs may offer clues to the polysystemic nature of the toxicity. In the instance when the intoxication is known, consultation of a toxicity reference center should be helpful to clarify clinical signs and treatments for these toxicities.

Table 5.6. Common toxicities of the central nervous system

Toxicities associated with seizures or CNS stimulation
- Strychnine
- Metaldehyde
- Fluoroacetate/fluoroacetamide
- Taxus (yew)
- 4-Aminopyridine
- Theobromine
- Caffeine
- Organochlorines
- 4-methylimidazole
- Amphetamines
- Cocaine
- DEET (diethyltoluamide)
- Zinc phosphide
- Tremorgenic mycotoxins (penitrem A, roquefortine)
- Nicotine

Toxicity with mixed clinical effects
- Lead
- Pyrethrins
- Pyrethroids
- Rotenone
- Bromethalin
- DEET
- Mushrooms
- Ethylene glycol
- Phenothiazines
- Tricyclic antidepressants

Toxicities associated with CNS depression
- Opiates
- Marijuana
- Ivermectin
- Piperazine
- Benzodiazepines
- Phenothiazines
- Tranquilizers
- Barbiturates
- Ethylene glycol
- Ethanol

Lead toxicity usually results from ingestion of lead-containing products. Removal of lead-containing paint via sanding may allow for lead-laden dust to be produced. If this dust contaminates the animal's fur or adheres to the feet, enough lead may be ingested during normal grooming to cause toxicity. Initial signs of toxicity are usually nonspecific and include lethargy, inappetence, and weight loss. Gastrointestinal signs (vomiting, diarrhea) and hematologic abnormalities (obvious basophilic stippling or nucleated red cells) may accompany the CNS signs.

Nervous system signs include alterations in mental acuity, behavioral changes such as hysteria, jaw champing, tremors, seizures, ataxia, blindness, laryngeal paralysis, megaesophagus, and weight loss.

Chlorinated hydrocarbon toxicity involves an insecticide and a nonspecific CNS stimulant. Clinical signs include anxiety, hysteria, facial muscle spasms, jaw champing, spastic gait, ataxia, mydriasis, salivation, and seizures.

Hexachlorophene toxicity results in a spongiform change in the white matter of the brain, cerebellum, and spinal cord. Clinical signs include head tremors, muscle spasms, opisthotonus, ataxia, weakness, paresis, and seizures. Tremors are an important clinical sign.

Strychnine poisoning and *metaldehyde toxicity* may result in stimulation of the nervous system. Clinical signs of strychnine intoxication include retraction of the corners of the mouth, drawing together of the ears, a sawhorse stance, hypersensitivity to stimulation, opisthotonus, seizurelike episodes, and apnea. Metaldehyde toxicity can result in seizurelike activity and tremor.

Numerous *therapeutic drugs* as well as exposure to illegal drugs may also have toxic side effects involving the nervous system. If the toxicity is known, product information should be reviewed for specific associated clinical signs. Of the currently used drugs, *metronidazole toxicity* is commonly associated with neural toxicity in dogs and cats. Dogs tend to have vestibular signs, whereas cats may have supratentorial or cerebral signs (blindness). Clinical signs may result with excessive doses of metronidazole, but may occur even with doses within the established safe range. This is especially true in animals with liver dysfunction, as metronidazole is metabolized via the liver. *Metaclopromide* may be associated with seizures and involuntary movements. *Doxorubicin* administration may result in acute, usually side-to-side head tremor. As all drugs have the potential to affect the nervous system, if clinical signs of neurologic dysfunction in an animal receiving a therapeutic drug are noted, drug label or insert information regarding side effects of the drug should be consulted.

CEREBROVASCULAR DISEASES

Cerebrovascular diseases, while reportedly uncommon in animals, are being diagnosed with increasing frequency in dogs and cats (see bibliography under Cerebrovascular Disease). Clinically, cerebrovascular disease has been recognized in animals for a number of years (Thomas 1996; Joseph et al. 1988; Fankhauser et al. 1965). Underlying causes for cerebrovascular disease are many. Atherosclerosis, a potential associated cause of cerebrovascular disease in humans, is uncommon in dogs but may be associated with hypothyroidism (Liu et al. 1986). Idiopathic thrombosis of intracranial vessels has also been reported in dogs. Diseases of the cerebral vasculature may result from excessive blood flow through cerebral vessels (hypertension), transmural extravasation of blood, ischemia, thrombosis, and embolization. Hypertension, associated with a variety of diseases in animals, such as renal disease and hyperadrenocorticism, can result in increases in cerebrovascular hydrostatic forces leading to intracranial hemorrhages. Hypertensive encephalopathy is an increasingly recognized clinical entity in animals now that blood pressure measurements are being more commonly performed in animals. Disorders of coagulation (coagulopathies, DIC) and platelet function (thrombocytopenia and thrombopathies) can also result in cerebral hemorrhage. Diseases that predispose to hypercoagulability, such as glomerulonephritis, may result in intramural emboli and subsequent thrombosis of cerebral vessels. Bacteremias (endocarditis) may predispose to septic embolization of intracranial vessels. Vessel wall integrity can be disrupted by neoplastic infiltration, or inflammatory diseases, including vasculitis syndromes, resulting in thrombosis and hemorrhage. Thrombosis, infarction, and hemorrhage can occur spontaneously or secondary to drug therapies such as L-asparaginase and anticoagulants. Less commonly, arteriovenous malformations and aneurysms have been reported in dogs. All of these intracranial vascular abnormalities may predispose to cerebral hypoxia and ischemia as well as intracranial hemorrhage.

Ischemic damage, regardless of cause, results in endothelial cell damage predisposing to thrombosis, necrosis, and hemorrhage. One of the most devastating effects of severe intracranial vascular disease is intracranial hemorrhage. Hemorrhage into and around the brain can result in an associated inflammatory reaction, increases in overall intracranial volume, and increases in intracranial pressure (fig. 5.15; also see fig. 10.18). Intraventricular bleeding and bleeding into the cerebrospinal fluid are irritating to local nervous tissue and may result in inflammation (meningitis, myelitis, or encephalitis). Hemorrhage into the third ventricle is often associated with fever, most likely due to local alterations in the thermoregulatory center. If bleeding is substantial, hematomas may subsequently form. This additional volume within the intracranial space can alter CNS volume/pressure relationships with pathogenic effects of increasing intracranial pressure and decreasing cerebral blood flow.

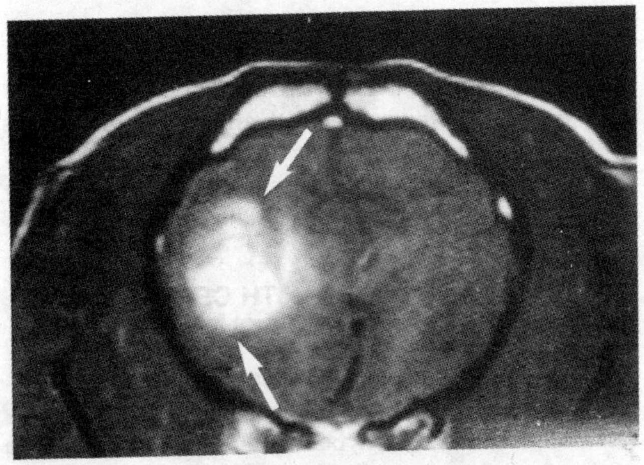

Fig. 5.15. Transverse, T1-weighted MR images following intravenous contrast administration from a dog with a cerebral hematoma (*arrows*).

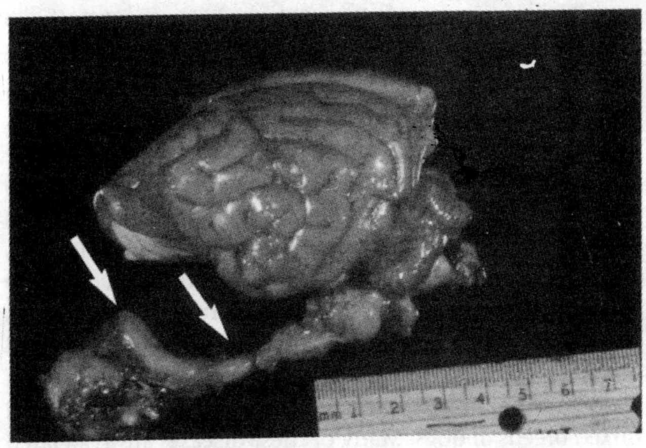

Fig. 5.16. Gross pathologic appearance of a nerve sheath tumor of the trigeminal nerve.

Cerebrovascular disease primarily results in ischemia and hemorrhage. Other secondary consequences include edema formation, mass effect, and increases in intracranial pressure. A variety of clinical signs may be seen in animals with cerebrovascular disease, depending upon which region of the CNS is involved. Behavioral alterations, changes in consciousness, seizures, salivation, and cranial nerve abnormalities are most often present. Focal hemorrhage or ischemia may result in hemiparesis, vestibular signs, or visual deficits. As cerebrovascular disease can evolve rapidly, clinical signs will most often occur acutely. If the disease is relatively mild, clinical signs may stabilize within the first 48 hours. If the degree of ischemia and its associated pathophysiologic sequelae are more severe, clinical signs may be rapidly progressive and often fatal.

Feline ischemic encephalopathy is an ischemic necrosis of the cerebral hemisphere of cats. The distribution of the infarction is usually in the area supplied by the middle cerebral artery. Vascular lesions, however, are infrequently found at necropsy. Clinical signs reflect a supratentorial or forebrain abnormality. Some have speculated that this disease is the result of a *Cuterebra* migration. A 7-year-old Siamese cat has been reported with an intravascular malignant T-cell lymphoma occluding the middle cerebral artery. Cats that survive the initial clinical period (48 to 72 hours) often improve. Seizures may be a residual complication.

DISEASES ASSOCIATED WITH CEREBELLUM OR CEREBELLAR PATHWAY CLINICAL SIGNS

This discussion will include diseases of the cerebellum as well as diseases that result in clinical signs of cerebellar dysfunction, such as ataxia, hypermetria, and tremors. Disease of the cerebellum may also be associated with vestibular signs, however, these diseases are discussed under vestibular disease.

Degenerative Diseases

Cerebellar abiotrophies result from loss of a vital substance necessary for continued life of the neuron (see bibliography under Cerebellar Degeneration). These diseases are seen most notably in the Kerry blue terrier, Gordon setter, rough-coated collie, border collie, bullmastiffs, and rarely, in Samoyeds, Airedales, Finnish harriers, Labrador retrievers, golden retrievers, beagles, cocker spaniels, cairn terriers, Great Danes, and Staffordshire terriers (table 5.7). Isolated cases have been described in German shepherds, English Springer spaniels, pit bull terriers, Portuguese spaniels, golden retrievers, cocker spaniels, Great Danes, Akitas, Clumber spaniels, fox terriers, Scottish terriers, and mixed breeds. Cerebellar degeneration may be seen sporadically in other breeds, such as the Doberman pinscher and mixed breeds of dogs. Many of these diseases are associated with loss of Purkinje cells.

Clinical signs are of a progressive cerebellar disease. Common signs of cerebellar dysfunction include ataxia, dysmetria, hypermetria, and lack of a menace response (with concurrent normal vision, pupillary light, and palpebral reflexes). In some instances, there are accompanying vestibular signs, such as nystagmus and head tilting.

The majority of these cerebellar degenerative diseases are suspected to be genetic and inherited. In Kerry blue terriers, clinical signs begin around 8 to 16 weeks of age. Pelvic limb stiffness and head tremors associated with hypermetria are seen. Clinical signs of cerebellar dysfunction are progressive with animals usually being unable to stand by 1 year of age. Degeneration is seen in the Purkinje cells and olivary nuclei, and as the disease progresses, the substantia nigra and caudate nucleus may be involved.

In Gordon setters, clinical signs often begin in slightly older animals between 6 and 30 months. Between 9 and 18 months, they develop thoracic limb stiffness, hypermetria, broad-based stance, nystagmus, and stumbling. Menace response is often absent with normal vision. Clinical signs are usually slowly progressive over several years. A similar onset of clinical signs has been seen in Old English sheepdogs. These dogs have been described with an adult-onset

Table 5.7. Animals with cerebellar abiotrophy

Dogs
Airedale terrier
Australian Kelpie
Beagle
Bernese mountain dog
Border collie
Brittany spaniel
Bullmastiff
Coton de Tulear
Finnish Harrier
Gorden setter
Irish setter
Jack Russell terrier
Kerry blue terrier
Labrador retriever
Miniature poodle
Old English sheepdog
Rhodesian ridgeback
Rough coated collie
Samoyed
Cats
Siamese
Domestic shorthair
Mixed breed

cerebellar abiotrophy. Clinical signs begin in animals aged 6 to 40 months.

In rough-coated collies, the disease is suspected to be autosomal recessive in inheritance. Pelvic limb ataxia begins at 1 to 2 months of age. Dogs develop a broad-based stance, hypermetria, head tremors, and occasionally a bunny-hopping gait. Dogs may fall into a lateral recumbency position with the legs in extension. Clinical signs are progressive but may stabilize by 1 year of age.

Cerebellar degeneration in Australian kelpies is also thought to be autosomal recessive. Clinical signs develop around 6 to 12 weeks of age. Ataxia, hypermetria, head tremor, and proprioceptive deficits are common. The menace response may be absent.

Cerebellar disease has been reported in some dogs from a litter of Labrador retrievers. Clinical signs began at 12 weeks of age. Pelvic limb ataxia, hypermetria, and wide-based stance were initially present and progressed rapidly to thoracic limb involvement, falling, and inability to walk. The cerebellum was grossly smaller than normal at necropsy.

Similarly, some animals from a litter of beagles in Japan had cerebellar degeneration. Clinical signs were present from 3 weeks of age. Affected animals would fall frequently. Clinical signs were progressive. The cerebellum was also grossly smaller in these dogs.

Two males from a litter of three miniature poodles had cerebellar degeneration. Clinical signs began from 3 to 4 weeks of age. Dogs were rolling from side to side, were unable to remain in a sternal position, had periodic opisthotonus and intention tremors, were absent menace responses, and had vertical nystagmus.

A cerebellar disease in bullmastiffs is also thought to be inherited in an autosomal recessive pattern. Clinical signs were present in dogs aged 4 and 9 weeks up to 7 months. These dogs also had hydrocephalus. Clinical signs included pelvic limb ataxia, hypermetria, proprioceptive deficits, head tremor, visual deficits, and decreased menace responses. Occasionally dogs had hysterical behavior, compulsive movements, circling, decreased mental acuity, and nystagmus. The cerebellum in these dogs was grossly smaller than normal.

Other cerebellar degenerations have affected Samoyeds, Coton de Tulear dogs, Airedale terriers, Finnish harriers, Bern running dogs, Akita, Clumber spaniels, golden retrievers, cocker spaniels, cairn terriers, fox terriers, Great Danes, mixed breeds, German shepherds, English Springer spaniels, miniature poodles, and pit bull terriers suggesting that the majority of breeds may be affected with some type of cerebellar disease. Cerebellar signs are a common theme clinically.

An hereditary cerebellar degeneration has been described in Japan in cats. An autosomal recessive mode of inheritance was presumed. Clinical signs of this hereditary cerebellar degeneration begin in 7- to 8-week-old cats. Clinical signs included head tremor along with ataxia, dysmetria, and intention tremor.

Storage diseases may also affect the cerebellum. Breeds affected and associated clinical signs are described in the degenerative intracranial disease section of this chapter. In cats with sphingomyelinosis (Niemann-Pick type C disease), clinical signs begin early in life (<6 months) and progress to ataxia and hypermetria, absent menace responses, and occasionally positional nystagmus. Death usually occurs by 8 to 10 months of age. Niemann-Pick type A disease occurs in Siamese and Balinese cats. Head tremor, head bobbing, and dysmetria begin at 3 to 4 months of age. Clinical signs progress to ataxia and paresis, which is worse in the pelvic limbs.

It is rarer to have primary cerebellar degeneration in *adult* or *older dogs*. In dogs, an adult-onset cerebellar degeneration has been found in Brittany spaniels. Animals are usually between 7 and 13 years of age when clinical signs begin. Clinical signs may progress for months to years. Usually female spayed animals are affected. Clinical signs include mild spasticity and hypermetria progressing to ataxia, head tremor, falling, and inability to stand. Affected dogs are often described as having unusual "lurching" or forward-falling movements. Histologically, this disease is associated with loss of Purkinje cells. An adult-onset cerebellar degeneration has also been reported with clinical signs beginning in a 6-year-old male schnauzer-beagle mixed-breed dog. Clinical signs progressed over a 5-year period until eventually the dog was unable to stand. In some American Staffordshire terriers, cerebellar degeneration also occurs in older animals. Clinical signs may be less severe when the animals are stressed, making clinical recognition more difficult. In human beings, cerebellar degeneration has been found as a paraneoplastic phenomenon associated with a variety of tumor types. A similar phenomenon may occur in dogs but has not been definitively proved.

There are diseases referred to as *neuroaxonal dystrophies* that are occasionally seen in animals. *Feline hereditary neuroaxonal dystrophy* has been reported in domestic tricolored cats and is thought to be inherited as an autosomal-recessive trait (Woodard et al. 1974). Affected kittens have a lilac coat color, which darkens with age. Unaffected kittens are black in coat color. Clinical signs begin in 5- to 6-week-old animals. Clinical signs include head tremors and head shaking, incoordination of gait, and hypermetria. At necropsy, atrophy of the cerebellal vermis is seen.

Neuroaxonal dystrophy of collie sheepdogs has been reported in 2- to 4-month-old dogs with cerebellar signs including ataxia and hypermetria. A similar disease has also been reported in bullmastiffs, Jack Russell terriers, and Chihuahuas (Summers et al. 1995).

Neuroaxonal dystrophy of Rottweiler dogs is characterized by cerebellar signs (ataxia, hypermetria, loss of menace response, head tremor) beginning at 1 to 2 years (ataxia) and progressing over the next 2 to 4 years (menace deficits; nystagmus, resting and positional; intention tremor). Conscious proprioception remains intact. The cell bodies in the grey matter are affected (axonal spheroids) throughout the nervous system except the cerebral cortex. The most severe lesions are in the spinocerebellar tracts and the Purkinje cells.

Leukoencephalomyelopathy has been seen in young Rottweilers aged 1.5 to 4 years of age with progressive ataxia, tetraparesis, hypermetria, normal to exaggerated reflexes, and increased muscle tone. Bilateral lesions are found primarily in the spinal cord, most severe in the dorsal and lateral funiculi. No signs suggestive of intracranial or cranial nerve dysfunction are seen, even though pathologically the deep cerebellar white matter is abnormal (demyelination). The menace response is unaffected. Clinical signs are initially more suggestive of a cervical spinal cord problem and are progressive over 6 to 12 months.

A *spongiform degeneration* has been described in Labrador retrievers (O'Brien and Zachary 1985; Zachary and O'Brien 1985, under Spongiform Degeneration). Clinical signs began between 4 and 6 months. Clinical abnormalities include extensor rigidity of the limbs, opisthotonus, and ataxia. Signs were worsened by external stimulation or excitement. This may be similar to Canavan disease of children.

Some diseases involve both central and peripheral nerve structures, and clinical signs may reflect multiple locations of nervous system involvement. As an example, a *leukoencephalomyelopathy* has been recognized in Birman cats with both central and peripheral nervous system degeneration (Moreau et al. 1989; Moreau et al. 1991). Cats were between 8 and 10 weeks when affected. Predominant clinical signs included pelvic limb ataxia, proprioceptive deficits, and hypermetria. Cats, most likely because of the associated peripheral nerve involvement, also walked plantigrade with their hocks splayed out. These types of diseases are sometimes referred to as central-peripheral distal axonopathy or dying-back axonopathy.

Anomalous Diseases. Congenital malformations of the cerebellum are occasionally seen (see bibliography under Anomalous Diseases). Caudal vermian hypoplasia is described, with some dogs having associated ventricular dilation (Dandy-Walker malformation) (Kornegay 1986). This is a rare congenital malformation that shares similarities with the human form of the disease. It consists of a triad of congenital anomalies including cerebellar vermian hypoplasia, communicating hydrocephalus, and the presence of a fluid-filled cyst (syrinx) within the posterior fossa. It has been reported in several dogs with no breed or sex predilection. The clinical signs are typical of cerebellar disease (ataxia, hypermetria, absent menace, and tremors). Some dogs have also displayed a head tilt and circling. It is unknown if the vestibular signs are due to the cerebellar disease or manifestations of the other developmental abnormalities. The clinical signs are usually not progressive. The condition has been reported in one kitten. Affected animals present early (3 months of age) in life.

Cerebellar hypoplasia has been recognized in Chow Chows, Airedale terriers, Boston terriers, Irish setters, and wirehaired fox terriers. The latter two breeds may have concurrent lissencephaly. Cerebellar aplasia has been reported in Siberian huskies.

Feline cerebellar hypoplasia is caused by in utero or immediately postnatal infection with the panleukopenia virus (parvovirus), which affects the external germinal layer of the cerebellum and prevents the formation of the granular layer. Infection of the fetus may occur when a pregnant queen is vaccinated with a modified-live panleukopenia virus. This virus destroys the external germinal layer of the cerebellum and prevents the formation of the granular layer. Some affected cats have a concurrent hydrocephalus and hydrencephaly. Clinical signs are most apparent when the animal begins purposeful movement and attempts to walk. Tremor accompanying the disease usually has a slower frequency (2–6 times/second) and larger amplitude. The tremor worsens (increases in frequency or amplitude), when the cat moves in a goal-oriented way (e.g., bends down to eat), which is termed an intention tremor. Other signs include ataxia, hypermetria, menace deficits (with normal vision and pupillary light reflexes), head tilt, and nystagmus. Clinical signs usually remain static or improve with growth as the cat compensates, causing the tremor to become less apparent.

Hydrocephalus that involves the fourth ventricle may result in cerebellar signs. Hydrocephalus is a component of Dandy-Walker syndrome. Hydrocephalus may also be acquired from ventricular obstruction secondary to neoplastic or inflammatory diseases. In some animals, hydrocephalus is limited *exclusively* or *primarily to the fourth ventricle*. Many of these animals have associated fluid caviations of the spinal cord called syringomyelia or hydromyelia. Signs of cerebellar dysfunction may be minimal or absent. This abnormality may represent a congenital obstruction of the lateral apertures, however, this is unproven.

Epidermoid or dermoid cysts are structural abnormalities that may result in cerebellar dysfunction. These abnormalities most often are present in the fourth ventricle and cerebellomedullary junction (see further discussion under intracranial anomalous disease in this chapter; fig. 5.7). Cystic abnormalities resembling arachnoid cysts may also involve the cerebellum (see fig. 10.19).

Hypomyelination or *dysmyelination* of the CNS is seen in many dog breeds, including the Chow Chow, Lurcher hound, Springer spaniel, Samoyed, Dalmation, Weimaraner, and Bernese mountain dog, cats, and others. This disease is inherited in an X-linked manner in Springer spaniels. Individual cases are reported in a Dalmatian and a mixed-breed dog. Clinical signs consist of tremor, which may appear to be cerebellar in origin. Often, affected animals appear to be "bouncing." This tremor usually worsens with excitement. Abnormal oligodendrocyte numbers or function is the suggested pathogenic mechanism. Tremor usually begins in these dogs by weeks of age. The majority of dogs are affected between 2 and 8 weeks of age. It is most commonly a generalized tremor, which may distinguish itself from the predominant intention tremor of the head seen with cerebellar disease. Spontaneous improvements can occur in clinical signs in Chow Chows, Lurcher hounds, and Weimaraners. These dogs may eventually become clinically normal. In Bernese mountain dogs, tremors may improve but not abate. The majority of affected Springer spaniels were euthanized so life-long disease course is not determined.

Hypomyelination or dysmyelination of the CNS has been reported in two Siamese cats (Stoffregen et al. 1993). Pathologically, there was a deficiency of myelin primarily in the ventral and lateral aspects of the spinal cord. Abnormal oligodendrocyte numbers or function is the suggested pathogenic mechanism. Clinical signs consisted of diffuse tremor accompanied by frenzied behavior and indiscriminate biting. Clinical signs worsen with activity. Reported cats were young (<1 year of age).

Occipital dysplasia is an anatomical abnormality of the occipital bone. The condition primarily affects small-breed dogs. In cases of occipital dysplasia, the ventral aspect of the occipital bone is malformed and replaced by a membranous band of tissue. Oftentimes, the caudal aspect of the cerebellum and the dorsal aspect of the cranial cervical spinal cord and caudal brain stem are exposed. It remains controversial whether this abnormality is primarily associated with clinical signs. However, this may be a manifestation of abnormalities of the infratentorial and foramen magnum area in human beings referred to as Chiari malformation (see syringomyelia discussion under anomalous diseases of the spinal cord in chapter 6). It has been proposed that fluid-filled cavities in the spinal cord, such as syringomyelia or hydromyelia, are secondary to abnormal pulsation of cerebrospinal fluid within or around the foramen magnum.

Neoplastic Diseases. Primary or secondary *neoplasia* may involve the cerebellum. *Meningiomas* and *choroid plexus tumors* are most common. *Medulloblastoma* is a primary brain tumor that rarely involves the cerebellum in dogs. Neoplastic diseases that involve the cerebellum and brain stem are discussed further in the neoplastic intracranial disease section in this chapter.

Medulloblastomas are highly metastatic brain tumors, usually occurring in the cerebellum of dogs and cats, usually between 3 and 10 years old. These tumors share many characteristics with the same tumor type in people. They are classified as a primitive neuroectodermal tumor. They arise from a population of cells thought to be present during the development of the cerebellum. Animals may present early or later in life with signs of cerebellar disease and possibly signs of brain stem compression. As the tumors grow into the fourth ventricle, they will often cause hydrocephalus. Tumor cells will invade the adjacent meninges. Metastasis along CSF pathways is also common.

Choroid plexus tumors and ependymal tumors arise from the ventricles. These tissues are related embryologically and function in the production and movement of cerebrospinal fluid. Tumors of ependymal origin are rare. The fourth ventricle is a common site for choroid plexus papillomas. Both of these tumor types can shed cells into the normal CSF pathways, which can eventually lodge and expand in other regions of the nervous system such as the spinal cord. Metastases of these tumors into the spinal cord via CSF pathways are referred to as "drop mets."

Inflammatory Diseases. Inflammatory diseases of the intracranial space may also involve the cerebellum (see Inflammatory Diseases previously within this chapter). The source of the inflammatory reaction includes both infectious and noninfectious etiologies.

An *encephalomyelopathy of young cats* has been reported in the United Kingdom (Palmer and Cavanagh 1995). Wallerian degeneration was noted primarily involving the spinocerebellar pathways and the ventral funiculus of the spinal cord. A viral etiology was suggested but not proven. Cats 3 to 12 months old were affected, however, the disease was seen in cats up to 3 years of age. Clinical signs usually are progressive over weeks to months. Ataxia of the pelvic limbs was the initial clinical sign noted. Other signs include paresis and "head shaking."

Trauma. The cerebellum may be damaged from *exogenous injury* to the head. These injuries most often occur from automobile trauma, although gunshot wounds and falls may also occur. Clinical signs of cerebellar or associated intracranial disease are usually acute in onset following the trauma. Evidence of external trauma to the head and face, such as facial lacerations, bleeding from the nose and mouth, bruising, or hemorrhage in the external ear canals, may be clues to the traumatic etiology. Some animals, however, with an acute onset of a variety of cerebellar (and vestibular) diseases may be so incoordinated that they fall (from their primary disease) and injury themselves secondarily.

Vascular Disease. Cerebellum *infarction* is an increasingly diagnosed abnormality. Similar to other cerebrovascular diseases, a multitude of etiologies is possible. Affected animals are usually middle-aged to older, and tend to have an acute onset of cerebellar or vestibular signs.

Diseases of Cranial Nerves. Cranial nerve dysfunction can result from disease of the intracranial region involving cranial nerve nuclei, or can involve the cranial nerves distal to the central nervous system. Clinical signs of individual cranial nerve dysfunction are discussed under neurologic examination abnormalities in chapter 3. Some cranial nerves, such as CNs VII (facial) and VIII (vestibular), are more commonly affected, while other cranial nerves (such as CN IV) are apparently rarely affected with specific disease processes.

Abnormalities of Smell. Anosmia (loss of smell) is most often recognized secondary to bilateral nasal passage disease. Unilateral lesions in the supratentorial structure will not cause anosmia as the integration of smell is a bilateral function. Bilateral olfactory lobe disease, however, can result in anosmia. Viral infections such as distemper and parainfluenza may also cause anosmia. Clinically, dysosmia (abnormal smell) is almost impossible to determine unless further objective testing with various smells is performed.

Abnormalities of Vision and Pupils. Abnormalities of vision can occur due to disease of the ocular structures, optic nerves, or central projecting and integrating pathways. Diseases of the central pathways for projection and integration of vision are discussed in the diseases of the intracranial structures of this chapter.

Optic nerve hypoplasia occurs in beagles, dachshunds, German shepherds, miniature schnauzers, rough-coated collies, Saint Bernards, toy poodles, Russian wolfhounds, Pekingeses, and Great Pyrenees. This may result in unilateral blindness and pupillary dilation.

Neoplastic diseases can affect the optic nerve. These may be primary diseases of the nerve, such as *meningiomas,* or may involve the optic nerve through extension from the periorbital tissues.

Inflammatory diseases can affect any portion of the nervous system including the optic nerve or visual system. Canine *distemper, granulomatous meningoencephalitis (GME),* and optic neuritis are possible. In the ocular form of GME, animals are often presented for unilateral blindness with reduced or absent pupillary light reflexes. On fundic examination, the optic disk may be protruded into the vitreous, and be hyperemic and edematous. Retinal vessels may be dilated and focal retinal hemorrhages may be present.

Optic neuritis is a primary inflammation of the optic nerves. Animals often present for blindness or visual difficulty, usually with associated absent or decreased pupillary light reflexes. Upon retinal examination, an edematous, elevated optic disk may be seen. Retinal vessels may be engorged and there may be associated focal retina hemorrhages. As no specific etiology is often identified, optic neuritis may be associated with other disease processes, such as granulomatous meningoencephalomyelitis, distemper virus, toxoplasmosis, fungal infections, and acute lead toxicity.

Protothecosis has been reported to cause central nervous system disease and also involve the eye. This may primarily be the result of an anterior uveitis. The organism has a predilection for the eyes, and ocular changes may therefore accompany signs of multifocal neurologic disease. The combination of acute blindness and deafness with this organism is possible.

Abnormalities of *pupils* may result from abnormalities of vision, the ocular structures, or the central visual pathways. Efferent abnormalities of the iris include diseases of the parasympathetic system through cranial nerve III, the sympathetic system, and the iris muscle.

Miotic pupils that do not dilate in the dark can result from a variety of disorders. Pupils may be small with anterior uveitis and apparently sluggish to respond to light due to iridic vascular congestion and edema. Painful conditions of the cornea may cause a miosis. This is a bilateral phenomenon mediated through cranial nerve V constrictor center (oculosensory pupillary reflex). Instillation of parasympathomimetic drugs into the eye may cause miosis.

The spastic pupil syndrome is a static anisocoria of cats that remains essentially unchanged during dark adaptation. Many of these cats are positive for the feline leukemia virus.

Abnormalities of sympathetic innervation to the eye can result in a miotic pupil alone (Horner's pupil) or in signs of complete sympathetic denervation of the orbit (Horner's syndrome). A lesion anywhere along the sympathetic pathway can result in these clinical signs including the intracranial region. Damage can occur to the vagosympathetic trunk in the cervical area from trauma or tumor. Lymphoma infiltrating the sympathetic nerves has resulted in Horner's syndrome in cats. Disease of the middle and inner ear can affect the sympathetic innervation to the pupil. Over 50% of cases of sympathetic abnormalities of the pupil do not have a defined cause. An idiopathic Horner's syndrome has also been reported in golden retrievers

With severe cerebrocortical disease, the pupils will often be smaller than normal (miotic). Two theories exist to explain this finding (deLahunta 1983). One is that there is a bilateral central sympathetic system abnormality, possibly at the hypothalamus or brain stem level. Alternatively, it appears as though systems of the supratentorial area normally provide descending inhibitory influences on the parasympathetic nucleus of CN III. It may be useful to have the pupils relatively larger to increase the amount of information presented to the supratentorial structure in the normal state of wakefulness. If the supratentorial systems responsible for this descending inhibitory influence are damaged, there is a release of this inhibitory influence over the parasympathetic pupillary constriction and it becomes hyperresponsive (excessive parasympathetic tone). Rarely, a miotic pupil is found with unilateral, usually severe cerebrocortical disease.

A large, poorly responsive or unresponsive pupil(s) (*mydriatic*) may indicate parasympathetic denervation of the iris. This can result from disease of cranial nerve III or its nucleus. Parasympathetic lesions affecting the nucleus in the midbrain have been discussed under intracranial diseases. Parasympatholytic drugs instilled in the eye will dilate the pupil (i.e., atropine). The affect of this drug may last for several days after one instillation.

Primary disease of the iris, such as iris atrophy, is common in older dogs. Iris atrophy is an age-related degeneration of the iris. The iris margin is irregular. When severe, a dyscoric pupil may be present. Upon viewing a tapedal reflection, thin slits or tears may be found in the iris. Primary disease of the eye such as synechia or glaucoma can also result in a dilated pupil.

A suspected idiopathic postganglionic parasympathetic denervation of the pupil is referred to as Adie's syndrome. This is rare in dogs.

Dysautonomia is a disease characterized by dysfunction of the autonomic system. In addition to other clinical signs, such as vomiting and constipation, dilated, poorly responsive to unresponsive pupils may be seen.

Disease of the cerebellum may rarely result in pupillary abnormalities. With unilateral lesions of the fastigial or interpositál nuclei, a *pupillary dilation,* which is slowly responsive to light, may be seen (Holliday 1979/1980). Occasionally, the third eyelid may protrude and the palpebral fissure may be enlarged. The pupillary dilation occurs in the eye ipsilateral to an interpositál nuclear lesion and contralateral to a fastigial nuclear lesion.

Regardless of the primary intracranial disease, if a *unilateral transtentorial herniation* occurs, the ipsilateral pupil can dilate and become nonresponsive to light either directly or indirectly. If unilateral transtentorial herniation occurs, pressure from the herniated parahippocampal gyrus may be exerted ventrally onto the brain stem. As the brain stem is compressed, cranial nerve III may be compressed along the floor of the skull. Compression on this nerve may result in parasympathetic dysfunction and the ipsilateral pupil will dilate and become nonresponsive to light (Kornegay 1983) (fig. 2.14). As the midbrain is compressed, fixed midrange pupils will occur (deLahunta 1983).

Cavernous Sinus Syndrome. The cavernous sinus is an intracranial venous structure that encircles the pituitary. A number of cranial nerves and nerves innervating the extra- and intraocular muscles traverse or travel near the cavernous sinus. These include cranial nerves III, IV, VI, and the ophthalmic branch of V as well as sympathetic input to the eye. With lesions in or around the cavernous sinus on the floor of the skull, abnormalities of one or more of these nerves may be seen (Lewis et al. 1984). Usually, there is a combination of abnormalities present. Clinical signs may include strabismus, lack of normal ocular movements, and pupillary abnormalities (dilation or constriction). Granulomatous disease and neoplastic involvement are the most common causes of this clinical presentation.

Trigeminal Nerve Disease. *Trigeminal neuritis* is a poorly characterized disease of the mandibular branches of cranial nerve V bilaterally. Dogs present with a dropped jaw and inability to close the mouth (see chapter 3 and fig. 3.51). Animals may drool and appear to be unable to swallow, however, swallowing is usually unaffected. The etiology of this disease is unknown but it is suspected to be an inflammatory disease of the mandibular nerves. No consistent cause for this inflammation has been identified. Most dogs improve with time. No treatment has shown beneficial.

A *primarily sensory trigeminal neuropathy* has been reported in a 2-year-old female rough-coated collie and infrequently seen accompanying other sensory neuropathies. Clinical signs included acute-onset excessive salivation, coughing, dysphagia, and bilateral loss of sensation in the face, tongue, and oral mucosa.

Tumors may arise on or around the trigmenial nerve. Trigeminal nerve abnormalities can occur with infiltrating neoplasia (*lymphosarcomas*) that involve a branch or the entire nerve. *Myelomonocytic leukemias* and other hematocellular neoplasia may affect this nerve. Other cranial nerves (such as CN VII) and the sympathetic system may be involved concurrently (Carpenter et al. 1987). The ophthalmic branch of the trigeminal nerve may be affected with cavernous sinus syndrome.

Tumors of the coverings of the nerve (*nerve sheath tumors*) may arise on or around the trigeminal nerve (fig. 5.16). These tumors can infiltrate or compress the nerve resulting in dysfunction. Unilateral muscle atrophy of the temporalis and masseter muscles is suggestive of an isolated disease of this cranial nerve.

Facial Nerve. Facial paralysis is the most common abnormality seen with facial nerve disease. This can occur as an *idiopathic* condition (especially in cocker spaniels), as a result of *otitis media/interna,* with *trauma,* and with *tumor* of the middle ear canal. Speculation in humans has focused on a chronic herpes virus infection as a cause of idiopathic facial nerve (Bell's) palsy. *Hypothyroidism* is a weakly associated cause in some dogs. Other neurologic abnormalities, in addition to facial paralysis, associated with hypothyroidism include head tilt, ventrolateral strabismus, nystagmus, hemiparesis, circling, and decreased corneal or facial sensation.

Hyperinsulinism (islet cell tumor) and other metabolic abnormalities such as hyperadrenocorticism are also possibly associated with facial nerve palsy. Rarely, primary tumor of CN VII (nerve sheath tumor, LSA or meningioma) is seen. Trauma may affect an isolated portion of the nerve. The facial nerve may also be affected concurrently with diseases that diffusely affect the peripheral nervous system.

Hemifacial spasm is suspected to be due to hypersensitivity of the facial nerve. Neoplastic, inflammatory, and traumatic causes are possible, however, these are not associated with hemifacial spasm in human beings.

Vestibulocochlear Nerve. Disease can affect the components of the vestibular nerve peripherally or centrally in the brain stem. Disease processes differ depending upon which location of the nerve is involved.

Congenital peripheral vestibular disease is seen in German shepherds, Doberman pinschers, English cocker spaniels, and Siamese and Burmese cats. While often this is an idiopathic condition, congenital peripheral vestibular disease has been associated with lymphocytic labyrinthitis in young Doberman pinschers (Forbes and Cook 1991). *Bilateral congenital vestibular disease* is seen in beagles and Akitas. Clinical signs include head tilt, ataxia, and, in some, deafness. Animals often have a wide-based stance and wide, swinging excursions of the head (also see chapter 3 and fig. 3.60). These animals do not have a normal oculovestibular response or normal physiologic nystagmus. Signs may remain persistent throughout life or may improve spontaneously.

Hypothyroidism has been a proposed cause of vestibular dysfunction in some dogs. Other neurologic abnormalities, in addition to facial paralysis, associated with hypothyroidism include head tilt, ventrolateral strabismus, nystagmus, hemiparesis, circling, and decreased corneal or facial sensation.

Tumors of the ear more often occur in older animals. Squamous cell carcinoma and adenocarcinoma are most common. Inflammatory polyps occur in cats. Tumors that extend through the tympanic membrane may be seen during otoscopic examination. Skull radiographs or advanced imaging is necessary to assess the middle and inner ear. Abnormalities seen with these studies, however, are not always definitive for neoplasia, and tissue diagnosis at surgery is often necessary for accurate assessment.

Otitis media/interna is a common cause of vestibular dysfunction. Most often this is due to a bacterial infection, either from extension from the external ear or auditory tube or, less commonly, from hematogenous spread. Foreign bodies such as grass awn migration may predispose to severe ear infections.

Clinical signs may reflect either primary ear, vestibular, or auditory dysfunction. A painful external ear and or pain on opening the mouth is often present. It has been suggested that up to 50% of animals with otitis media/interna have associated facial nerve involvement. Otoscopic examination should be used to examine the tympanic membrane. This may be difficult in animals with severe otitis externa prior to cleansing. The tympanic membrane is often discolored (hyperemic), opaque, and bulging outward with middle ear disease. Clear to yellow fluid may be seen behind the membrane.

Idiopathic peripheral vestibular disease occurs in both dogs and cats (Schunk 1988). Older dogs (*canine geriatric vestibular disease*) and young to middle-aged cats are most commonly affected. Cats in the Northeast are commonly affected in late summer and early fall. No cause is defined. In the Southeast, a similar syndrome is suspected to be caused in cats by eating the tail of the blue tail lizard.

Clinical signs are an acute peripheral vestibular disorder with nystagmus (horizontal or rotary), head tilt (usually toward the side of the lesion), rolling, and falling. No other neurological signs are seen. Often these animals are initially so incapacitated that they are misdiagnosed with cerebrovascular accidents. Clinical signs, while initially severe, are restricted to the vestibular system. If Horner's syndrome or facial nerve paresis is also present, other differentials should be considered. Differential diagnosis of peripheral vestibular disease includes otitis interna in dogs and cats, middle ear polyps in cats, and neoplasia (squamous cell carcinoma of the middle ear) in both species.

Clinical signs of idiopathic vestibular disease usually improve dramatically in 1 to 2 weeks. The nystagmus usually resolves quickly (within the first few days). Improvements in posture and walking occur within 5 to 7 days, whereas a mild head tilt may remain persistent. While most animals compensate well, some may have episodic ataxia when performing tasks such as jumping up on furniture. No treatment has proved beneficial and recurrence is possible.

Toxicity with *metronidazole* may result in central vestibular signs in both dogs and cats (Dow et al. 1989; Saxon and Magne 1993). Usually, this is associated with relatively elevated doses of the drug. As metronidazole is metabolized by the liver, however, toxic serum levels can occur with appropriate doses in animals with liver dysfunction. Ataxia is usually the initial clinical sign, progressing to nystagmus and more severe vestibular dysfunction. Clinical signs in dogs often reflect central vestibular dysfunction, and morphological lesions have been found in the brain stem of affected dogs. Central blindness may be seen in cats.

Aminoglycosides, administered either systemically or topically, may cause deafness and vestibular signs. This class of drug may concentrate in the perilymph and endolymph and is toxic to the hair cells. Streptomycin and gentamicin have the most pronounced effects on the vestibular receptors, while neomycin, kanamycin, and amikacin preferentially damage auditory receptors. Chlorhexidine solution used to clean the external ear may result in vestibular abnormalities.

Other idiopathic or inflammatory neuropathies may affect the vestibular nerve. Overall, these diseases are poorly described and difficult to definitively diagnose. Similarly, a possible relationship exists between some metabolic diseases, such as hypothyroidism, and a vestibular neuropathy. A cause and effect relationship, however, is not commonly established.

Deafness can be both acquired and congenital. Numerous breeds have been associated with congenital deafness (table 5.8). Deafness in these dogs is usually associated with developmental abnormalities of the peripheral cochlear structures including total or partial agenesis of the organ of Corti, spiral ganglion, and cochlear nucleus. Affected animals sometimes have color coat abnormalities (white hair colors) and iris coloring abnormalities associated with deafness due to the merle color gene. Deafness can be unilateral or bilateral.

Deafness may be acquired to both central and peripheral auditory pathway abnormalities. Congenital abnormalities of the temporal lobe have been suggested to result in deafness, however, this is unclear. Congenital deafness and vestibular disease is seen in Akita and Doberman dogs and Siamese cats. Tumor, infection, and trauma of the inner ear can result in unilateral deafness. Aminoglycosides may concentrate in the perilymph and endolymph and are toxic to the hair cells. Neomycin, kanamycin, tobramycin, and amikacin more commonly result in damage to auditory receptors. Other drugs that may be toxic to the auditory receptors include disinfecting agents such as chlorohex, antimicrobials such as polymyxin B and chloramphenicol, diuretics such as furosemide, and chemotherapeutic agents such as cisplantin. Central nervous system inflammatory diseases (encephalitis and meningitis) can also occasionally result in deafness.

Table 5.8. Breeds of dogs and cats with congenital deafness

Dogs	
Akita	Italian greyhound
American-Canadian shepherd	Jack Russell terrier
American Eskimo	Kuvasz
American Staffordshire terrier	Labrador retriever
Australian blue heeler	Maltese
Austrian cattle dog	Miniature pinscher
Australian shepherd	Miniature poodle
Beagle	Mixed breed dogs
Bichon frise	Norwegian dunkerhound
Border collie	Nova Scotia duck trolling retriever
Borzoi	
Boston terrier	Old English sheepdog
Boxer	Papillion
Bull terrier	Pit bull terrier
Cardigan Welsh corgi	Pointer
Catahoula leopard dog	Puli
Cavalier King Charles spaniel	Rhodesia ridgeback
Chihuahua	Rottweiler
Chow Chow	Saint Bernard
Cocker spaniel	Schnauzer
Collie	Scottish terrier
Dalmatian	Sealyham terrier
Dappled dachshund	Shetland sheepdog
Doberman pinscher	Shropshire terrier
Dogo Argentino	Siberian husky
English bulldog	Soft coated Wheaten terrier
English cocker spaniel	Springer spaniel
English setter	Sussex spaniel
French bulldog	Tibetan terrier
German shepherd	Toy poodle
Great Dane	Walker American foxhound
Great Pyrenees	West Highland white terrier
Ibizan hound	Whippet Yorkshire terrier
Cats	
European white	Scottish fold
Foreign white	Turkish Angora
White Cornish rex	American shorthair
White Devon rex	British shorthair
White Manx	Oriental shorthair
Persian	

Source: Dewey 2003.

Central Vestibular Diseases. Tumors of the infratentorial space, such as meningiomas and choroid plexus tumors, may cause vestibular signs due to infiltration or compression of the vestibular nerve. Meningiomas may form a mass or grow in a sheetlike configuration ("en plaque"). Choroid plexus tumors arise around the fourth ventricle, often at the level of the lateral apertures.

Thiamine deficiency is the most common nutritional deficiency affecting the central nervous system. This deficiency most often affects cats and results in lesions in the oculomotor and vestibular nuclei, the caudal colliculus and lateral geniculate. The earliest clinical sign is vestibular ataxia, progressing to seizures with ventral neck flexion and dilated, nonresponsive pupils.

Inflammatory disease can affect the vestibular nuclei in the brain stem as well as other areas of the nervous system. These include both infectious and noninfectious etiologies. The incidence of infectious diseases associated with meningitis varies with geographic location. Most meningitis syndromes (approximately 60%) in small animals, however, do not have a definable infectious cause.

Specifically, the rickettsia associated with *Rocky Mountain spotted fever* commonly involves the brain stem, particularly the vestibular system (Greene et al. 1985). Usually there is a history of systemic illness (usually with thrombocytopenia) 5 to 10 days prior to development of neurological signs. As the animal's fever is decreasing, neurological signs appear. Clinical features of vestibular disease after a systemic febrile illness associated with thrombocytopenia should raise the suspicion for RMSF.

Brain stem trauma usually occurs secondary to being hit by a car. Brain stem function can be assessed by evaluation of cranial nerve function, particularly the oculovestibular response. Occasionally, dogs have brain stem signs with cranial cervical lesions, therefore, manipulation for the oculovestibular response should be made only after assessing for unstable cervical fracture or luxations. Also, an otoscopic examination may reveal hemorrhage in the ear canals.

Vascular diseases that involve the central vestibular structures are possible. Infarction, thrombosis, and hemorrhage may affect the vestibular system.

Cranial Nerve IX and X Disease. Disease of cranial nerves IX and X results primarily in dysphagia and laryngeal/pharyngeal problems. Dysphagia may be seen with myopathy, peripheral neuropathy, and NMJ disease. Central causes are rarer, but disease involving these cranial nerve nuclei may result in dysphagia. Hydrocephalus, tumor, and inflammatory diseases are possible.

Laryngeal paralysis occurs without obvious cause in numerous animals. A tenuous association has been seen with hypothyroidism. Laryngeal paralysis may be a component of a diffuse peripheral neuropathy. Idiopathic laryngeal paralysis occurs as an inherited abnormality in Bouvier des Flandres, Siberian huskies, and Dalmatians. Cricopharyngeal dysphagia may represent a myopathy or neuropathy involving the cricopharyngeal muscle or its innervation.

Cranial Nerve XII Disease. Disease of hypoglossal nerves is extremely rare. Diseases of the brain stem may result in signs of tongue paralysis and atrophy. Iatrogenic cranial nerve XII nuclear trauma secondary to a cisterna magnum CSF collection was suspected in a dog.

6 Clinical Features of Important and Common Diseases Involving the Spinal Cord of Dogs and Cats

There are numerous diseases that primarily affect the spinal cord of dogs and cats. Some diseases can occur at any spinal cord level, while others are found only in specific localized regions of the spinal cord. Still other diseases diffusely affect the central nervous system and involve both the brain and spinal cord concurrently. Some of these diseases are also discussed under intracranial diseases in chapter 5. Important diseases affecting the spinal cord are discussed below under the major *DAMNNIITT (V)* disease categories beginning with primary degenerative spinal cord diseases.

DEGENERATIVE DISEASE

Primary degenerative spinal cord disease occurs in two general clinical scenarios. In one of these, degenerative spinal disease is found in younger animals and is a breed-associated abnormality. Breed associations are important initial clues to many disease processes. Breed-associated neurologic problems are described in appendix 2. This disease category includes many genetic-associated disease processes. Examples of degenerative spinal cord diseases primarily affecting younger animals include *Afghan myelomalacia, hereditary ataxia of smooth-haired fox terriers and Jack Russell terriers,* and *miniature poodle demyelination.* The specific etiology that results in many of these primary degenerative spinal diseases is often not identified or established. Selected examples are discussed in more detail to illustrate the clinical spectrum of spinal degenerative diseases reported. While reported in specific breeds currently, other primary degenerative spinal cord diseases with similar clinical features may be identified in the future prompting the astute clinicians to be familiar with the spectrum of clinical presentations associated with these disease processes. Important clinical hallmarks of primary degenerative spinal diseases of younger animals include progressive clinical signs and lack of associated spinal pain.

Afghan hound myelopathy is thought to be of autosomal-recessive inheritance. A similar disorder is described for *Dutch Kooiker* dogs (Averill and Bronson 1977; Cockrell et al. 1973; Cummings and deLahunta 1984; Mandigers et al. 1993). Clinical signs begin in dogs between 3 and 13 months of age. Pelvic limb ataxia and paresis is seen initially. A bunny-hopping gait is also possible. Signs rapidly progress to paralysis over the ensuing weeks. Death ultimately results from respiratory paralysis. Histologically, there is cavitation of spinal cord white matter from caudal cervical to midlumbar region.

Clinical signs of a *Labrador retriever axonopathy* usually begin in 3- to 4-week-old dogs (deLahunta et al. 1994). Steps are shortened in the pelvic limbs. The pelvic limbs are adducted and there is a crouched appearance. Dogs tend to fall, collapse, and have pelvic limb ataxia. The thoracic limbs are also abnormal, appearing stiff and abducted. Hypermetria eventually becomes pronounced. Some dogs have intention tremors suggestive of cerebellar system involvement. Signs usually progress with dogs becoming unable to stand by 3 to 5 months of age. In some dogs, signs may stabilize over time. Associated abnormalities in a few dogs included aplasia or hypoplasia of the corpus callosum and spina bifida supporting a congenital basis for the disease process.

Clinical signs of a *demyelinating myelopathy of miniature poodles* begin at 2 to 4 months of age in this breed (Douglas and Palmer 1961; Matthews and deLahunta 1985). Pelvic limb signs were seen initially, which then progressed to involve all limbs (tetraplegia).

Cats may also be affected with primary degenerative spinal conditions. Feline polioencephalomyelitis is a chronic, slowly progressive disease of cats (Vandevelde and Braund 1979). Five of six affected cats in one report were females. Clinical signs include incoordination, paresis, and hypermetria. Cranial nerve functions are usually normal except for decreased pupillary light reflexes. Occasionally, hyperesthesia is noted as well as psycomotor seizures, apparent hallucinations, wild stares, clawing, hissing, and biting at imaginary objects. Pathological alterations were most severe in the thoracic spinal cord, but were also present in the cerebral cortex, basal and diencephalic nuclei, midbrain, periaqueductal grey, oculomotor, and pontomedullary nuclei. This disease is characterized pathologically by demyelination and axonal necrosis of the white matter. This disease process may have an infectious etiology such as an associated viral infection rather than a genetic basis.

Many primary degenerative conditions involve specific spinal cord pathways. For example, diseases that affect the central cerebellar pathways may initially result in clinical signs attributable to spinal cord dysfunction. In cats an encephalomyelopathy has been reported in the United Kingdom with primary involvement of the spinocerebellar pathways (Palmer and Cavanagh 1995). Cats were affected between 3 and 12 months of age, however, the disease was seen in cats up to 3 years of age. Clinical signs usually are progressive over weeks to months. Signs include ataxia, paresis, and "head shaking." Ataxia of the pelvic limbs was the initial clinical sign noted. Wallerian degeneration was noted primarily involving the spinocerebellar pathways and the ventral funiculus of the spinal cord. A viral etiology for the primary degeneration was suggested but not proven.

Leukoencephalomyelopathy has been seen in young Rottweilers aged 1.5 to 4 years of age with progressive ataxia, tetraparesis, hypermetria, normal to exaggerated reflexes, and increased muscle tone (see cerebellar disease and references in chapter 5 intracranial diseases; Chrisman 1986). Clinical signs are initially more reflective of a cervical spinal cord problem and are progressive. Affected dogs often have ataxia, overstepping, and possibly hypermetria involving all limbs. Clinical signs are usually slowly progressive over months to years. Importantly, these animals show no evidence of spinal pain. Initially clinical signs may be more obvious in the pelvic limbs. Pathologically, bilateral lesions are primarily found in the spinal cord with the most severe changes in the dorsal and lateral funiculi. Cranial nerve abnormalities are not evident (menace response is unaffected), even though pathologically the deep cerebellar white matter is abnormal (demyelination).

A similar disease termed neuroaxonal dystrophy of Rottweiler dogs is characterized by cerebellar signs (ataxia, hypermetria, loss of menace response, head tremor) beginning at 1 to 2 years (ataxia) and progressing over the next 2 to 4 years (menace deficits; nystagmus, resting and positional; intention tremor). Conscious proprioception remains intact. The cell bodies in the grey matter are affected (axonal spheroids) throughout the nervous system except the cerebral cortex. The most severe lesions are in the spinocerebellar tracts and the Purkinje cells.

Hereditary ataxia of smooth-haired fox terriers and Jack Russell terriers is a disease primarily of historical interest (Bjorck et al. 1962; Hartley and Palmer 1973). Affected smooth-haired fox terriers were described in Sweden and affected Jack Russell terriers in Britain. Affected animals tended to have clinical signs beginning between 2 and 6 months of age. Weakness and pelvic limb incoordination was seen initially with progression of clinical signs to involve all limbs. Some animals had a prancing or dancing type of gait. Clinical signs stabilized after a number of months. Pathologic abnormalities were primarily present in the dorsolateral and ventromedial white matter of the cervical and thoracic spinal cord. In Jack Russell terriers, changes were also seen in the central auditory pathways and peripheral nerves.

Clinical Clues to Primary Degenerative Myelopathies

- Dogs less than 1 year of age most commonly affected
- Paresis or ataxia of the pelvic or all limbs
- Usually progressive clinical signs
- Nonpainful myelopathy

Degenerative Myelopathy

The term "degenerative myelopathy" is used to describe a specific degenerative spinal cord disease of mature dogs that results initially in paraparesis but eventually evolves to tetraparesis and cranial nerve signs (see bibliography under Degenerative Myelopathy , including Averill 1973; Braund and Vandevelde 1978; Clemmons 1989). This disease most commonly is reported to affect mature German shepherds, but can affect other breeds of dogs as well. Cats are rarely reported to be affected (Mesfin et al. 1980). The cause of this myelopathy is unknown. Historically, this disease was initially thought to be associated with a deficiency of vitamin (B and E) concentrations, however, this was subsequently not supported scientifically. Recent speculation has centered on immune mechanisms such as disregulation of suppressor T-cell function as assessed by decreased lymphocyte blastogenesis in affected dogs (Waxman et al. 1980a and 1980b). Inflammation, however, is often not present in pathologically specimens.

German shepherds have historically been diagnosed with this disease most commonly, however, other breeds may also be affected. For example, a similar disease is increasingly recognized in the Corgi breed. In most affected dogs, clinical signs usually begin in middle-aged to older dogs. Occasionally, very young dogs including German shepherds and Siberian huskies are affected (Bichsel and Vandevelde 1983; Longhofer et al. 1990). Clinical signs are usually chronic in duration and progressively worsen. Clinical features initially and most notably are reflective of a T3–L3 spinal cord lesion, however, the actual histopathological lesions may be more severe in the caudal cervical area. Pathologic changes may also occur in the brain stem in long-standing instances (Johnston et al. 2000).

In the mature dogs, upper motor neuron (UMN) signs in the pelvic limbs are the rule, with the exception that the patellar reflexes may be decreased due to dorsal sensory nerve root involvement in approximately 10% of cases (Griffiths and Duncan 1975). Pelvic limb withdrawal reflexes, however, are maintained throughout the clinical course. Symmetrical paraparesis is common. Occasionally, one limb or side of the body is more obviously affected. Dogs are usually more paretic than ataxic and may drag the feet causing excessive nail wear of the longest toenails. Importantly, there is no spinal pain upon palpation. As the disease progresses, the thoracic limbs and (much later) the brain stem will become involved. The degree of paresis is usually much worse, however, in the pelvic limbs. Animals are often to the point of being paralyzed in the pelvic limbs prior to signs of thoracic limb involvement. Bladder and bowel function is maintained throughout the course of the disease. Histologically, the most severe lesions are found in the dorsolateral and ventromedial funiculi thoracic spinal cord. Degenerating axons, swollen myelin sheaths, gliosis, macrophage infiltration are reported.

Degenerative myelopathy should be differentiated from the other common diseases that affect the pelvic limbs of older German shepherds including hip dysplasia and lumbosacral compression/stenosis. In contradistinction to degenerative myelopathy, hip dysplasia is not associated with conscious proprioceptive deficits, and lumbosacral disease is associated with LMN rather than UMN signs (see below, Degenerative Lumbosacral Disease). In the current era, many dogs diagnosed clinically with degenerative myelopathy may, in fact, have other disease processes such as chronic intervertebral disk protrusions, which may also result in a nonpainful, progressive myelopathy with similar initial clinical features. Therefore, it is impossible to diagnose degenerative myelopathy by assessment of clinical signs alone.

Clinical Clues to Degenerative Myelopathy

- Middle-age to older German shepherds commonly reported to be affected
- Progressive paraparesis
- Usually progressive clinical signs
- Nonpainful
- UMN paraparesis
- Smaller percentage of dogs with decreased patellar reflexes
- Normal urinary and fecal continence

Intervertebral Disk Disease

Intervertebral disks are present between adjacent vertebral bodies from the C2–3 intervertebral space through the lumbosacral region. The intervertebral disk (IVD) consists of an inner portion, the nucleus pulposus, and an outer fibrous portion, the annulus fibrosis (fig. 6.1). On cut section, the annulus appears as interwoven linear fibers. The annulus fibrosis is also thicker ventrally (approximately 2/3 of the annulus) compared with dorsally (approximately 1/3 of the annulus). The disk elements contain collagenous and noncollagenous proteins, including, proteoglycan subunits of glycosaminoglycans such as hyaluronic acid, chondroitin sulfate 4 and 6, and keratin sulfate.

Intervertebral disks serve to support the vertebral structures lending stability, but also flexibility to the spinal column. These structures are responsible for at least 50% of the rotation strength of the spine as well as aiding in distraction and alignment between the vertebral elements. The degree of stability afforded the spinal column from the intervertebral disks is often underappreciated when considering the overall strength of the spinal column. Intervertebral disks are also often thought of as cushions or shock absorbers for the spine.

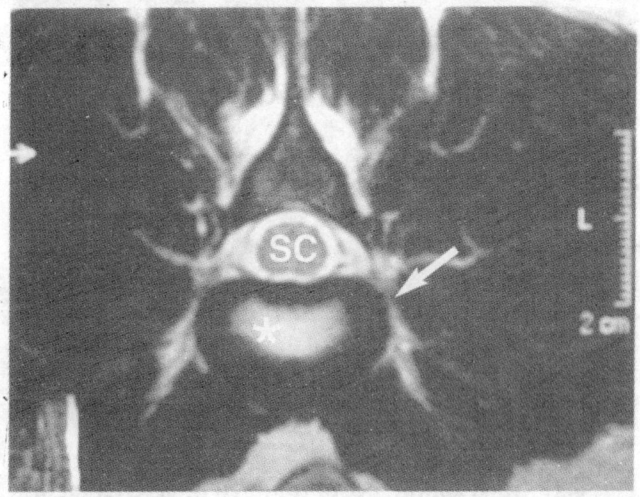

Fig. 6.1. Transverse, T2-weighted magnetic resonance images from a dog showing the intervertebral disk. Note the inner nucleus pulposus (*) and the outer annulus fibrosis (*arrow*). The spinal cord (SC) is present dorsal to the intervertebral disk space.

There are 26 intervertebral disks in the neck and back regions of the spinal column. Intervertebral disk abnormalities, therefore, can occur in any area of the spine from C2–3 caudally to the lumbosacral region. Normally there is not an intervertebral disk at the C1–2 vertebral articulation. A rudimentary intervertebral disk, however, may be present at the C1–2 space as a congenital abnormality in some animals.

Intervertebral disk disease (IVDD) is the term commonly used to describe a multitude of degenerative processes of the intervertebral disks (see bibliography under Intervertebral Disk Disease). Some of these alterations are age or trauma related. However, much of the inherent intervertebral disk abnormality is most likely a genetic-related predisposition for disk degeneration. Disk degeneration subsequently predisposes the disk elements to damage and injury. In some breeds of dogs, the intervertebral disks will undergo degeneration prematurely compared to what would be expected during the normal aging process. Degenerative processes within the disk ultimately result in a loss of water content of the disk elements (usually the nucleus pulposus), decreasing the ability of the disk to deform when pressurized and support the inherent forces that are placed on the disk structure. When forces are applied to the disk via a spinal column, the disk elements may fail, resulting in structural damage to the disk. In these instances, portions of the intervertebral disks may prolapse or rupture. If the disk elements prolapse or rupture dorsally or laterally, spinal cord or exiting nerve root compression, respectively, may result.

While the spectrum of clinical intervertebral disk disease is diverse, two basic types of intervertebral disk damage or injury can occur resulting in clinical signs of spinal cord disease. With tearing of the annulus, free or partially attached fragments of annulus may be released or become

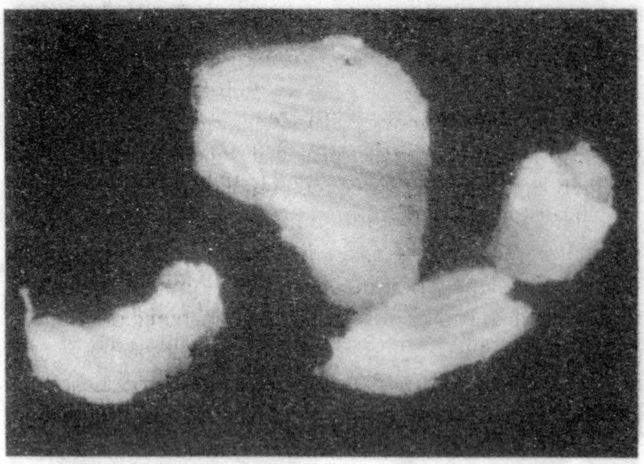

Fig. 6.2. Gross appearance of ruptured intervertebral disk material (annulus fibrosis).

directed into the spinal canal and impact the spinal cord or associated nerves (fig. 6.2). This tearing of annular structures may be associated with disruption of other ligamentous structures such as the dorsal longitudinal ligament. In some instances, rather than tearing free, the annulus fibrosis may weaken and bulge or protrude into the spinal canal. This is referred to as an intervertebral disk *protrusion*. In addition to this type of disk pathology, portions of the nucleus pulposus may be released into the spinal canal from within the center of the intervertebral disk. This latter type of damage results in what is referred to as *extrusion* of nucleus pulposus material. Similarly, nuclear material may impact or compress the spinal cord, as well as incite a local inflammatory reaction in or around the adjacent spinal region. In many instances, intervertebral disk disease is the result of some combination of intervertebral disk protrusion and extrusion.

Similarly, two basic types of disk degeneration have been described pathologically, referred to as Hansen's type disk degeneration (type I and type II) (Hansen 1952). These descriptions were originally based on pathologic features of disk degeneration, however, these terms have been modified over time to also have a clinical connotation.

Hansen's type I intervertebral disk degeneration is described as a pathologic change primarily in chondrodystrophic breeds of dogs such as dachshunds. In these animals, the nucleus pulposus degenerates via a process of chondroid metaplasia and may subsequently calcify. At gross observation, this nuclear material appears as a pasty white substance. Conversely, healthy nucleus pulposus has the appearance and consistency of gelatin or mucus. Clinically, type I degeneration of nuclear material usually predisposes to an extrusion of nucleus pulposus through a tear in the annulus resulting in clinical disease. As it is common that this extrusion of material occurs rapidly, clinical signs in dogs affected with this type of disk pathology often have an acute onset.

Hansen's description of type II IVDD results more from a fibroid metaplasia of the disk and, primarily, the annulus fibrosis. This disk pathology is often associated with the anatomical protrusion or "bulging" of annular elements into the spinal canal. This protruding IVD material may compress the spinal cord or nerve roots. Classically, clinically affected dogs with type II IVDD are older and are the nonchondrodystrophoid breeds of dogs. This group of affected dogs also tends to have greater body weights, for example German shepherds and Labrador retrievers, but this is not an exclusive feature of clinically affected animals. Breeds of dogs like Corgis, schnauzers, basset hounds, and pugs often have similar types of disk change. Older cats also often have this type of disk abnormality. Protrusion of the intervertebral disk material in affected animals tends to occur temporally more slowly. Clinical signs, therefore, are usually more gradual in onset and more slowly progressive and chronic in duration.

Within these two general categories there is much pathological and clinical diversity with IVDD. Some animals with type I pathological abnormalities of the disk may have more protrusion of disk material, whereas animals with type II pathological change may acutely have a tear or rupture of the annulus or extrusion of the nucleus pulposus. Additionally, a histologically normal disk may be anatomically damaged if excessive forces are placed on the disk structure. This traumatic damage to an otherwise healthy disk often results in rapid release of nuclear material into the spinal canal (traumatic intervertebral disk extrusion). The type, extent, and character of IVDD present influences treatment options as well as the prognosis in animals with IVDD.

Any breed of dog may potentially have clinical abnormalities due to damage or disease of the intervertebral disk. Some have more disk extrusions, whereas others are more likely to have disk protrusions. In other cases, a combination of disk extrusions and protrusions occurs. Dachshunds are the most common breed affected overall with intervertebral disk disease (fig. 6.3). Being chondrodystrophoid, dachshunds more often have type I pathologic changes in their intervertebral disks, and often clinically acute signs associated with extrusions of nuclear material. In dachshunds, because of the inherent and rapid degeneration involving their disks, intervertebral disk disease may occur in animals as young as 1 year of age. Some breeds are more likely to have IVDD in various regions of the spinal column. For example, beagles have a relatively high incidence (second to dachshunds) of cervical intervertebral disk disease. Overall, intervertebral disk disease is rare in all animals less than 1 year of age and is most often a clinical problem in adult animals. Common breeds affected with intervertebral disk disease include dachshunds, beagles, poodles, Lhasa Apsos, basset hounds, German shepherds, and Labrador retrievers. Intervertebral disk disease is also an important component of other spinal cord compressive diseases, such as wobbler syndrome and lumbosacral stenosis (see below, Wobbler Syndrome and Degenerative Lumbosacral Disease).

In cats, intervertebral disk disease was historically not felt to be a clinically important cause of spinal cord disease

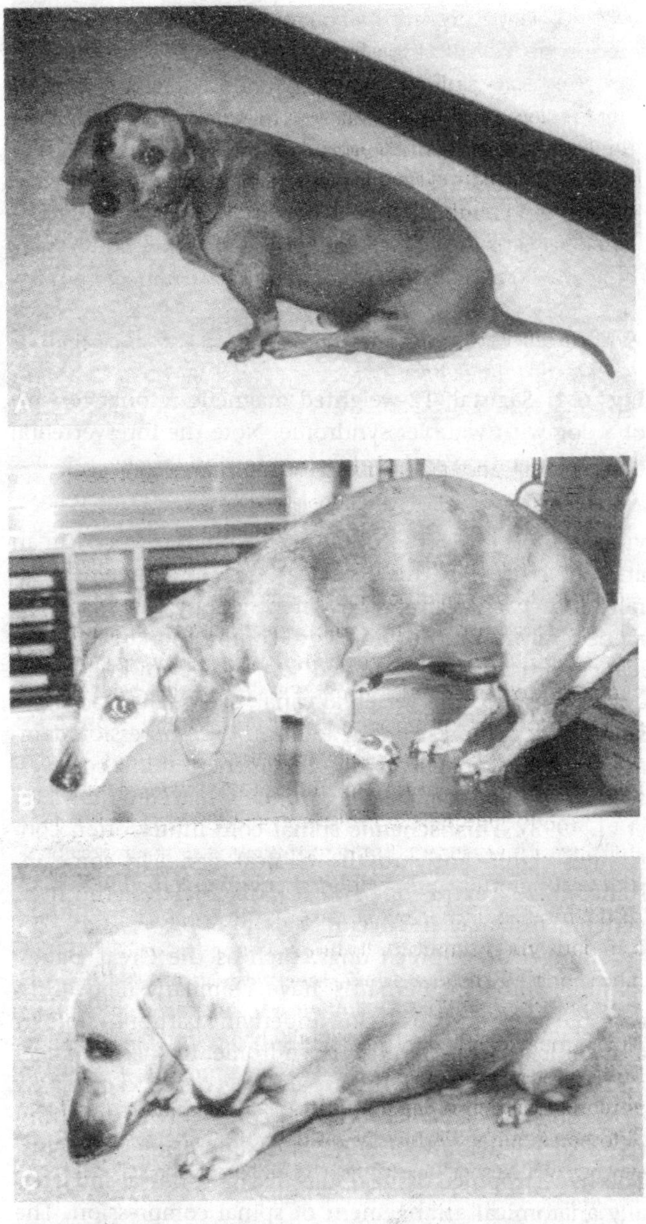

Fig. 6.3. "Classic" appearance of dachshunds with (A) paraplegia, (B) tetraparesis, and (C) cervical pain.

even though many older cats at necropsy had protrusions of the intervertebral disks (King et al. 1958; King and Smith 1960a and 1960b; Munana 2000). Clinical disease of the IVD disease in cats is still uncommon but is being recognized with increasing frequency. While older cats may more often have protrusions of the intervertebral disk, acute extrusion of nuclear material resulting in acute clinical signs of myelopathy may also occur.

Although intervertebral disk disease may occur at any site along the spine, certain regions have been more commonly affected. The region affected may also be influenced by the type of pathologic alteration present in the disk. In the thoracolumbar area, the disk spaces between T11 and L2 appear at the greatest risk for having extrusion of intervertebral disk material. In the cervical region, both C2–3 and C4–5 have been suggested as commonly affected again primarily with extrusions of nuclear material. On the other hand, some regions of the spinal cord such as the cranial and midthoracic regions have historically been rarely associated with intervertebral disk disease. This has most often been explained by the extra ligamentous support from the intercapital ligaments between the rib heads in this area. Occasionally, however, both intervertebral disk extrusions and protrusions occur in this region of the spinal column. There is an increasingly recognized incidence of intervertebral disk protrusions in this area, specifically in large-breed dogs such as German shepherds with progressive myelopathic signs.

Clinical signs of IVDD most often include spinal pain and varying degrees of paresis (fig. 6.3). Depending upon the rapidity with which the intervertebral disk elements are released into the spinal canal, clinical signs may be more acute in onset, or more chronic and progressive. In general, extrusions of material more often result in acute onset of clinical signs, whereas protrusions more often result in a more chronic clinical course. Intervertebral disk disease in the cervical and cervicothoracic areas often results in paresis of both the thoracic and pelvic limbs. In some instances of cervical IVDD, the pelvic limbs are exclusively or predominantly affected. The degree of impairment of limb function may vary from mild (paresis) to severe (plegia). As clinical signs of intervertebral disk disease may mimic those of other spinal disease, clinical signs of spinal cord dysfunction are not pathognomonic for IVD.

As animals with a predisposition for IVDD may have the disease present in multiple disks, clinical signs may be recurrent as these disks degenerate over time. Surprisingly, though, many animals with recurrent clinical signs are eventually found to have only one site of IVDD, which is responsible for the repeated clinical episodes.

As the majority of intervertebral disk pathologies results in shifting of vertebral elements, or direct compression and inflammation of the spinal cord, meninges, or nerve roots, IVDD often results in varying degrees of spinal pain. In some animals spinal pain is severe and incapacitating even without additional signs of paresis or paralysis. Oftentimes, spinal pain is localized in or immediately around the region of IVDD. The presence and location of spinal pain becomes an important aid in localization of the spinal disease. Importantly, in some instances, IVDD is not associated with spinal pain. This may be more common with chronic IVD spinal cord and nerve root compression, but spinal pain is occasionally absent even in acute IVD extrusions. While often associated with spinal pain, IVDD should not be excluded from consideration as a cause of myelopathy if spinal pain is not present clinically.

Nerve root signature, wherein a limb is held in a flexed position, may be a clinical sign associated with IVDD. This clinical feature is thought to result from meningeal or nerve root compression. Pain either in the paraspinal location or apparently emanating from the limb itself may result in the flexed limb posture. This has commonly been equated as a "pinched nerve." Nerve root signature may also result from other painful spinal cord conditions in addition to IVDD. Bladder and bowel dysfunction can occur with some spinal lesions depending upon the severity and location of those spinal lesions. As clinical signs of spinal cord dysfunction reflect only the location of the disease, not the etiology, IVDD may result in clinical signs similar to other spinal disease processes.

Clinical Clues to Intervertebral Disk Disease

- Any region of the spine can be affected from cervical to thoracolumbar and lumbosacral regions.
- Breed associations with IVDD are important clues as certain breeds of dogs such as dachshunds have a greater incidence of IVDD.
- Clinical signs can be acute or chronic.
- Spinal pain and paresis usually result with IVDD.

Wobbler Syndrome

The term "wobbler syndrome" encompasses a number of cervical vertebral abnormalities (see bibliography under Wobbler Syndrome). These include vertebral malarticulation/malformation, intervertebral disk extrusion and protrusion, articular facet disease, and spinal ligamentous disease. These abnormalities often result in ataxia or a wobbly gait, hence the clinically descriptive term used. The constellation of these pathologic alterations contribute to the diverse clinical and pathologic conditions grouped together under the heading wobbler syndrome. Hence, wobbler syndrome does not describe a single specific disease entity.

While the pathophysiologic processes associated with these clinical abnormalities are complex, two general clinical manifestations predominate under the wobbler syndrome label. One clinical form is classically noted in middle-aged to older Doberman pinschers. Other breeds of dogs including both large and small body types can also be affected by a similar disease process. The form of wobbler syndrome as epitomized in the middle-aged to older Doberman is characterized by ventral compressive spinal cord lesions primarily in the caudal cervical area. These lesions result primarily from ligamentous hypertrophy and intervertebral disk (usually annulus fibrosis) protrusion (fig. 6.4). While the pathophysiology of this disease is not entirely understood, some degree of caudal cervical instability possibly coupled with increased flexion force (due to the pull of gravity in a comparatively large head size) predisposes to damage to the intervertebral disk elements and the associated vertebral articulations. The associated vertebral abnormalities are more often a secondary change associated with the consequences of IVDD and the subsequent pathological forces placed upon the vertebral elements. It is also possible that an inherent degeneration occurs in the intervertebral disk as an initiating factor as the disk itself provides significant stability to the spinal column. It is also possible that some degree of vertebral malformation predisposes to the IVDD. Hypertrophy of the associated ligamentous supporting structures (dorsal longitudinal ligament, dorsal intervertebral ligament—ligamentum flavum) is most likely a secondary reaction of the body in an attempt to decrease this instability and strengthen or naturally fuse these vertebral segments. Bony malformation alone rarely results in spinal cord compression in this clinical condition. Hypertrophied soft tissue, however, often encroaches into the vertebral canal, eventually leading to spinal cord compression. In addition to compression damage to axons and neurons, impingement of spinal cord vessels results in ischemic damage to the spinal cord (Al-Mefty et al. 1993). This ischemic spinal cord injury often contributes significantly to the clinical signs. In some instances, actual extrusion of nuclear material from the intervertebral disk may also occur.

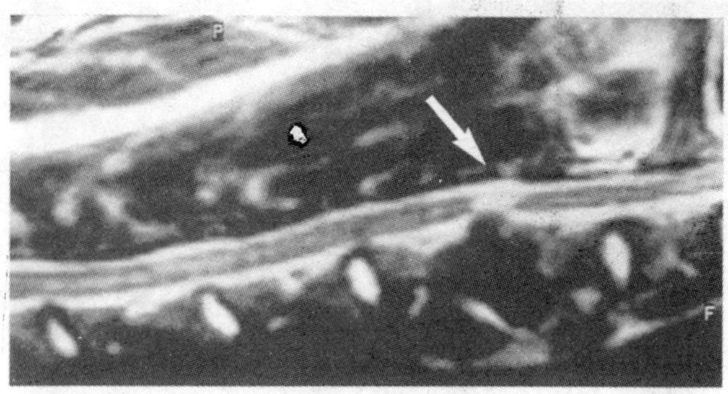

Fig. 6.4. Sagittal, T2-weighted magnetic resonance view of a dog with wobbler syndrome. Note the intervertebral disk degeneration and spinal compression (*arrow*).

Younger, large-breed dogs, such as the Great Danes, mastiffs, and Saint Bernards, have a similarly named disease, but apparently differing underlying pathophysiologic and clinical form of wobbler syndrome. In these younger and larger dogs, there is disease and degeneration primarily of the dorsal articular facets with secondary hypertrophy of the associated joint capsules and supporting ligaments. This hypertrophied tissue results in a more dorsal and laterally anatomical arrangement of spinal compression. The articular facet joints may inherently degenerate, or may be damaged due to ineffectual ability to support the weight of the head (fig. 6.5). Some animals may have congenital bony malformations of the articular facets predisposing to a stenotic vertebral canal associated bony compression of the spinal cord. In still other instances, small portions of synovial tissue containing synovial fluid may become entrapped and "pinched off." These sacs of inspissated synovial fluid are known as synovial cysts. These cysts may compress the spinal cord, either statically or with vertebral movement (dynamic compression). A similar type of spinal compression from hypertrophied dorsal ligaments and abnormal articular facet joints is possible in older dogs. As with many spinal cord syndromes, there is overlap in the pathologic changes present in the spinal column and IVD.

The clinical presentation of the broad group of animals with wobbler syndrome may differ depending upon the underlying pathologic alterations within and around the spinal cord. Clinical signs in affected dogs, however, are usually reflective of a progressive spinal cord dysfunction

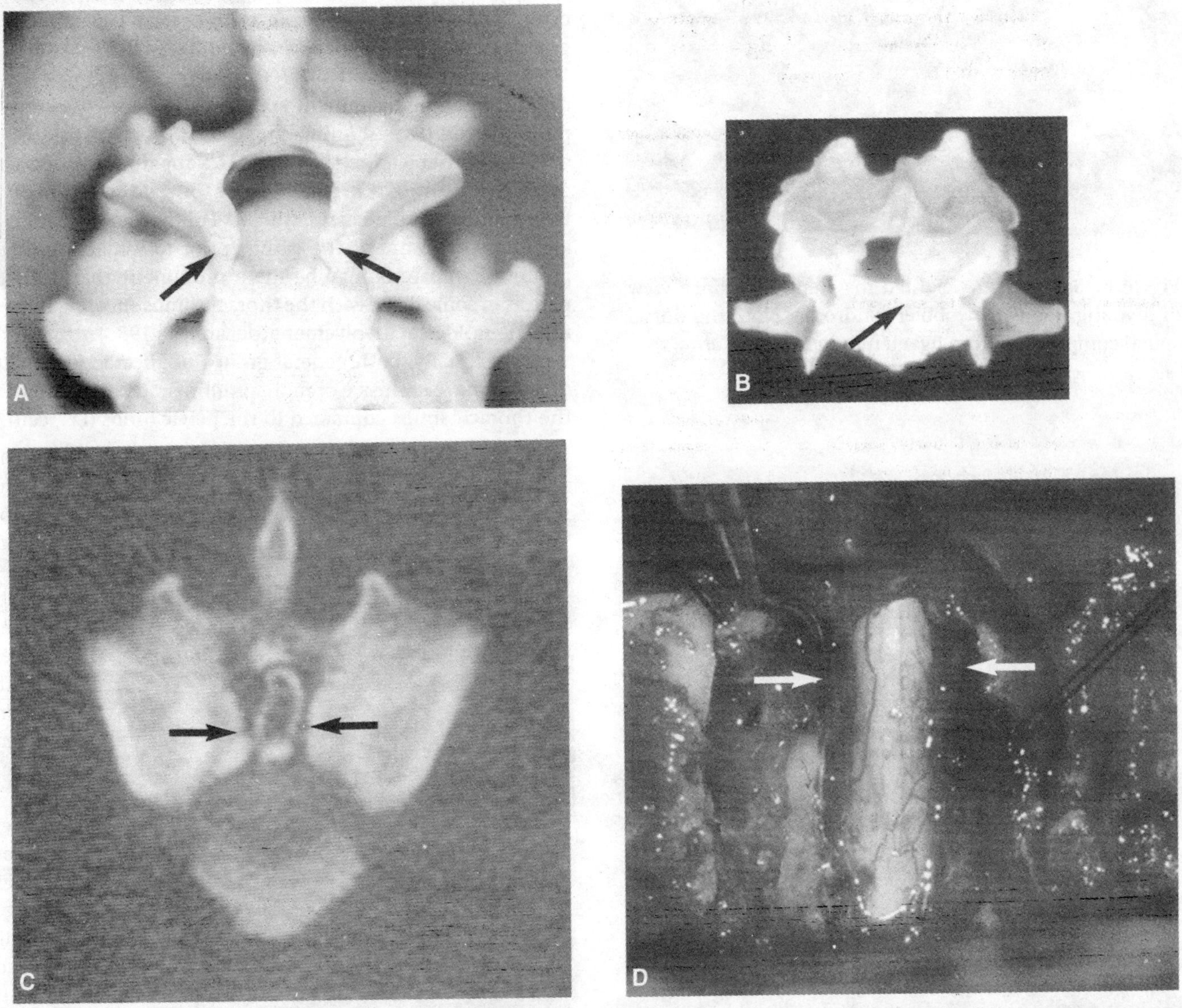

Fig. 6.5. (A) Gross appearance of the cervical vertebrae from a young dog with wobbler syndrome showing spinal canal stenosis from bone (*arrows*). (B) Gross appearance of the cervical vertebra from a young dog with wobbler syndrome with malformation of the facet joint (*arrow*). (C) Transverse, CT view of the cervical spine of a young dog with wobbler syndrome. Note the lateral spinal cord compression (*arrows*). (D) View at surgery of the dorsal cervical area in a young dog with wobbler syndrome showing dorsolateral spinal cord compression (*arrows*).

involving the cervical region. Signs are usually progressive relatively slowly over weeks to months. Occasionally, acute exacerbation of clinical signs may occur. Doberman pinschers, for example, may have concurrent acute extrusions of nucleus pulposus into the spinal canal similar to what is seen with Hansen's type I IVDD, which may result in an acute onset or exacerbation of clinical signs.

Underappreciated with this disease syndrome is the degree of instability of the spinal column present. As this group of diseases may be associated with significant spinal column instability, the spinal cord may be dynamically compressed with changes in neck position. Therefore, the degree and location of spinal cord compression may vary with the associated position of the head and neck. An acute "pinching" of the spinal cord may result in acute worsening of clinical signs (figs. 6.6, 6.7).

Tetraparesis and trunkal ataxia are frequently present as clinical signs in all clinical forms of wobbler syndrome. Animals may drag the limbs along the ground, which may be audible during walking especially on hard surfaces. Additionally, this dragging may result in scuffing of the toenails and associated abnormal toenail wear (see the conscious proprioceptive section of chapter 3). The longest toes of the limb are more often affected with this abnormal toenail wear. When clinical signs of the disease are early or mild, only the pelvic limbs may be affected. This may be due to the overall smaller numbers of motor tracts projecting to the pelvic limbs, the location of the tracts projecting

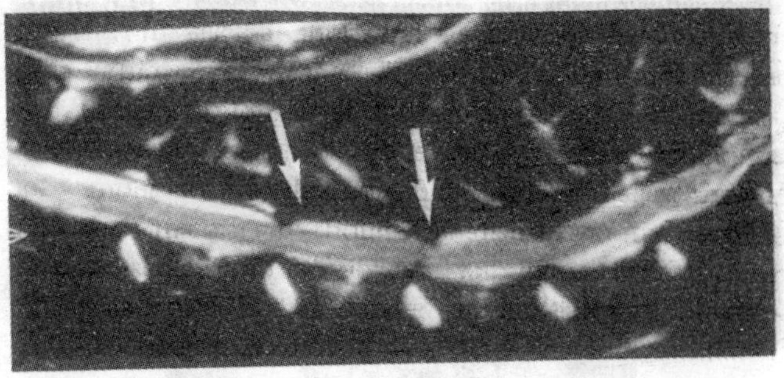

Fig. 6.6. Sagittal, T2-weighted magnetic resonance view of a young dog with wobbler syndrome. Note the dorsal spinal compression from ligament hypertrophy (*arrows*).

to the pelvic limbs being more laterally (somotopically) located, or the distance of the pelvic limbs from the center of gravity (which is over the thoracic limb area).

Young, larger-breed dogs with cervical compression often have more prominent ataxia and hypermetria compared to overt paresis. Animals may also have a spastic, stiff, or floating character to the limbs. The apparent stiffness is often the result of a degree of extensor rigidity of the affected limbs. In some cases, the paws of the thoracic limbs are flipped forward at the carpus prior to impacting the ground. Paraparesis may be more prominent than tetraparesis in some dogs, with the thoracic limbs showing minimal neurological involvement (deLahunta 1983).

Occasionally, both general groups of affected wobbler dogs will have exclusive or more prominent dysfunction of the thoracic limbs compared to the pelvic limbs (i.e., cen-

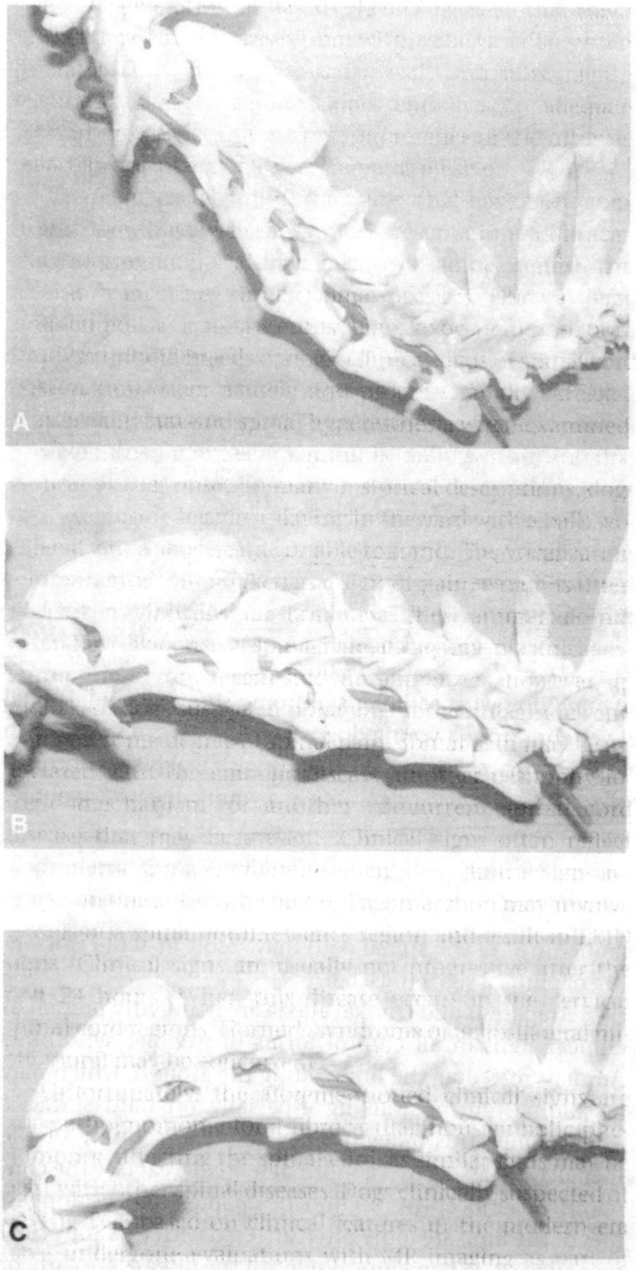

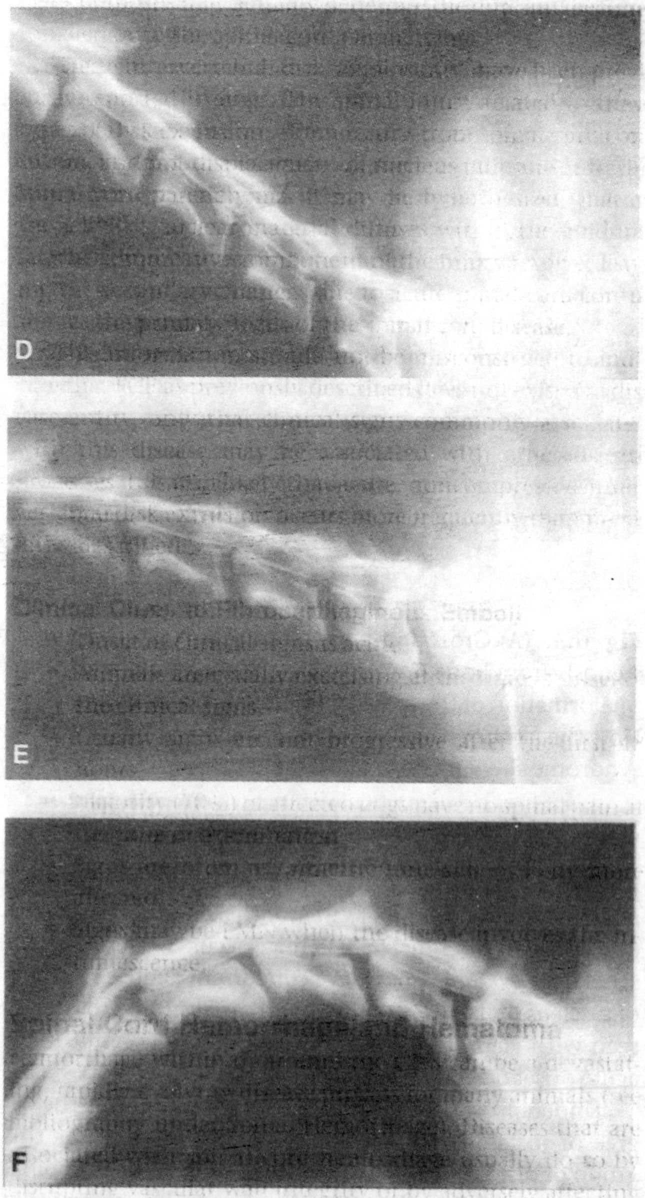

Fig. 6.7. (A, B, C) Gross appearance and (D, E, F) lateral myelographic appearance of the cervical vertebrae showing the position appearance of the vertebrae in (A, D) extension, (B, E) neutral, and (C, F) flexed positions.

tral cord syndrome). Spasticity of the thoracic limbs at gait may be noted. This is recognized as a stiff, straight-legged movement of the thoracic limbs with a normal to increased step length.

Cervical pain is not always obvious, however, affected dogs tend to hold their heads downward in a more flexed position. Evidence from dynamic spinal cord contrast injection studies (myelography) suggests that this posture is associated with relief of spinal cord compression in some affected animals such as those with ventral spinal cord compression. Affected animals may not have normal range of motion of the neck either in an extended position or laterally. Atrophy of the supraspinatus and infraspinatus muscles may be noted due to LMN involvement of the caudal cervical nerves such as the suprascapular.

Clinical Clues to Wobbler Syndrome

- Middle-age to older Doberman pinschers
- Younger, giant-breed dogs such as Great Danes, mastiffs, and Saint Bernards
- Ataxia and paresis of all limbs, which may be worse in the pelvic or, occasionally, the thoracic limbs
- Usually progressive clinical signs
- Cervical pain variable and may not be clinically apparent
- Affected animals may hold their head in a more flexed position or may be unable to extend their head fully.

Degenerative Lumbosacral Disease

Various spinal diseases can involve the lumbosacral region of the spine. Many of these conditions exist under the *lumbosacral disease* or *cauda equine syndrome* labels. Degenerative lumbosacral (LS) disease is often the cumulative result of malarticulation, malformation, or, most commonly, intervertebral disk degeneration and protrusion at the lumbosacral joint space (see bibliography under Lumbosacral Disease). In some instances, this abnormality is associated with occult osteochondritis dessicans (OCD) lesions of the L7 vertebrae or sacrum. Similar to what was described with some aspects of wobbler's syndrome, damage and degeneration of supporting elements of the lumbosacral vertebral structures may result in intervertebral disk damage, annulus protrusion, tearing of the annulus, or nucleus extrusion. Conversely, primary disease of the IVD may be the inciting pathologic feature of this disease process. Hypertrophy of supporting ligamentous elements and joint capsule may also occur concurrently. In some instances, primary vertebral abnormalities of either the L7 vertebrae or the sacrum may be present. These pathologic processes may predispose this area to instability.

Hypertrophy of ligamentous tissue and synovial elements, as well as intervertebral disk protrusion/extrusion may result in spinal cord or nerve compression. The associated spinal nerve compression usually affects the L7 peripheral nerve and nerve roots as well as the sacral and caudal nerve roots as these nerves traverse through the lumbosacral area (fig. 6.8). Nervous tissue compression can result from a dorsal direction from the interarcuate ligament and joint capsule, or ventrally from the bulging or tearing of the anulus fibrosis or occasionally, from extrusion of the nucleus pulposus. The L7 nerve roots are often also compressed from a ventral and lateral direction as they exit the vertebral canal at the intervertebral foramen either from collapse of the foraminal area or from osteophyte proliferation.

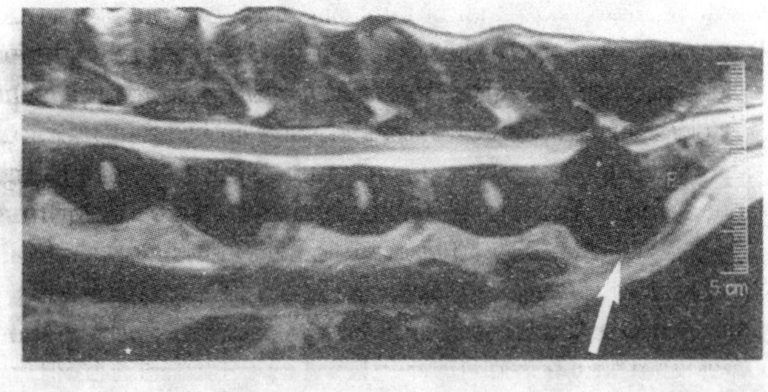

Fig. 6.8. Sagittal, T2-weighted magnetic resonance view of an animal with a lumbosacral spinal cord compression (*arrow*).

Occasionally, other diseases such as neoplasia, fracture, or diskospondylitis (see further discussions of this specific disease in this chapter) can result in nerve compression in the lumbosacral regions of the spine. Primary inflammation of these nerves (cauda equina neuritis) similar to the disease seen in horses is rare (Griffiths et al. 1983; Summers 1995).

Degenerative lumbosacral disease and compression occur most often in larger breeds of dogs such as German shepherds. Many of these dogs are also working breeds whose performance activity may place added strains on the lumbosacral articulation and associated IVD elements. In some breeds, a congenital stenosis of this region may also contribute to spinal and nerve root compression and is the primary pathological feature of the disease.

Of the clinical signs associated with LS disease, spinal pain is one of the more common initial signs. A painful response may be elicited upon palpation dorsally over the LS area. In more severe instances fecal and/or urinary incontinence and decreases in withdrawal or flexion reflexes (sciatic nerve involvement) may be present. Often the tail will be dysfunctional and will be positioned in a downward direction (fig. 6.9). This tail position sometimes gives the appearance of a protrusion or hump at the tail base. Movement of the tail as it is hung in a downward direction may only be noted distally.

It is unusual for degenerative LS disease to result in an inability to stand and walk, and very rare for this type of LS disease to result in paraplegia. In some cases where LS pain is very severe, animals may be reluctant to stand and walk. This is most often the case with spinal fractures or diskospondylitis of the LS region.

In other instances, the patellar reflexes will appear exaggerated due to the loss of muscle function in the antagonistic muscles to this reflex, which are innervated by the sciatic nerve. Muscle atrophy, primarily of the cranial tibial, gastrocnemius, semimembranosus, semitendinosus, and

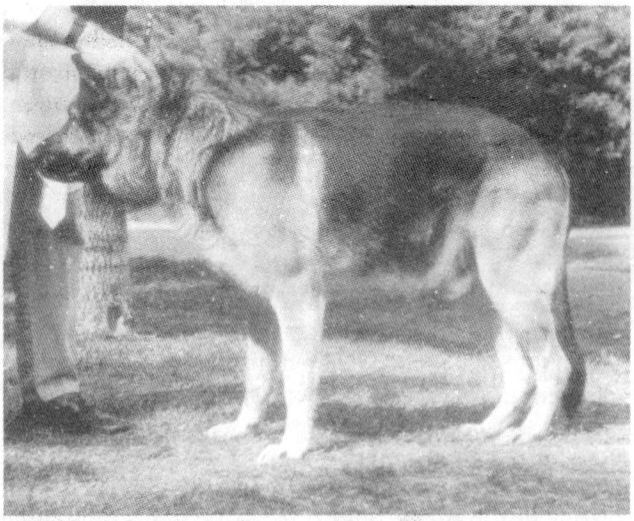

Fig. 6.9. Appearance of a German shepherd with lumbosacral disease showing lack of tail movement. The tail hangs ventrally.

gluteal muscles, is often present. In severe instances, the anal sphincter may be dilated with poor contraction and the bladder dilated and easily expressed (LMN bladder). Animals may continually release urine ("dribbling") while walking, or at other times, when lying down. In some instances, urine and feces will result in skin irritation in and around the perianal region. A pelvic limb tremor may be a reflection of either weakness or pain from LS disease. A painful response may be elicited with dorsal extension or direct palpation of the LS joint, however, it can also be seen with hip dysplasia and other lumbar abnormalities. It is important to palpate the LS area when the animal is laterally recumbent, as pressure placed here in a standing animal with, for example, coxofemoral joint disease, may also result in apparent pain. This painful response to pressure distributed though the coxofemoral area may be misinterpreted as LS joint pain. A digital rectal examination is also warranted to exclude intrapelvic masses and can also be important when assessing the strength of anal sphincter contraction.

Clinical Clues to Degenerative Lumbosacral Disease

- Middle-aged to older dogs
- Pain in the lumbosacral region
- Dysfunction of the tail
- Fecal or urinary incontinence
- Decreased withdrawal reflexes
- Cranial tibial muscle atrophy

Spondylosis Deformans/Ventral Bridging Spondylosis

Spondylosis deformans or ventral bridging spondylosis is commonly encountered in middle-aged to older dogs (fig. 6.10, also see fig. 11.23). This pathologic change is thought to be the result of an age-related, degenerative vertebral and paravertebral abnormality. Spondylosis may be found at all

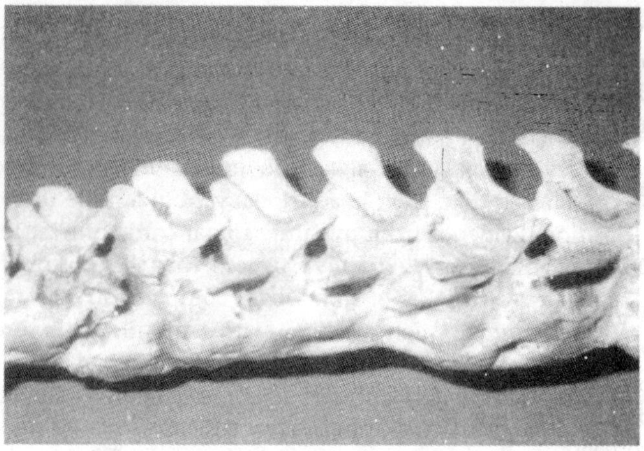

Fig. 6.10. Gross appearance of the vertebrae from a dog with bridging spondylosis.

vertebral levels (Langeland and Lingaas 1995; Larsen and Selby 1981; Morgan et al. 1989; Morgan and Biery 1985). While these bony abnormalities can be evident in younger animals (disseminated skeletal hyperostosis), bony proliferations are most often found in middle-aged to older dogs and cats (Morgan and Stavenborn 1991; Woodard et al. 1985). In cats, hypervitaminosis A results in severe spondylitic change in the vertebrae, usually affecting the cervical region (Goldman 1992).

The etiology of spondylosis deformans in adult and older animals is not always determined, however, chronic, mild vertebral instability and associated intervertebral disk damage, specifically of the annulus fibrosis, are probable causes. This spondylitic change may, in fact, be a result of a ventral intervertebral disk extrusion or protrusion with associated peridiskal calcification.

In many older animals, spondylosis deformans is found incidentally and is without clinical significance. Debate continues as to its clinical significance in animals with vertebral pain. While often this bony change does not cause obvious clinical disease, if the proliferative bone extends dorsally and laterally to compress exiting peripheral nerves, pain and limb dysfunction may result (Bagley and Tucker 1996; Morgan et al. 1989; Morgan and Biery 1985; Morgan et al. 1967). If spondylosis results secondarily to intervertebral disk disease, alterations in vertebral articulation associated with intervertebral disk degeneration may result in spinal pain concurrently.

Dural Ossification

Ossification of the dura can be seen in older animals, more commonly in the cervical area (Morgan 1969; Wilson et al. 1975). A radiopaque linear density is noted on radiographs in the area where the dura (meninges) would normally be found (see fig. 11.25). The pathologic significance of this radiographic finding is unknown, however, most feel that this abnormality is not associated with clinical signs of spinal or peripheral nerve disease. Occasionally, mineralized dura plaques will be adherent to the underlying spinal cord, which could result in a spinal cord abnormality. Some of these mineralized plaques occur focally in areas where the dura (chronically) chafes or rubs against a vertebral element (such as the articular facet). These focal dural mineralizations may occur secondary to other spinal cord compressive or instability disorders such as chronic IVDD.

ANOMALOUS DISEASES

A variety of spinal cord congenital abnormalities may involve the vertebrae, the meninges, or the spinal cord proper (see anomalous spinal diseases references). As many of these disorders are present from birth, congenital spinal cord abnormalities are more often identified as clinical problems in younger animals.

Spina bifida is a failure of the dorsal aspect of the vertebrae to fuse during development (see bibliography under Spina Bifida). This abnormality is most often encountered in the caudal lumbar and lumbosacral regions and may be a component of sacrococcygeal dysgenesis (see bibliography under Sacrococcygeal Dysgenesis). English bulldogs and Manx cats are most commonly affected. These defects may be associated with protrusion or adhesion of the meninges (meningocele) or meninges and spinal cord (meningomyelocele). With meningocele or meningomyelocele, there may be an associated, usually soft, fluctuant, swelling or enlargement involving the skin dorsal to the affected spinal area. Included in these defects may be a multitude of tissue types such as fat (lipoma) or even skin elements. These tissues may resemble a teratoma pathologically. The spinal cord may be attached, adhered, or tethered to the skin resulting in traction on the spinal cord and cauda equina nerves. Associated spinal cord defects such as myelodysplasias may also be present.

Abnormalities of the vertebral structures may sometimes be associated with clinical signs of spinal cord dysfunction. This most commonly results from a failure of the vertebrae to form normally during development. *Hemivertebrae* are vertebral abnormalities wherein only portions of the vertebral segment are present (see bibliography under Vertebral Anomalies). These may also be referred to, based upon the radiographic appearance of the vertebral segment, as "butterfly vertebrae" (fig. 6.11). In some instances, the developing vertebral segments do not separate normally resulting in a fusion of two adjacent vertebral segments referred to as a block vertebrae (fig. 11.26). In still other animals, vertebrae at or adjacent to transition zones of the vertebral column, as between the last thoracic and the first lumbar vertebrae or between the last lumbar (L7) vertebrae and the sacrum, may form similarly to this adjacent segment rather than to the segment of origin. These vertebral abnormalities are referred to as transitional vertebrae. In these situations, the last lumbar segment (L7) may have the characteristics and appearance of the first sacral segment (sacralization of the last lumbar segment). Conversely, the first sacral segment may have the characteristics and appearance of the last lumbar segment (lumborization of the first sacral segment). By themselves, these defects may not result in clinical signs, but may predispose to premature failure of the associated vertebral segment. In other animals, these vertebral defects result in no associated clinical signs.

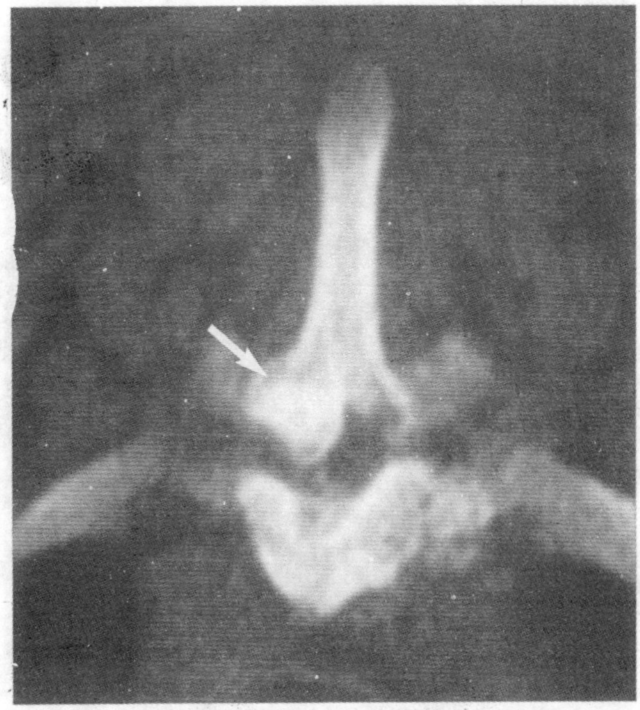

Fig. 6.11. Transverse CT image of a dog with hemivertebrae. Note the misshapen appearance of the vertebrae (*arrow*).

The aforementioned types of vertebral abnormalities are more commonly seen in certain breeds of dogs such as English bulldogs, pugs, and Boston terriers. Congenital vertebral abnormalities are possible in cats but are more infrequently encountered. It is important to remember that there may be concurrent, underlying congenital spinal cord abnormalities in association with a congenital vertebral abnormality.

Animals affected with sacrococcygeal dysgenesis often present with varying degrees of pelvic limb paresis, urinary and fecal incontinence, dilation of the anal sphincter, and irritation of the surrounding skin (urine and fecal scalding). Some animals may have a bunny-hopping gait. A plantigrade stance and decreased withdrawal reflexes may be found. There may also be associated deficits of the perianal sensation.

Myelodysplasia or other forms of abnormal spinal cord development are occasionally seen as a congenital abnormality. These defects are sometimes placed under specific headings such as spinal dysraphism (of Weimaraners) or even syringomyelia and hydromyelia. Primary abnormalities of spinal cord development may result in portions of the spinal cord being structurally abnormal, undeveloped, or in some cases, a duplication or multiplication of spinal cord elements.

Rhodesian ridgeback dogs and occasionally other

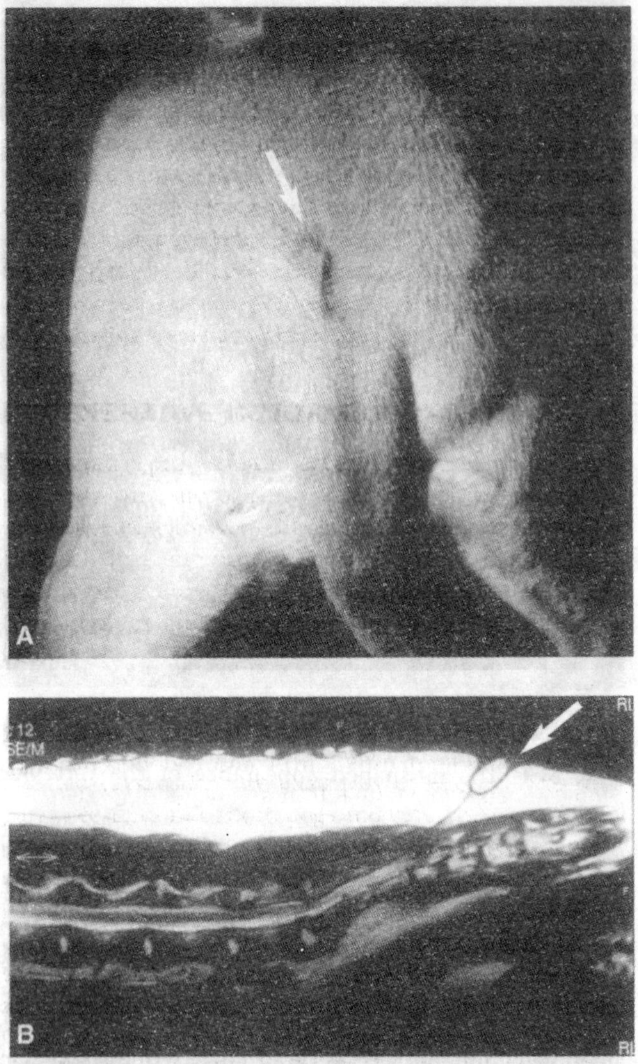

Fig. 6.12. (A) Appearance of a dog with a dermoid sinus (*arrow*). (B) Sagittal, T2-weighted magnetic resonance view of the same dog with a dermoid sinus. There is a vitamin E capsule placed in the external dermal opening for contrast (*arrow*).

breeds of dogs such as Shih tzus and boxers may have a congenital connection from the spinal cord to the skin referred to as a *dermoid sinus* (fig. 6.12) (Antin 1970; Hofmeyr 1963; Gammie 1986; Selcer et al. 1984). This is an embryological defect with resultant failure of separation of the skin during normal developmental closure of neural tube. The characteristic unusual hair pattern on the dorsal neck and back of Rhodesian rigdeback dogs is a dermal reflection of the defect, however, these dermal abnormalities are not always connected to the spinal cord. A dermoid sinus may appear as small indentations or openings in the skin, often associated with an abnormal hair pattern. In some instances, fluid will exude from the abnormal skin area and may be associated with local dermatitis. Dermoid sinuses usually occur on midline in the cervical, thoracic, or sacrococcygeal regions. The associated adhesion between the spinal cord elements and the overlying skin may result in a tethering of these tissues together. The tethering effect or associated spinal cord damage may result in paresis and pain. If the nerves of the lumbosacral area are involved, the animal may be painful on walking, sitting, or standing as these movements result in sliding of the skin and traction on the adherent nerves or nerve roots. Additional abnormalities of urination and defecation may result.

Most congenital diseases of the spinal cord are identified and recognized in younger animals. Occasionally, congenital vertebral defects do not result in spinal abnormalities until adulthood or later in life. Some spinal defects may be subclinical, but leave the spinal cord and vertebrae vulnerable to damage from trauma and other diseases that may occur throughout the animal's lifetime. Instability of the vertebral column resulting from vertebral abnormalities may predispose to failure of these vertebral segments at a later time.

Similarly, intraspinal anomalous defects such as syringo/hydromyelia are evident in younger animals (Bagley et al. 1997; Child et al. 1986). Some of these intraspinal cystic abnormalities, however, can be acquired later in life due to intraspinal disease such as trauma, intraspinal hemorrhage, tumors, or in the instance of syringomyelia, abnormalities of the foramen magnum region. Suspicion for all of the anomalous spinal diseases should be higher in a younger animal with a spinal cord condition.

Clinical Clues to Spinal Cord Anomalies

- Affected animals usually younger (less than 1 year of age at onset of clinical signs)
- Abnormalities may be found in the overlying skin or spinal column
- Anomalies usually breed associated

Atlantoaxial Subluxation. Atlantoaxial (AA) instability is a form of spinal anomaly that occurs usually in small, but occasionally large, dog breeds (fig. 6.13) (see bibliography under Atlantoaxial Subluxation). Yorkshire terriers, Chihuahuas, Lhasa Apsos, miniature poodles, and Pomeranians are most often affected. Other breeds affected include the Japanese Chin, toy poodle, Pekingese, Rottweiler, and Doberman pinscher. This disease is occasionally reported in cats.

This disease is often the result of an abnormal articulation between the C1 and C2 vertebrae. This may be acquired as the result of exogenous trauma with either fracture of the occiput, axis, atlas, or disruption of the atlanto-occipital ligaments. More commonly there is a congenital abnormality of this vertebral articulation. Various combinations of ligamentous and joint capsule abnormalities may be present. The ventral, cranial aspect of C2 including the dens (odontoid process), which forms the caudal articulation of this joint is also commonly malformed. Atlantoaxial instability may also be associated with an abnormally shaped or absent dens. In some instances, there is a fracture of the dens. In still other cases, the dens is present but abnormally angulated in a dorsal direction to compress the spinal cord. Many of these ligamentous and bony abnor-

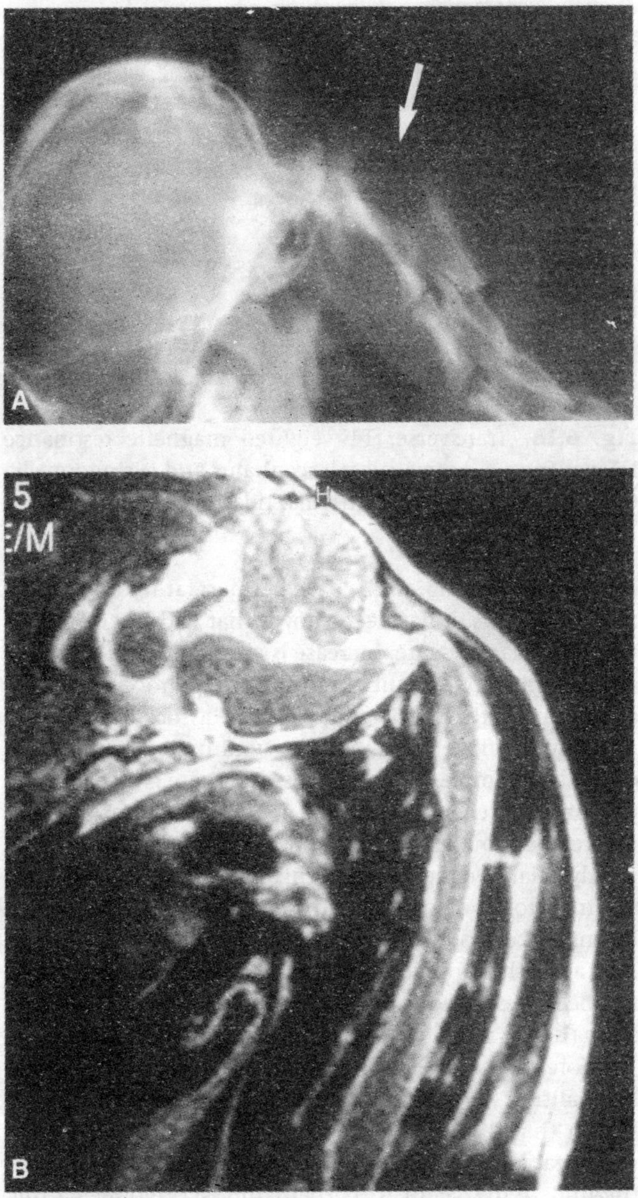

Fig. 6.13. (A) Lateral survey radiograph of a dog with atlantoaxial instability (*arrow*). (B) Sagittal, T2-weighted magnetic resonance image of a dog with atlantoaxial instability.

malities are assumed to affect the stability of C1 and C2 articulation or result in direct spinal cord compression.

Clinical signs result from direct or dynamic spinal cord compression. Spinal cord compression may also result in alterations in spinal cord blood flow. As AA abnormalities result in vertebral instability, spinal cord compression may be dynamic depending on the position of the head and neck. In most instances in dogs, spinal compression is worsened in a flexed neck position.

Common clinical signs associated with this disease process usually include varying degrees of cervical pain, abnormal head carriage (usually held low), and varying degrees of ataxia, spasticity, and tetraparesis. In many instances, ataxia and hypermetria are initial signs, with paresis or plegia occurring as the disease progresses. Flexion of the neck may exacerbate the clinical signs and should be avoided. In some animals, AA instability is present but does not result in obvious clinical signs until a secondary event such as a spinal trauma or injury occurs. This may be why some animals with AA disease do not have clinical signs associated with this abnormality until later in life.

Syringomyelia and Hydromyelia. Syringomyelia refers to abnormal cavities filled with fluid in the parenchyma of the spinal cord (see bibliography under Syringomyelia). A syrinx refers to one of these cavities (fig. 6.14). Hydromyelia refers to a pathologic condition characterized by accumulation of fluid within an enlarged central canal of the spinal cord. In both of these instances, the fluid that accumulates is similar, if not identical, to cerebrospinal fluid (CSF). Some authors refer to hydromyelia as a communicating syringomyelia and use the term "syringomyelia" to describe all intraspinal abnormal fluid accumulations.

Clinically and diagnostically, it is often difficult to differentiate between syringomyelia and hydromyelia. The terms "syringo-/hydromyelia" or "syringomyelia" alone are, therefore, used. Ultimately, the diagnosis is made at a

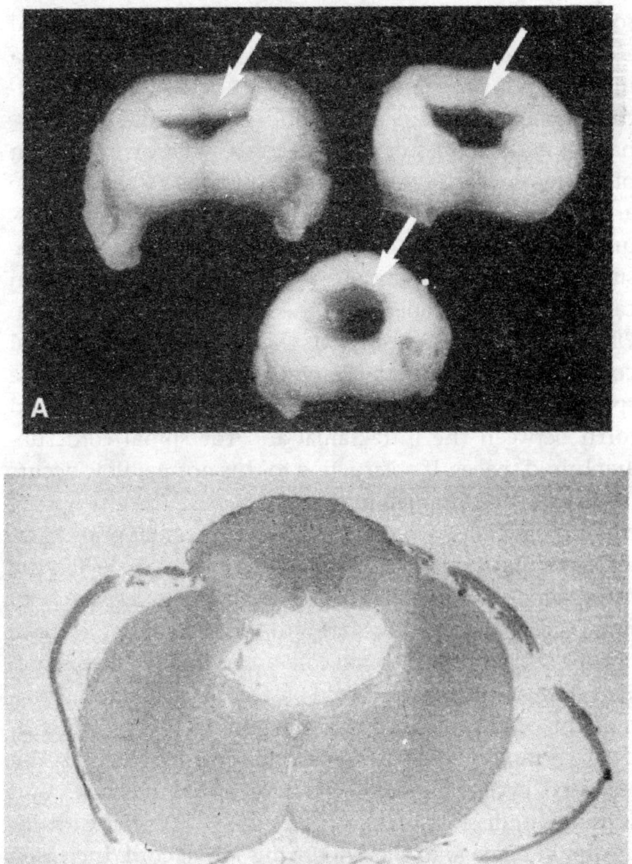

Fig. 6.14. (A) Gross and (B) histologic appearance of a spinal cord from an animal with syringomyelia and hydromyelia (*arrows*).

histologic examination wherein the fluid cavity in hydromyelia is identified as being lined by ependymal cells characteristic of the central canal. A syringomyelic cavity, on the other hand, is usually present within the spinal cord external to the central canal and is often lined by glial cells. In many instances these abnormalities are present concurrently.

The pathophysiologic mechanisms that result in syringomyelia and hydromyelia are many and varied and no single pathologic mechanism adequately explains all instances of the diseases. Possible pathogenic mechanisms of cyst formation include changes in CSF pressure relationships within the spinal cord (as occurs with hydrocephalus or foramen magnum abnormalities), loss of spinal parenchyma, stenosis of the central canal, and obstruction to CSF flow via inflammation or tumor. Each of these mechanisms is possible in dogs and cats but has yet to be definitively proved. In many instances where syringomyelia exists, there are associated abnormalities of the infratentorial or foramen magnum regions.

Syrinxes that do not communicate with the central canal (extracanalicular syrinxes) are often acquired due to spinal injury or damage from disease (hemorrhage and inflammation). These syrinxes tend to occur in the central grey matter or dorsal and lateral white matter, possibly associated with changes in vascular distribution ("watershed zones"). Another important cause of syringo-/hydromyelia in humans is abnormal CSF dynamics at the fourth ventricle/foramen magnum area. Abnormal pressure/fluid dynamics may then result in spinal cord cavitation or dilation of the central canal. Proposed explanations for this include arterial pulsation of CSF with pressure waves being transmitted to the cervical cord and increased CSF pressures resulting in transmedullary passage of CSF from the central canal and epidural space into the spinal cord parenchyma. Obstruction of CSF flow from the cranium to the spinal cord may result in pressure differentials that impact the spinal cord. With each heartbeat, CSF moves back and forth between the intracranial and the spinal cord subarachnoid spaces. If obstruction to this normal flow occurs (such as with a foramen magnum stenosis), the CSF within the intracranial space reaches a higher pressure prior to release within the spinal cord subarachnoid space. When the intracranial CSF pressure is greater than the resistance to flow, CSF is propelled or shot into the subarachnoid space of the cranial cervical spinal cord under increased pressure. This increase in subarachnoid pressure may result in compression of the spinal cord. Ultimately, as this pressure increase is rapidly dissipated, the spinal cord is released. The repeated cycle of increased subarachnoid pressures and subsequent dissipation of this pressure with each heartbeat results in damage to the underlying spinal cord. Increased or pulsatile differential CSF pressure external to or within the spinal cord parenchyma may result in vascular compromise to the cord, impairing venous drainage and predisposing to parenchymal damage.

Hydromyelia as well as syringomyelia are often, but not consistently, associated with hydrocephalus in both humans and dogs (fig. 6.15). In experimental hydrocephalic models in dogs, it has been shown that with increased intraventricular pressure, increase is also found in the syrinx cavity. Other abnormalities resulting in hydrocephalus and a dilated fourth ventricle may also be associated with syringomyelia. The Dandy-Walker syndrome in humans is one such example. With this disease, there is a malformation of the cerebellum resulting in a cystlike abnormality in the cerebellum. The lateral and third ventricles are commonly dilated concurrently. This is a congenital problem assumed to be associated with abnormal embryogenesis. Examples of a similar syndrome have been described in dogs and other animals. The spinal cord abnormalities have not been described, however, the spinal cords of affected animals may not have been examined pathologically.

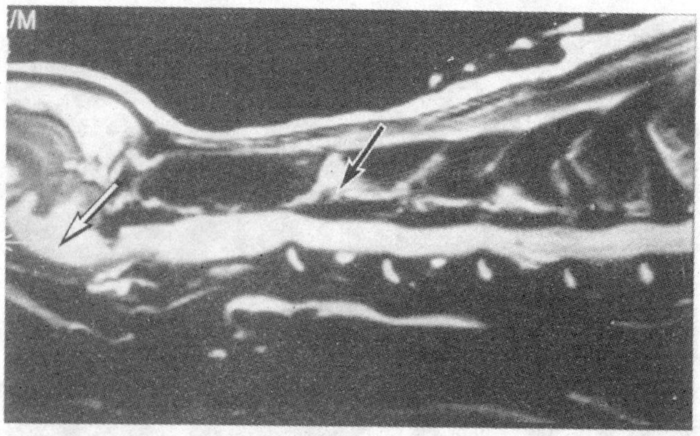

Fig. 6.15. Transverse, T1-weighted magnetic resonance images from a dog with hydrocephalus and syringomyelia (*right arrow*). Note the ventricular dilation (*left arrow*).

More recent studies of humans with posterior fossa abnormalities (referred to as Chiari malformations) have shown that disequilibration and movement of CSF from the intracranial to the spinal subarachnoid space may be the underlying factor in perpetuating syringomyelia (fig. 6.16). If the back and forth flow of CSF at the foramen magnum is obstructed due to caudal displacement of the cerebellum or some other anatomical abnormality, CSF cannot move in either direction. Cerebrospinal fluid, which cannot freely flow from the intracranial space during systole, may evidently be released under increased pressure. The pulsatile increase in pressure is transmitted into the spinal cord subarachnoid space and appears to be an important factor in perpetuating the syrinx cavity. We have shown previously in normal dogs via measurement of CSF pressures that there are CSF pulsations concurrently with the heartbeat, and that there is an increase in CSF pressure from the caudal to cranial cervical area. Also, using a similar CSF pressure monitoring system, we have shown that ICP pressures are significantly higher than cervical spinal cord pressures. These data combined would indirectly suggest that there may normally be a pressure differential (step-down) at the foramen magnum area.

There is evidence that the initial structural change in the spinal cord prior to the formation of overt syrinx is

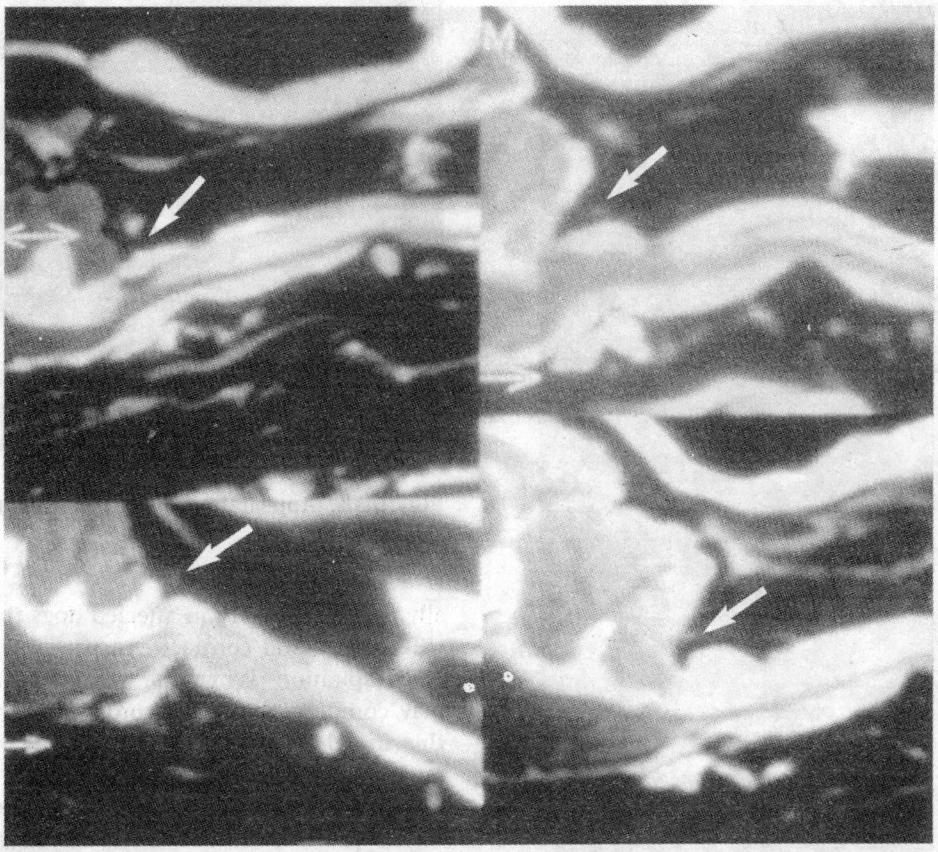

Fig. 6.16. Sagittal, T1-weighted MR images from four dogs with abnormalities of the foramen magnum region and syringomyelia (*arrow*).

edema. Cerebrospinal fluid may enter the syrinx by multiple microscopic connections of the syrinx with the subarachnoid space. Cerebrospinal fluid may then accumulate, coalesce, and expand. Additionally, the effects of gravitation flow of these CSF pockets may contribute to the expansion of these fluid-filled regions more caudally in the spinal cord.

Syringomyelia and hydromyelia may be more common in smaller breeds of dogs, however, large breeds can also be affected. A variety of clinical signs of spinal cord abnormality may be found including ataxia, paresis, and pain. Some Cavalier King Charles spaniels affected with syringomyelia in association with a malformation of the caudal aspects of the foramen magnum and brain stem (Chiari malformation) have an unusual facial scratching or rubbing behavior.

Signs of syringomyelia reflect spinal cord dysfunction. Signs may include spinal pain, paresis, and ataxia. Severely affected animals may be plegic and unable to stand, but this is unusual. If the cervical region is the site of the main pathologic abnormality, clinical signs are often seen affecting all limbs. If the thoracolumbar region is affected, only pelvic limb signs may be present. Bladder and bowel dysfunction may also be found. Interestingly, a number of dogs with syringomyelia have associated scoliosis.

Scoliosis. Scoliosis is lateral deviation of the vertebral column, the etiology of which is not always discernible (fig. 6.17). In humans with scoliosis that occurs prior to skeletal maturity, abnormalities of vertebrae, ribs, and associated ligaments may result in this abnormal spinal configuration. These bony and ligamentous abnormalities may contribute to spinal bending due to the associated loss of stability of the spinal column. Previous spinal surgery, such as hemilaminectomy, may contribute to abnormal spinal curvature. In addition, and possibly most importantly, abnormal paraspinal muscular support has been suggested as a contributing factor to some spinal deformities such as kyphosis. Similar etiologies for scoliosis in dogs and cats are less clearly defined.

The lateral deviation of the spine can contribute to abnormal gait, changes in weight bearing, and chronic pain. Associated spinal cord compression can result in ataxia and paresis. Pain may be the result of damage to vertebrae or the associated ligamentous support structures, but it often occurs due to damage to the intervertebral disks and other supporting ligamentous structures. Scoliosis present prior to skeletal maturity is often progressive with further vertebral growth. For younger human patients, prevention of further structural deformity and associated problems such as abnormal posture, decreased pulmonary compliance, and improved appearance are often indications for surgical correction.

Intramedullary cystic spinal lesions such as syringomyelia and hydromyelia have most commonly been associ-

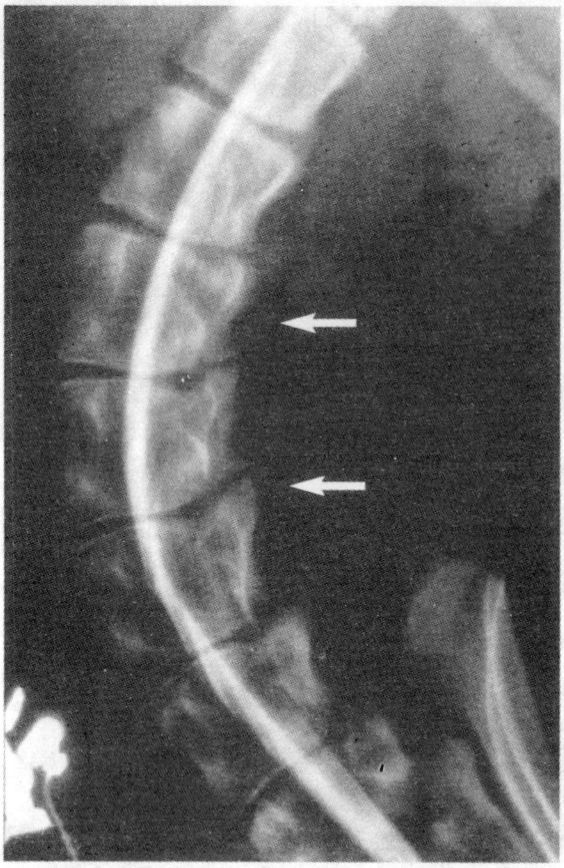

Fig. 6.17. Ventrodorsal myelographic view from a dog with scoliosis (*arrows*).

ated with scoliosis and other spinal deformities in dogs (Bagley et al. 1997; Child et al. 1986). While association between these types of lesions and scoliosis is not fully understood, it has been theorized that local lower motor neuron (LMN) cell bodies are damaged or destroyed in association with or secondary to the cyst formation. This cell body damage then results in denervation of the associated paraspinal musculature and contributing asymmetrical lateral muscle tension and subsequent vertebral deviation.

Arachnoid Cysts. Spinal arachnoid cysts are reported with increasing frequency in dogs (fig. 6.18) (see bibliography under Arachnoid Cysts). The term "cyst" is misleading as the tissue bordering the fluid pocket is not lined by a secretory cell layer and there is no epithelial lining to the cyst. A congenital etiology for this lesion is most likely, although trauma has been implicated in both human beings and dogs. Scarring of the pia or other meninges may result in the creations of pockets of CSF accumulation. Oftentimes there is a weblike configuration of aberrant arachnoid and similar tissues that form pockets where CSF can be trapped and accumulated. It is also possible that abnormal cerebrospinal fluid dynamics contribute to cyst formation. The superficial spinal cord vascular structures are also often abnormal in the region of the cyst, and are often prominent at the borders of the abnormality. We have occasionally noted at surgery in affected dogs that the cyst cavity will expand and contract concurrent with the heartbeat and respiration. When the cyst is expanded, this region may compress the spinal cord. Similar to syringomyelia, this spinal cord compression may be dynamic and pulsatile. With situations associated with increases in subarachnoid CSF pressure such as during the Valsalva maneuver, the pressure within this cyst may increase dramatically.

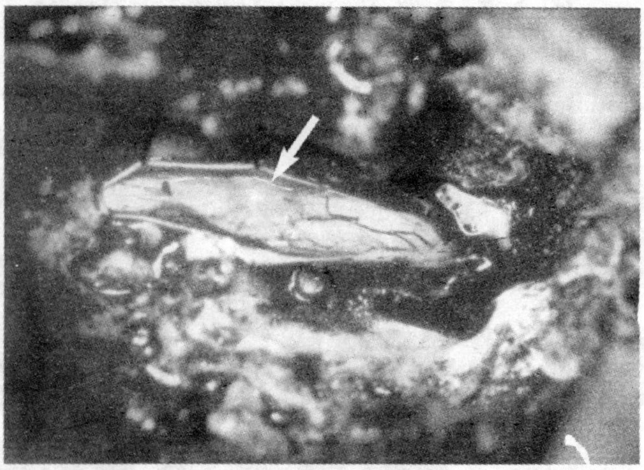

Fig. 6.18. Appearance at surgery of an arachnoid cyst (*arrow*) in a dog.

A variety of breeds is affected including Weimaraners, Chow Chows, Doberman pinschers, Rhodesian ridgebacks, and Lhasa Apsos. Two of the more commonly affected breeds of dogs, however, are Rottweilers and pugs. Clinical signs result from the focal cord compression or associated spinal cord damage. Spinal pain is not typically present. Arachnoid cysts have also been found in dogs with no associated clinical signs. The majority of cases reported have been in dogs less than 18 months old but older animals can be affected. The cysts have been present in the cervical spinal cord area approximately 40% of the time, and also in the thoracolumbar regions. Large breeds of dogs tend to be affected. This disease is rare in cats. In older animals, these cysts may more likely be acquired as a result of recurrent spinal trauma, intervertebral disk compression, or inflammation. Many affected older animals have concurrent chronic disk protrusion. In younger animals, arachnoid cysts may reflect a congenital diverticulum of the subarachnoid space possibly associated with abnormal development of the arachnoid, dural, and pial tissues.

Clinical signs will reflect the region of spinal cord involvement. Paresis and ataxia are common. Infrequently, pain on spinal manipulation or palpation will be present. In some cases of disease in the cervical area, the thoracic limbs are more obviously affected compared to the pelvic (central cord syndrome). This clinical finding suggests that the central nervous system tracts projecting to the thoracic limbs are more affected than those tracts projecting to the pelvic limbs. A number of animals with arachnoid cysts and other cystic spinal cord abnormalities also have an apparently associated fecal incontinence. The fecal incontinence is characterized by defecation of normal stool in inappropriate locations and without the normal behavior posturing associated with defecation.

Additionally, we have evaluated a number of pug dogs with focal cystic abnormalities of the dorsal and lateral subarachnoid space. Lesions are usually in the thoracolumbar area of the spinal cord and may be in a location dorsal to an area of chronic disk protrusion. Clinical signs are reflective of a thoracolumbar myelopathy with progressive paraparesis. Interestingly, some of these affected animals have fecal incontinence as a predominant presenting complaint. In many of these dogs, the gross appearance of the lesion is that of a focal *cicatrix* or *scarring* involving the pia mater and subarachnoid structures. Fibrous adhesion to the spinal cord is common. In some situations, these abnormalities resemble arachnoid cysts and may, in fact, be a variant of this disease. It is also possible that some arachnoid cysts are actually the result of arachnoid and pial scarring, adhesion, and fibrosis from an inflammatory or chronic irritation etiology.

Metabolic. *Metabolic diseases* generally are more often associated with signs of either intracranial or LMN dysfunction. Associated muscle weakness or limb dysfunction may sometimes be misinterpreted as occurring from spinal cord disease. *Hypoadrenocorticism* (Addison's disease) primarily results in clinical signs of the weakness (possible muscle and peripheral nervous system dysfunction) but occasionally results in limb paresis with apparently normal spinal reflex function. The classic nonspecific signs of this disease and its associated metabolic imbalances (hyperkalemia, hypoglycemia) can result in apparent alterations in mental acuity.

NEOPLASIA

Spinal neoplasms are often categorized based upon the anatomical area, in relation to the dura and spinal cord, of spinal involvement or tumor proliferation (see bibliography under Spinal Tumor). Tumors are grouped in this way into those primarily arising from an extradural location (extradural), arising within the dura but outside the spinal cord proper (intradural/extramedullary), or arising within the spinal cord parenchyma proper (intramedullary). Obviously, depending upon growth characteristics and tumor aggressiveness, tumors can expand and extend from one of these anatomical regions to involve another. This is most often seen with peripheral nerve sheath tumors that may begin in an extradural location but may traverse the dura into the intradural/extramedullary space and, eventually, infiltrate into the spinal cord grey matter.

Spinal tumors may also be categorized by their cell of origin into primary tumors (those tumors that arise from cells native to the spinal, dural, and perispinal tissues) or secondary tumors (those tumors that have metastasized from another location within the body). This system lends information as to whether the disease is localized or systemic and influences treatment and prognosis.

Understanding the initial anatomical location of the

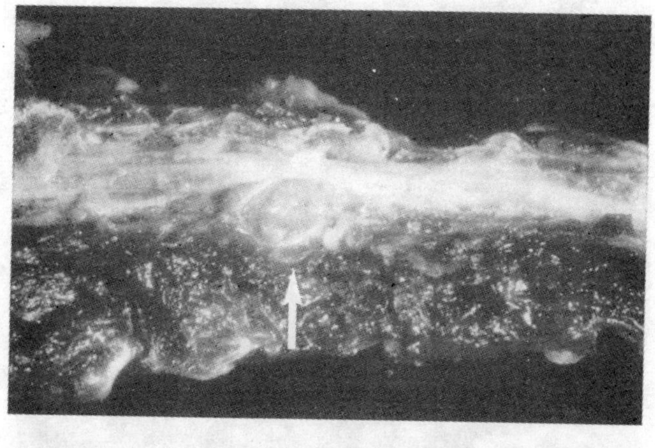

Fig. 6.19. Gross pathologic specimen of a spine from a dog with an extradural tumor (*arrow*).

cell of origin of the tumor aids in predicting the type of tumor present. Extradural tumors are most common of all spinal tumors in dogs and cats (fig. 6.19). These tumors include primary and secondary bone tumors (osteosarcoma, fibrosarcoma, chondrosarcoma), hemangiosarcoma, multiple myeloma and other plasma cell tumors, liposarcomas, and lymphosarcoma. Carcinomas from other locations within the body often are commonly found to metastasize to the extradural spinal location. Epidural lymphosarcoma is the most common spinal tumor in cats.

Less commonly, benign neoplasms of bone such as osteomas, fibromas, chrondromas, and lipomas may occur. Vascular expansile lesions have been seen in cats. In some instances, proliferations of bone and connective tissues mimic tumors but are not neoplastic. One example is multiple cartilaginous exostoses (MCE). These abnormalities are proliferations of bone and cartilage that are thought to result from aberrant growth of displaced chondrocytes from the metaphyseal growth plates of bone (see bibliography under Multiple Cartilaginous Exostoses). Subquently, this disease is most often seen in younger animals (<12 months of age) prior to skeletal maturity. Dogs, cats, and other species have been reported with this disease. The bony and cartilaginous proliferations often are numerous and can affect other bony structures such as long bones and ribs in addition to the vertebrae. The bony protuberances may be palpable, especially on long bones. If the bony proliferations affect the vertebrae, varying degrees of spinal pain, paresis, and/or paralysis may result. Radiographs of the affected bones often show proliferations of bone that are smooth contoured, irregular, and multilobulated. While usually benign, occasionally these bony proliferations may become malignant later in life.

Intradural but extramedullary tumors include meningiomas and nerve sheath tumors. Meningiomas are most often found in the cervical area followed by the lumbar area. These tumors are infrequently found in the thoracic area. In the lumbar area meningiomas often proliferate around, entwine with, and become adherent to exiting peripheral nerves.

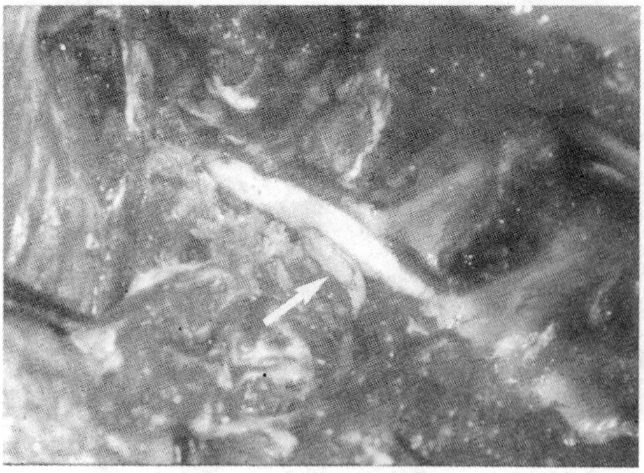

Fig. 6.20. Appearance at surgery of nerve sheath tumor (*arrow*) in a cat.

Primary neoplasia may involve numerous peripheral nerves within or around the spinal cord. Nerve sheath tumors are the most common type of primary neoplasia of the peripheral nervous system (fig. 6.20). These tumor types include Schwannomas, neurofibromas, and neurofibrosarcomas. Accordingly, these tumor types can arise from the Schwann (myelinating) cells of the peripheral nervous system, from connective tissue elements associated with the peripheral nerve, or from the axon and cell body. As histological differentiation of these tumor types is sometimes difficult, and the biological behavior is similar, the generic term "nerve sheath tumor" is often used to describe this category of tumor types. Tumors occur most commonly in nerves of the thoracic limbs, less so in other spinal peripheral nerves. These tumor types may also occur in cranial nerves (see chapter 5).

Additionally, there is an unusual intradural but extramedullary tumor that has been referred to by various terms including neuroepithelioma and spinal cord blastoma. This tumor tends to occur in younger animals (less than 1 year of age), and often occurs in the T11 to L2 area of the spinal cord. German shepherds may be overrepresented with this tumor type. Clinical signs are often of a progressive paraparesis in younger animals.

Intramedullary tumors include astrocytomas, oligodendrogliomas, and ependymomas. These tumors arise from cells within the spinal cord parenchyma. Intramedullary tumors are often poorly encapsulated and sometimes difficult to differentiate from normal spinal cord tissue. In some instances, however, the tumors are well encapsulated and firm, making differentiation easier.

Neoplasia may also metastasize from other locations within the body to affect the spinal cord. Metastasis both to the extradural and intramedullary spinal locations are possible. The most common tumors associated with extradural metastasis are carcinomas. In some instances, clinical signs of the metastasis may be apparent prior to clinical signs of the primary tumor. Hemangiosarcoma has a propensity for intramedullary spinal cord metastasis.

Clinical Features

Clinical signs of spinal tumor are rarely pathognomonic and typically reflect spinal cord dysfunction (paresis) and pain. Clinical signs will be reflective of the region of tumor involvement.

If the tumor begins in a peripheral nerve prior to spinal cord involvement, clinical signs are related to dysfunction of the involved peripheral nerves. General clinical signs reflect lower motor neuron dysfunction. These include hyporeflexia or areflexia, hypotonia or atonia, neurogenic atrophy, and abnormal proprioception. Primary neoplasia involving the peripheral nervous system usually results in clinical dysfunction localized to one body area or nerve segment. Due to the location and involvement of peripheral nerve elements, animals with nerve sheath tumors often appear painful either locally in the affected limb or around the spinal cord in the area of the lesion.

Clinical signs of nerve sheath tumors usually involve a nonlocalizable lameness, monoparesis, localized appendicular muscle atrophy, or pain. Dogs with nerve sheath tumor of the brachial plexus initially may present for lameness and may be presumptively diagnosed as having an orthopedic or musculoskeletal cause for the dysfunction. Complicating the ultimate diagnosis, many animals concurrently have minor orthopedic or musculoskeletal abnormalities. Progression of signs that more obviously are reflective of LMN dysfunction ultimately suggests a nervous system origin of the problem. Pain upon axillary palpation may be present, with some dogs requiring sedation or anesthesia for adequate palpation of this area. Some animals, even at seemingly adequate depths of anesthesia, will awaken quickly during palpation of the axilla indicative of a painful reaction. Occasionally, a mass is palpatable in the affected area. These masses may be linear and oblong as they course along the involved nerve.

Nerve sheath tumors are often associated with chronically painful syndromes. In some animals, the only sign of chronic pain may be a behavioral change as a focally painful region may not be found on physical examination. Associated behavior abnormalities include aggression toward owners, unwillingness to play, and general lethargy. These clinical signs could reflect a variety of clinical diseases and may prompt pursuit of diagnostic evaluations for systemic disease.

If the nerve roots involved are not associated with the cervical or lumbar intumescence, the animal may only have spinal pain. Nerve root signature is possible. Clinical signs may eventually progress to paresis or paralysis. Occasionally, an animal will present with acute para- or tetraplegia due to spinal cord compression. This compression may result from the effects of the mass itself or from associated spinal cord swelling, ischemia, or hemorrhage as a consequence of the mass. These latter pathophysiologic abnormalities could account for the acuity of onset of clinical signs that often accompany spinal tumors. Importantly, a spinal tumor should not be overlooked as a cause of acute spinal cord dysfunction.

Clinical signs of all spinal tumor types are ultimately

the result of the level of spinal cord involvement. Tumors of the C6–T2 segments or brachial plexus nerves may be associated with ipsilateral Horner's syndrome or ipsilateral loss of cutaneous trunci contraction. The extradural and intradural extramedullary tumors usually result in pain, whereas the intramedullary tumors are classically described as nonpainful. If, however, the tumor causes expansion of the spinal cord resulting in stretching of nerve roots or compression of the dura (which often occurs with intramedullary tumors), hyperesthesia may be present. The progression of clinical signs is often more chronic with the extradural tumors, and more acute with the intramedullary tumors. Importantly, a spinal tumor should never be excluded from consideration just because the clinical signs occurred acutely. Oftentimes spinal tumors result in an acute onset of clinical abnormalities.

Clinical Clues to Spinal Tumor

- Spinal cord tumors can affect any region of the spinal cord.
- Clinical signs can occur acutely or may be chronically progressive.

NUTRITIONAL

Nutrition-related spinal cord diseases are reportedly uncommon in dogs and cats. A disease referred to as *Hound ataxia* has been described in adult foxhounds, harrier hounds, and beagles primarily in Britain (Palmer et al. 1984; Palmer 1988; Sheahan et al. 1991). Dogs were affected anywhere from 2 to 7 years of age. Clinical signs included pelvic limb weakness and ataxia as well as an exaggerated elevation of the pelvic limbs. The cutaneous trunic reflex was absent caudal to the T12 to L2 spinal segments, however other spinal reflexes were normal. Dogs had been fed a diet of ruminant (cow and sheep) stomachs. Degeneration was present in the majority of spinal tracts except in the dorsal funiculus. Animals had decreased serum methionine levels and abnormally elevated liver methionine synthetase levels, which may have contributed to the pathologic changes.

Hypervitaminosis A may be found in cats fed whole liver (usually beef or sheep). Affected cats are usually between 2 and 10 years of age. This toxicity results in proliferation of bone resembling spondylosis along the spine, often in the cervical region. Clinical signs include lameness and flexed pelvic limbs, and the head may be held ventroflexed compared to normal. Even with dietary correction, resolution of signs is unlikely.

Degenerative myelopathy was initially thought to be due possibly to a deficiency of B vitamin concentrations. This was not, however, scientifically supported with repeated evaluations.

IDIOPATHIC

Calcinosis circumscripta is a disease typically of German Shepherds, Great Danes, and vizslas but has also been reported in breeds such as English Springer spaniels and Rottweilers. Regions of mineralization and degeneration in a fibrous tissue matrix are present in subcutaneous tissues. Often these masses are found in the cranial cervical region between the C1 and C2 vertebrae. In some instances, these masses will compress the spinal cord. Intramuscular hemorrhage secondary to abnormalities of coagulation may result in calcification of the axial or appendicular muscles. This may occur secondary to systemic bleeding disorders such as von Willebrand's disease and other coagulation factor deficiencies.

Spinal epidural lipomatosis is associated with abnormal accumulations of fat in the spinal canal. This is most often the result of release of excessive endogenous corticosteroids or excessive administration of exogenous corticosteroids. The normal amount of epidural fat in some locations of the spine, and especially in large breeds of dogs, is often underappreciated by clinicians. These normal accumulations of fat, however, should not be misinterpreted as epidural lipomatosis.

INFECTIOUS/INFLAMMATORY DISEASES

Meningitis /Myelitis

Central nervous system inflammatory diseases affecting the spinal cord are often referred to as *meningitis and myelitis*. Meningitis refers to inflammation of the meninges, where *myelitis* is used to describe an inflammation of the spinal cord parenchyma. A diffuse inflammation of the brain and spinal cord may be referred to as an *encephalomyelitis* or *meninigoencephalomyelitis*. Some of these diseases that diffusely affect both the brain and spinal cord are also discussed under the intracranial inflammatory diseases (see chapter 5 under inflammatory brain disease section).

Inflammation may occur anywhere along the spinal cord, and can be focal or diffuse. Meningitis frequently results in clinical signs suggestive of cervical spinal cord involvement, however, diffuse spinal pain may also be evident. Less commonly, focal myelopathies (myelitis) can result from inflammatory diseases. Meningitis and myelitis is more common in young to middle-aged animals, but may affect older dogs and cats.

Inflammatory diseases of the central nervous system are often separated into those that are associated with an *infectious* organism and those that are *noninfectious* in origin (see bibliography under Myelitis). Numerous infectious agents have been incriminated as causing inflammation of the central nervous system. Incidence of infectious agents causing meningitis varies with geographic location. In general, most encephalitis and meningitis syndromes (~ 60% or greater) in small animals do not have a definable infectious cause. This may indicate that an infectious cause was present at some point in the course of the disease and is either no longer actively present or escapes clinical detection.

Infectious agents causing spinal disease primarily include *viral* (distemper, feline infectious peritonitis), *bacterial, fungal* (blastomycosis, histoplasmosis, cryptococcosis, coccidiomycosis, aspergillosis), and *protozoal* (toxoplasmosis, neosporosis)etiologies. Parasitic migration may also affect the spinal cord.

As inflammatory CNS diseases may affect the nervous system at multiple levels, clinical signs may reflect multiple levels of neurological involvement. Systemic signs may accompany the neurologic signs and reflect diffuse body sys tem involvement. Joint, skin, heart, liver, kidney, and bone marrow are examples of other commonly affected body systems. Associated organ dysfunction is often different for differing disease processes.

Spinal cord signs (paresis, ataxia) are common. If the myelitis is focal, clinical signs may mimic other focal spinal cord disorders such as intervertebral disk disease. Spinal pain may also result from inflammation of the vertebrae (osteitis), vertebral joint (polyarthritis), or muscle (myositis) and be clinically indistinguishable from spinal or nerve root pain. Cervical pain is a prominent clinical feature of meningitis, but may be less obvious with pure parenchymal involvement (e.g., myelitis). Pain may be recognized by vocalization during direct palpation or by reluctance to move the head and neck freely or with manipulation (decreased range of motion). Some animals will react as if painful to minimal palpation anywhere on the body, especially of the limbs and face. Many animals become irritable and uncharacteristically aggressive. As chorioretinitis is often concurrently present, fundic examination may yield important clues to the polysystemic nature of the problem.

Clinical Clues to Myelitis

- Clinical signs may be diffuse or focal.
- Often affected animals have spinal pain including cervical pain.
- Other signs of systemic illness (fever, organ dysfunction) may be present.

Specific Inflammatory Diseases

Viral. *Viral myelitis* may result from systemic viral infections. *Canine distemper* remains a surprisingly common cause of neurologic dysfunction in dogs. This disease is caused by a paramyxovirus. Clinical signs can occur in any aged dog, regardless of vaccination status. Most commonly, young dogs with inadequate vaccinations are affected with the polysystemic signs (i.e., gastrointestinal, respiratory) as well as the neurologic signs of infection. Hyperkeratotic pads that sometimes accompany systemic distemper infection have been suggested to occur preemptively to CNS involvement. In the modern era of prophylactic vaccination for distemper, however, distemper infection may result only in clinical signs of nervous systemic abnormality. Nervous system disease associated with distemper is characterized pathologically by two main forms: neuronal and glial cell death (polioencephalomyelopathy) and demyelination (leukoencephalomyelopathy). It has been suggested that those animals with a less adequate antibody response to the virus tend to have the former form, and those with an adequate immune response to the virus tend to have the latter, immune-mediated demyelination. Any region of the nervous system can be involved. A chronically relapsing encephalomyelitis has been reported in a dog attributed to distemper virus infection.

Canine distemper virus may affect dogs of any age, however, the pattern of destruction of nervous system tissue is age dependent. Those dogs affected with the disease early in life suffer from a polioencephalomyelopathy (grey matter disease), usually have a history of seizures, and rarely survive. Dogs affected by the disease later in life may have brain stem, cerebellar, and vestibular signs. They typically have a leukoencephalomyelopathy (white matter disease) or a combination of grey and white matter disease and in most cases the disease is less severe.

Myoclonus, a rhythmic, shocklike contraction of a muscle or group of muscles, is usually the result of previous or concurrent distemper infection and is a clue to presence of the virus. Muscles of the limbs are commonly involved (suggesting ventral spinal motor neuron involvement), but other muscles, including the tongue, may be affected. Clinical signs of a prior or concurrent systemic illness (respiratory, gastrointestinal) are not always found in dogs with neurologic signs associated with distemper.

Feline infectious peritonitis (FIP) results from a coronavirus-induced vasculitis. This disease can involve various areas of the nervous system, primarily the intracranial structures and spinal cord. Both very young and very old cats seem predisposed. Of the two forms of FIP that exist, the "dry" form commonly affects the nervous system. This viral infection results in an immune complex vasculitis, which is responsible for most of the pathological effects.

The pyogranulomatous (dry) form of feline infectious peritonitis virus can affect the central nervous system and may result in inflammation of the ependyma, choroid plexus, or meninges that surround the brain stem and junction of the cerebellum and medulla. This disease can be a challenge to diagnose, as there is no definitive antemortem test to prove a cat has the disease. It has been reported that over 45% of cats affected with the dry form of the disease will have signs of central nervous system dysfunction. This results from an inflammatory response to the virus but a lack of a protective cell-mediated immune response. Because the disease occurs as a multifocal pyogranulomatous meningoencephalomyelitis in the CNS, the neuroanatomical localization can be diverse. The disease is usually fatal. When this disease involves the spinal cord, paraparesis or paraplegia is most often encountered.

Feline leukemia virus may result in lymphoma that can affect the central nervous system. Lymphoma in cats often occurs in the extradural spinal locations. Infection with the feline leukemia virus, however, has also been associated with a myelopathy independent of the presence of lymphoma. *Feline Borna disease*, thought to be associated with a viral cause, results in progressive pelvic limb ataxia, sacral hyperesthesia, fever, loss of appetite, aggressiveness, staring, seizure, hypersensitivity to light and sound, inability to retract claws, and increased affection toward owners (Berg 2000; Lundgren and Ludwig 1993). This disease has not been currently described in the United States.

Feline polioencephalomyelitis is a chronic, slowly progressive disease with primary spinal cord clinical signs (Vandevelde and Braund 1979). A viral etiology has been suspected but not proven. Five of six affected cats were female. Pathology was most severe in the thoracic spinal cord, but was also present in the cerebral cortex, basal and diencephalic nuclei, midbrain, and periaqueductal grey, oculomotor, and pontomedullary nuclei. This disease is characterized by demyelination and axonal necrosis of the white matter.

Clinical signs include incoordination, paresis, and hypermetria. Cranial nerve functions are usually normal except for decreased pupillary light reflexes. Occasionally, hyperesthesia is noted, as well as psychomotor seizures, apparent hallucinations, wild stares, clawing, and hissing and biting at imaginary objects.

Bacteria. Bacterial meningitis and myelitis is rare in dogs and cats. Diseases that are associated with significant bacteremia may cause secondary infection of the CNS. Examples include endocarditis and pyometra. Direct inoculation of bacteria, most commonly from wounds, may also be a possible cause. This may occur in cats from cat bite injury. Immunosuppression, either naturally or as the result of iatrogenic steroid administration, may play a role in establishment and perpetuation of CNS infection.

Rarely in dogs, a bacterial spinal abscess will form. This is usually associated with a penetrating trauma, or extension from diskospondylitis or a vertebral osteomyelitis. This may also occur as a result of a foreign body such as a porcupine quill or grass awn in the vicinity of the spinal canal.

A variety of causative bacteria may be present. Most commonly, *Staphylococcus*, *Escherichia*, *Streptococcus*, and *Klebsiella* species are causative. Other organisms include *Pasteurella multocida*, *Actinomyces*, and *Nocardia*. Anaerobic infections with *Bacteroides*, *Peptostreptococcus*, *Fusobacterium*, and *Eubacterium* have been noted. Often there are multiple bacteria species present.

Protozoal

Toxoplasma gondii and *Neospora caninum* are protozoal organisms that can affect any area of the nervous system resulting in encephalitis, myelitis, peripheral neuropathy, or myositis in dogs. The organism damages the nerve and muscle either primarily or secondarily through associated inflammation. Cats also commonly have toxoplasmosis within the nervous system, however, neosporosis has been established only experimentally in this species. Cats are more likely to have systemic illness from toxoplasmosis. Signs are most severe in cats under 1 year of age, especially young kittens, although any age of cat can be affected. Lethargy, anorexia, and dyspnea due to pneumonia are the most frequent signs of generalized infection. Fever may be present. Gastrointestinal or hepatic signs, such as icterus, vomiting, diarrhea, and abdominal effusion may occur as a result of diffuse organ involvement or from a granuloma.

Limb weakness, paresis, or plegia may be present if the spinal cord, peripheral nerves, or muscles are involved. Hyperesthesia on muscle palpation, stiff gait, or shifting leg lameness may also be due to an associated myositis. Spinal pain may be focal or diffuse. Pain also may involve limb and spinal muscles. A classic sign of the either toxoplasmosis or neosporosis infection in young dogs is a rigidly hyperextended pelvic limb(s) (see postural abnormalities in chapter 3). Other systemic signs such as chorioretinitis may be present.

Fungal. Of the fungal diseases that can affect the nervous system, cryptococcus, blastomycosis, coccidiomycosis, candidiasis, and aspergillosis are most common. Immunodeficiency may play a role in these uncommon nervous system infections. In some instances, a history of respiratory, gastrointestinal or nasal signs accompany signs of neurologic dysfunction. Oftentimes these organisms involve the vertebrae or intervertebral disk space compared to the spinal cord. Associated granuloma formation or associated vertebral fracture may result in spinal cord compression (see diskospondylitis and vertebral osteomyelitis below).

Parasites. Involvement of the spinal cord can occur with parasites such as *Cuterebra* larvae, toxocara, and aberrant heartworm migration. Migration of *Angiostongylus cantonensis* in puppies between 6 and 16 weeks of age has resulted in lumbosacral pain and paresis of tail, bladder, and pelvic limbs. *Cuterebra* migration has been seen in the spinal cord of cats.

NONINFECTIOUS DISEASES

Although a number of inflammatory diseases can affect the CNS, often the cause of an inflammation goes undetermined or is not associated with an established infectious agent. Some primary, noninfectious, CNS as well as spinal cord inflammatory diseases have been described. While clinical signs may be reflective of diffuse CNS involvement, in some situations, spinal cord signs are predominant.

A *steroid-responsive meningitis* is found primarily in young (<2 years of age) large-breed dogs, such as Labrador retrievers. Clinical signs are usually acute to subacute in onset. Dogs often have severe cervical or diffuse spinal pain. Fever may occasionally be present. No specific etiology has been identified as causative. This may be an immune-mediated meningitis as some dogs have abnormalities on some immunologic testing (LE preparations).

Spinal cord vasculitis syndrome is seen in beagles (beagle pain syndrome), German short-haired pointers, Bernese mountain dogs, Nova Scotia duck trolling retrievers, and others. Clinical signs often include cervical pain and paresis. Intracranial signs are uncommon but possible. Aseptic meningitis and polyarthritis have been reported in Akita dogs.

Granulomatous meningoencephalitis (GME) is a disease of the brain and eye that may sometimes involve the spinal cord primarily. A specific etiology for this disease is not yet identified. Some animals initially thought to have this disease have been shown, upon further study, to have lymphoma, but this is not true of all cases. This disease has been reported in two related Afghan hounds suggesting a genetic influence or a common environmental (possibly infectious) cause.

Young to middle-aged (6 months to 10 years, mean age slightly less than 5 years) animals are most commonly affected. Of reported cases, 80% are in small breeds of dogs, with 30% being poodles.

Clinical signs can vary. Spinal cord signs may be present exclusively or in combination with other intracranial or ocular signs (also see noninfectious inflammatory brain disease in chapter 5). The spinal cord may be affected diffusely, or focal mass lesions within the spinal cord may be identified. Paresis and hyperesthesia are common. Clinical signs will ultimately depend upon which region of the spinal cord is affected.

Allergic encephalomyelitis is primarily a historical entity following rabies *vaccination* with phenolized brain tissue. This disease was a disseminated, demyelinating encephalitis or encephalomyelitis, which resulted as an allergic reaction to vaccine components. Clinical signs are usually of an ascending paralysis with initial signs in the pelvic limbs. This disease does serve to suggest reactions to a variety of antigens. Some types of noninfectious encephalitis may have an allergic or immune-mediated initiation. Other vaccines have also been incriminated in immune-mediated or direct infection of the nervous system.

Diskospondylitis

Diskospondylitis is characterized by infection in the IVD space and surrounding vertebral end plates or bodies (see bibliography under Diskospondylitis). This infection can occur focally in any IVD of the spinal column or be present in multiple sites. The most common organisms associated with this disease are bacteria, specifically *Staphylococcus intermedius*, *Brucella canis*, and *Escherichia coli* (table 6.1). Rarely, fungal infections such as paecilomycosis and aspergillosis, may be causative. The role of immunodeficiency in this disease is unclear but has been speculated. Many of these dogs have abnormal lymphocyte blastogenesis tests, but this may be a nonspecific finding secondary to the underlying chronic infection. In other instances, iatrogenic immunosuppression as a result of exogenously administered corticosteroids may contribute to disease process.

Many dogs with diskospondylitis have persistent bacteremia. This is often the result of a chronic infection somewhere in the body. Areas of chronic infection include those in the bladder and urinary system, the prostate, or the skin. In some of these cases, concurrent treatment with corticosteroids may contribute to the length and severity of the bacteremia. As a prime example, animals with bacterial folliculitis of the skin may be initially misdiagnosed as having allergic skin disease and inappropriately treated with corticosteroids such as prednisolone. The immune response generated subsequent to the bacterial dermatitis may be blunted in efficacy due to the corticosteroid administration allowing an otherwise containable and localized infection to become systemic. In other animals, the persistent infections within the body may secondarily result from the chronic bacteremia associated with diskospondylitis.

Table 6.1. Organisms associated with diskospondylitis

Organisms
Bacterial
Staphylococcus
S. aureus
S. intermedius
Brucella canis
Nocardia
Streptococcus
Escherichia coli
Alcaligenes
Micrococcus
Proteus
Corynebacterium
Mycobacterium avium
Fungal
Aspergillus
Paecilomyces

Young to middle-aged dogs are most commonly affected with diskospondylitis, with males more affected by a 2:1 compared to females. Large breeds of dogs are more commonly affected than small breeds of dogs. Cats are rarely affected with diskospondylitis, and often have the infection because of an associated wound overlying the spine. Usually, a predisposing factor such as a history of chronic infections (of the skin, urinary tract, or prostate) or administration of immunosuppressive drugs (corticosteroids) is found in most dogs. A history of reproductive problems such as infertility and excessive fetal deaths may be noted with *Brucella* infections.

Spinal pain is the most consistent clinical sign of diskospondylitis. Paresis is usually mild unless the infectious process extends into the spinal canal or the infection weakens the vertebrae and results in vertebral fracture (pathological fracture). The dura, however, is usually an effective barrier to prevent extension of the infection into the spinal cord itself. Paraspinal muscle atrophy, most likely due to local denervation or associated myositis, around the affected area may be severe (fig. 6.21). Fever and other signs of a systemic infectious process may be present but are surprisingly inconsistent clinical findings.

Vertebral body osteomyelitis may result in clinical features similar to diskospondylitis. When present in the midlumbar vertebrae, osteomyelitis is often associated with a foreign body migration of, for example, a grass awn. This foreign body may enter the body through the respiratory tract and subsequently migrate toward the diaphragm. At the diaphragm, migration continues dorsally toward the attachment of the diaphragm ventral to the midlumbar vertebral bodies where an inflammatory focus is generated. In severe cases of both vertebral body osteomyelitis or diskospondylitis, a fistula may be formed from the paraspinal regions and vertebrae to the skin (fig. 6.21). In the lumbar area, this fistula often is present in the flank.

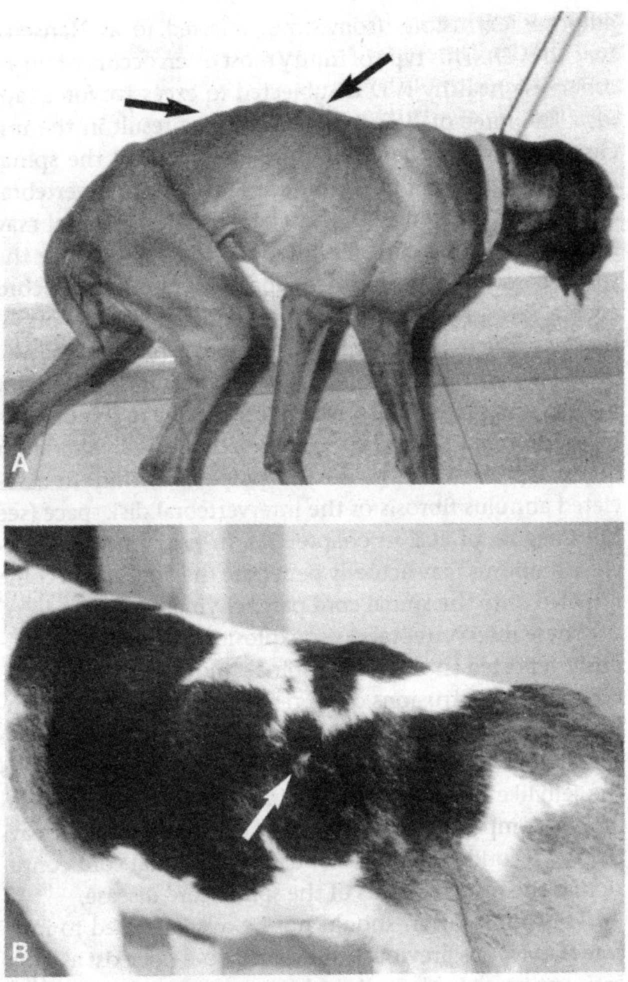

Fig. 6.21. (A) Appearance of a dog with diskospondylitis and paraspinal muscle atrophy (*arrows*). (B) Appearance of a dog with diskospondylitis and a fistula in the flank area (*arrow*).

Clinical Clues to Diskospondylitis

- Spinal pain is common.
- Paraspinal muscle atrophy may occur.
- Fever and other systemic signs may occur.
- Paresis is usually mild unless a spinal abscess or associated pathologic fracture occurs.

Spinal abscessation is rare in dogs and cats but can result from hematogenous infection or local penetrating trauma. Grass awn and porcupine quill migration may enter the spinal canal and result in focal infection. *Actinomyces* and *Nocardia* may be present in these locations. Fungal granulomas also occur in the spinal canal. In some instances of diskospondylitis, the infectious process may extend from the disk into the perispinal tissues and fat.

Animals with *paraspinal muscle abscess* may present for stiffness and reluctance to move. When palpating, the dorsal or lateral paraspinal muscles are firm and may be warm to the touch. The skin often feels taut over this area. Softer indentations may be found in focal areas of the muscle. In some dogs, a fistula tract extends through the skin, usually in the flank region (fig. 6.21). Discharge from this fistula may have a foul odor depending upon the organism present. In some instances, the paraspinal abscessation will extend into the retroperineal space or even the abdominal cavity (peritonitis).

TRAUMA

Spinal cord trauma is relatively common in small animals (see bibliography under Trauma; also see chapter 22 for a complete clinical discussion). Spinal injury is often either from exogenous or endogenous injury. Automobile-induced injury is the most common exogenous cause of trauma to the spine in small animals, with falls, damage resulting from falling objects, and projectile missile damage also possible. Intervertebral disk extrusion is the most common endogenous cause.

Because the spinal cord is encircled by a rigid, inelastic bony encasement (vertebrae) and because of the relatively delicate substance of spinal parenchyma, changes in the vertebral alignment and vertebral canal diameter result in spinal cord displacement and compression. Often, spinal cord compression is the result of bony malalignment or disk extrusion/protrusion. Additional pathologic consequences of spinal injury include edema, hemorrhage, and ischemia. These pathologic entities can predispose to or result in a self-perpetuating process of damage to the spinal cord that often is equally if not more detrimental to the spinal cord than the initial mechanical injury. This is often referred to as the secondary spinal injury. Suggested mediators of this self-perpetuating process include excitatory neurotransmitters, endorphins, catecholamines, and free radicals released after the initial insult. It is commonly agreed, however, that this secondary injury is primarily mediated through spinal cord ischemia.

Clinical signs of spinal trauma usually have an acute onset. Rarely, a prolonged delay (days to weeks) is seen following a spinal trauma. When this happens, this most likely reflects persistent spinal instability and repeated spinal compression, or proliferation and hypertrophy of ligaments, intervertebral disks, or vertebral elements in response to vertebral healing (callous formation). Signs of internal or external trauma, such as lacerations or skin bruising, may help in determining the presence of a prior injury.

Clinical Clues to Spinal Trauma with Fracture or Luxation

- There may be a witnessed traumatic event such as being struck by a car.
- Clinically, signs usually begin acutely.
- Affected animals often have spinal pain.
- Animals may have external evidence of injury such as skin lacerations or superficial hemorrhages.

Vascular Spinal Diseases

While many spinal cord diseases may be associated with ischemia, some spinal conditions are the result of primary spinal cord vascular abnormalities. *Ischemic myelopathy,* or *fibrocartilaginous emboli (FCE),* has been a hallmark disease in this category of spinal diseases diagnosed with increasing frequency in dogs over the last 15 years (see bibliography under Fibrocartilaginous Emboli). This disease process has been historically thought to result secondary to primary vascular embolization and subsequent infarction of the spinal cord. The speculated cause of the emboli material has focused around fibrocartilage material, similar to that found in intervertebral disks. It has been assumed that this material enters the spinal cord vascular system and results in the embolization. How this fibrocartilage actually enters the vascular system remains unclear. Theories include extrusion of disk material into the vascular system, either directly or through neovascularization of the IVD due to degeneration. It has also been suggested that the fibrocartilage actually arises from within the vascular system (metaplasia of the inner vascular wall) and subsequently becomes dislodged and becomes embolic. An adequate pathophysiologic explanation for presence of the intravascular fibrocartilage, however, remains elusive.

There are certain clinical features that have been commonly identified with the clinical presentation of fibrocartilaginous emboli and have been used to distinguish this disease from other similar spinal diseases. Fibrocartilaginous emboli, as a disease entity, tends to occur in nonchondrodystrophoid breeds of dogs. Clinical signs of spinal cord dysfunction occur acutely and progress rapidly. Affected dogs usually have no spinal hyperesthesia when examined, however, they may seem painful initially (within the first 24 hours) after onset. In many historical descriptions, dogs were exercising heavily (playing in the yard with a ball), vocalized, and then became unable to stand. The vocalization component is often taken as a sign of pain, which is often difficult to clinically substantiate as these animals do not often have evidence of spinal pain at the time of clinical examination. In one recent study in schnauzers, however, up to 30% of dogs suspected of having fibrocartilaginous emboli had some degree of spinal pain. Spinal pain may be associated with the embolic disease, another pathophysiologic mechanism, or another concurrent spinal cord disease that may be present. Clinical signs often reflect asymmetric spinal cord involvement (i.e., clinical signs are worse on one side of the body). The infarction may involve vessels of a spinal intumescence region and result in LMN signs. Clinical signs are usually not progressive after the first 24 hours. When this disease occurs in the cervical spinal cord regions, Horner's syndrome or an ipsilateral miotic pupil may be concurrent.

Unfortunately, the aforementioned clinical signs are not pathognomonic for a fibrocartilaginous embolic phenomenon affecting the spinal cord, as similar signs may be seen with other spinal diseases. Dogs clinically suspected of having FCE based on clinical features in the modern era have undergone evaluations with MR imaging as part of their diagnostic evaluation. In a surprising number of these dogs, diseases other than FCE were present. The most common of these diseases are acute, noncompressing nucleus pulposus extrusions (sometimes referred to as Hansen's type III IVD). This type of injury most often occurs when an otherwise healthy IVD is subjected to excessive force rapidly. The force of IVD compression may result in the nucleus pulposus to be rapidly projected toward the spinal cord through a rent in the annulus (also see intervertebral disk disease previously in this chapter). This material may impact the spinal cord with enough force to contuse the spinal cord. In these instances, local associated spinal cord edema, hemorrhage, and vascular damage may be found, however, the extruded intervertebral disk material may be dissipated within the spinal canal and therefore does not form a compressive mass. An important clue to this disease, in addition to the focal spinal cord disease, is an alteration in the appearance of the nucleus pulposus within the associated annulus fibrosis of the intervertebral disk space (see MR imaging of FCE in chapter 11). In rarer instances, nucleus pulposus may actually penetrate the dura and become impaled onto the spinal cord parenchyma.

These intervertebral disk "explosions" have been previously reported in dogs. The spinal injury related to these types of disk extrusions often results from spinal cord contusion, and not displacement of nucleus pulposus into the spinal cord parenchyma. It may be hypothesized that as the jellylike nuclear material diffuses within the epidural fat, the compressive component of the injury resolves leaving the secondary changes due to acute spinal cord contusion as the primary focus of the spinal cord disease.

This information should not be misconstrued to indicate that FCE as previously described does not exist as a disease entity, only that clinical signs commonly associated with this disease may be associated with other disease processes. It is also likely that acute, noncompressive intervertebral disk extrusion occurs more frequently than previously described.

Clinical Clues to Fibrocartilaginous Emboli

- Onset of clinical signs is acute.
- Animals are usually exercising at the time of onset of the clinical signs.
- Usually signs are not progressive after the first 48 hours.
- Majority (70%) of affected dogs have no spinal pain at the time of examination.
- Signs are often asymmetric (one side of body more affected).
- Signs may be LMN when the disease involves the intumescence.

Spinal Cord Hemorrhage and Hematoma

Hemorrhage within or around the CNS can be a devastating, rapidly evolving disease process for many animals (see bibliography under Spinal Hemorrhage). Diseases that are associated with spinal cord hemorrhage usually do so by disrupting vascular wall integrity or by adversely affecting hemostatic mechanisms. Vessel wall integrity can be disrupted by traumatic injury, neoplastic infiltration, or inflammatory diseases. Spinal cord tumors, for example, that destroy vessel integrity initiate bleeding within or around the tumor forming a hematoma. Metastatic tumor may be more apt to be associated with hemorrhage either because of their more aggressive behavior (hence the metastasis) or because the vasculature is the route of the metastasis. Metastatic hemangiosarcoma is an example. Acute hemorrhage is often associated with a rapid clinical decline in these instances.

While uncommon, primary vascular abnormalities such as arteriovenous malformations and aneurysm are also possible. These may mimic, primarily because of their appearance on imaging studies and creation of mass effect, neoplastic diseases. Ischemic damage is another way in which vessel wall damage may result. Endothelial cell damage may result, predisposing to thrombosis, necrosis, and hemorrhage. Thrombosis and embolization are possible in animals, especially with hypercoagulability syndromes, bacteremias (endocarditis), and septicemia. Trauma may also mechanically disrupt spinal cord vascular integrity resulting in hemorrhage and hematoma formation. Primary injury to the vascular system may occur during mechanical shearing associated with rapid acceleration/deceleration of the intraspinal contents. Iatrogenic trauma from cerebrospinal fluid collection is also possible, especially in animals with underlying bleeding tendencies. This is also a possible complication of epidural anesthesia administration.

Most commonly, however, complications of systemic hemostatic diseases can affect the spinal cord. Examples include thrombocytopenias and coagulopathies. Animals being given anticoagulant drugs (Heparin, Coumadin) may have apparent spontaneous hemorrhagic episodes in or around the nervous system. Disseminated intravascular coagulopathy, anticoagulant rodenticide intoxication, and hemophilia and other congenital hemostatic diseases may also be associated with spinal cord bleeding.

Hemorrhage into and around the spinal cord can adversely affect nervous tissue. Bleeding into the cerebrospinal fluid is irritating to local nervous tissue and may result in inflammation (meningitis, myelitis, or encephalitis). Most devastating, however, is when the bleeding is substantial enough to form excessive additional volume within the spinal canal or cord. Hematomas may subsequently form. Spinal cord hematomas have been seen primarily in the cervical, caudal cervical, and thoracolumbar regions, often in younger animals. Clinical signs with intraspinal cord hematomas usually are progressive over 5 to 15 days.

Clinical signs of any spinal cord hemorrhagic disorder vary in onset, but are usually peracute to acute. Many affected animals have paresis or paralysis, and often have regions of spinal pain. Paresis can rapidly evolve to plegia. Animals may also have evidence of active systemic hemorrhage through hemorrhage from body orifices, such as the nose, mouth, rectum, or urinary tract. Some animals have melena or other evidence of gastrointestinal hemorrhage. Still other animals may have petechia and ecchymosis of the skin or mucous membranes.

7 Clinical Features of Important and Common Diseases Involving the Peripheral Nervous System, Neuromuscular Junction, and Muscle of Dogs and Cats

There are numerous diseases that can affect the peripheral nerves, neuromuscular junction, or muscle resulting in clinical signs of lower motor neuron (LMN) disease. Clinical signs commonly associated with such diseases include abnormalities in standing and walking, loss of muscle strength, diminished or absent spinal reflexes, and diminished or absent muscle tone. Additionally, abnormalities of LMN function may result in irregularities of visceral functions such as regurgitation from megaesophagus. Cranial nerves may also be affected by diseases of the peripheral nerves. Diseases of cranial nerves are discussed in chapter 5.

As with intracranial and spinal diseases, there are recognized breed-associated diseases of LMN structures, the knowledge of which may provide an initial clue to the underlying diagnosis (see appendix 2). Examples of specific disease processes are discussed as representatives of the clinical spectrum of disease possible.

DEGENERATIVE NEUROPATHIES

Many diseases that result in primary degeneration of peripheral nerve elements do so by as yet unrecognized mechanisms and etiologies (see bibliography under Degenerative Neuropathies; also Neuropathies and Myopathies Without Known Cause). These diseases are associated with primary degeneration of the peripheral nervous structures and may be categorized as degenerative neuropathies. As an etiological diagnosis is lacking, some of these diseases may also be categorized as idiopathic neuropathies. The pathologic spectrum of disease processes range from demyelination and other myelination abnormalities to axonal and neuronal cell body changes. Some diseases concurrently affect both peripheral nerves and central nervous system elements. Examples of representative disease processes include giant axonal neuropathy, hypertrophic neuropathies, degenerative polyneuropathies, storage diseases, and motorneuronopathies.

A *giant axonal neuropathy* has been reported in German shepherds as an autosomal recessive disease (Duncan 1977; Duncan et al. 1981). Dogs were usually affected between 14 and 16 months of age. Clinical signs included paresis, proprioceptive loss, decreased patellar reflexes, and pelvic limb hypotonia. The bark was occasionally decreased or absent. Fecal incontinence and megaesophagus were also present in some instances. Dogs became tetraparetic by 18 to 24 months of age.

Hypertrophic neuropathy is an apparent autosomal recessive inherited disease of Tibetan mastiffs (Cooper et al. 1984; Cummings et al. 1981; Sponenberg and deLahunta 1981). Animals were usually affected by 7 to 10 weeks of age. Clinical signs included weakness, hyporeflexia, hypotonia, and dysphonia. Animals usually progressed to a state of recumbency in 3 weeks and some developed limb contracture. Repeated demyelination and remyelination ("onion-bulb" formation) most likely contributed to the enlargement of nerves seen pathologically.

Birman cat distal polyneuropathy is suspected to be a gene-associated neuropathy with a recessive mode of inheritance (Moreau et al. 1991). Affected cats showed signs beginning at 8 to 10 weeks of age. Cats tended to stand and walk on the hocks (plantigrade stance) and the hocks were held in an adducted fashion. Cats tended to fall from side to side in the pelvic limbs when walking. At gait there was mild hypermetria of all limbs and progressive pelvic limb ataxia. While there was sciatic nerve degeneration, pathological lesions were most prominent in the lateral pyramidal tracts of the lumbar cord, the fasciculi gracilis of the dorsal funiculus in the cervical spinal cord, and the cerebellar vermian white matter. This disease is an example where both the peripheral and central nervous systems are involved with apparently the same disease process.

Some *storage diseases* are associated with peripheral nerve pathology and clinical signs. Cats with *Niemann-Pick type-A storage disease* may have alterations in peripheral nerves (Cuddon et al. 1989). Tetraparesis, hypotonia, and areflexia were present in affected cats. Norwegian forest cats with glycogen storage disease type IV may have a multitude of clinical signs, which may include tetraparesis and decreased spinal reflexes. Globoid cell leukodystrophy may involve peripheral nerves (Blakemore et al. 1974; Vicini et al. 1988). For more clinical features of storage diseases, see degenerative intracranial diseases in chapter 5.

DEGENERATIVE MOTORNEURONOPATHIES

Degenerative processes can occur primarily in the neuronal cell body, and subsequently affect associated axonal and synaptic elements (see bibliography under Motor Neuron Disease). These motorneuronopathies often do not have an established cause, and are discussed further under Neuropathies and Myopathies Without Known Cause, below.

PRIMARY DEGENERATIVE MYOPATHIES

Muscular dystrophies are examples of degenerative myopathic conditions of both dogs and cats. These diseases are exemplified by an X-linked disease of golden retrievers and other breeds (see bibliography under Degenerative Myopathies; Muscular Dystrophy). In humans this type of muscular dystrophy is referred to as Duchenne's muscular dystrophy. These disease processes result from gene-associated abnormalities of a muscle membrane protein (dystrophin). Clinical signs are usually evident in dogs by 6 to 9 weeks of age. Weakness, stiffness, shuffling gait, abduction of elbows, bunny-hopping, exercise intolerance, and atrophy of head and limb muscles are noted. Other signs include a plantigrade stance, enlargement of base of tongue, inability to fully open the jaw, pharyngeal and esophageal dysfunction, salivation, weak barking, and kyphosis that may develop into lordosis. Clinical signs may plateau after 6 months of progressive deterioration. Other breeds affected with muscular dystrophies include Irish terriers, Samoyeds, Rottweilers, Welsh corgis, and Bouvier des Flandres dogs.

An *X-linked muscular dystrophy* similar to Duchenne's and golden retriever myopathy has been described in male cats. Similar to these other diseases, a membrane-associated protein (dystrophin) is deficient or absent. Signs generally develop before 2 years of age beginning with hypertrophy of the proximal limb muscles, which may be evident as early as 10 weeks of age. In addition to the limb musculature, cardiac muscle may also be affected in this disorder. Clinical signs of X-linked muscular dystrophy in cats are similar to those in dogs. The gait is mildly stiff or stilted, and cats tend to bunny hop when running. Occasionally, there is marked stiffness and reluctance to move. Cats often appear to have increased muscle mass, especially of the neck and proximal limb muscles, and stand with adducted hocks. The tongue is hypertrophied and may protrude partially. Excessive drooling of saliva occurs. Dehydration may be a recurring problem because the tongue hypertrophy makes it difficult to drink and eat. There may be a history of gagging, regurgitation, or vomiting of food. Additionally, these cats may have fatal complications when undergoing general anesthesia or from manual restraint as a result of peracute rhabdomyolysis.

A myopathy of *Labrador retrievers* is associated with a deficiency of selected (type II) muscle fibers. This disease has an autosomal recessive mode of inheritance. Both male and female dogs can be affected. Animals can have either yellow or black hair coats. Clinical signs begin between 6 weeks and 8 months of age. Muscle weakness is prominent, resulting in short steps and occasionally a bunny hopping gait in the pelvic limbs. The head may be positioned closer to the ground and posture is often kyphotic (see fig. 3.21). Carpal overextension and carpal valgus and well as a "cow-hocked" appearance can be present. Clinical signs may be worse in cold environments. Conscious proprioception is usually normal, however, tendon reflexes such as the patellar reflex are reduced or absent. Signs are usually progressive but may plateau after some months.

A *hereditary myopathy* occurs in *Devon Rex cats* (Malik et al. 1993). Cats are usually younger (3–23 months of age). Clinical signs include generalized muscle weakness, ventroflexion of the neck, and dorsal protrusion of the scapula. Difficulty maintaining the normal head position when eating may result in obstruction of the pharynx with food and laryngospasm, which may be fatal. Megaesophagus may be present in some cats. Progression of clinical signs occurs until 6 to 9 months of age. Clinical signs may stabilize or plateau after this time. Four of the six cats in one instance died suddenly of laryngospasm due to obstruction of the pharynx with food.

Nemaline rod myopathy of cats is named based on the characteristic pathologic features in peripheral nerves. Clinical signs of weakness begin between 6 and 18 months of age (Cooper et al. 1986; DeLauche et al. 1998). Clinical signs progress to a choppy, hypermetric gait. The patellar reflex is decreased, however, flexion reflexes are present. Signs usually progress slowly over the first year of life.

METABOLIC NEUROPATHIES AND MYOPATHIES

Diabetic neuropathy commonly affects the peripheral nerves of cats and dogs (see bibliography under Metabolic Neuropathy; Diabetic Neuropathy). The clinical abnormalities, however, are usually more recognizable in cats compared to dogs. Clinical signs in cats are most reflective of tibial nerve dysfunction even though other nerves may be abnormal. Classically, cats have a "dropped hock" or plantigrade pelvic limb stance (fig. 7.1). This appearance, however, is not pathognomonic for diabetes as other causes of LMN weakness as well as mechanical damage to the gastrocnemius tendon may result in a similar clinical appearance. Diabetic cats are most often affected prior to initiation of treatment or if they have poorly controlled diabetes mellitus. Other clinical signs include generalized weakness

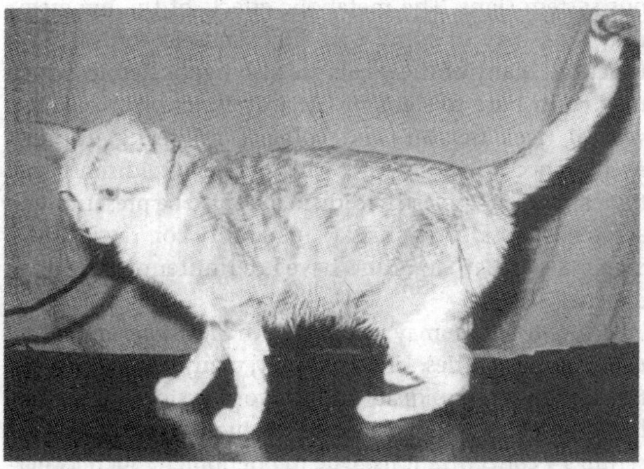

Fig. 7.1. Cat with "dropped hock" appearance.

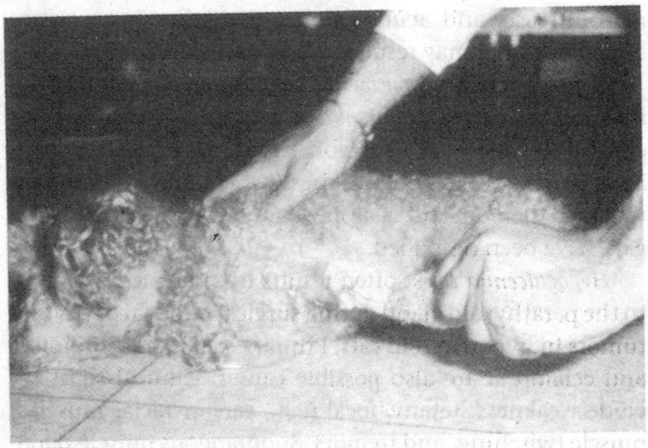

Fig. 7.2. Dog with hypokalemia and muscle weakness showing decreased thoracic limb withdrawal reflexes.

usually evident as reduced activity, reluctance to move, and difficulty jumping. The pathogenesis of diabetic neuropathy is most likely multifactorial including metabolic derangements in nerve, microvascular changes possibly resulting in ischemia, and inflammation. Diabetic neuropathy can also occur in dogs but is less clinically apparent. Lesions in peripheral nerves have also been described in very young dogs with congenital diabetes mellitus.

Hypoglycemia in adult animals can occur secondary to some endocrine disorders such as hypoadrenocorticism, insulin overdose, and lack of glucose production associated with liver failure, and with some tumors (liver, spleen, GI), which may produce hypoglycemia most likely through excess IGF-2 production. Hypoglycemia is most often associated with insulinoma in older dogs. In addition to the central nervous system (CNS) signs of hypoglycemia, a *peripheral neuropathy* has commonly been recognized in dogs with insulinoma (Braund et al. 1987; Bergman et al. 1994; Dyer et al. 1986; Schrauwen et al. 1996; Shahar et al. 1985). Both peripheral nerves and cranial nerves (CN VII) may be affected. In some instances, the nerve alterations are subclinical. Whether this neuropathy is a result of the hypoglycemia, insulin, or some other paraneoplastic effect is unknown. Clinical signs of a diffuse LMN nature include muscle weakness and decreased spinal reflexes.

Potassium is important for maintenance of normal muscle cell membrane potentials. Potassium depletion can result in alterations in muscle cell membrane potentials, muscle cell glycogen content and synthesis, and blood flow to muscle. Hypokalemia results in hyperpolarization of muscle cell membranes, which then require greater stimulus for depolarization. This may lead to generalized muscle weakness. *Hypokalemia myopathy* has been described primarily in cats, although it can occasionally occur in dogs (fig. 7.2) (see bibliography under Hypokalemic Myopathy). It is commonly thought that some historically described *polymyopathies of cats* such as that reported in Burmese cats (see below) may have been the result of unrecognized hypokalemia. Cats with hypokalemic myopathy are usually older (greater than 8 years) and have associated or underlying renal disease and excessive urinary losses of potassium. Acidification of diets to prevent struvite urolithiasis increases renal and fecal potassium loss. Hypokalemia occurs when the dietary intake is insufficient to replace urinary and fecal loss. Clinical signs occurred in one group of cats fed a vegetarian diet.

Muscle weakness is a prominent clinical sign of hypokalemia and may result in ventroflexion of the neck (see fig. 3.13). Concurrently, there is often an acute onset of a stiff gait, reluctance to move, exercise intolerance, and muscle pain. Postural reactions and pain perception are normal. The clinical signs can also be episodic.

Burmese cats have an *inherited hypokalemic myopathy* producing signs of periodic muscle weakness. Clinical signs are usually first evident before 12 months of age, and usually between 4 and 12 weeks of age. Cats most commonly show clinical signs somewhere between 2 and 6 months of age. Potassium depletion may have played a role in the previously described myopathy of these cats. Transient episodes of acute weakness may be seen. However, decreased activity and inappetence are often present for weeks to months prior to presentation to a veterinarian. Clinical signs include ventral neck flexion; stiff, stilted gaits; and a reluctance to walk or jump. Typically, weak cats do not walk far and sit or lie by flopping down instead of carefully sitting. Palpation of larger muscle groups may result in a painful reaction. Dyspnea, most likely the result of respiratory muscle weakness, occurs when the serum potassium is substantially low (2.0–2.5 mmol/L). Hypokalemic myopathic signs may also occur or be exacerbated after intravenous fluid administration due to volume dilution and increased urinary potassium loss.

Primary *hyperkalemic myopathy,* sometimes referred to as *hyperkalemic periodic paralysis,* is much less commonly recognized in dogs and cats compared to horses (Jezyk 1982). Intermittent signs of muscle weakness or fasciculation and collapse with exercise may result. Hyperkalemia secondary to other disease processes such as hypoadrenocorticism, renal disease, and acute cellular disruption (e.g., tumor lysis syndrome) may result in muscle weakness.

Hypernatremic myopathy has been reported in young domestic cats (<1 year). This is a much rarer disease but has clinical signs similar to hypokalemic myopathy. Generalized, progressive muscle weakness, which may include ventral neck flexion and a dropped hock appearance to the gait, have been described.

Hypocalcemia most often results from iatrogenic injury to the parathyroid gland during surgical removal of thyroid tumors in hyperthyroid cats. Primary hypoparathyroidism and eclampsia are also possible causes. Clinical signs include weakness, tetany, focal (e.g., ears or facial muscles) muscle twitching, and tremors. Spontaneous muscle depolarization can manifest as muscle fasciculation, cramping, rigidity, and twitching. Animals with preparturient hypocalcemia present with anorexia, lethargy, trembling, muscle twitching, and weakness.

Hyperadrenocortical myopathy most commonly occurs in dogs. Affected dogs often have a stiff, stilted, and shuffling gait (fig. 7.3). In some instances, there is increased muscle mass and animals may have well-defined muscle groups similar to those affected with myotonia. This myopathy is most commonly found in dogs with chronic, untreated instances of hyperadrenocorticism. There is also occasionally a neuropathy reported with hyperadrenocorticism that may contribute to the clinical features.

Hypoadrenocorticism (Addison's disease) primarily results in clinical signs of weakness (possible muscle and peripheral nervous system dysfunction), but occasionally results in limb paresis for unknown reasons. The classic nonspecific signs of this disease and its associated metabolic imbalances (hyperkalemia, hypoglycemia) can result in muscle weakness.

Cats with *hyperthyroidism* may have a variety of nervous system signs. The metabolic effects of the hyperthyroid state may in some way affect muscle and/or nerve function. Many of these cats are also hypokalemic, which may contribute to signs of LMN dysfunction. Weakness, ventral neck flexion, and collapse following minimal exercise occur in some cats with hyperthyroidism. Other typical signs of hyperthyroidism may also be present, such as weight loss, polyphagia, irritability, or restlessness. Some cats are lethargic and have intermittent vomiting or diarrhea.

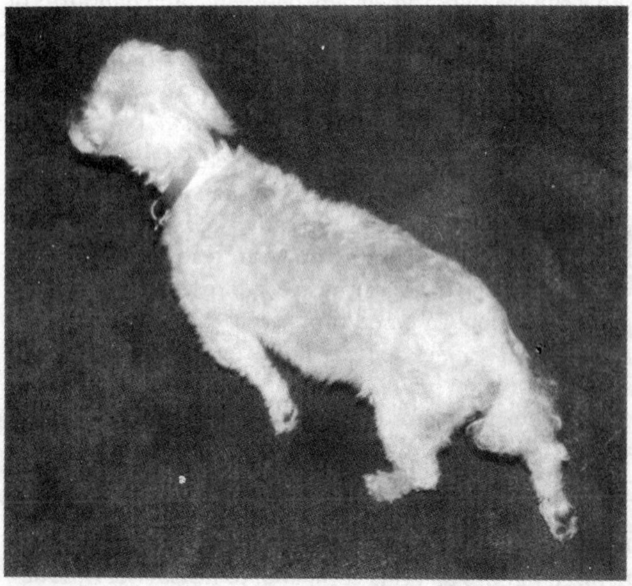

Fig. 7.3. Dog with hyperadrenocorticism and myotonia with a stiff thoracic limb appearance.

Hypothyroidism may result in both *myopathic* and *neuropathic* abnormalities. Unfortunately, many clinical associations of hypothyroidism and nervous system disease are based solely on the diagnosis of hypothyroidism from serum T4 concentrations. Due to phenomena such as sick-euthyroid syndrome, some of these animals with neurologic signs may not have, in fact, had concurrent hypothyroidism. In other instances, clinical improvement in neurologic signs following thyroid hormone replacement therapy was taken to indicate a cause and effect relationship between nervous system signs and hypothyroidism. These caveats make the true relationship between hypothyroidism and neurologic disease unclear. In some instances, however, the evidence of a causative relationship is much stronger.

A hypothyroid-associated neuropathy has been described involving the facial and limb muscles. Cranial nerve signs are described commonly including facial paralysis, ventrolateral strabismus, nystagmus, hemiparesis, circling, and decreased corneal or facial sensation. The pathophysiologic cause of the peripheral neuropathy associated with hypothyroidism is uncertain. Peripheral nerve compression from myxedema has also been a speculated cause.

Hyperchylomicronemia is seen in cats due to an inherited reduction in lipoprotein lipase activity (Jones et al. 1986). Clinical signs occur around 8 months of age. Xanthomata (lipid granulomas) that compress peripheral nerves apparently cause the peripheral nerve disease. Clinical abnormalities include Horner's syndrome, facial paralysis, tibial nerve paralysis, femoral nerve paralysis, trigeminal nerve abnormalities, radial nerve (inability to extend digits) abnormalities, and recurrent laryngeal disease.

Hyperoxaluria (L-glyceric aciduria) is thought to be inherited as an autosomal recessive disease in cats (McKerrell et al. 1989). Domestic shorthaired cats are affected with this disease. Cats reportedly developed clinical signs between 5 and 9 months of age. Renal failure and neurologic signs were the most prominent abnormalities. In some instances, clinical signs of weakness occurred prior to the onset of renal failure. Neurologic signs included crouching, cow-hocked appearance, reluctance to walk, conscious proprioceptive deficits, decreased patellar and withdrawal reflexes, and decreased pain responses. The cutaneous trunci reflex was absent in most cats. Cats usually died prior to 1 year of age.

Mitochondrial myopathy has been reported in Clumber and Sussex spaniels and Old English sheepdogs. The latter dogs were presented at 1 and 2.5 years of age. Animals may be affected as young as 3 months of age, however. Animals tend to tire easily. Their step distance may become increasingly shortened similar to signs commonly associated with myasthenia gravis. Similarly, affected animals may eventually collapse to sternal recumbency during exercise.

Numerous other myopathies associated with inherent intracellular metabolic abnormalities exist. Some have associated deficiencies of carnitine or vitamins or other metabolic substrates. Clarification of these muscle abnormalities is ongoing.

NEOPLASTIC NEUROPATHIES AND MYOPATHIES

Lymphoma can affect either the central or peripheral nervous system. In cats, lymphoid neoplasia commonly occurs in the extradural spinal location and can involve nerve roots. Occasionally, only peripheral nerve involvement is seen in both dogs and cats (Presthus and Teige 1986). Cranial nerves (V, VII) are often involved with lymphosarcoma and other hematogenous neoplasia (monocytic leukemias) due to direct involvement with the tumor cells (Carpenter et al. 1987) (see also the cranial nerve section of chapter 5). A paraneoplastic effect associated with this type of neoplasia is also possible.

Nerve sheath tumors (Schwannoma, neurofibroma, neurofibrosarcoma) commonly involve the peripheral nerves of dogs (fig. 7.4). With brachial plexus tumors, a unilateral thoracic limb lameness is common. Pelvic limb nerves may also be involved. Affected dogs usually present for a chronic, undiagnosed lameness. Often dogs are presumptively diagnosed with occult arthritis or another orthopedic disease. Clinical signs in some animals are persistent for up to a year or more suggesting a relatively slower growth pattern of some tumors. Clinical clues to the presence of a nerve sheath tumor include atrophy of isolated or focal muscle groups and pain upon direct palpation in the region of the tumor. In animals with nerve sheath tumors involving nerves of the brachial plexus, pain is often present on direct palpation of the axillary region. In some instances, a discrete mass can be palpated in the axilla. Dogs that are extremely painful may require general anesthesia for adequate palpation. If the depth of anesthesia is minimal, animals may wake up rapidly during palpation if they are painful. Tumors of the sciatic nerve may be palpated per rectally in some dogs.

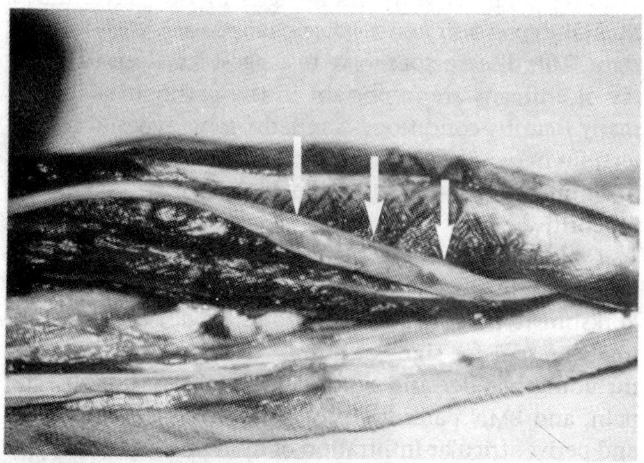

Fig. 7.4. Peripheral nerve tumor in the thoracic limb of a dog (*arrows*).

Both *paraneoplastic neuropathies* and occasionally *paraneoplastic myopathies* have been described in dogs. These abnormalities may contribute to the clinical weakness often present in animals with systemic neoplastic disease. There are many paraneoplastic neuropathies identified in humans. In some instances, clinical signs of peripheral neuropathy may precede those associated with the primary tumor. While numerous tumors may be associated with paraneoplastic effects involving the peripheral nerves, lung tumors have a common association with paraneoplastic peripheral nerve disease. It is most often thought that there is a shared antigen between the tumor and the peripheral nerve, and if the body's immune system reacts to the tumor antigen, the peripheral nerve may be damaged as a bystander in the immunologic reaction to the tumor. Consideration should be given to an underlying neuropathy or myopathy in animals with cancer and weakness or muscle atrophy, such as with "cancer cachexia."

NUTRITIONAL MYOPATHIES

Nutritional myopathies are uncommon in dogs and cats (deLahunta 1983) (see bibliography under Nutritional Myopathy). Selenium deficiency has been suspected in some of these disorders. Dogs may have stiff movements of the limbs and take short steps. Exercise may exacerbate muscle weakness. Disorders of other important muscle electrolytes such as potassium and calcium may affect muscle function. If these elements are deficient in the diet the potential exists for associated muscle dysfunction and damage. Disorders of the muscle and peripheral nerve associated with these electrolyte imbalances have been discussed under the Metabolic Neuropathies and Myopathies in this chapter.

INFECTIOUS AND INFLAMMATORY NEUROPATHIES AND MYOPATHIES

Consequences of infectious diseases on the peripheral nervous system may result from direct damage from an organism, from the associated immune response of the body in response to the presence of the organism, or from the effects of a product of the organism. The clinical presentation of *Botulism,* for example, is the result of an exotoxin of *Clostridium botulinum* (see bibliography under Toxic Neuropathies and Myopathies). The clinical presentation of *Tetanus* results from a neurotoxin (tetanospasmin) secreted by the organism *Clostridium tetani*. These diseases associated with infectious organisms that secrete neurotoxic products are discussed further below under Toxic Neuropathies and Myopathies.

NEURITIS

Toxoplasma gondii and *Neospora caninum* are protozoal organisms that can affect any area of the nervous system resulting in encephalitis, myelitis, peripheral neuropathy, or myositis. Clinical signs may include peripheral nerve or muscle dysfunction. Muscle weakness, paresis, and muscle pain may be found if the LMN is more predominantly involved with the disease processes. These diseases are also classically associated with a hyperextended pelvic limb(s) abnormality in young dogs (see fig. 3.10).

Hepatozoon canis is a protozoan present in some parts of the United States (Texas). This organism is transmitted by the tick *Rhipicephalus sanguineus*. Clinical signs include muscular hyperesthesia, weight loss, paraparesis or paralysis, and bloody diarrhea. Other abnormalities may include mild anemia and purulent ocular and nasal discharges. Periosteal bone proliferation can occur on any bone but the skull. If this bony proliferation involves the vertebrae, exiting peripheral nerves may be entrapped in this reaction and damaged. If this occurs in the lumbar vertebrae, LMN paresis may result. Additionally, there may be myositis and muscle pyogranulomas present, which contribute to muscle weakness.

Noninfectious Neuritis

Coonhound paralysis or *polyradiculoneuritis* is a disease of dogs similar to Guillain-Barré syndrome in human beings. A suspected antigen (in the case of coonhound paralysis from raccoon saliva) results in an immunologic-mediated reaction with inflammation directed primarily toward the nerve root and proximal nerves of the limb. In essence, this is an autoimmune disease with self-destruction of peripheral nerve elements. Other antigens, such as bacterial and viral infections, may also initiate this disease, as raccoon exposure is not associated with the disease in all animals. Campylobacter infection may be a cause in humans. Hence, the more general term "polyradiculoneuritis" is used to describe the disease when the inciting cause is not known.

Clinical signs are of a diffuse LMN disease usually with dysfunction of all limbs. There is most often an acute to subacute progressive paresis and paralysis, often within hours. It is common that clinical signs are initially observed in the pelvic limbs but usually progress to involve the thoracic limbs within the first 24 to 48 hours. If the animals can still walk during the initial phases of the disease, the gait is stiff and stilted due to resultant decreases in step distance. A clinical hallmark of this disease is that animals seem hyperesthetic to minimal pressure such as minimal pressure toe pinching. This is often most obvious when the limbs are palpated during assessment of the withdrawal reflexes. Cranial nerve functions usually remain normal, however, some dogs may have decreases in their palpebral reflex possibly associated with decreased facial nerve function.

Once an animal becomes paralyzed, clinical signs usually persist for weeks. Death can occur as a result of respiratory muscle paralysis. Abdominal breathing and a "whispering" sound during barking are clues to respiratory compromise. Muscle atrophy may occur and become severe. This may be a combination of disuse and neurogenic atrophy as some affected animals have evidence of denervation electrophysiologically. This finding suggests underlying axonal damage. Dogs with associated axonal damage also appear to be those that take longer to recover (i.e., weeks).

In cats there is a suspected similar disease reported and referred to as *idiopathic peripheral neuropathy*. Clinical signs were similar to those dogs reported with polyradiculoneuropathy, or coonhound paralysis. In affected cats, there was a rapid onset of paraparesis progressing to tetraparesis with loss of spinal reflexes. Muscle atrophy was evident within 7 to 10 days. In a similar disease of cats referred to as *chronic relapsing polyneuropathy*, there was a marked lower motor neuron tetraparesis that spontaneously regressed and reoccurred months later. Conscious proprioceptive abnormalities, depressed spinal reflexes, and muscle atrophy were present in the limbs. One cat was reported with a severe, acute polyneuritis, which had weakness, conscious proprioceptive deficits, and decreased spinal reflexes. Icterus and anemia were associated systemic abnormalities.

Brachial plexus neuritis is suspected also to be an immune-mediated neuritis but one that preferentially affects the nerves of the thoracic limbs. Clinical signs reflect LMN dysfunction involving the thoracic limbs. The limbs are often affected bilaterally, however, the disease may also occur in an single limb. Decreased spinal reflexes and neurogenic muscle atrophy are common clinical features. This disease is thought to result from an allergic or hypersensitivity reaction that is directed primarily at the peripheral nerves. In one dog, horse meat in the diet was thought to be the inciting antigen (deLahunta 1983).

Postvaccinal (allergic) encephalomyelitis is primarily an historical entity following rabies vaccination with phenolized brain tissue. This disease was a disseminated, demyelinating encephalitis or encephalomyelitis, which resulted as consequence of an allergic immune-mediated reaction to vaccine components. Clinical signs were usually of an ascending paralysis with initial signs in the pelvic limbs. Mental depression and a voice change were other clinical signs. This disease does serve to suggest reactions to a variety of antigens are important in the pathophysiology of many neuritis conditions. Similarly, some types of noninfectious nervous system inflammation may have an allergic or immune-mediated initiation such as with polyradiculoneuritis.

Cauda equina polyradiculoneuritis has been reported infrequently in dogs in breeds such as Labrador retrievers, Yorkshire terriers, and Bernese mountain dogs. Affected animals present for signs of lumbosacral nerve dysfunction including bladder and bowel abnormalities, lumbosacral pain, and LMN paresis. Histologically, there is interstitial and periventricular infiltration of mononuclear cells (lymphocytes, plasma cells, and macrophages) suggesting an immune-mediated inflammation directed specifically toward these nerves.

MYOSITIS

Polymyositis may occur without obvious cause, be an immune-mediated primary myositis, or result from muscle infections with infectious organisms such as protozoa including *Toxoplasma gondii* and *Neospora caninum* (see bibliography under Myositis). Occasionally, other infectious myopathies, such as from viral infections, may result in muscle inflammation. A subclinical myopathy has been shown to occur in experimentally infected FIV cats. Primary bacterial and fungal myositis is extremely rare in small animals. Cats with leptospirosis surprisingly will often present with muscle pain as a primary clinical problem. Infectious myositis has also been associated with *Leptospira australis* in a 10-year-old greyhound. *Trichinella* has also resulted in muscle inflammation in a dog. In some instances, muscle damage and associated inflammation may result from excessive use (exercise) or muscle trauma.

Classically clinical signs of *polymyositis* include muscle pain, muscle atrophy, and generalized muscle weakness. Degree of muscle pain in response to palpation is a sometimes difficult and subjective clinical assessment to make, however. In cats, neck ventroflexion is common. In young dogs, toxoplasmosis and neosporosis may result in an extended pelvic limb appearance (see fig 3.10). The limb often cannot be manually flexed, and there is associated muscle atrophy and fibrosis. This appearance may be the result of direct muscle damage or chronic denervation. Megaesophagus may occur with inflammatory myopathies.

Myositis, usually immune-mediated, may also affect only selected muscle groups or regions of the body. For example, muscle inflammation purely of the masticatory muscles (masticatory myositis) is a reasonably common entity in dogs. This disease is thought to result from an immune-mediated destruction of the type 2 M fibers found selectively in these muscles (Gilmour et al. 1992). This is most likely another example of an autoimmune destruction of these structures. Clinical signs can occur acutely with animals presenting for enlarged, painful temporalis and masseter muscles. Animals may be reluctant or unable to open the mandible and consequently may not eat and drink. Masticatory muscles are most commonly bilaterally affected. As the disease progresses, the muscle of the head may become atrophic and fibrotic with increasing definition of the bony landmarks of the skull. Muscle fibrosis at this stage also often results in an inability to open the jaw. Similar clinical findings may be present in dogs with trauma to the skull and jaw that results in fibrosis or bony fusion of the mandible to the skull.

Extraocular polymyositis has been reported primarily in young dogs between 6 and 18 months. Golden retrievers have been the most common breed affected, however, other breeds including Doberman pinschers, German shepherds, and mixed breeds may also have this problem. Bilateral exophthalmos is the most common clinical sign present, along with inability to move the globe through the various phases of gaze. If the extraocular muscle enlarges significantly, compression of the optic nerve may result, subsequently affecting vision and causing blindness.

Laryngeal myositis is a rarely reported clinical entity. Breeds affected include Boykin spaniel, Malamute, and Bouvier des Flandres.

Dermatomyositis is primarily a disease of collie and Shetland sheepdogs. Clinical signs are most often of a chronic dermatitis of the nose and face. While the deep muscle layers may be affected by the inflammation, there are no clinically significant effects on muscle or nerve function.

Myositis ossificans is a disease reported primarily in cats. Muscle alterations include fibrosis, muscle necrosis, dystrophic mineralization, and ossification. Clinically affected animals may show weakness and swollen, painful muscles.

NEUROMUSCULAR JUNCTION DISEASE

Myasthenia gravis is a disease associated with muscle weakness (see bibliography under Myasthenia Gravis). There are two forms of this disease: a *congenital form* due to a developmental abnormality resulting in a deficiency or abnormality of acetylcholine receptors on the postsynaptic membrane of the neuromuscular junction, and an acquired form that is associated with antibodies being produced against the acetylcholine receptor. The congenital form occurs in dogs such as smooth-haired fox terriers, Springer spaniels, Samoyeds, and Jack Russell terriers, and cats such as the Siamese. The acquired form can occur without obvious cause or secondary to a variety of tumors (thymoma, cholangiosarcoma, osteosarcoma). With thymoma, the tumor either produces excess antibody or the antibody is produced against a similar antigen within the tumor and in muscle within the tumor. In many instances, a shared antigen is suspected between the tumor and the NMJ. Acquired myasthenia gravis is another example of an autoimmune disease process involving a component of the nervous system.

The clinical diagnosis of myasthenia gravis is suggested by the classic signs of exercise-induced muscle weakness. Animals that can walk will usually have a progressive shortening of the step distance as they continue to walk or run (fig. 7.5). The steps also get quicker as the step distance becomes shorter. Often these animals will progressively bring the pelvic limbs in a more forward position sometimes giving the appearance that they are trying to stop or even back up. This commonly also results in a kyphotic posture. If observed closely, the facial muscles will also show progressive weakness with many dogs having a "droopy" or tragic facial expression (figs. 7.5, 7.6, 7.7). The jaw may open concurrently, and salivation may occur. As the step distance becomes progressively shorter, the tail will often remain in an upright position, and may be "swished" back and forth, directed away from the pelvic limb that contacts the ground.

In other dogs, only evidence of focal muscle involvement will occur with myasthenia gravis. Megaesophagus may be the only clinical manifestation of the disease in

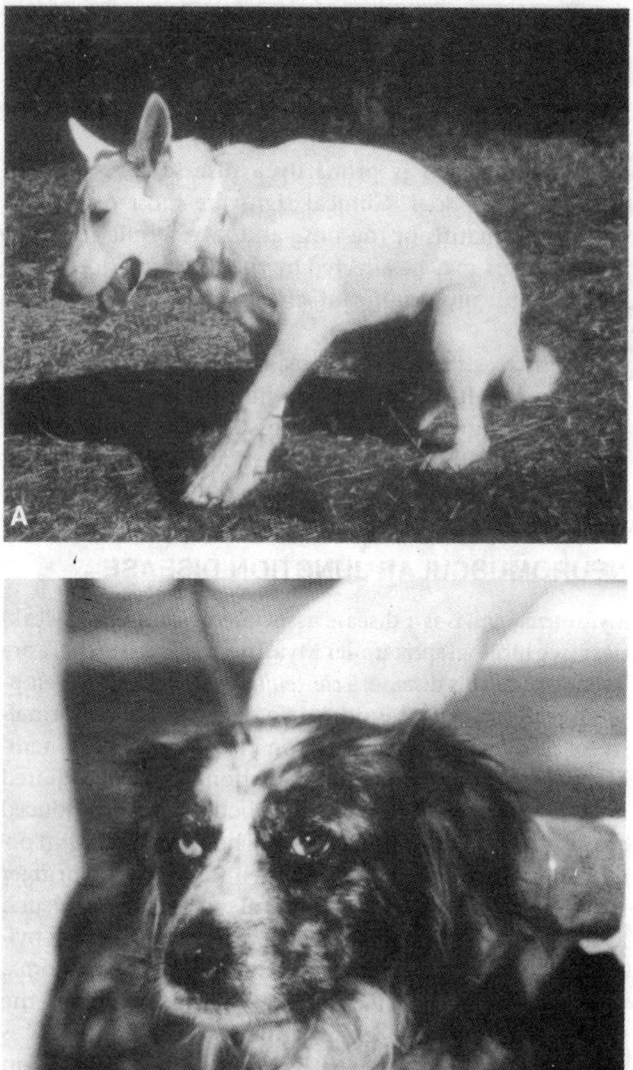

Fig. 7.5. (A) Dog with myasthenia gravis showing kyphotic posture and drooping of the facial muscles. (B) Dog with myasthenia gravis showing ptosis. (C) Dog with myasthenia gravis showing excessive salivation.

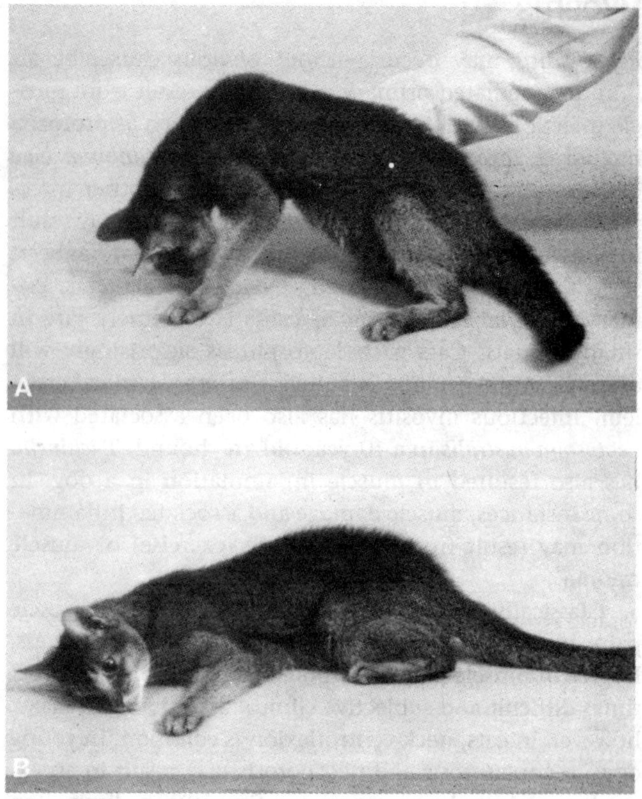

Fig. 7.6. (A, B), Cat with muscle weakness that is unable to support its own body weight and is "floppy."

many dogs (Shelton et al. 1990). Complicating factors include respiratory abnormalities and aspiration pneumonia secondary to megaesophagus. In other dogs, the laryngeal muscles are primarily affected resulting in stridor and upper respiratory inspiratory distress. Upper airway obstruction from paralysis of the vocal folds can result in a rapidly fatal situation.

Myasthenia gravis also occurs in cats similar to dogs (Joseph et al. 1988). A congenital form occurs in Siamese cats. Abyssinian cats and possibly Somalis may be predisposed to the acquired form. The acquired form can occur without obvious inciting cause, as in dogs, or as a secondary consequence of a variety of tumors (thymoma). With thymoma, the tumor either produces excess antibody or the antibody produced is directed against a similar antigen both within the tumor and in muscle. In addition, an associated myositis may occur concurrently with acquired myasthenia gravis.

Generally, myasthenia gravis in cats is a disease of adult animals. In the congenital form in Siamese, affected cats have signs from a young age (usually beginning at less than 6 months of age). Exercise intolerance and episodic weakness induced by walking or playing are typical signs. Affected cats may walk a few steps and "flop" or lie down in a sternal position (fig. 7.6). Cats that tend to lie sternally rest one side of their head on the thoracic limbs (fig. 7.7). This appearance may also be seen with chronic organophosphate toxicity (see below, Toxic Neuropathies and Myopathies) and other diseases of cats associated with

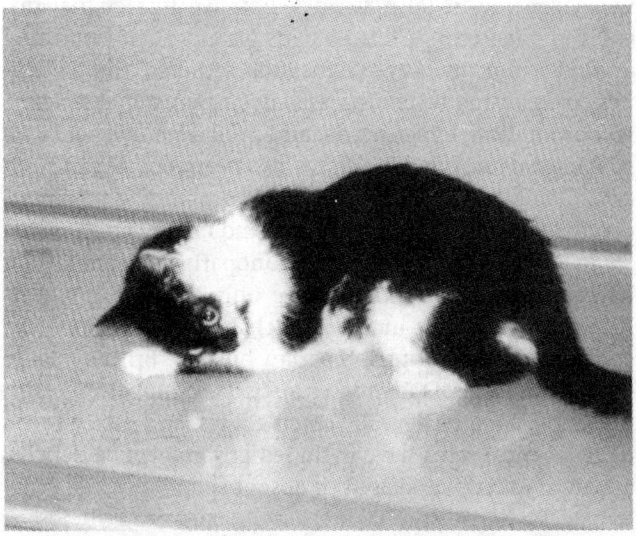

Fig. 7.7. Cat with muscle weakness resting its head on its thoracic limbs.

muscle of NMJ weakness. Improvement in clinical signs often occurs after a period of rest. Muscle tremors may be present but are usually episodic with a short duration and occur in muscles that are actively being used. A stiff, stilted gait is often noted prior to collapse. Weakness of facial muscle may also be seen, and this is most evident as a decrease in the palpebral reflex and narrowing of the palpebral fissure. This sign appears to be a consistent finding in cats with acquired myasthenia gravis. An associated megaesophagus is uncommon in cats but may lead to aspiration pneumonia. One cat has been reported with a jaw drop and dysphagia as the only clinical signs of myasthenia gravis.

NEUROPATHIES AND MYOPATHIES WITHOUT A KNOWN CAUSE

The clinical spectrum of neuropathies and myopathies of dogs and cats are just beginning to be recognized and clarified. Many different disease types have been reported, however, many of these diseases are without established specific etiologic cause (see bibliography under Idiopathic Neuropathies and Myopathies). Additional diseases are discussed above under Degenerative Neuropathies.

Distal denervating disease is a disease of dogs most notably in the United Kingdom. This polyneuropathy results in progressive tetraparesis over 1 week to 1 month with associated muscle atrophy. Spinal reflexes are decreased, and atrophy of limb muscles may be prominent, especially proximally. Animals may also have neck muscle weakness and decreased barking. Most dogs recover, however, in 4 to 6 weeks.

A *distal symmetrical polyneuropathy* has been reported in dogs aged 1.5 to 5 years. Pelvic limb paresis progressing to involve the thoracic limbs and bilateral atrophy of masticatory muscles were predominant clinical signs. Great Danes have been more commonly reported with this disease. Other breeds suspected with a similar disease are Chesapeake Bay retrievers, Saint Bernards, Newfoundlands, collies, Labrador retrievers, and Rottweilers.

Rottweiler distal sensorimotor polyneuropathy occurs in 1.5- to 4-year-old dogs. Clinical signs include paraparesis progressing to tetraparesis, decreased spinal reflexes, hypotonia, and muscle atrophy. The distal limbs appear flaccid during walking.

A *hereditary polyneuropathy* has been described in Alaskan Malamutes in Norway and in the United States. In both instances, dogs are usually affected between 7 and 18 months of age. Disease characteristics were different in these two populations of dogs. In the dogs from Norway, proprioception was normal, however, patellar reflexes were decreased. Megaesophagus was also prominent. In affected dogs from the United States, progressive paraparesis, with decreased spinal reflexes and hyperesthesia without megaesophagus, was seen. Occasionally, affected malamutes may also have tetraparesis.

Hypomyelination of peripheral nervous system has been reported in golden retrievers with clinical signs beginning around 7 weeks of age. Clinical signs included pelvic limb ataxia, a crouched stance, mild pelvic limb atrophy, and limb weakness. Circumduction of the limbs was evident during walking. Some bunny hopping also was apparent. Improvement, but not resolution of signs, occurred as the animals matured.

Walker hound mononeuropathy is an unusual clinical problem that affected a single pelvic limb in a kennel of walker hounds from North Carolina. Monoparesis progressing to self-mutilation was evident. An environmental toxin cause was suspected to be causative.

Laryngeal paralysis has been reported as an autosomal dominant inherited disease in Bouvier des Flandres. Other breeds, such as Siberian huskies, husky crossbreeds, and bull terriers, have also been described with laryngeal paralysis. In cats, laryngeal paralysis may result from lymphoma infiltration of these nerves or lead toxicity.

Inspiratory stridor and dyspnea are the primary clinical signs associated with laryngeal paralysis in animals. Stridor may be exacerbated by lightly externally compressing the larynx with fingers during the physical examination. While sometimes being an isolated disease entity, laryngeal paralysis may also be a component of a more diffuse polyneuropathy or myopathy. In Dalmatians, for example, there is a *laryngeal-polyneuropathy complex*. In addition to laryngeal paralysis, there may be limb paresis, hyporeflexia, exercise intolerance, and voice change. In addition to Dalmatians, Rottweilers, and male Leonberger dogs have been reported with a disease of similar clinical features. The latter dogs may have associated hip and stifle extension. Cataracts may be seen in Rottweilers.

Motor neuronopathies are diseases that affect the cell bodies of the lower motor neuron leading to degeneration of the cell in the ventral horn of the spinal cord and occasionally the cranial nerve nuclei. These may also be referred to as *spinal muscle atrophy* conditions (fig. 7.8). Histologic lesions are most severe in the ventral spinal grey matter and consist of neuronal cell loss and gliosis.

Spinal muscular atrophy in Brittany spaniels is described

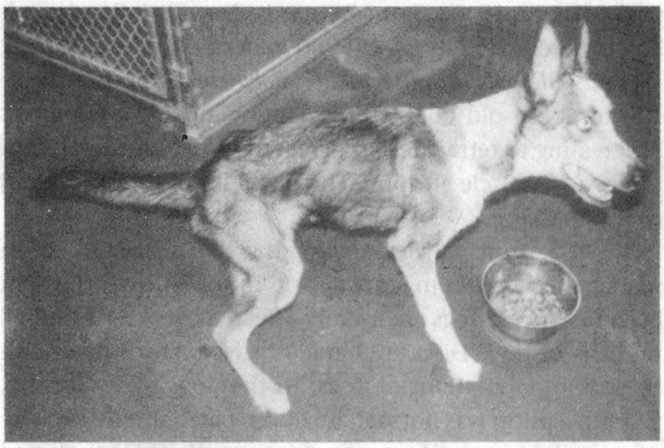

Fig. 7.8. Dog with spinal muscle atrophy showing diffuse muscle atrophy.

in three main clinical forms. An early-onset accelerated form may result in clinical signs in affected dogs as young as 6 to 8 weeks of age. Clinical signs include generalized muscle weakness, a slow tremor of the head, weakness of the muscles of mastication and the tongue, and a depressed gag reflex. Dogs progress to tetraplegia after a few months. An intermediate form of the disease is seen in dogs 6 to 12 months of age. Clinical signs include weakness of proximal muscle of limb and trunk, walking in a waddling fashion, and respiratory muscle involvement. Finally, there is a more chronic form of this disease wherein signs of LMN dysfunction can be present over months to years.

Spinal muscle atrophy is reported in *Swedish Lapland dogs* with apparent autosomal recessive inheritance. Dogs are affected from 5 to 7 weeks of age. Clinical signs include thoracic and pelvic limb weakness that rapidly progresses to tetraparesis. Dogs had decreased spinal reflexes, muscle atrophy, and limb deformities (acquired). A similar disease has been suspected in a collie sheep dog, collie, and a cat.

Spinal muscle atrophy of Great Danes, bloodhounds, and Saint Bernard crossbred dogs, referred to as Stockard's paralysis, has not been observed since the 1930s. This is primarily only of historical significance. Spinal muscle atrophy has also been reported in 2 German shepherds with primarily thoracic limb weakness from 2 weeks following birth. There were associated limb deformities (carpal valgus deformity and carpal flexion contracture).

Spinal muscle atrophy is also described in *Rottweilers.* Dogs at 4 weeks of age showed pelvic limb ataxia rapidly progressing to tetraparesis and tetraplegia. Spinal reflexes were decreased or absent, there was mild intention tremor and limb tremor after exercise, decreased conscious proprioception, megaesophagus, inability to hold up the head, generalized muscle atrophy, and pelvic limb extensor rigidity.

Spinal muscle atrophy has been reported in English pointers in Japan. Dysphonia and decreased tendon reflexes were found.

A *neuronopathy in cairn terriers* is a progressive neuronopathy also known as multisystemic chromatolytic neuronal degeneration (also see degenerative intracranial diseases in chapter 5). Clinical signs were present beginning around 5 months of age. Signs included pelvic limb weakness progressing to tetraparesis, decreased spinal reflexes, incoordination, hypermetria, and head tremor.

Motor neuronopathies have also been reported in adult cats. Clinical signs included tremor, progressive weakness, cervical ventroflexion, dysphagia, and muscle atrophy.

In addition to the motorneuronopathies, neuropathies have been reported that involve only the *sensory nerves.* Breeds affected have included dachshunds, boxers, border collies, English pointers, Siberian huskies, Brittany spaniels, Welsh corgis, Doberman pinschers, Whippets, Scottish terriers, golden retrievers, Scotch collies, and mixed breed dogs. Clinical signs have included proprioceptive deficits, apparent ataxia, decreased or absent spinal reflexes, facial hypalgesia or paresthesia, megaesophagus, head tilt, loss of hearing and voice, anisocoria, dysphagia, a stiff gait, and self-mutilation. Dogs often have a characteristic "paddling" gait, in which the distal palmar and plantar aspects of the feet are flipped forward to impact the ground. Dogs may also "sink" on these limbs during impact. This may also be associated with a jerky movement from side to side that may be misidentified as ataxia.

Sensory neuropathy of boxers (progressive axonopathy) is thought to be a disease of autosomal recessive inheritance. Dogs are usually affected beginning at 2 months of age. There is progressive ataxia and weakness, initially in pelvic limbs, which progresses to involve the thoracic limbs. Muscle tone and spinal reflexes are decreased or absent. Absent patellar reflexes are found by 1 month of age. Signs tend to progress until 12 to 18 months of age, then plateau.

Sensory neuropathy of *long-haired dachshunds* is also thought to be of autosomal recessive inheritance. Dogs are affected beginning between 8 and 12 weeks of age. There is progressive ataxia and weakness (initially in pelvic limbs), decreased pain sensation, dribbling of urine, self-mutilation of the penis, and intermittent vomiting. The pelvic limbs may splay out when dogs are lying down. Patellar reflexes are normal to decreased. A similar disease has been reported in *border collies.*

A sensory neuropathy was seen in a 6-year-old *Jack Russell terrier.* Clinical signs included abnormal pelvic limb posture and biting at one pelvic limb. The dog stood with one pelvic limb flexed and one extended. Conscious proprioceptive deficits were present in the pelvic limbs and one thoracic limb. The dog dribbled urine following voiding. Pain perception was decreased in pelvic limbs distal to the stifle. Patellar reflexes were exaggerated.

Sensory neuropathy of *English pointers* and *Czechoslovakian short-haired pointers* has a suspected autosomal recessive mode of inheritance. Animals were affected between 3 and 8 months of age. Nociceptive loss and self-mutilation usually of the paws are characteristic. This self-mutilation may represent a paresthesia or abnormal sensory impulses.

Sensory neuropathies may also primarily involve the *cranial nerves.* A sensory *trigeminal neuropathy* is reported in a 2-year-old female *rough-coated collie.* Clinical signs included acute onset excessive salivation, coughing, dysphagia, and bilateral loss of sensation in the face, tongue, and oral mucosa. Clinical signs remained unchanged over 18 months.

Other neuropathic diseases primarily affect *autonomic nerves*. *Dysautonomia* is an idiopathic autonomic nervous system disease primarily seen in cats and, with surprising frequency in some part of the United States, in dogs (see bibliography under Dysautonomia). Clinical signs reflect autonomic system dysfunction. This disease is regional in the United States in dogs, with primary concentrations of disease in Kansas and Missouri (the Midwest). Dogs are often presented for vomiting and other gastrointestinal abnormalities. Other clinical signs are poor gastrointestinal motility, megacolon, dilated pupils, xerostomia, and keratoconjunctivitis sicca. Affected dogs may have a dilated anal sphincter. Dogs may also have LMN signs of a peripheral neuropathy affecting the limb muscles. A common environmental toxin or bacteria such as *Clostridium* is suspected.

In cats, dysautonomia has historically been confined to Europe (primarily the United Kingdom) or occurs in imported cats from Europe. The prevalence has decreased markedly and it is now uncommon. Younger cats (<3 years) were more often affected. Clinical signs are often acute in onset over 48 hours with all cats showing depression and anorexia. Other signs reflect autonomic system dysfunction and included ocular signs such as fixed, dilated pupils without blindness, prolapsed third eyelids, and dry eyes (keratoconjunctivitis sicca develops). Gastrointestinal signs include regurgitation, megaesophagus, constipation and megacolon, loss of the anal reflexes, dry mouth (xerostomia), bradycardia (90–120 beats/minute), dysuria and/or distended bladder or incontinence with an easily expressive bladder, and generalized weakness.

MYOPATHIES

Some of the important myopathies of dogs and cats have previously been discussed under the degenerative section (see bibliography under Neuropathies and Myopathies Without Known Cause; Degenerative Myopathies). Many myopathic diseases of dogs and cats exist and are in the process of being recognized and reported.

Muscular dystrophy is an X-linked disease of golden retrievers and other breeds such as Irish terriers, Samoyeds, Rottweilers, Welsh corgis, and Bouvier des Flandres (see above under degenerative myopathies). Clinical signs are usually evident in dogs by 6 to 9 weeks of age. Weakness, stiffness, shuffling gait, abduction of elbows, bunny-hopping, exercise intolerance, and atrophy of head and limb muscles are noted. Other signs include a plantigrade stance, enlargement of base of tongue, inability to fully open the jaw, pharyngeal and esophageal dysfunction, salivation, weak barking, and kyphosis that may develop into lordosis. Clinical signs may plateau after 6 months of progressive deterioration. *Feline muscular dystrophy* is seen in males and is probably also an X-linked genetic trait. Clinical signs occur around 5 to 6 months of age. Signs include skeletal muscle hypertrophy, excessive salivation, exercise intolerance, a stiff gait, bunny-hopping, difficulty jumping, adducted hocks, cervical rigidity, vomiting or regurgitation, partial protrusion of the tongue, multifocal lingual calcification, hepatosplenomegaly, and megaesophagus.

Labrador retriever myopathy is associated with a deficiency of type II muscle fibers. Both male and female dogs can be affected. Animals can have either yellow or black coats. Clinical signs begin between 6 weeks and 8 months of age. Absent patellar reflexes are a clinical clue.

A *hereditary myopathy* occurs in Devon Rex cats. Cats are usually young (3–23 months of age). Clinical signs include generalized muscle weakness, ventroflexion of the neck, and dorsal protrusion of the scapula.

Nemaline rod myopathy is reported in cats from 6 months to 1.5 years of age. Clinical signs include weakness; reluctance to move; a crouched, jerky, hypermetric gait; skin and muscle twitching; and depressed or absent patellar reflexes. *Corelike myopathy* was described in an 18-month-old Great Dane with clinical signs from 6 months of age. Clinical signs included generalized weakness and exercise intolerance.

With *Bouvier des Flandres myopathy*, dogs approximately 2 years of age are affected. Clinical signs included regurgitation, exercise intolerance, generalized muscle atrophy, weakness, and a paddling gait characterized by overextension of the paws during walking. Cranial nerves, conscious proprioception, and spinal reflexes were normal. Dysphagia associated with megaesophagus was reported in older animals (6 months to 9 years).

Exertional myopathy occurs primarily in racing greyhounds. Clinical signs include muscle pain and stiffness. Myoglobinuria is usually present within the first 48 hours.

Labrador retievers have a curious exercise-induced dysfunction, which appears independent of the previously discussed type II muscle fiber deficiency (Taylor and Shelton 2002; Shelton and Taylor 2002). Field trial dogs are most often affected. Dogs tend to be high-strung and active. After variable periods of intense activity, the animals fall down and are unable to perform. Clinical signs may progress even after lying down. Rectal temperatures are elevated, but in a similar range as unaffected animals under similar exercise conditions. It is unknown if this is an occult myopathy or possibly even a central nerve system problem.

Fibrotic myopathy occurs primarily in German shepherds between 2 and 7 years of age. The gait is characteristic in the pelvic limb and aids in identification of this condition. Immediately following the zenith of the flight phase of the pelvic limb, the paw is rapidly directed (jerked) medially before impacting the ground. During the initial flight phase, the distal paw may be in a more extended position compared to a normal dog. A fibrous band of tissue may be palpated from the tuber ischii to the tibia with the semitendinous muscle. A similar condition occurred in a Himalayan cat.

Other types of muscle fibrosis may occur following trauma, myopathic disease, or denervation. Muscle fibrosis can occur secondary to toxoplasmosis and neosporosis in dogs resulting in a rigid extension of one or both pelvic limbs (see figure 3.10). Following muscle trauma, disuse, or injury secondary to musculoskeletal or orthopedic abnormalities, limbs may be positioned in abnormal positions.

Infraspinatous muscle contraction usually occurs in active, medium to large breeds, and usually hunting breeds (Montgomery and Fitch 2003). Possibly the result of muscle trauma, compartmental syndrome, or damage to the infraspinatous nerve, the infraspinatous muscle will become atrophied and fibrotic. The limb is held externally rotated and slightly abducted (see fig. 3.19). When the dog is placed on its nonaffected side, the limb may be held in an upward position and cannot be pushed downward. At gait there is circumduction of the affected limb. The infraspinatous muscle is atrophic on palpation.

Iliopsoas muscle injury may result in lameness of the pelvic limb. The iliopsoas muscle may be painful when palpated during a rectal examination.

Rupture of the *gastrocnemius tendon* may result in a dropped hock appearance. The toes are often flexed caudally giving the limb a characteristic appearance (see fig. 3.14).

Scotty Cramp is characterized by paroxysms of muscular hypertonicity, usually precipitated by excitement or exercise. The disease is believed to be inherited as a recessive trait. The underlying mechanism for these episodes is thought to be the result of decreased central serotonin effects. Initially during movement there is abduction of the thoracic limbs. Arching of back, pelvic limb stiffness, jumping into the air, falling, and curling into a ball may follow. Respirations may cease and facial muscles may be contracted. A similar syndrome is seen in Dalmatians and Norwich terriers.

Episodic falling of Cavalier King Charles is seen mostly in dogs from the United Kingdom. Dogs are affected by 3 to 4 months of age. During exercise, dogs develop a bounding pelvic limb gait with stiff pelvic limbs, falling, and extensor rigidity of the limbs. The episodes are usually life-long in duration.

Myotonia occurs as a congenital problem in various breeds of dogs including the Chow Chow and also in cats (fig. 7.9). The excessive muscle contraction is thought to be due to an abnormal muscle cell membrane that supports persistent depolarization. Animals with myotonia have sustained muscle contraction, which is initiated voluntarily or with stimulation, and sustained involuntarily. Myotonia most often occurs as a congenital problem, however, the disease can be acquired with some toxicities (some herbicides) and secondary to hyperadrenocorticism (see fig. 7.3). Signs are first evident in young dogs and cats less than 1–2 years of age. Animals with myotonia may have a short-stilted gait and apparent stiffness or extensor rigidity of the limbs. Affected animals may also have large, bulky muscles on palpation. Muscle dimpling may occur with direct muscle percussion.

A *myotonic myopathy* has been reported in Chow Chows, Staffordshire terriers, Great Danes, and others. Animals are affected around 2 to 3 months of age. Stiffness and bunny-hopping with rigid limb hyperextension is common. Dysphagia and respiratory difficulty may also be present.

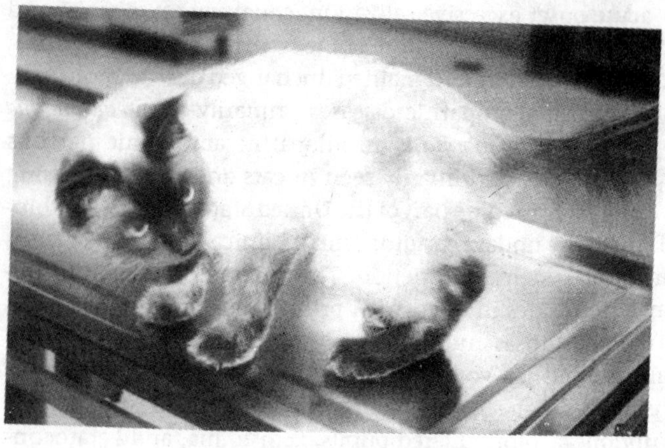

Fig. 7.9. Cat with congenital myotonia.

An acquired myotonia is also present in Rhodesian ridgebacks and cats. Toxicity from some herbicides may also result in acquired myotonia as stated previously.

Familial myoclonus (reflex myoclonus) of Labrador retrievers is a disease of marked, intermittent muscular hypertonicity that occurs in young dogs usually around 3 weeks of age (Fox et al. 1984). Extensor muscle rigidity is usually initially episodic, but can progress to become more frequent. Muscle contractions are worsened by stimulation and handling. Other breeds (Dalmatian) are occasionally affected. The cause is unknown but is suspected to be an inhibitory neurotransmitter abnormality of neurons in the spinal cord, possibly similar to spastic paresis of cattle. Previous treatment with diazepam does not appear helpful.

Dancing Doberman syndrome is a disease characterized by alternating pelvic limb flexion when the animal is standing (Chrisman 1990). Dobermans between 6 months and 7 years may be affected. Flexion of one or both pelvic limbs when standing is the characteristic clinical feature. There is usually associated atrophy of pelvic limb muscles, especially the gastrocnemius. Some dogs with partial rupture of the gastrocnemius tendon may also present similarly and are commonly misdiagnosed with Dancing Doberman syndrome (see fig. 3.14).

Cold tail may be the same as "limber tail" or "limp tail" and has been described as a myopathy of the tail muscles. This syndrome is usually an acute onset of the flaccid tail and is seen as a clinical entity primarily in working breeds of dogs such as Labrador retrievers and pointers.

Some animals will *self-mutilate* or excessively chew their tails without apparent cause. Breeds affected are often described as high-strung including Siamese, Burmese, Himalayan, and Abyssinian cats. In dogs, Doberman pinschers, bull terriers, German shepherds, Great Danes, Irish setters, and spitzes are often affected. Animals usually self-mutilate the tail, limbs, or flank. Bull terriers may spin in circles and chase their tails. It is unknown if this is a behavior abnormally (obsessive compulsive disorder) or whether these animals are reacting to pain or other abnormal sensations. With the latter, peripheral neuropathies with paraesthesia have been suggested.

Many *older dogs* develop significant muscle atrophy in the temporalis muscles without apparent cause. While this muscle atrophy results in an abnormal appearance, no clinically apparent dysfunction of these muscles is apparent.

TRAUMATIC NEUROPATHIES AND MYOPATHIES

Trauma can occur to a single nerve (misplaced injection into the sciatic nerve) or multiple nerves (brachial plexus avulsion) (see bibliography under Peripheral Nerve Trauma). The severity of involvement clinically usually will aid in determining the prognosis for return of clinically useful function. *Neuropraxia* (least severe injury) is an interruption in function and conduction in the nerve, usually associated with a lesion of the myelin without severe axonal involvement. *Axonotmesis* suggests separation and damage of axons, where *neurotmesis* (most severe injury) is complete severance of all structures of the nerve. The likelihood of regeneration is less with neurotmesis as compared to neuropraxia.

Brachial plexus avulsion usually occurs as a result of a trauma to the thoracic limb, which results in a rapid and nonphysiologic abduction of the limb. The force of this movement can result in the nerve rootlets in the cervicothoracic spinal cord, which contribute to the peripheral nerves of the limb, to be avulsed or torn from the spinal cord. The avulsion usually then results in LMN paresis/plegia in the affected thoracic limb. Ipsilateral loss of the cutaneous trunci reflex (due to damage to the lateral thoracic nerve that exits the spinal cord at C8–T1 area) and/or Horner's syndrome (sympathetic nerves exit the spinal cord at T1–3) may be associated signs (see fig. 3.39). Severe damage to a significant portion of the nerve or nerves may result in lack of sensation in the limb. Animals with severe impairment of limb function or decreased sensation may drag the limb along the ground or cause other excoriations to the skin on the limb. In some instances, a suspected paresthesia from the limb may cause animals to bite, chew, or otherwise self-mutilate the limb. Some have even speculated that primary dermatologic disorders such as lick granulomas may result from animals licking and biting of the skin secondary to some paresthesia. Obviously, underlying sensory phenomena are impossible to determine definitively in animals, as animals cannot verbally communicate these sensations to us.

Exiting peripheral nerves or spinal nerves may also be damaged from compression in association with spinal or vertebral diseases. Osteoarthritis and osteophyte proliferation may entrap or compress peripheral nerves that travel in close proximity to bones or joints. For example, *sciatic nerve entrapment* from coxofemoral osteophyte and arthritis associated with hip dysplasia and other coxofemoral degenerative processes has been described.

TOXIC NEUROPATHIES AND MYOPATHIES

There are numerous chemical and biologic toxicities that can result in signs of nervous system dysfunction (see bibliography under Toxicity). Many intoxications result in multifocal neurologic dysfunctions. Some toxicities are primarily associated with signs of peripheral nerve or muscle dysfunction (table 7.1).

Table 7.1. Chemical and environment toxicities associated signs of peripheral nerve or muscle dysfunction

- Heavy metals
  - Lead
  - Mercury
  - Arsenic
- Chemotherapeutic agents
  - Vincritine
  - Doxorubicin
  - Cisplantin
- Herbicides (myotonia)
  - Organophosphate

Toxicants Affecting Autonomic Nervous System

- Cholinergic blockers
  - Atropine
  - Scopolamine
  - Belladonna (Atropa)
  - Glycopyrrolate
- Muscarinic effects
  - Pilocarpine
  - Bethanecol
- Cholinesterase inhibitors
  - Organophosphorus
  - Carbamate insecticides
  - Blue-green algae (Anabaena)

Botulism is due to the exotoxin of *Clostridium botulinum*. Many botulism toxin types have been identified, however, C toxin appears to most often cause the disease in dogs. This exotoxin blocks the presynaptic release of acetylcholine from the neuromuscular junction. This toxin is usually ingested as a preformed toxin rather than being produced from the organism actively proliferating in the body. Dogs are most often exposed to this toxin by eating decaying flesh or other spoiled foods.

Clinical signs are usually acute to subacute in onset and appear as diffuse LMN signs. Early in the disease, animals may have a stiff, stilted, or even bunny-hopping gait. Signs include weakness of the limbs, face, jaw, pharynx, and esophagus, dysponia, dysphagia, facial paralysis, and megaesophagus. Keratoconjunctivitis in some dogs suggests autonomic dysfunction. The predominant clinical signs are of a flaccid paralysis of all limbs. Cranial nerve involvement is common and can be used as a differentiating feature of botulism from tick or coonhound paralysis. This may be reflected in alterations in voice, megaesophagus, or facial muscle weakness. Cranial nerve abnormalities are rare with the other diseases (polyradiculoneuritis—coonhound paralysis—and tick paralysis) that have similar clinical features involving the LMN.

Tick paralysis is due to infestation with ticks. In North America, *Dermacentor andersoni*, *Dermacentor variabilis*, and *Argas* (*Persicargas*) *radiatus* are the species of ticks most commonly associated with paralysis. In general, these ticks secret a toxin that prevents release of ACH from the neuromuscular junction. Clinical signs are those of a diffuse LMN disease. Diagnosis depends upon clinical signs and the presence of ticks. One should be sure to look in hard to find places such as the ear canals, anus, between the toes, and in regions of heavy hair growth. Usually a single adult female tick will cause disease; rarely, large numbers of larvae or nymphs will cause disease. The tick usually will feed on the host for at least 5 days before disease develops. The toxin produced by the tick acts to inhibit the release of acetylcholine from the neuromuscular junction to produce flaccid paralysis. Acute onset of paresis of the pelvic limbs is the most consistent clinical sign. This rapidly progresses (over several hours) to flaccid paralysis and ascends to involve the thoracic limbs and results in lateral recumbency. Dyspnea accompanies paralysis and severe dyspnea with forced expiration and cyanosis occurs terminally.

In Australia, the tick resulting in paralysis is usually *Ixodes holocyclus,* which is found along the eastern coast of this country. Clinical signs of the disease are also more severe and often life-threatening. In addition to the LMN signs, a change in voice and inappetence may occur early in the course of disease. Pupils are dilated and become nonresponsive to light. The nictitating membrane may protrude across the globe. The gag reflex is impaired and drooling of saliva occurs. Regurgitation/ vomiting can occur rarely at any stage. Death may occur within 24 to 48 hours of onset of signs.

Toxicity from *heavy metal* exposure such as mercury, arsenic, and lead has been associated with peripheral neuropathies. These products are usually ingested, inhaled, or absorbed across the skin or mucous membranes. Clinical signs are reflective of a peripheral nerve disease with weakness, muscle atrophy, and decreased reflexes.

Organophosphate intoxication potentiates the effect of acetylcholine at the neuromuscular junction and other synapses, by binding with and inactivating acetylcholinesterase. This leads to increased acetylcholine concentrations at the neuromuscular junction, increased receptor stimulation, and fatigue. Chronic exposure can result in peripheral neuropathies. Cats are one of the species most prone to delayed neurotoxicosis. Organophosphate and carbamate toxicity can result in a multitude of clinical signs including muscle weakness. Muscarinic signs classically include salivation, lacrimation, bradycardia, and pupillary constriction. Nicotinic signs include muscle fasciculations, tremors, and twitching.

Chronic organophosphate toxicity can result in weakness, primarily in cats (Jaggy and Oliver 1990). Cats may attempt to walk a few steps then collapse in sternal recumbency mimicking clinical signs of catoplexy/narcolepsy and myasthenia gravis. Cats may lie down frequently during movement. Ventroflexion of the neck and muscle tremors may be evident. Acute signs of fenthion toxicity are muscle weakness with minimal autonomic signs.

A *delayed neurotoxicity* in cats is reported associated with the use of *chlorpyrifos* spray for household application against fleas. There is individual variation in sensitivity to chlorpyrifos, and signs of toxicity have occurred even when used according to label instructions. Toxicity has also been reported with the flea collars containing chlorpyrifos.

Envenomation from insects and reptiles can result in a variety of signs of nervous system dysfunction. Bites from brown snakes (*Pseudonaja* sp.), coral snakes (*Micrurus fulvius*), tiger snakes (*Notechnis scutatus*), and death adders (*Acanthophis antarcticus*) can cause ataxia, paralysis, and dilated pupils. Additionally, bites from the red-back spider (*Latrodectus* sp.) and ingestion of the tetrodotoxin from toadfish (*Sphaeroides hamiltoni*) may also result in weakness. Red-back spider venom results in depletion of acetylcholine reserves at the motor endplate. Coral snake envenomation may result in acute, flaccid paralysis especially in cats.

A variety of drugs, environmental organisms, and plants may have effects on neurotransmitters and synaptic functions. Ivermectin increases GABA (inhibitory neurotransmitter) concentrations and effects in the CNS. Antibiotics such as aminoglycosides, lincomycin, penicillamine, polymyxins, and tetracyclines have been associated with neuromuscular blockade. Blue-green algae toxicity may result in neurologic dysfunction and weakness.

Tetanus is due to the effects of a neurotoxin (tetanospasmin) secreted by the organism *Clostridium tetani*. This toxin binds to interneurons and inhibits the release of inhibitory neurotransmitter (glycine) in inhibitory interneurons (Renshaw cells). The organism gains access to the body through a wound. Dogs and cats are inherently resistant to this disease, with cats being more resistant than dogs. Therefore, as the wound on a dog may be undetectable, the wound on a cat is usually obvious.

Clinical signs include extensor rigidity, inability to open the mouth, salivation, prolapsed nictitating membrane, inability to urinate, and seizures (see fig. 3.9). Bradycardia (Panciera et al. 1988), megaesophagus, and hiatal hernia (Dieringer and Wolf 1991) may be seen. Tetanus localized to one part of the body such as a single thoracic limb is occasionally found, and appears more commonly in cats possibly related to the overall resistance to tetanus toxin of this species (Malik et al. 1989).

VASCULAR NEUROPATHIES AND MYOPATHIES

Ischemia neuropathy is most often associated with aortic thromboembolism, but may occur with any condition that prevents adequate blood flow to the peripheral nerves or muscles. In cats, aortic thrombosis is the consequence of cardiomyopathy (hypertrophic) (see bibliography under Vascular Neuropathies and Myopathies). Occasionally, these thrombi can lodge in vessels supplying a thoracic limb. In dogs, aortic thrombosis is associated with diseases of hypercoagulability such as protein-losing nephropathies (glomerular disease) and hyperadrenocorticism.

Clinical signs include acute onset paraplegia, with firm,

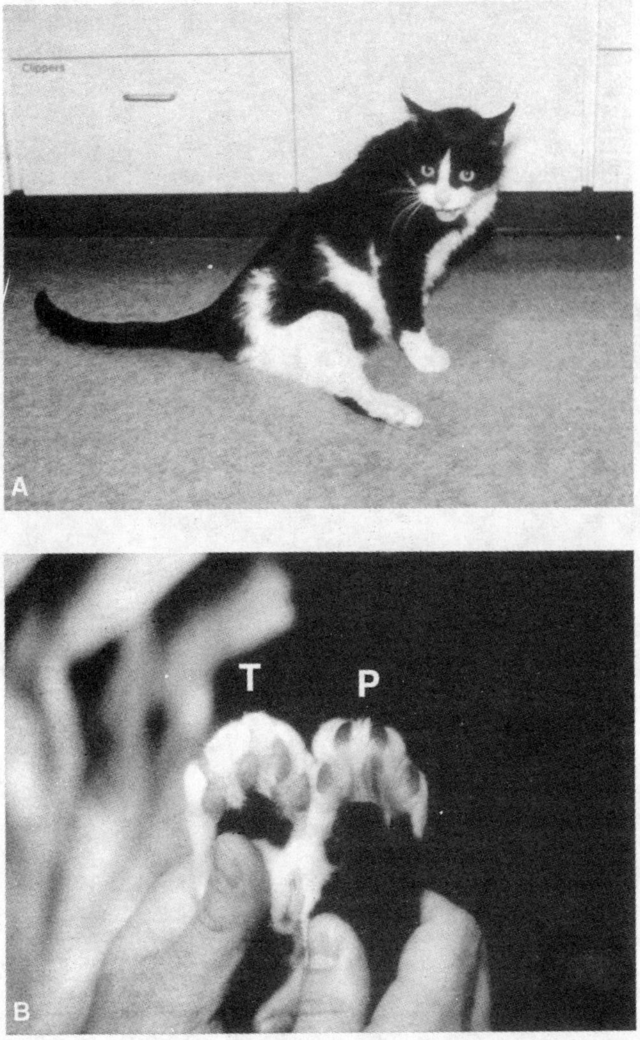

Fig. 7.10. Cat with paralysis from aortic thromboembolus. (A) The cat was vocalizing and had firm, painful pelvic limb muscles. (B) Comparison of the appearance of the thoracic (T) versus the pelvic (P) limbs. The pelvic limbs are discolored due to poor perfusion.

hard painful muscles in the affected limb(s) (Griffiths and Duncan 1979d). Spinal reflexes will usually be decreased or absent. Cats invariably show apparent distress usually with associated vocalizing (fig. 7.10). Absent femoral pulses, cold cyanotic extremities, and absent bleeding when a toenail is cut are also found.

8 Formulation of the Differential Diagnosis of Animals with Neurologic Disease

The ultimate goal of any clinical evaluation is to determine the exact disease process that is adversely affecting the patient. Once the neuroanatomical diagnosis is established, the location of the lesion and other clinical features of the disease process are considered to determine, ideally, which disease process is most likely. In many instances, however, multiple disease processes may have similar clinical features making the separation between them based solely on clinical information difficult if not impossible.

Some disease processes have characteristic clinical signs that help in the identification of that particular disease. If disease characteristics are pathognomonic, the most likely cause of the disease can be rendered based on clinical features alone. This is referred to as a *presumptive diagnosis.* More often, however, a variety of diseases may affect the same area of the nervous system. The clinical signs present reflect the region of the nervous system that is involved with the disease process, but not the individual disease. Therefore, multiple diseases may need to be considered as the cause of a localized neurologic deficit. This is referred to as the *differential diagnosis.* It is important to always initially consider as many disease processes as possible to avoid overlooking a disease process that may be present. Formulation of an accurate differential diagnosis also is important when deciding which diagnostic tests to perform to definitively diagnosis the disease present.

A differential diagnosis can be formulated in a variety of ways. Diseases may be considered based on those associated with specific clinical abnormalities, such as seizures or lameness. Commonly, diseases are considered based on the specific neuroanatomical regions of the nervous system that those particular diseases affect. Finally, differentials may be considered based on which diagnostic tests will be helpful in clarifying the disease process. In many instances, formulation of an accurate differential diagnosis is the key to the successful diagnosis of a disease process in an individual patient.

DIFFERENTIAL DIAGNOSIS BASED ON SPECIFIC NEUROLOGIC ABNORMALITIES

Specific clinical abnormalities may provide clues to the neuroanatomical location, and in some instances, the underlying disease process. The following lists contain common clinical problems along with the general disease processes that are associated with these clinical signs. In some instances the clinical signs may result from specific disease processes, but in most, the clinical signs may only generally indicate the presence of a pathologic process.

CLINICAL MANIFESTATIONS OF DISEASE OF THE NERVOUS SYSTEM

Abnormalities of Cognition and Awareness

Abnormal mentation, stupor, or coma: Consider supratentorial and infratentorial diseases. Also consider systemic disease processes that may secondarily affect intracranial functions.

Aimless wandering or walking: Consider supratentorial and infratentorial diseases. Also consider systemic disease processes that may secondarily affect intracranial functions. Sometimes occurs in animals with pain such as from the abdominal cavity.

Circling, compulsive and unidirectional: May result from either supratentorial or vestibular disease. Animals usually, but not always, circle in the direction of either a supratentorial or vestibular abnormality.

Compulsive (stereotypic) behavior: Consider primary behavioral abnormalities, seizure activity, localized pain in the region of the animal's attention, or intracranial diseases.

Head pressing: Usually indicates abnormalities of cognition, awareness, or consciousness. Consider supratentorial and infratentorial diseases. Also consider systemic disease processes that may secondarily affect intracranial functions.

Hemiinattention: Usually associated with supratentorial disease.

Narcolepsy/cataplexy: Usually occurs without a definable pathologic abnormality. Rarely associated with anatomical disease of the brain stem. Some toxicities, such as organophosphate toxicity in cats, can result in similar appearing episodes.

Pacing: Consider supratentorial and infratentorial diseases. Also consider systemic disease processes that may secondarily affect intracranial functions. Sometimes occurs in animals with pain such as in the abdominal cavity.

Seizures: Consider diseases of the supratentorial structures. Also consider systemic metabolic diseases that secondarily alter intracranial function.

Syncope: Short, episodic loss of consciousness that results from transient cerebral hypoxia or anoxia. Consider diseases of the cardiopulmonary and vascular systems, or autonomic nervous system.

Vocalizing: May be indicative of a disorder of cognition, consider intracranial diseases and metabolic encephalopathies. Also consider as a reaction to pain, especially if associated with abnormal posturing, limb carriage, or movement.

Involuntary or Repetitive Movements

Dyskinesias: Impairment of the power of voluntary movements resulting in fragmented or incomplete movements. Usually result from central nervous system disease. Similar episodes can occur as a result of muscle disorders ("cramping syndromes").

Face rubbing: Consider abnormal sensation or pain (paresthesia, sensory neuropathy). Also may be seen with Chiari malformation (Cavalier King Charles spaniels). Consider xerostomia and other abnormalities of mouth sensation.

Fasciculations: Consider diffuse CNS, peripheral nerve, or muscle diseases; muscle weakness, pain.

Fly-biting: Consider ocular (visual), hearing, and other sensation (taste, smell, touch) disorders, cognition abnormalities (supratentorial disease), behavioral abnormality, seizure activity.

Myoclonus: Suggestive of distemper virus infection of the CNS in dogs. Rarely associated with other forms of inflammatory brain disease, also lead toxicity.

Myoclonus, reflex: Consider diffuse CNS or muscle disease. Congenital disease in some breeds of dogs, such as Labrador retrievers.

Tail chasing or biting: Consider a primary behavior abnormality, pain in the tail or pelvic/lumbosacral region, perianal disease, seizure activity, cognition abnormality.

Tremor, generalized: Consider diffuse neurologic diseases. Inflammatory central nervous system disease is common in adult dogs with generalized tremor. Toxicity with mycotoxins and others possible. In animals less than 1 year of age, consider hypo- or dysmyelination, some storage diseases.

Tremor, head: Consider idiopathic head tremor disorder, cerebellar disease (intention tremor), vestibular disease.

Tremor, limbs: Consider muscle weakness or pain.

Seizures: Consider diseases of the supratentorial structures. Also consider systemic metabolic diseases that secondarily alter intracranial function.

Shivering: Assess for underlying tremor disorder. Animals may be apprehensive or hypothermic.

Sleep (excessive) movements: Consider sleep disorders, seizure activity.

Abnormalities of Posture

"Dropped hock": Consider diseases of the peripheral nerve (sciatic), gastrocnemius muscle, calcaneon tendon, or calcaneus. Often seen with diabetic neuropathy in cats.

Decerebellate rigidity: Characterized by opisthotonus with thoracic limb extension and flexion of the pelvic limbs up under the body due to contraction of the sublumbar muscles. Mental status is normal. Associated with diseases of the cerebellum.

Decerebrate rigidity: Characterized by opisthotonus (extreme dorsal extension of the head and neck toward the back) and extension of all limbs; usually the animal is stuporous or comatose. Associated with midbrain lesions.

Extension (rigid, fixed) of a limb: Consider myopathic or LMN disease. Seen in pelvic limbs with toxoplasmosis and neospora infection in young animals. Also consider UMN spasticity.

Falling: Consider diseases that result in weakness or ataxia. Often associated with vestibular or cerebellar dysfunction if animals fall to the side rather than straight ventrally. Can sometimes be associated with dysfunction of the intracranial structures, spinal cord, or peripheral nerves. Falling directly ventrally and becoming sternally recumbent may indicate syncope, cataplexy, other forms of muscle weakness.

Flexing of a limb: Most often associated with a painful reaction in or around the limb. Consider lameness, musculoskeletal or orthopedic abnormalities, nerve root signature (from spinal or peripheral nerve pain). If in the pelvic limbs of a Doberman pinscher, also consider Dancing Doberman syndrome.

Head tilt: Assess for vestibular (central or peripheral) or cerebellar disease. Rarely associated with primary ear pain. Tilting is usually, but not always, toward the side of the lesion.

Head turn: Usually associated with supratentorial diseases, usually structural. Head usually turns in the direction of the side of the lesion.

Kyphosis: An abnormal flexion primarily of the thoracolumbar spine, results in a "hunched-back" appearance. Associated with cervical, abdominal, back pain; diseases of the spine or vertebrae; paraspinal muscle abscess. If occurs during walking may be associated with weakness.

Lordosis: Abnormal extension of the vertebral column particularly in the thoracolumbar region; this results in a concave appearance of the vertebral column when the animal is viewed from the side. May be associated with muscle weakness, spinal disease, possibly abdominal pain.

Opisthotonus: May be associated with decerebrate or decerebellate posture. Diseases of the central nervous system and brain stem.

Schiff-Sherrington posture: Characterized by thoracic limb extension with normal tone and reflexes in the pelvic limbs; this results from a severe lesion between the third thoracic (T3) to lumbar spinal cord segments that interrupts the ascending inhibitory impulses to the extensor muscles of the thoracic limbs.

Scoliosis: An abnormal lateral deviation of the vertebral column usually associated with spinal cord or vertebral diseases. Often associated with syringomyelia and other cystic spinal cord defects in animals.

Tetanus/tetany: Extensor rigidity of the limbs, neck, trunk, and/or tail. If persistent, consider tetanus, other forms of muscle rigidity (myotonia). If episodic, consider muscle cramping, muscle depolarization, reflex myoclonus.

Torticollis: A contracted state of the cervical muscles producing twisting of the neck and head. Usually associated with brain stem or cranial cervical abnormalities.

Ventral flexion of the neck: Consider diseases associated with muscle weakness. In cats, consider diseases such as hypokalemic myopathy, myasthenia gravis, organophosphate toxicity, hyperthyroidism.

Abnormalities of Voluntary Movement and Gait

Ataxia: Usually associated with diseases of the cerebellum, vestibular system, or spinocerebellar tracts in spinal cord. Possibly associated with disease in other intracranial structures.

"Bunny-hopping": Seen with various diseases of the spinal cord, peripheral nerves, NMJ, and muscle. May also be seen with musculoskeletal diseases of the pelvic region and limbs. Occasionally seen with diseases that affect vascular perfusion to the pelvic limbs (right to left PDA).

Dragging of the feet on dorsal aspect of paw: Consider abnormalities of conscious proprioception. May be associated with either UMN or LMN diseases. Could be indicative of the lesion in either the intracranial structures, spinal cord, or peripheral nerves.

Dysmetria: Improper measurement of range and force in muscular act, usually associated with diseases of the cerebellum, vestibular system, or spinocerebellar tracts in spinal cord. Possibly associated with disease in other intracranial structures.

Hypermetria: Voluntary muscular movement results in overreaching of the intended goal, often resulting in high-stepping. Usually associated with diseases of the cerebellum, vestibular system, or spinocerebellar tracts in spinal cord. Possibly associated with disease in other intracranial structures.

Hypometria: Voluntary movement falls short of the intended goal. Similar concerns as in hypermetria.

Lameness: Reduced ability or desire to bear weight on a limb due to pain or a mechanical restriction of normal joint movement. In severe instances the limb may be held in a flexed position. Usually indicative of a pain in or around the limb. May be associated with musculoskeletal or soft tissue disease of the limb. May also be associated with pain from a peripheral nerve or spinal cord condition.

Myotonia: Consider diseases of muscle including congenital abnormalities, muscular dystrophies, nutritional myopathies, toxicity (herbicide), and hyperadrenocorticism.

Nerve root signature: A persistent or episodic non-weight-bearing lameness, presumably the result of nerve irritation and pain. Consider diseases that involve peripheral nerves or spinal cord segments in or around the affected limb.

Overstepping or overreaching with a limb: Consider UMN diseases of either the spinal cord or intracranial structures, including vestibular and cerebellar disease. May be seen with supratentorial diseases primarily in the thoracic limb contralateral to the supratentorial abnormality.

Paralysis (-plegia): Inability to voluntarily move. Usually associated with severe lesions of the spinal cord or peripheral nerves.

Paresis: May be associated with UMN or LMN diseases.

Shortened step distance: Consider diseases associated with muscle weakness, pain (limbs or spine), and other LMN (peripheral nerve, NMJ, or muscle) weakness.

Spasticity: Increased extensor tone of muscles, most often seen in the limbs. Usually indicative of a UMN abnormality (intracranial or spinal cord).

Stiffness: Decreased range of motion and step length when moving. Consider diseases associated with muscle rigidity. If associated with a decreased step distance, consider pain, and LMN (peripheral nerve, NMJ, or muscle) weakness.

Wide-based stance: Standing with the limbs placed more lateral than usual. Usually indicative of a UMN proprioceptive deficit. If involving the thoracic limbs, consider cervical or intracranial disease. If involving the pelvic limbs, consider spinal cord diseases.

Abnormalities in Appearance of the Head and Face

Anisocoria: Consider diseases of the eyes, pupils, visual system, intracranial neurologic system, parasympathetic and sympathetic innervation to the pupils. Can occasionally be associated with cerebellar disease. The miotic pupil may be too small, or the mydriatic pupil may be too large.

Anosomia: Usually associated with nasal diseases, viral infections. Rarely occurs with intracranial diseases (olfactory bulb area).

Blindness (visual deficit): Consider diseases of the eye, ocular pathways, and intracranial structures necessary for visual integration.

Corneal ulcer: Consider primary corneal disease, often the result of poor corneal sensation (cranial nerve V), corneal dryness (cranial nerves V and VII), or inability to protect the eye through blinking (cranial nerve VII).

"Dropped jaw": Inability to close the jaw—usually due to bilateral trigeminal nerve disease, possibly due to TMJ locking or jaw fracture.

Dysomia: Usually associated with nasal diseases, viral infections. Rarely occurs with intracranial diseases (olfactory bulb area).

Facial asymmetry: Unequal facial expression; usually due to disease of the facial nerve.

Hemifacial spasm: Persistent contraction of the muscles of facial expression on one side; most often associated with disease of the facial nerve, internal ear disease.

Megaesophagus: Dilated esophagus due to numerous causes; often seen with cranial nerve, muscle, and neuromuscular junction disease; esophagitis; myasthenia gravis; esophageal parasites; esophageal reflux; vascular ring anomalies; lead toxicity; hypothyroidism; hypoadrenocorticism.

Miosis: Consider diseases of the eye (painful eye, uveitis), abnormalities of sympathetic innervation to eye (Horner's syndrome or pupil), parasympathomimetic drug therapies or toxicity (pilocarpine, organophosphate intoxication), supratentorial diseases.

Muscle atrophy (temporalis and masseter): Bilateral—consider disease of muscles such as masticatory myositis, age-related degeneration, disuse if associated with abnormalities of jaw movement or pain; *Unilateral*—consider disease of cranial nerve V.

Mydriasis: With blindness—consider diseases of the eye, retina, and optic nerve. Possibly intracranial disorders such as brain herniation if the animal has concurrent severe alteration of consciousness; *With normal vision*—consider diseases of the pupil (iris atrophy, parasympatholytic drug therapies), abnormalities of parasympathetic innervation to eye (cranial nerve III abnormalities), supratentorial diseases, dysautonomia.

Neurotropic keratitis: Loss of corneal integrity due to loss of innervation from the trigeminal nerve; suggests disease of the ophthalmic branch of CN V.

Nystagmus(spontaneous or positional): Consider vestibular or cerebellar disorders, inner ear disease.

Poor blinking, inability to close the eyelids: Usually associated with poor palpebral reflex function and cranial nerve V or VII disease. Possibly muscle weakness.

Ptosis: Consider abnormalities of cranial nerve III or the sympathetic innervation to the eyelid. Gravitational ptosis may occur with facial nerve disease.

Regurgitation: Usually indicates megaesophagus.

Salivation, excessive: Consider local problems with the mouth (inflammation, tumor, toxicity, burn); hepatic encephalopathy (especially in cats); swallowing problems; cranial nerve V, VII, IX, and X disease; megaesophagus; nausea; facial muscle weakness.

Strabismus: Positional—consider abnormalities of the vestibular system, possibly other intracranial structures; *Spontaneous or resting*—consider abnormalities of cranial nerves III, IV, or VI, or the extraocular muscles.

Swallowing abnormality: Usually the result of cranial nerve IX and X dysfunction; can also be associated with some intracranial abnormalities and muscle lesions; Cricopharyngeal dysphagia.

Tongue paresis/paralysis: Inability to use the tongue normally; often associated with disease of the hypoglossal nerve, occasionally seen with supratentorial abnormality.

Vomiting: Rarely a reflex of seizure activity; may be associated with vestibular disease.

Abnormalities of Spinal Reflexes

Areflexia: Lack of reflex action indicative of abnormality of either the spinal nerve cell body (in spinal intumescences), peripheral nerve, NMJ, or muscles.

Atonia: Absent muscle tone; limbs are often limp or flaccid. Indicative of abnormality of either the spinal nerve cell body (in spinal intumescences), peripheral nerve, NMJ, or muscles.

Crossed-extensor reflex: When the animal is in lateral recumbency, eliciting a flexion reflex in the up limb results in extension of the down limb. Seen with disease of the upper motor neuron (spinal cord or intracranial abnormalities).

Hyperreflexia: May be associated with UMN diseases (spinal cord or intracranial); may be normal in an excited animal.

Hyporeflexia: Indicative of abnormality of either the spinal nerve cell body (in spinal intumescences), peripheral nerve, NMJ, or muscles.

Hypertonia: Increase in muscle tone; often results in extension of the limbs. Usually associated with UMN diseases (spinal cord or intracranial) if not due to local muscle fibrosis and contracture. Tetanus possible.

Hypotonia: Decrease in muscle tone; often results in flaccidity of the limbs. Indicative of abnormality of either the spinal nerve cell body (in spinal intumescences), peripheral nerve, NMJ, or muscles.

Muscle atrophy: Disuse—loss of muscle mass due to lack of appropriate use of a muscle. Associated with UMN or orthopedic disease. Usually less severe and more slowly evolving than neurogenic atrophy; *Myopathic*—loss of muscle mass due primary muscle disease; *Neurogenic*—loss of muscle mass due to lack of lower motor neuron innervation of the muscle. Usually severe atrophy that evolves quickly after a LMN lesion.

Spasticity: Increased extensor tone of muscles, most often seen in the limbs. Usually indicative of an UMN abnormality (intracranial or spinal cord).

Weakness: Nonspecific term meaning inability to perform normally; can result from disease of variety of systems within the body. Consider neurologic, muscle, musculoskeletal, metabolic, and cardiovascular systems.

Abnormalities of Urination

Incontinence: Can be due to neurologic abnormalities, or primary diseases of the urinary system.

Increased frequency: In addition to causes of polyuria, may rarely be associated with cerebellar disease.

Lower motor neuron bladder: Bladder characteristics seen with a lesion affecting the lower motor neuron system; characterized by a large bladder, with poor detrusor and sphincter tone, therefore, easy to manually express.

Upper motor neuron bladder: Bladder characteristics seen with a lesion affecting the upper motor neuron system; characterized by a large bladder, with good detrusor and sphincter tone, therefore, difficult to manually express. Consider diseases of the spinal cord and intracranial nervous system.

Abnormalities of Sensation

Hyperesthesia: Increased sensitivity to stimulation; painful. If diffuse, may be associated with inflammatory CNS (meningitis), polyarthritis, polymyositis, abnormal cognition, polyradiculoneuritis (coonhound paralysis).

Pain: Can be associated with diseases of the dura, nerve root, peripheral nerve, muscle, bones, joints, ligaments, and tendons.

Abnormalities of Vital Functions

Adipsia: Consider intracranial (supratentorial; diencephalic) disease.

Bradycardia: Consider increased intracranial pressure.

Ventricular premature contractions: Consider increased intracranial pressure and brain-heart syndrome.

Irregular respiration: Consider brain stem or spinal cord disease; associated whispering bark may indicate lack of tidal volume; increased abdominal effort may indicate respiratory muscle (intercostals and diaphragm) weakness or paralysis; may also be associated with abnormalities of the phrenic nerve.

DISEASES OF INTRACRANIAL STRUCTURES

Certain neurologic diseases primarily or exclusively affect the intracranial structures (table 8.1–8.4). These diseases are considered more or less likely in relation to the clinical features of the disease, the age, and breed of the animal, or whether these diseases affect the gross anatomical structure of the intracranial structures. Some of these diseases are found exclusively or more commonly in selected breeds of animals (table 8.5 and 8.6). Some diseases are found more commonly in younger versus older animals (table 8.7 and 8.8).

Table 8.1. Important diseases that affect the supratentorial and infratentorial nervous system

Degenerative	Abiotrophies (channelopathies?) Leukodystrophies Spongiform encephalopathies Feline spongiform encephalopathy Neuronopathies (multisystemic neuronal degeneration) Polioencephalopathies Storage diseases Cognitive dysfunction
Anomalous	Arachnoid cysts Dermoid or epidermoid cysts Hydrocephalus Hydrencephaly Lissencephaly
Metabolic	Electrolyte imbalances (sodium, calcium, potassium) Glucose abnormalities Hypo-/hyperthyroidism Hyperadrenocorticism Lipid (hypertriglyceridemia) Liver disease (hepatic encephalopathy) Mitochondrial encephalopathies Pancreatic disease Renal encephalopathy
Neoplastic	Primary brain tumor Metastatic tumors Local Extension from skull, nose, or ears
Nutritional	Thiamine deficiency
Inflammatory/Infectious	
Viral	Distemper (dog) Herpes virus Parvovirus Parainfluenza virus (hydrocephalus) Feline infectious peritonitis (cat) Rabies
Fungal, Protozoal	Toxoplasmosis Neospora
Rickettsial	Rocky Mountain spotted fever (vestibular) Ehrlichia
Bacteria	
Parasites	
Protothecosis	
Prions–spongiform encephalopathy	
Inflammatory/ Noninfectious	Granulomatous meningoencephalitis Breed-specific meningitis Pug encephalitis Maltese encephalitis Yorkshire terrier encephalitis Idiopathic encephalitis
Trauma	Head trauma Intracranial hemorrhage Subdural hematoma
Toxicity	Metronidazole (vestibular) Lead
Vascular	Arteriovenous malformation Feline ischemic encephalopathy Hemorrhage Hypertension Infarction Thrombosis

Table 8.2. Important and common diseases that affect the peripheral vestibular structures

Anomalous
- Congenital peripheral vestibular disease
  - Akitas, beagles (bilateral)
  - German shepherd, Doberman, English cocker
  - Siamese, Burmese cats

Metabolic
- Hypothyroidism (possibly but significance uncertain)

Neoplastic
- Middle/inner ear tumor
  - Squamous cell tumor
  - Adenocarcinoma

Idiopathic
- Canine geriatric vestibular disease
- Feline idiopathic vestibular disease

Inflammatory/Infectious
- Otitis media/interna

Inflammatory/Noninfectious
- Idiopathic vestibulitis

Trauma
- Trauma to internal ear structures
- Foreign material in ear

Toxicity
- Ototoxic drugs (aminoglycosides, furosemide, chlorhexidine, cisplatin)
- Metronidazole (may initially have peripheral nerve signs)

It is important from a diagnostic standpoint to recognize which of these diseases affect the gross anatomical *structure* of the nervous system (*structural diseases*), compared to those that alter the inherent cellular functions of the neurons (table 8.9). Diseases that affect the gross central nervous system structure often result in focal neurologic abnormalities. When considering diagnostic testing, diseases that affect CNS structural integrity often require diagnostic tests that show anatomical structural elements, such as magnetic resonance (MR) imaging, for appropriate diagnosis.

DIFFERENTIAL DIAGNOSIS OF SPINAL CORD DISEASE

Certain spinal cord diseases may affect any region of the spinal cord, whereas others affect only specific anatomical regions (table 8.10). An important piece of physical diagnosis information that assists in formulating this differential diagnosis is whether the animal seems painful upon palpation of the spinal area. If there is spinal pain, the five main differentials to consider include:

1. Intervertebral disk disease
2. Fracture/luxation (trauma)
3. Tumor
4. Diskospondylitis/vertebral osteomyelitis
5. Myelitis

Additional differentials may be considered based on breed incidence (table 8.11), time course of the disease, or age of onset of clinical signs (tables 8.12 and 8.13).

Table 8.3. Central diseases more commonly associated with vestibular signs

Anomalous
- Arachnoid cysts
- Dermoid or epidermoid cysts
- Hydrocephalus
- Dandy-Walker syndrome

Metabolic
- Hypothyroidism (possibly but significance uncertain)

Neoplastic
- Meningioma
- Choroid plexus tumor

Nutritional
- Thiamine deficiency (cat and dog)

Inflammatory brain diseases
- Infectious
  - Viral
    - Distemper (Dog)
    - Herpes virus
    - Parvovirus
    - Parainfluenza virus
    - Feline infectious peritonitis (cat)
  - Fungal
  - Protozoal
    - Toxoplasmosis
  - Rickettsial
    - Rocky Mountain spotted fever
    - Ehrlichia
  - Bacteria
  - Parasites
- Noninfectious encephalitis
  - GME
  - Breed-specific meningitis
  - Generalized tremor syndrome
  - Numerous idiopathic apparently noninfectious encephalitides

Trauma
- Head trauma
- Intracranial hemorrhage
- Subdural hematoma

Toxicity
- Metronidazole

Vascular
- Infarction
- Primary Hemorrhage (coagulopathies or platelet disorders)
- Hypertension

Note: Also see infratentorial diseases in table 8.1.

Table 8.4. Important diseases that affect the cerebellum (or result in signs of cerebellar disease)

Degenerative
- Abiotrophies (Channelopathies?)
- Spongiform encephalopathies
  - Feline spongiform encephalopathy
- Neuroaxonal dystrophy
- Leukocephalomyelopathy
- Storage diseases

Anomalous
- Arachnoid cysts
- Dermoid or epidermoid cysts
- Hydrocephalus
- Hypoplasia (panleukopenia infection in cats)
- Dandy-Walker syndrome

Metabolic

Neoplastic
- Meningioma
- Choroid plexus tumor
- Medulloblastoma
- Glioma

Nutritional
- Thiamine deficiency (dog)

Inflammatory diseases

Infectious

Viral
- Distemper (dog)
- Herpes virus
- Parvovirus
- Parainfluenza virus
- Feline infectious peritonitis (cat)

Fungal

Protozoal
- Toxoplasmosis

Rickettsial
- Rocky Mountain spotted fever
- Ehrlichia

Bacteria

Parasites

Noninfectious encephalitis
- GME
- Breed-specific meningitis
- Generalized tremor syndrome

Trauma
- Head trauma
- Intracranial hemorrhage
- Subdural hematoma

Toxicity
- Metronidazole

Vascular
- Infarction
- Primary hemorrhage (coagulopathies or platelet disorders)
- Hypertension

Table 8.5. Common breed associations for intracranial neurologic disease in dogs

Breed	Disease
Afghan hound	Narcolepsy, cataplexy
Airedale	Cerebellar hypoplasia Cerebellar degeneration Granulomatous meningoencephalomyelitis (possible association)
Alaskan husky	Subacute necrotizing encephalopathy
Alaskan Malamute	Mitochondrial encephalopathy
Australian cattle dogs	Polioencephalomyelopathy Ceroid lipofuscinosis
Australian Kelpies	Cerebellar degeneration
Australian shepherd	Deafness
Basset hound	Globoid cell leukodystrophy Glycoproteinosis
Bernese mountain Dog	Hypomyelinogenesis Histiocytosis
Beagle	Bilateral peripheral vestibular disease Cerebellar cortical degeneration Glycoproteinosis Idiopathic epilepsy Globoid cell leukodystrophy Narcolepsy
Beagle mixed	Gangliosidosis GM_1
Belgian sheepdog	Congenital Nystagmus
Belgian Tervuren	Idiopathic Epilepsy
Belgian Malinois	Neuronal degeneration
Bern running dog	Cerebellar degeneration
Bichon frise	Generalized tremors
Blue heeler	Ceroid lipofuscinosis
Blue tick hound	Globoid cell leukodystrophy
Border collie	Cerebellar degeneration Deafness Ceroid lipofuscinosis
Boston Terrier	Hydrocephalus Cerebellar hypoplasia Arachnoid cyst
Boxer	Progressive axonopathy Primary brain tumor (glioma)
Brittany spaniel	Cerebellar degeneration (late onset)
Bullmastiff	Cerebellar degeneration
Bull terrier	Deafness Cerebellar degeneration
Cairn terrier	Globoid cell leukodystrophy Multisystem neuronal degeneration
Catahoula	Deafness
Cavalier King Charles spaniel	"Fly-biting" Chiari malformation Syringomyelia
Chihuahua	Hydrocephalus Ceroid lipofuscinosis
Chow Chow	Cerebellar hypoplasia Hypomyelination
Cocker spaniel	Deafness Idiopathic facial nerve paralysis Multisystem neuronal degeneration Ceroid lipofuscinosis
Collie (rough-coated)	Cerebellar abiotrophy Optic nerve hypoplasia
Collie (Scotch)	Deafness
Collie (sheepdog)	Neuroaxonal dystrophy
Coton de Tulear dogs	Cerebellar disease
Dachshund	Ceroid lipofuscinosis Narcolepsy /Cataplexy
Dachshund (dapple)	Deafness
Dalmatian	Cavitating leukodystrophy Deafness

(continued)

Table 8.5. Common breed associations for intracranial neurologic disease in dogs (*continued*)

Breed	Disease
Dalmatian	Hypomyelination
	Ceroid lipofuscinosis
Doberman	Congenital vestibular disease
	Deafness
	Idiopathic head tremor
	Narcolepsy/cataplexy
English bulldog	Head tremor
English cocker spaniel	Congenital peripheral vestibular abnormality
English setter	Deafness
	Ceroid lipofuscinosis
Finnish Harrier	Cerebellar degeneration
Foxhound (English)	Hound ataxia
Fox terrier	Deafness
	Congenital vestibular disease
German shepherd	Congenital vestibular disease
	Deafness
	Masticatory myositis
German short-haired pointer	Gangliosidosis GM_2
	Pyogranulomatous meningoencephalomyelitis
Golden retriever	Eosinophilic meningitis (possible association)
	Primary brain tumor (meningioma)
Gorden setter	Cerebellar degeneration
Great Pyrenees	Deafness
	Optic nerve hypoplasia
Greyhound	Deafness
Ibizan hound	Deafness
Irish setter	Cerebellar hypoplasia
	Hereditary quadriplegia and amblyopia
	Idiopathic epilepsy
	Lissencephaly
Japanese Akita	Deafness
	Congenital vestibular disease (Bilateral)
Japanese spaniel	Gangliosidosis GM_2
Keeshond	Idiopathic epilepsy
Kerry blue terrier	Cerebellar abiotrophy
Kuvasz	Deafness
Labrador retriever	Cerebellar degeneration
	Narcolepsy/Cataplexy
	Reflex myoclonus
	Spongiform degeneration
	Central axonopathy
Lapland dogs	Gycogenesis Type II
Lhasa Apso	Hydrocephalus
	Lissencephaly
Lurcher hound	Hypomyelination
Malinois shepherd	Spongiform encephalopathy
Maltese terrier	Hydrocephalus
	Generalized tremor syndrome
	Necrotizing meningoencephalitis
Mastiff	Cerebellar disease
	Neuronal degeneration
Miniature pinscher	Generalized tremors
	Mucopolysaccharidosis
Nova Scotia duck trolling retrievers	Meningitis syndrome
Old English sheepdog	Deafness
	Cerebellar degeneration
Papillon	Deafness
	Neuroaxonal dystrophy
Pekingese	Optic nerve hypoplasia
	Hydrocephalus
Plott hound	Mucopolysaccharidosis
Poodle (miniature)	Cerebellar and cerebral cortical degeneration
	Fibrinoid encephalomyelopathy
	Glycoproteinosis
	Sphingomyelinosis
	Narcolepsy/Cataplexy
	Optic nerve hypoplasia
Poodle (toy)	Hydrocephalus
Pomeranian	Hydrocephalus
	Globoid cell leukodystrophy
Portuguese water dogs	Gangliosidosis GM_1
Pug	Pug encephalitis
Rottweiler	Deafness
	Leukoencephalomyelopathy
	Neuroaxonal dystrophy
	Neuronal vacuolation
Russian wolfhound	Optic nerve hypoplasia
Saluki	Ceroid lipofuscinosis
Samoyed	Cerebellar atrophy
	Hypomyelination
	Spongiform degeneration
	Lissencephaly
St. Bernard	Narcolepsy /cataplexy
	Idiopathic epilepsy
Schnauzer (giant)	Narcolepsy /cataplexy
Schnauzer (miniature)	Idiopathic adipsia
	Hyperlipidemia (seizures)
	Idiopathic epilepsy
Scottish terrier	Fibrinoid encephalomyelopathy
	Cerebellar degeneration
Sealyham terrier	Deafness
Sheltie	Hyperlipidemia (seizures)
Shetland sheepdog	Leukodystrophy
Shropshire terrier	Deafness
Siberian husky	Cerebellar agenesis
Silky terrier	Spongiform degeneration
Spitz	Generalized tremor
Springer spaniel	Hypomyelination
	Fucosidosis
Staffordshire terrier	Cerebellar degeneration
Standard poodle	Polymicrogyria and Hydrocephalus
Swedish Lapland	Gycogenesis type II
Sydney silky terrier	Glucocerebrosidosis
Weimaraner	Hypomyelination
Welsh Pembroke corgi	Narcolepsy /cataplexy
West Highland white terrier	Globoid cell leukodystrophy
Wire-haired fox terrier	Cerebellar hypoplasia
	Lissencephaly
Wire-haired griffon	Narcolepsy/Cataplexy
Yorkshire terrier	Hepatic encephalopathy (portosystemic shunt)
	Microvascular dysplasia (liver)
	Hydrocephalus
	Necrotizing encephalitis
Yugoslavian sheepdog	Ceroid lipofuscinosis

Table 8.6. Common breed-associated intracranial neurological abnormalities of cats

Breed	Abnormality
Balinese	Sphingomyelinosis
Birman	Spongiform encephalopathy
Burmese	Congenital vestibular disease
	Deafness
Domestic short-haired	Gangliosidosis GM_1
	Gangliosidosis GM_2
	Globoid cell leukodystrophy
	Mannosidosis
	Metachromatic leukodystrophy
	Mucopolysaccharidosis
	Gycogenesis type II
	Ceroid lipofuscinosis
Domestic tricolor	Neuroaxonal dystrophy
Egyptian Mau	Spongiform encephalopathy
Korat	Gangliosidosis GM_1
Norwegian Forest cats	Glycogenosis type IV
Persian	Mannosidosis
Siamese	Congenital strabismus/nystagmus
	Congenital visual pathway abnormal
	Deafness
	Sphingomyelinosis
	Peripheral vestibular disease
	Gangliosidosis GM_1
	Mucopolysaccharidosis
	Ceroid lipofuscinosis

Table 8.7. Important diseases of the intracranial nervous system that affect younger animals

Degenerative
- Storage diseases
- Abiotrophies

Anomalous
- Hydrocephalus
- Hydrencephaly
- Lissencephaly

Metabolic (secondary affect on brain function)
- Liver disease (hepatic encephalopathy)
- Renal encephalopathy
- Pancreatic disease
- Glucose abnormalities
- Hypo-/Hyperthyroidism
- Electrolyte imbalances (Sodium)

Nutritional
- Thiamine deficiency

Infectious
- Distemper (dog)
- Herpes virus
- Parvovirus
- Parainfluenza virus (hydrocephalus)
- Feline infectious peritonitis (cat)
- Feline panleukopenia virus (cat, cerebellum)
- Fungal disease
- Toxoplasmosis
- Rickettsial
  - Rocky Mountain spotted fever (vestibular)
  - Ehrlichia
- Bacteria
- Parasites

Trauma
- Head trauma
- Intracranial hemorrhage
- Subdural hematoma

Toxicity
- Metronidazole (vestibular)
- Lead

Table 8.8. Important diseases of the intracranial nervous system that primarily affect older animals

Anomalous
- Acquired hydrocephalus

Metabolic (secondary affect on brain function)
- Liver disease (hepatic encephalopathy)
- Renal encephalopathy
- Pancreatic disease
- Glucose abnormalities
- Hypo-/Hyperthyroidism

Neoplastic
- Primary brain tumor
- Metastatic tumors
- Local extension

Infectious
- Distemper (dog)
- Herpes virus
- Parvovirus
- Parainfluenza virus (hydrocephalus)
- Feline infectious peritonitis (cat)
- Fungal disease
- Toxoplasmosis
- Rickettsial
  - Rocky Mountain spotted fever (vestibular)
  - Ehrlichia
- Bacteria
- Parasites

Trauma
- Head trauma
- Intracranial hemorrhage
- Subdural hematoma

Toxicity
- Metronidazole (vestibular)
- Lead

Vascular
- Arteriovenous malformation
- Infarction
- Feline ischemic encephalopathy
- Hemorrhage
- Hypertension

Table 8.9. Diseases that often affect the gross anatomical structure of the intracranial nervous

Anomalous
- Hydrocephalus
- Hydrencephaly
- Lissencephaly

Neoplastic
- Primary brain tumor
- Metastatic tumors
- Local extension

Nutritional
- Thiamine deficiency

Inflammatory/Infectious
- Various encephalitis
- Parasite migration

Trauma
- Head trauma
- Intracranial hemorrhage
- Subdural hematoma

Vascular
- Arteriovenous malformation
- Infarction
- Feline ischemic encephalopathy
- Hemorrhage
- Hypertension

Table 8.10. Location of diseases along the spinal cord

Spinal cord, any region
- Intervertebral disk disease
- Diskospondylitis/vertebral osteomyelitis
- Tumor
- Trauma (vertebral fracture, luxation)
- Myelitis
- Fibrocartilaginous emboli and other vascular-associated diseases
- Congenital defects
  - Vertebral defects (e.g., hemivertebrae, block vertebrae)
  - Cystic Spinal cord defects (syringo-/hydromyelia, arachnoid cysts)

Spinal cord, cervical region
- Cervical vertebral malformation/malarticulation (wobbler syndrome)
- Atlantoaxial instability

Spinal cord, lumbosacral region
- Lumbosacral instability
- Cauda equina syndrome

Spinal cord, thoracolumbar region
- Degenerative myelopathy
- Spinal cord blastoma

DIFFERENTIAL DIAGNOSIS OF PERIPHERAL NERVE, NEUROMUSCULAR JUNCTION, AND MUSCLE

Diseases that affect the peripheral nerve, neuromuscular junction, or muscle are also numerous and variable (table 8.14). Many of these diseases are found in specific breeds (tables 8.15, 8.16).

MULTIFOCAL DISEASE OF THE NERVOUS SYSTEM

Multifocal disease of the nervous system implies that more than one functional area is involved (table 8. 17). Some diseases can affect multiple regions of the spinal cord simultaneously. Or two or more different diseases can affect the nervous system in differing areas. If the clinical signs cannot be adequately explained by a single focal abnormality, then consideration should be give to a single disease with multifocal or diffuse lesions or multiple disease processes present.

Table 8.11. Common breed-associated spinal cord diseases

Breed	Disease
Afghan hound	Myelomalacia
Airedale	Lumbosacral disease
Alaskan Malamute	Myelodysplasia
Basset hound	Cervical vertebral malformation
	Intervertebral disk disease
Bernese mountain dog	Spinal cord vasculitis
Beagle	Intervertebral disk disease (cervical)
	Spinal cord vasculitis (Beagle pain syndrome)
Belgian Malinois	Degenerative myelopathy
	Lumbosacral disease
Bichon frise	Atlantoaxial subluxation
Borzoi	Cervical vertebral malformation/malarticulation
Boston terrier	Vertebral anomalies
	Arachnoid cyst
Boxer	Progressive axonopathy
	Dermoid sinus
Bullmastiff	Cervical vertebral articular facet disease
Cavalier King Charles spaniel	Chiari malformation
	Syringomyelia
Chihuahua	Atlantoaxial subluxation
Chow Chow	Arachnoid cyst
Cocker spaniel	Intervertebral disk disease
Corgi	Intervertebral disk disease
	Degenerative myelopathy
Dachshund	Intervertebral disk disease
Dalmatian	Wobbler syndrome
Doberman	Cervicalvertebral malformation/malarticulation
English bulldog	Spina bifida
	Hemivertebrae
	Sacrococcygeal malformation
Foxhound (English)	Hound ataxia
German shepherd	Calcinosis circumscripta
	Degenerative myelopathy
	Lumbosacral instability/stenosis
	Multiple cartilaginous exostosis
	Spinal cord blastoma (neuroepithelioma)
	Intervertebral disk disease
German short-haired pointer	Hemivertebrae
	Pyogranulomatous meningoencephalomyelitis
Great Dane	Cervicalvertebral malformation/malarticulation
	Fibrocartilaginous emboli
	Disseminated idiopathic skeletal hyperostosis
Harriers	Myelopathy
Hounds	Hound ataxia (United Kingdom)
Irish wolfhound	Cervical vertebral malformation/malarticulation
Japanese chin	Atlantoaxial subluxation
Kooiker dogs (Dutch)	Hereditary necrotizing myelopathy
Labrador retriever	Intervertebral disk disease
	Traumatic intervertebral disk rupture
	Fibrocartilaginous emboli
Malamute	Multiple cartilaginous exostosis
Mastiff	Cervical stenosis
Nova Scotia duck trolling retrievers	Meningitis syndrome
Pekingese	Intervertebral disk disease
	Atlantoaxial subluxation
Poodle (miniature)	Demyelinating myelopathy
	Intervertebral disk disease
	Sacrococcygeal dysgenesis
	Atlantoaxial subluxation
Poodle (toy)	Atlantoaxial subluxation
Pomeranian	Atlantoaxial subluxation
Pug	Spinal scarring
	Arachnoid cysts
Rhodesian ridgeback	Dermoid sinus
Rottweiler	Aplasia of the dens
Schnauzer (miniature)	Fibrocartilaginous emboli
	Intervertebral disk disease
Shih Tzu	Intervertebral disk disease
	Atlantoaxial subluxation
	Dermoid sinus
Siberian husky	Degenerative myelopathy
Smooth-coated fox terrier	Hereditary ataxia
Weimaraner	Spinal dysraphism
Welsh Pembroke corgi	Intervertebral disk disease
Yorkshire terrier	Atlantoaxial subluxation
	Intervertebral disk disease
	Multiple cartilaginous exostosis

Table 8.12. Time course and progression of the spinal disease

Acute onset of signs, rapidly progressive courses
- Intervertebral disk disease (type I)
- Trauma (Fracture/luxation)
- Fibrocartilaginous emboli

Slower onset of signs, chronic courses
- Intervertebral disk disease (type II)
- Lumbosacral instability
- Cauda equina syndrome
- Degenerative myelopathy
- Diskospondylitis
- Tumors

Table 8.13. Age of onset of clinical signs of spinal disease

Diseases in young dogs
- Atlantoaxial instability
- Trauma
- Myelitis
- Congenital defects
  - Vertebral defects (e.g., hemivertebrae, block vertebrae)
  - Spinal cord defects (e.g., syringo-/hydromyelia)
- Scoliosis
- Degenerative myelopathy (German shepherd and Siberian huskies)
- Spinal cord blastoma
- Multiple cartilaginous exostoses
- Diskospondylitis
- Cervical vertebral malformation/malarticulation (wobbler syndrome) (in Great Danes, mastiffs)

Diseases in older dogs
- Lumbosacral instability
- Cauda equina syndrome
- Degenerative myelopathy
- Tumors

Table 8.14. Diseases of the peripheral nervous system, neuromuscular junction, and muscle

Degenerative	Various Myopathies
	Labrador retriever myopathy
	Mitochondrial myopathies
	Muscular dystrophies
	Nemaline rod myopathy
	Various Neuropathies
	Peripheral neuropathies
	Axonal neuropathy
	Hypertrophic neuropathy
	Storage diseases
	Motor neuron diseases
Metabolic	Neuropathies
	Diabetic neuropathy
	Insulinoma neuropathy
	Myopathies
	Polymyopathy (hypokalemic)
	Hyperadrenocorticism
Neoplastic	Lymphoma
	Nerve sheath tumors (Schwannoma, neurofibroma, neurofibrosarcoma)
	Paraneoplastic neuropathy
Nutritional myopathies	
Inflammatory/ Infectious	Brachial plexus neuritis
	Chronic relapsing neuropathy
	Coonhound paralysis or polyradiculoneuritis
	Masseter muscle myositis
	Myasthenia gravis
	Tetanus
	Toxoplasma gondii and *Neospora caninum*
Idiopathic	Laryngeal paralysis
	Myotonia
	Idiopathic neuropathies
	Motor neuronopathies
	Polyneuropathies (sensory or motor) nerves
	Scotty Cramp and other cramping syndromes
	Familial myoclonus of Labrador
	Dancing Doberman syndrome
	Dysautonomia
Trauma	Brachial plexus avulsion
Toxic	Botulism
	Heavy metals
	Organophosphate toxicity
	Tick paralysis
Vascular	Aortic thromboembolism

Table 8.15. Common breed-associated peripheral nerve, nmj, or muscle diseases

Alaskan Malamute	Peripheral neuropathy
Basset hound	Globoid cell leukodystrophy
Bouvier des Flandres	Laryngeal paralysis
	Degenerative myopathy
Boxer	Progressive axonopathy
Brittany spaniel	Spinal muscle atrophy
	Sensory ganglioradiculitis
	Dystrophy-like myopathy
Bull terrier	Laryngeal paralysis
Cairn terrier	Spinal muscle atrophy
Chesapeake Bay retriever	Distal polyneuropathy
	Laryngeal paralysis
Chow Chow	Hypomyelination
	Myotonia
Clumber spaniel	Mitochondrial myopathy
Collie (rough-coated)	Sensory trigeminal neuropathy
Collie (Scotch)	Dermatomyositis
	Distal polyneuropathy
Collie (sheepdog)	Neuroaxonal dystrophy
	Spinal muscle atrophy
Dachshund	Myasthenia gravis
	Sensory neuropathy
Dachshund (long-haired)	Sensory neuropathy
Dalmatian	Hypomyelination
	Laryngeal paralysis-polyneuropathy
	Cramping syndrome
Doberman	Dancing Doberman syndrome
	Sensory neuropathy
English pointer	Sensory neuropathy (self-mutilation)
	Motorneuron degeneration
English springer spaniel	Muscular dystrophy
Gammel Dansk honsehund	Myasthenia gravis
German shepherd	Fibrotic myopathy
	Giant axonal neuropathy
	Masticatory myositis
	Motorneuron degeneration
Golden retriever	Extraocular polymyositis
	Hypomyelination (peripheral)
	Muscular dystrophy)
	Hypomyelination polyneuropathy
Great Dane	Corelike myopathy
	Distal symmetrical polyneuropathy hyperostosis
	Myotonia
Greyhound	Exertional myopathy
Griffon Briquet Vendeen	Spinal muscle atrophy
Hounds	Polyradiculoneuritis
Irish setter	Laryngeal paralysis
Irish terrier	Muscular dystrophy
Jack Russell terrier	Congenital myasthenia gravis
	Sensory neuropathy
Labrador retriever	Distal polyneuropathy/Laryngeal paralysis
	Hereditary myopathy
	Reflex myoclonus
	Myotonia
Leonberger dogs	Polyneuropathy and laryngeal paralysis
Lurcher hound	Hypomyelination
Malamute	Neuropathy
Mongrel	Myasthenialike syndrome
Norwich terrier	Cramping syndrome
Old English sheepdog	Mitochondrial myopathy
Rhodesian ridgeback	Myotonialike syndrome
Rottweiler	Distal sensorimotor polyneuropathy
	Motorneuron degeneration
	Neuroaxonal dystrophy
	Laryngeal paralysis-polyneuropathy
Saluki	Spinal muscle atrophy
Samoyed	Hypomyelination
	Myopathy
	Myotonia
Schnauzer (miniature)	Muscular dystrophy
	Myotonia
Shar pei	Megaesophagus
Sheltie	Dermatomyositis
Siberian husky	Laryngeal paralysis
	Sensory neuropathy
Silky terrier	Myopathy
Smooth-coated fox terrier	Congenital myasthenia gravis
	Hereditary ataxia
Springer spaniel	Congenital myasthenia Gravis
	Hypomyelination
Staffordshire terrier	Myotonia
Sussex spaniel	Mitochondrial myopathy
Swedish Lapland	Motorneuron degeneration
Tibetan mastiff	Hypertrophic neuropathy
Walker hound	Mononeuropathy
Welsh Pembroke corgi	Muscular dystrophy
	Narcolepsy/cataplexy
Whippet	Sensory ganglioradiculitis

Table 8.16. Breed-associated neurological abnormalities of cats involving the peripheral nerve, NMJ, or muscle

Abyssinian	Myasthenia gravis
Birman	Distal polyneuropathy
Domestic short-hair	Hyperoxaluria
	Myasthenia gravis
	Muscular dystrophy
	Spinal muscle atrophy
Domestic tricolor	Neuroaxonal dystrophy
Himalayan	Fibrotic myopathy
Manx	Sacrococcygeal dysgenesis
Norwegian forest cats	Glycogenosis type IV
Rex	Myopathy
Siamese	Hyperchylomicronemia
	Myasthenia gravis
	Spinal muscular atrophy
Somali	Myasthenia gravis

Note: Also see storage diseases in table 5.4.

Table 8.17. Diseases that commonly result in multifocal nervous system signs

Degenerative
- Storage disease
- Multineuronal degeneration

Anomalous
- Hydrocephalus/syringo-/hydromyelia complex

Metabolic
- Hepatic
- Renal
- Hypoglycemia
- Thyroid (hypo and hyper)
- Hyperadrenocorticism
- Hyperosmolar syndromes
- Adipsia

Neoplastic
- Lymphoma
- Leukemias
- Metastatic tumors

Nutritional
- Thiamine

Inflammatory
- Infectious
  - Viral
    - Distemper
    - Herpes
    - Parvovirus
    - Parainfluenza
    - FIP
    - FIV
  - Bacterial
    - Tetanus
  - Fungal
    - Cryptococcosis
    - Blastomycosis
    - Coccidiomycosis
    - Candidiasis
    - Aspergillosis
  - Protozoal
    - Toxoplasmosis
    - Neosporosis
  - Parasitic
    - Toxocara
  - Rickettsial
    - Rocky Mountain spotted fever
    - Ehrlichia
  - Unclassified
    - Protothecosis
- Noninfectious
  - Granulomatous-meningoencephalitis (GME)
  - Pug Encephalitis
  - Maltese Encephalitis
  - Spinal Cord Vasculitis
  - Nonclassified
  - Steroid-responsive meningitis

Idiopathic
- Dysautonomia

Toxins

Vascular disease
- Thromboembolism
- Hypertension
- Cerebral hemorrhage

9 Options for Diagnostic Testing in Animals with Neurologic Disease

Clinical evaluation of animals with neurologic disease is based firmly upon physical diagnosis (*neurologic examination, neuroanatomic diagnosis*) and establishment of a list of possible diseases that could result in the clinical signs present (*differential diagnosis*) (table 9.1). Appropriate *diagnostic tests* are then performed that will prove (or disprove) whether each differential diagnosis or the presumptive diagnosis is the cause of the clinical abnormality. The true diagnosis is referred to as the *definitive diagnosis*. As diagnostic tests are often used to evaluate a specific area of the nervous system based on the neuroanatomic diagnosis, it is imperative that the clinician knows, prior to performing a diagnostic test, where to look for the disease process. Equally important in the choice, but also in the interpretation and clinical significance, of a diagnostic test is to have a preconceived idea of what diseases to look for (see chapters 5,6, and 7). The importance of these aspects of clinical evaluation (i.e., *neuroanatomic diagnosis* and *differential diagnosis*) cannot be overemphasized when choosing or performing diagnostic tests. No diagnostic test can be substituted for a thorough and accurate clinical evaluation!

While the scope of disease affecting the nervous system is broad, the number of diagnostic tests that are most helpful in definitive antemortem diagnosis of neurologic disease is surprisingly limited. Diagnostic tests are chosen based on a logical process following physical assessments. A *diagnostic plan* is the formulation of diagnostic tests to definitively diagnose a disease process.

A particular diagnostic test is chosen as part of the diagnostic plan primarily based on the *cost/benefit ratio* of the diagnostic test for diagnosis of a particular disease process (see below). Performing and interpreting this analysis accurately requires a knowledge of the utility of the diagnostic test for the particular disease in question, as well as disease characteristics that may be identified with the particular diagnostic test.

Table 9.1. Steps in formulating a diagnostic plan for animals with neurologic disease

- Collect physical and neurologic examination clues
- Establish a list of clinical problems
- Determine the neuroanatomical diagnosis
- Consider diseases that may result in the clinical findings (differential diagnosis)
- Decide if the suspected disease processes are likely to alter gross nervous system structure or disrupt physiologic function
- Chose diagnostic tests that will identify the disease process

In general, disease of the nervous system either will alter the gross *structural integrity* (*anatomy*) of the nervous system, or will cause dysfunction at a *cellular metabolic level* (*function* or *physiology*) of neurons. If alterations in the gross anatomic structure of the nervous system are likely in association with a specific disease process, then it is most appropriate to choose a diagnostic test that will allow for assessment of gross neuroanatomy. The advent and increasing use of sophisticated imaging studies for viewing internal body structures, such as *magnetic resonance imaging*, have revolutionized the antemortem diagnosis of central nervous system disease simply by providing a better "picture" of the internal gross structure of the nervous system in a live animal. If the disease does not affect the nervous system structure but results in a cellular physiologic dysfunction, *electrophysiological, clinical pathologic*, and *biochemical* tests may be more helpful in establishing the definitive diagnosis. Ultimately, histologic assessment of abnormal tissue is often the "gold standard" for most diagnosis in medicine but may not always be possible with nervous system disease due to the associated morbidity.

This chapter provides an overview of diagnostic tests commonly used in the antemortem diagnosis of neurologic disease. Necropsy along with histologic diagnosis of neurologic diseases have been reviewed previously (Summers 1995). Unfortunately, many of the diagnostic tests helpful in the diagnosis of animals with neurologic disease will not be available in the general veterinary practice. However, for the practicing clinician, it is important to understand when it is appropriate to employ a given diagnostic test, such as electrodiagnostics or magnetic resonance imaging, in the diagnostic process as these diagnostic tests are increasing becoming available in university, private, and specialty practice settings. Providing the patient and the client with the best diagnostic options available requires a fundamental understanding of neurological disease process (see chapters 5 through 7) as well as a fundamental understanding of the neurodiagnostic testing procedures, indications, complications, and utilities.

COST BENEFIT ANALYSIS OF NEUROLOGIC DIAGNOSTIC TESTING

As with all diagnostic tests, an understanding of the *cost/benefit* of a diagnostic test is crucial. The "cost" portion of this ratio includes both the *financial cost* to the client (or the hospital) and, most importantly, the *risks* or the potential for patient morbidity associated with that procedure. The overall "benefit" of any diagnostic test is, in essence, the likelihood that that particular test will provide the definitive diagnosis (true disease), or, at the very least, the test will provide supporting information in clarifying the definitive diagnosis by excluding other disease processes from further consideration. Costs and benefits of an individual diagnostic test will vary depending upon individual patient characteristics, the overall systemic health of the animal and, most importantly, upon the disease process present. As these aspects change, so may the cost/benefit of a particular diagnostic test.

Clinical practice commonly revolves around "playing the odds" during formulation of the different diagnosis and establishing a diagnostic plan. A reasonable question to ask during formulation of the diagnostic plan is, "What is the chance that a particular diagnostic test will reveal or definitively determine the presence of the disease process?" The answer to this question depends upon the disease that the patient actually has as well as the ability of the particular diagnostic test to reveal that the disease is, in fact, present.

Financial costs associated with performing an individual diagnostic test may vary with geographic location, access to a particular diagnostic test, and charging philosophy of the hospital (e.g., cost-based pricing versus historical pricing). Obviously, the quality of the diagnostic procedure will influence the likelihood of providing for an appropriate diagnosis. A poorly performed or interpreted test is less likely to yield a diagnosis regardless of its inherent likelihood of establishing a diagnosis. The cost/benefit of any diagnostic test, therefore, is dynamic and changes with the individual clinical situations.

BASELINE DATA FOR ANIMALS WITH NEUROLOGIC DISEASE

It is commonplace when evaluating animals for any significant disease process that a general (routine) database of overall systemic health be determined (table 9.2). Some of these tests are used as a screen for abnormalities or dysfunction of body systems. These tests include, but are not limited to, blood cellular and chemistry assessments, such as CBC and serum chemistries, urinalysis, and thoracic and abdominal radiographs. While these particular types of tests rarely provide specific information regarding nervous system disease, they may provide clues to underlying systemic diseases that may also involve the nervous system or affect nervous system function. Additional test evaluations will vary depending upon the type and severity of the patient impairment, and depending upon clues collected from the basic physical examination. Blood pressure measurements, for example, are being used with increasing frequency as a routine measure of systemic health. As hypertension can result in central nervous system abnormalities, blood pressure measurements should become more routine in the evaluation of animals with neurologic disease, especially in animals with derangements of intracranial function. As hepatic encephalopathy is a reasonably common cause of intracranial dysfunction, particularly in younger animals, bile acids determination or another type of liver function testing should also be a routine part of the baseline evaluations in animals with intracranial neurologic dysfunction.

Table 9.2. Minimum database for animals with intracranial signs

- CBC
- Serum biochemistry including CK analysis
- Urinalysis
- Bile acids or other liver function testing
- Blood pressure measurement
- Heartworm testing (dog)
- FeLV/FIV testing (cat)

Expanded database for animals with intracranial signs

- Assessment of coagulation status (buccal mucosal bleeding time, PT, PTT, FDPs, platelet count)
- Thoracic radiograph
- Abdominal radiograph
- Abdominal ultrasound

SPECIFIC DIAGNOSTIC TESTING FOR ANIMALS WITH NEUROLOGIC DISEASE

There are a relatively finite number of clinically helpful antemortem diagnostic tests to identify disease processes in animals with neurologic dysfunction. These tests may be used to assess the anatomical integrity, the cerebrospinal fluid circulating in the subarachnoid space, or the physiological (electrical) integrity of the nervous system.

In determining the anatomical integrity of the nervous system, an *anatomical imaging study* is often necessary. In the modern era, the two most commonly used advanced imaging studies are *computed tomography* (*CT*) scanning and *magnetic resonance* (*MR*) *imaging*. *Survey radiographic* evaluations are often performed of the spine and skull, however, these evaluations do not allow for assessment of nervous system parenchyma. If disease is suspected to involve the *spinal cord*, subarachnoid injections of contrast media during *myelography* have been a historical standard for lesion clarification. Advanced imaging studies, such as *CT* and *MR* imaging, however, yield much more anatomically useful information and are currently the gold standard for evaluation of both intracranial and spinal disease. Analysis of *cerebrospinal fluid (CSF)* is used primarily to identify disease that does not alter gross nervous system structure but may alter the microscopic anatomy or physiology. Inflammatory nervous system diseases would be an example of the type of processes CSF evaluation is helpful in identifying.

Electrodiagnostic studies may be performed to assess certain electrical (physiologic) properties or functions of nerves and muscles. Biopsy of abnormal tissues with associated histologic evaluation is often necessary to establish the presence of a specific disease process.

DIAGNOSTIC TESTING FOR INTRACRANIAL DISEASE

Neuroimaging Studies

Skull Radiographs. In animals with suspected intracranial disease, skull radiographs can be used to assess the bony integrity of the skull, but they obviously have limited utility in the evaluation of the intracranial cavity (Forrest 2002). If the disease alters the cranial bones, as is the case with tumors or skull fractures, this information may be obtained with skull radiography (fig. 9.1). The complexity in radiographic appearance of the skull, however, makes evaluation and interpretation of the cranial structures sometimes difficult. The most obvious limitation of skull radiography in intracranial nervous system assessment is the inability of radiographs to provide information regarding soft tissue structural detail of the brain and cranial nerves.

Proper radiographic technique and positioning are important when performing skull radiographs, as accurate interpretation depends primarily upon the evaluation of symmetry of the bony structures. To achieve the degree of positioning necessary, sedation or anesthesia is often required, both of which increase patient risk and client expense. Exposure of personnel and the patient to ionizing radiation is also of concern, but is usually not of a significant dose for individual patients or for individual studies.

Skull radiographs are primarily used for evaluation of animals with head trauma resulting in skull fracture, tumors involving the head, nasal disease including the frontal sinus area, and bulla disease. Most commonly the clinically significant question associated with these disease processes is the degree of associated disease or disruption of the integrity of the underlying nervous system. This determination cannot be made through interpretation of skull radiographs alone.

In some situations, such as in cats with meningiomas, a brain tumor may result in a hyperostosis of the overlying skull that will be apparent on high-quality skull radiography. In immature animals with hydrocephalus, the normal contour of the skull may be less apparent on a radiograph providing for a "ground-glass" appearance to the calvarium. Fontanels may also be present and be apparent on skull radiographs. While a fontanel that persists into maturity is often associated with an underlying hydrocephalus, this finding is not pathognomonic for this disease.

Abnormalities of the caudal portions of the skull are referred to as forms of occipital dysplasia. These caudal skull and foramen magnum abnormalities are commonly found in smaller breeds of dogs such as poodles, Pomeranians, and Chihuahuas. The clinical consequences of this anatomical abnormality have been debatable. These types of defects, however, may be associated with spinal cord abnormalities such as syringomyelia and hydromyelia. Whether the relationship between these types of abnormalities is cause and effect or serendipitous is not known. Radiographic studies of the foramen magnum, such as using an open-mouth rostral-caudal view, can show the bony appearance of the foramen magnum.

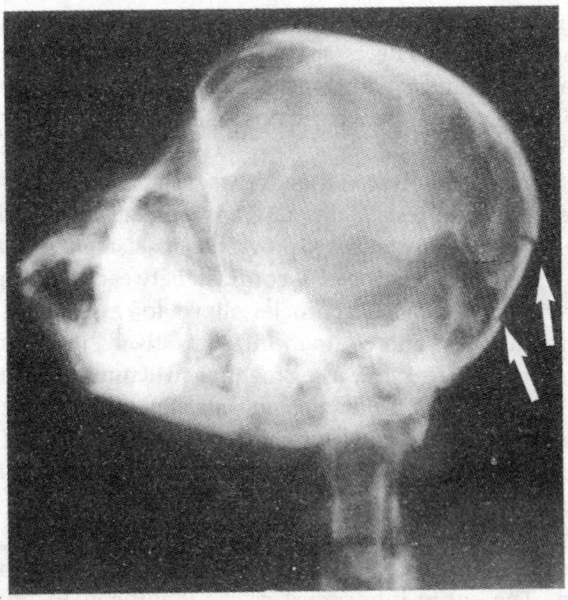

Fig. 9.1. Skull radiograph from a young dog with a fracture (*arrows*).

Ultrasound. Ultrasonographic evaluation of the intracranial structures is possible in some selected situations (fig. 9.2) (Gallagher et al. 1995; Tucker et al. 1996). As the ultrasonic waves are impeded by bone, the overlying skull makes routine diagnostic ultrasonographic imaging of the

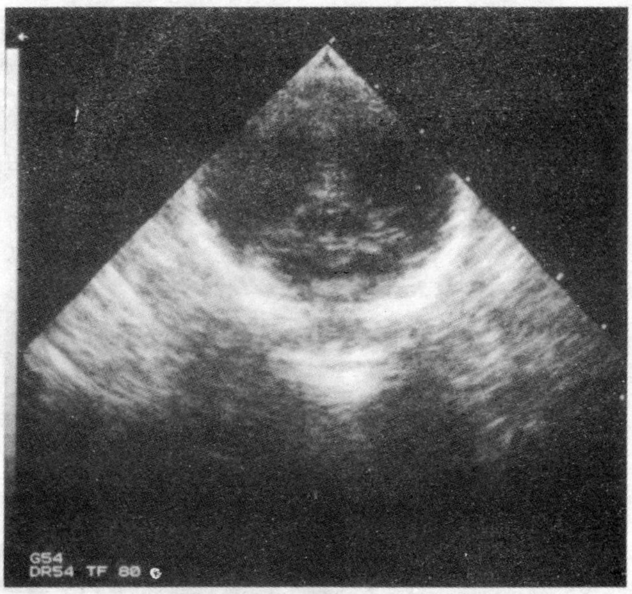

Fig. 9.2. Ultrasonic image of the brain of a dog.

brain difficult. Therefore, bone removal, for example, at the time of surgery is necessary to obtain a diagnostic quality image. In animals with fontanels, ultrasound imaging of the brain can be performed through these natural skull openings.

Ultrasonography has the advantage of being a noninvasive diagnostic test. Ultrasonographic imaging has been used in selected instances to provide an assessment of brain structure. Specifically, the contrast between the brain parenchyma and the ventricles allows for assessment of ventricular size and contour. Intraoperatively, ultrasound can provide a real time assessment of structures below the surface of the brain allowing more accurate surgical dissection. Intraparenchymal tumors often are hyperechoic to normal brain tissue. Cystic structures and those containing fluid cavities may show up as hypoechoic.

Disadvantages of ultrasonography for assessment of intracranial tissues center around image quality and resolution. The entire intracranial cavity is difficult to image through a relatively small fontanel, and resolution through all levels of the image is relatively poor compared to advanced imaging studies such as MR imaging. As ultrasound waves do not penetrate bone, ultrasonic imaging of the brain can only be formed through natural skull opening, fontanels, or following surgical skull removal (craniectomy or craniotomy).

Doppler imaging, conversely, can be performed even through the intact skull in animals. This technique is referred to as transcranial Doppler (TCD) imaging (fig. 9.3) (Bagley, Tucker et al. 1997). This ultrasonic technique is most useful in evaluation of cerebral blood flow. Doppler signal can be obtained across the intact skull through the relatively thinner (ventral) portions of the temporal bone (temporal window) and through the foramen magnum. Through the temporal window, blood flow in the circle of Willis and its associated branches can be evaluated. Flow in the middle cerebral artery is most consistently recorded. Through the foramen magnum, flow in the vertebral and basilar arteries can be recorded. Unfortunately, the range of normal flow velocities for dogs has not been well established and data have been taken primarily from dogs in experimental settings under controlled physiologic conditions. Spontaneously occurring abnormalities of cerebral blood flow still require clarification with Doppler evaluations.

Scintigraphy. Prior to advanced imaging modalities such as MR, nuclear medicine (gamma scintigraphy) was used for diagnostic brain imaging in animals (fig. 9.4) (Daniel et al. 1992; Dykes et al. 1994; Tucker 1996). This imaging modality is based on changes in uptake of a radiopharmaceutical within the brain following intravenous administration of a radiopharmaceutical. Areas where the injected radiopharmaceutical accumulates outside the vascular system are assessed. As the blood-brain barrier (BBB) normally is responsible for preventing certain molecules from leaving the vascular system and entering the brain, accumulation of the radiopharmaceutical is indicative of a loss of the integrity of the BBB in the affected area. Scintigraphic evaluations result in an anatomically crude image of the intracranial structures and associated disease. Disadvantages to this imaging modality are the use of radiopharmaceuticals and associated radiation concerns, and the poor overall anatomical image quality. Also, as not all intracranial disease results in a breakdown of the BBB, many intracranial disease processes are not apparent with this imaging modality. These limitations are significant enough that routine neuroscintigraphy has largely been replaced with CT and MR imaging in the modern era evaluation of structural intracranial disease in animals.

Single photon emission computed tomography (SPECT) and positron emission tomography (PET) are tomographic neuroscintigraphy imaging modalities that pro-

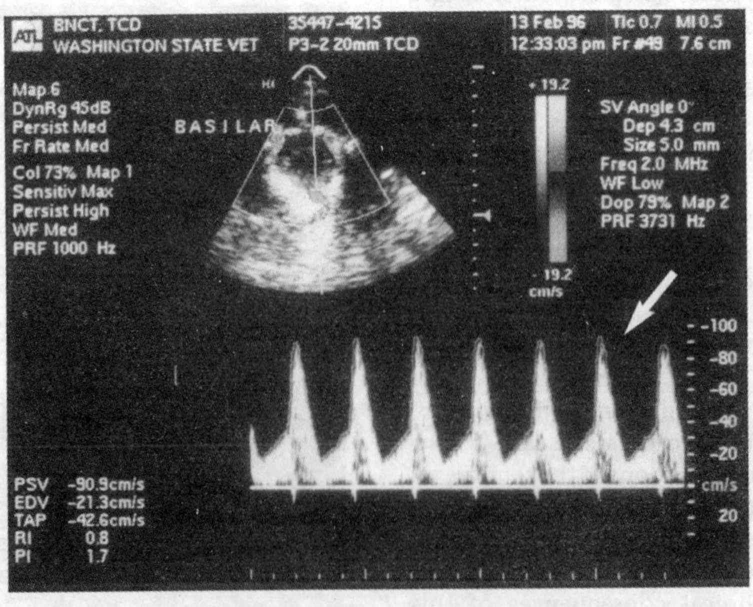

Fig. 9.3. Transcranial Doppler assessment of intracranial blood flow in the basilar artery (*arrow*).

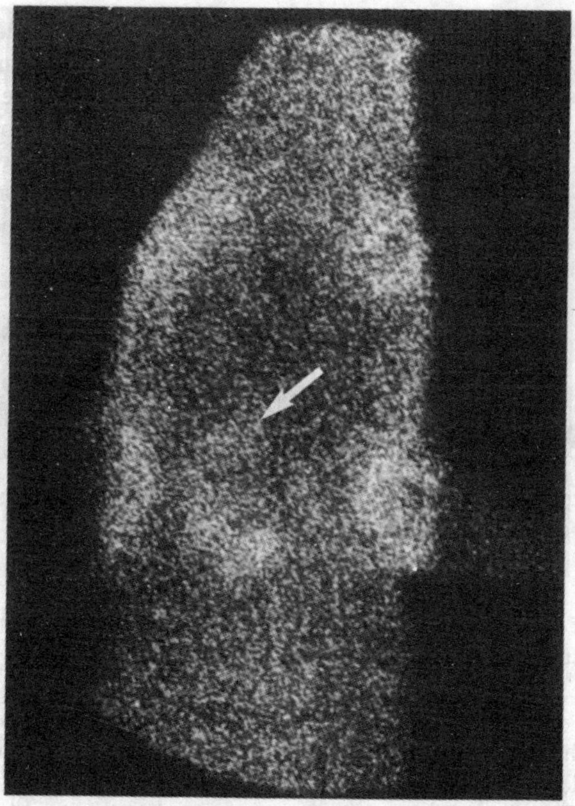

Fig. 9.4. Dorsal view brain scintigraphic image of a dog with a brain hemorrhage (*arrow*).

vide multiple image projections summed to generate cross sectional images of the brain (Tucker et al. 1996). SPECT can be performed so that only information from the brain and not peripheral tissues is assessed. Similar to routine neuroscintigraphy, intracranial lesions that disrupt the BBB are primarily evaluated.

PET scanning has utility in assessment of functional activity as compared to anatomical information in the brain. This imaging may be helpful by determining physiologic changes associated with intracranial diseases. Areas of abnormal cellular metabolism may be identified. These abnormal areas may be associated with seizure or ischemic foci. Unfortunately, PET scanning is not routinely available for clinical evaluation in animals.

Computed Tomography (CT). Computed tomography revolutionized both human and veterinary neurology in the 1970s and 1980s, and continues to be an important diagnostic tool in assessment of the central nervous system and associated structures. With CT, information is collected from the relative penetration of a number of X-ray beams projected in a circumferential manner around the head (or other body part) (Berry 2002). These individual pieces of information are then arranged through computer data processing to form a two-dimensional image of structures within the cranial cavity or spine. The images can be reformatted in differing planes corresponding to major anatomical planes (i.e., sagittal, transverse, dorsal).

When interpreting information from the advanced imaging modalities (CT or MR imaging), knowledge of cross-sectional and planar anatomy is very helpful (see also appendix 1). This knowledge aids in correlating information seen with the suspected area of dysfunction based on clinical examination. As it is common to find anatomical imaging abnormalities that may not result in clinical signs, interpretation of anatomical findings generated with these types of imaging modalities is correlated with clinical abnormalities found during examination.

When evaluating CT (or MR) images of the central nervous system, the most important characteristic to look for is symmetry. For example, a mass on one side of the brain may impinge on the ipsilateral lateral ventricle, causing collapse of that ventricle. A shift of structures from their normal anatomic location due to a space-occupying mass within the intracranial space is often referred to as a *mass effect*.

On a CT image, just as with a radiograph, black colors are associated with tissue such as air or fluid. Nervous and other soft tissues appear as varying shades of gray with bone appearing whiter in color. The relative color of the image is dependent on its CT number (a relative representation of tissue density). Tissues are represented on a scale ranging from +1000 to -1000 Hounsfield units (HU). Tissues of varying densities are shown in table 9.3.

A finite scale of CT HU values within this +1000 to -1000 range can be chosen to be viewed in order to highlight certain structures more than others. For example, if information is needed regarding bone integrity, the viewing scale could be adjusted to concentrate more in the higher CT numbers closer to those associated with bone density. In this example, CT viewing would be referred to as a "bone window." The outline and integrity of the bone are more easily viewed; however, the contrast between other soft tissues is less distinct.

With CT, tissues seen on the image can be assessed as being isodense (same color as a reference brain tissue), hyperdense (whiter than brain tissue), and hypodense (blacker than brain tissue) on either the pre- or postcontrast scan. Depending upon the quality of the scan, a reference soft tissue such as the brain (i.e., grey matter compared to white matter) can be used for comparison. Areas in the brain that are hyperdense (whiter) than normal brain parenchyma on the image prior to administering any exogenous contrast agent include mineralization (i.e., mineralized tumor) or hemorrhage. Areas that are hypodense

Table 9.3. Approximate CT numbers of differing tissues

Tissue	CT number	Relative color
Bone	+1000	White
Blood	+100	
Brain matter	+30	Grey
CSF	+5	
Water	0	
Fat	−100	
Air	−1000	Black

(blacker) compared to normal brain parenchyma generally contain increased fluid (i.e., edema). Normal brain grey matter has a HU value between 25 and 50 compared to white matter, which is 20–35. Cerebrospinal fluid is in the range of 0–15, and fat is around -100. Edema within brain tissue, because of the increased water content, is ~10–20 HU. Solid tumors are usually >45, heterogenous tumors range from 15 to 45, and tumors with necrosis or edema are between 20 and 45. Flowing blood has an HU value of 20–50. Hemorrhage, depending on whether acute or chronic, will vary from near 0 to greater than 80 HU.

A series of CT images are performed before and after intravenous injection of an iodinated contrast material. Abnormalities disrupting the blood-brain barrier (BBB) may become more apparent with this technique. Loss of integrity of the BBB or increased vascularity may result in an area of increased whiteness ("enhancement") after intravenous contrast enhancement. Contrast enhancement is most often seen with tumors, vascular abnormalities, and inflammatory foci.

The major advantage of both CT and MR imaging techniques is the ability to noninvasively view structures deep to the surface of the body (fig. 9.5, 9.6, 9.7). Advantages of CT imaging include the ability to image in planes giving a spatial orientation to abnormalities seen. Computed tomography is an ideal imaging modality for evaluation of abnormalities of the bone within the vertebrae or skull. Disadvantages of CT include the use of ionizing radiation (radiation exposure), the need for general anesthesia, and its sometimes poor definition of intracranial abnormalities, especially those in the posterior fossa. Artifacts in this area due to the larger mass of bone are present as linear hypodense stripes referred to as beam-hardening artifact. These artifacts can easily obscure relatively small lesions in the posterior fossa in animals. Spatial resolution, especially for small animals like cats, may not be adequate to determine small (<5 mm) lesions.

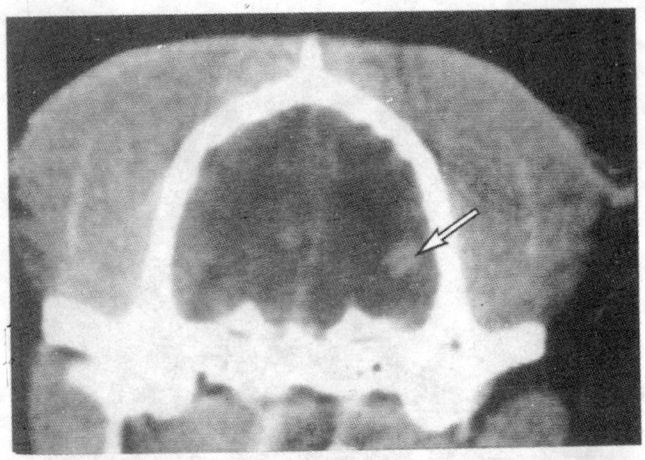

Fig. 9.5. Computed tomographic image from the brain of a dog with an intracranial hemorrhage (*arrow*).

Magnetic Resonance (MR) Imaging. The use of MR imaging has revolutionized the diagnosis of animals with neurologic disease. As this imaging modality was originally developed for use in human medicine, access to these modalities for diagnostic imaging in animals has been an historical stumbling block. Access to MR imaging, however, is becoming less of an obstacle as more MR imaging facilities dedicated to imaging animals are being established. The sophisticated and expensive equipment required for MR is now available in many veterinary teaching institutions and referral centers, and is also found in private practice situations. Other general practices often utilize the facilities of human hospitals or various mobile MR imaging facilities.

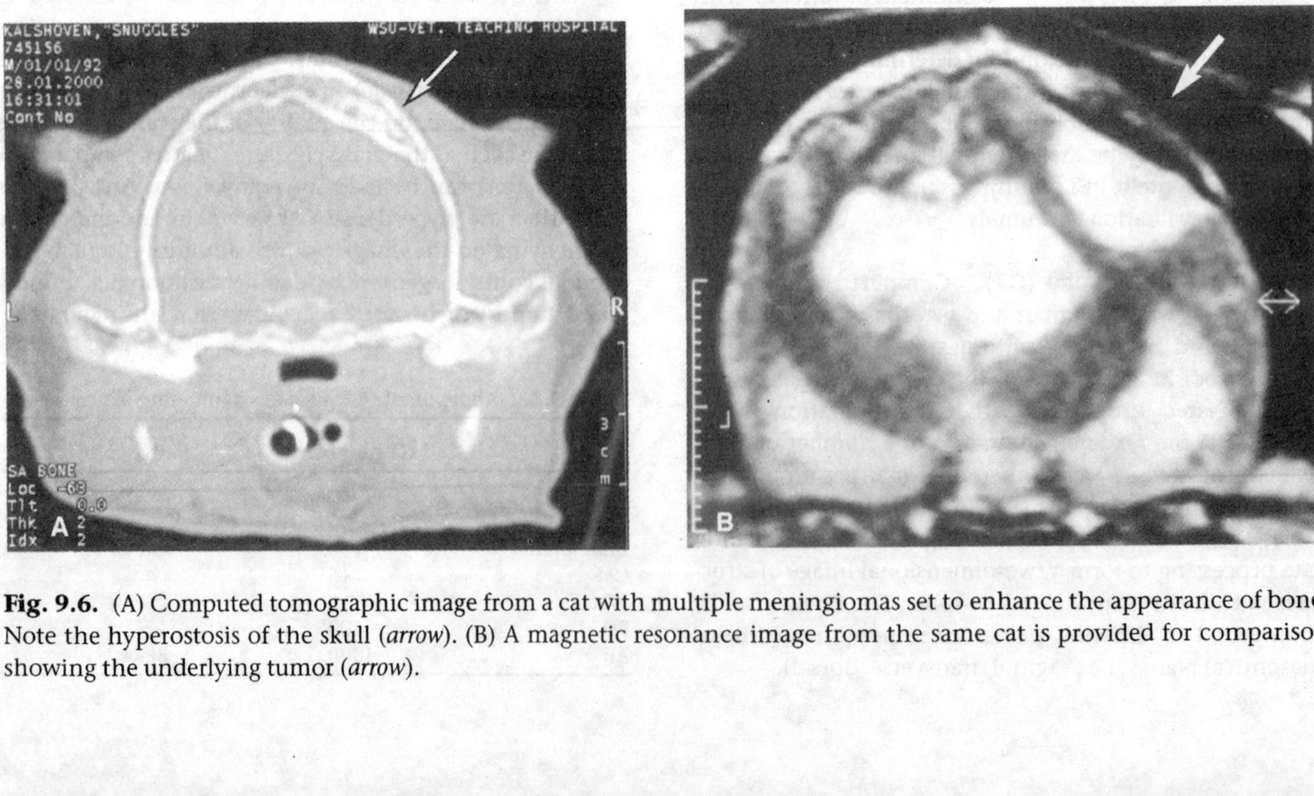

Fig. 9.6. (A) Computed tomographic image from a cat with multiple meningiomas set to enhance the appearance of bone. Note the hyperostosis of the skull (*arrow*). (B) A magnetic resonance image from the same cat is provided for comparison showing the underlying tumor (*arrow*).

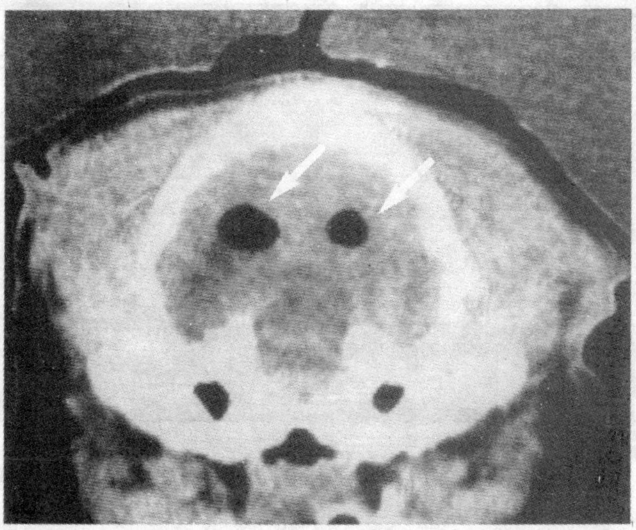

Fig. 9.7. Computed tomographic image from the brain of a dog with air in the lateral ventricles following head trauma (*arrows*).

Similar to CT imaging, MR imaging is a noninvasive anatomical imaging modality. Unlike CT, MR imaging does not require ionizing radiation. The physical principles associated with MR imaging are complex and have been reviewed (Berry 2002). An MR image represents the response of various nuclei to absorb radio frequency energy. Magnetic resonance relies on the magnetic environment of cellular nuclei. Currently, magnetic properties of hydrogen nuclei (which consist of one proton) are used most commonly to produce medical magnetic resonance images. The MR properties of body tissues may result in various degrees of signal intensity. Images are commonly produced with colors on a black/white/gray scale.

All soft tissues are usually visualized with MR imaging. The appearance of a tissue type is described as hypointense (blacker), hyperintense (whiter), or isointense (the same color) relative to some reference tissue. Dense bone and air, for example, lack MR signal due to the inability of the protons to relax (change energy states) in the dense bone matrix. These tissues appear black on MR imaging. In air there is a relative lack of hydrogen nuclei from which a signal can be produced. All other structures appear as various shades of grey to bright white due to signal intensity variations.

Numerous excitation and detection sequences are available. The various sequences provide images of the proton density, and the two basic forms of relaxation, named longitudinal (T1) and transverse (T2). The most commonly used imaging sequence to date has been a spin-echo sequence yielding a proton density and a T2-weighted image followed by T1-weighted sequence before and following the administration of a paramagnetic contrast agent. The most commonly used contrast agent to date utilizes the paramagnetic material gadolinium (Gd) in the form of Gd-DTPA. This paramagnetic material does not pass the intact blood-brain barrier (BBB), and, therefore, the only enhanced areas in the normal brain are those that lack a blood-brain barrier including the pituitary and choroid plexus. Most diseases of the central nervous system (CNS) disrupt the BBB resulting in a hyperintense (whiter) signal intensity in the presence of the contrast agent.

Magnetic resonance imaging initially was used primarily for diagnosis of animals with intracranial disease. As compared to CT scanning, MR provides superior anatomical detail of the intracranial nervous system and associated structures, such as cranial nerves (fig. 9.8, 9.9, 9.10, 9.11). A variety of structural intracranial diseases is readily apparent with MR imaging. This includes brain tumors, hemorrhage, hydrocephalus, infarctions, and encephalitis. The spinal cord is also readily imaged with MR techniques.

As with all anatomical diagnostic tests, it is important to have knowledge of the appearance of the neuroanatomical

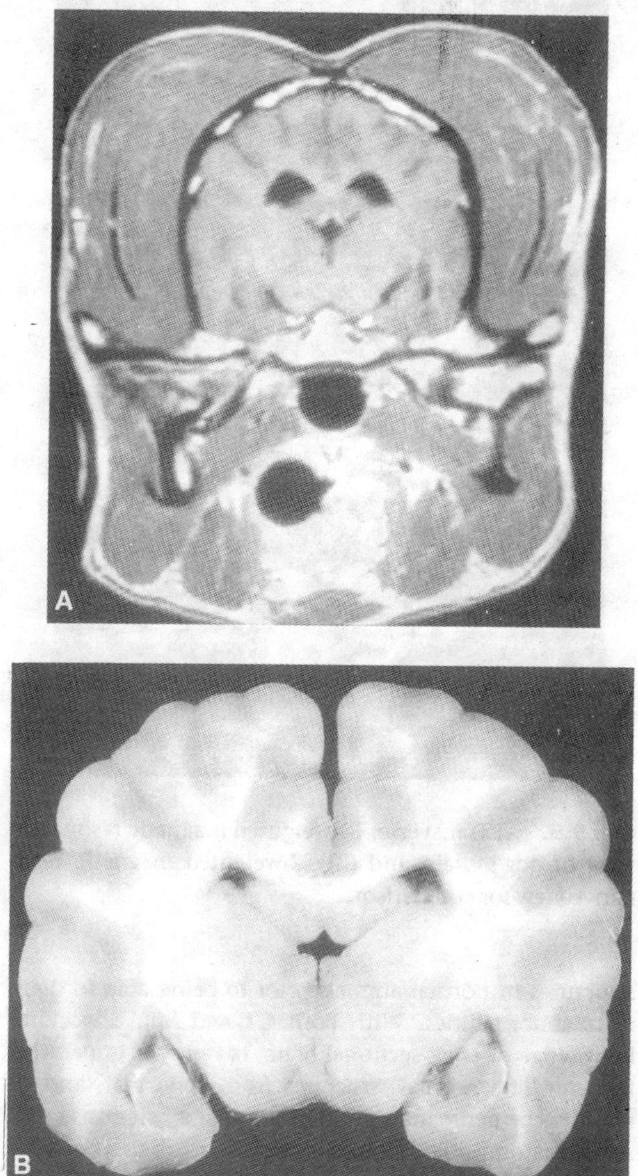

Fig. 9.8. (A) Transverse, T1-weighted magnetic resonance view of dog's brain. (B) An anatomical specimen at the same level is provided for comparison.

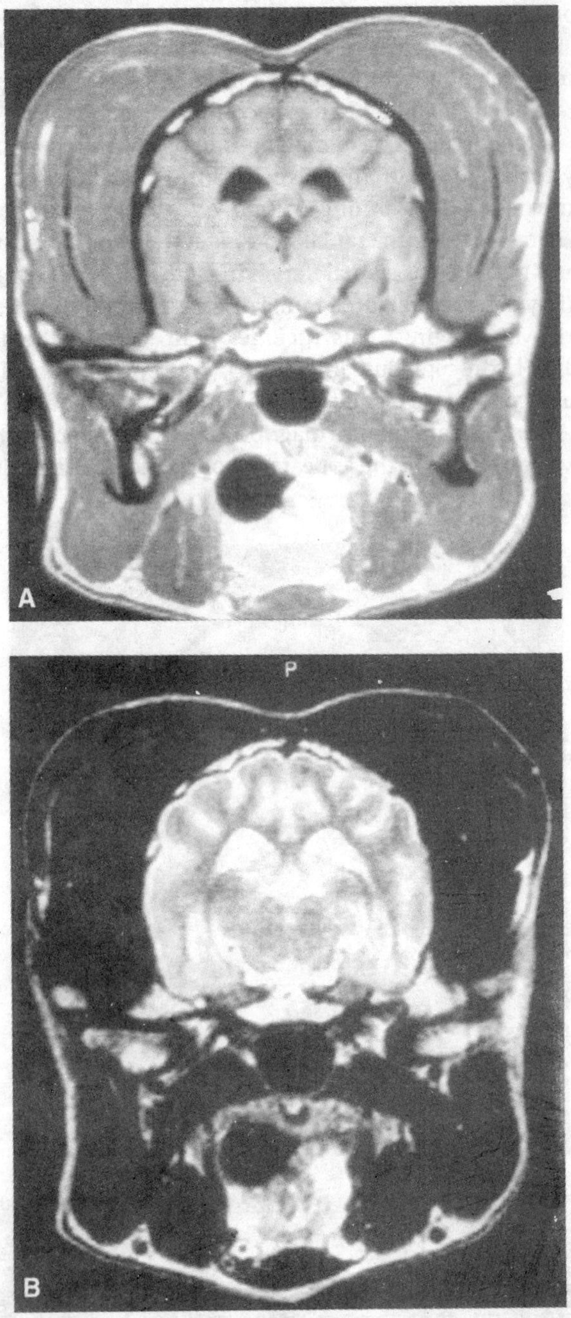

Fig. 9.9. (A) Transverse, T1-weighted magnetic resonance view of dog's brain and (B) T2-weighted magnetic resonance view for comparison.

structures in normal animals prior to being able to diagnose abnormalities. With both CT and MR, a working knowledge of cross-sectional brain anatomy is imperative to determine normal structures from abnormal, and to identify the neuroanatomical location of any lesions seen. A MR anatomy atlas is found in appendix 1 of this book for comparison of the MR appearance of the gross brain compared with the MR appearance of the brain.

Similar to CT, MR diagnoses are based on imaging features such as mass effect, displacement and disruption of normal structures, and abnormally contrast-enhanced

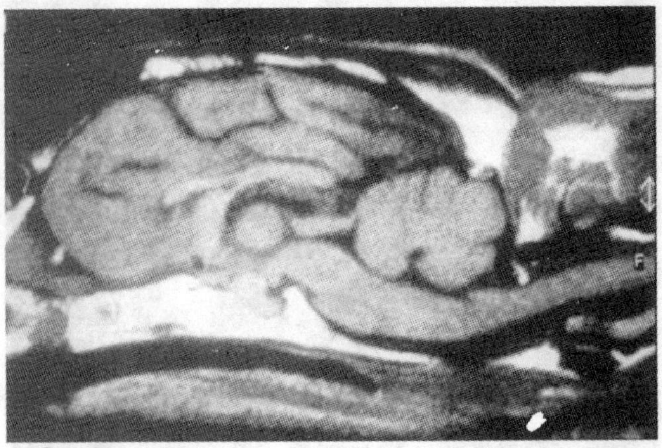

Fig. 9.10. Sagittal, T1-weighted MR image of the brain of a dog.

areas. Loss of symmetry, changes in signal intensity, and displacement of normal structures are extremely helpful in arriving at a diagnosis. The improved resolution afforded by MR imaging often allows for a determination of whether lesions are inside (intra-) or outside (extra-) the axis (axial) of the nervous system parenchyma. The location of a lesion helps determine potential tissues of origin, as does the shape of the lesion and characteristics of its edges. In general, signal intensity is increased (hyperintense or whiter) in or around brain tumors, especially on the T2-weighted images. Depending on the image sequence, however, tumors may be hypointense (blacker), isointense (the same intensity as the reference tissue), hyperintense (whiter), or of a heterogeneous (regions of either hypo-, hyper-, or isointensity) character as compared to normal surrounding tissue. Because nonneoplastic lesions can mimic the appearance of tumors, biopsy of the abnormal tissue is often required for determination of appropriate therapy. Specific MR imaging features and abnormalities associated with diseases of the brain and the spinal cord are discussed further in chapters 10 and 11, respectively.

Additional MR imaging sequences have been developed that allow cerebral vessels (angiography) to be imaged without the use of any exogenously administered contrast material (fig. 9.13). Assessments of arterial and venous structures can be obtained with this technique.

Imaging artifacts occur with MR and need to be recognized to avoid inadvertent misdiagnosis of these artifacts as pathological processes (fig. 9.14). The main causes of artifacts in images of the CNS are generally motion and deformations in the magnetic field from implanted metallic objects. Since the time required for MR studies is 10 to 60 minutes, general anesthesia must be utilized to avoid animal movement during the study sequences. Occasionally, animals have implanted metallic objects that are ferromagnetic enough to perturb the image field. Microchips and other steel objects (BB pellets) can create artifacts with MR that affect image quality.

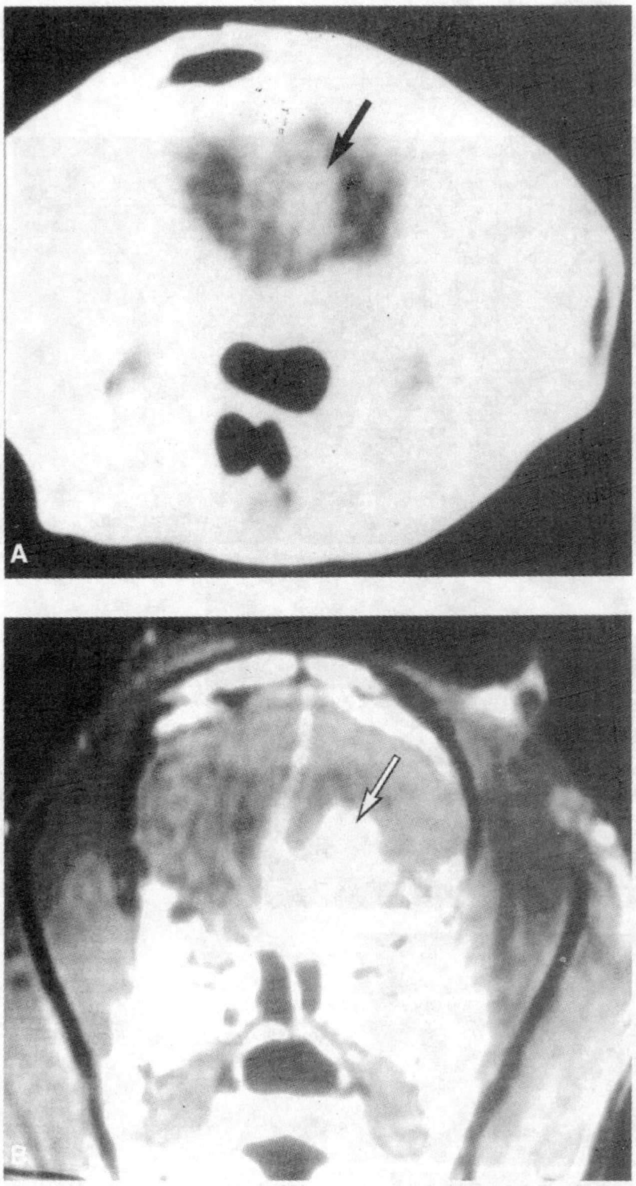

Fig. 9.11. (A) Computed tomographic and (B) magnetic resonance image at approximately the same level of a cat with a brain tumor (*arrows*).

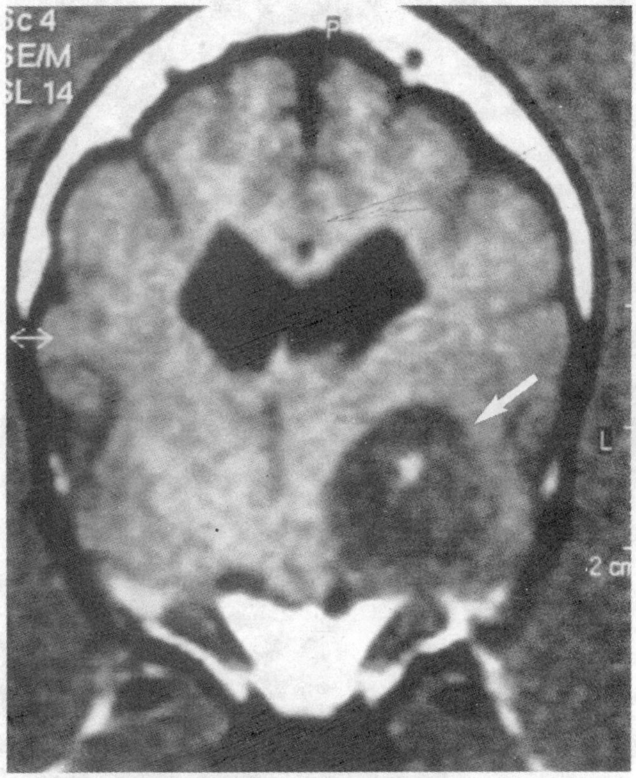

Fig. 9.12. Transverse, T1-weighted MR image from a dog with a glioma (*arrow*).

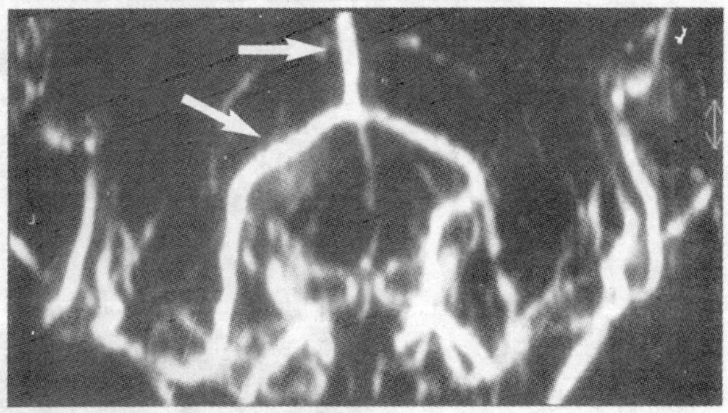

Fig. 9.13. Magnetic resonance angiogram of the cerebral venous system (caudal view). Note the dorsal sagittal and transverse venous sinuses (*arrows*).

CEREBROSPINAL FLUID COLLECTION AND ANALYSIS IN DOGS AND CATS

Cerebrospinal fluid (CSF) collection and analysis is often performed as a component of diagnostic evaluation of animals with neurologic disease. CSF analysis can contribute to the antemortem understanding of many disease processes affecting the central nervous system.

Cerebrospinal Fluid Collection

For CSF collection, anesthesia is necessary in all but the comatose animal as this is a painful procedure (Bagley 2003b). Even some animals not overtly responsive to external stimuli will move or twitch when the needle is advanced through skin, subcutaneous tissues, muscles, or the dura. Anesthesia is usually only for a short duration of time for CSF collection unless additional diagnostics are to be performed concurrently. If a cisterna magna collection is to be attempted, tracheal intubation is necessary to avoid obstruction of the airways during positioning of the head. Intubation is recommended for all animals with potential neurologic disease to maintain control of breathing if necessary.

Cerebrospinal fluid collection may be detrimental in animals that may have increased intracranial pressure, however, this clinical observation is debatable (Speciale et al. 1995). If CSF collection is deemed necessary in such animals, attempts to lower or stabilize intracranial pressure by

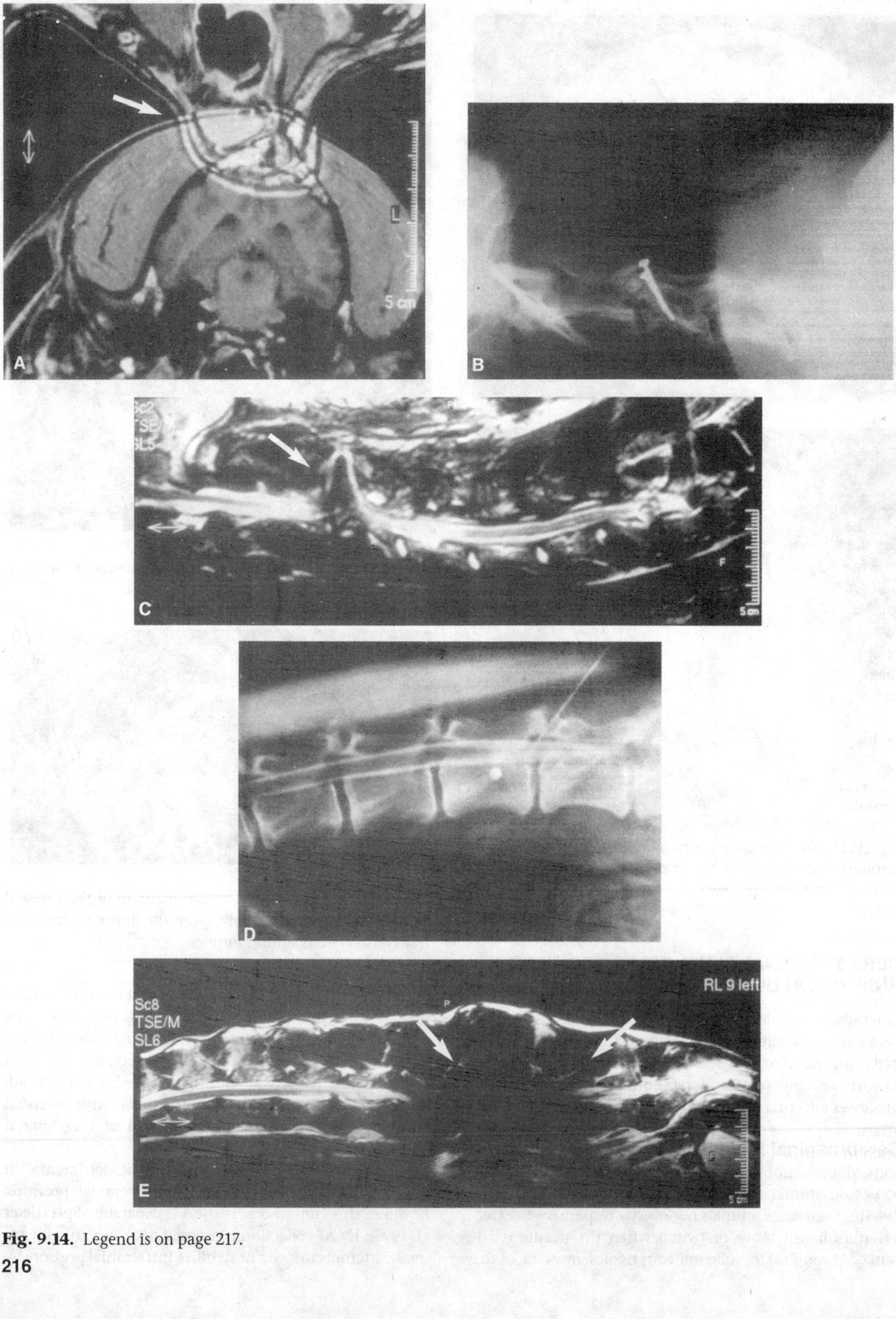

Fig. 9.14. Legend is on page 217.

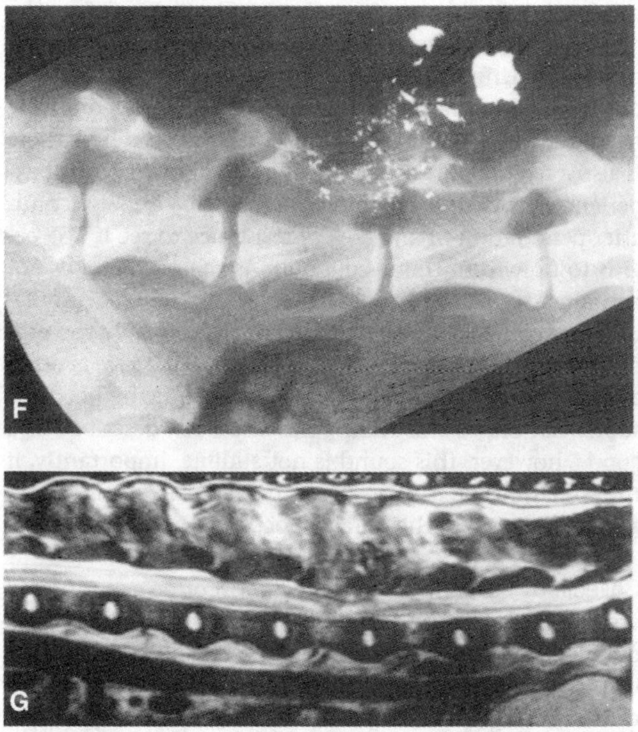

Fig. 9.14. Transverse, T1-weighted MR images from a dog showing (A) a wrapping artifact (*arrow*). (B) Lateral survey radiograph and (C) sagittal, T2-weighted MR image from a dog with metal implants in the cervical vertebrae. Note the distortion of the image (*arrow*). (D) Lumbar survey radiograph from a dog with a BB shot. (E) On the sagittal MR image, note the distortion of the image (*arrows*). (F) Lumbar survey radiograph from a dog with a lead gun shot injury. (G) On the sagittal MR image, note the lack of distortion of the image.

administering diuretics (mannitol 0.25 to 1 gram/kg IV bolus; furosemide 0.7 mg/kg IV bolus), maintaining systemic blood pressure, and preventing hypercapnia are important.

Cisterna Magna CSF Collection. Cerebrospinal fluid can be collected from two main areas in dogs and cats: the cisterna magna and the lumbar spinal cord area. The cisterna magna is a dilated area of the subarachnoid space found dorsal to the caudal brain stem and cranial cervical spinal cord at the level between the foramen magnum and the dorsal arch of the first cervical vertebrae. For collection of CSF in this area, the animal is anesthetized and placed in a lateral recumbent position on a flat, stable surface such as a table or gurney (fig. 9.15). Tabletops with a slight concave surface may result in subtle malposition of the animal, which may make CSF collection more difficult. The animal can be placed in either a right or left lateral recumbent position depending upon the preference of the collector.

A square-shaped area over the foramen magnum area is shaved and surgically scrubbed. The size of the shaved area varies depending upon preference; however, a reasonable

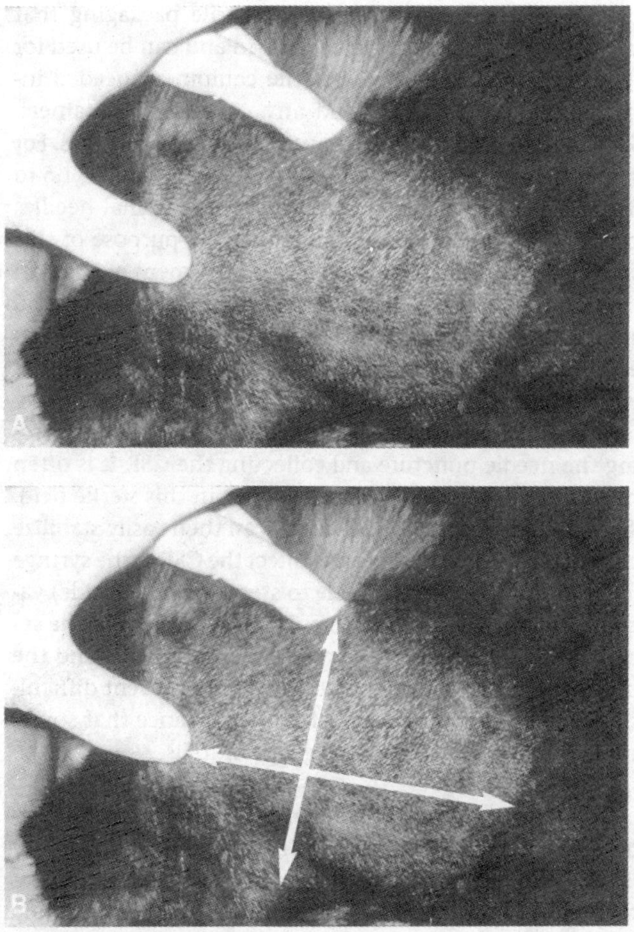

Fig. 9.15. (A) View of a dog in lateral recumbency in preparation for a cisterna magnum CSF collection. (B) Landmarks (*arrows*) for cisterna magnum CSF collection.

length extends hair removal from approximately 2 cm rostral to the external occipital protuberance to approximately 2 cm caudal to the cranial aspect of the wings of C1. In a lateral dimension, the hair is removal from the base of ear medially on either side. Surprisingly, clipping the hair off-centered can create enough of a visual illusion to make landmark determination and subsequent collection of CSF difficult. Once the hair is removed, the area is surgically scrubbed as for any sterile procedure.

The animal is then positioned so that an imaginary plane drawn sagittally from the bridge of the nose through the external occipital protuberance and caudally to the dorsal spinous process of C2 is parallel with the surface of the table. The bridge of the nose is then flexed ventrally toward the xyphoid process of the sternum; an imaginary line traveling transversely along the cranial aspect of the wings of C1 forms a 90° angle with the line draw sagittally along the dorsal spinous process of C2. A person holding the animal in this position most easily stands across the table (i.e., on the sternal side of the animal) from the person collecting the sample.

Once the animal is in the appropriate position, the sterile field, which contains the equipment necessary for CSF collection, is prepared. The inner sterile packaging that contains the surgical gloves is opened and can be used for this sterile field. Additional sterile equipment needed includes the spinal needle and any collection containers. Spinal needles are available in various sizes and gauges. For small animal CSF collection, 20 to 22 gauge needles, 1.5 to 3 cm in length, are most commonly used. Spinal needles contain an appropriately sized stylet. The purpose of this stylet is to prevent laceration and displacement of the skin inward as the needle is advanced into the subarachnoid space. There is the potential for growth of displaced skin elements in the subarachnoid space resulting in dermoid or epidermoid abnormalities.

If a single individual (i.e., no assistant) is to be performing the needle puncture and collecting the CSF, it is often helpful to include a sterile 3 cc syringe in this sterile field. The collector, once CSF is flowing, can then easily stabilize the needle with one hand and collect the CSF in the syringe for later transfer of the sample to sterile (on the inside) vacutainers or similar containers. The plunger seal of the syringe should be broken down between the casing and the barrel of the syringe prior to collection to prevent difficulties encountered due to the plunger resistance that sometimes is present in sterile syringes prior to use.

Landmarks for Needle Insertion. The landmarks for needle insertion are next defined. In general, two imaginary lines that bisect at 90° angles are determined over the foramen magnum area (fig. 9.15). One line is drawn on midline from the external occipital protuberance to the dorsal spinous process of C2. The second line is drawn between the cranial borders of the wings of C1 and perpendicular to the first line. The needle is inserted approximately 2 to 4 mm cranial to the point where these lines bisect and is directed caudoventrally toward the ramus of the mandible.

It is important to keep the needle directed in the sagittal plane on midline to access the cisterna magna. It is often helpful in maintaining this orientation during needle puncture and advancement for the person collecting the sample to kneel on the floor so that the point of needle insertion is at eye level for the collector. Importantly, the collector should be in a comfortable position to avoid any unnecessary distractions during collection. Foam knee rests, such as those a gardener would use, or a similar device placed in the floor helps in preventing knee pain during kneeling for prolonged periods. Additionally, if the CSF is to be collected by a single person, the equipment necessary for collection should be placed easily within arm's reach of the kneeling person. This is often facilitated by having a stool or stand available to rest a sterile field upon within arm's reach of the collector.

An appropriate-sized needle is chosen. For almost all dogs, even those with large heads and necks, a 22 g, 1 1/2 inch needle is the size of choice for CSF collection at the cisterna magna. Once the landmarks are defined, the collector will often rest one hand on the animal's head, keeping the fingers sterile while the skin is penetrated with the needle. As the stylet is no longer necessary after the skin has been traversed, it is removed from the needle at this point. The needle is then advanced cautiously toward the cisterna magna. Depending upon the sharpness of the needle, various fascial and muscle planes may be encountered during needle advancement. When the dura is encountered, there is also a feeling of resistance. It is a good practice, until experienced with the technique, to stop for a few seconds after penetration of any area of resistance to see if CSF begins to flow from the needle hub. As the needle does not contain a stylet at this point, if an area of fluid accumulation is encountered, it will usually freely flow from the needle. When the cisterna magna is penetrated, there is often a feeling of a "give and go" of the needle. If the needle is somewhat blunt, this feeling has also been described as a "pop," however, this sound is not audible. Importantly, if the spinal needle is very sharp, less resistance may be felt and penetration of the dura will occur with less force.

Collection. The three substances most often encountered during CSF collection at the cisterna magna are CSF, blood, or bone (fig. 9.16). If bone is encountered, and it is felt that this is the bone dorsal to the spinal cord area, the needle can be redirected in a sagittal plane either cranially or caudally in an attempt to enter the cisterna magna. If this is not successful after a few redirections, it is often best to remove the needle, reestablish the external landmarks, and try again. If the needle has not been contaminated by the procedure, the stylet can be replaced and the same needle used. If any concerns exist regarding sterility of the needle, it should be discarded and a sterile needle obtained.

If the needle is directed just lateral to the cisterna magna, free-flowing blood may accumulate in the needle hub. This blood is often from venous structures external to the dura, and, therefore, uncontaminated CSF can still be collected even following this situation. Of course, a new spinal needle should be used and new landmarks should be established.

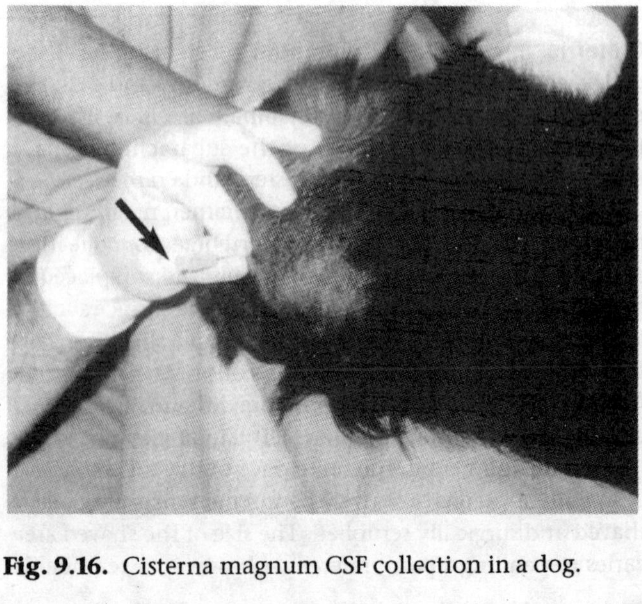

Fig. 9.16. Cisterna magnum CSF collection in a dog.

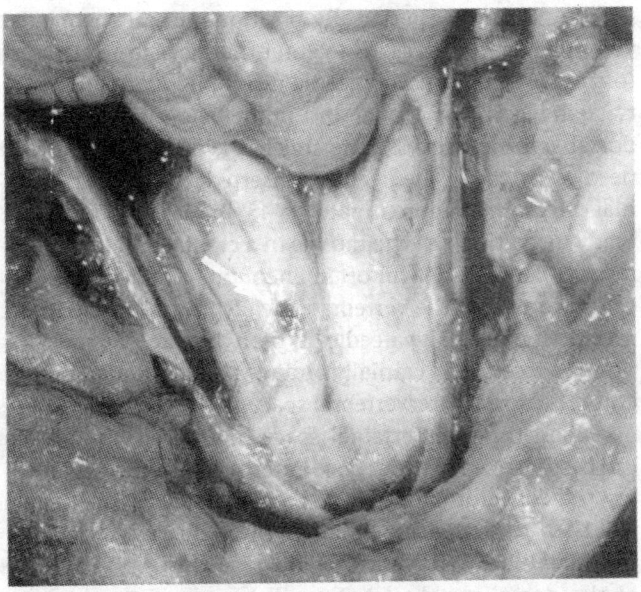

Fig. 9.17. Pathologic specimen showing needle penetration of the brain stem during CSF collection (*arrow*).

Obviously, if the dura is penetrated unknowingly and the needle is advanced too far ventrally, the underlying nervous system parenchyma can be damaged (fig. 9.17). After the "give and go" feeling is encountered, needle advancement is stopped, and, if successful, the CSF will begin freely flowing from the spinal needle. Drops of CSF can be aspirated into the syringe as they are produced. The syringe should not be attached to the spinal needle for aspiration to avoid either unintentional advancement of the needle into the neural tissue or aspiration of the neural tissue into the needle tip due the pressure produced by syringe aspiration. Cerebrospinal fluid will often continue to flow so that 2 to 3 cc of fluid can be collected from the cisterna magna. Depending upon the analysis methodology, as little as 0.5 cc of fluid is needed for routine (cytology and protein determination) analysis. The additional volumes collected are often necessary for further serological testing or culture of the CSF.

If the CSF is to be submitted to a commercial laboratory for analysis, the laboratory may have instructions regarding sample transport and storage. Cerebrospinal fluid submitted in a purple-top vacutainer is sometimes used to preserve cells for cytologic analysis. The Ca EDTA present in these tubes, however, may impede bacterial growth and therefore be an inadequate way to submit CSF for culture. If an adequate volume of CSF is obtained, the sample can be divided, with some being submitted in a purple-top vacutainer for routine analysis, and the remaining portion submitted in a sterile tube with preservative (red-top tube) for culture. If it will take 24 to 48 hours for the laboratory to obtain the CSF, serum may be mixed with a separate portion of the sample to preserve the integrity of the cells present. Obviously, however, this may affect subsequent CSF protein determinations.

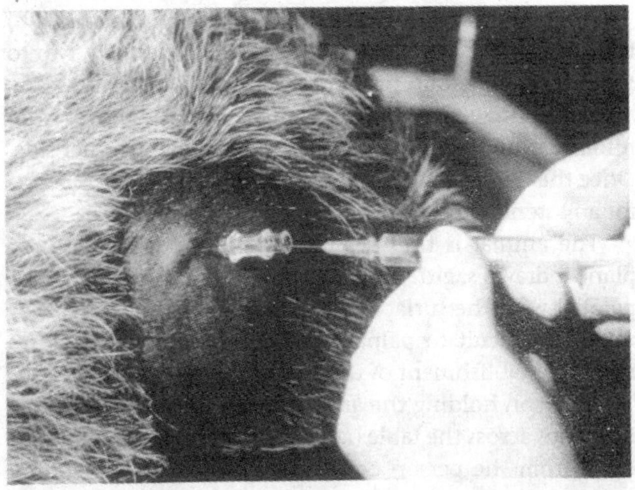

Fig. 9.18. Aspiration of CSF with a syringe following lumbar collection.

Lumbar CSF Collection. For many diseases of the central nervous system, especially those involving the spinal cord, collection of CSF from the lumbar area (i.e., caudal to the level of the lesion) is more likely to provide an accurate reflection of the disease process present (fig. 9.18) (Thomson et al. 1990). With spinal disease, if CSF is collected at the cisterna magna (essentially "above" the abnormality), the sample may not reflect the nature and extent of the disease present. There is information to suggest that CSF collected in the lumbar area accurately reflects disease in both the intracranial and spinal areas. In some instances, such as when mild inflammatory disease is present in the intracranial space, a cisterna magna CSF sample will reflect these changes while a lumbar sample will be normal. It is also suggested that lumbar collection of CSF may be less likely to result in brain herniation if there is significant increased intracranial pressure. This has not been definitively proven, and herniation can still occur with lumbar collection in animals with increased intracranial pressure. If the nervous system is damaged inadvertently through needle puncture, the clinical consequences are often more devastating if this occurs in the cisterna magna area. Bleeding subsequent to vessel laceration with the spinal needle can be substantial enough to cause clinically significant spinal cord compression.

For collection of CSF in the lumbar area, the animal is anesthetized, and placed in a lateral recumbent position on a flat, stable surface such as a table. Tabletops with a slight concave surface may result in subtle malposition of the animal that may make CSF collection more difficult. The animal can be placed in either a right or left lateral recumbent position depending upon the preference of the collector. Some prefer to perform lumbar CSF collection with the animal in sternal recumbency. When the pelvic limbs are extended and directed cranially, the size of the space dorsally between subsequent vertebrae in the lumbar region may be increased and allow for improved ease of entering the spinal canal with the needle.

A square-shaped region extending from 2 cm caudal to the cranial borders of the wings of ilium cranially two to four dorsal spinous processes is shaved and surgically scrubbed. In a lateral dimension, the hair is removal from midline to approximately 2 to 4 cm laterally on either side. Once the hair is removed, the area is surgically scrubbed as for any sterile procedure.

The animal is then positioned so that an imaginary plane is drawn sagittally along the dorsal spinous processes parallel with the surface of the table. In obese animals, if may be difficult to palpate the dorsal spinous processes making establishment of these landmarks difficult.

A person holding the animal in this position most easily stands across the table (i.e., on the sternal side of the animal) from the person collecting the sample. Depending upon the collector's preference, the pelvic limbs are held in a flexed position or, more commonly, extended cranially so that the caudal lumbar spine assumes a kyphotic position.

Once the animal is in the appropriate position, the sterile field is prepared, which contains the equipment necessary for CSF collection. The inner sterile packaging that contains the surgical gloves is opened and used for this sterile field. Additional sterile equipment needed includes the spinal needle and any additional collection containers. If a single individual (i.e., no assistant) is to be performing the needle puncture as well as collecting the CSF, it is often helpful to include a sterile 3 cc syringe in this sterile field. The collector, once CSF is flowing, can then easily stabilize the needle with one hand and collect the CSF in the syringe and later transfer the sample to sterile (on the inside) vacutainers or similar containers with the other. The plunger should be pulled down the barrel of the syringe prior to use to break any seal and prevent difficulties encountered due to the plunger resistance that sometimes is present in sterile syringes prior to use.

Importantly, the collector should be in a comfortable position to avoid any unnecessary distractions during collection. Foam knee rests, such as those a gardener would use, or a similar device placed in the floor helps in preventing knee pain during kneeling for prolonged periods. It is often easier, however, for the collector to sit on a stool at eye level with the lumbar spine. Additionally, if the CSF is to be collected by a single person, the equipment necessary for collection should be placed easily within arm's reach of the kneeling person. This is often facilitated by having a second stool or stand available to rest a sterile field upon.

Landmarks for Needle Insertion. The landmarks for needle insertion are next identified. In general, establishing imaginary lines that bisect at 90° angles are determined over the lumbar area. One line is drawn on midline connecting the dorsal spinous processes of the lumbar vertebrae. The cranial aspects of the wings of the ilium are palpated, and the first dorsal spinous process felt on midline is usually L6. The intervertebral space cranial to this area should be L5–6. The dorsal intervertebral space is slightly caudal but more medial than the point where the spinous process is palpated. Since the lamina of the cranial vertebrae is slightly more dorsally positioned than the caudal vertebrae, it is often easier to enter the space from a caudal to cranial direction. The needle is initially placed to penetrate the skin just caudal and immediately lateral to the dorsal spinous process. The stylet is kept in place during needle puncture. The needle is inserted in a caudal to cranial direction at approximately a 45° angle to midline and is advanced through the muscle in a cranial and medial direction. The needle will often encounter the dorsal aspect of the lamina of the vertebrae, ideally caudal to the intervertebral space. The needle is then "walked" or repositioned successively cranially and medially in an attempt to enter the dorsal intervertebral space.

When the intervertebral space in entered, the needle can be advanced without encountering bone, again providing the collector with a "give and go" feeling. The needle will then penetrate the dura and often be passed through the dural tube to the ventral epidural space, where the bone of the dorsal vertebral body will be encountered. Commonly, when the dura is entered, the animal will twitch or jump slightly.

The needle is then removed slightly (2 to 3 mm) so that the bevel will lie within the subarachnoid space. The stylet is removed, and CSF is then collected into a syringe or sterile container.

In some instances, due to excessive osteophytes or collapsed bone structure, the dorsal intervertebral space cannot be entered or significant resistance is encountered. The needle may have to be "drilled" through this bony tissue to enter the spinal canal. This is accomplished by aggressively twisting the needle in a rotational direction both clockwise and counterclockwise until the needle can be advanced. Obviously, if the collector is not sure of the location of the needle, this procedure may result in damage to other important structures in the immediate area. If significant resistance to needle advancement is still encountered, or if repeated attempts to enter the space are not successful, performing a lateral survey radiograph of the area may help in determining correct needle placement or direction. Additionally, when the needle is advanced into the epidural space, the venous sinus may be penetrated and result in excessive hemorrhage. If only hemorrhage is encountered during stylet removal, a reattempt at a CSF collection may be necessary. If the CSF is contaminated with some free-flowing hemorrhage, the CSF can be aspirated from the hub of the needle with a second syringe and hypodermic needle until this hemorrhage ceases. In some instance, turning the bevel of the needle may result in encountering a less-contaminated area of CSF. Blood-contaminated CSF may alter the CSF analysis results, however, it can often still be used for culture if indicated. In some instance, cytology of blood-contaminated CSF may reveal important data such as the presence of neoplastic cells.

After the appropriate samples have been collected, these are submitted for a cytologic evaluation, as well as a protein concentration determination. Additional testing, such as electrophoresis evaluation, may be performed in selected instances.

Analysis Techniques

CSF Sample Handling and Examination. Cerebrospinal fluid can be analyzed at many commercial and human hospital laboratories, but is occasionally analyzed in the private veterinary hospital (Bohn et al. 2003). In most instances, for the most consistent and accurate CSF assessments, it is recommended that CSF be analyzed in a commercial laboratory to avoid errors results from inappropriate sample processing. It is always a good practice to check with the laboratory that will perform the analysis about special handling and shipment protocols prior to CSF collection and sample submission. This avoids sample loss through improper handling.

Cerebrospinal fluid has historically been analyzed as soon after collection (within 30 minutes) as possible to ensure the integrity of the cellular elements present. Because of the low protein content of the sample, a delay in CSF analysis may result in rupture of the cells present, making accurate analysis difficult (Bienzle et al. 2000). If a sample cannot be analyzed within 30 minutes, it should be refrigerated or placed on ice until analysis. If there is to be a prolonged (i.e., >1 hour) delay in CSF analysis, a portion of the sample can be mixed with serum to preserve the integrity of the cells. Obviously, due to the addition of the serum, this portion of the CSF sample would yield inaccurate results if analyzed for protein content.

Analysis of CSF usually includes an assessment of the gross appearance of the sample, total protein concentration, total nucleated cell and erythrocyte counts, and cytological examination. Further testing can be performed to measure chemical constituents and protein fractions, detect specific antibodies or specific organisms using molecular techniques, or culture infectious agents.

Normal CSF. Normal CSF is colorless and clear. A reddish-colored sample may indicate recent hemorrhage, either reflecting hemorrhage into the subarachnoid space or iatrogenic hemorrhage at the time of sample collection. A yellowish sample may indicate previous hemorrhage in the subarachnoid space (xanthochromia) or icterus. A cloudy sample may indicate increases in cell numbers or protein content. Even a visually clear sample, however, may contain increases in nucleated cells and protein. Therefore, a subjectively clear sample cannot be automatically regarded as normal.

Total Nucleated Cell and Erythrocyte Counts. The number and type of cells present in CSF are important determinates of whether the sample is deemed normal or not. In addition to the total nucleated cell count, a cytological examination should be performed for differential cell counts and assessment of the sample for the presence of atypical cells. Common cell types seen include red blood cells, lymphocytes, monocytes, and neutrophils. Due to the relatively low numbers of cells in CSF even in disease processes, the cells need to be concentrated for most accurate assessment.

Protein Concentration and Electrophoresis. Normal CSF usually contains a relatively low amount of protein (normally approximately 200–400X less concentrated than serum). Evaluation of the different protein components of cerebrospinal fluid can also be measured. Since CSF albumin and globulin are somewhat proportional to concentrations in the blood, alterations in plasma albumin or globulin concentrations can be reflected in the CSF. Therefore, ratios have been developed to better assess albumin and globulin concentrations in CSF (Bichsel 1984; Chrisman 1992; Tipold et al. 1994).

$$\text{Albumin quotient} = \frac{\text{CSF albumin (mg/dl)}}{\text{Serum albumin (g/dl)} \times 10}$$

$$\text{IgG index} = \frac{\text{CSF IgG/serum IgG}}{\text{CSF albumin/serum albumin}}$$

Since albumin is exclusively of serum origin, an increase in the albumin quotient suggests that the blood-brain barrier has been disturbed. An increase in the IgG index is an indication that intrathecal production of immunoglobulins has occurred because of local antigenic stimulation.

Most chemical constituents of CSF other than protein can be measured using the same techniques that are used for serum. For concentrations of substances that are normally in equilibrium with serum concentrations (such as glucose), it is important to concurrently measure the concentration in serum for proper interpretation. Other chemical substances such as neurotransmitters may sometimes provide important clues to underlying central nervous system disease (Vaughn et al. 1988a, 1988b). In addition to the more routine CSF evaluations, culture of CSF and assessment for the presence of antibody titers are important if infectious nervous system disease is suspected. Aerobic, anaerobic bacterial, or fungal cultures may be indicated depending on clinical findings and results of CSF analysis. CSF collected in an EDTA tube, however, should not be used for culture, as EDTA is bacteriostatic.

Immunologic testing is available for many infectious agents, including viral, protozoal, fungal, and some bacterial organisms. CSF can be tested for antibodies to distemper, herpes, parainfluenza, adenoviruses, and parvoviruses. A serum sample should always be submitted along with the CSF. CSF can be tested for protozoal infections. CSF and serum should both be submitted when testing for immunoglobulins to *Toxoplasma* or *Neospora* organisms. It is best to measure both IgM and IgG antibodies to *Toxoplasma gondii*.

Interpretation of Routine Cerebrospinal Fluid Analysis. As with all diagnostic tests, the results of CSF evaluation should be interpreted in association with the clinical examination findings and results of additional diagnostic tests. In the modern era of advanced imaging studies such as MR imaging for neurologic diagnosis, CSF has a limited utility due to its relative sensitivity and nonspecific changes in the presence of disease. While CSF may yield abnormal results in central nervous system disease processes, often these results are not pathognomonic for a specific neurologic disease. Additionally, CSF evaluations may be normal even in the presence of significant structural nervous system abnormalities.

Normal CSF contains no red blood cells. It is common, however, to introduce a small amount of blood contamination to the sample at the time of collection (Chrisman 1992; Chrisman 1983; Cook and DeNicola 1988; deLahunta 1983; Hoerlein 1978; Jamison and Lumsden 1988; Kornegay 1981; Mayhew and Beal 1980; Parker 1972; Vandevelde and Spano 1977). A minimal amount of blood contamination that is not visibly detectable usually is associated with the presence of 50 to 500 RBCs/μl when the sample is analyzed. These relatively minimal amounts of iatrogenic blood contamination (<500 RBCs/μl) are expected at the time of sample collection and while absolute correlations are not established, iatrogenic red blood cell contamination of less that 500 cells/μl usually does not hinder interpretation of associated nucleated cell counts and protein concentrations. In normal cats, blood contamination of CSF in the range of 500 to 1700 RBCs/μl results in increases of CSF WBC counts up to 15 WBC/μl (Rand 1990). Obviously, some assessment of suspected iatrogenic blood contamination can be made and should be recorded at the time of CSF collection. As no accurate correction formula exists for determination of the degree of increased nucleated cells and protein concentration present from iatrogenic hemorrhage at time of collection, the clinician is forced to interpret blood contaminated CSF results without objective limits for nucleated cell counts and protein concentration (Hurtt and Smith 1997; Wilson and Stevens 1977). A general rule of thumb used clinically is that approximately 700 red blood cells will result in an increase of one additional nucleated cell from contamination if the peripheral WBC count is normal, however, this association is variable and is often inconsistent (Adams 1989). In the presence of a systemic leukocytosis, neutrophilia, or elevated serum protein concentration, this rule of thumb may be invalid.

Red blood cells may also be present in CSF from spontaneous subarachnoid hemorrhage. Additionally, inflammation of the meninges may result in vascular engorgement of meningeal vessels with resultant increased meningeal hemorrhage as the needle penetrates and traverses the dura. This is especially true with some of the so-called steroid-responsive meningitis and spinal cord vasculitis syndromes (Meric et al. 1985; Meric 1988). When the CSF sample is collected during the acute phase of the disease (<12–24 hours in duration), a true hemorrhagic disease process may be difficult to separate from iatrogenic hemorrhage at sample collection. Xanthochromia of the supernatant of a centrifuged CSF sample and cytologic evidence of erythrophagocytosis would suggest the presence of hemorrhage in the CSF prior to CSF collection. Disease processes that result in rupture of spinal and meningeal vessels such as trauma, vascular disorders (infarction), and inflammation as well as primary bleeding disorders such as thrombocytopenias and coagulopathies may result in hemorrhage in the CSF.

Normal cell counts for nucleated cells or WBCs in CSF vary between laboratories and possibly among species. In general, nucleated cell counts from normal dogs are less than 5 to 6 nucleated cells/μl. In cats, normal nucleated cell counts are slightly lower (<3 nucleated cells/μl) (Rand et al. 1990). Slightly higher nucleated cell counts were found in cats with some evidence of blood contamination of the sample. In CSF from normal cats with <500 RBCs, no more than 2 nucleated cells were present. If, however, RBC counts were between 501 and 1700 RBCs, nucleated cells counts as high as 15 cells/μl were present (Rand et al. 1990). It would be reasonable to conclude from this information that a CSF sample from a cat with up to 1700 RBC/μl, nucleated cells counts greater than 15 cells/μl may indicate a CNS inflammatory process if the peripheral WBC count is normal.

Increases in nucleated cell counts above the expected normal range in CSF are useful in determining the presence of an associated meningeal, central nervous tissue, or proximal nerve root inflammatory process (fig. 9.19) (Chrisman 1992; Chrisman 1983; Cook and DeNicola 1988; deLahunta 1983; Hoerlein 1978; Jamison and Lumsden 1988; Kornegay 1981; Mayhew and Beal 1980; Parker 1972; Rand et al. 1990; Rand et al. 1994; Tipold 1995; Vandevelde and Spano 1977). No strong correlations exist between magnitude of nucleated cell count increase or the type of nucleated cell present and the disease process or prognosis. Additionally, as any disease process that effects the nervous tissues can result in a secondary inflammatory process, the presence of increased numbers of nucleated cells in CSF is not indicative of a primary inflammatory central nervous system disease. As an example, in instances of dogs with brain tumor, increases in CSF WBC counts have been found in up to 50% of these animals (Bailey and Higgins 1986; Carrillo et al. 1986). Cerebrospinal fluid analysis, if used alone for a diagnosis of the intracranial disease process in these dogs, would potentially be misinterpreted as being reflective of a primary meningitis or encephalitis. Elevations in CSF nucleated cell counts can be most accurately interpreted, therefore, as evidence of a central nervous inflammatory response occurring either primarily or secondarily to a variety of underlying central nervous system disease processes. Many diseases that affect the central nervous system, including trauma, tumor, infarction, hemorrhage, and primary encephalitis, may increase nucleated cell count in CSF. In some instances, only elevations in either protein concentration or nucleated cell counts can occur making etiologic diagnoses from routine CSF analysis difficult if not impossible. As an example, in a study of 30 dogs with distemper who had CSF evaluations, only 50% (15/30) had abnormal nucleated cell counts, whereas 83% (25/30) had elevations in protein concentrations (Thomas et al. 1993b).

The site of CSF collection relative to the location of the primary disease process may also influence the analysis results. While CSF may flow in both a cranial and caudal direction, there seems to be a predominant cranial to caudal

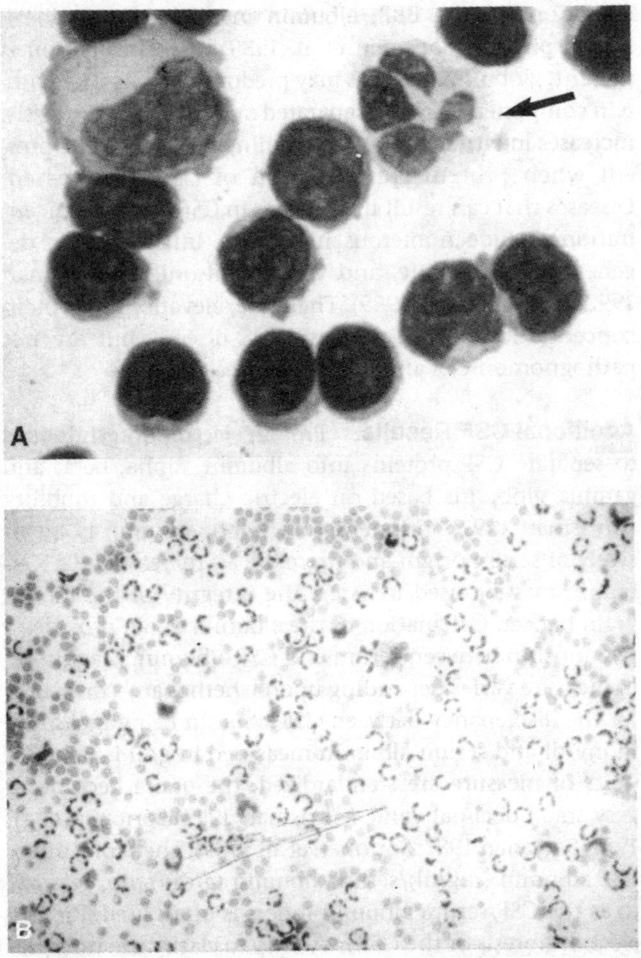

Fig. 9.19. (A) CSF cytology showing small and large mononuclear cells and one neutrophil (*arrow*). (B) CSF cytology showing predominantly neutrophils.

flow of CSF from the intracranial space following caudally in the subarachnoid space of the spinal cord (Chrisman 1992). CSF samples collected cranial (i.e., at the cisterna magna) relative to a focal lesion spinal cord lesion, therefore, may not be reflective of the disease process present occurring more caudal. It is common that if a disease process is primarily located in the thoracolumbar spinal cord and the CSF sample is collected at the cisterna magna, the results of the CSF analysis are often normal. It has been suggested that CSF sampling from the lumbar area is most diagnostic in establishing the presence of either intracranial or spinal cord neurologic disease (Thomson et al. 1990). In a few instances, however, when intracranial CNS disease results in a mild increase in CSF nucleated cell counts (usually 15 or < cell/μl), CSF collected at the cisterna magna will reflect this change, however, CSF collected in the lumbar area will be normal. In general, therefore, CSF should be collected as close to, but caudal to, the location of the suspected disease process. For intracranial disease, cisterna magna CSF should be diagnostic. Lumbar CSF may also be helpful for determination of intracranial disease, except in some instances of mild encephalitis. In the presence of spinal disease, lumbar CSF should be collected and analyzed to provide the most accurate assessment of disease characteristics. Normal results of a cisterna magna CSF sample in an animal with thoracolumbar spinal cord disease may not be reflective of the disease process.

In some instances, animals have neurologic signs that indicate disease in multiple areas within the nervous system. In these situations, collection of CSF from both the cisterna magnum and the lumbosacral area may be helpful. If the cisterna magnum sample is normal and the lumbosacral sample is abnormal, these findings would suggest that the predominant neurologic abnormality is in the spinal cord. With cervical spinal cord disease, however, the cisterna magnum CSF may be abnormal (Thomson et al. 1990).

As important as the number of cells present may be the morphology of those cells (Christopher et al. 1988), in dogs, the predominant nucleated cell in normal CSF is a monocytoid cell with a smaller percentage of lymphocytes. This is also true for cats (Rand et al. 1990). Small numbers of neutrophils and eosinophils may be present in CSF from clinically healthy animals and probably result from systemic blood contamination at the time of sampling. Some authors, however, have suggested that the presence of neutrophils or eosinophils in the CSF is indicative of an abnormality (Christopher et al. 1988). In cats, conversely, up to 8% of the nucleated cells can be neutrophils in non-blood-contaminated CSF (Rand et al. 1990). With increasing amounts of blood contamination of CSF from clinically healthy cats, neutrophils can account for 40% or more of the nucleated cells present. It is reasonable, therefore, to conclude that neutrophils may be present in normal CSF if some blood contamination is present. Additionally, there has been no correlation established between the degree and cell type of pleocytosis and a specific disease process making the rendering of specific diagnoses from CSF cell count and cytologic evaluations alone almost impossible.

Increases in nucleated cells that cannot be accounted for by contamination with blood at the time of sample collection indicate central nervous system disease. A variety of central nervous system diseases are associated with inflammation. These include diseases in which the inflammation is primary, such as infectious encephalitis, and those diseases where the inflammation is secondary to another primary disease, such as trauma or tumors. Regardless of etiology, inflammation in the CNS is reflected in increases in monocytoid and lymphoid cells in the CSF. In some situations, neutrophils are the predominant cell present. While increases in neutrophils are classically seen with bacteria encephalitis in humans, this is not necessarily the case in animals, as neutrophils may be present in a number of CNS inflammation situations.

Abnormal elevations of eosinophils in the CSF are uncommon in CNS inflammatory diseases (Bennett et al. 1997; Schultze et al. 1986; Smith-Maxie et al. 1989; Tyler et al. 1980). Eosinophilic meningitis is most often associated with parasitic or allergic reactions within or around the nervous system. Eosinophils have also been found associated with CNS infectious with other organisms such as cryptococcal meningoencephalitis, protothecal meningoencephalomyelitis, distemper virus, toxoplasmosis, rabies, and bacterial infections. Eosinophilic meningitis has also been reported to occur without an obvious infectious cause. Some breed of dogs, such as golden retrievers and Rottweilers, may be predisposed (Bennett et al. 1997; Smith Maxie et al. 1989).

With knowledge of the inherent variability of CSF findings and disease, some disease processes have more consistent and somewhat characteristic CSF cytological abnormalities. For example, dogs with generalized tremor syndrome almost always have a mild mononuclear pleocytosis (<20 nucleated cells/µl) and a normal to mildly elevated protein concentration (Bagley et al. 1993). Dogs with steroid-responsive meningitis and spinal cord vasculitis often have a primary neutrophilic pleocytosis, often with associated hemorrhage (Meric et al. 1985; Meric 1988). In cats with FIP, CSF samples tend to have increases in protein and nucleated cell counts, with neutrophils being the predominant cell type present (Baroni and Heinold 1995; Rand et al. 1994).

Neoplastic cells may also be present within the CSF, even in small numbers. Choroid plexus cells may break free from these tumors and be found on CSF evaluation (Chrisman 1992). Other neoplastic diseases that more commonly contribute to neoplastic cells in the CSF circulation include lymphoma and carcinomatosis. Infectious organisms are rarely present in CSF. If identified, the presence of these organisms is helpful in definitive diagnosis. Special techniques, such as India ink staining, may be necessary to enhance the viewing of these organisms. Therefore, even if overall nucleated cell counts are within the normal range, cytologic analysis of any cells present is important.

Protein Concentration. The normal protein content of CSF varies between species, laboratories, and also with site of collection. Slightly higher protein content is present in CSF collected from the lumbar area compared to the cisterna magna. In general, CSF collected from the cisterna magna of clinically healthy dogs contains protein concentrations less than 25 mg/dl, whereas samples collected in the lumbar area of clinically healthy dogs contains protein concentrations less than 35 mg/dl. Again, blood contamination may influence the protein concentration. Blood contamination of <500 RBC/µl usually does not increase protein concentrations. As a rule of thumb, 1000 red blood cells will iatrogenically increase the CSF protein concentration by 1 mg/dl if the serum protein concentration is normal (Adams and Victor 1993). Again, this rule of thumb is only a general guideline and does not hold true in all instances.

Cerebrospinal fluid protein concentrations can be elevated in numerous diseases of the nervous system. Any disease that alters the blood-brain barrier (BBB) or results in exudation or escape of protein from tissue and vessels into the CSF can result in protein elevations in CSF (Chrisman 1992). Proteins present may be albumin or globulin. With alterations in the BBB, albumin increases are predominantly present (Sorjonen et al. 1989). If inflammation is present, globulin increases may predominate. As these protein components are not separated on routine CSF analysis, increases in either albumin, globulin, or both may be present when protein concentration of CSF is increased. Diseases that can result in increases in CSF protein concentration include numerous neoplastic, inflammatory, degenerative, traumatic, and vascular disorders (Chrisman 1992; Sorjonen et al. 1989). Therefore, elevations in protein concentration in CSF suggest CNS disease, but are not pathognomonic of any particular disease process.

Additional CSF Results. Protein electrophoresis is used to separate CSF proteins into albumin, alpha, beta, and gamma globulins based on electric charge and mobility (Chrisman 1992; Sorjonen et al. 1989). Albumin is exclusively of serum origin and therefore an increase in CSF albumin may be used to assess the integrity of the blood-brain barrier. Calculation of the albumin quota provides a relationship between serum and CSF albumin. Magnitude of measure varies depending upon whether any correction for the discrepancy between CSF albumin being measured in mg/dl and serum albumin measured in g/dl is made. If units of measure are standardized, the quota becomes a very small decimal value (Chrisman 1992; Sorjonen et al. 1981; Sorjonen 1987; Sorjonen et al. 1989). Therefore, direct CSF albumin (mg/dl)/serum albumin (g/dl) ratio, referred to as the CSF/serum albumin index, is often used. Protein electrophoresis of the CSF may help to clarify the interpretation of CSF titer results.

Chemistry and enzyme concentration are variable in CSF and have rarely been used for correlation of specific clinical diseases (Chrisman 1992; deLahunta 1983). Glucose content of CSF is approximately 80% of plasma values. Decreases in CSF glucose have been a consistent consequence of bacterial meningitis in humans. AST and CK values may increase when extensive myelin degeneration has occurred. LDH levels have been stated to be increased with lymphosarcoma (deLahunta 1983). Unfortunately, all of these CSF chemistry abnormalities have not been routinely evaluated in clinically affected animals. Conclusions, therefore, as to their utility are unproven and await further evaluation.

Serological evidence of antibodies, primarily to infectious organisms, in the CSF has also been inconsistently evaluated to determine their clinical utility. Theoretically, the presence of antibodies to specific organisms indicates the presence of that organism and an associated immunologic reaction in the CSF. Detection of intrathecal antibodies, however, is inconsistent. In two studies of dogs with distemper virus infection, one detected the presence of antibody in 56% (9/16) dogs, whereas antibody was present in only 1 of 13 dogs in another study (Thomas et al. 1993b; Sorjonen et al. 1989). With nonspecific encephalitis, however, antibodies present in the serum may cross the damaged blood-brain (CSF) barrier and be detected in the CSF. Comparison of serum and CSF titers may help in determining the presence of intrathecal production of antibody. If, for example, the concentration of a particular antibody is greater in the CSF than serum, this suggests intrathecal production of this antibody. Protein electrophoresis may be helpful in this determination of the presence of BBB breakdown and increases in albumin compared to intrathecal production of antibody and subsequent increases in globulins. Unfortunately, electophoretic patterns on CSF may overlap between differing diseases, and, therefore, are not pathognomonic for specific disease etiologies.

Cerebrospinal fluid analysis can provide important diagnostic information in some animals with nervous system disorders, however, it should be interpreted with knowledge of the previously discussed nuances. The clinical examination remains important in determining clues to the presence of a neurologic problem. Cerebrospinal fluid results are then assessed in consideration of the (1) clinical suspicion of the presence of a suspected neurologic problem after completion of the neurologic examination and (2) the suspected disease or diseases present.

Interpretation and Evaluation

Interpretation of a Normal CSF Sample. Cerebrospinal fluid analysis is sometimes used to determine if a neurologic disease process exists in an individual animal (Bagley and Bohn 2003b). A neurologically normal animal would be expected to have a normal cerebrospinal fluid analysis. Unfortunately, some animals with central nervous system disease have a normal CSF analysis. A normal CSF analysis alone, therefore, does not exclude the possibility of an associated central nervous system disease process. As an example, in one study of dogs with seizures, slightly greater than 25% of dogs with lesions detected with MR imaging had normal CSF evaluations (Bush et al. 2002). With focal disease, the location of CSF collection relative to the disease location is also important. If CSF is collected cranial to the level of the lesion in the spinal cord, CSF may not be reflective of the associated disease process and is often normal (Thomson et al. 1990).

If the disease process involves the nervous tissue parenchyma and does not communicate with the CSF, CSF may be normal. This is often the case with metabolic and degenerative neurologic diseases. In some instances, primarily with mild CSF inflammatory changes, prior corticosteroid administration can decreased the inflammatory response and result in a normal CSF evaluation.

A normal CSF result, therefore, may be found both in normal animals and in animals with neurologic disease. A normal CSF result cannot be taken to mean that an animal is neurologically normal, nor does this indicate that a neurologic disease is not present.

Interpretation of an Abnormal CSF Sample. Abnormalities on routine CSF analysis indicate the presence of some nervous system disease process. Increases in nucleated cell counts and protein concentration are indicative of CNS disease if the sample has not been contaminated with iatrogenic hemorrhage at the time of collection. Cerebrospinal fluid alterations are, unfortunately, rarely characteristic of a specific disease. If a neoplastic cell or infectious organism is found, or a specific antibody suggestive of intrathecal production is detected, CSF can provide a more definitive diagnosis for these diseases. The overall incidence of these specific cytologic and immunologic findings, however, is low. Pragmatically, this means that CSF evaluation has reasonable specificity but poorer sensitivity. Cerebrospinal fluid analysis is helpful in determining the presence of disease affecting the nervous system, but it is unreliable in determining specific disease entities.

As with many diagnostic tests, the sensitivity and specificity of CSF testing is variable depending upon the disease present. Additional diagnostic tests, such as titers for infectious agents, are often needed for a more accurate etiologic diagnosis to be determined. CSF analysis should not be used as a replacement for advanced neuroimaging, such as MR imaging, if structural CNS disease is suspected. Given the array of diseases that affect the central nervous system, a combination of diagnostic tests may be the most practical approach when evaluating animals with suspected neurologic disease.

It would be a mistake, therefore, to diagnose diseases such as granulomatous meningoencephalitis, toxoplasmosis, distemper, feline infectious peritonitis, and numerous other primary inflammatory diseases based on results of CSF alone as there is overlap in the CSF results from numerous diseases. Even within specific diseases, CSF results may vary depending upon the location and severity of the disease process.

CSF Pressure Evaluations. Intracranial pressure (ICP) is the pressure exerted between the skull and the intracranial tissue. Because the skull is relatively inelastic as compared to the other intracranial tissue, ICP is determined primarily by changes in intracranial tissue volume and the compensatory ability of these tissue to accommodate for volume changes (Germon 1988; Lyons and Meyer 1990; Shapiro 1975). The major volume components residing within the intracranial space are the brain tissue (intracranial cellular elements), CSF, and blood. Cerebrospinal fluid is, therefore, a component of intracranial pressure, and it also exerts a certain pressure. With production of CSF being independent of intracranial pressure, absorption is the primary homeostatic mechanism for maintenance of intracranial pressure with regard to CSF.

Cerebrospinal fluid pressure (CSFP) is sometimes used as an assessment of ICP. Cerebral fluid pressure changes, however, are dynamic and pulsatile, with a small pressure wave occurring almost simultaneously with each heart beat (Cardoso et al. 1983; Germon 1988; Lundberg 1960; Rosner and Becker 1984). This waveform is referred to as the intracranial pulse pressure wave (ICPPW). Periodic fluctuations of CSFP and ICP may occur in response to normal body functions such as coughing or abdominal straining, through increases in intrathoracic pressure and venous pressure impairing venous return from the intracranial space. With intracranial disease, CSF pressure may increase persistently or episodically, thereby resulting in persistent or episodic clinical abnormalities.

Historically, in animals, measurements of CSFP have been used to infer ICP (deLahunta 1983; Hoerlein 1965; Novak et al. 1974; Parker 1972; Schirmer 1958; Simpson and Reed 1987). Needle puncture and manometer readings have been employed to provide this information, however, this method does not lend itself easily to long-term measurement of ICP. As ICP is dynamic, fluctuations are important to recognize and objectively measure. Also, to perform needle puncture safely, anesthesia is required in all but the comatose animal. If ventricular obstruction or herniation occurs, the CSF spaces may become compartmentalized. In this situation, depending upon where CSFP is measured, CSFP may not accurately reflect global ICP. Evidence from humans with unilateral structural brain lesions suggests that the most accurate assessment of ICP occurs when measured ipsilateral to the lesion (Weaver et al. 1982).

A summary of CSFPs and ICP values for clinically healthy dogs is given in tables 9.4 and 9.5. Most of CSFPs fall between 5 and 12 mm Hg.

To address the need for long-term recording of ICP, a fiberoptic ICP monitoring system has been developed for use in humans and adapted for dogs and cats. With this system, pressures can be measured from the CSF or the brain tissue (BTP). This system yields accurate measurements long-term in humans and has gained acceptance in clinical practice. The same system has been used by us and others to monitor ICP in dogs and cats (Bagley et al. 1995b, 1995c; Bagley et al. 1996; Keegan et al. 1995; Harrington et al. 1996; Iannotti et al. 1984; Pluhar et al. 1994).

Brain tissue pressure in clinically healthy dogs measured with this fiberoptic system is presented in table 9.5. Previous measurements of CSFP are similar to BTP measured, however, there is a tendency for BTP measured with the fiberoptic system to be slightly higher than CSFP. When BTP measurements obtained with this fiberoptic system are compared with intraventricular pressure measured with conventional transducers in dogs, the fiberoptic system is accurate to +/- 3 mm Hg. Very similar degrees of change in ICP, however, were noted regardless of the type of transducer used. Because of this variability of ICP inherent within the monitoring devices, absolute values of ICP may not be as important as the establishment of trends suggesting persistent increases in ICP. This may be also why a specific upper limit where normal ICP becomes pathologically increased is unclear.

Previous studies have reported the potential for fiberoptic intracranial pressure monitoring in dogs (Bagley et al. 1995; Keegan et al. 1995; Harrington et al. 1996; Iannotti et al. 1984; Pluhar et al. 1994; Shores et al. 1991). The use of a fiberoptic ICP monitor in establishing changes in ICP under anesthesia and during intracranial surgery has been shown. In one study, using isoflurane as a maintenance anesthetic, mean intracranial pressure was found to ~ 10 mm Hg (range 8–13 mm Hg) (Shores et al. 1991). Mean ICP in dogs we have evaluated has been slightly higher, but the range of pressures measured were similar (table 9.5) (Bagley et al. 1995; Keegan et al. 1995; Harrington et al. 1996; Iannotti et al. 1984; Pluhar et al. 1994). Again, values obtained with this fiberoptic method of ICP monitoring are slightly higher overall in comparison to results from previous studies looking at CSF pressure determined by a cisterna magna puncture and manometer readings (deLahunta 1983; Hoerlein 1965; Novak et al. 1974; Parker 1972; Schirmer 1958; Simpson 1987).

An absolute level wherein ICP is pathologically increased has not been established (Lyons and Meyer 1990; Hassler et al. 1988; Johnston et al. 1970; Obrist et al. 1984.). Some of this may be the result of the inherent inaccuracies of the monitoring equipment and the variation in baseline ICP normally. Most information from humans suggests that ICP >15–20 mm Hg is pathologically increased. Cerebral blood flow may not be significantly decreased until ICP reaches ~ 30 mm Hg. Experimentally, however, ICP has been raised to very high levels (>100 mm Hg) before brain death occurred (van Loon et al. 1993). We have seen ICP as high as 30–40 mm Hg in dogs that subsequently have recovered from brain injury.

Table 9.4. Reported normal CSF pressures in various species

Dog	< 170 mm H_2O (8–12 mm Hg)
Cat	< 100 mm H_2O (~7 mm Hg)
Ox	< 200 mm H_2O (~14 mm Hg)
Sheep	< 270 mm H_2O (~19 mm Hg)
Pig	< 145 mm H_2O (~10 mm Hg)
Horse	< 400 mm H_2O (~28 mm Hg)
	(~1.4 cm H_2O = 1 mm Hg)

Sources: deLahunta 1983; Hoerlein 1985; Novak et al. 1974; Parker 1972; Schirmer 1958; Simpson 1987.

Table 9.5. Summary of CSFPs and ICP values for dogs

Cerebrospinal fluid pressure in clinically healthy dogs (in mm Hg)		
	Mean[1]	Range[1]
Schirmer (1958)	5	NA
Horlein (1965)	7	NA
Parker (1972)	NA	5–10
Novak (1974)	9	4–16
Simpson (1987)	6	4–10

Brain tissue pressure in clinically healthy dogs (in mm Hg)[2]		
	Mean[3]	Range
Shores (1991)	9.8	8–13
Keegan (1995)	10.0	8–12
Bagley (1995)	11.0	8–14
Pluhar (1995)	9.6	8–12

[1]Pressures converted from mm CSF to mm Hg and rounded to nearest whole number.

[2]Measured under isoflurane anesthesia with a fiberoptic ICP monitoring system.

[3]Values rounded to nearest whole number.

ELECTRICAL DIAGNOSTIC TESTING

As nervous system activity is based on alterations in transmembrane potentials, recording of spontaneous and evoked nervous system electrical activity can be helpful in the identification of nervous system dysfunction (Braund 1994; Chrisman 1991; Dewey 2003; Holliday 1992; Oliver et al. 1987; Oliver et al. 1997). The electrical studies used in the diagnosis of nervous system disease are under the umbrella of what are generally referred to as *electrodiagnostic evaluations* or *electrodiagnostics.*

There are a number of ways that the electrical activity of the nervous system can be measured. In general, spontaneous activity can be recorded, from the surface (skin) of the body or from structures within the body (such as muscles). Conversely, the nervous system can be stimulated and the resultant nervous or muscle electrical activity can then be recorded. These latter techniques are often referred to as "evoked" potentials, as an electrical stimulus is necessary for their production. Evoked activity is an attempt to mimic the normal stimulated electrical activity of the nervous system.

Electrodiagnostic techniques require electrodiagnostic measuring equipment as well as experience in recording and interpreting any resultant activity. The following discussion is an introduction to electrodiagnostic testing procedures and their clinical utility. While electrodiagnostic evaluations will usually not be performed in general clinical practice, familiarity with the techniques will allow the astute clinician to determine the appropriateness of these diagnostic techniques for diagnosis of an individual patient disease.

Intracranial Electrodiagnostic Testing

Electrical information from the brain can be recorded and analyzed in an attempt to determine functional abnormalities of nervous tissues. While a number of electrodiagnostic techniques have been used, two of the more commonly utilized tests for evaluation of intracranial disease are electroencephalography (EEG) and brain stem auditory evoked potential or response (BAEP, BAER).

Electroencephalography

The EEG is a surface recording of the electrical activity of the cerebral hemispheres (fig. 9.20) (Redding 1990). Electrical activity of cortical neurons is occurring spontaneously and continually. This electrical activity may propagate through the skull, muscles, and tissues of the head, to the skin. By placing recording electrodes on the skin surface or immediately beneath the skin of the head, this spontaneous electrical activity can be recorded. Depending upon the number of electrodes and where these electrodes are placed, summated activity from differing areas of the cerebral hemispheres can be recorded. This electrical activity is the overall representation of the activity of the cerebral hemispheres.

The random activity of the numerous cortical neurons is recorded through a number of electrodes. The location of placement of the electrodes on the head is referred to as a montage. In normal animals, the amount of activity will vary depending upon the activity and number of cortical neurons that are depolarizing at any one moment. The activity level of these neurons will depend upon the level of arousal (alertness) and responses to stimuli. Anesthesia, for example, may affect the spontaneous activity of cortical neurons. However, many of the recordings of EEG activity in animals have been collected under sedation or anesthesia. It in important, therefore, to determine the potential influences on normal cortical activity due to the testing conditions and any sedative or anesthetic drug therapies. The relatively large size of the temporalis muscles in dogs may dampen the propagation of the cortical signal. As the electrodes record all electrical activity, muscle electrical activity such as from twitching or blinking of the eye will also be recorded. This muscle activity can create artifacts in the EEG tracing that may mimic abnormal cortical electrical activity. The recognition of these artifacts and testing procedure influences is important to avoid inaccurate conclusions after analysis of the EEG recording.

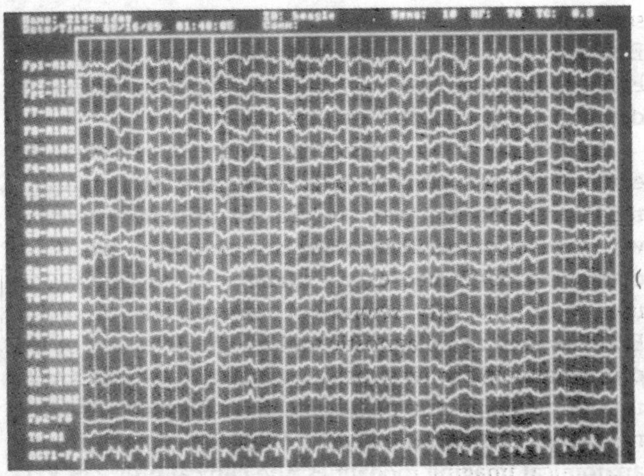

Fig. 9.20. Electroencephalographic recording from a dog.

Cortical activity is recorded on a paper chart or via computer over a certain time period. The EEG tracing will visually appear as a number of connected waveforms of varying sizes (amplitudes). The number of waveforms present per second is referred to as the frequency. The frequency is reported as waveforms or cycles/second or hertz (Hz). The size (height usually measured in millivolts) of the waveforms is referred to as the amplitude of the potential.

Alterations in cortical activity measured with the EEG may occur with a number of diseases of the central nervous system (Redding 1990; Steiss et al. 1990). For example, hydrocephalus commonly results in a decreased number of waveforms/second, with a concurrent increase in the size of the waveforms (high amplitude slow wave activity). This EEG pattern, however, may be seen in other instances of cortical neuron damage or loss. Therefore, alterations in the pattern of EEG activity are rarely pathognomonic for a particular cortical disease. Also, as the EEG is a reflection of the larger activity of groups of neurons, focal and relatively smaller lesions may not be identified through abnormal EEG activity. EEG evaluations, however, may be useful in establishing seizure activity, patterns or foci, evaluation of depth of anesthesia, and disorders of sleep.

In clinical practice, considering the need for specialized equipment and experience in recording and interpretation, the important artifacts and procedural influences, coupled with the lack of specificity as to disease etiology, EEG is uncommonly performed except under selected conditions, usually in university, referral, or research environments. EEG was used as a diagnostic tool for the detection of hydrocephalus and other structural intracranial diseases prior to the development of advanced anatomical imaging modalities such as MR imaging. With the advent of these anatomical imaging modalities, the clinical utility of EEG has become of lesser importance in the diagnosis of intracranial diseases. In the modern era, EEG collection and analysis are relegated primarily as a diagnostic component of some seizure disorders and in experimental settings.

Brain Stem Auditory Evoked Potential or Response (BAEP, BAER, BSEP). The brain stem auditory response (potential) is a surface (far field) recording of the electrical activity of brain stem neuronal element activity following auditory stimulation (Fischer and Obermaier 1994; Steiss et al. 1994). Most commonly, a series of clicks is generated into the ear canal through tubing in ear plugs or via headphones. Following this auditory stimulation, a series of neuronal depolarizations occur along the neuroanatomical pathways associated with the sensation of hearing. When various pathways or neurons are depolarized in groups, an electrical potential is generated and radiates from the associated nervous tissue to the skin surface (fig. 9.21). These potentials can be recorded with electrodes placed on the surface of the head.

Potentials generated are numbered with Roman numerals (from I to VII or in some instances, more). The exact anatomical structures generating the BSEP are not confirmed, but wave I is thought to be due primarily to activity in the auditory nerve. The subsequent waves are generated along the pathway for hearing (cochlear nucleus, dorsal nucleus of the trapezoid body, lateral lemniscus, and caudal colliculus).

The BSEP is primarily useful in evaluating animals for deafness, as deaf animals will show no activated potentials in the deaf ear (Strain et al. 1992). As the hearing pathways travel through the brain stem, in some instances, the BSEP will also be abnormal in the presence of brain stem disease. The location of the abnormality may be identified within the brain stem or peripheral auditory receptors.

SURGICAL DIAGNOSIS

In many instances, even with anatomically accurate imaging studies of the CNS, a definitive diagnosis cannot be rendered based on noninvasive diagnostic techniques alone. In these situations, a biopsy of the affected tissue for histologic assessment is imperative for diagnosis.

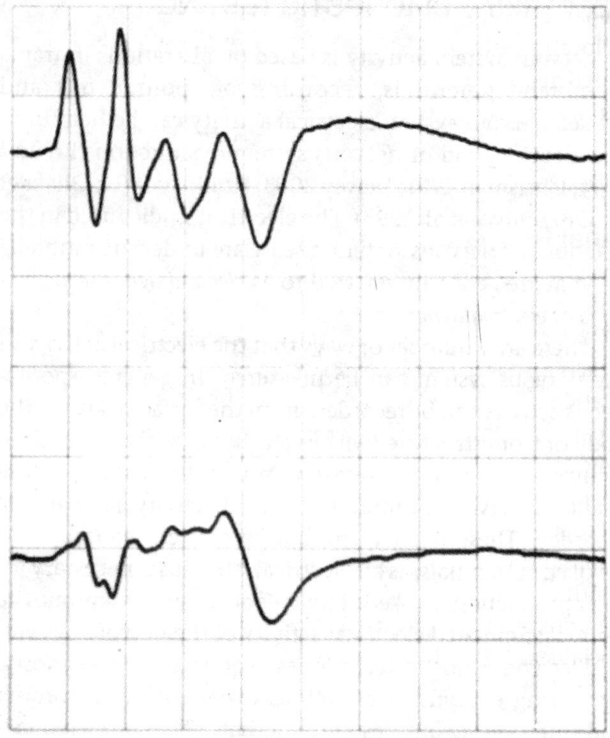

Fig. 9.21. BAEP (BSEP) recording from a dog.

Intracranial Surgery

Biopsy of intracranial lesions can be performed at the time of a craniotomy (removal of the skull for access to the intracranial structures) (Bagley 2003a). This might also be referred to as an "open" surgical biopsy implying the surgical exposure of the intracranial nervous tissues. In many instances, a craniotomy is performed for both diagnostic as well as therapeutic reasons. Tissues collected at the time of the intracranial surgery are submitted for histologic evaluation, immunologic studies, or culture for infectious organisms. A craniotomy may also allow for decompression of the intracranial contents and provide short-term control of elevations in intracranial pressure.

Intracranial tissues can also be collected for histologic evaluation by making only a small hole in the skull for entrance of a biopsy instrument or needle. This is often referred to as a "closed" biopsy. As it is important to be precise with the location of the biopsy, surgical systems have been developed to allow for accurate placement of the biopsy instrument. These are referred to as stereotactic biopsy systems. The process is referred to as collection of a stereotactic biopsy specimen.

Obviously, the benefit of a histologic diagnosis becomes important to accurately plan appropriate therapy. Because of the need for expertise and some surgical equipment, there are obviously additional financial costs to the owner for surgical biopsy. Most important, as a surgical biopsy is an invasive procedure, the potential for iatrogenic damage to the brain including intracranial hemorrhage is increased compared to a nonsurgical diagnosis. In some instances, the location of the lesion within the nervous system (i.e., located in a vital region for life) may preclude the collection of an intracranial biopsy sample.

DIAGNOSTIC TESTING FOR SPINAL DISEASES

Spinal Radiography

Survey radiographs are often performed during the diagnostic evaluation of animals with spinal diseases (Walker 2002). The risks to the patient are minimal if general anesthesia is not needed. There is a small amount of exposure to radiation, which is usually inconsequential for the individual patient. Compared to other anatomical spinal diagnostic modalities, financial costs are relatively less for performance of spinal radiographs.

Proper radiographic technique and patient positioning for spinal radiography are important factors that influence the utility of this diagnostic test (fig. 9.22). Poor quality radiographs are less likely to yield a diagnosis regardless of the associated costs. For the most accurate assessments to be rendered, the spine should be straight and the radiographic beam centered directly over the area of interest to avoid misinterpretation of vertebral alignment, intervertebral foraminal size, as well as intervertebral disk size and shape. For appropriate patient positioning, anesthesia or heavy sedation is often necessary. In some disease conditions, such as in the instance of spinal trauma, the effects of anesthesia may be detrimental to spinal cord health. If the traumatized spinal cord becomes ischemic during anesthesia-induced hypotension, or if an unstable vertebral segment (i.e., fracture) is excessively manipulated or moves during patient positioning, the spinal cord can be further damaged. Cautious manipulation of the spine is always a good practice when positioning any animal for spinal radiography.

Vertebrae are complex bony structures and have many nuances and protuberances that may be mistaken for abnormalities by the inexperienced observer. Interpretation of vertebral abnormalities is more difficult if the vertebrae are not positioned correctly.

While spinal radiographs are associated with relatively low costs, the beneficial aspects of these diagnostic tests ultimately depend upon the disease process present. Spinal radiographs are most likely to yield helpful diagnostic information in diseases that affect the vertebral structures. Spinal fracture, vertebral neoplasia, and vertebral infections such as diskospondylitis and vertebral osteomyelitis are most likely to be associated with radiographic abnormalities. If these diseases are present, the cost/benefit of spinal radiographs is relatively good. The most obvious limitation of survey spinal radiography is that the spinal cord is not evident on these radiographic studies (fig. 9.23). Spinal radiographs can be normal in the presence of significant inherent spinal cord disease or with soft tissue spinal compressive diseases such as intervertebral disk extrusion.

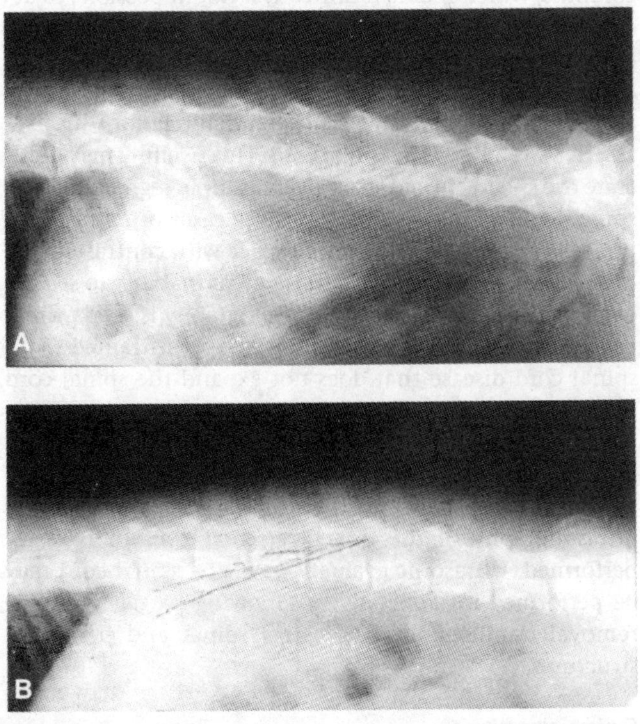

Fig. 9.22. Lateral survey radiograph of (A)the lumbar spine of a dog that is rotated and (B) properly positioned.

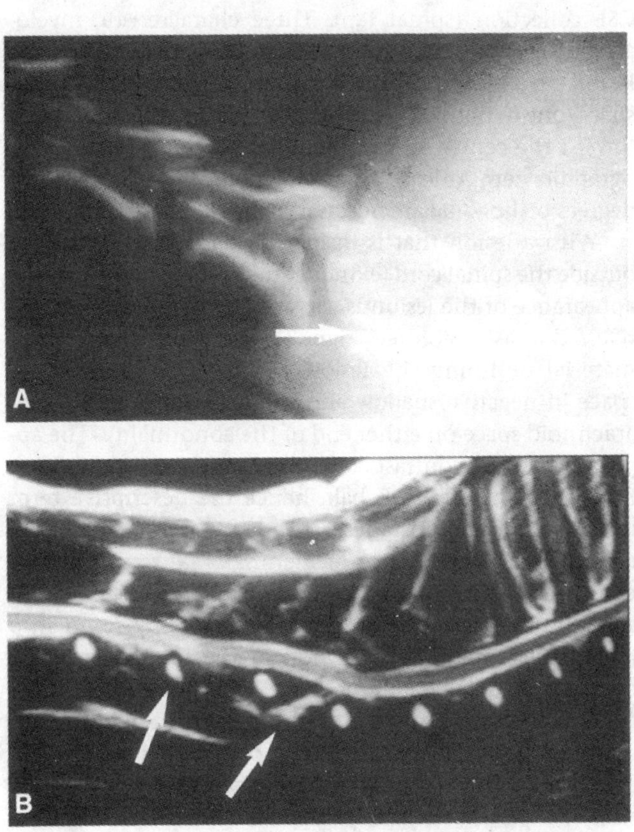

Fig. 9.23. (A) Lateral survey radiograph of the cervical spine of a dog showing a fracture of C5 vertebra (*arrow*). (B) Transverse, T2-weighted MR images of the same dog showing no spinal compression at C5, but rather a traumatic disk herniation at C3–4 (*arrows*).

The specific utility of spinal radiographs in the diagnosis of individual spinal cord diseases is discussed further in chapter 11. To most accurately determine if spinal cord compression or other primary spinal cord diseases are present, an advanced imaging modality that allows for identification of the spinal cord structure such as myelography, CT scanning, or magnetic resonance imaging must be performed for most accurate diagnosis.

Myelography

Myelography has historically been the most commonly employed spinal imaging procedure to determine if a compressive or expansile lesion of the spinal cord exists (Olby et al 1994; Roberts and Selcer 1993; Widmer and Thrall 2002). Myelography provides an "outline" of the spinal cord through an injection of a contrast agent (media) into the subarachnoid space surrounding the spinal cord (fig. 9.24, 9.25). This technique allows for localization and confirmation of spinal cord compression or enlargement by radiographing the spine from two or more directions with this subarachnoid contrast media present. The outline of the spinal cord will be represented by two approximately parallel lines of contrast media (contrast columns).

The contrast agent (e.g., Iohexol, Iopamidal—0.3 up to 0.5 ml/kg for Iohexol 300) is injected into the subarachnoid space by penetrating the subarachnoid space as for CSF collection (spinal tap). Three characteristic myelographic patterns can be seen with spinal cord lesions. If the lesion is extradural and compresses the subarachnoid space, one or both of the contrast columns will be deviated toward the center of the spinal cord in at least one radiographic view. At least two radiographic views taken at 90 degrees orthogonal are necessary to make this distinction.

With a lesion that is inside the dura (intradural) but outside the spinal cord (extramedullary), the myelographic appearance of the lesion is classically described as what is referred to as a "golf tee" sign. This is due to the contrast material outlining the lesion within the subarachnoid space in negative shadow and the distension of the subarachnoid space on either end of the abnormality. The appearance of the contrast columns is similar to the tee used for placement of a golf ball, hence the descriptive term used. In almost all instances, a tumor of the subarachnoid area (nerve sheath tumor or meningioma) results in this characteristic myelographic pattern. Intramedullary lesions (lesions within the spinal cord) usually result in a focal enlargement or expansion of the spinal cord. The contrast-filled subarachnoid space will, therefore, diverge from midline or the center of the spinal cord in both radiographic views taken at 90 degrees orthogonal planes.

Myelography is used primarily to demonstrate compression or expansion of the spinal cord as evidenced by alterations in the subarachnoid space surrounding the spinal cord. In this way, many structural spinal cord diseases can be identified.

Unfortunately, myelography is an invasive procedure. Contrast is injected in the subarachnoid space via a lumbar (L5–L6) or cisterna magna penetration with a spinal needle (spinal tap). Potential complications of subarachnoid needle puncture include iatrogenic trauma to the nervous tissue and iatrogenic introduction of infectious organisms to the CNS. Histologic evidence of edema, cystic necrosis, myelomalacia, demyelination, and axonal necrosis have been described in the spinal cord following needle passage through the spinal cord, with or without contrast injection. These same abnormalities were noted when there were multiple cord punctures during the examination and in those single punctures in which contrast medium was injected into the central canal. These complications may have devastating consequences for the patient in some instances.

The most commonly used radiographic contrast media in animals for myelography in the modern era are the nonionic tri-iodinated phenolic compounds iopamidol and iohexol. These media have replaced the previously used compounds such as metrizamide. Although iopamidol and iohexol are much safer than previously available myelographic contrast agents, their use during myelography is accompanied by a number of potential adverse reactions ranging from decreases in mental acuity to seizures. Seizure activity appears more common when contrast is injected into the cisterna magna compared to the lumbar region subarachnoid space and may occur in between 10 and 30% of animals. Side effects of these compounds have been attributed to a number of possible mechanisms, including leakage of cerebrospinal fluid, the osmolarity of the solutions, and the direct cytotoxicity of the contrast media.

Technical aspects of myelography also influence the diagnostic test. If the contrast medium is injected in the epidural space instead of the subarachnoid space, the result (an epiduragram) is a scalloping appearance of the contrast columns, which makes it difficult, if not impossible, to accurately interpret the location of the subarachnoid space, and subsequently, determine if a compressive spinal cord abnormality exists. Intramedullary neoplastic, traumatic, inflammatory, cystic and acute traumatic lesions may result in a swelling of the spinal cord. This swelling may obliterate the subarachnoid space over multiple segments of the spine. Myelographic studies in these cases often result in poor filling of the subarachnoid space with contrast media over the swollen area with a subsequent inability to see the extent of the actual lesion. As myelography is used primarily to image the subarachnoid space, intramedullary spinal cord disease that does not expand the spinal cord will also not be evident with myelography.

Ultrasound

Due to the impedance of the ultrasound signal by bone, ultrasongraphy of the intact vertebral column is rarely performed. Ultrasonic evaluations of the spinal cord may be performed intraoperatively following partial vertebrae removal (laminectomy) to assess spinal and perispinal structures.

Scintigraphy

Scintigraphy has been used in the diagnosis of spinal disease primarily to assess activity in vertebrae (bone scan-

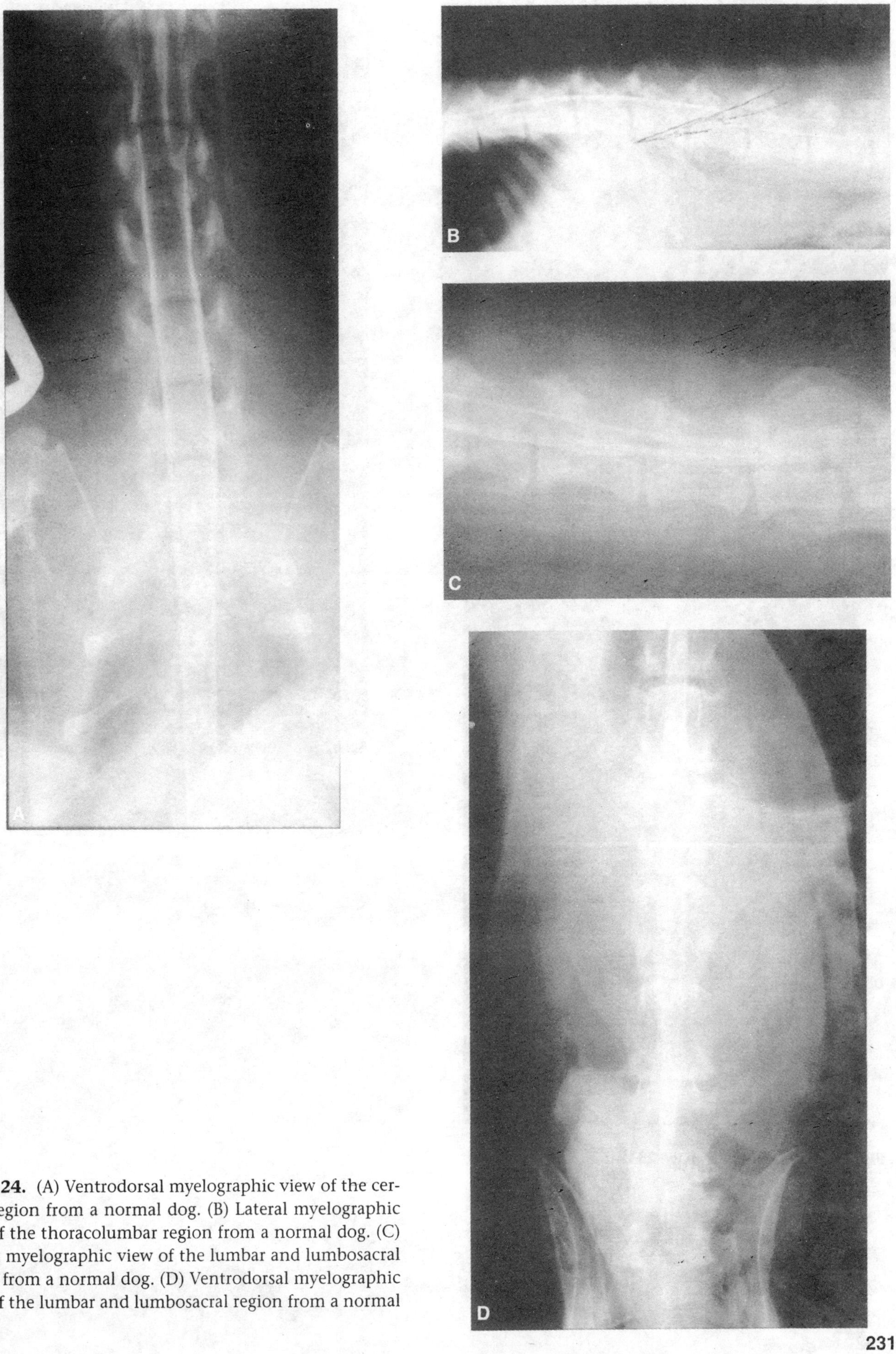

Fig. 9.24. (A) Ventrodorsal myelographic view of the cervical region from a normal dog. (B) Lateral myelographic view of the thoracolumbar region from a normal dog. (C) Lateral myelographic view of the lumbar and lumbosacral region from a normal dog. (D) Ventrodorsal myelographic view of the lumbar and lumbosacral region from a normal dog.

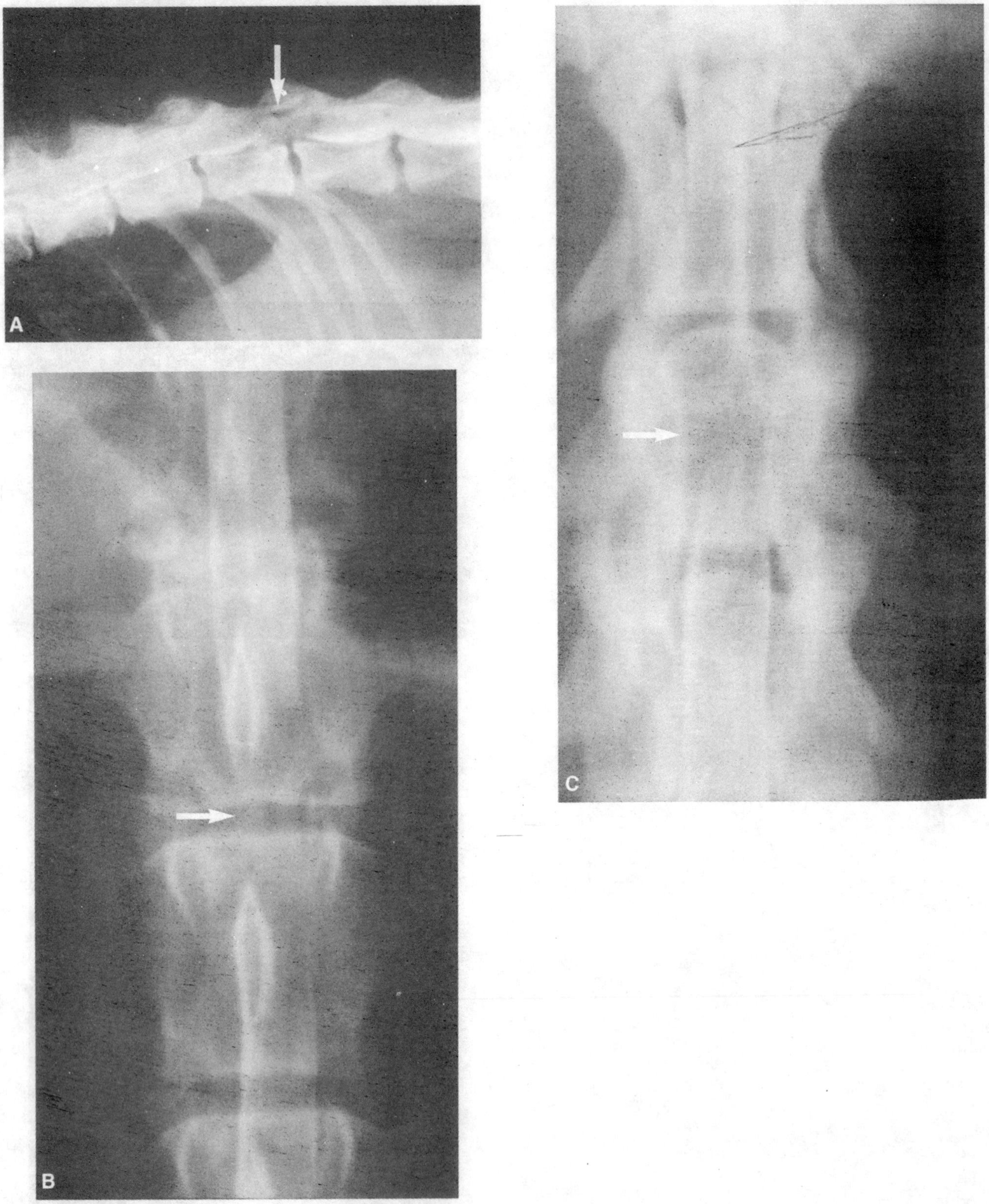

Fig. 9.25. Legend is on page 233.

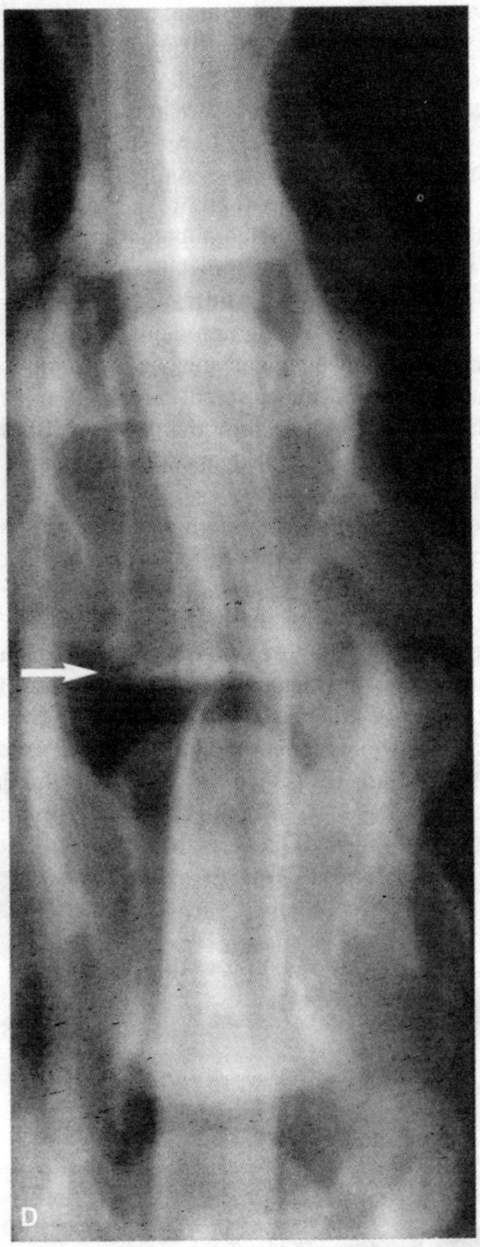

Fig. 9.25. (A) Lateral view of a myelogram in a cat with an extradural spinal cord compression (*arrow*). (B,C,D) Ventrodorsal views of myelograms in dogs with a lateral extradural spinal cord compression (*arrows*).

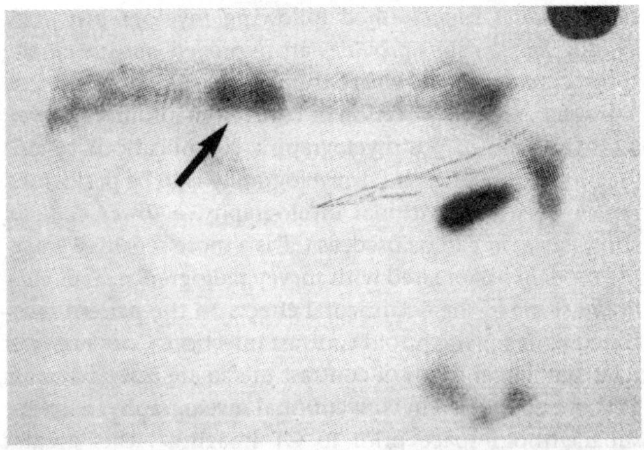

Fig. 9.26. Scintigraphic image of the lumbar spine of a dog with diskospondylitis showing uptake of the radioactive tracer (*arrow*).

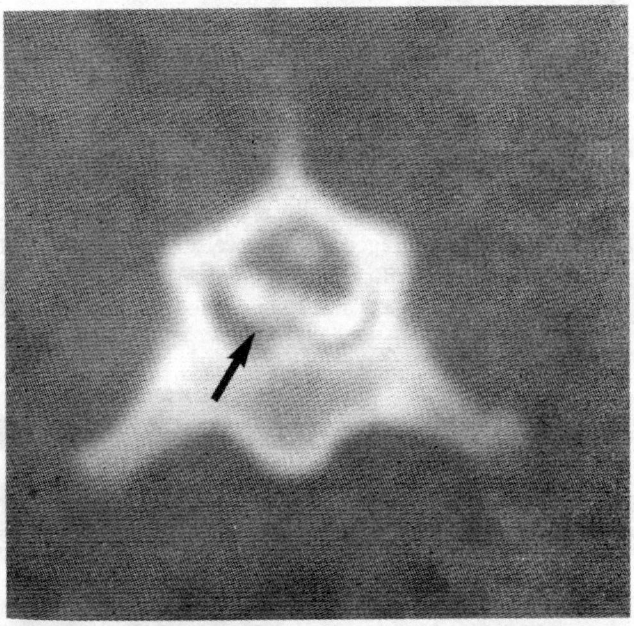

Fig. 9.27. Transverse, spinal CT images (following subarachnoid injection of contrast) showing spinal cord compression (*arrow*).

ning). While anatomical image quality is poor, the radiopharmaceutical may be concentrated in regions of bone production, growth, or remolding. Scintigraphy is most often used to identify radiographically occult tumors and infections of the vertebrae (fig. 9.26).

Computed Tomography (CT)

Computed tomography can be used in evaluation of spinal cord and vertebral disease. In general, CT is an excellent diagnostic modality for showing the vertebral structures. Abnormalities such as intervertebral disk extrusions that are mineralized are usually also apparent on CT spinal imaging. Compared to myelography, a significant advantage of CT (and MR) for spinal imaging is the ability to view the vertebrae in a transverse orientation (fig. 9.27). This view allows for improved localization of spinal cord lesions in a circumferential dimension compared to conventional myelography. As the spinal cord is usually evident, the anatomical relationship of the lesion to the spinal cord can be assessed. CT images can be reformatted in differing planes corresponding to major anatomical planes (i.e., sagittal, transverse, dorsal).

The main disadvantage of CT spinal imaging is the relatively poor image of the spinal cord parenchyma. Also, the delineation of a perispinal lesion from the spinal cord is difficult. CT performed following myelography (CT-myelography) often provides an improved outline of the spinal cord compared with either of these modalities alone. The subarachnoid injection of contrast medium, however, adds the risks of postmyelographic complications to this diagnostic modality. If CT-myelography is to be performed rather than conventional myelography, a lower dose of contrast agent can be used, as CT is a more sensitive imaging modality compared with survey radiographs. This may lessen some of the detrimental effects on the patient associated with subarachnoid contrast injection. Conversely, if relatively larger doses of contrast media are injected (such as those doses used in conventional myelography) into the subarachnoid space prior to CT imaging , this greater amount may make it more difficult to detect spinal cord lesions.

Spinal Magnetic Resonance (MR) Imaging

Spinal MR imaging provides images of vertebrae, intervertebral disks, the spinal cord, exiting spinal nerves, and paraspinal soft tissue anatomy (fig. 9.28, 9.29, 9.30, 9.31). Similar to intracranial MR imaging, a number of image acquisition sequences and imaging planes can be performed to order to clarify spinal cord lesions.

Sagittal images are often initially performed and provide a longitudinal view of a spinal cord region. Abnormal areas identified are imaged in a transverse plane and dorsal plane for further clarification. As cortical bone is dark or hypointense on both T1- and T2-weighted images, the MR appearance of the vertebral column depends mainly on the signal from bone marrow. Medullary bone, rich in fat and blood, is moderately intense (grey) on the T1-weighted images and less intense on the T2-weighted images. The ultimate appearance of marrow, however, depends upon the composition of the numerous components that may be present. The spinal cord tends to be isointense to the medullary bone of the vertebral bodies in the T1-weighed study and is typically surrounded by epidural fat, which is hyperintense to the spinal cord. This hyperintense outline can be seen on the T1-weighted sagittal and axial images. Epidural fat is easily displaced and hence may not be visible in conditions that result in spinal cord swelling. The intervertebral disks on T1-weighted images are slightly hypointense to isointense to the medullary cavity of the vertebral bodies.

The spinal cord on T2-weighted images is also isointense to the vertebral bodies, however the CSF surrounding the spinal cord emits a bright white (hyperintense) signal. The normal anatomy of the intervertebral disk is best appreciated on a T2-weighted sagittal MR image. Due to its high water content, the normal nucleus pulposus is bright (hyperintense) while the outer layers of the normal annulus fibrosis are homogeneously dark (hypointense).

By intensifying the CSF signal on a T2-weighted study, a "myelogram effect" can be achieved. This, in essence, provides for an exclusive image of the subarachnoid space. Abnormalities on MR images associated with specific spinal disease processes are discussed in chapter 11.

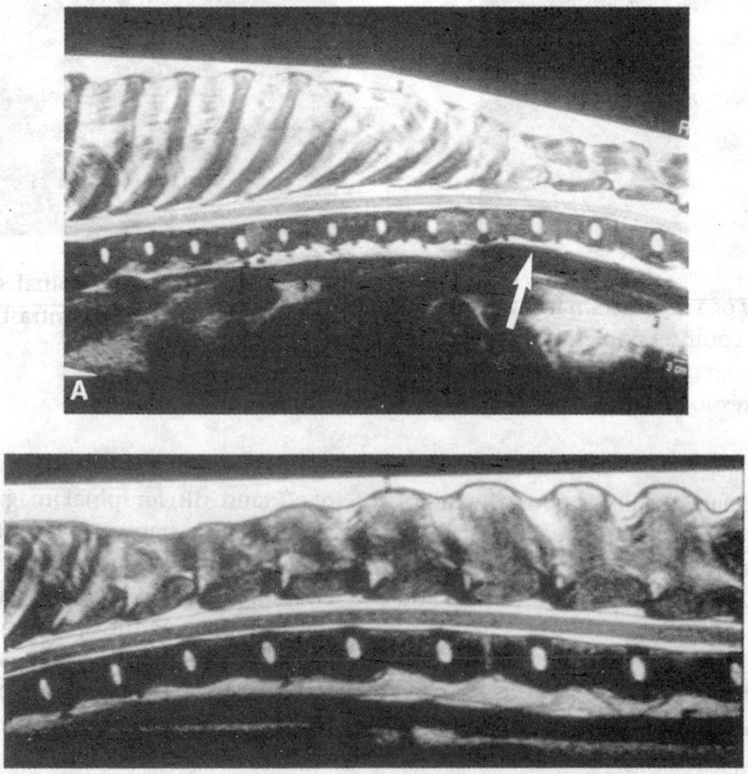

Fig. 9.28. Sagittal, T2-weighted MR images of (A,B) the thoracolumbar spine of two dogs. Note the hyperintense appearance of the nucleus pulposus of the intervertebral disk (*arrow*).

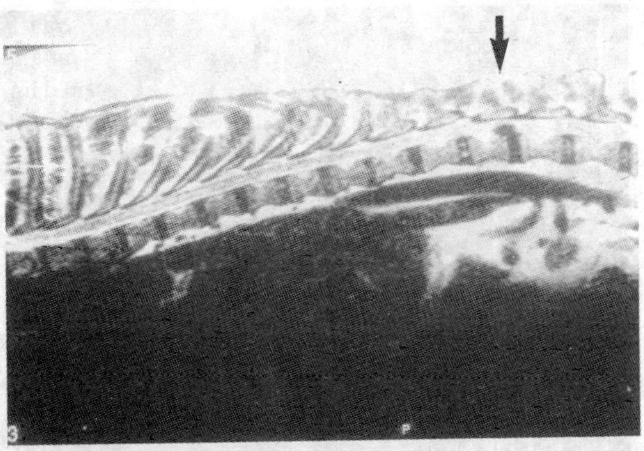

Fig. 9.29. Sagittal, T2-weighted MR images of the thoracolumbar spine of a dog with an intervertebral disk herniation (*arrow*).

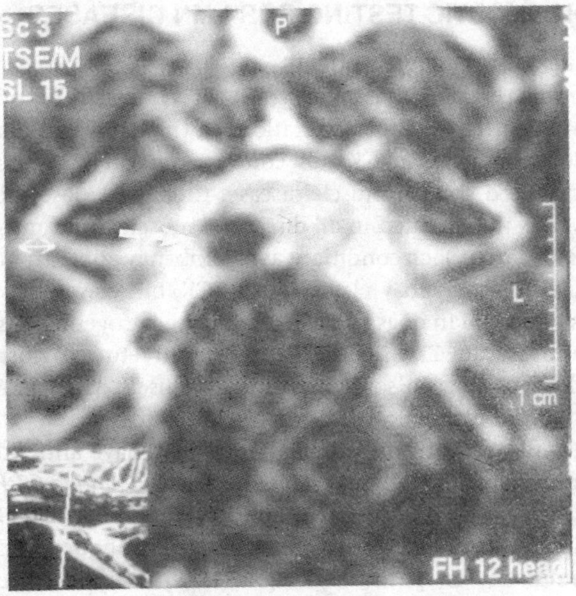

Fig. 9.30. Transverse, T2-weighted MR image from a dog with an intervertebral disk herniation (*arrow*).

CSF Analysis

Cerebrospinal fluid analysis is helpful primarily to determine the presence of inflammatory diseases of the spinal cord. In general, collection of spinal fluid caudal to the level of the lesion is most accurate for diagnosis. Fluid is analyzed for cellularity, protein content, and cell morphology. While CSF analysis is often useful in identifying the presence of nervous system disease, evaluated alone, this test does not often lend a specific etiologic diagnosis. Titers to specific infectious agents can be measured in CSF to assess for intrathecal production of antibody. In the presence of blood-brain barrier breakdown, however, antibodies may nonspecifically cross into the CSF from the systemic circulation. In this instance, correlation of the CSF to serum titer may be necessary. An increased antibody titer in the CSF relative to the serum antibody titer implies local production of antibodies within the CNS suggestive of actual CNS infection. Protein electrophoresis on CSF can give additional information concerning integrity of the blood-brain barrier and local production of immunoglobulins. Additional information regarding collection, analysis, and interpretation of CSF results is discussed under the diagnosis of intracranial disease section of this chapter. Obviously, CSF should be collected prior to injection of any contrast agent into the subarachnoid space such as during myelography as these contrast agents may alter the results of CSF analysis.

Spinal Cord Surgery

Surgery of the spinal cord is often performed for treatment and diagnosis of spinal diseases. Technical aspects of spinal surgery are described in chapter 14. In most instances, specimens for biopsy and culture are collected via a laminectomy. In general, biopsy of extradural abnormalities results in the least amount of surgical morbidity whereas biopsy of intraspinal disease has the potential for the greatest morbidity. Percutaneous fine needle aspirates of the spinal cord and perispinal structures including the vertebrae have been performed in some situations (Irving and McMillan 1990; Schulz et al. 1994). In most instances, associated radiographic imaging (fluoroscopy) is required to ensure accuracy of the location of the biopsy.

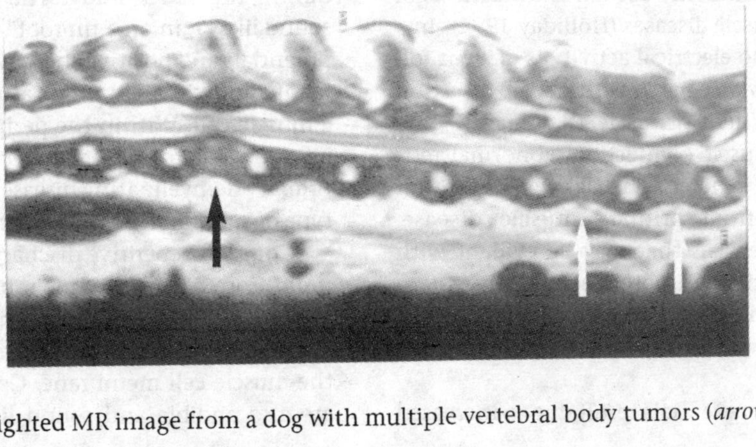

Fig. 9.31. Sagittal, T2-weighted MR image from a dog with multiple vertebral body tumors (*arrows*).

DIAGNOSTIC TESTING FOR LMN DISEASES

Laboratory Evaluations

Creatine kinase (CK) is an enzyme that is normally found in muscle with lesser concentrations in the brain and heart. Elevations in serum CK most commonly occur as a result of associated skeletal muscle disease. Creatine kinase, however, is not elevated in all disease of muscle. Mild muscle trauma from such conditions as recumbency and intramuscular injection may elevate serum CK, but elevations are usually mild in dogs and cats. Following iatrogenic muscle injury, serum CK will usually increase but return to normal within 5 days. In some instances of muscle damage, AST and ALT biochemical tests will also be increased.

Animals with myasthenia gravis may have antibodies produced against the acetylcholine receptor (*antiacetylcholine receptor antibodies*) (see chapter 7) (Shelton et al. 1990). Many infectious diseases involving the cell body are presumptively or specifically diagnosed with serum or cerebrospinal fluid titers revealing antibodies to, or antigen from, these infectious organisms. Specific antibody or antigen testing will depend upon the suspected infectious organism present.

Cerebrospinal Fluid Collection

Cerebrospinal fluid analysis may be useful for diseases that involve the central nervous system and spinal cord. If a primary peripheral nerve disease also involves the associated spinal nerves present within the subarachnoid space, collection of CSF from the lumbar area (i.e., caudal to the level of the lesion) may add information as to the nature of the disease involving these nerve roots or proximal peripheral nerves. Disease of the proximal nerve roots within the dura may be associated with both changes in CSF cytology and protein concentration. Cerebrospinal fluid abnormalities are most likely to be found in inflammatory peripheral nerve diseases such as polyradiculoneuritis or coonhound paralysis. In diseases that primarily involve the more distal portions of the peripheral nervous system, NMJ, and muscle, CSF will be normal.

Electromyography (EMG) and Nerve Conduction Velocity (NCV) Testing

The electromyogram (EMG) is a recording of the resting activity of muscle and is commonly used in the diagnosis of peripheral nerve and muscle diseases (Holliday 1992). In a normal resting muscle, no electrical activity is evident following the initial activity associated with needle insertion (insertional activity). When a muscle is damaged, and specifically, the nerve/muscle connection, abnormal resting spontaneous activity is noted. This damage may result from denervation or from primary muscle disease. Abnormal electrical potentials that may be evident with EMG testing include fibrillation potentials, positive sharp waves, myotonic potentials, and complex repetitive discharges (previously referred to as bizarre high-frequency activity) (fig. 9.32).

All of these abnormal potentials result due to increased

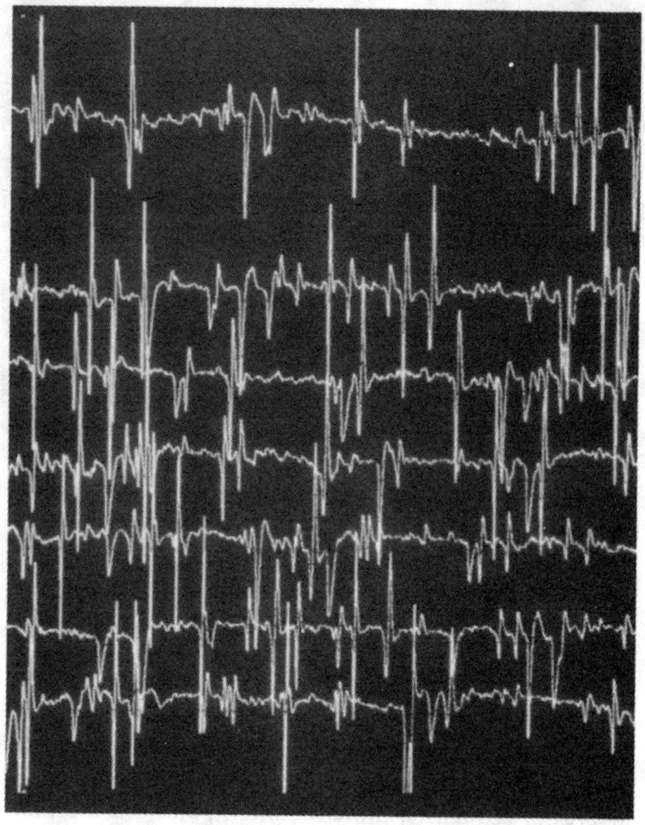

Fig. 9.32. Abnormal spontaneous electrical activity (fibrillation potentials) during an EMG evaluation from a dog.

excitability in a damaged or abnormal muscle membrane. When a muscle cell is denervated, the number of acetylcholine receptors increases on the membrane away from the NMJ. Therefore, small amounts of circulating acetylcholine (ACH) may result in individual muscle cells depolarizing independently of nervous stimulation or activation. Because this abnormal electrical activity reflects activity in single muscle fibers, these potentials are relatively small in amplitude. Fibrillation potentials are reflective of spontaneous depolarization of single muscle cells. Positive sharp waves result from the same basic pathophysiologic process, but occur in single muscle cells that have been physically damaged by the act of inserting the needle during the EMG study. The potentials are audible and sound like "rain on a tin roof" or "frying eggs." Fibrillation potentials and positive sharp waves will usually become evident approximately 5 days after significant denervation of a muscle cell. Within the peripheral nerve, the axon must be damaged for these denervation potentials to occur. Primary demyelinating diseases usually do not result in this type of spontaneous muscle activity.

Complex repetitive discharges and myotonic potentials result from more than one muscle cell or groups of muscle cells that spontaneously or continuously abnormally depolarize. Both of these types of activity reflect instability of the muscle cell membrane. Complex repetitive discharges are also audible and sound like a dive bomber airplane.

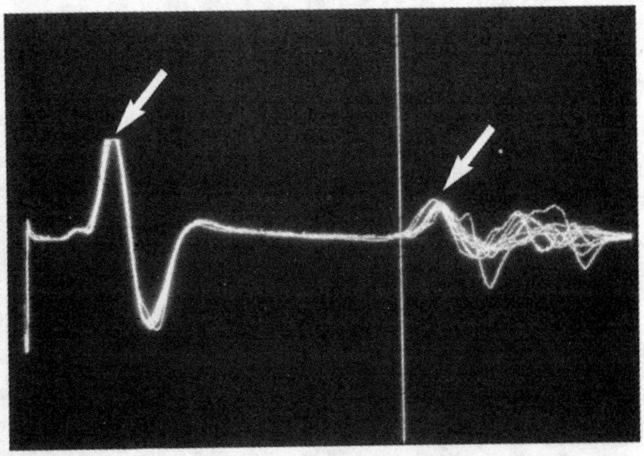

Fig. 9.33. Evoked motor unit potential (*left arrow*) during the performance of an NCV study and associated F waves (*right arrow*).

These potentials have an abrupt termination. Myotonic potentials are more continuous and sound like a motorcycle engine being continually revved. These potentials, therefore, have sounds that wax and wane.

Cranial nerves, similar to other peripheral nerves, innervate the muscle in and around the head including the larynx and pharynx. If these nerves are abnormal, the affected muscles may show spontaneous muscle activity that may be recorded with an EMG.

A peripheral nerve may also be stimulated along its length with electrodes that are placed near the nerve. The electrical activity activates the nerve, with subsequent generation of an axon potential within the nerve. This action potential then travels along the nerve to its termination. If the nerve terminates on a muscle, the nervous impulse depolarizes the neuromuscular junction, which ultimately results in a depolarization of the muscle. The electrical activity, either generated within the nerve, or within the muscle at the termination of the nerve can then be recorded and analyzed (fig. 9.33). These data can be used to calculate the nerve conduction velocity or speed of electrical propagation along a nerve segment.

By determining the time that it takes for the impulse to travel along the nerve and by measuring the distance the impulse travels over that time period, a velocity can be calculated referred to as the nerve conduction velocity (NCV). The speed of conduction in a peripheral nerve is dependent primarily upon the degree of myelination in the nerve. Primary axonal disease may result in mild slowing of the NCV, whereas demyelination will result in significant slowing of the NCV. The NCV is most commonly recorded and measured along peripheral nerves of the limbs, however, some cranial nerves have been tested in a similar way.

Other electrodiagnostic techniques have been developed to assess the function in the proximal portions of the peripheral nerve. For example, F waves and H waves can be obtained during the NCV study and give information about conduction in the proximal portions of the spinal nerves and nerve roots (Cuddon 1998; Knecht et al. 1985; Sims and Selcer 1981; Steiss et al. 1984). These studies may be abnormal in diseases that preferentially affect the nerve root over the peripheral nerve, such as coonhound paralysis or polyradiculoneuritis. In still other instances of electrodiagnostic testing, as when a peripheral nerve in a limb is stimulated, the resultant electrical activity that is evoked either at the spinal cord level or the cerebral cortex is recorded. This is referred to as spinal-cord-evoked potentials or cord dorsum potentials if recorded over the spinal cord, or somatosensory-evoked potentials, if recorded overlying the cerebral cortex. These tests may aid in determining conduction primarily of sensory pathways in the CNS. Similar potentials evoked by stimulation of the cerebral cortex and recorded from limb muscles may aid in determining conduction along motor pathways (motor evoked potentials).

Single fiber EMG is a relatively new technique of looking at impulses evoked in single muscle fibers (Hopkins et al. 1993; Lavely et al. 2003). This test is useful to define abnormalities of the neuromuscular junction, such as myasthenia gravis.

Nerve and Muscle Biopsy

Biopsy of a peripheral nerve or muscle is often necessary to clarify the disease process within these tissues (fig. 9.34). Peripheral nerves that are more commonly biopsied include the peroneal and the tibial nerves of the pelvic limb and the cutaneous radial and ulnar nerves of the thoracic limb. When selecting a nerve for biopsy, the criteria listed in table 9.6 should be considered (Braund 1991).

If the nerve can be sacrificed (i.e., a sensory nerve), a small segment of the nerve is removed (segmental biopsy).

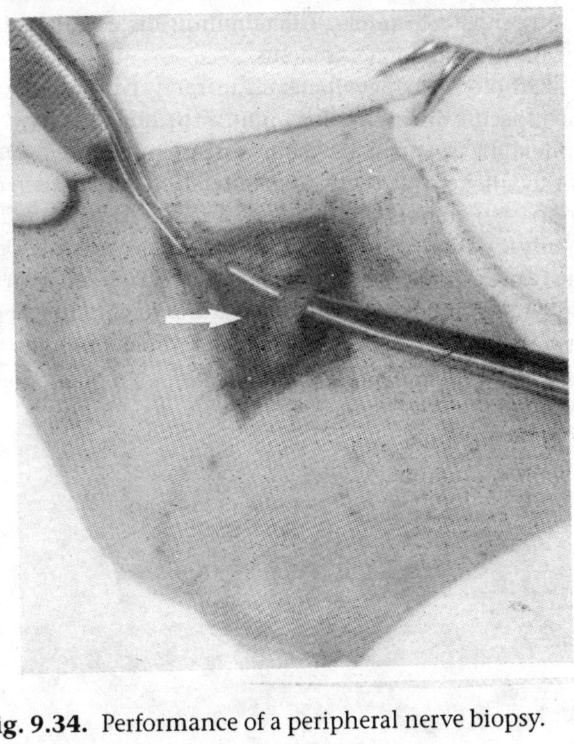

Fig. 9.34. Performance of a peripheral nerve biopsy.

Table 9.6. Criteria for selection of a peripheral nerve for biopsy

- The nerve should perform a nonessential function
- The nerve should be affected by the disease
- The nerve should be constant in its anatomical location
- The nerve should normally be protected from entrapment and recurrent nerve trauma
- The surgical approach should not damage nearby blood vessel, tendons or joints
- The area should be apt to heal well following surgery
- Normal quantitative data about the nerve morphology should exist

Source: Braund 1991.

Table 9.7. Criteria for selection of a muscle for biopsy

- Biopsy of the muscle should not affect muscle function.
- The muscle should be affected by the disease.
- Normal quantitative data should exist about the muscle morphology.
- Muscle groups not penetrated by a needle, such as during electrodiagnostic evaluation, should be biopsied to avoid misinterpretation of iatrogenic muscle damage.
- The surgical approach to the muscle should not interfere with any vital structure or function.
- The biopsy site should result in minimal postoperative pain.

Source: Braund 1991.

More commonly, a portion of the nerve is removed to avoid deficits of function following biopsy. This is referred to as a fascicular biopsy, as some fascicules of the nerve, but not the entire nerve, are removed and used for the evaluation. When performing a fascicular biopsy, approximately one-third of the diameter of the nerve can usually be removed without severe clinical consequences. After removal, the nerve is placed in a fixation such as gluteraldehyde for electron microscopic (EM) evaluation.

As pathologic alterations in the nerve can be difficult to detect with routine histologic processing and evaluation, it is recommended that peripheral nerve specimens be evaluated by an individual experienced in the microscopic evaluation of peripheral nerve disease. Appropriate analysis of peripheral nerve usually requires an EM evaluation. A more sophisticated analysis may include morphometric analysis, which determines the percentage of fibers of a certain diameter within the nerve. As disease may alter the number of a selective type of nerve fibers, morphometric analysis can aid in determining abnormalities of peripheral nerve axons. Teased fiber analysis is another evaluation technique used to examine individual nerve fibers. This analysis is useful, for example, in determining diseases that affect the myelination of nerve axons.

Pathologic changes in nerves are rarely pathognomonic for a specific disease etiology. Similar to kidney or liver, peripheral nerves are damaged by disease in a finite number of ways. In general, there can be alterations in the axon (axonopathy), abnormalities of myelination (demyelination, dysmyelination, or hypomyelination), or a combination of the two. Pathologic changes in the nerve, coupled with signalment of the animal and the features of the clinical disease are used to clarify or diagnose the disease process.

Muscle Biopsy

Muscle biopsy provides diagnostic information in a variety of congenital, degenerative, inflammatory, and metabolic muscle disorders. Muscle biopsy is useful for eliminating potential causes of myopathy. Muscle biopsy is indicated if there is a suspicion of primary muscle disease, denervation of muscle, animals with persistent and unexplained increases in CK, or animals with abnormal electrodiagnostic studies. Criteria for selecting a muscle for biopsy are similar to those for selecting a nerve for nerve biopsy and are listed in table 9.7 (Braund 1991).

Muscle samples collected at biopsy are also analyzed differently compared to routine histologic evaluation of other tissues. Consultation with a muscle pathologist will help the surgeon determine the best way to collect and store the muscle prior to analysis.

Muscle biopsy analysis is usually performed on fresh, nonfixed muscle samples. Enzyme histochemical evaluations for fiber type determination require fresh frozen muscle. Refrigeration of the muscle is used for transport, with the muscle frozen at the analysis laboratory. Formalin fixation limits the degree of muscle analysis. Muscle is frozen, sectioned, and stained to assess muscle morphology and muscle fiber types. Myopathic processes such as degeneration, inflammation, denervation, and necrosis can be determined. As with peripheral nerve biopsy, in some instances, muscle pathologic features are pathognomonic for a specific myopathic disease. In other instances, a finite number of pathologic processes occur in abnormal muscle in similar disease processes. Pathologic changes in the muscle coupled with signalment of the animal and the features of the clinical disease are used to clarify the diagnosis of the disease process.

10 Diagnostic Testing in Animals with Intracranial Neurologic Disease

Once a disease is suspected to be involving the intracranial nervous system, diagnostic testing is performed to elucidate or clarify the disease process. Surprisingly, there is a limited number of helpful antemortem diagnostic tests available and useful for identifying intracranial disease processes in animals (Braund 1994; Chrisman 1991; Dewey 2003; Oliver et al. 1987; Oliver et al. 1997). Some of these diagnostic tests are used to assess anatomical structural elements of the intracranial nervous system, while others are used to assess physiologic or functional integrity.

If the suspected disease is likely to alter the *anatomical structure* of the brain or intracranial nervous system, an *anatomical imaging study* is most likely to yield important information that will be helpful in revealing these types of pathological processes. In the modern era, the two most commonly employed antemortem anatomical imaging studies are *computed tomography (CT)* scanning and *magnetic resonance (MR) imaging*. The indications for, and utility of, these tests will be discussed further in this chapter. Survey radiographs of the skull are usually useful only in some instances of cranial disease. Skull radiographs may provide some indication of skull fracture or middle ear (bulla) disease, however, these studies do not allow for assessment of the underlying nervous system parenchyma. If peripheral ear disease is suspected, a thorough otoscopic examination, preferably while the animal is anesthetized, is indicated.

Analysis of *cerebrospinal fluid (CSF)* is used to elucidate disease that may currently involve the subarachnoid spaces of the brain cavity. Inflammatory brain diseases would be an example of the type of process CSF evaluation is helpful in identifying.

Electroencephalography (EEG) records electrical activity associated with intracranial and primarily supratentorial structures. This test may yield information regarding some aspects of brain electrical activity. The EEG may also be helpful in defining episodic brain dysfunction such as narcolepsy and seizure. Another electrophysiologic test, a *brain stem auditory potential (BAEP, BAER, or BSEP)*, may be useful in determining the presence and function of pathways for hearing including the integrity of central brain stem projection pathways (Steiss et al. 1994; Fischer and Obermaier 1994).

If a cranial nerve abnormality is suspected, *electromyography (EMG)* as a measure of the spontaneous electrical activity of muscle can be helpful in identifying abnormalities of innervation of the facial or head muscles (Holliday et al. 1992). Magnetic resonance imaging is utilized to show the anatomical location and structure of individual cranial nerves. Contrast radiographic studies, such as cavernous sinus venography, have been historically used to assess the cavernous sinus area, but are rarely necessary in the modern era as MR evaluations will provide a better anatomical evaluation of these structures and associated intracranial regions (Oliver et al. 1987). Other forms of intravascular contrast angiography to identify disease of the cerebrovascular structures are rarely performed in the modern era.

DIAGNOSIS OF INTRACRANIAL DISEASES

Degenerative Diseases

Many primary degenerative intracranial diseases of dogs and cats are inherited or congenital, and occur primarily in young animals (see discussion of degenerative intracranial disease in chapter 5). The majority of these diseases result in neurologic dysfunction without alterations in gross anatomical structure of the brain (Braund 1987; Coates and Mine 1995; March 1996). Therefore, advanced intracranial imaging studies, such CT or MR imaging, are invariably normal in affected animals. If the degenerative process results in atrophy or loss of intracranial cells and structural elements, this atrophy may be evident with MR imaging. For example, with some cerebellar diseases, the cerebellum is hypoplastic or becomes atrophied. A smaller than normal or absent cerebellum compared to an age-matched control animal might be found in MR evaluations of these animals. In some instances, the cerebellum will be reduced to a fluid-filled cyst (fig. 5.3). Other diseases may result in diffuse alterations in either white matter or grey matter of the brain (Vite et al. 2001). Some degenerative diseases in dogs, such as those similar to Leigh's syndrome in humans, may show bilateral hyperintense lesions (T2-weighted sequences) on MR imaging of the intracranial structures. These abnormalities may be present in various regions of the intracranial structures, but often involve the supratentorial (thalamic) structures.

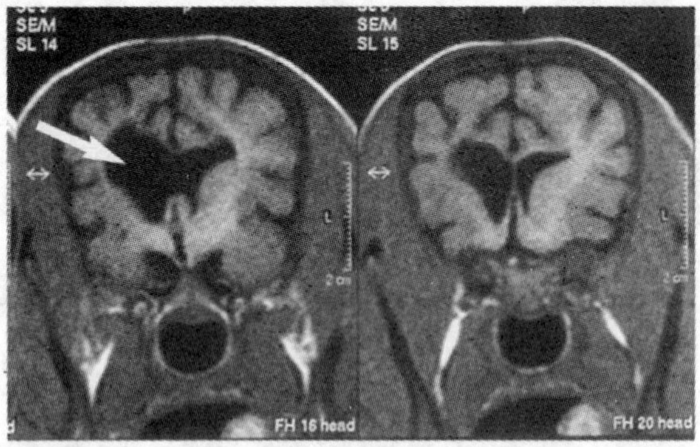

Fig. 10.1. Transverse MR image from a dog with a congenital malformation of the supratentorial structure. There is unilateral ventricular enlargement and lack of central cerebral white matter (*arrow*). The gyri and sulci are prominent.

As these processes are primary degenerative conditions without associated inflammation, routine CSF evaluations will often be normal. In some instances, protein elevations without concurrent increases in nucleated cells will be present in CSF, however, this is a nonspecific abnormality associated with a variety of nervous system diseases. Rarely, such as with globoid cell leukodystrophy (storage disease), an abnormal cell distended with a metabolic by-product may be apparent with cytologic evaluation of CSF. Additionally, in some instances, a more advanced evaluation of CSF for abnormal enzyme products or neurotransmitter analysis may be possible (see bibliography under Storage Diseases).

With many degenerative diseases, it is important to exclude underlying systemic abnormalities. A routine evaluation for systemic metabolic diseases of the heart, liver, and adrenals, for example, is necessary to ensure a primary cause for the central nervous system (CNS) degeneration. As primary intracranial degenerative diseases are usually isolated to the nervous system, routine blood work testing is normal.

Older animals with intracranial signs often have an underlying structural intracranial disease such as a brain tumor or systemic metabolic disorders as a cause of their clinical signs (Bagley 1997). Older animals (usually older than 10 to 12 years depending upon the breed) if evaluated with CT or MR imaging may show decreased size of the cortical layers of the hemispheres and resultant increases in cerebral ventricular dimensions. It is important to recognize that a degree of ventriculomegaly is a normal age-related change within the intracranial structures, most likely the result of cortical atrophy with increasing age. Occasionally on MR images in these older animals there will be concurrent increased signal intensity on T2-weighted images immediately adjacent to the ventricular walls. This may be an aging change in many of these dogs, however, the significance of this finding is under investigation.

For definitive diagnosis of many degenerative intracranial disorders, a biopsy is required. This is, however, rarely performed antemortem in animals. For diagnosis of storage diseases, biopsy of affected tissue or identification of metabolic products in serum or urine may support the diagnosis. Determination of lysosomal enzyme activities of brain and other cells may be helpful. Of note, in animals with globoid cell leukodystrophy, peripheral nerve biopsy may show characteristic pathologic changes of this disease (Vicini et al. 1988).

Anomalous Disease

Development anomalies such as aplasia, hypoplasia, or dysplasia may alter the normal intracranial anatomical relationships and be evident as anatomically abnormal regions within the nervous system on MR studies (Fig. 10.1) (Jeffery et al. 2003). As an example, with lissencephaly, the cortical gyri may be more prominent and thicker than normal (Dewey 2003). Cerebrospinal fluid analysis is usually normal unless there is associated neural degeneration or inflammation.

Intracranial arachnoid cysts may be congenital in origin, or may result as out-pocketing of the cerebral ventricles (fig. 10.2). These abnormalities are usually readily apparent with MR imaging.

Epidermoid and dermoid cysts result from abnormal development of the neural tube. These abnormalities are often found in the fourth ventricle and foramen magnum area as irregular, multilobulated, fluid-containing structures on CT and MR imaging (fig. 10.3). Contrast enhancement (following intravenous administration of contrast media) may be present in the tissues on the periphery of the cystic structures.

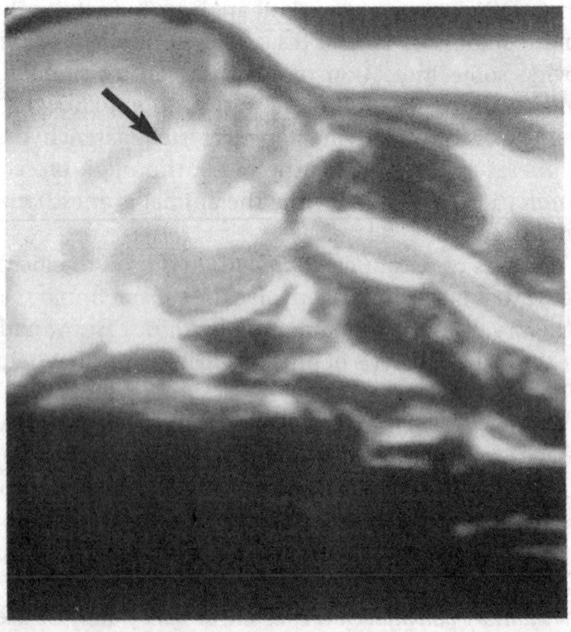

Fig. 10.2. Sagittal, T2-weighted magnetic resonance view of an animal with an intracranial arachnoid cyst (*arrow*) and associated hydrocephalus. This dog also has an atlantoaxial subluxation.

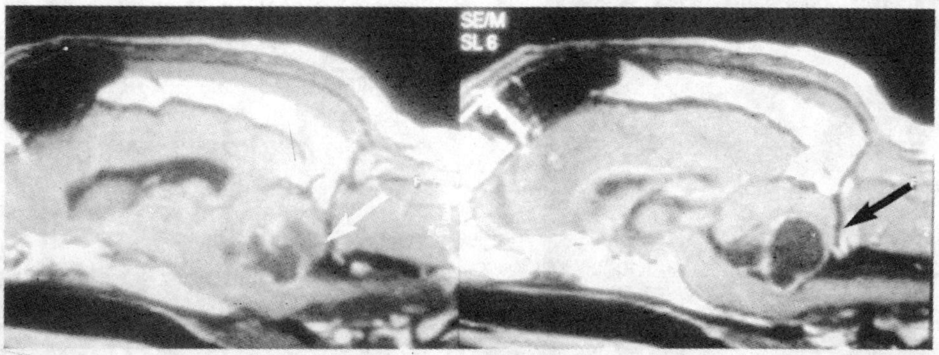

Fig. 10.3. Sagittal, T2-weighted magnetic resonance views of an animal with an epidermoid cyst (*arrows*).

Hydrocephalus

Hydrocephalus can result from obstruction of the ventricular system, irritation of the ventricle (from inflammation or hemorrhage), and increased size of the ventricles due to loss of brain parenchyma (hydrocephalus ex vacuo). Diagnosis of hydrocephalus can be supported by information obtained from a variety of imaging and electrophysiologic modalities (see bibliography under Hydrocephalus). Survey radiographs of the skull may be abnormal in instances of congenital hydrocephalus, however, these are usually not helpful for definitive diagnosis. Findings associated with congenital hydrocephalus include loss of gyral striations, separation of cranial sutures (diastasis), and persistent fontanels (Few 1966). If hydrocephalus is acquired after the skull has formed, abnormalities are rarely demonstrated with skull radiographic evaluation.

Historically, invasive techniques such as pneumo- or contrast ventriculography where air or a radiologic contrast agent is directly injected into the ventricular system were used to anatomically diagnose hydrocephalus (deLahunta 1983). These tests, however, have been replaced by noninvasive evaluations, such as MR imaging in the modern era. Electroencephalography has been used historically to support the diagnosis of hydrocephalus. This study was primarily used prior to the utilization of advanced imaging studies such as MR imaging. Classically, slow frequency, high voltage (amplitude) activity is noted on the EEG in animals with hydrocephalus (Klemm and Hall 1971). This pattern, however, can be seen with other encephalopathies that destroy cortical parenchyma. Because of the poor specificity of this diagnosis test, EEG is rarely used as the sole means of diagnosis of hydrocephalus.

Ultrasound can be used to support a diagnosis of hydrocephalus (Hudson et al. 1989; Hudson et al. 1990; Hudson et al. 1991; Spaulding and Sharp 1990). This is most readily accomplished when a fontanel is present providing an "acoustic window" as ultrasound waves do not usually penetrate the skull well enough to provide a reasonable anatomical image. Measurements of ventricle size have been recorded for normal neonatal dogs and dogs with hydrocephalus using ultrasound imaging, however, the correlation between the degree of ventricular enlargement and clinical signs is poor. Also, ultrasonic ventricular evaluation does not always provide for a global view of the ventricular system, and, therefore, some obstructive lesions may be missed.

Computed tomography is often useful in defining ventricular size (fig. 10.4). As CSF has a lower CT number than brain parenchyma, the ventricular system is usually readily identified due to the relative blackness of CSF in comparison to brain parenchyma. Computed tomographic evaluation also affords the ability to examine the majority of the ventricular system as well as additional intracranial structures (Kay et al. 1986). As stated previously, however, ventricular size does not correlate with the presence or degree of clinical signs.

Magnetic resonance imaging also affords evaluation of the ventricular system (figs. 10.4 and 10.5) (Harrington et al. 1996). The ventricular system filled with CSF will appear hypointense (blacker) on a T1-weighted, and hyperintense (whiter) on a T2-weighted imaging sequence. The ability of MR imaging to provide anatomical views in multiple planes without reductions in image quality allows for a more thorough assessment of the ventricular system. Focal dilation of portions of the ventricular system are also readily determined.

Cerebrospinal fluid analysis in instances of hydrocephalus is performed to exclude an underlying inflammatory cause for hydrocephalus. As parainfluenza infection in young animals has been associated with dilation of the ventricles, specific evaluation for this and other infectious agents with serum or CSF titers may be currently necessary. Intraventricular hemorrhage, either as a cause or effect of hydrocephalus, may result in xanthochromia and cytologic evidence of erthyrophagocytosis.

Metabolic Encephalopathies

Numerous metabolic abnormalities may alter intracranial functions (Cuddon 1996). Clues to the diagnosis of many of these diseases can be present on routine database blood and urine assessments. A diagnosis of hepatic encephalopathy is supported by clinical signs and abnormal liver function studies such as bile acids testing (see bibliography under Hepatic Encephalopathy). Various ultrasound, scin-

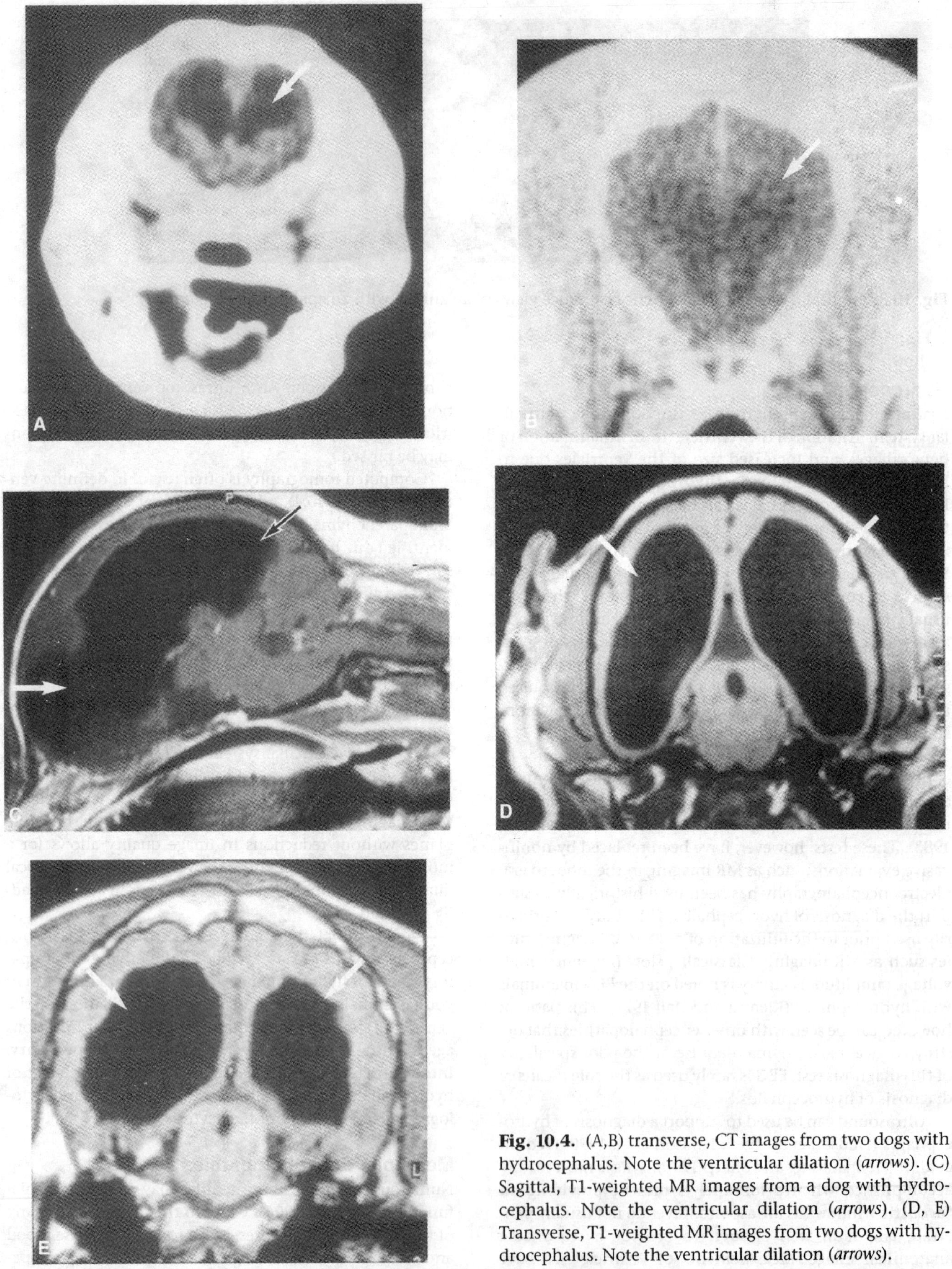

Fig. 10.4. (A,B) transverse, CT images from two dogs with hydrocephalus. Note the ventricular dilation (*arrows*). (C) Sagittal, T1-weighted MR images from a dog with hydrocephalus. Note the ventricular dilation (*arrows*). (D, E) Transverse, T1-weighted MR images from two dogs with hydrocephalus. Note the ventricular dilation (*arrows*).

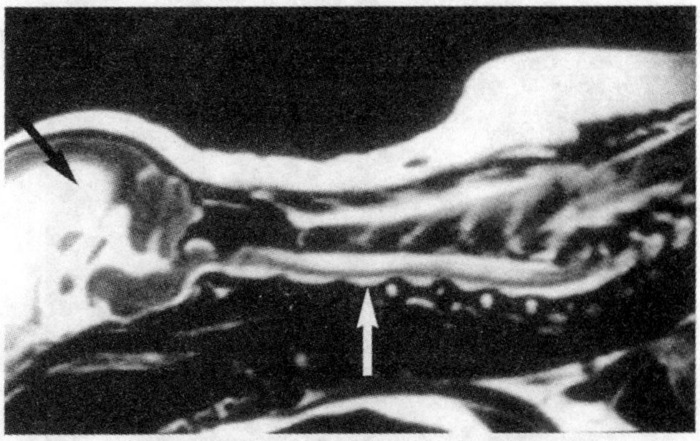

Fig. 10.5. Sagittal, T2-weighted MR image from a dog showing hydrocephalus and syringomyelia (*arrows*).

tigraphic, portal angiography, and MR-angiography studies of the liver and abdominal vasculature may show the anatomical vascular abnormalities of the liver and portal system. Liver biopsy and direct visualization of the liver and portal system at laparotomy may be used for diagnosis of abnormalities of the portal system and liver parenchyma.

The diagnosis of hypoglycemia as a cause of neurologic dysfunction is based upon finding hypoglycemia (blood glucose <60 mg/dl) in association with clinical signs (Howerton and Shell 1992). Concurrent serum insulin concentration will help in determining the presence of an insulin-secreting tumor. Insulinomas will be associated with relatively increased serum insulin compared to serum glucose, whereas extrapancreatic neoplasia will be associated with low insulin concentrations in the face of hypoglycemia. Ultrasound of the pancreas may show larger tumors or may detect evidence of metastasis to lymph nodes or liver. Extrapancreatic neoplasms are usually relatively large and are palpable or found on survey abdominal radiographs. As hypoglycemia associated with insulinoma often results in an associated peripheral neuropathy, peripheral nerve biopsy may be used to diagnose underlying peripheral nerve pathology.

Persistent, insulin-resistant hyperglycemia may suggest acromegaly from a pituitary tumor, especially in cats. Computed tomography or MR imaging of the intracranial structures may reveal a pituitary mass in these animals.

Diseases such as hyperthyroidism, hypothyroidism, and hyperadrenocorticism (Cushing's disease) are diagnosed based on appropriate clinical signs and concurrent abnormalities on blood, urine, or endocrine testing. Similarly, electrolyte disorders such as hypernatremia and hyponatremia are diagnosed through evaluation of blood and serum electrolyte concentrations. Osmotic myelinolysis, which can result from too rapid correction of hyponatremia, can result in characteristic bilateral lesions on MR imaging of the intracranial structures. Lesions are most notable as hyperintense (whiter) lesions on T2-weighted sequences that are bilaterally symmetrical, usually round or oval abnormalities primarily located in the thalamus of dogs. The degree of T2-weighted MR signal intensity is often correlated with the duration of the abnormality (more hyperintense earlier in the disease). Some of the animals may have associated cerebrovascular disease and evidence of cerebral infarction on MR studies. These lesions may persist on MR imaging for weeks even with associated clinical improvement.

With some of the primary *metabolic encephalopathies,* such as mitochondrial encephalopathies, there is increased CSF lactate and pyruvates in humans, however, this is not established in dogs (Dewey 2003). Cerebrospinal fluid analysis is usually normal. CT or MR may show bilaterally symmetric, cavitary lesions of brain and spinal cord. With MR, these lesions are hypointense on T1-weighted images and hyperintense on T2-weighted images.

Neoplasia

Neoplastic diseases affecting the intracranial space will often alter the anatomical structure of the affected intracranial structures. The diagnosis of an intracranial mass is readily made using advanced imaging modalities such as CT or MR imaging (figs. 10.6, 10.7, 10.8, 10.9, 10.10) (see bibliography under Brain Tumor). Imaging features of primary brain tumor have been reviewed (Tucker and Gavin 1996; Turrel et al. 1986). Cats and, rarely, dogs may have multiple tumors (fig. 10.9). Meningiomas most commonly appear as a broad-based, extra-axial (arising outside and pushing into the parenchyma) contrast-enhancing mass on CT or MR imaging (fig. 10.6). These tumors may contain hemorrhagic regions or be mineralized (calcified). With CT, these two components result in a hyperdense (more white) appearance on precontrast studies. Hemorrhage may have a varied appearance with MR depending on the duration of the hemorrhage.

The CT and MR appearance of gliomas is varied and enhancement after contrast administration is inconsistent (fig. 10.7). In general, gliomas are hypodense to isodense on CT images. Gliomas may be difficult to detect on some CT studies. With MR imaging, gliomas often appear hyperintense (whiter) on T2-weighted images and hypointense (blacker) on T1-weighted imaging sequences. A tumor confined within the parenchyma of the brain is characteristic of a glioma on both CT and MR imaging. Diffuse gliomas may result in multiple abnormal areas within the intracranial space mimicking an inflammatory process or cerebrovascular disease.

Choroid plexus tumors, because of the concentration of blood vessels within the tumor, are often markedly enhanced after intravenous contrast administration (fig. 10.8). Obstruction of the ventricle system may result in hydrocephalus in association with these tumors. Pituitary tumors may be found in the sella or suprasellar location and expand into the diencephalon (fig. 10.10). Smaller tumors are more readily seen with MR imaging especially with dynamic contrast studies. Macroadenomas may enlarge dorsally and invade or compress the diencephalon.

Cerebrospinal fluid analysis may be abnormal in ani-

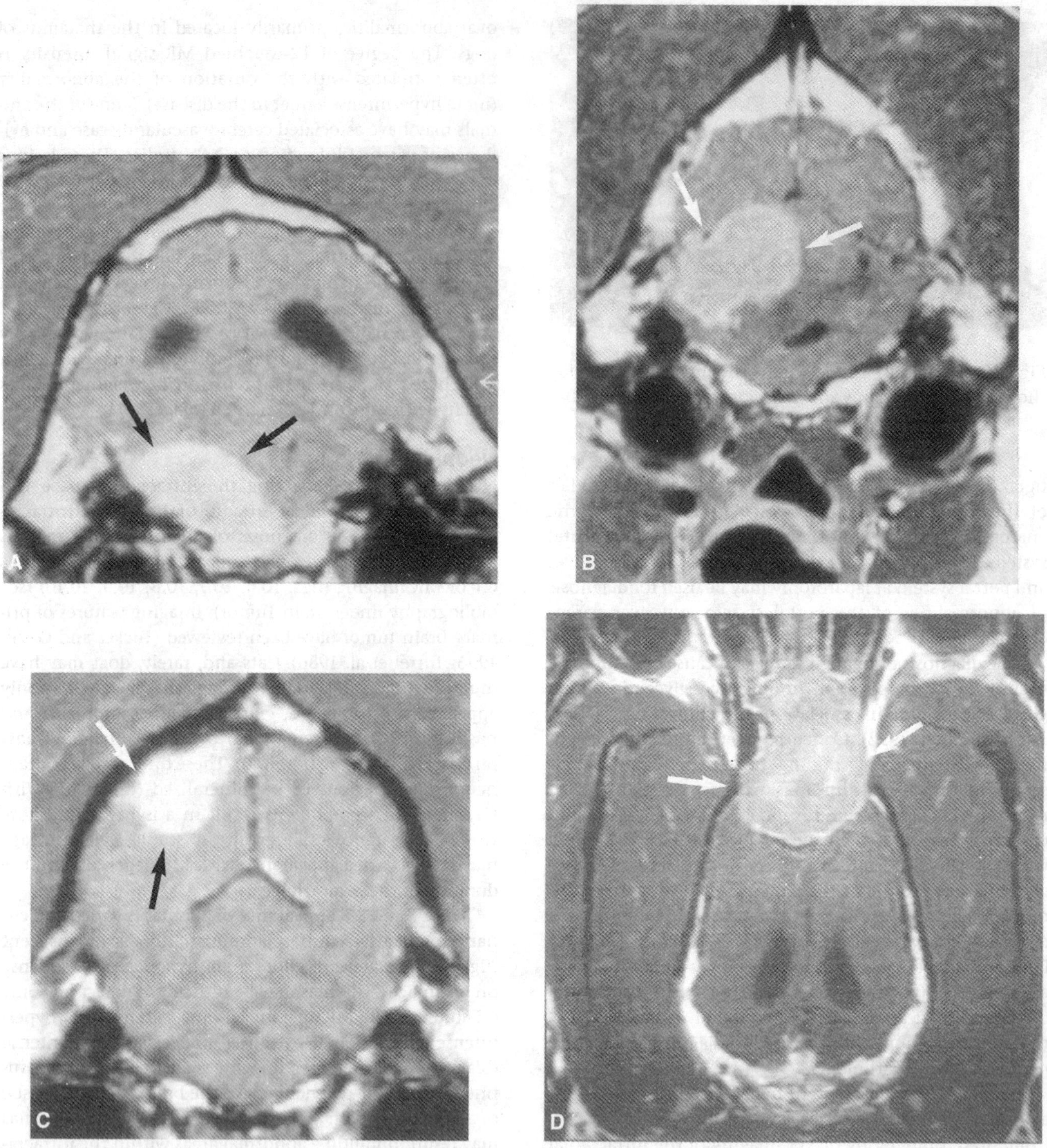

Fig. 10.6. (A,B,C) Transverse and (D)dorsal, T1-weighted MR images following intravenous contrast administration from dogs with brain tumors (*arrows*). Histologic diagnosis for all of these tumors was meningioma.

mals with brain tumor, but results are often not helpful for definitive diagnosis. Classically, CSF in dogs with brain tumor contains increased protein without a concurrent pleocytosis (albuminocytologic dissociation). In a significant proportion of dogs with brain tumors, however, cellular changes consistent with inflammation are present and, interpreted in isolation, may falsely suggest a primary inflammatory disease (encephalitis or meningitis) (Bailey and Higgins 1986; Carrillo et al. 1986). Occasionally, CSF in a dog with a brain tumor will be normal. The presence of neoplastic cells in the CSF is specific for certain neoplastic diseases, however, neoplastic cells are rarely (<2% of cases) found in CSF from animals with primary brain tumors. Neoplastic cells in CSF are more readily present with neoplastic disease such as lymphoma, carcinomatosis, and choroid plexus tumors.

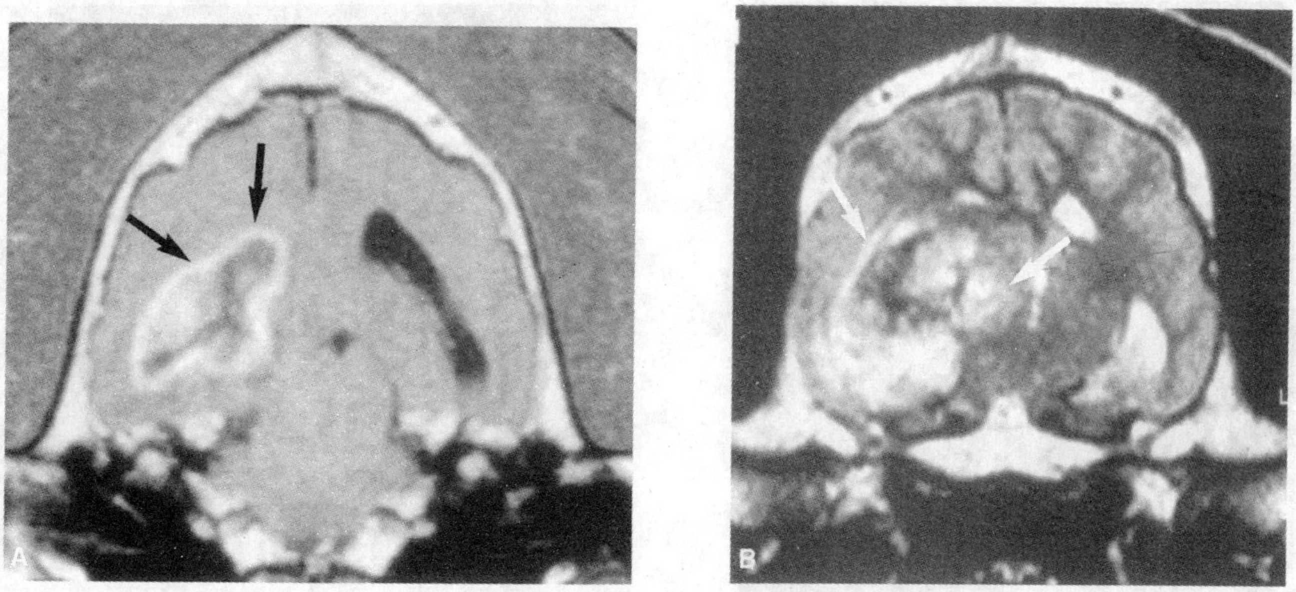

Fig. 10.7. (A) Transverse, T1-weighted MR image following intravenous contrast administration from a dog with a brain tumor (*arrows*). Histologic diagnosis was a glioma. (B) Transverse, T2-weighted MR image from a dog with a brain tumor (arrows). Histologic diagnosis was a glioma.

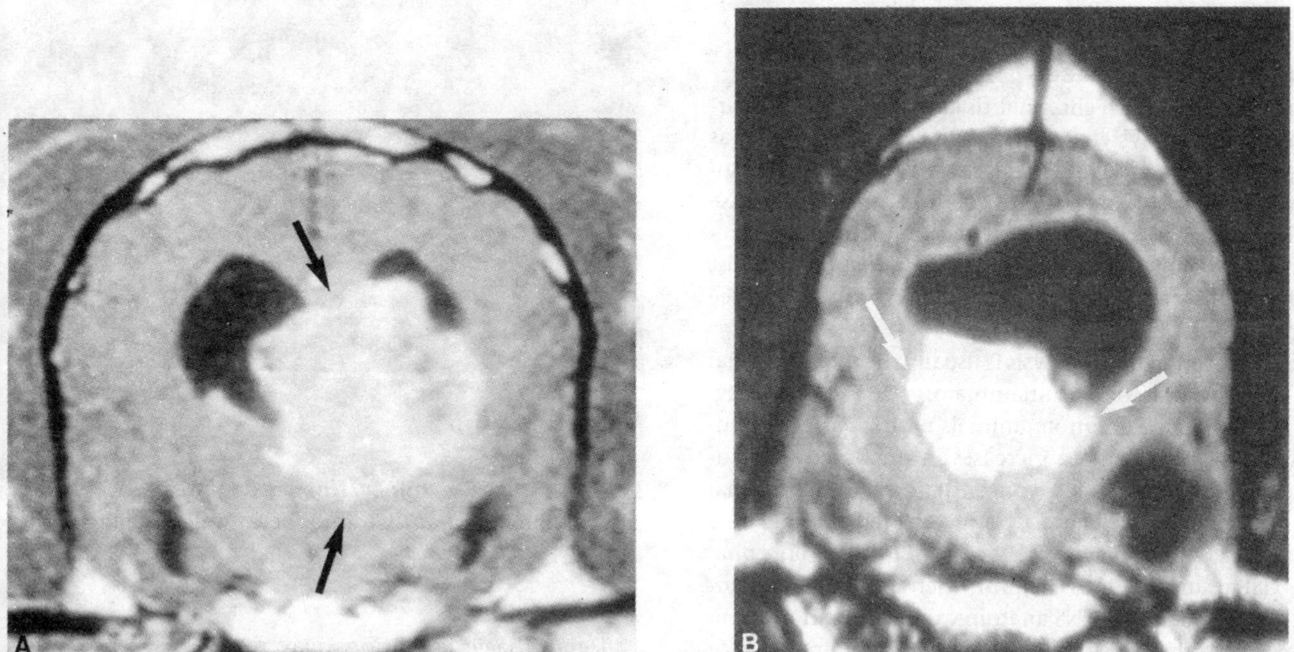

Fig. 10.8. (A,B) Transverse, T1-weighted MR images following intravenous contrast administration from two dogs with brain tumors within the ventricles (*arrows*). Histologic diagnosis from both dogs was a choroid plexus tumor.

Definitive diagnosis of a brain tumor requires a biopsy, as all masses seen with MR and CT imaging are not neoplastic. Biopsy of a brain mass may occur at the time of a craniotomy or be performed percutaneously with a stereotaxic brain biopsy system (stereotaxic biopsy). As this may not be performed for a variety of reasons, a brain tumor is often diagnosed presumptively based on characteristic imaging features.

Nutrition

Thiamine deficiency is the most commonly recognized nutritional abnormality affecting the intracranial structures of animals. Bilaterally symmetrical hyperintense (whiter) abnormalities may be seen in brain stem nuclear areas, and possibly the cerebellum (in dogs) with MR imaging of affected animals (Garosi et al. 2003).

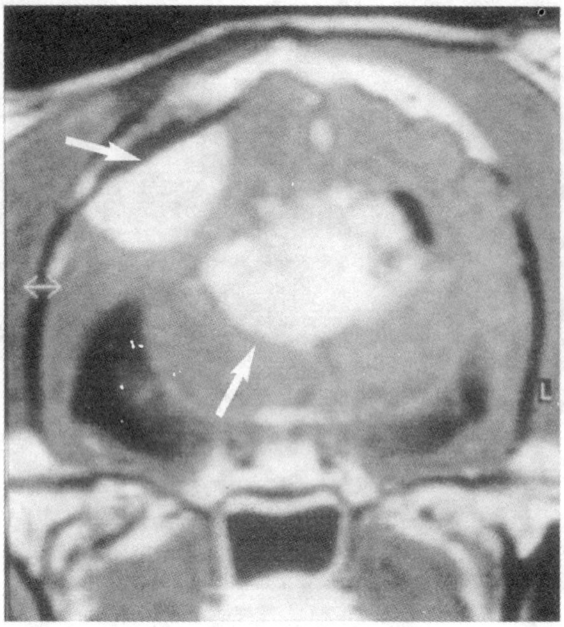

Fig. 10.9. Transverse, T1-weighted MR image following intravenous contrast administration from a cat with multiple meningiomas (*arrows*).

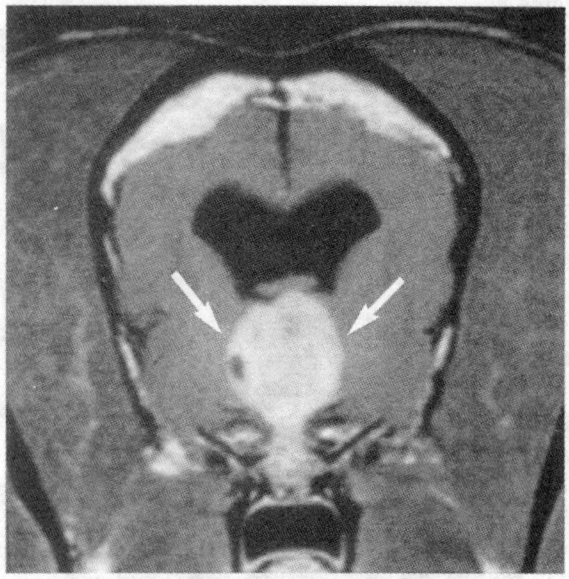

Fig. 10.10. Transverse, T1-weighted MR image following intravenous contrast administration from a dog with a pituitary tumor (*arrows*).

Inflammatory Diseases

In many animals with encephalitis and meningitis the cardinal signs of an systemic inflammatory processes such as the presence of a fever and increases in WBCs in the leukogram may not be found as localized inflammatory disease in the CNS may not elicit a systemic inflammatory response (see bibliography under Encephalitis). Classically, clinical signs are diffuse within the nervous system (see chapter 5).

Cerebrospinal fluid analysis is usually the most essential test for diagnosis of an inflammatory CNS disease (fig. 10.11). Classically, CSF from animals with a variety of encephalitidies will contain increases in nucleated (inflammatory) cells and protein concentrations. Cerebrospinal fluid results used in isolation, however, rarely provide for a definitive etiologic diagnosis. In cases of primary encephalitis, CSF results are most helpful when evaluated concurrently with results of CNS anatomical imaging in order to exclude underlying primary diseases such as brain tumor or hemorrhage that may secondarily result in intracranial inflammation. Increased numbers of nucleated cells and increased protein concentrations are commonly present in CSF from animals with inflammatory CNS disease.

Nucleated cell numbers and types are variable in instances of encephalitis depending upon the underlying etiology. In most primary inflammatory CNS conditions in dogs and cats, however, mononuclear cells and neutrophils are the predominant cell types present. Eosinophils may indicate an inflammatory response to a parasite or allergen, however, these cell types may also be predominant in certain infection conditions such as cryptococcus in cats and protothecosis in dogs.

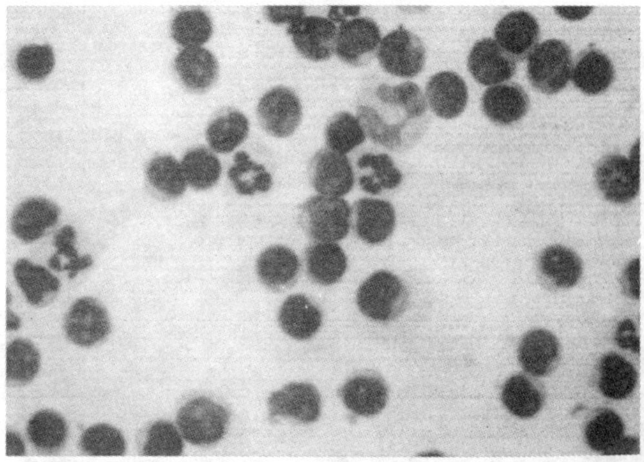

Fig. 10.11. CSF cytology from a dog with encephalitis showing predominantly mononuclear cells and a few neutrophils.

Hemorrhagic conditions may result in secondary inflammation in the CSF. Conversely, inflammation of the CNS may secondarily result in hemorrhage. If prior CNS hemorrhage has occurred, CSF may have a xanthochromic or hemorrhagic appearance and contain cytologic evidence of erythrophagocytosis with cytologic evaluation of a sample. If the clinician is not certain that a hemorrhagic appearance to CSF is the result of iatrogenic hemorrhage, it is reasonable to have the sample analyzed for possible associated or underlying inflammation.

Unfortunately, evidence of inflammation on CSF evaluation alone is not specific for primary encephalitis as other CNS diseases (e.g., neoplasia, trauma, infarction) may result in a CSF pleocytosis and protein elevations (Bailey and

Higgins 1986; Carillo et al. 1986). Evaluation of serum or CSF titers for the multiple infectious diseases is often necessary to establish associated infectious diseases. Common infectious etiologies for dogs include toxoplasmosis, neospora, distemper, and some types of fungi. Common infectious etiologies in cats include toxoplasmosis, feline infectious peritonitis, cryptococcus, and other as yet unclassified but suspected viral agents. In up to 60% or more of cases of encephalitis in dogs and cats, however, an infectious etiology is not identified.

Occasionally, CSF from an animal with inflammatory CNS disease may be normal at a single sampling. This is especially true when the disease is primarily intraparenchymal and sometimes occurs following corticosteroid administration prior to CSF collection.

For specific diagnosis, imaging studies such as MR imaging and CT are helpful in providing information regarding anatomical lesions associated with primary inflammation (fig. 10.12). Multifocal discrete, anatomical lesions may be present within the nervous system, and these lesions may be especially conspicuous after intravenous contrast medium administration suggesting alterations in the blood-brain barrier or the cerebral vasculature. Areas of inflammation may appear as either hyperintense (whiter) or hypointense (blacker) areas depending upon the underlying pathological process. As inflammation is often associated with edema formation, areas of inflammation are often apparent as hyperintense (whiter) regions on T2-weighted MR imaging sequences.

Biopsy, either via craniotomy or percutaneously with stereotactic devices, of any structural abnormalities associated with inflammatory CNS processes has the potential to result in a definitive diagnosis. Culture (aerobic, anaerobic, and fungal) should also be performed of any biopsied material to exclude common infectious organisms.

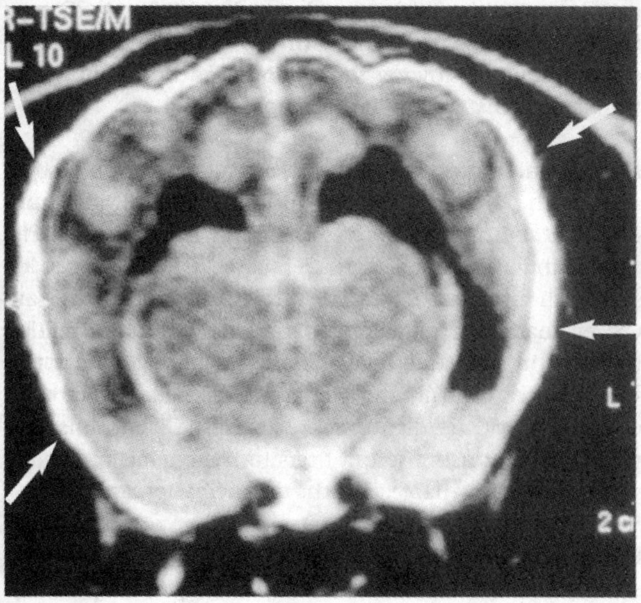

Fig. 10.12. Transverse, T1-weighted MR image following intravenous contrast administration from a dog with meningitis. Note the contrast enhancement of the meninges (*arrows*).

Diagnosis of Specific Inflammatory Diseases

Bacteria. The diagnosis of bacterial meningitis is aided by CSF analysis. Cerebrospinal fluid collection should be performed with caution, however, as the intracranial alterations associated with bacterial encephalitis may result in significant increases in intracranial pressure and resultant brain herniation. A cerebral abscess may also form (fig. 10.13). While attempts have been made to classify CSF changes commonly associated with septic inflammatory CNS diseases, the degree of overlap in CSF nucleated cell counts and types makes it difficult to diagnose a specific inflammatory disease using routine CSF results alone. One clue to the presence of a bacterial component is a decreased glucose concentration in CSF as compared to plasma, presumably due to consumption of glucose by the organism. If bacterial encephalitis is suspected, additional CSF should be collected in a sterile container without fixative or other chemicals for culturing and sensitivity testing. Glass tubes containing EDTA, commonly used for submission of CSF for cytological analysis, are not appropriate for culture as the EDTA is bacteriostatic and may hinder organism growth. As the number of organisms in CSF can be small, the greater amount of CSF cultured the more likely an organism will be isolated. As identification of the organism through culturing may take a few days and the clinical signs are often rapidly progressive, treatment is often initiated prior to culture analysis (see chapter 13).

If a cerebral abscess forms, acute surgical decompression is often warranted. The associated inflammation and increased ICP with cerebral abscessation often is rapidly fatal. Debridement and decompression of the abscess can be performed more effectively with a craniotomy. Occasionally,

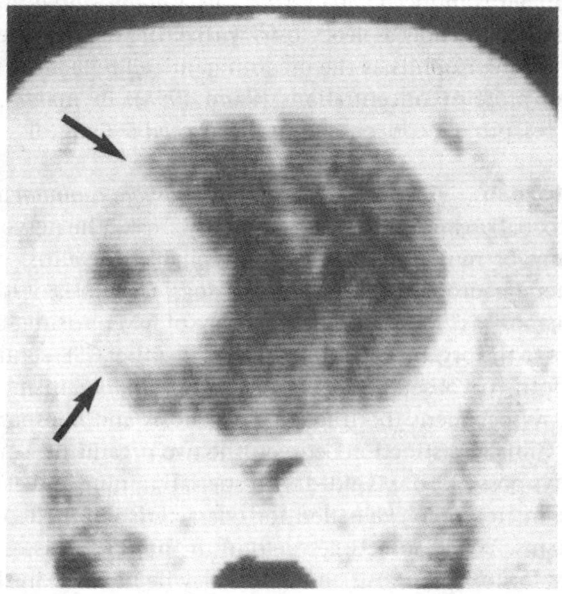

Fig. 10.13. Transverse, CT images from a dog with a cerebral abscess (*arrows*).

epidural or subdural localized infection (abscessation) may occur and also may require surgical drainage and decompression.

Virus. Viral encephalitis is often associated with increases in mononuclear cells and protein on CSF evaluation. A presumptive diagnosis of viral encephalitis is suggested by finding inclusion bodies in CSF cellular elements. Elevated CSF antibody titer (IgG and IgM) against distemper virus is supportive of a diagnosis especially if concurrent serum distemper titers are not elevated or if a CSF electrophoresis suggests intrathecal antibody production. As many dogs are either exposed to, or vaccinated for, canine distemper, dogs commonly have serum titer evidence of distemper antibodies. Cerebrospinal fluid from vaccinated dogs should not contain antibody to this virus. If, however, there is disruption of the blood-brain barrier, serum antibodies may "leak" from the serum to the CSF and be detected on CSF distemper titers even if those antibodies were not produced in the CSF. Therefore, in evaluation for evidence of distemper antibody in CSF, it is common to measure both CSF and serum distemper antibody titers. An antibody titer for distemper virus in the CSF that equals or exceeds a concurrent antibody titer in the serum is suggestive of local (intrathecal) antibody production in the CSF. Protein electrophoresis of the CSF sample may also give an indication of the presence of intrathecal antibody production in response to distemper virus infection. Occasionally, dogs with CNS distemper do not have positive CSF distemper titers.

Other viruses of dogs that result in encephalitis and meningitis do so primarily in very young animals. Diagnosis of these viral etiologies requires supportive evidence such as the presence of antibodies to these viral agents in CSF.

Feline infectious peritonitis (FIP) results from a coronavirus-induced vasculitis in cats. Cerebrospinal fluid analysis may show a pleocytosis, with either mononuclear cells or neutrophils as the predominant cell type and elevated protein concentrations (Rand 1994). In many instances, protein concentrations will exceed 500 mg/dl.

Protozoan. *Toxoplasma gondii* and *Neospora caninum* are protozoal organisms that can affect any area of the nervous system or muscle resulting in encephalitis, myelitis, peripheral neuropathy, or myositis in dogs. Diagnosis of toxoplasmosis is based upon the presence of IgM or rising IgG titers to the organism (toxoplasmosis) in either CSF, serum, or both, or observation of the protozoan organism in biopsy specimens (both for toxoplasmosis and neosporosis). Clinical distinction between the two organisms is not always possible, but is aided with special staining and electron microscopic evaluation for characteristics of the organisms. While sometimes helpful in the diagnosis, CSF titers for toxoplasmosis antibodies may be negative in the presence of CNS toxoplasmosis infection.

Cerebrospinal fluid may show a pleocytosis, usually with mononuclear cells, and occasionally, eosinophils. Increasing IgG or a single positive IgM serum antibody titer is diagnostic of active infection (Lappin et al. 1989). Serum titers may be more often positive compared to CSF titers with CNS toxoplasmosis. Serological titers to the presence of *Neospora* antibodies are also available to support the diagnosis of this infection. As with most systemic titer results, the presence of antibodies against these organisms does not ensure but rather suggests the presence of active CNS infection.

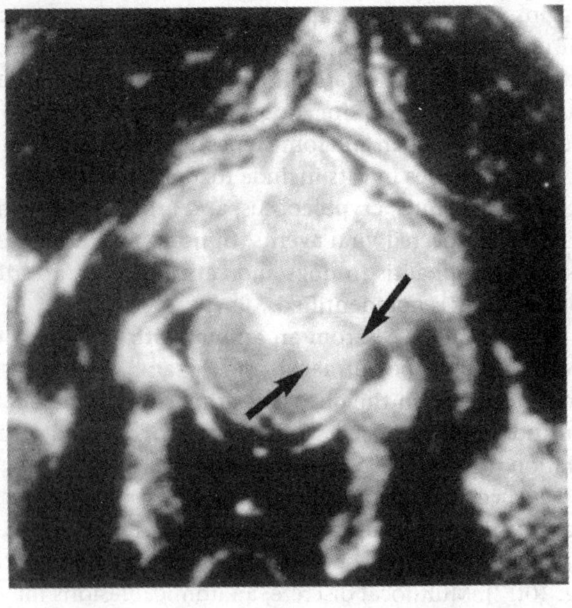

Fig. 10.14. Transverse, T2-weighted MR images from a cat with focal brain stem abnormality (*arrows*). Histologic diagnosis was a toxoplasmosis.

Imaging studies such as MR may show focal or multifocal abnormalities with toxoplasmosis (fig. 10.14). Often, there is evidence of edema within these lesions, however, enhancement following intravenous contrast administration is inconsistent and is often not found.

Rickettsia. Infection with rickettsial organisms associated with Rocky Mountain spotted fever (RMSF) and *Ehrlichia* commonly involves the brain stem, particularly the vestibular system. Diagnosis is based on lack of mass lesion with intracranial imaging studies and a pleocytosis on CSF evaluation. Cerebrospinal fluid usually contains milder increases in nucleated cells (<50 nucleated cells/µl; normal <5 nucleated cells/µl) and milder increases in protein concentration (<50 mg/dl; normal <25 mg/dl). Diagnosis is supported by increasing serum titers to the organism, but results often are available after the disease has progressed.

Fungus. Definitive diagnosis is often made through observing the fungal organism in CSF or biopsy samples and fungal culture of infected nervous tissues. Advanced imaging studies may show focal or diffuse, usually contrast-enhancing abnormalities.

With cryptococcosis, identification of the organism from cytological evaluation of samples such as CSF, nasal discharge, and skin lesions supports the diagnosis. A neutrophilic pleocytosis, and occasionally an eosinophilic pleocytosis, may be found on CSF analysis. Specialized CSF testing, such as India ink, may reveal the organism. Positive detection of the cryptococcal capsular antigen in serum or CSF is usually diagnostic. Tissue biopsy and fungal culture or fungal culture of CSF may be more definitive in the diagnosis as occasionally the serum titer is negative.

Parasites. Disease of the intracranial nervous structures can occur secondary to the effects of parasites such as *Cuterebra* larvae, *Toxocara*, and aberrant heartworm migration. Imaging studies have been rarely reported with parasitic migrations, but they may reveal abnormalities of anatomical intracranial structure if the parasite creates a large enough abnormality. With cystic parasites, such as *Echinococcus*, multifocal cystic abnormalities may be present within the brain and apparent with MR or CT imaging. These lesions are usually more diffuse and uniformly round in appearance compared to other cystic intracranial structural diseases, such as tumor, vascular disease, or encephalitis. With parasitic infection, CSF may classically contain inflammation with eosinophils, but this is inconsistent. Evidence of CSF inflammation with increases in other inflammatory cells (mononuclear cells, neutrophils) and protein may also be present in parasitic disease.

Noninfectious Diseases. *Granulomatous meningoencephalitis* (*GME*) is histologically characterized by dense aggregations of mesenchymal cells arranged in a whirling perivascular pattern. Cerebrospinal fluid analysis in affected animals usually contains increases in nucleated cell counts with concurrent increases in protein concentrations (40 to 400+ mg/gl). Lymphocytes or monocytes are usually the predominant cell type, but these cells are often the predominant cell type with a variety of intracranial inflammatory disease processes. Sometimes large anaplastic mononuclear cells are found that might be more suggestive of GME, however, neoplasia and other conditions that can result in increased reactivity of cells should be considered with these cell types. Occasionally, CSF from affected dogs will be normal or contain only elevated protein. Computed tomography or MR imaging may show diffuse inflammatory changes or a mass lesion (Plummer et al. 1992). When GME forms a focal mass lesion, this abnormality can be difficult to distinguish from a focal neoplasm on advanced imaging studies (fig. 10.15). Biopsy of the abnormal tissue is needed for definitive diagnosis.

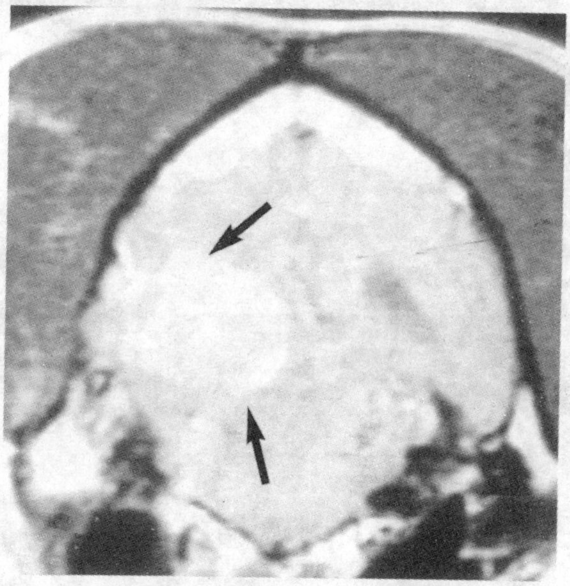

Fig. 10.15. Transverse, T1-weighted MR image following intravenous contrast administration from a dog with GME forming a focal mass (*arrows*).

There are a number of CNS inflammatory diseases that occur in specific breeds of animals, referred to as breed-specific meningitis (fig. 10.16). Cerebrospinal fluid in these dogs may contain elevations in protein concentration and increases in nucleated cell counts. Usually lymphocytes or monocytes predominate, however, neutrophils may occasionally be present. Magnetic resonance and other advanced imaging studies may show edema, focal mass effect, diffuse hyperintense abnormalities on T2-studies, or focal or multifocal contrast-enhancing lesions. Abnormalities apparent on MR images, however, are not pathognomonic for these diseases.

There is a unique clinical syndrome associated with generalized tremoring (generalized tremor syndrome; white shaker dog syndrome), which is commonly the result of an encephalitis. Cerebrospinal fluid usually is abnormal containing a mild lymphocytic pleocytosis. Protein concentration may be normal or mildly increased. Occasionally, CSF analysis is normal. Computed tomography has been reported in only a few cases. In one group of seven Maltese terriers with this disease, four of four evaluated with CT had ventricular enlargement (Bagley et al. 1993). The significance of this finding is unknown, however, as there is a high incidence of ventricular enlargement in Maltese terriers without this concurrent tremor disorder.

Idiopathic Disease. Any disease that doesn't have a specific etiology is referred to as idiopathic. With some disease processes, even with exhaustive clinical, biochemical, and histologic evaluations over years of observation, no etiology has been established. Idiopathic epilepsy, for example, would fulfill these diagnostic criteria. Some dogs with idiopathic epilepsy when imaged with MR following their seizure (usually more than one) will have structural alterations in the intracranial structures (fig. 10.17). Persistent structural alterations in brain tissue due to chronic seizures and associated brain atrophy may also be evident on MR imaging.

Narcolepsy (excessive daytime sleepiness) and cataplexy (periods of acute muscular hypotonia) usually occur without underlying structural brain disease (Thomas 2003). Acute onset of REM sleep , usually occurring with stimulation such as eating, is characteristic of narcolepsy.

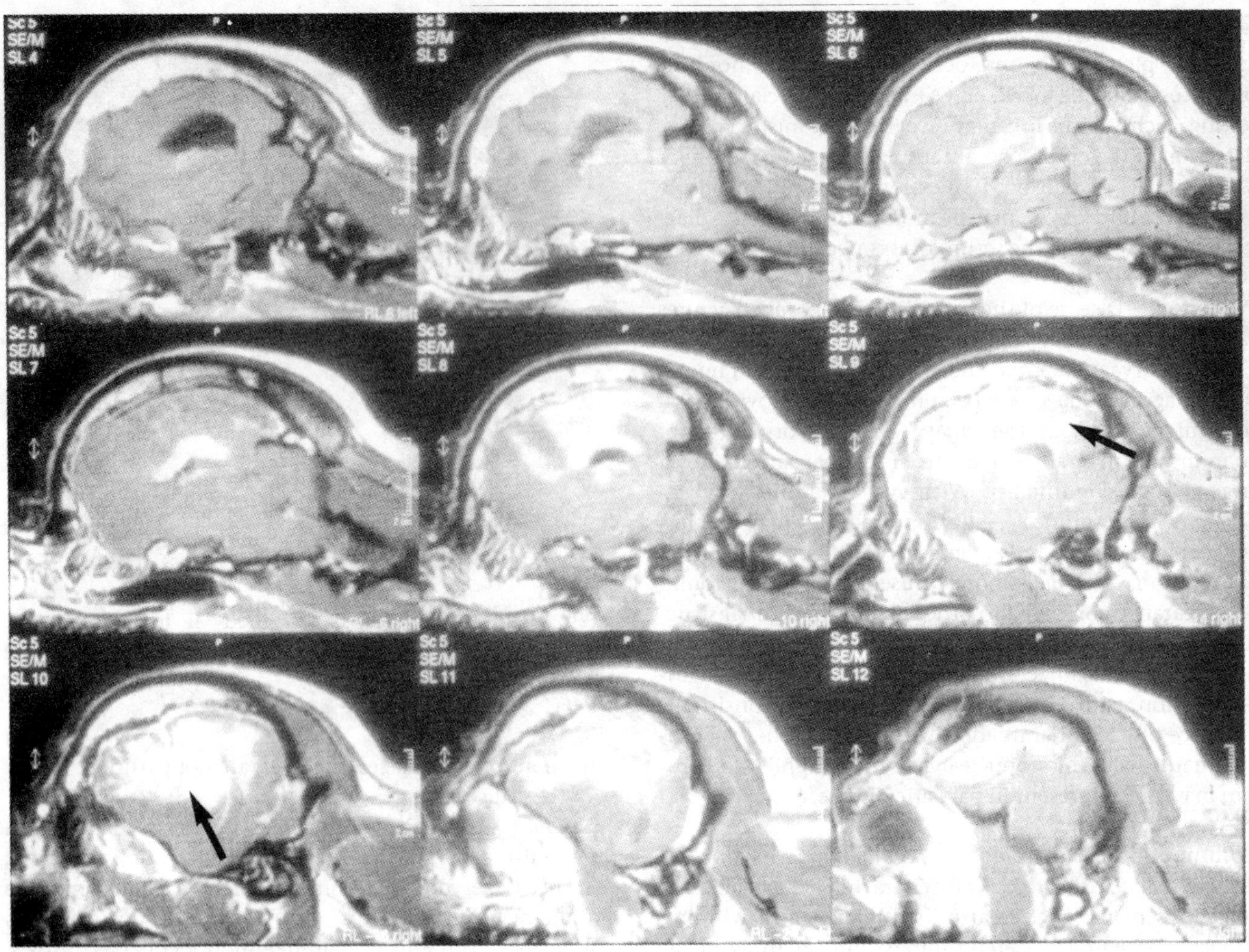

Fig. 10.16. Parasagittal, T2-weighted MR images from a pug dog with encephalitis. Note the cortical abnormalities *(arrows)*.

Physostigmine (0.025–0.1 mg/kg IV) potentiates the attacks for up to 45 minutes. The tricylic antidepressant, imipramine , which potentiates serotonin, may be helpful as both a diagnostic test and as therapy for narcolepsy. Electroencephalography may reveal inappropriate periods of brain electrical activity characteristic of REM sleep activity.

Feline hyperesthesia syndrome has been associated with both seizures and a behavior abnormality (Chrisman 1991; March et al. 1999; Quesnel and Parent 1997). Diagnosis is usually made solely on clinical signs. A complete neurological examination should be performed to identify pain or deficits suggesting an underlying spinal lesion. Spinal radiographs are performed to rule out lumbar and lumbosacral lesions. Biopsy of the paraspinal muscles should be used to rule out vacuolar myopathy. Cerebrospinal analysis and titers for infectious organisms such as *Toxoplasma*, FeLV, and FIP are used to exclude central nervous system inflammatory disorders.

Trauma

Traumatic injury remains a common cause of brain dysfunction in dogs and cats (see bibliography under Trauma). Survey radiographs of the skull may aid in determining whether fractures are present. This information may allow for assumptions about underlying brain injury, but it does not determine the extent of that injury. Cervical spinal radiographs should be included to rule out a cranial cervical lesion that may result in clinical signs similar to a caudal brain stem lesion. Structural anatomical abnormalities associated with a traumatic intracranial injury are most readily determined with either CT or MR imaging.

Evidence of cerebral edema or hemorrhage is most often apparent with these imaging studies. Occasionally, a subdural or extradural hematoma or focal intraparenchymal hematoma is found. Cerebrospinal fluid analysis is often unrewarding and may be detrimental, especially with elevated ICP. Withdrawal of CSF may alter intracranial fluid dynamics resulting in brain herniation . Therefore, unless a preexisting disease is suspected prior to the trauma, it is best to avoid CSF collection.

Electrophysiological evaluations, such as brain stem auditory evoked potentials and electroencephalography, have the potential to provide localization as well as prognostic information. Often, however, these tests often yield nonspecific information, and results may not correlate with recovery.

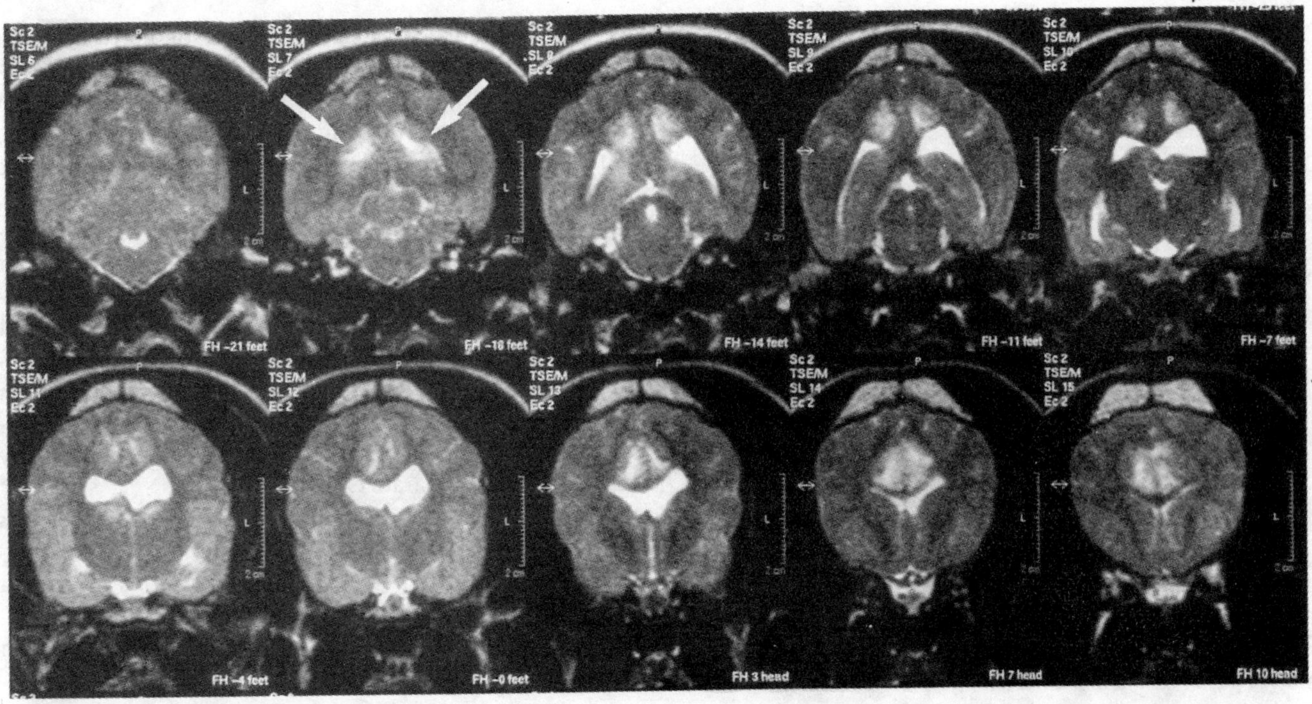

Fig. 10.17. Transverse, T1-weighted MR images from a dog with previous seizures. Note the abnormal MR signal dorsal to the lateral ventricles bilaterally (*arrows*).

Toxicity

Numerous toxins can affect the nervous system either primarily or secondarily (see bibliography under Toxicity). Diagnosis of a toxicity is most easily accomplished if an animal has been exposed to a known toxic product. Specific tests for known toxins in serum, urine, or vomitus may then be performed through a toxicologic testing laboratory. Animal poison information centers should be contacted to determine the most accurate samples needed for diagnosis.

Cerebrovascular Diseases

Cerebrovascular disease should be suspected in any animal with acute neurologic signs (see bibliography under Cerebrovascular Disease) (Joseph et al. 1988; Thomas 1996; Thomas 2001). A thorough examination of the body for petechia is important, including the mucous membranes (especially of the penis, prepuce, and vulva) and the retina. Pallor, low-grade heart murmurs, weakness, and tachycardia are hallmark signs of anemia, which may be associated with coagulopathies. These signs may result with significant amounts of bleeding into body cavities. Thoracic auscultation for pleural fluid and abdominal palpation for hemoperitoneum is important. Radiographs and ultrasound may help when the physical examination is unrewarding but large amounts of internal bleeding are suspected. Large amounts of blood can be lost through the gastrointestinal tract and examination of the stool for hematochezia or melena is important.

Besides documenting any hypertension via either direct or indirect methods, complete blood cell count, with special attention to red cell and platelet counts, are often helpful. Specific coagulation testing (bleeding time, PT, PTT, FDPs) is also commonly evaluated. Biochemical evidence of a predisposition to hypercoagulability such as proteinuria should be collected. Diseases associated with hypertension such as renal disease and hyperthyroidism should also be considered.

As cerebrovascular disease often alters the structural integrity of the brain, clarification of the cause of the clinical signs often requires some advanced imaging modality to evaluate brain structure, such as CT or MR imaging. Depending upon the degree of the cerebral disease (i.e., ischemia versus overt hemorrhage), and the relationship between onset of the disease and time of imaging, the characteristics of cerebrovascular disease may vary. With CT images, acute to subacute intraparenchymal hemorrhage is most often hyperdense (whiter) compared to normal brain parenchyma, but may be either isodense (the same appearance as), or hypodense (blacker) compared to brain parenchyma at various stages following the hemorrhagic event. Hemorrhage in the extradural or subdural area often is hypodense (blacker) in appearance and has a crescent-shaped appearance between the skull and the intracranial tissues.

With MR imaging, hemorrhage can have a varied appearance, primarily based on the duration of the hemorrhage and alterations in blood hemoglobin (Thomas 1996). As different regions within hemorrhagic focus may contain differing stages of hemoglobin breakdown, a heterogenous appearance to the lesion may be encountered. In addition to the form of hemoglobin present, the signal intensities of a blood clot may vary depending on the operating field strength and the type of sequence used for imaging. Hem-

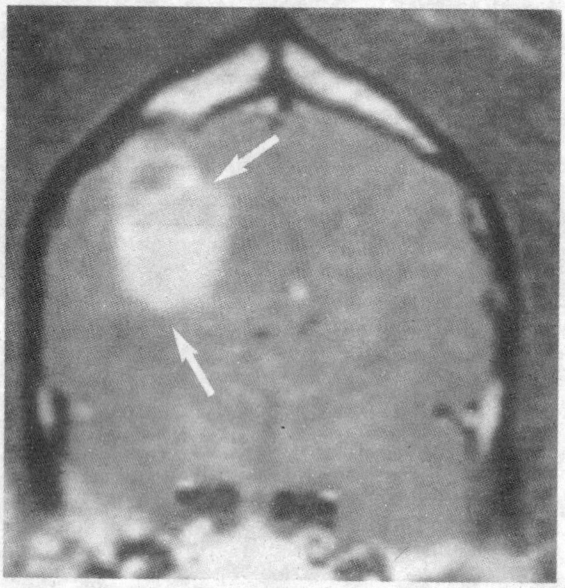

Fig. 10.18. Transverse, T1-weighted MR images following intravenous contrast administration from a dog with a cerebral hematoma (*arrows*).

orrhage may also vary in appearance depending on the cavity (subdural, intraparenchymal, or subarachnoid) where the bleed occurred (fig. 10.18). With MR imaging, cerebrovascular disease may vary from evidence of a focal mass to diffuse or multifocal changes. Often there is evidence of edema, which may be cytotoxic or vasogenic, in the area of the cerebrovascular damage. Classically, a wedge-shaped lesion may be encountered with the point of the wedge being directed more centrally. The common sites of infarction are the corona radiata, internal capsule, or periventricular white matter of the cerebrum. The white matter of the cerebellum is another common site. Contrast enhancement following gadolinium administration will depend on the interval between the time of the vascular damage and the MRI examination, the resulting inflammatory response, and the degree of vascular disruption (break in the blood-brain barrier). Most cases are imaged within 48 hours after the insult due to the severity of signs, and therefore contrast enhancement is uncommon. When present, contrast enhancement in cerebrovascular lesions is minimal, heterogenous, or peripheral to ringlike. Also, depending on the imaging characteristics, focal inflammatory brain diseases and some neoplastic processes such as gliomas may have a similar appearance on MR images.

Feline ischemic encephalopathy is an ischemic necrosis of the cerebral hemisphere of cats (deLahunta 1983). Cerebrospinal fluid often contains mild elevations in protein and occasionally increases in nucleated cells. Computed tomography and MR imaging abnormalities have not been specifically described.

Diseases of the Cerebellum

Diseases of the cerebellum are diagnosed in a manner similar to other parenchymal diseases of the intracranial structures (see bibliography under Cerebellar Disease). Advanced imaging studies such as MR or CT are used to assess the anatomic structure of the cerebellum (fig. 10.19). In most instances, as with other intracranial anatomic imaging, MR imaging provides a superior anatomical assessment compared to CT scanning. Diseases such as tumor, infarction, hemorrhage, and hydrocephalus (fourth ventricle) are usually apparent on MR imaging. Abnormalities

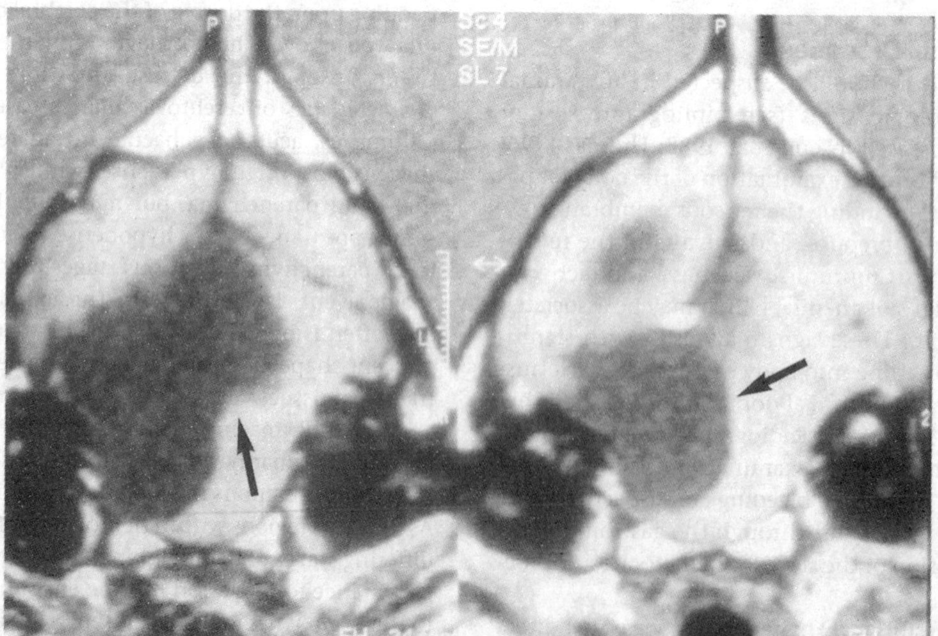

Fig. 10.19. Transverse, T1-weighted MR images from a dog with a cerebellar and brain stem cystic abnormality (*arrows*).

of the foramen magnum and brain stem such as Chiari malformations may result in prolapse or herniation of the caudal cerebellar structures caudally into the foramen magnum dorsal to the cranial cervical spinal cord. This abnormality is most obvious on a sagittal MR view of the caudal brain stem and cerebellum. Associated abnormalities such as syringomyelia may also be apparent in the cranial cervical spinal cord with MR imaging (fig. 10.5).

Cerebrospinal fluid analysis may provide evidence of inflammatory diseases affecting the cerebellum. Alterations in CSF with inflammatory intracranial diseases are discussed under diagnosis of encephalitis in this chapter.

Diseases of Cranial Nerves

Anatomical abnormalities of the cranial nerves are most often apparent with MR imaging. Tumors and inflammation of cranial nerves often result in enlargement of the affected nerves. Nerves may be more hyperintense (whiter) on T2-weighted MR sequences, and may enhance following intravenous contrast administration. Occasionally, however, animals with no apparent clinical abnormalities will show contrast enhancement of some cranial nerves, most often the trigeminal nerve. The significance of this contrast enhancement is unknown, and may represent normal variations in blood flow or occult cranial nerve pathology.

Cerebrospinal fluid analysis may reveal evidence of inflammation of cranial nerves. Nonspecific increases in nucleated cells and or protein concentrations may be found. Commonly, only increases in CSF protein concentration alone are apparent.

Surprisingly common, cranial nerves are often infiltrated with diffuse neoplastic diseases such as myelomonocytic leukemias or lymphoma. In these animals, cytologic evaluation of CSF may reveal the neoplastic cells.

With lesions of the cavernous sinus, intravenous contrast studies such as venography were historically performed to outline this region. These intravenous contrast studies have been replaced in the modern era with advanced imaging modalities such as MR imaging.

The facial nerve and vestibular nerve may be affected with disease of the middle and inner ear. Otoscopic examination and bulla radiographs are used in the assessment of the ear structures. Otoscopic examination may be difficult in animals with severe otitis externa prior to cleansing. The tympanic membrane is often discolored (hyperemic), opaque, and bulging outward with middle ear disease. Clear to yellow fluid may be seen behind the membrane. Diagnosis may also be supported by bulla radiographs or advanced imaging studies (figs. 10.20, 10.21) (Remedios et al. 1991). Definitive diagnosis is made through culture of the organism via a myringotomy or at surgical exploration.

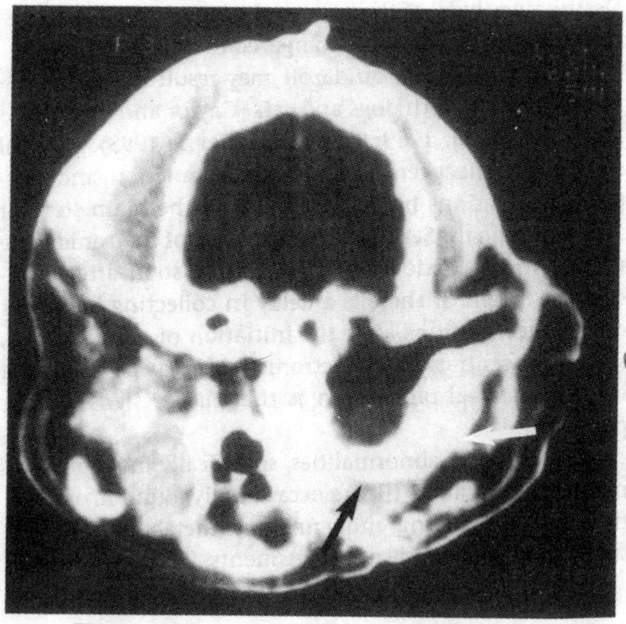

Fig. 10.20. Transverse, CT images from a dog with otitis interna. Note the proliferation of the tympanic bulla (*arrow*).

Computed tomography and MR imaging provide superior anatomical evaluations of the middle and inner ear, and concurrently have an advantage of allowing for anatomical assessment of the brain stem for evaluation of the nuclear regions associated with these cranial nerves. Lesions and associated brain stem structures, however, are often better seen with MR imaging as compared to CT as beam-hardening artifact with the latter commonly obscures structural detail in this area.

Tumors of the ear that extend through the tympanic membrane may be seen during otoscopic examination. This, however, is rare. Skull radiographs or advanced imaging is necessary to assess the middle and inner ear (figs. 10.20, 10.21). Abnormalities seen with these studies, however, are not always definitive for neoplasia, and tissue diagnosis at surgery is often necessary for accurate assessment.

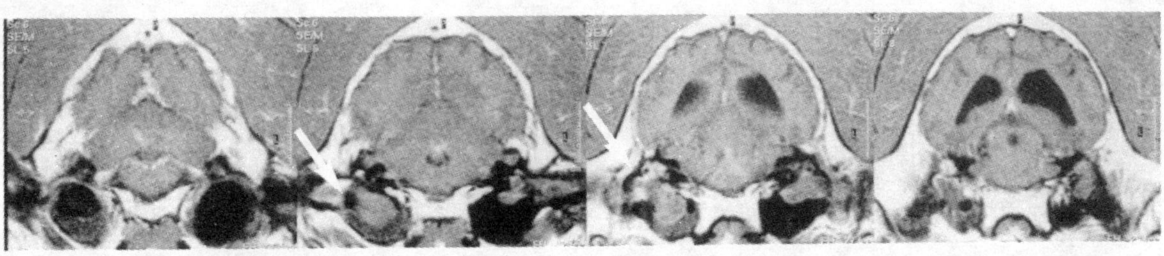

Fig. 10.21. Transverse, T1-weighted MR images following intravenous contrast administration from a dog with otitis interna. Note the material within the bulla (*arrows*).

Destruction (lysis) of the bone of the bulla is more often associated with neoplasia as compared to inflammation.

Toxicity with metronidazole may result in central vestibular signs in both dogs and cats (Caylor and Cassimatis 2001; Dow et al. 1989; Saxon and Magne 1993). Clinical signs often reflect central vestibular dysfunction, and morphological lesions have been found in the brain stem of affected animals. Serum concentrations of metronidazole will be in the toxic range if measured soon after clinical signs begin. If there is a delay in collecting blood for drug concentrations after the initiation of clinical signs, serum concentrations of metronidazole may be decreased into the normal range even as the clinical signs remain persistent.

Cranial nerve abnormalities, specifically involving cranial nerves VII and VIII, are occasionally found in association with underlying endocrine and metabolic disorders such as hypothyroidism. Assessments for these diseases through evaluation of thyroid hormone activity may be helpful in the diagnosis of these abnormalities.

Dysfunction of the cochlear portion of CN VIII commonly results in deafness. Brain stem auditory potential testing can be used to assess the integrity of the auditory pathways and the peripheral auditory function. With this test, an auditory stimulus (usually a clicking sound) is provided to the ear, and the electrical potentials generated from the neural structures of the peripheral auditory receptors in the ear and the central brain stem projection pathways are recorded. With abnormalities of the peripheral auditory receptors that result in deafness, no BSEP activity may be elicitable. As this test can evaluate each individual ear, unilateral deafness that is not clinically apparent may be revealed. As the BSEP contains potentials that are associated with the brain stem projection pathways for hearing, occasionally the BSEP will be abnormal in animals with brain stem disease.

11 Diagnostic Testing in Animals with Spinal Disease

Similar to intracranial disease processes, spinal diseases may result in anatomical alterations of spinal tissues or affect spinal cord elements at a microscopic, physiologic, or functional level. Diagnostic tests for detection of spinal cord disease are used to determine either structural or functional alterations in spinal cord function.

In addition to the routine baseline data for assessment of systemic health (table 11.1), *radiology* of the spine and *myelography* have been the historical standards for clarification of structural spinal cord disease. With myelography, a radiopaque contrast medium is injected into the subarachnoid space to outline the spinal cord so that this structure will be apparent on radiographic studies. Advanced imaging modalities, such as computed tomography (CT) and magnetic resonance (MR) imaging, however, yield much greater anatomical information, and are currently the gold standard for evaluation of the spine and spinal cord. Magnetic resonance imaging, compared to CT, yields superior images of the soft tissue such as the spinal cord, intervertebral disks, and nerve roots or peripheral nerves in close proximity to the spinal cord. *Cerebrospinal fluid (CSF)* collected from the subarachnoid space surrounding the spinal cord can be analyzed to identify microscopic and intraparenchymal diseases such as myelitis and meningitis. Ideally, CSF should be collected caudal to the suspected lesion for the most accurate assessment of spinal cord disease (Thompson et al. 1990). *Electrodiagnostic studies* of spinal cord electrical transmission, such as evoked potentials, provide supportive information as to lesion location and possible severity but are rarely used in routine clinical practice (Holliday 1992). As the lower motor neuron (LMN) cell bodies reside in the ventral grey matter of the spinal cord, spinal diseases that damage these LMN cell bodies may result in denervation of muscles of the axial (paraspinal) or appendicular (limb). This denervation may be evident on electromyography (EMG) studies of these muscles.

Some diseases are not readily identifiable with the currently available diagnostic tests as these diseases are the result of physiologic abnormalities of the spinal cord structures. In general, these diseases tend to be the primary degenerative diseases of the spinal cord (see chapter 6 under Degenerative Disease). These diseases may only be definitively diagnosed at necropsy examination.

It is important to consider the possibility that more than one spinal disease may be present in the same animal. For example, an underlying cellular microscopic dysfunction process may be present in an animal with a concurrent structural disease, as the structural disease is more apt to be identified with the currently available diagnostic tests. If, a compressive spinal condition occurs in association with a degenerative spinal condition, the compressive problem may be revealed with diagnostic testing, however, the degenerative process may remain unidentified. A high index of suspicion for selected underlying degenerative spinal diseases based on clinical features and breed association will help in remaining cognizant of the potential presence of these underlying functional disorders of the spinal cord.

DIAGNOSIS OF SPINAL CORD DISEASE PROCESSES

Degenerative Disease

Primary degenerative spinal cord disease usually occurs in specific breeds of animals, and younger animals are more often affected (chapter 6 and see appendix 2). An exception to this rule is the specific entity referred to as "degenerative myelopathy," which usually occurs in middle-aged to older dogs (see below). Examples of primary degenerative spinal cord diseases of younger animals include Afghan myeloma-

Table 11.1. Minimum database for animals with spinal cord signs

- CBC
- Serum biochemistry
- Urinalysis
- Bile acids or other liver function testing
- Blood pressure
- Heartworm testing (dog)
- FeLV/FIV testing (cat)

Expanded database for animals with spinal cord signs

- Assessment of coagulation status (buccal mucosal bleeding time, PT, PTT, FDPs, platelet count)
- Thoracic radiograph
- Abdominal radiograph
- Abdominal ultrasound

lacia, hereditary ataxia of smooth-haired fox terriers and Jack Russell terriers, Labrador retriever axonopathy, encephalomyelopathy of young cats, leukoencephalomyelopathy of Rottweilers, and miniature poodle demyelination. An etiology for the neural element degeneration in many of these diseases has not been established.

A presumptive diagnosis of a primary degenerative spinal cord disease is based on known breed associations with specific spinal cord degenerative processes and presence of the established, appropriate clinical signs. Antemortem diagnostics either have not been consistently performed or are invariably normal in animals with primary degenerative spinal cord disease. Cerebrospinal fluid may contain elevated protein without increase in cells, but this analysis is usually normal. Myelography has been reportedly normal in instances where this diagnostic test has been performed. Magnetic resonance imaging features of many of these primary degenerative diseases have not been described. Definitive diagnosis is ultimately made at necropsy for many of these degenerative spinal conditions.

Clinical Clues to Primary Degenerative Spinal Cord Diseases

- Dogs less than 1 year of age
- Progressive paresis or ataxia of the pelvic or all limbs
- Usually progressive clinical signs
- Nonpainful
- Antemortem diagnostic testing normal

Degenerative Myelopathy

Degenerative myelopathy is the name commonly used to describe a specific degenerative spinal cord disease of mature dogs and cats that results in paraparesis, eventually evolving to tetraparesis and, possibly, cranial nerve signs. Dogs most often become paralyzed in the pelvic limbs prior to clinically detectable thoracic limb abnormalities. This disease most commonly is reported in middle-aged to older *German shepherds,* but also affects other breeds of dogs and has been occasionally reported in cats. Similar disease processes have been described in very young dogs including *German shepherds* and *Siberian huskies.* Clinical signs are usually gradual in onset, chronic in duration, and progressively worsen. Clinical features most notably reflect an abnormality of the T3–L3 spinal cord segments, however, the actual histopathological lesions may be more severe in the caudal cervical area.

A presumptive diagnosis is made based on breed-associated clinical features (Clemmons 1992). Diagnosis of this disease process based on clinical features alone, however, is often found to be in error as other disease processes may result in similar clinical signs and disease course. Routine tests of systemic health (CBC, serum chemistry panel, urinalysis) are normal. Cerebrospinal fluid may be normal (especially if collected at the cisterna magna) or may contain elevated protein without increase in cells. More specific CSF and blood tests are being evaluated as an aid in the diagnosis of this disease process, but none to date offer a definitive diagnosis or are consistently available. Antemortem imaging studies such as myelography are usually normal as this is an intramedullary degenerative process that does not result in swelling or compression of the spinal cord. Magnetic resonance images from affected dogs are also normal.

In many dogs with clinical features suggestive of degenerative myelopathy evaluated in the modern era with MR spinal imaging, there is evidence of disk protrusion affecting various regions of the spinal cord. In some instances, this protrusion occurs at a single disk, or in other instances compression is present at multiple intervertebral disk spaces. The relationship between the presence of intervertebral disk protrusion and degenerative myelopathy is currently unknown. Most likely, these are separate disease entities with, unfortunately, similar clinical features. Concurrent disease processes such as spinal cord compression (i.e., with intervertebral disk disease—IVDD) may occur in association with degenerative myelopathy in the same animal. This creates a diagnostic dilemma, as there are no currently established pathognomonic magnetic resonance imaging features that will indicate the presence of degenerative disease. Electrodiagnostic studies of the paraspinal and limb muscles should be normal, however, spinal cord evoked potentials have not been evaluated universally. Definitive diagnosis of a true degenerative myelopathic condition is made only at necropsy (Summers et al. 1995).

Clinical Clues to Degenerative Myelopathy

- Middle-aged to older German shepherd
- Progressive paraparesis
- Invariably progressive clinical signs
- Nonpainful
- Antemortem diagnostic testing normal

Intervertebral Disk Disease

Intervertebral disk disease is one of the most common abnormalities seen in clinical practice in animals with spinal disease (see bibliography under Intervertebral Disk Disease). Selected breeds of dogs such as dachshunds often have a greater incidence of IVDD. Clinical features such as spinal pain, paresis, or paralysis are suggestive of IVDD but also are associated with other spinal cord conditions. Importantly, there is no pathognomonic clinical feature of IVDD.

For further clarification of suspected IVDD, survey spinal radiographs are often performed during the diagnostic evaluation process of animals with possible IVDD (figs. 11.1, 11.2). There are survey radiographic features that have been described in animals with IVDD. The term "intervertebral disk disease" is often used synonymously with intervertebral disk herniation, extrusion, or protrusion. The intervertebral disk, however, may undergo degeneration without herniating or protruding into the spinal canal (fig. 11.1). When the nucleus pulposus of a disk degenerates, this region of the disk may become calcified and therefore be apparent on spinal radiographic evaluations. This degenerative change occurs most commonly in the intervertebral disk in chondrodystrophoid breeds (Hansen's Type I IVDD) of dogs such as dachshunds. Calcification of the nu-

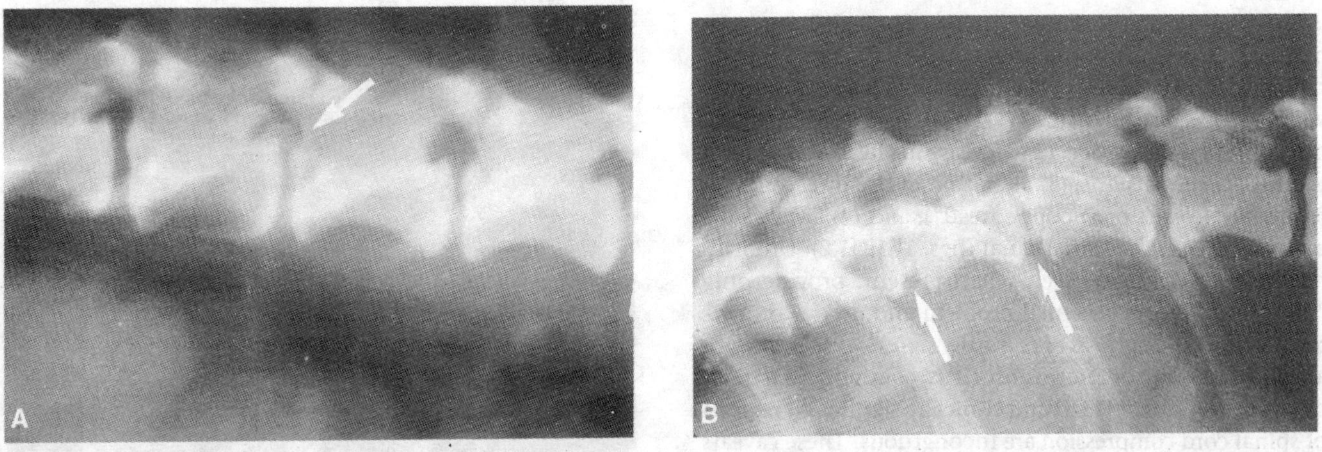

Fig. 11.1. (A) Lateral survey radiograph of the lumbar area of dog with an intervertebral disk herniation. Note the radiopaque material within the spinal canal (*arrow*). (B) Lateral survey radiograph of the thoracolumbar region of a dog showing calcification of the nucleus pulposus of the intervertebral disk (*arrows*).

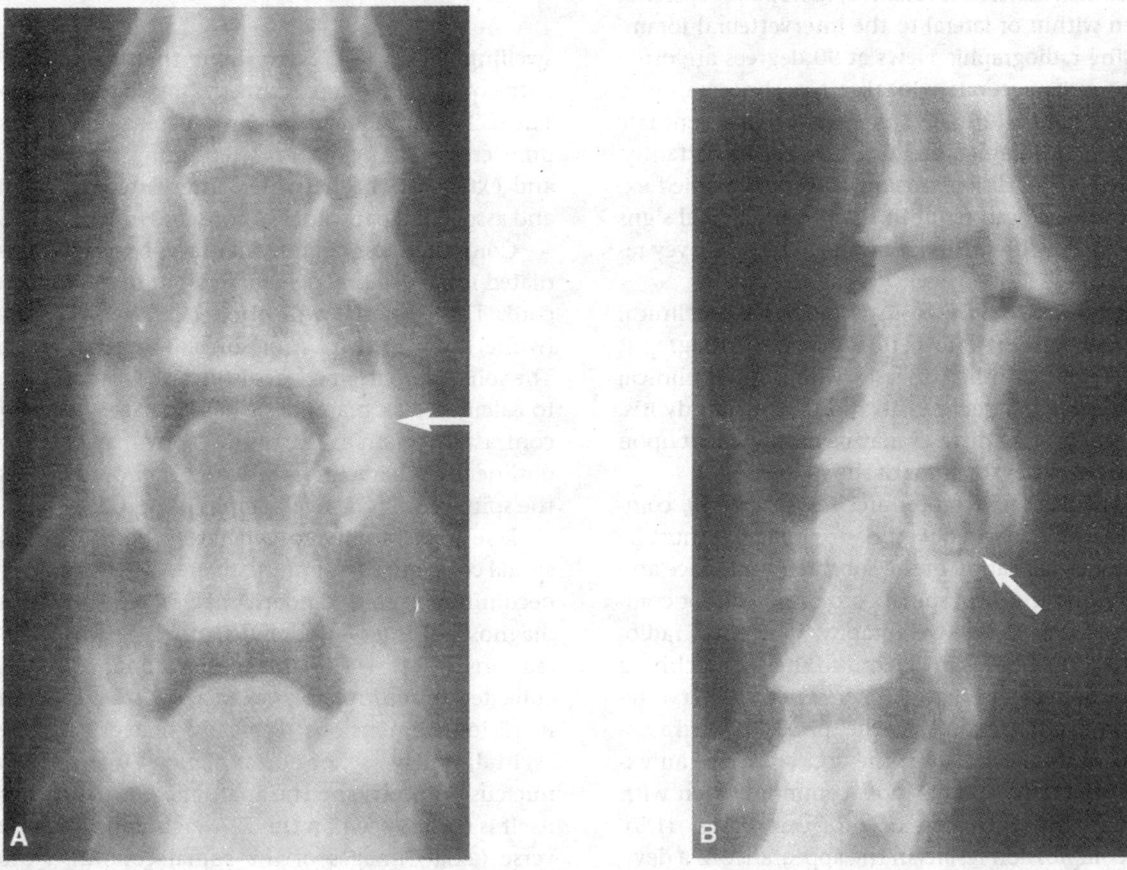

Fig. 11.2. (A) Ventrodorsal and (B) oblique survey radiographic views of the cervical spine of a dog with neck pain. Note the calcified intervertebral disk material within the intervertebral foramen (*arrows*).

cleus pulposus in association with disk degeneration, however, should not be interpreted as disk material herniation into the spinal canal. If the calcification remains within the limits of the normal nucleus pulposus region, this is referred to as intervertebral disk calcification *in situ*. Calcification in situ of the nucleus pulposus of an intervertebral disk space is evidence of disk degeneration, but not necessarily herniation of nucleus pulposus or annulus fibrosis. The presence of this calcified material outside the limits of the healthy nucleus pulposus region and either within or surrounding the spinal canal is more likely to be associated with clinical signs of spinal or nerve root disease.

Herniation or rupture of intervertebral disk material may also result in abnormalities apparent on survey spinal radiography. These "classic" radiographic features of intervertebral disk disease include (1) collapse or wedging of the intervertebral disk space, (2) decrease in the articular facet joint space dimensions, (3) alteration in the intervertebral foramen ("horse's or Snoopy's head"), and (4) radiopaque material within the spinal canal (figs. 11.1, 11.2). Unfortunately, these features, even when present, provide only "footprints" of the potential problem and do not provide for a definitive diagnosis of clinically significant disk herniation, extrusion, or protrusion. It is common that radiographic features of IVDD and clinically significant regions of spinal cord compression are incongruous. These caveats limit the diagnostic utility of survey radiographs in the definitive diagnosis of intervertebral disk herniation.

Herniation of disk material may occur in numerous directions from the disk space. Lateral or foraminal intervertebral disk extrusions are being recognized frequently. If the extruded disk material is calcified, radiopaque material may be seen within or lateral to the intervertebral foramina. Opposing radiographic views at 90 degrees are often necessary to more accurately localize the abnormality to the lateral or foraminal area. Oblique views that accentuate the intervertebral foramen are also helpful. Importantly, even relatively small disk extrusions and noncalcified extruded disk material can result in significant clinical signs and these abnormalities will not be apparent on survey radiographs.

In instances where IVDD is suspected based on clinical features, it is appropriate to perform survey radiographs primarily to exclude other diseases with similar clinical signs such as vertebral fracture, luxation, diskospondylitis, and tumor. These latter diseases may be more evident upon survey radiographic evaluations of the spine.

Additional diagnostic procedures (myelography, computed tomography, magnetic resonance imaging) must be performed for visualization of the subarachnoid space and spinal cord and to confirm spinal cord or nerve root compression (figs. 11.3–11.8). Myelography, wherein a radiopaque contrast medium is injected into the subarachnoid space, can be used to determine the presence of intervertebral disk material that compresses the spinal cord and associated dura. With myelography, the appearance of an extradural spinal compression is most commonly seen with intervertebral disk extrusion or protrusion (fig. 11.3). Extradural compression results in the appearance of a deviation of the myelographic columns toward the center of the spinal canal in one or both opposing radiographic views at 90 degree angles from one another. Herniated disk material is commonly found ventral or lateral to the spinal cord, but also may be found dorsal to the spinal cord. In rare instances, intervertebral disk material may actually rupture through the dura and enter the spinal cord proper.

With acute intervertebral disk herniation, spinal cord swelling associated with the spinal injury may be severe, resulting in focal enlargement of the spinal cord that subsequently obliterates the subarachnoid space. Spinal cord swelling will then prevent filling the subarachnoid space with contrast medium during the myelographic procedure. The lack of a radiographically apparent subarachnoid column creates difficulty in determining the exact location and extent of the herniated intervertebral disk material and associated pathological consequences.

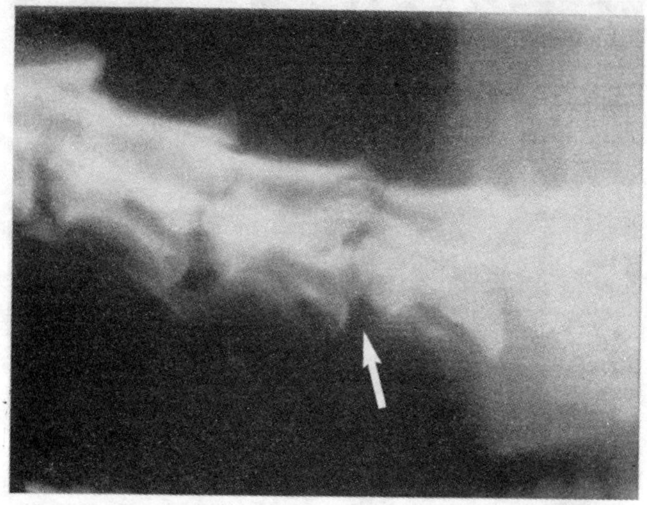

Fig. 11.3. Lateral myelographic of the cervical region from a dog with an intervertebral disk herniation (*arrow*).

Computed tomography may also be used to image herniated intervertebral disk material in or around the spinal cord. This material will often be seen as a hyperdense (whiter) density within or surrounding the spinal canal. The spinal cord itself is less distinct on CT images compared to calcified disk material or hemorrhage. A subarachnoid contrast injection as for myelography may be necessary to outline the subarachnoid space for improved delineation of the spinal cord (CT-myelography).

Due to its ability to generate superior images of the spinal cord and surrounding tissues, MR imaging is rapidly becoming the gold standard imaging modality for accurate diagnosis of intervertebral disk disease, extrusion, or protrusion (figs. 11.4–11.8). Magnetic resonance images can be collected in multiple planes to allow for viewing of IVDD in various dimensions. Typically, images are collected in sagittal, transverse, or dorsal planes. Degeneration of the nucleus pulposus and the anatomical structure of the disk itself is readily seen on the T2-weighted sagittal and transverse (axial) images of the spinal column. Normal hydrated nucleus pulposus has a hyperintense (whiter) signal compared to the annulus fibrosis. As the nucleus pulposus loses hydration (seen in chondroid metaplasia—Hansen's type I disk disease), the signal becomes less intense and may appear iso- or hypointense relative to the annulus fibrosis. Most acute disk extrusions of this type of degenerated disk material appear as a hypointense lesion within or surrounding the spinal cord on the T2-weighted sagittal image. Traumatic rupture of previously healthy nucleus pulposus results in a high signal intensity (hyperintense or whiter) material in or around the spinal cord as this mate-

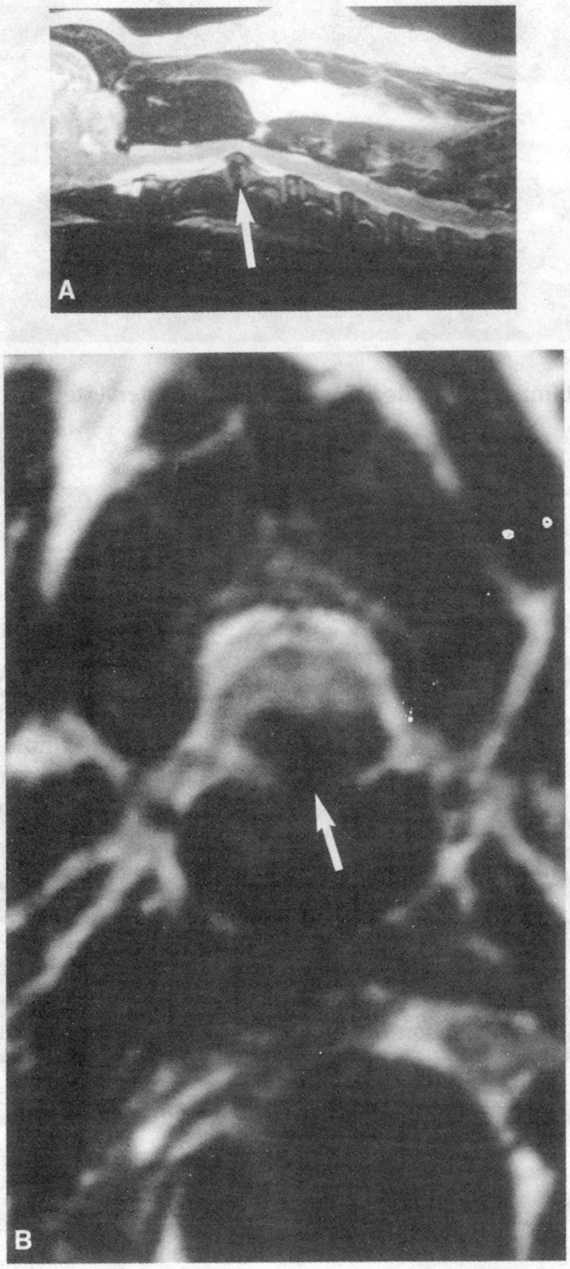

Fig. 11.4. (A) Sagittal and (B) transverse, T2-weighted MR images from a dog showing the intervertebral disk herniation (*arrow*) at the C2–3 IVD space.

rial is usually (at least initially) hydrated. The transverse MR view provides important information regarding the location of any compressive material surrounding the spinal cord in a cross-sectional dimension. If one area (side) of the spinal cord is exclusively or more compressive than others, this can readily be determined with spinal MR imaging.

Oftentimes and especially with acute IVD extrusions, there is associated hemorrhage and inflammation in the region of the IVD rupture. Hemorrhage usually is the result of damage or rupture of the ventral vertebral venous sinus (venous blood). In some instances, epidural hematomas may form as a result of this hemorrhage. This hemorrhage or hematoma formation can extend for multiple disk space

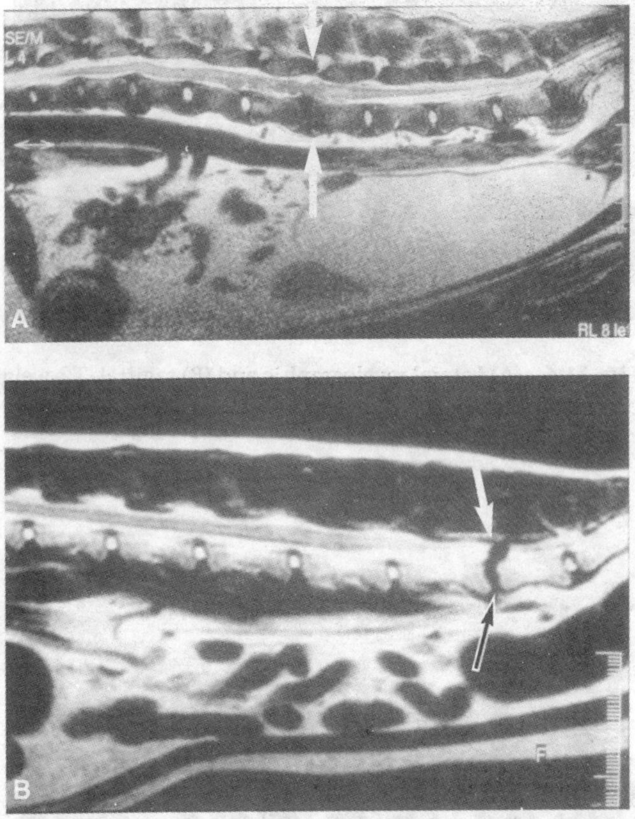

Fig. 11.5. (A) Sagittal, T2-weighted MR images from a dog showing the intervertebral disk herniation (*arrows*). Note the normal white appearance of the nucleus pulposus is absent in the affected intervertebral disk space (*arrow*). (B) Sagittal, T2-weighted MR images from a cat with an IVD herniation at L6–7 (*arrows*).

levels in or around the regions of the acute disk rupture. Hemorrhage associated with IVD extrusion may be present in the ventral, lateral, or even dorsal aspects of the spinal canal. Also commonly, the acutely extruded IVD material will become admixed with hemorrhage to result in spinal cord compression. The combination of varying consistencies of extruded intervertebral disk material and/or stages of hemorrhage mixed with disk material may create a spectrum of MR imaging characteristics of disk material herniation. Most often, the combination of herniated intervertebral disk material and hemorrhage often results in a mixed or heterogeneous signal intensity on T2-weighted MR images.

In instances of lateral disk extrusion, the location of the lesion may not be identified with myelography, especially if the extruded disk material is either within or lateral to the intervertebral foramen (fig. 11.8). In these situations, however, the degenerative disk is generally identifiable on the T2-sagittal MR image as decreased signal intensity and an abnormally shaped (smaller) nucleus pulposus. The transverse (axial) image often confirms the laterally extruded disk impinging on a nerve root.

Occasionally, and especially with more chronic IVD extrusion or protrusion, IVD material within or around the

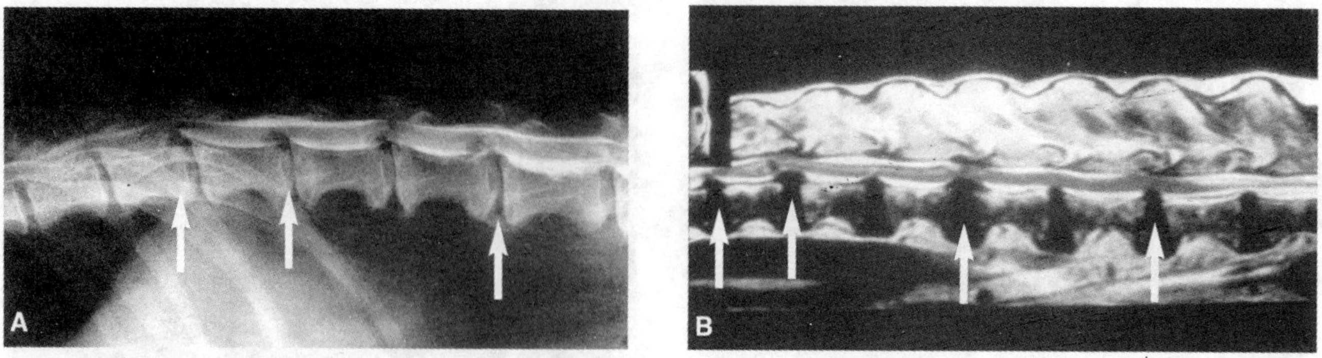

Fig. 11.6. (A) Lateral myelographic and (B) sagittal, T2-weighted MR image from a dog showing multiple intervertebral disk protrusions (*arrows*).

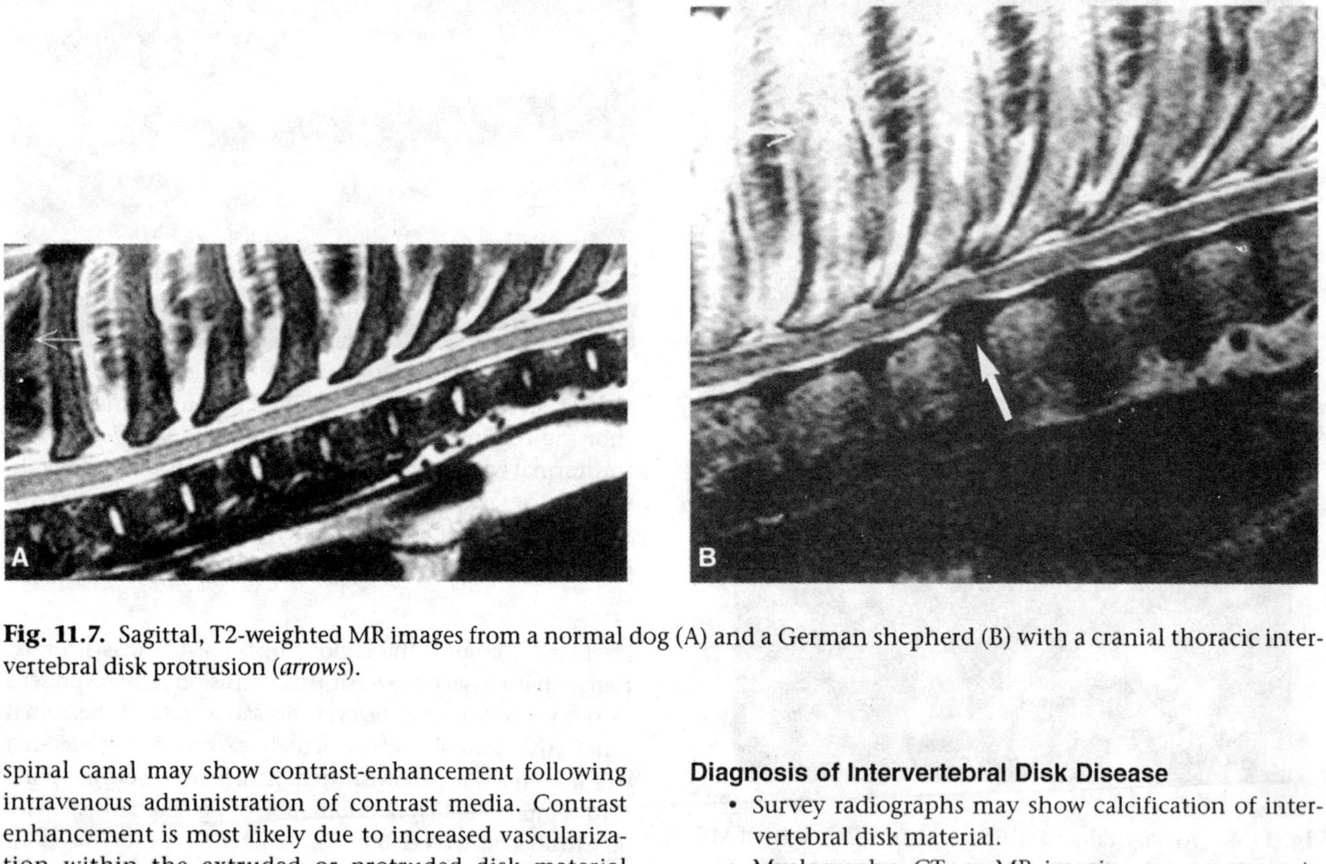

Fig. 11.7. Sagittal, T2-weighted MR images from a normal dog (A) and a German shepherd (B) with a cranial thoracic intervertebral disk protrusion (*arrows*).

spinal canal may show contrast-enhancement following intravenous administration of contrast media. Contrast enhancement is most likely due to increased vascularization within the extruded or protruded disk material and/or associated inflammation. This is true of both CT and MR images. In some instances, the contrast enhancement will occur at the peripheral edges of the IVD material (ring enhancement). It is important to recognize this feature of IVDD to avoid misdiagnosis of other disease processes showing contrast-enhancement such as spinal tumors.

As with all imaging studies, knowledge of the location of the lesion in a sagittal as well as transverse plane is imperative, especially if surgical correction is to occur. Localization can be slightly more difficult using MR imaging as body landmarks such as ribs are not always present within the plane of section. Additional views, such as a dorsal (coronal image), may be helpful in establishing lesion location and normal anatomical variations.

Diagnosis of Intervertebral Disk Disease

- Survey radiographs may show calcification of intervertebral disk material.
- Myelography, CT, or MR imaging are necessary to demonstrate spinal cord compression.
- CSF may show alterations associated with spinal injury or compression.

Cerebrospinal fluid collected cranial (at the cisterna magna) to an intervertebral disk herniation in the thoracolumbar region will invariably be normal due to the predominant caudal flow of CSF. Cerebrospinal fluid is ideally collected caudal to the location of any intervertebral disk lesion. Depending upon the severity and acuity of the disk herniation, CSF may show a variety of abnormalities including increases in protein content, increases in nucleated cell counts, or evidence of hemorrhage (increases in red blood cells, xanthochromia, and erythrophagocytosis). Increases in protein and in nucleated cell counts in CSF are

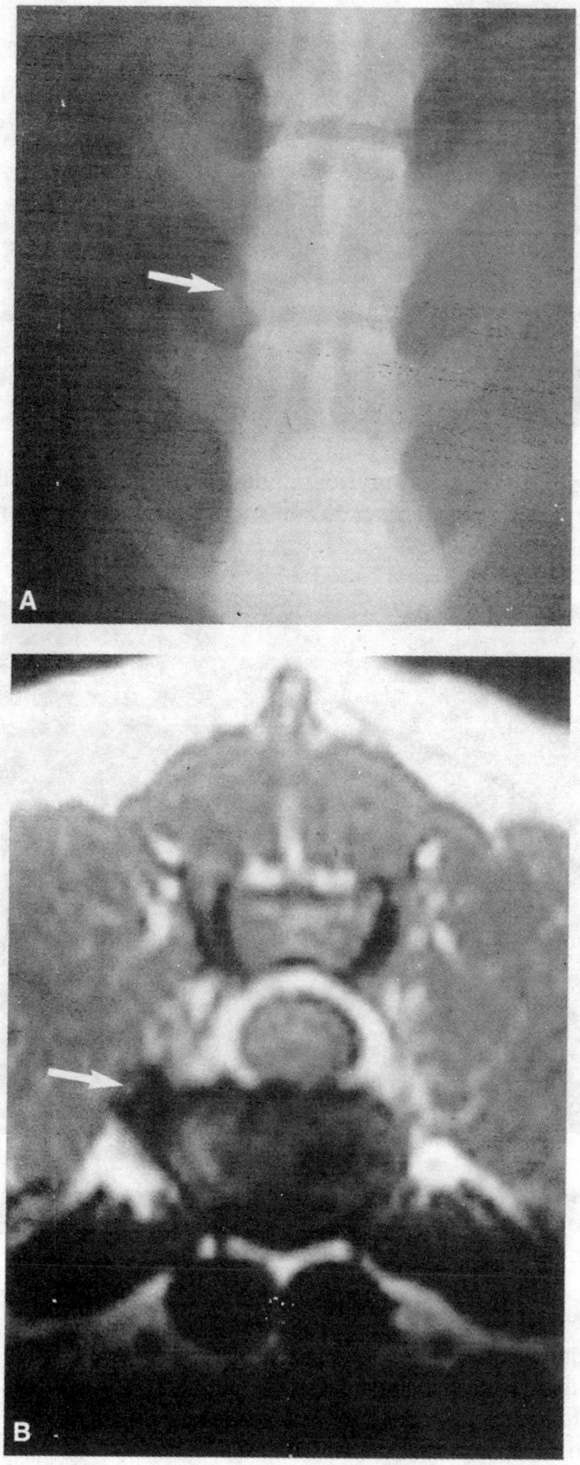

Fig. 11.8. (A) Ventrodorsal survey radiographic view from a dog with a lateral extrusion of intervertebral disk material (*arrow*). (B) Transverse, T2-weighted MR image of a dog with a lateral extrusion of intervertebral disk material (*arrow*).

a nonspecific reflection of inflammation and degeneration, or a combination of these pathological processes. Lymphocytes and monocytes are the predominant cell types present in instances of intervertebral disk herniation, however, neutrophils may also occasionally be present. In some situations, the number of nucleated cells present in CSF associated with intervertebral disk herniation can be sizable. A xanthochromic appearance of the CSF may accompany intervertebral disk herniation and associated spinal or subarachnoid hemorrhage and be a consequence of spinal cord contusion.

Electrodiagnostic studies may be helpful if the intervertebral disk involves spinal segments or spinal nerves resulting in denervation of either paraspinal or limb musculature. If the disk herniation involves segments or nerves associated with the limbs (affects nerves from cell bodies within the cervicothoracic or lumbar intumescences of the spinal cord), limb muscles may show evidence of spontaneous electrical muscle activity (fibrillation potentials and positive sharp waves). If the disk herniation affects spinal segments or spinal nerves that innervate the paraspinal muscles, similar abnormal electrical activity may be present in these muscles. Electromyographic abnormalities may be present focally providing additional information regarding the location of the IVDD. Following an acute denervation injury, abnormal EMG activity may not be evident for 5 or more days following the injury. Experimentally, and in some specialty practices, spinal-evoked or motor-evoked potentials (electrical activity generated along the spinal cord) may be used to determine the location of a spinal lesion. This is rarely performed, however, in routine clinical practice.

Ultimately, gross inspection and or biopsy at the time of decompressive laminectomy of herniated material is used to confirm the presence of intervertebral disk material affecting the spinal cord. If any question exists as to the origin and character of the material present, histological evaluation and culturing for aerobic, anaerobic, and fungal organisms should be performed.

Wobbler Syndrome

The term "wobbler syndrome" encompasses a number of cervical vertebral abnormalities (figs. 11.9–11.18) (see bibliography under Wobbler Syndrome). These include vertebral malarticulation/malformation, intervertebral disk extrusion and protrusion, articular facet hypertrophy, and spinal ligament hypertrophy. Two general clinical presentations of this disease exist (see chapter 6 discussion of wobbler syndrome for more details). One of these is classically seen in middle-aged to older Doberman pinschers. Other breeds, however, including both large and small body types, can also be affected. The disease in these animals is characterized primarily by ventral compressive lesions of the caudal cervical area resulting from ligamentous hypertrophy and intervertebral disk (usually annulus fibrosis) protrusion. While the pathophysiology of this disease is not fully understood, some caudal cervical instability coupled with increased flexion force due to the pull of gravity in a comparatively large head size predisposes to damage to the intervertebral disk space and the associated articulations. Hypertrophy of the associated ligamentous supporting structures (dorsal longitudinal ligament, dorsal intervertebral ligament—ligamentum flavum) is most likely an attempt by the body to decrease this instability

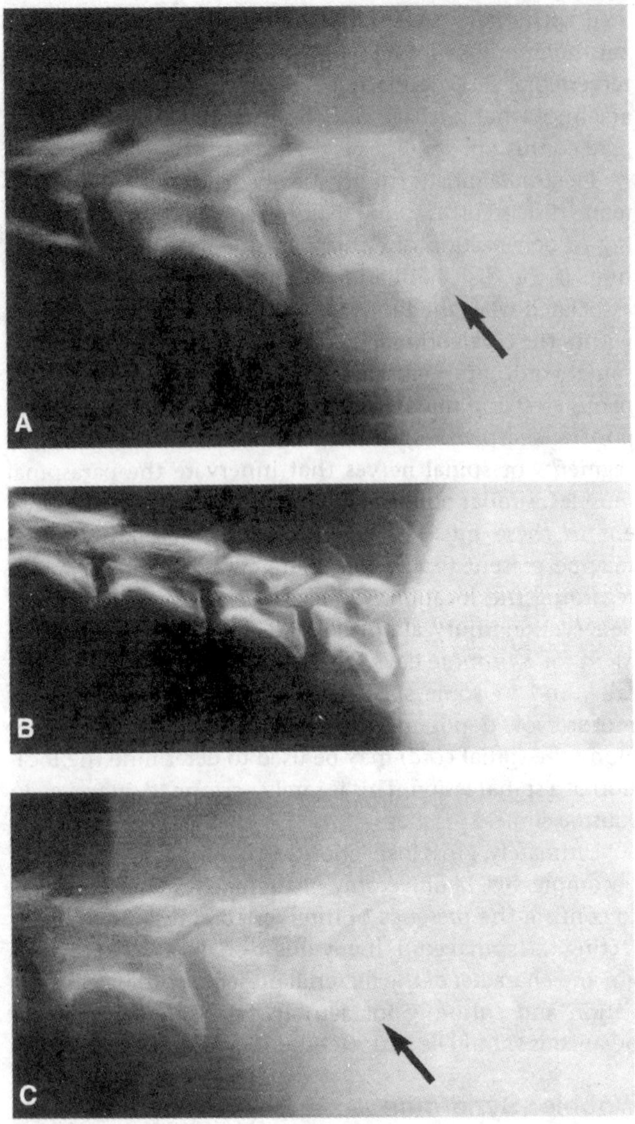

Fig. 11.9. (A,B) Lateral, survey radiograph from two Doberman pinschers with wobbler syndrome showing collapse of the intervertebral disk space (*arrow*). (C) Lateral, survey radiograph from a Doberman pinscher with a calcified intervertebral disk (*arrow*).

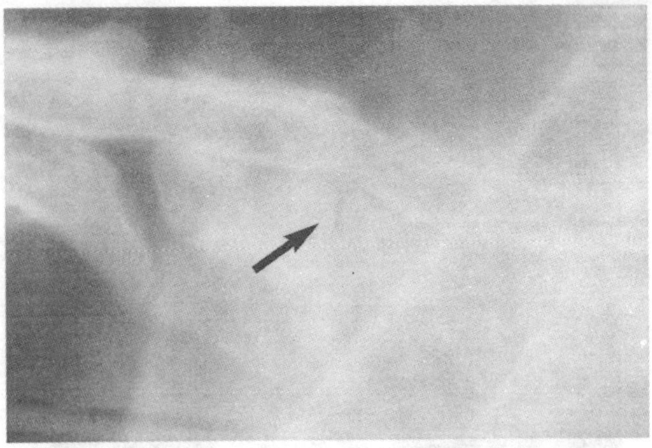

Fig. 11.10. Lateral myelographic from a Doberman pinscher with wobbler syndrome showing spinal cord compression (*arrow*).

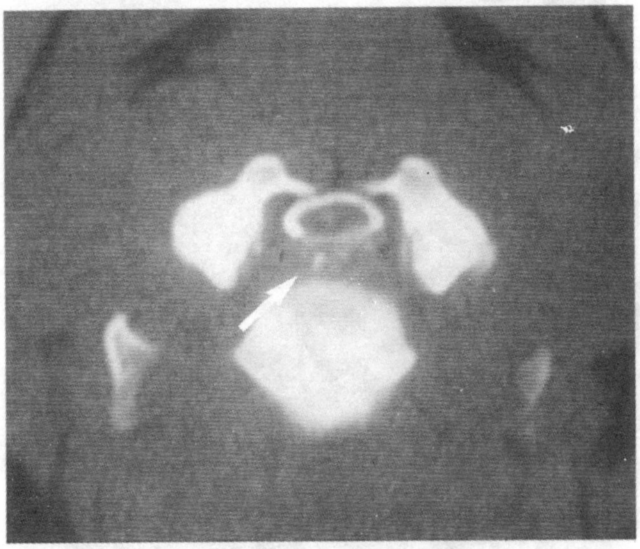

Fig. 11.11. Transverse CT image following subarachnoid contrast injection from a dog with wobbler syndrome and ventral spinal cord compression (*arrow*).

and to naturally fuse these articulations. This hypertrophied tissue, however, encroaches into the vertebral canal leading eventually to spinal cord compression. In addition to compressive damage to axons and neurons, impingement of spinal cord vessels can result in ischemic damage to the spinal cord.

Younger, large-breed dogs, such as Great Danes, mastiffs, and Saint Bernards, have a similarly named disease, but with a differing pathophysiology. In these younger and larger dogs, the disease involves the dorsal articular facets with secondary hypertrophy of the associated joint capsules and ligaments. This hypertrophy results in a more dorsal and lateral anatomical location of spinal compression. The articular facet joints may inherently degenerate, or may be damaged due to ineffectual ability to support the weight of the head. Some animals may have congenital bony malformations of the articular facets predisposing to a stenotic vertebral canal. In still other instances, small portions of synovial tissue may become entrapped and "pinched off" containing synovial fluid. These sacs of inspissated synovial fluid are known as synovial cysts. These cysts may also compress the spinal cord, either statically or with vertebral movement (dynamic compression). A similar-type spinal compression from hypertrophied dorsal ligaments and abnormal articular facet joints is possible in older dogs.

Survey radiographs may show malalignment of the vertebral elements, abnormal vertebral configuration, or collapse and other abnormalities of the intervertebral disk space (fig. 11.9). The appearance of the vertebrae may differ depending upon the position of the animal's neck when

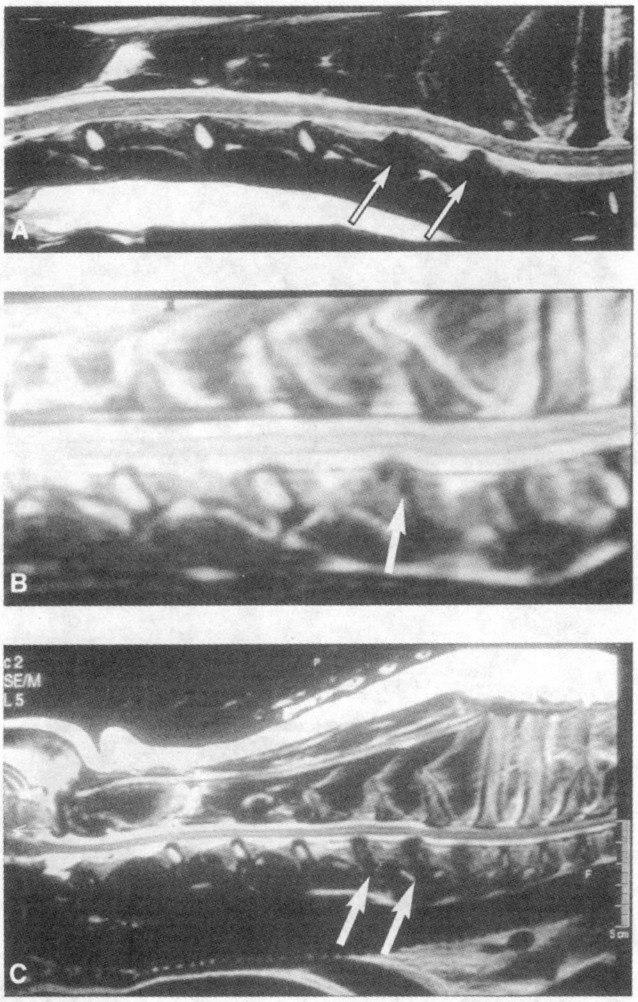

Fig. 11.12. (A,B,C) Sagittal, T2-weighted magnetic resonance views of three dogs with wobbler syndrome. Note the intervertebral disk degeneration and spinal compression (*arrows*).

the radiograph was performed. It has been suggested that evidence of survey radiographic abnormalities in the cervical vertebrae may be predictive later in life of the development of wobbler syndrome (Lewis 1989, 1991). In young, large-breed dogs, there may be enlarged and poorly defined articular facets on survey radiographs of the cervical area (fig. 11.14). The articular facets may have irregular margins. In some ways it appears that someone has smeared a thumbprint over the area of these facets on the lateral radiographic view.

Myelography, CT-myelography, or MR imaging is necessary to determine the exact location of any spinal cord compressed segments. As both dynamic and static spinal cord compression may be present with these diseases, flexed and extended myelographic or advanced imaging views may be needed to reveal the dynamic nature of the compressive lesion (fig. 11.13). Commonly in dogs with lesions such as those classically seen in Doberman pinschers ventral compression is worse when the head (and neck) is extended dorsally. Magnetic resonance imaging or CT may be helpful in assessing vertebral changes, spinal cord atrophy, and the degree of spinal cord compression (figs. 11.16, 11.17) (Lipsitz et al. 2001). The transverse imaging view afforded by these imaging modalities provides for the most accurate visualization of spinal cord compression in a 360 degree orientation surrounding the spinal cord. With ventral compression from annulus fibrosis or hypertrophied spinal ligaments, a ventral extradural compressive lesion is more apparent. With articular facet disease or vertebral stenosis, compression of dorsal and lateral aspects of the spinal cord is more often present. Soft tissue hypertrophy and synovial cysts are more easily seen with MR imaging compared with myelography or CT imaging.

Cerebrospinal fluid abnormalities, if present, are nonspecific indicators of CNS disease. If CSF is collected cranial to the lesion (i.e., at the cisterna magna), CSF may be, and often is, normal. Cerebrospinal fluid collected from the lumbar region is usually more reflective of any spinal cord damage, degeneration, or inflammation. Most commonly, increases in CSF protein concentration are present without concurrent increases in nucleated cell counts with this type of spinal cord compression. Occasionally, increases in lymphocytes and mononuclear cells are seen. Again, as with the majority of spinal diseases, CSF should be collected caudal to the level of the lesion to provide the most accurate reflection of the associated spinal cord disease process. In some instances, even if collected in the lumbar region, CSF will be normal in dogs with this constellation of diseases.

Diagnosis of Wobbler Syndrome

- Clinical signs are consistent with this disease (see chapter 6 under Wobbler Syndrome).
- Survey radiographs may show collapsed or abnormal intervertebral disk spaces or malalignment of the vertebral canal.
- Younger, giant-breed dogs may have proliferation of cervical articular facets on survey radiographs.
- Myelography, CT, or MR imaging is necessary to document spinal cord compression.
- CSF may contain nonspecific evidence of spinal compressive disease such as increases in protein content.

Lumbosacral Disease

Lumbosacral (LS) disease can occur as a congenital stenosis of the lumbosacral region or be acquired due to malarticulation, malformation, occult osteochondritis dessicans (OCD) lesions, or, most commonly, IVD degeneration and protrusion (figs. 11.19–11.22) (see bibliography under Lumbosacral Disease). The associated spinal nerve compression usually affects the L7, sacral, and caudal nerve roots as these traverse through the lumbosacral area. Compression can result dorsally from the interarcuate ligament, or ventrally from the bulging or tearing of the annulus fibrosis. The L7 nerves are often also compressed from a ventral and lateral direction as they exit the vertebral canal at the intervertebral foramen from collapse of the foraminal area or secondary osteophyte production (fig. 11.20). Occasionally, other diseases such as neoplasia, fracture, or diskospondylitis can result in lumbosacral nerve compres-

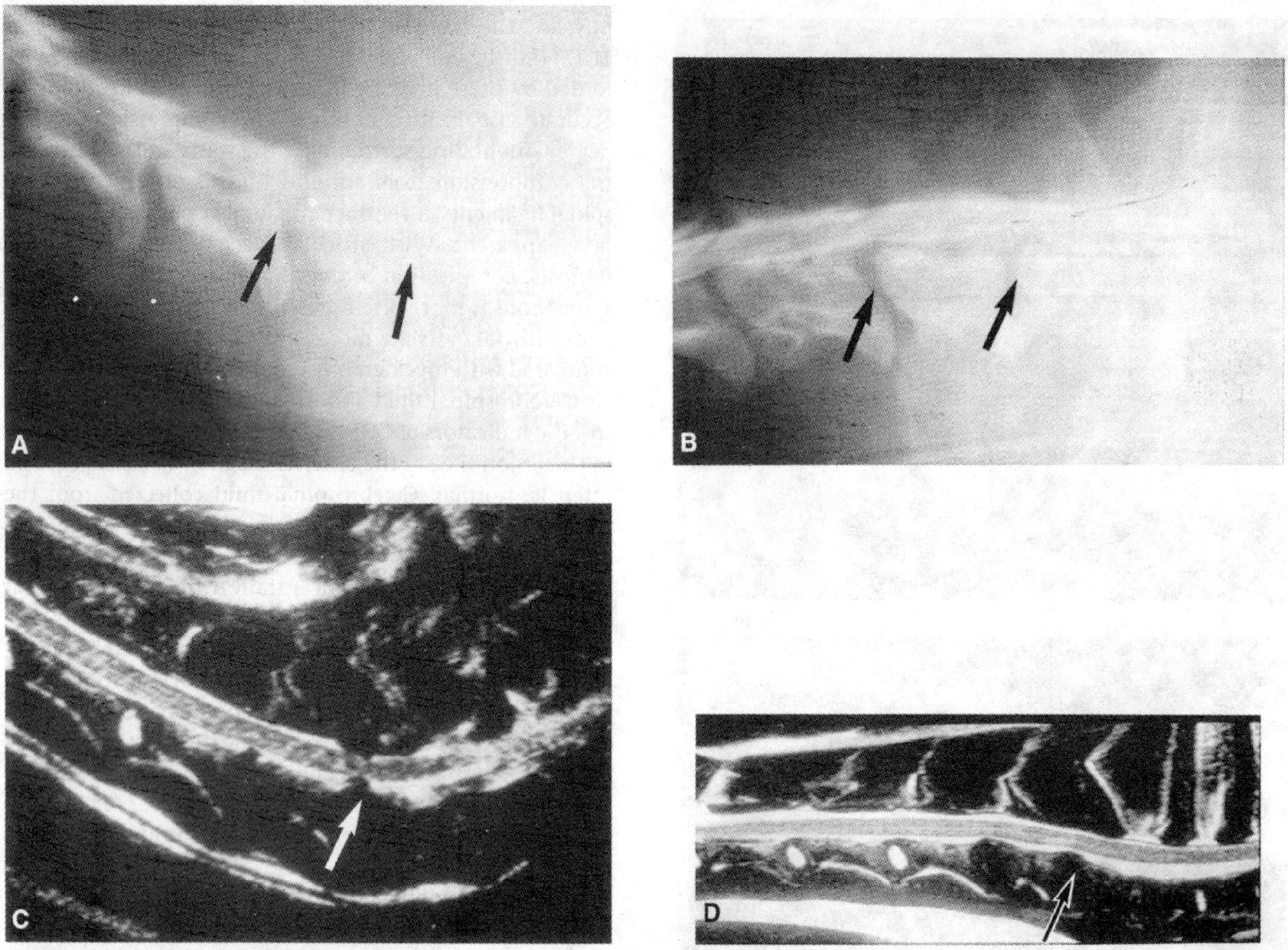

Fig. 11.13. Lateral myelographic appearance of the cervical spine from a dog with wobbler syndrome in (A) an extended and (B) flexed neck position. Note the compression on the spinal cord is lessened in the flexed-neck position. (C) Sagittal, T2-weighted MR images from a dog with cervical compression showing lessening of the compression in a flexed (D) compared to extended (C) neck position (*arrows*).

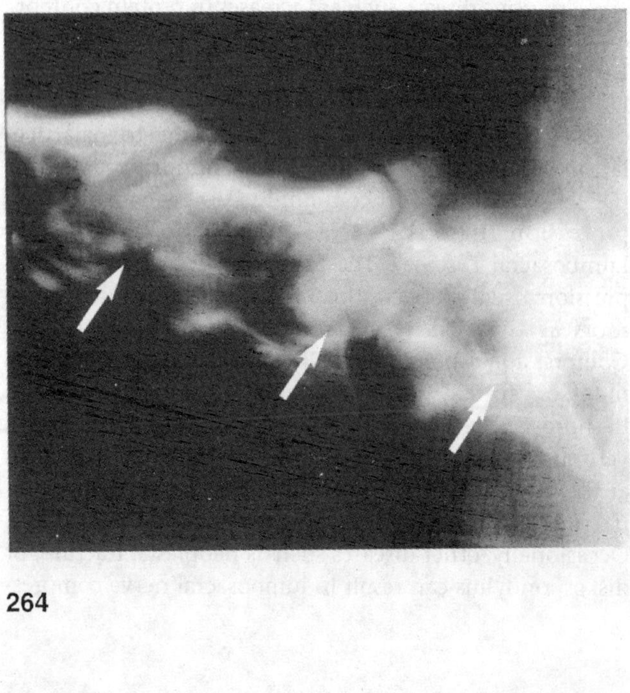

Fig. 11.14. Lateral survey radiographic view from a young dog with wobbler syndrome showing proliferation of the dorsal articular facet joints (*arrows*).

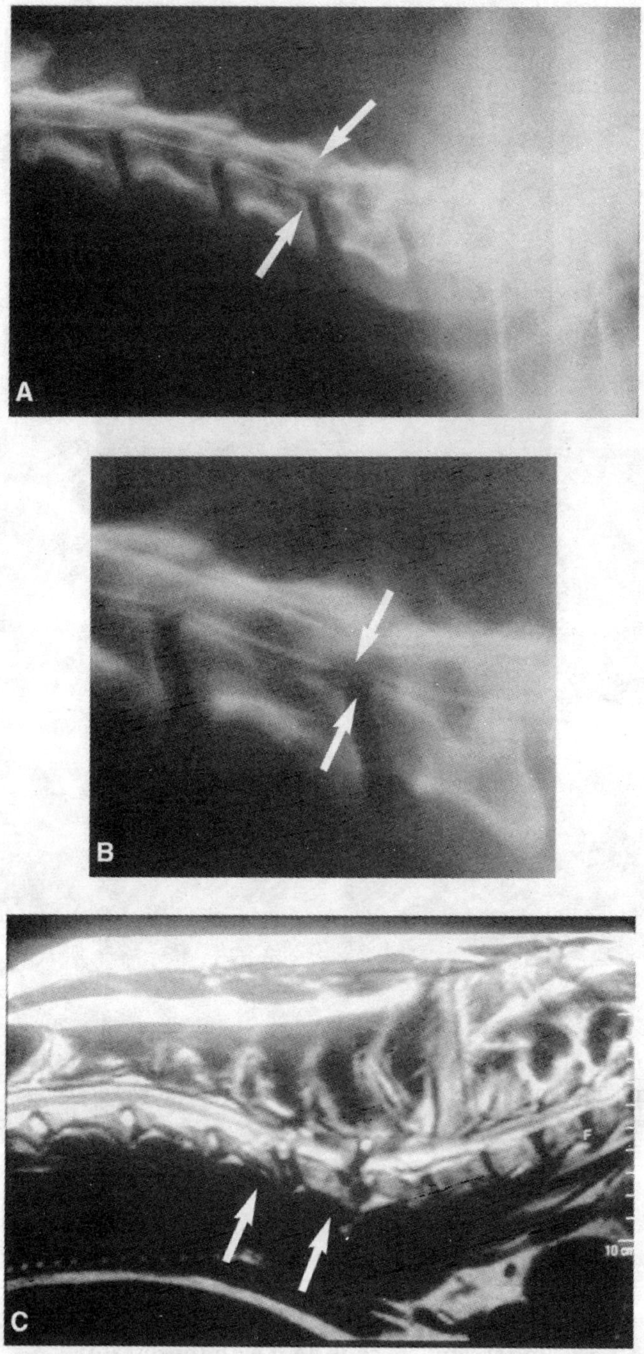

Fig. 11.15. (A) Lateral myelographic appearance of the cervical spine from a dog with wobbler syndrome. Note the spinal cord compressions (*arrows*). (B) Close-up view. (C) Sagittal, T2-weighted view of a young dog with lateral spinal cord compression (*arrows*).

sion. Primary inflammation of these nerves (cauda equina neuritis) is rare (Griffiths et al. 1983; Summers et al. 1995).

With degenerative lumbosacral disease, other diseases with similar clinical signs, such as diskospondylitis, should be excluded initially with survey spinal radiographs. Survey radiographs in animals with degenerative lumbosacral degenerative disease may show collapse or wedging of the intervertebral disk space, sclerosis of the vertebral end plates, and possibly malalignment of the L7 and sacral vertebral structures. In some situations it appears that the sacrum is ventrally subluxated compared to the L7 vertebrae. Malalignment of the L7 and sacral vertebrae may affect the appearance of the associated intervertebral disk space. Oftentimes spondylosis deformans is also present ventral to, and sometimes lateral to, the vertebral body at the L7-sacral intervertebral disk space. However, all of these survey radiographic abnormalities may also be found on radiographic evaluation of older dogs without clinical signs of lumbosacral disease. Therefore, survey radiographic evaluation alone cannot be used exclusively to diagnose clinically significant lumbosacral disease. Diseases such as diskospondylitis, tumors, and fractures that involve the lumbosacral vertebrae may be evident on survey radiographs (see below under these specific diseases) (fig. 11.19).

Diagnosis of caudal spinal or lumbosacral nerve compression is based upon documentation of such compression with myelography, epidurography, diskography, CT, or MR studies. Myelography is often not helpful in the diagnosis of lumbosacral disease as the subarachnoid space will terminate prior to the lumbosacral articulation. In some dogs, the dural sac will terminate caudal to the LS intervertebral space and compression in this area may be apparent with myelographic imaging. Myelography may be helpful to exclude spinal lesions of the thoracolumbar spinal cord and lumbosacral intumescence. As often there is only nerve root compression with lumbosacral compressive diseases, myelographic studies do not adequately document the extent and location of nerve root compression. Other radiographic contrast studies historically used for diagnosis of LS disease include epidurography, intervertebral osseous venography, or discography. These studies are inconsistent at best in yielding information helpful for the diagnosis of LS disease and have been essentially abandoned. In the modern era, these studies have been replaced by advanced imaging modalities such as CT and MR for the diagnosis of LS disease.

Advanced imaging diagnostic modalities (MR, CT) have the advantage of providing for a transverse view of the LS joint, allowing an assessment of the foraminal areas where exiting nerves are often compressed as well as the spinal cord and associated paraspinal vertebral, ligament, and joint structure (figs. 11.20–11.22). However, interpretation of these advanced imaging studies may be associated with both over- and underrepresentation of spinal and nerve compression. It is important in the diagnosis of LS disease, as with any disease, to correlate any imaging abnormality with the appropriate clinical signs.

There is both clinical and radiological evidence that instability exists in many instances of LS disease (Bagley 2003). Dynamic imaging studies of the LS joint tend to show that the LS joint is movable and that LS compression is worse in most instances when the joint is in a neutral or extended position as compared to a flexed position. We have had similar experiences when using MR imaging to

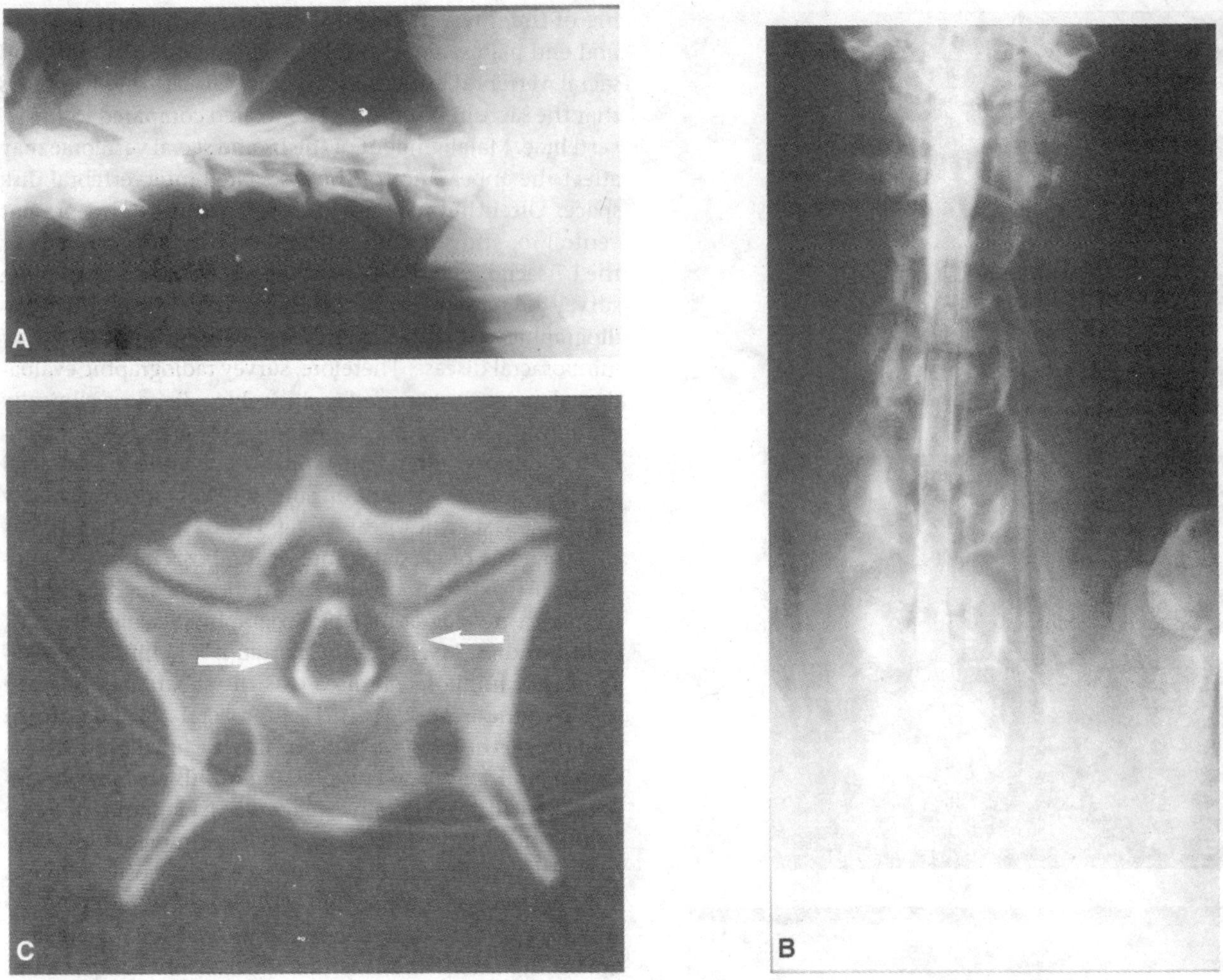

Fig. 11.16. (A) Lateral and (B) ventrodorsal myelographic view and (C) transverse CT image following subarachnoid contrast injection of a young dog with wobbler syndrome. The lateral myelogram shows no spinal compression, however, the CT shows dorsal lateral compression (*arrows*).

image the LS articulation in various positions (fig. 11.22). Compression of the spinal cord is worsened when the animal's lower spine is dorsally extended, and improved when the spine is in a ventrally flexed position. Because of this dynamic compression, the position that the animal is placed in at the time of imaging study may influence the detection of any LS compression.

Electromyography may be used to determine evidence of denervation of nerves compressed in the lumbosacral region (Sisson et al. 1992). Denervation of the tail, of the perianal area, and in the distribution of the sciatically innervated muscles may be present with damage of the nerves in the lumbosacral area. Electromyographic studies in these instances will reveal spontaneous muscle activity (fibrillation potentials or positive sharp waves) in the affected muscles. Cerebrospinal fluid analysis is usually not helpful in the diagnosis of LS degenerative disease as the disease process exists caudal to the site of CSF collection. If a diffuse inflammation of the nerves of the cauda equina is present, CSF collected in this region may contain increased numbers of inflammatory cells or increased protein concentration.

Diagnosis of Lumbosacral Disease

- Clinical signs are consistent with the disease.
- Survey radiographs may show diseases such as diskospondylitis, vertebral tumor, or vertebral fracture.
- Contrast radiography is invariably poor for establishing nerve compression.
- MR or CT imaging is used to document nerve compression.
- EMG may reveal evidence of denervation.

Spondylosis Deformans/Ventral Bridging Spondylosis

Spondylosis deformans or ventral bridging spondylosis is commonly encountered on survey radiographic spinal evaluation in dogs (fig. 11.23). This bony proliferation is thought to be the result of an age-related, degenerative vertebral and paravertebral abnormality and most likely initi-

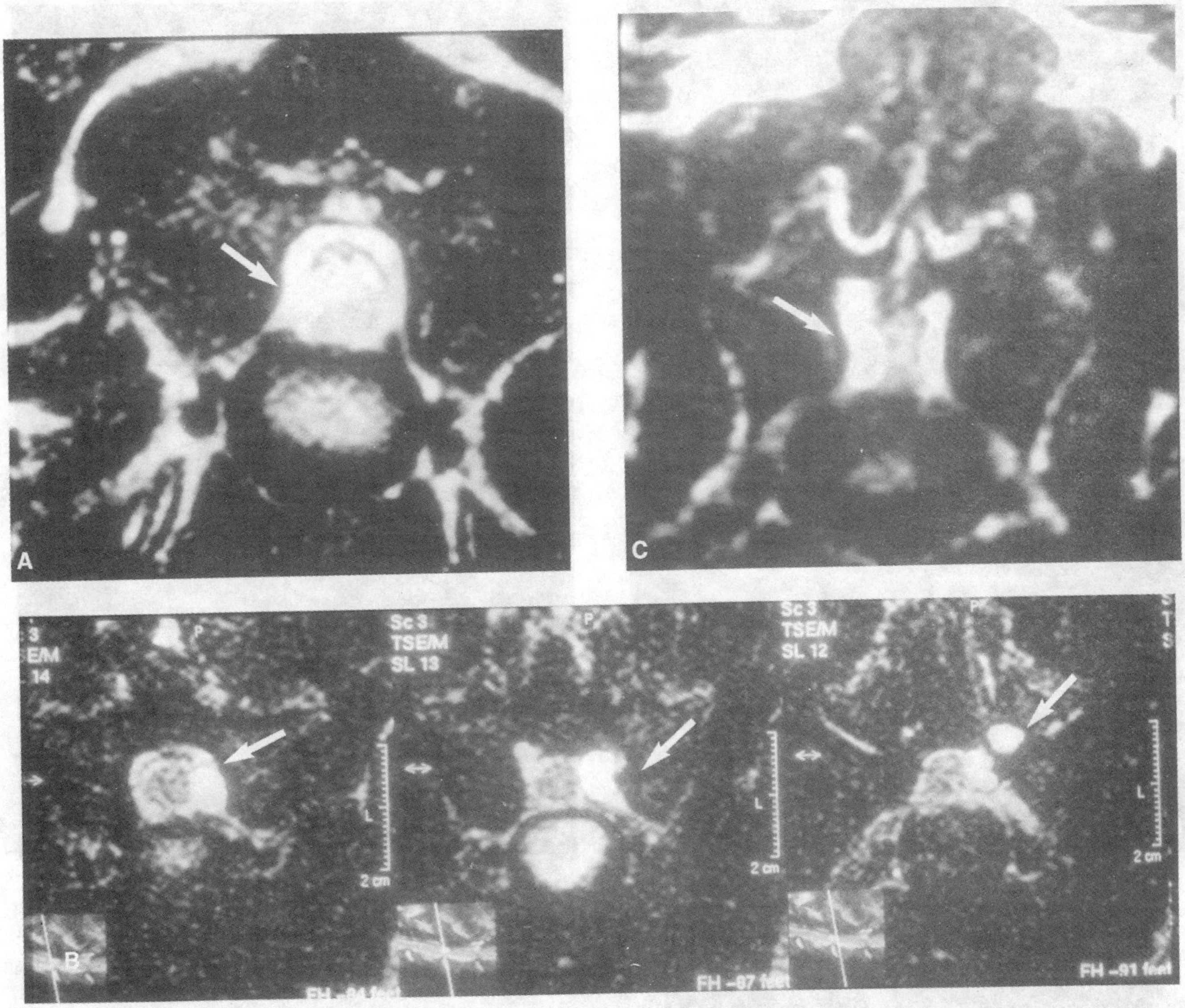

Fig. 11.17. (A,B,C) Transverse, T2-weighted magnetic resonance views of three young dogs with wobbler syndrome. Note the lateral spinal compression from a synovial cyst (*arrows*).

ated by ventral extrusions or protrusions if IVD components. Spondylosis can be found at all vertebral levels (Morgan et al. 1989, 1991). While it can be acquired in younger animals (disseminated skeletal hyperostosis), it is most often found in middle-aged to older dogs and cats (Woodard et al. 1985). In cats, hypervitaminosis A results in severe spondylitic change in the vertebrae, usually affecting the cervical region (see bibliography under Nutrition).

In many older animals, spondylosis deformans is found incidentally on spinal radiographic evaluation. The clinical ramifications of spondylosis deformans are much harder to determine. Bony proliferation is seen in an arching pattern, usually ventral or lateral to the affected intervertebral disk space. Bony proliferations extend from the vertebral end plates and may form a bridge of bone between adjacent vertebral bodies. In some instances, incomplete bony prolifer-

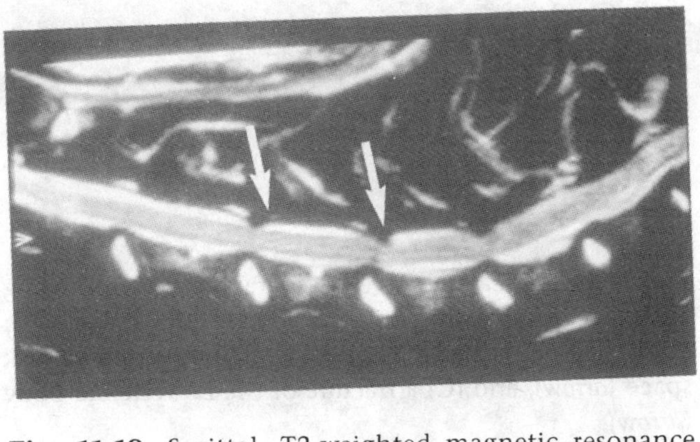

Fig. 11.18. Sagittal, T2-weighted magnetic resonance views of a young dog with wobbler syndrome. Note the dorsal spinal compression from ligament hypertrophy (*arrows*).

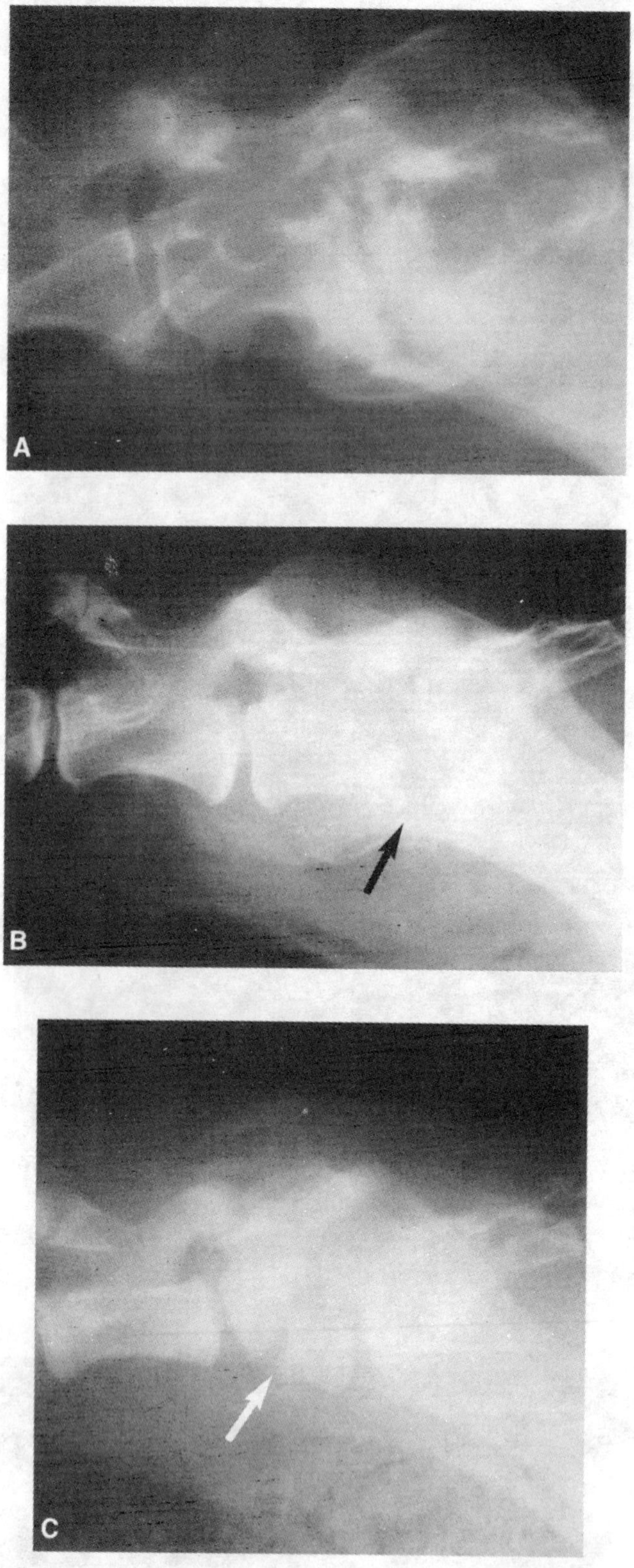

Fig. 11.19. (A) Lateral survey radiographic view from a dog with degenerative lumbosacral disease, (B) a dog with diskospondylitis of the lumbosacral intervertebral disk space (*arrow*), and (C) a fracture of the L7 vertebral body (*arrow*).

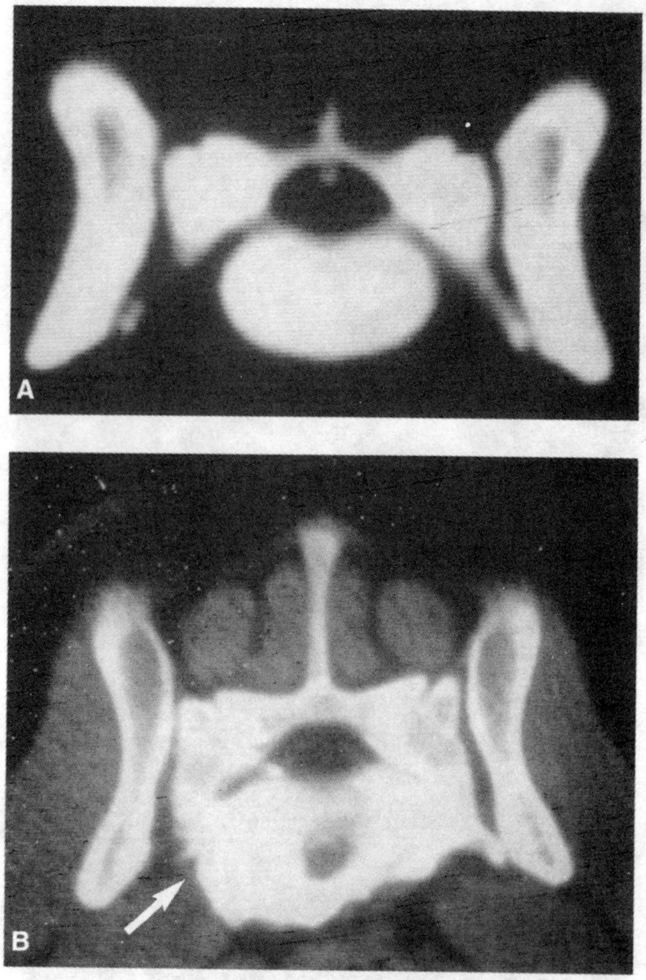

Fig. 11.20. Transverse CT image from (A) a normal dog and (B) a dog with lumbosacral disease. Note the compression of the intervertebral foramen (*arrow*).

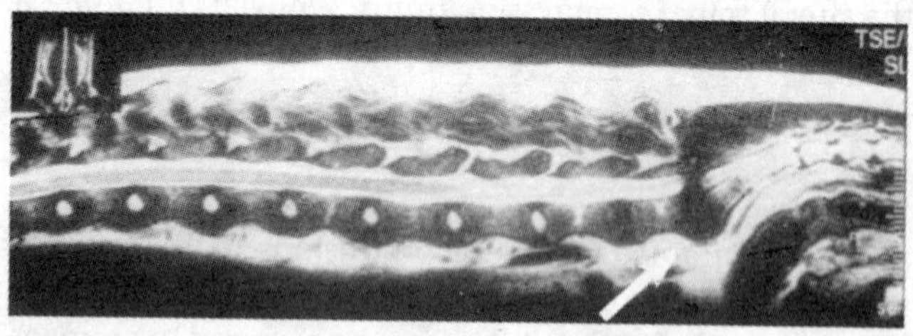

Fig. 11.21. Sagittal, T2-weighted magnetic resonance view of an animal with a lumbosacral spinal cord compression (*arrow*).

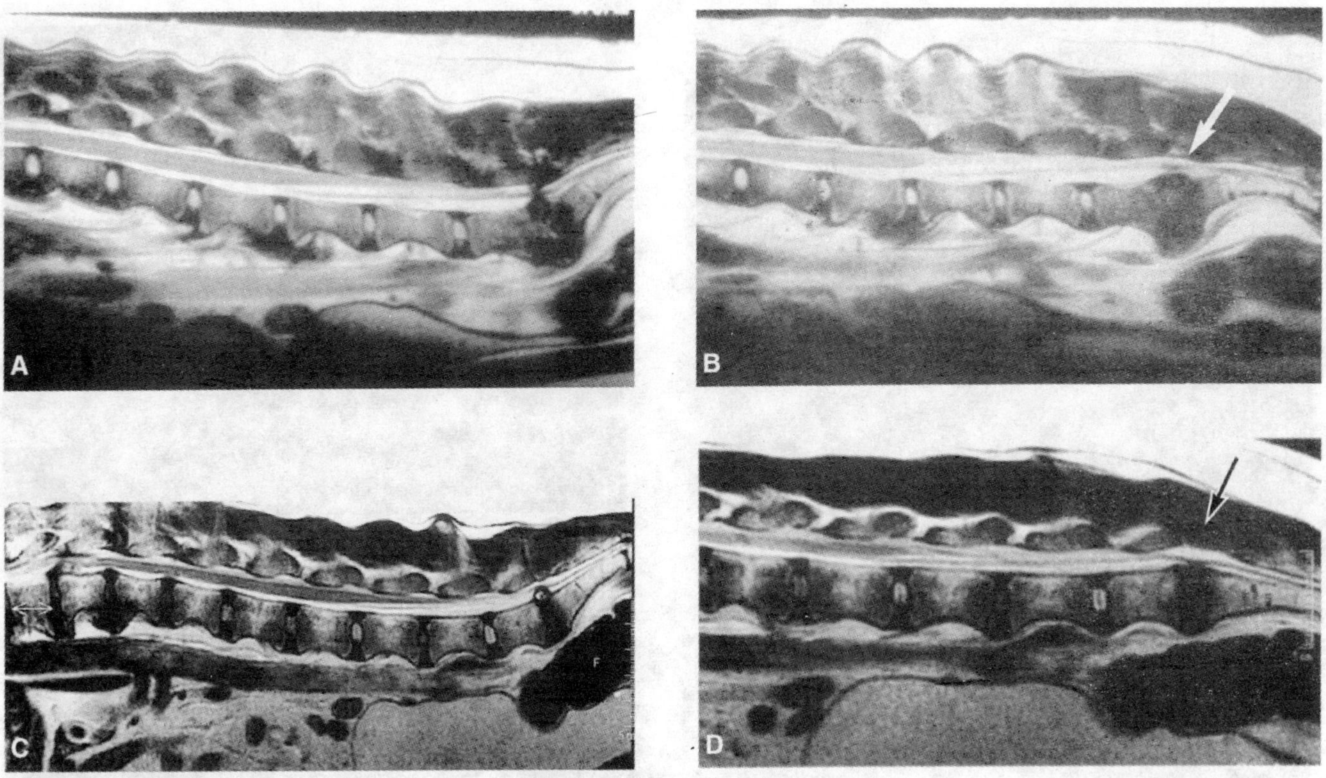

Fig. 11.22. Sagittal, T2-weighted MR images from two dog with lumbosacral disease in (A,C) a neutral and (B,D) flexed position. Note the lumbosacral compression is lessened in the flexed position (*arrow*).

ation will be evident as lucency between areas of spondylosis. This radiographic feature is often misinterpreted as a fracture of the spondylosis. If spondylosis results secondarily to intervertebral disk disease, alterations in vertebral articulation resulting in pain may also occur. Additionally, spondylosis may extend into or around the intervertebral foramen and compress the exiting spinal nerves. In these instances, transverse spinal imaging studies such as CT or MR are the best way to reveal bony proliferation into or around exiting spinal nerve (fig. 11.24). Electromyographic studies may reveal evidence of denervation from spinal nerve compression.

Dural Ossification

Ossification of the dura can occur in older animals, more commonly in the cervical area. (Morgan 1969; Wilson et al. 1975). A radiopaque, usually relatively thin, linear density is noted on radiographs in the area where the dura would normally be found (fig. 11.25). The pathologic significance of this radiographic finding is unknown, however, most feel that this abnormality is not associated with clinical signs of spinal or peripheral nerve disease. Occasionally, mineralized dura plaques will be adherent to the underlying spinal cord, which could result in a spinal cord abnormality. These focal dura mineralizations are rarely evident on survey spinal radiographs. Dural ossification has been difficult to determine with MR imaging if the lesion does not increase the size of the dura. Computed tomography may be more likely to show this radiopaque density in the region of the dura.

Anomalous Diseases

A variety of spinal cord congenital abnormalities may involve the vertebrae, the meninges, or the spinal cord proper. Spina bifida is a failure of the dorsal aspect of the vertebrae to fuse during development. This may be seen on a dorsal ventral survey spinal radiograph as an ununited dorsal lamina and spinous process (Dewey 2003). A dorsal spinous process may not be apparent on a survey radiograph in affected animals. Protrusion or adhesion of the meninges (meningocele), or meninges and spinal cord (meningomyelocele), through an associated vertebral defect may be seen with myelography but is best clarified with MR or CT imaging (Fingeroth et al. 1989; Plummer et al. 1993). Myelography may show communication of these meningeal structures with the spinal cord. Myelodysplasia or abnormal spinal cord development are best evaluated with MR imaging. Abnormalities of the normal spinal architecture usually result in a distortion of the anatomical appearance of the spinal cord. Often, on T2-weighted imaging sequences, the spinal cord contains abnormal hyperintense regions suggesting increases in fluid, malacia, or possibly, hemorrhage.

Vertebral abnormalities such as hemivertebrae, block vertebrae, or transitional vertebrae are often evident on survey radiographs (figs. 11.26, 11.27). These abnormalities

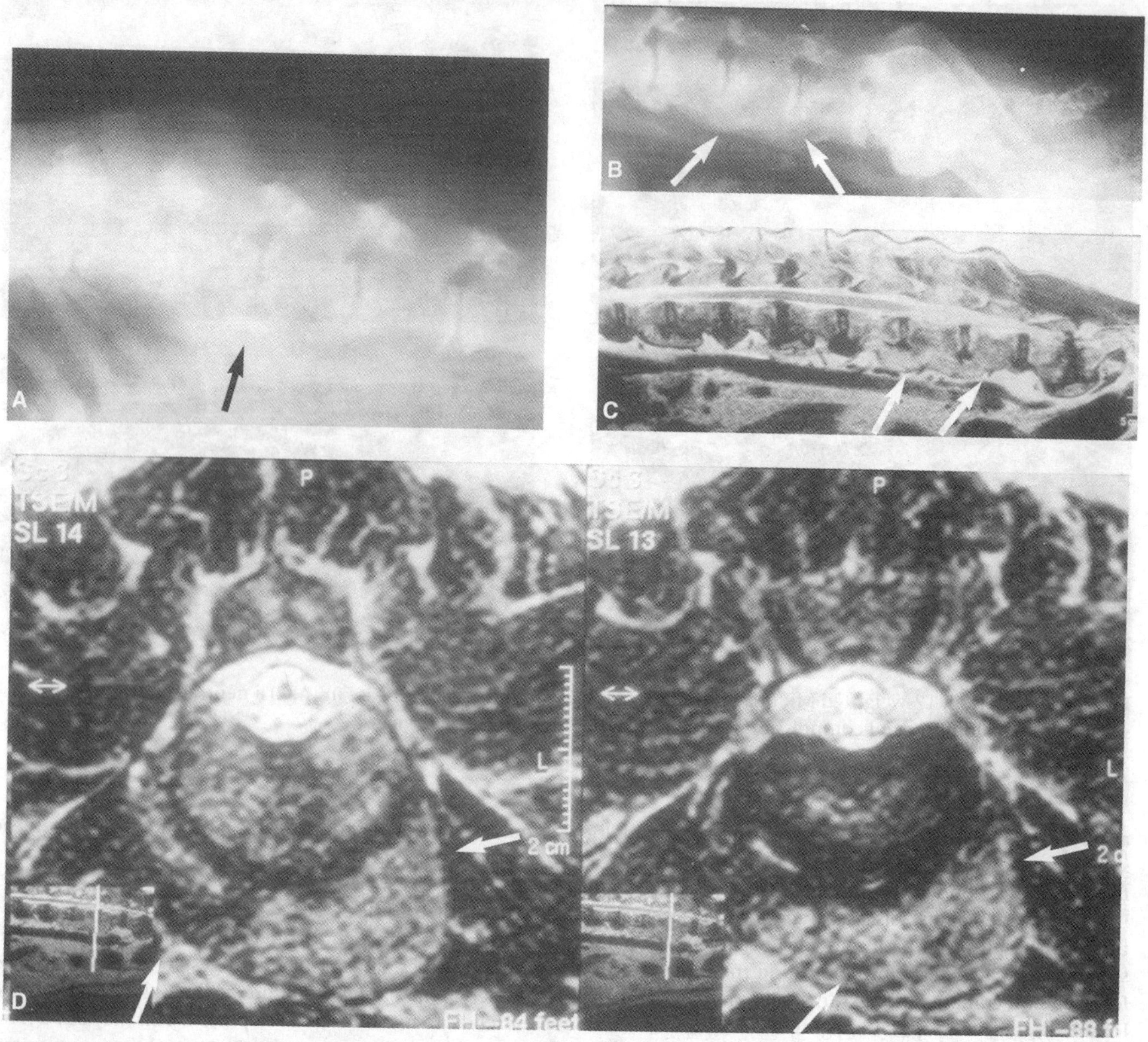

Fig. 11.23. (A,B)Lateral survey radiographic views of the lumbar spine of two dogs with bridging spondylosis (*arrows*). (C) Sagittal, T2-weighted MR image of the dog in (B). Note the spondylosis (*arrows*). (D) Transverse, T2-weighted MR image of the dog in (B). Note the spondylosis (*arrows*).

result in abnormally shaped vertebrae. Vertebral defects may result in malalignment of the vertebral segments with associated scoliosis, kyphosis, or lordosis. Spinal cord compression is only determined with myelography, CT, or MR imaging. Associated spinal cord defects such as myelodysplasia or syringomyelia are most obviously evident on spinal MR imaging as distortions of normal spinal cord architecture. In instances where the spine is permanently deviated, proper alignment of the patient for MR imaging may be difficult and subsequently affect image quality by creating positional artifacts. Cerebrospinal fluid may be normal or contain nonspecific increases in protein, nucleated cell counts, or both.

Rhodesian ridgeback dogs, and occasionally other breeds of dogs such as Shih tzus, Yorkshire terriers, and boxers, have a congenital connection from the spinal cord to the skin referred to as a *dermoid* sinus (see fig. 6.12) (Antin 1970; Hofmeyr 1963; Gammie 1986; Selcer 1984). This is the result of failure of separation of the skin from underlying tissues during closure of the neural tube. The characteristic unusual hair pattern on the dorsal neck and back of Rhodesian ridgeback dogs is a reflection of the defect, however, this abnormality does not always connect to the spinal cord. Dermoid sinus may appear as small indentations or openings in the skin. In some instances, fluid will be present from the abnormal skin area with an associated dermatitis. Dermoid sinuses usually occur on midline in the cervical, thoracic, or sacrococcygeal regions. Myelog-

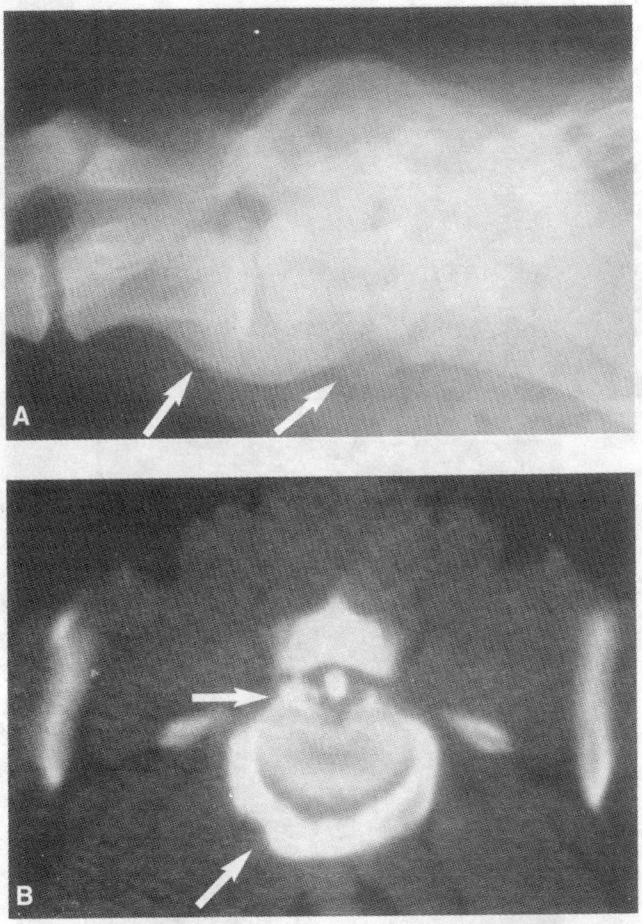

Fig. 11.24. (A) Lateral survey radiograph and (B) transverse, CT image from a dog with spondylosis deformans (*arrows*). Note the proliferation of the spondylosis into the foraminal area (*arrows*).

raphy, CT, or MR imaging is used for diagnosis of spinal cord involvement with this disease. Survey radiographs may show associated vertebral defects, but usually do not show any associated soft tissue defects. In instances where these abnormalities contain localized accumulations of fat, this abnormality may be more apparent than usual on survey radiographs alone. Injections of contrast media may show the connection between the skin and underlying nervous system (fistulogram), however, this technique is not recommended due to the increased risk of causing extension of infection and inflammation from the skin into the nervous system.

Scoliosis

Scoliosis is usually evident on physical evaluation. Survey radiographs of the affected spinal areas confirm the lateral deviation of the vertebral column (see fig. 6.17). This deviation is often associated with abnormalities of the vertebral structures. The vertebrae may be misshapen and irregular in appearance and contour. In animals that are still growing, abnormalities of the growth plates may be present. However, these vertebrae may not be inherently misshapen, but may develop abnormally due to abnormal

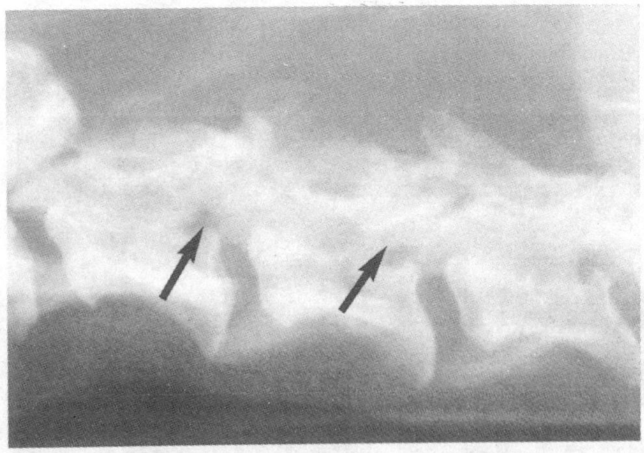

Fig. 11.25. Lateral survey radiographic view of the cervical spine of a dog with dural ossificans (*arrows*).

forces being placed on the vertebral unit from the pressures associated with spinal bending.

Scoliosis has most commonly been associated with intramedullary cystic spinal lesions such as syringomyelia and hydromyelia in dogs (Bagley et al. 1997; Child et al. 1986). Evaluation for underlying spinal cord defects in association with scoliosis is most accurately performed with CT or MR spinal evaluations. With MR imaging, the lateral deviation of the vertebral column may make it difficult to achieve acceptable positioning for sagittal imaging. This may create positional artifacts in the images produced. Electromyography of the paraspinal muscles may show abnormal spontaneous activity suggesting denervation of these muscles. Cerebrospinal fluid may be normal or reveal nonspecific alterations such as increases in protein concentration, nucleated cells, or both.

Atlantoaxial Subluxation

Atlantoaxial instability occurs in numerous, usually small, but occasionally large, dog breeds (see bibliography under Atlantoaxial Subluxation). Yorkshire terriers, Chihuahuas, Lhasa Apsos, and Pomeranians are most often affected. Other breeds affected include the Japanese Chin, toy poodle, Pekingese, Rottweiler, and Doberman pinscher. This disease is occasionally reported in cats.

This disease is often the result of some degree of abnormal articulation between the C1 and C2 vertebrae. This abnormal articulation may be the result of exogenous trauma with either fracture of the occiput, axis, or atlas, or disruption of the atlantooccipital ligaments. There may also be a congenital abnormality of the ligamentous or bony structures associated with this articulation. Various degrees of ligamentous and joint capsule abnormalities may be present. The ventral, cranial aspect of C2 forming the caudal articulation of this joint is also commonly malformed. Many of these ligamentous abnormalities are assumed to affect the stability of the odontoid process or dens. Atlantoaxial instability may also be associated with an abnormally shaped or absent dens. In some instances, there is a fracture

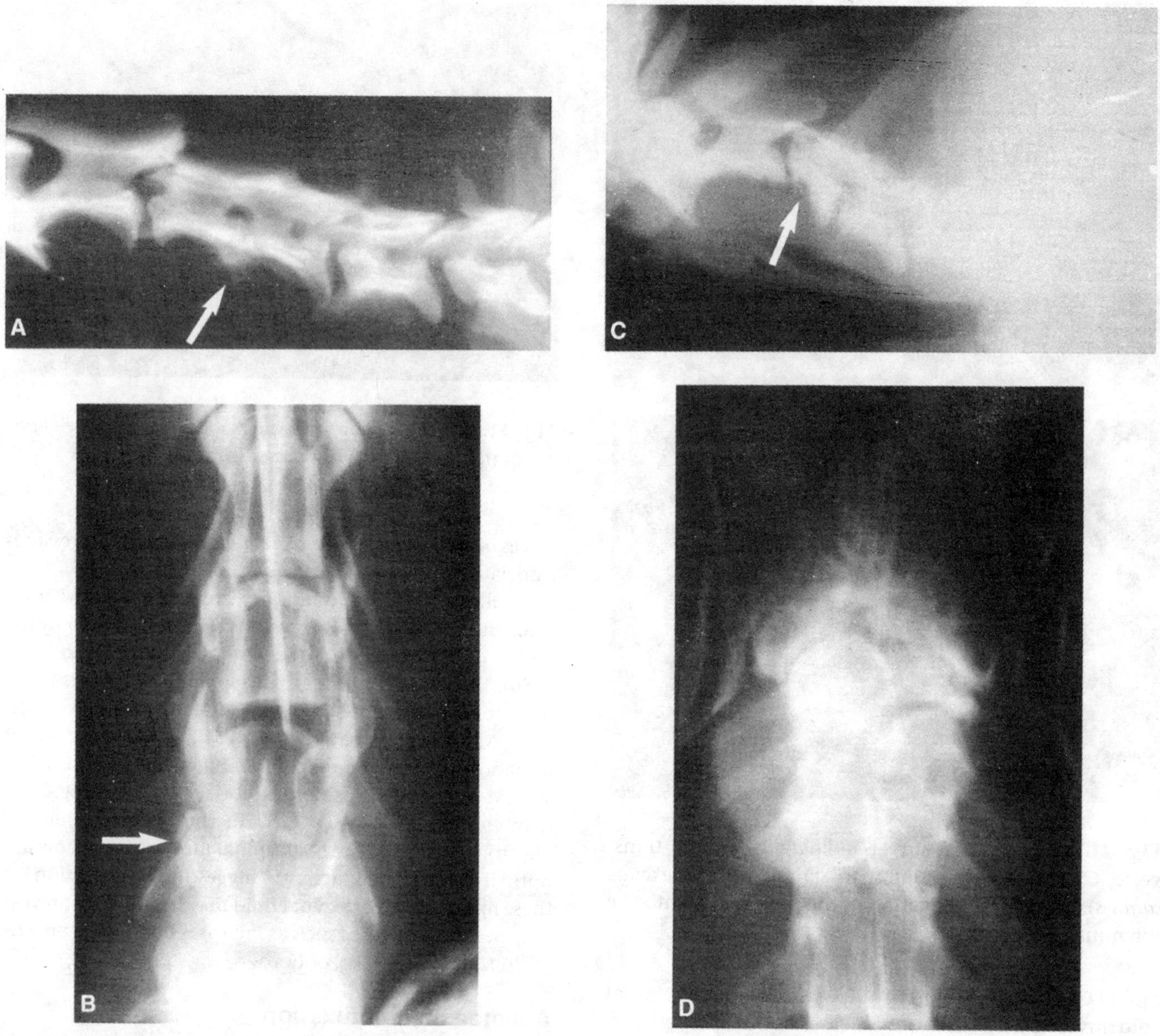

Fig. 11.26. (A) Lateral survey and (B) ventrodorsal radiographic view of the spine of a dog with congenitally fused (block) vertebral segments (*arrow*). (C) Lateral survey radiographic view of the spine of a basset hound with congenital abnormality of the third vertebral segment (*arrow*). (D) Ventrodorsal and survey radiograph from a dog with a congenital abnormality (hemivertebrae).

of the dens. In still other cases, the dens is present but abnormally angulated in a dorsal direction to compress the spinal cord. Clinical signs result from spinal cord compression or alterations in spinal cord blood flow. As this abnormality results in vertebral instability, spinal cord compression may be dynamic depending on the position of the head.

The diagnosis of AA instability is supported by demonstrating an increased distance (greater than a few millimeters) between the dorsal aspects of C1 and C2 when viewed on a lateral survey radiograph (fig. 11.28). Flexion of the neck may exacerbate the radiographic features, but may also exacerbate clinical signs so should be performed cautiously if not minimally. Atlantoaxial instability may also be associated with an abnormal or absent odontoid process (dens), which also may be evident on survey radiographs. Assessment for associated spinal cord compression or spinal cord parenchymal abnormalities is most accurately determined with myelography, MR imaging, or possible CT scanning (fig. 11.29). Syringomyelia is surprisingly common in association with atlantoaxial instability and may contribute to any associated clinical signs of spinal cord dysfunction. Imaging of the spinal cord with MR is the most accurate way to determine the presence of syringomyelia (fig. 11.30).

Cerebrospinal fluid may be normal or reveal nonspecific alterations associated with increases in protein concentration, nucleated cells, or both. Cerebrospinal fluid

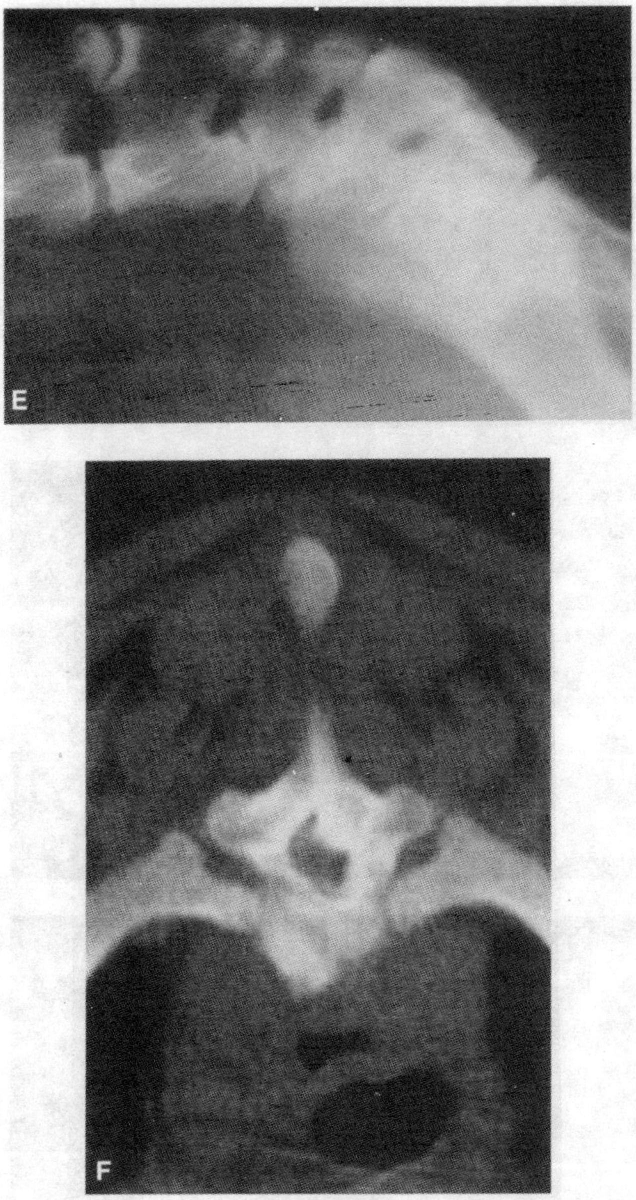

Fig. 11.26. (*continued*) (E) lateral radiographic view of a dog with congenital vertebral abnormalities. (F) Transverse, CT view from a dog with a congenital vertebral abnormality.

should be collected with caution or not at all from the cisterna magna region of animals with AA abnormalities as the associated anatomical abnormalities may result in an increased potential for iatrogenic nervous system injury from misplaced needle placement.

Syringomyelia and Hydromyelia

With the increased utilization of MR imaging for evaluation of animals with central nervous system disease, syringomyelia and hydromyelia are relatively common encountered spinal cord disease processes (Bagley et al. 2000; Lu et al. 2003; Tage et al. 2000). Syringomyelia refers to abnormal cavities filled with fluid in the substance of the spinal cord. A syrinx refers to one of these cavities. Hydro-

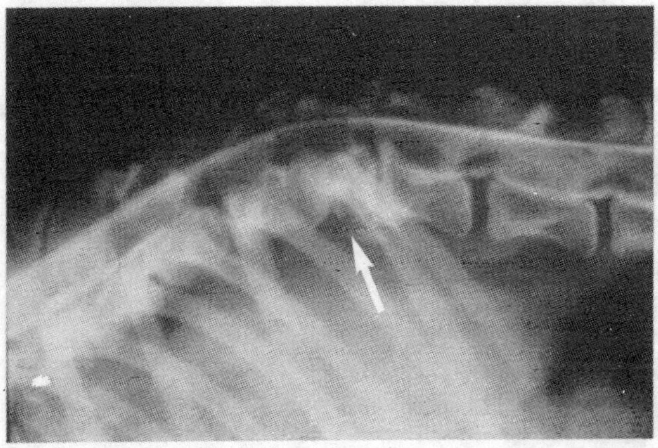

Fig. 11.27. Lateral myelographic appearance of the spine from a dog with spinal cord compression from a hemivertebra (*arrow*).

myelia refers to a pathologic condition characterized by accumulation of fluid within an enlarged central canal of the spinal cord. In both of these instances, the fluid that accumulates is similar, if not identical, to CSF. Some authors refer to hydromyelia as a communicating syringomyelia and use the term "syringomyelia" to describe all intraspinal abnormal fluid accumulations.

Clinically and diagnostically, it is often difficult to differentiate between syringomyelia and hydromyelia. Therefore, the term "syringo-/hydromyelia" is used. Ultimately, the diagnosis is made at a histologic evaluation. The fluid cavity within the spinal cord in hydromyelia is lined by ependymal cells characteristic of the central canal. A syringomyelic cavity, on the other hand, is located within the spinal cord external to the central canal and is lined by glial cells. Again, in many instances, these pathologic processes occur concurrently.

Malformations of the foramen magnum and infratentorial anatomical relationships (Chiari malformations) are frequently associated with both hydrocephalus and syringo- /hydromyelia in dogs. Obstruction of CSF flow at the foramen magnum and alterations in CSF pressure seem to be the primary mechanisms of these pathologic changes. Similar abnormalities may occur in dogs and other animals. Intracranial abnormalities resulting in hydrocephalus and a dilated fourth ventricle may also be associated with syringomyelia. The Dandy-Walker syndrome is one such example. With this disease there is a malformation of the cerebellum resulting in a cyst-like abnormality in the cerebellum. The lateral and third ventricles are commonly concurrently dilated. This is a congenital problem assumed to be associated with abnormal embryogenesis. Examples of a similar syndrome have been described in dogs and other animals. Spinal cord abnormalities have not been historically described. However, the spinal cords of affected animals may not have been examined pathologically. Interestingly, a number of dogs and humans with syringomyelia have associated scoliosis (see discussion above of scoliosis).

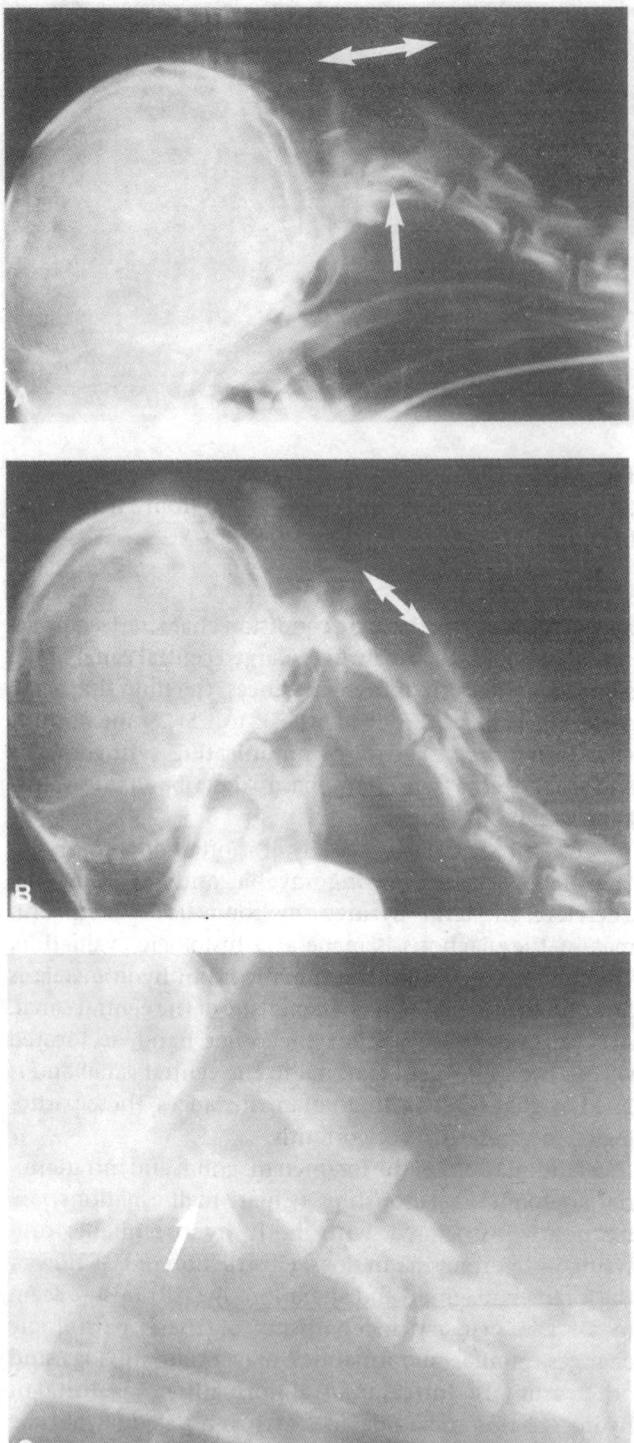

Fig. 11.28. (A,B,C) Lateral survey radiographs of three dogs with atlantoaxial instability (*arrow*).

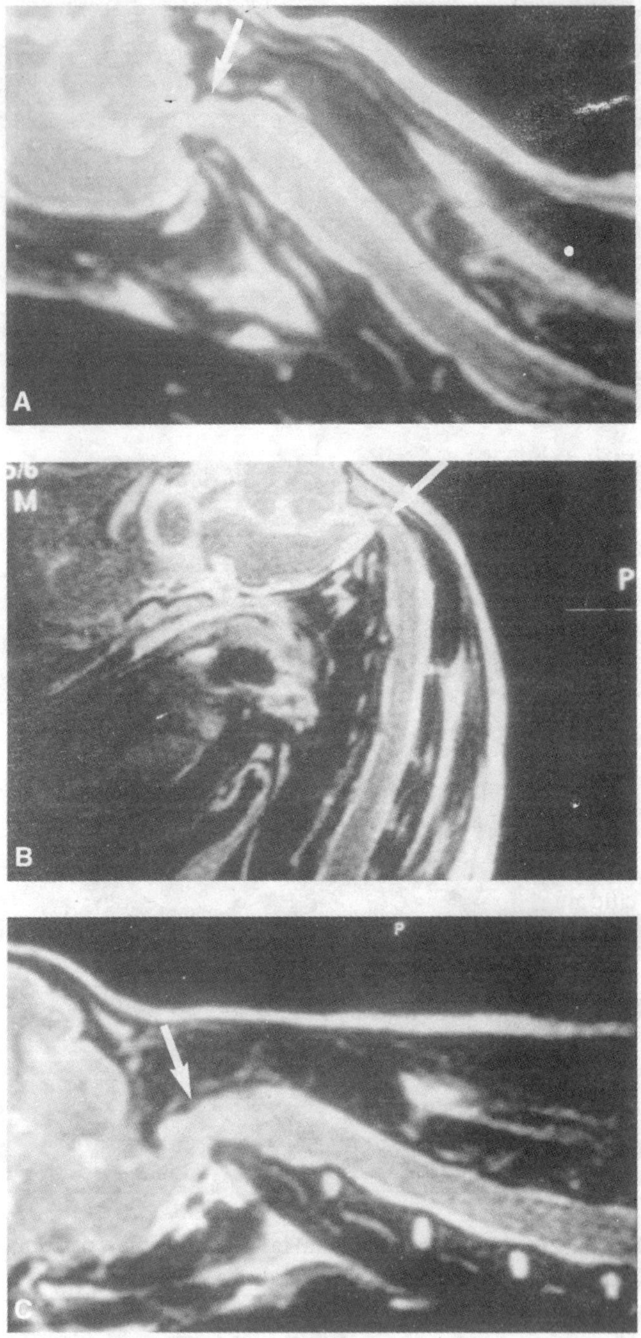

Fig. 11.29. (A,B,C) Sagittal, T2-weighted magnetic resonance views of three dogs with atlantoaxial instability. Note the spinal compression (*arrow*).

Syringomyelia is not apparent on survey spinal radiographic evaluation and usually also not apparent on myelography. If during myelography, contrast enters or is injected into the central canal of the spinal cord, hydromyelia may be evident. While this is sometimes attributed to the force of the injection, the enlarged central canal is usually present prior to the injection. That is, the injection is not the cause of the central canal dilation. If syringomyelia is associated with scoliosis, vertebral deviation may be evident on survey spinal radiographs.

Magnetic resonance imaging is the gold standard diagnostic test for detection of spinal intramedullary processes (figs. 11.30, 11.31, 11.32). These cavities are hyperintense or whiter regions compared to the spinal cord on T2 weighted MR images shown, while on T1-weighted MR images these cavities are hypointense or blacker compared to the spinal cord. Often these cavities are more conspicuous with T2-

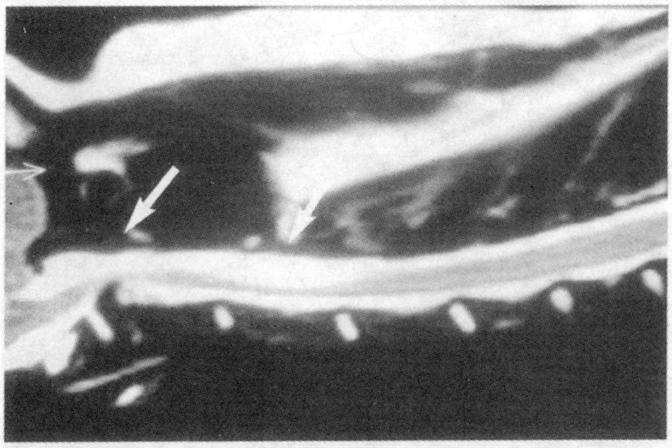

Fig. 11.30. Sagittal, T2-weighted magnetic resonance view of a dog with atlantoaxial instability and syringomyelia (*arrows*).

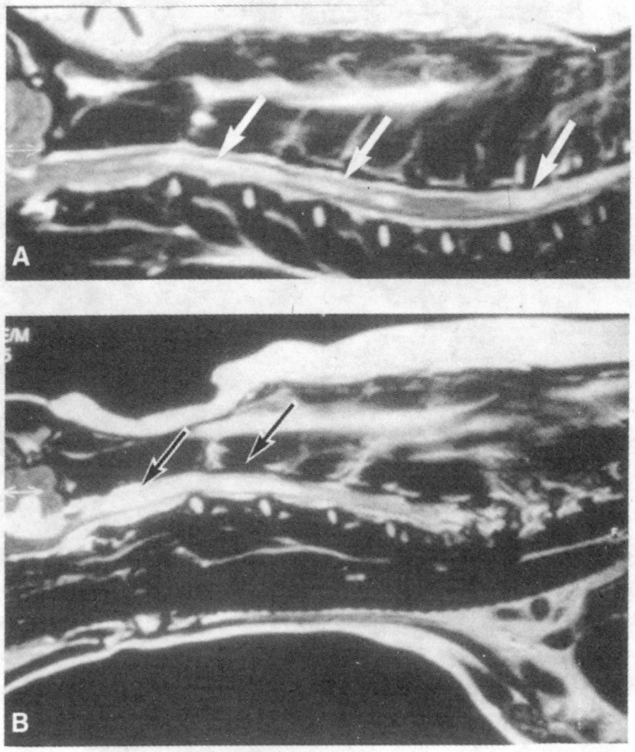

Fig. 11.31. (A,B) Sagittal, T2-weighted MR images from two dogs with syringomyelia (*arrows*).

weighted images, but the actual borders of the cavity with the associated spinal cord parenchyma may be indistinct. Magnetic resonance images of the caudal brain stem and cerebellum (infratentorial area) should be performed in any animal with syringomyelia as associated abnormalities of this portion of the nervous system and foramen magnum region are commonly associated with this disease process.

Cerebrospinal fluid may be normal or reveal nonspecific alterations such as increases in protein concentration, nucleated cells, or both. If syringomyelia results secondary to myelitis, more obvious evidence of inflammatory CNS disease may be found. Cerebrospinal fluid should be collected with caution or not at all from the cisterna magna region of animals with syringomyelia as the associated anatomical abnormalities may result in an increased potential for iatrogenic nervous system injury from misplaced needle penetration.

Arachnoid Cysts

Spinal arachnoid cysts have been reported with increasing frequency in dogs (figs. 11.33, 11.34, 11.35)(Cambridge et al. 1997, Dyce et al. 1991, Galloway et al. 1999, Rylander et al. 2002.) The term "arachnoid cyst" is misleading as these are extramedullary expansion and cord cavitation rather than cyst formation. Additionally, there is no epithelial lining to the cyst. A congenital etiology for lesion is most likely, although trauma has been implicated as a potential cause in both human beings and dogs. Scarring and local inflammation of the pia or other meninges may result in the creations of pockets of CSF accumulation. These cystic cavities may expand with each heartbeat and with respirations due to alteration in intracystic pressures. It is also possible that abnormal subarachnoid CSF dynamics contribute to cyst formation.

Arachnoid cysts are not apparent on survey spinal radiographs. Classically, an arachnoid cyst appears as a teardrop-shaped expansile abnormality of the dorsal, or occasionally ventral or lateral, subarachnoid space on myelography (figs. 11.33). With CT or MR, a similar expansile, fluid-filled structure with a teardrop shape (on a sagittal view) is seen. With MR, this cystic structure is hypointense (darker) and hyperintense (whiter) relative to the spinal cord parenchyma on T1-, and T2-weighted MR sequences, respectively. Cerebrospinal fluid may be normal or reveal nonspecific alterations associated with increases in protein concentration, nucleated cells, or both. Surgical biopsy confirms the type of abnormality present.

We have seen a number of *pug dogs* with focal cystic abnormalities of the dorsal and lateral subarachnoid space. Lesions are usually in the thoracolumbar area of the spinal cord, and may be in a location dorsal to an area of chronic disk protrusion. Clinical signs are reflective of a thoracolumbar myelopathy with progressive paraparesis. Interestingly, a number of affected animals with spinal cord scarring, arachnoid cysts, or other focally cystic spinal cord abnormalities have fecal incontinence as a predominant presenting complaint (see chapter 6 under Arachnoid Cysts). In many of these dogs, the gross appearance of the lesion is that of a focal *cicatrix* or *scarring* involving the pia mater and subarachnoid structures. Fibrous adhesion to the spinal cord is common. In some instances, these abnormalities resemble arachnoid cysts and may, in fact, be a variant of this disease. It is also possible that some arachnoid cysts are actually the result of arachnoid and pial scarring, adhesion, and fibrosis from an inflammatory or chronic irritation etiology. Diagnosis has been made with MR imaging to reveal the location and characteristics of these lesions and surgical biopsy of the offending tissue.

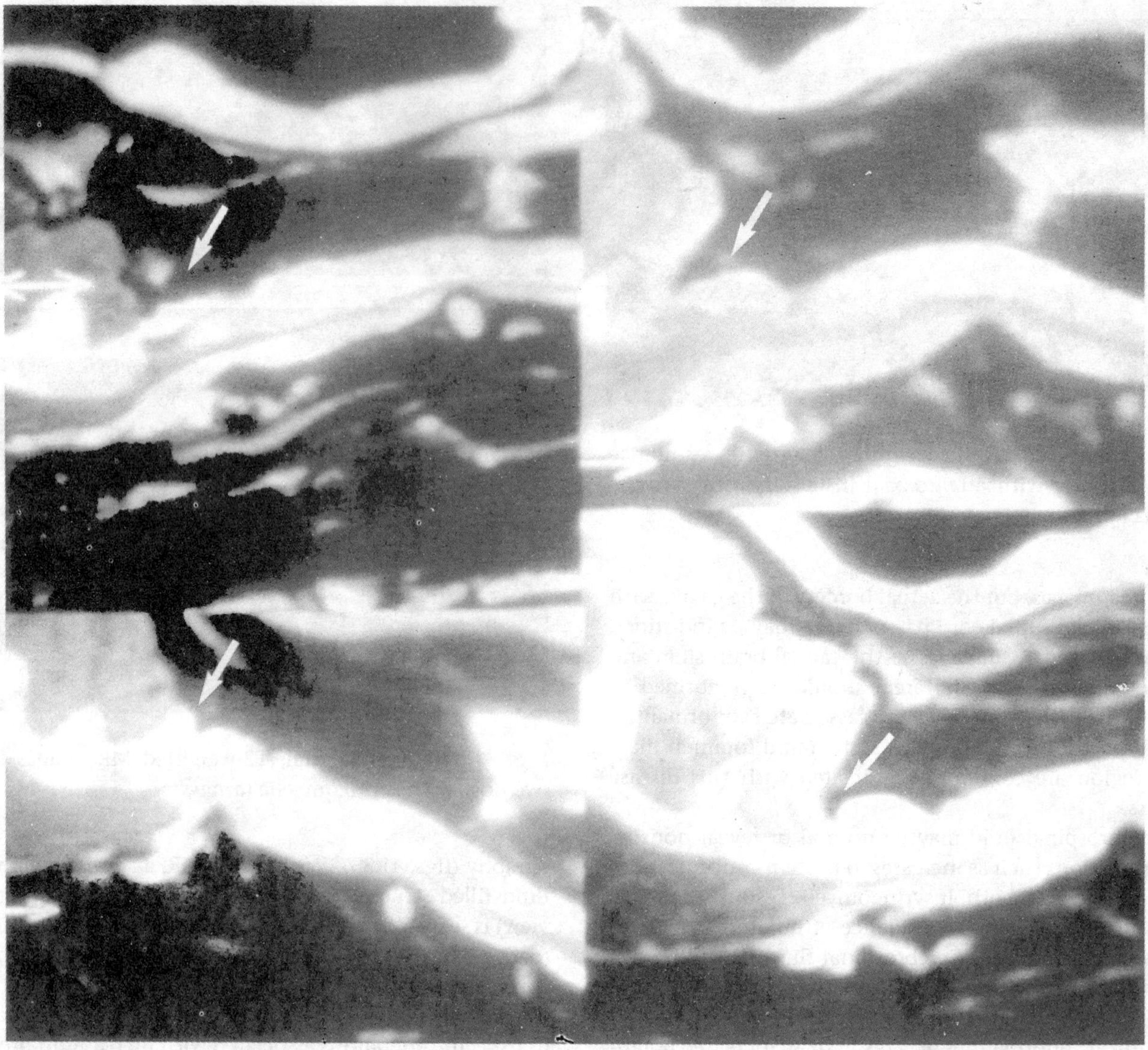

Fig. 11.32. Sagittal, T2-weighted MR images from four dogs with various abnormalities of the foramen magnum area (*arrows*) and concurrent syringomyelia.

Neoplasia

Spinal neoplasms are often categorized initially by the anatomical area, in relation to the dura and spinal cord, of spinal involvement (see bibliography under Spinal Tumor). Tumors are grouped into those primarily arising from an extradural location (extradural), within the dura but outside the spinal cord proper (intradural/extramedullary), or arising within the spinal cord parenchyma proper (intramedullary). Depending upon growth characteristics and tumor aggressiveness, a tumor can expand and extend from one of these strict anatomical areas to involve another. This is most often seen with peripheral nerve sheath tumors that may begin in an extradural location but may traverse the dura into the intradural/extramedullary space, and eventually, into the spinal cord grey matter.

Diagnosis of a spinal tumor is often presumptively made using survey spinal radiographs, myelography, or advanced imaging (CT, MR) (figs. 11.36, 11.37, 11.38, 11.39). Tumors involving the vertebral bone may be evident on survey radiographs as osteolytic and/or osteoproliferative processes. These bony changes need to be differentiated from diskospondylitis and vertebral body osteomyelitis. Classically, vertebral tumors do not traverse the joint space (intervertebral disk) from one vertebra into an adjacent one. Vertebral tumors are found, however, to invade adjacent vertebral bodies in some instances. Extradural compression of the spinal cord overlying the vertebral body rather than the intervertebral disk space is suspicious for, but not pathognomonic of, neoplastic disease.

Soft tissue tumors of the spinal cord or peripheral nerve tumors are usually not apparent on survey radiographs. Nerve sheath tumors, however, may involve exiting peripheral nerves within the intervertebral foramina. The foramen where the abnormal nerve is exiting may be enlarged due to associated bone atrophy and visible on survey radiographs.

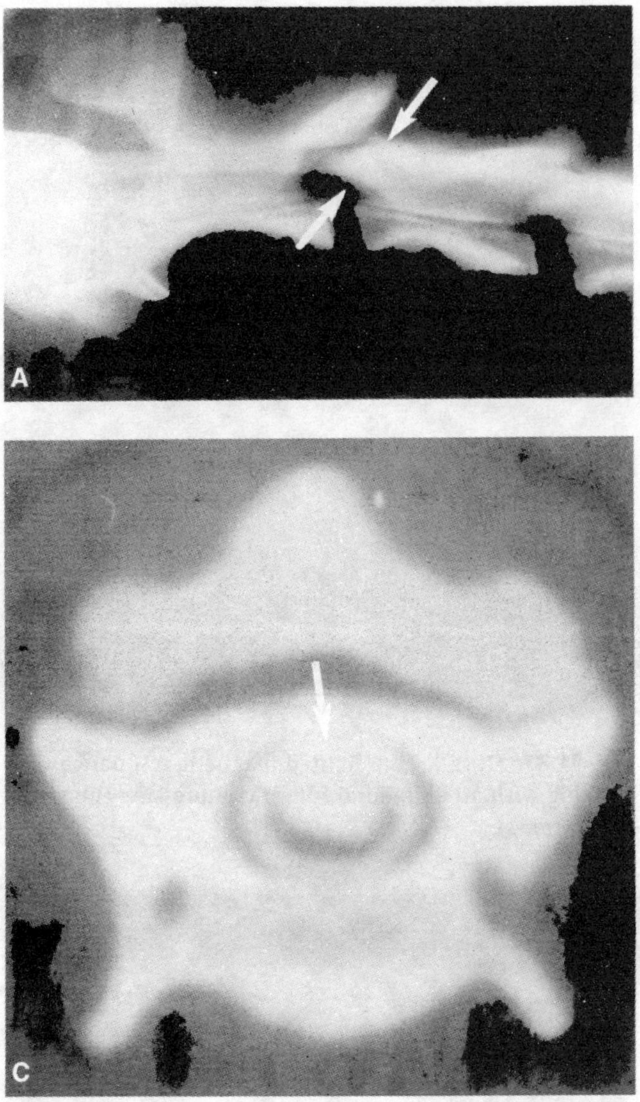

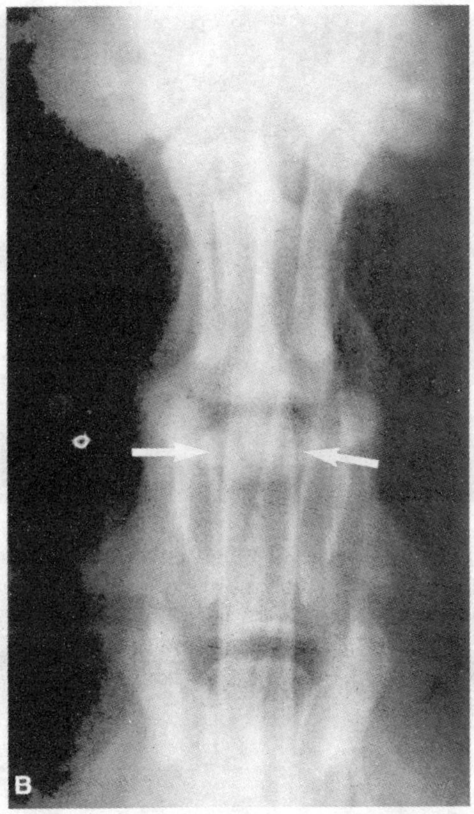

Fig. 11.33. (A) Lateral and (B) ventrodorsal myelographic appearance of the spine from a dog with an arachnoid cyst (*arrows*). (C) Transverse CT image following subarachnoid contrast injection in the same dog showing the dorsally located cyst (*arrow*).

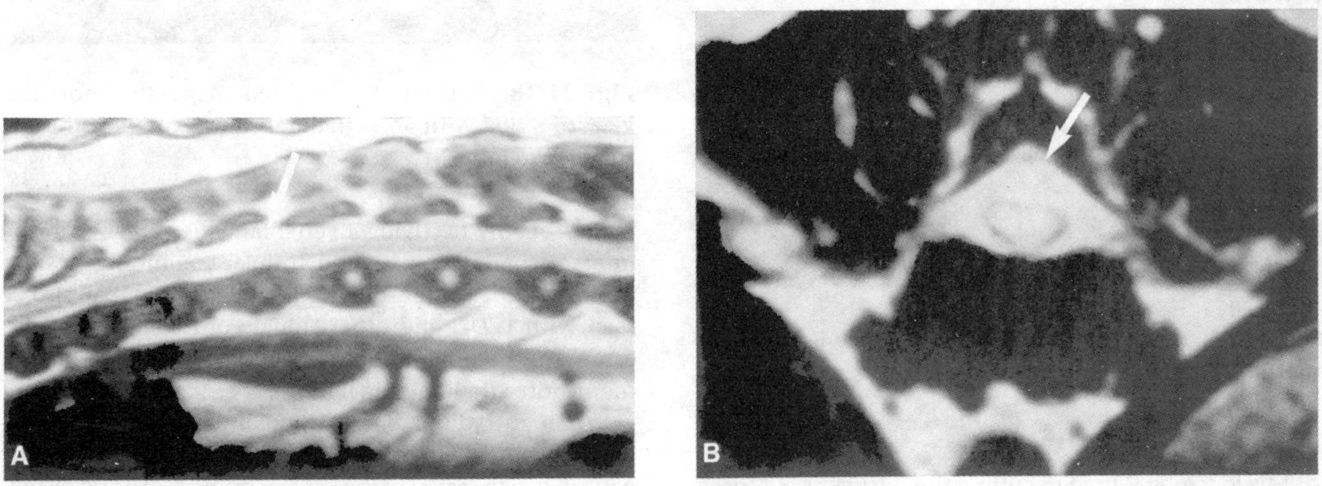

Fig. 11.34. (A) Sagittal and (B) transverse T2-weighted magnetic resonance views of a dog with an arachnoid cyst (*arrow*).

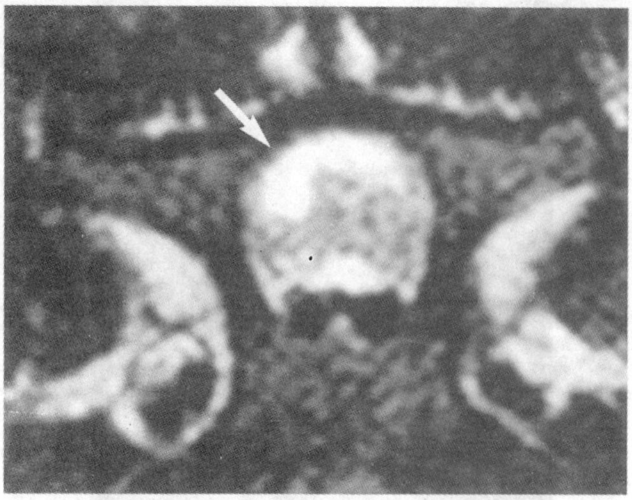

Fig. 11.35. Transverse T2-weighted magnetic resonance views of a dog with an arachnoid cyst (*arrow*).

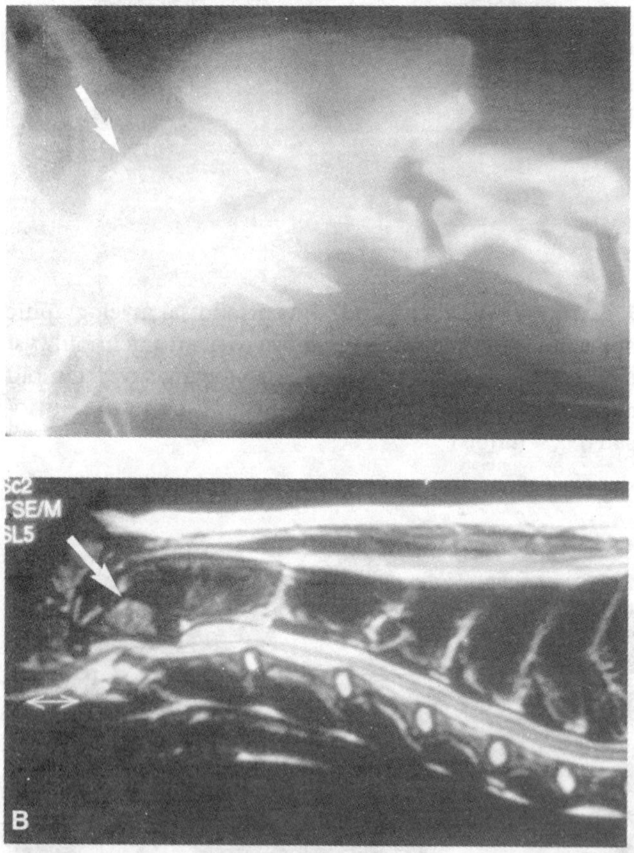

Fig. 11.36. (A) Lateral survey radiographic view and (B) sagittal, T2-weighted MR image of a dog with a bone tumor of C1 (*arrows*).

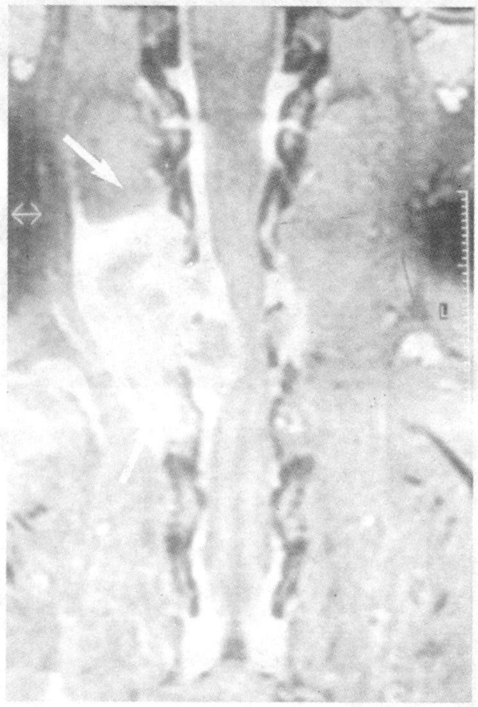

Fig. 11.37. Dorsal, T2-weighted magnetic resonance view of a dog with an extradural tumor compressing the spinal cord (*arrows*).

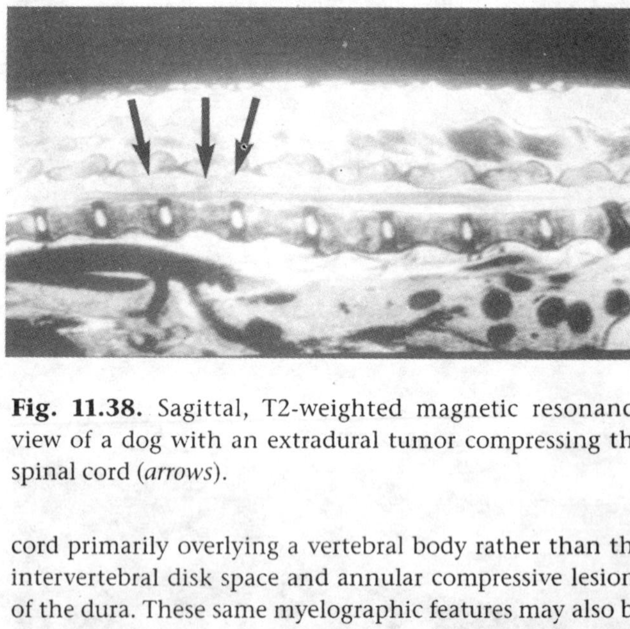

Fig. 11.38. Sagittal, T2-weighted magnetic resonance view of a dog with an extradural tumor compressing the spinal cord (*arrows*).

Myelography is used to outline the subarachnoid space and determine if spinal cord compression or expansion is present. With extradural tumors, one or both of the contrast columns may be deviated axially (toward the center of the spinal canal). Clues to the presence of an extradural tumor on myelography include compression of the spinal cord primarily overlying a vertebral body rather than the intervertebral disk space and annular compressive lesions of the dura. These same myelographic features may also be seen with IVDD and other spinal cord compressive diseases, and therefore should not be considered pathognomonic for extradural spinal tumor.

With intradural but extramedullary tumor, myelographic spinal imaging will often result in a characteristic pattern of expansion of the subarachnoid space and outlining of the tumor in negative shadow referred to as a "golf tee" (fig. 11.39). Nerve sheath tumors may also expand on either side of where the nerve traverses the dura, giving these tumors a dumbbell-shaped appearance. Conversely, expansion of the dural tube in 90° opposed radiographic

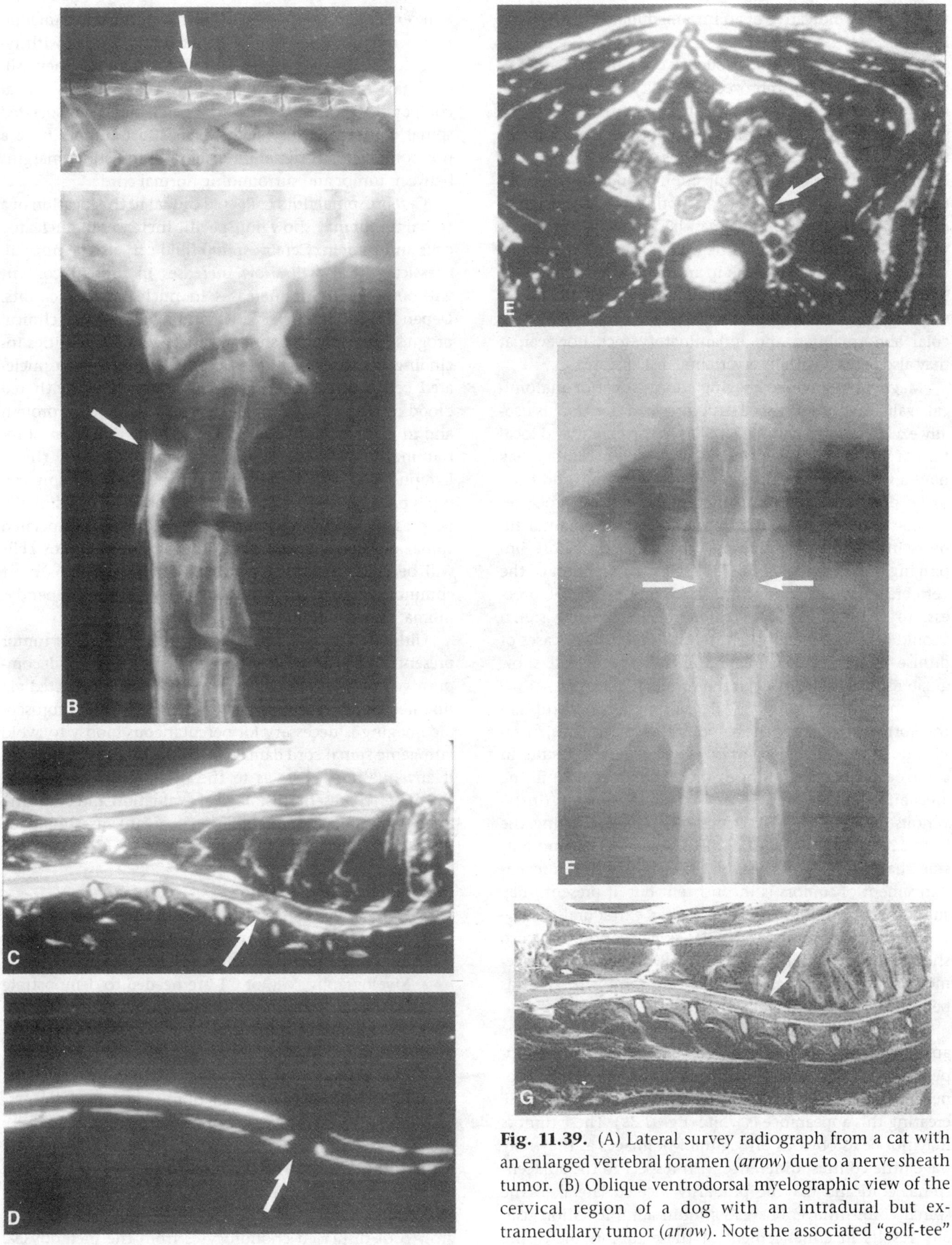

Fig. 11.39. (A) Lateral survey radiograph from a cat with an enlarged vertebral foramen (*arrow*) due to a nerve sheath tumor. (B) Oblique ventrodorsal myelographic view of the cervical region of a dog with an intradural but extramedullary tumor (*arrow*). Note the associated "golf-tee" appearance. (C) Sagittal, T2-weighted and (D) myelogram effect magnetic resonance views of a dog with an intradural but extramedullary spinal tumor ("golf-tee" sign) compressing the spinal cord (*arrow*). (E) Transverse, T2-weighted MR image from a dog with a nerve sheath tumor (*arrow*). (F) Dorsoventral myelographic image from a dog with an intramedullary tumor (*arrow*). (G) Sagittal, T2-weighted MR image from a dog with an intramedullary spinal cord lesion (*arrow*).

views is most indicative of an intramedullary or intradural lesion.

Advanced imaging studies such as computed CT and MR imaging have greatly improved the ability to determine the location and extent of any spinal tumor. With CT, a myelogram is often performed initially to outline the subarachnoid space. In some instances, a series of scans is performed before and after intravenous injection of an iodinated contrast material. Abnormalities disrupting the blood-spinal cord or blood-nerve barrier may become more apparent with this technique. Loss of integrity of these barriers or increased vascularity may result in an area of increased uptake (whiteness) after intravenous contrast enhancement. Contrast enhancement is most often seen with tumors, vascular abnormalities, and inflammatory foci, however, it may also be seen with intervertebral disk disease.

Magnetic resonance imaging affords superior anatomical evaluation of soft tissue structures and therefore is usually excellent in providing detail as to the extent and location of spinal tumors (Kippenes et al. 1999). Tumors may have a variety of appearances with MR imaging, and need to be differentiated from other spinal disease processes such as intervertebral disk herniation. Most epidural tumors invade the surrounding vertebral body before impinging on the spinal cord. Thus, bony destruction of the vertebrae may be a clue to an underlying neoplastic process. In general, on T1-weighted images marrow signal should be roughly equivalent to disk material. In cases of diffuse marrow involvement, the disk spaces will show greater signal intensity than the vertebral marrow.

Tumors are typically vascular and invasive, disrupting the normal integrity of the blood-brain barrier. Thus, intravenous injection of a contrast agent generally results in some degree of either diffuse or focal enhancement in the area affected by tumor. Contrast enhancement (intravenous gadolinium-DTPA) does not precisely define the tumor borders as neoplastic cells are generally found outside the enhanced portion of the mass. Gadolinium enhancement of tumors is inconsistent but, if present, may support a diagnosis of tumor. Other extradural disease processes, such as intervertebral disk herniation, may also show contrast enhancement on MR. Contrast enhancement characteristics alone, therefore, cannot be used as being pathognomonic for spinal neoplasia.

Intradural, extramedullary tumors often have a golf tee appearance in the subarachnoid space similar to the appearance of these tumors on myelography. This golf-tee appearance is most evident on T2-weighted images as the CSF creating this appearance is white (fig. 11.39). These tumors may not be as obvious on sagittal MR images as they may have little contrast difference with respect to the adjacent spinal cord and may be primarily located lateral to the spinal cord. Intravenous gadolinium administration usually results in enhancement of these tumors increasing their signal intensity on T1-weighted images. Dorsal and transverse contrast-enhanced images are often helpful to detect this category of tumors.

Intramedullary tumors generally cause the spinal cord to be expanded. On T1-weighted images, most intramedullary neoplasms have diminished signal intensity with respect to the spinal cord. On T2-weighted images, they usually have a brighter (hyperintense or whiter) signal compared to spinal cord, which often reflects associated spinal cord edema or hemorrhage. Most tumors have a nonhomogeneous signal intensity and indistinct margins between tumor and surrounding normal cord.

Cerebrospinal fluid collected caudal to the location of a spinal tumor may show nonspecific increases in nucleated cells and protein. Cerebrospinal fluid can also be normal. Classically, CSF will show increases in protein content without concurrent increases in nucleated cell counts. Depending upon the severity and acuity of the clinical progression, CSF may show a variety of abnormalities including increases in protein content, increases in nucleated cell counts, or evidence of hemorrhage (with red blood cells and erythrophagocytosis). Increases in protein and in nucleated cell counts in CSF are a reflection of inflammation, degeneration, or combination of these. Lymphocytes and monocytes are the predominant cell types present, however, neutrophils may also occasionally be present. Xanthochromia may accompany associated spinal or subarachnoid hemorrhage. Rarely, tumor cells will be evident on CSF cytologic analysis. This is most commonly found in instances of lymphoma, ependymoma, and carcinoma.

Ultimately, surgical biopsy confirms the type of tumor present. This is most often collected at the time of decompressive laminectomy, however, may also be collected via fine needle aspiration or percutaneous biopsy. Fluoroscopic imaging is necessary for percutaneous biopsy to avoid iatrogenic spinal cord damage with the biopsy instrument. If any question exists as to the origin and character of the material present, histological evaluation and culturing for aerobic, anaerobic, and fungal organisms should be performed.

Diagnosis of Spinal Tumor

- Clinical signs are consistent with the disease.
- Survey radiographs may show tumors that involve the bony structure of the vertebrae.
- Myelography, MR, or CT are needed to demonstrate soft tissue tumors and spinal compression.
- CSF may show alterations consistent with spinal disease but rarely contain neoplastic cells (except with lymphoma).
- EMG may reveal evidence of muscle denervation especially with nerve sheath tumors.

Multiple Cartilaginous Exostoses

Multiple cartilaginous exostoses are proliferations of bone and cartilage that are thought to result from aberrant growth of displaced chondrocytes from the metaphyseal growth plates of bone (fig. 11.40) (Caporn and Read 1996; Jacobson and Kirberger 1996). Subqeuently, this disease is most often seen in younger animals (<18 months of age). Dogs, cats, as well as other species including humans have been reported with this disease. The bony and catilaginous proliferations often are numerous and can affect the long bones, ribs, or vertebrae. The bony protruberences may be palpable. If this bony proliferation affect the vertebrae, varying degrees of spinal pain, paresis, and/or paralysis may result. Radiographs of the affected bones often show proliferations of bone that are smooth, contoured, irregular, multilobulated. Myelography will show an extradural compressive abnormality. With MR imaging, these vertebral lesions are expansile, irregular massses, and often involve the articular facets. The center of the mass has signal characteristics similar to medullary bone. A catilage cap (decreased signal intensity on a T2-weighted image) may be present at the periphery of the lesion. Surgical biopsy is necessary to definitively confirm the lesion.

Nutrition

Nutritional diseases of the spinal cord such as hound ataxia are usually confirmed histologically (Palmer et al. 1984; Palmer 1988; Sheahan et al. 1991). Affected animals did have decreased serum methionine levels and liver methionine synthetase levels abnormally elevated.

Hypervitaminosis A is usually found in cats fed whole liver (usually beef or sheep) (Clark et al. 1970; Goldman 1992; Lucke et al. 1968). Age of affected cats is usually between 2 and 10 years. This toxicity results in proliferation of bone resembling spondylosis along the spine, often in the cervical region. Survey spinal radiographs show the bony proliferation and spondylosis. Advanced imaging studies are necessary to document any associated spinal cord compression.

Idiopathic Disease

Calcinosis circumscripta is a disease of German shepherds, Great Danes, and vizslas but has been reported in English springer spaniels and Rottweilers (Bichsel et al. 1985; DeRisio and Olby 2000). Regions of mineralization and degeneration in a fibrous tissue matrix are present subcutaneously, which may extend into the spinal canal. These abnormalities are usually evident on survey spinal radiographic evaluations. Myelography, CT, or MR is necessary to confirm associated spinal cord compression. Cerebrospinal fluid may show nonspecific abnormalities associated with spinal cord compression including increases in protein concentration, nucleated cell counts, or both.

Spinal epidural lipomatosis is an abnormal accumulation of fat in the spinal canal. This is most often the result of release of excessive endogenous corticosteroids or excessive

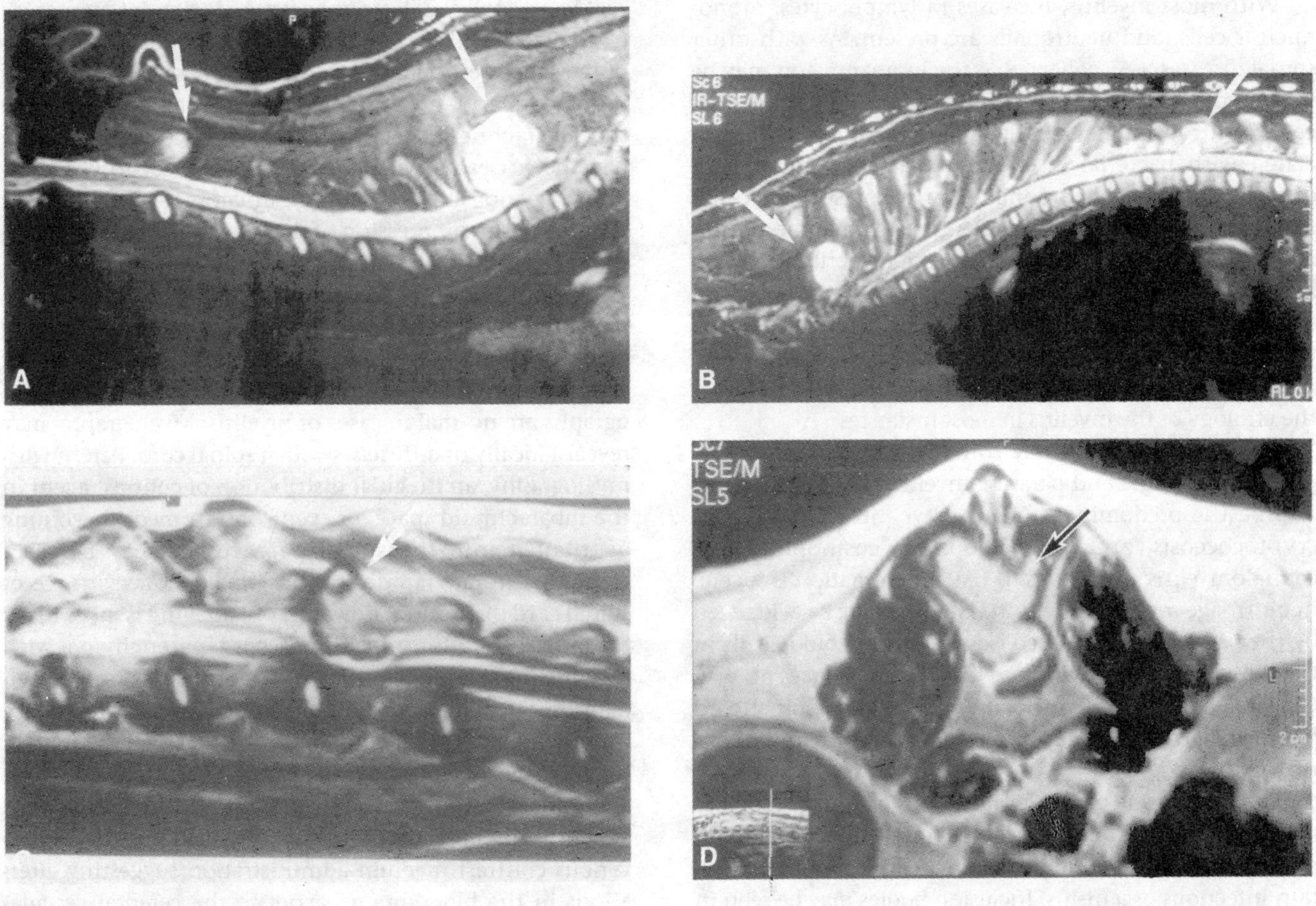

Fig. 11.40. (A)Sagittal, T2-weighted magnetic resonance views of the cervical and (B) thoracic regions of a young dog with multiple cartilaginous exostoses (*arrows*). (C) Sagittal and (D) transverse, T1-weighted MR image from a dog with a cartilaginous exostosis (*arrow*).

administration of exogenous corticosteroids. Myelography, CT, or MR is necessary to confirm associated spinal cord compression. Cerebrospinal fluid may show nonspecific abnormalities associated with spinal cord compression including increases in protein concentration, nucleated cell counts, or both.

Infectious/Inflammatory Diseases

Myelitis, encephalomyelitis, or *meningoencephalomyelitis* can result from a variety of infectious and noninfectious causes (see bibliography under Myelitis). Inflammation may occur anywhere along the spinal cord, and can be focal or diffuse. In many animals with encephalitis and meningitis, the cardinal signs of a systemic inflammatory processes such as the presence of a fever and increases in WBCs in the leukogram may not be found, as localized inflammatory disease in the CNS may not elicit a systemic inflammatory response.

The diagnosis of myelitis is most readily made through CSF analysis. Cerebrospinal fluid analysis contains increases in protein concentrations, nucleated cell counts, or both. A variety of CSF alterations may be present in association with myelitis. Unless a specific organism is observed on CSF cytology, it can be difficult, if not impossible, however, to separate the various causes of myelitis based on CSF analysis alone.

With most myelitis, increases in lymphocytes, mononuclear cells, and neutrophils are present. As with other spinal diseases, CSF collected in the lumbar region may be more representative of the disease process in the spinal cord. Neutrophils may be the predominant cell type associated with bacterial disease, but bacterial spinal cord diseases are rare. Neutrophils may be present in other instances of myelitis as well. Neutrophils may be prominent in CSF of cats with feline infectious peritonitis (FIP) and in dogs with spinal cord vasculitis syndromes and corticosteroid-responsive meningitis. Unfortunately, the type and distribution of CSF lymphocytes, monocytes, macrophages, and neutrophils cannot be used to predict the etiology of the myelitis in most instances.

Cerebrospinal fluid may contain increases in eosinophils with allergic and parasitic myelitis. Eosinophils may also be the predominant CSF cell type in protothecosis, cryptococcosis, and some idiopathic eosinophilic encephalomyelitis conditions. If CSF inflammation is severe, hemorrhage may be present in CSF. This may be evidenced by the presence of increased numbers of red blood cells in CSF, but is suggested more by the presence of erythrophagocytosis or xanthochromia. Primary spinal cord hemorrhagic disease may also result in secondary inflammatory CSF changes.

Special staining of CSF for infectious organisms, such as an India ink stain for cryptococcus (rarely involves the spinal cord), may be helpful in delineating the presence of certain infectious organisms. Inclusion bodies may be seen in CSF cellular elements in distemper and other viral diseases.

Unfortunately, evidence of inflammation on CSF evaluation alone is not specific for primary myelitis as other spinal cord diseases (e.g., neoplasia, trauma, infarction) may result in a CSF pleocytosis and protein elevations. Evaluation of serum or CSF titers for the evidence of infectious diseases is often necessary to establish specific infectious disease processes. Common infectious etiologies in dogs with myelitis include toxoplasmosis, neospora, distemper, and some fungal organisms. Common infectious etiologies in cats include toxoplasmosis, feline infectious peritonitis, and other as yet unclassified but suspected viral agents.

Toxoplasma gondii (dogs and cats) and *Neospora caninum* (dogs) are protozoal organisms that commonly are associated with myelitis. Diagnosis is based upon the presence of IgM antibodies to *Toxoplasma gondii* (usually appear in serum within 1 to 2 weeks of infection and persisting for 3 months, sometimes for years), or substantially increasing IgG titers, which appear by the fourth week of infection and increase over 2 to 3 weeks. IgG titers may remain persistent for months or years. Demonstration of the protozoan or other organisms in spinal cord biopsy specimens is also diagnostic.

In up to 60% or more of cases of myelitis, however, an infectious etiology is not identified. These noninfectious forms of myelitis may be associated with an occult inciting infectious cause, however, the presence of an infectious organism cannot be identified at the time of diagnosis.

Occasionally, CSF from an animal with inflammatory CNS disease will be normal at any individual single sampling. This is especially true when the disease is primarily intramedullary and inflammation is not associated with the subarachnoid space. In other instances, animals that have been treated with corticosteroids prior to CSF sampling may not show evidence of inflammatory changes on CSF due to the suppression of the infection due to administration of this class of drugs.

As some myelitis can result in or be associated with structural changes in the spinal cord, spinal cord imaging may be helpful in determining the extent and character of any regions of spinal cord inflammation. Survey radiographs are normal in cases of myelitis. Myelography may reveal a focally or diffusely swollen spinal cord. Rarely, with myelography, an irregular distribution of contrast agent in the subarachnoid space, or even contrast media becoming distributed into the spinal parenchyma may be seen. Computed tomographic scanning may show evidence of spinal cord disruption, however, MR imaging is more likely to show alterations in spinal cord parenchyma with myelitis (fig. 11.41). A variety of abnormalities may be evident on MR spinal imaging in cases of myelitis, including intramedullary spinal cord swelling (hyperintense signal), hemorrhage, or contrast enhancement. Multifocal discrete, anatomical lesions are often present within the nervous system, and may be especially conspicuous after intravenous contrast medium administration suggesting alterations in the blood-brain barrier to the cerebral vasculature. Occasionally, myelitis will appear as a focal mass lesion on MR spinal imaging mimicking a spinal tumor or hematoma. Surgical biopsy, with aerobic, anaerobic, and

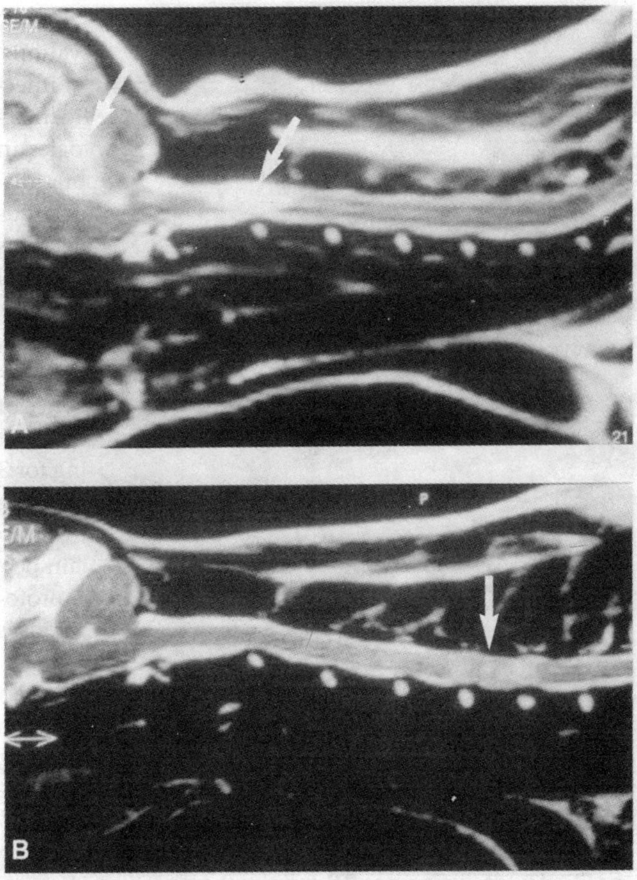

Fig. 11.41. (A,B) Sagittal, T2-weighted magnetic resonance view from two dogs with myelitis (*arrows*).

fungal culturing of any collected lesions should provide for a more definitive diagnosis.

Diskospondylitis

Diskospondylitis is infection in the IVD space and surrounding vertebral end plates and bodies (Johnson 1995; Kornegay and Barber 1980; Kornegay 1992). This disease can occur focally in any area of the spinal column or be present in multiple intervertebral disk sites. The most common class of infectious organisms associated with this disease are bacteria. Specific bacteria commonly associated with diskospondylitis are *Staphylococcus intermedius*, *Brucella canis*, and *Escherichia coli*. Rarely, fungal infections such as paecilomycosis and aspergillosis may be causative. Importantly, in situations of diskospondylitis, there are usually underlying processes that predispose to persistent bacteremia within the body. This may be persistent or recurrent infectious in parts of the body (such as the skin, urinary tract, and prostate). Additionally, animals may have suppressed or otherwise abnormal immune responses that allow for persistent or unresolved bacteremias to continue. Immunosuppression is commonly the result of exogenously administered corticosteroids (see chapter 6, Diskospondylitis).

Vertebral body osteomyelitis may result in similar clinical features. When present in the midlumbar vertebrae, osteomyelitis is often associated with a foreign body migration of a grass awn. In severe cases of osteomyelitis or diskospondylitis, a fistula may form from the vertebrae to the skin through the muscle and subcutaneous tissues. In the lumbar area, this fistula often is present in the lateral flank.

Diagnosis of Diskospondylitis

- Classic survey radiographic features of lysis of the vertebral end plates adjacent to the affected intervertebral disk space.
- Blood and urine cultures may establish the presence of a specific organism.
- Assessment of a brucellosis titer for supporting evidence of this disease.
- Occasionally, biopsy and culture of the affected intervertebral disk space are necessary for definitive organism identification.

As diskospondylitis is usually associated with an infectious etiology, it would be expected that routine laboratory assessments such as CBC, serum biochemical evaluations, and urinalysis might reflect evidence of the body's reaction to infection. Surprisingly, though, many animals with diskospondylitis do not have changes on their CBC evaluations that suggest an endogenous body reaction to an infectious organism (i.e., leukocytosis, neutrophilia). Animals with persistent infection of body organs such as the liver or urinary tract may have associated serum biochemical abnormalities reflecting damage or dysfunction of these organ systems.

Diskospondylitis is usually evident on survey radiographic evaluations of the spine(figs. 11.42, 11.43). Radiographic findings of lysis of the end plates of the vertebral bodies results in an irregular intervertebral disk, vertebral end plate margin. Within the surrounding vertebral structures, there is often sclerosis. Very early (i.e., <14 days) in the disease course, no radiographic abnormalities may be apparent. In the earlier stages of diskospondylitis, the intervertebral disk space appears widened as the disease erodes the vertebral end plate. As significant amounts of bone are damaged over time, the adjacent vertebrae may collapse resulting in decreases in the intervertebral disk space. In rare instances, this disease may predispose to vertebral luxation and fracture. These pathologic vertebral changes result in further collapse and malalignment of the spine.

Osteomyelitis can involve the vertebrae. On survey radiographs of affected animals, varying combinations of lysis and bony proliferation are present. These alterations primarily involve the vertebral body (fig. 11.44). The location of the vertebrae involvement (body versus end plate) is used in differentiating vertebral osteomyelitis from diskospondylitis. Osteomyelitis results in combinations of bone lysis, new bone proliferation, and sclerosis. It is common that the vertebral body, lamina, facets, or dorsal spinous processes are also involved. In areas where grass awn migrations are endemic, osteomyelitis is often found in the ventral aspect of the middle lumbar (L2 through L4) verte-

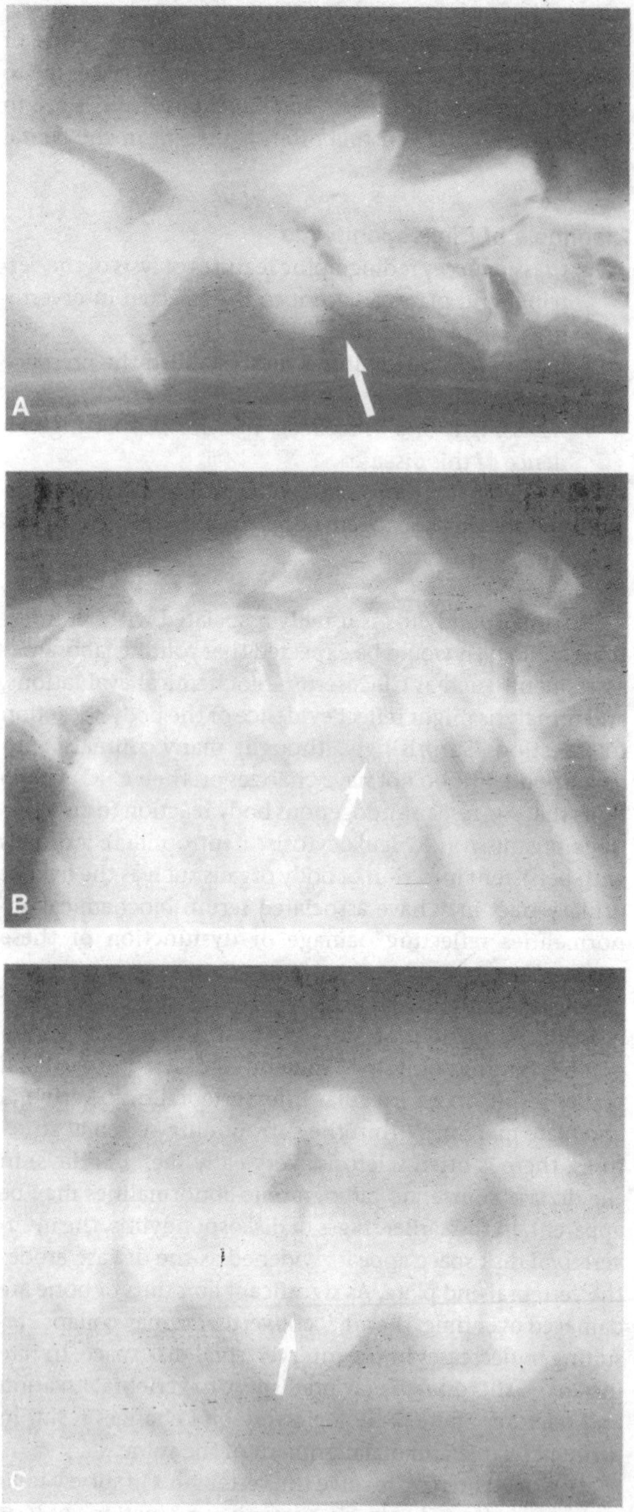

Fig. 11.42. (A) Lateral survey radiograph of a dog with diskospondylitis at the C2–3 intervertebral disk space (*arrow*). (B) Lateral survey radiograph of a dog with diskospondylitis at the T13–L1 intervertebral disk space (*arrow*). (C) Lateral survey radiograph of a dog with diskospondylitis at the L1–2 intervertebral disk space (*arrow*).

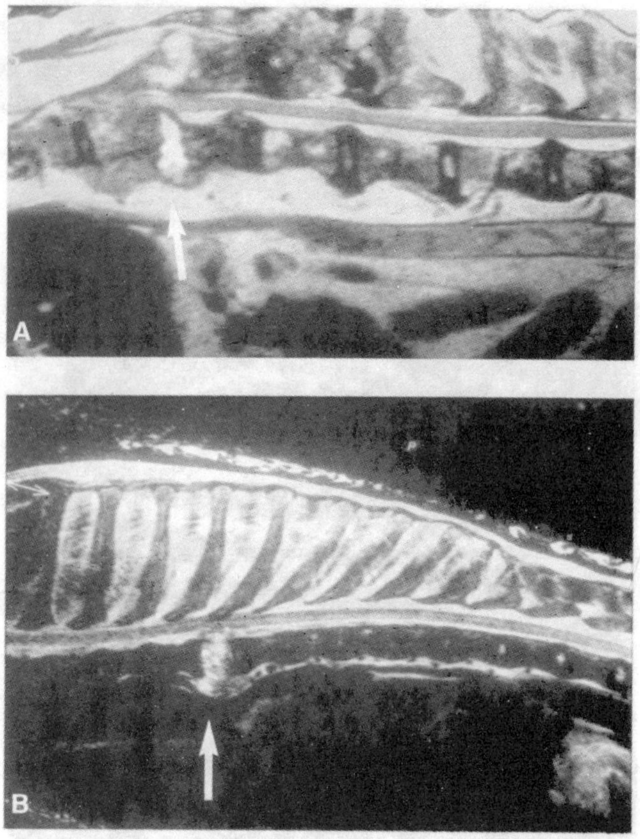

Fig. 11.43. (A,B) Sagittal, T2-weighted magnetic resonance view of the thoracolumbar spine of two dogs with diskospondylitis (*arrow*).

brae. This area is associated with the attachment of the diaphragm (and possible termination of foreign body migration) and is a common place for abscessation to occur.

If myelography is performed, an extradural, usually ventral compression of the spine may be present overlying the affected intervertebral disk space. As the infection is in the extradural location, CSF collected caudal to the lesion may show nonspecific signs of spinal cord disease or compression including increases in protein concentration, and rarely, increases in nucleated cells. Cerebrospinal fluid changes will usually not show the presence of a specific infectious organism as the primary infection resides outside of the dura (extradural). If the disease results in spinal abscessation and this process erodes through the dura, a septic meningitis may be evident on CSF analysis.

Vertebral diskospondylitis and osteomyelitis may also be evident on CT and MR studies (figs. 11.43, 11.44). With CT, vertebral end plate irregularity and lysis are present. On the T1-weighted MR images, the involved intervertebral disk space and involved adjacent vertebral bodies often have a decreased signal (hypointense). On the T2-weighted images, an increase in signal (hyperintense) is seen in the involved vertebral bodies or intervertebral disk area (fig. 11.43). Disruption of the low signal end plates on both T1 and T2 images is a hallmark of diskospondylitis/osteomyelitis that enables distinction of this entity from neo-

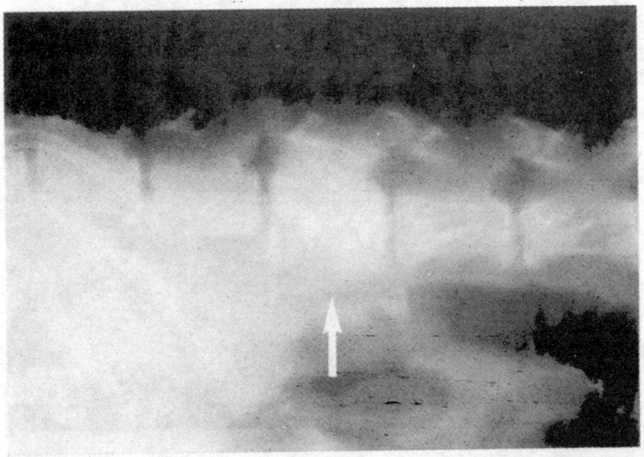

Fig. 11.44. Lateral survey radiograph of a dog with vertebral body osteomyelitis of the L3 vertebral body (*arrow*).

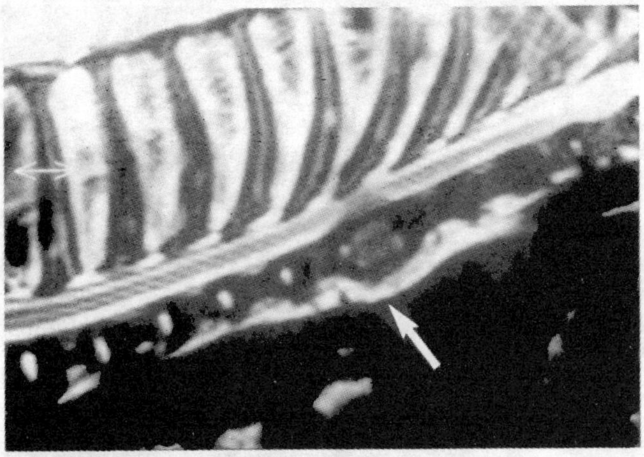

Fig. 11.45. Sagittal, T2-weighted magnetic resonance view of the thoracic spine of a dog with a fungal osteomyelitis of the vertebral body (*arrow*).

plasms, which rarely breach the end plates but frequently and extensively involve the marrow. Contrast enhancement is often present in the affected intervertebral disk space.

Spinal abscessation is rare in dogs and cats but can result from hematogenous infection or local penetrating trauma. Grass awn and porcupine quill migration may enter the spinal canal and result in focal infection. *Actinomyces* and *Nocardia* may be present in these locations. Fungal granulomas may also occur in the spinal canal. In some instances of diskospondylitis, the infectious process may extend from the disk into the perispinal tissues and fat. Diagnosis is supported by finding evidence of a compressive (most commonly extradural) or expansile lesion of the spinal cord on myelography, CT, or MR studies. Cerebrospinal fluid may show evidence of septic inflammation. If the abscess occurs extradurally, nonspecific increases in protein concentration and nucleated cell counts can occur. Occasionally, CSF will be normal.

External Trauma to the Spinal Cord

Spinal cord trauma is relatively common in small animals. This occurs either from exogenous or endogenous injury (Bagley 1999, 2000a, 2000b). Automobile-induced injury is the most common exogenous cause of trauma to the spine in small animals, with falls, trauma from falling objects, and projectile missile damage also occurring. Intervertebral disk extrusion remains the most common endogenous cause.

If, based upon initial historical and physical assessments, a vertebral injury is suspected, it is reasonable to cautiously perform survey radiographs of the affected area prior to additional manipulation to aid in identification of unstable vertebral segments (figs. 11.46, 11.47). As with any radiographic procedure, proper positioning is of utmost importance. Spinal trauma is associated with significant pain and in some instances anesthesia may be required if the animal is systemically stable and can tolerate the anesthesia. If, however, anesthesia is performed, the patient should be cautiously moved, transported, and manipulated to avoid iatrogenic injury to the patient. If further workup and therapy are not available at the immediate site and referral to a secondary care facility is probable, it may be more beneficial to forgo anesthesia for survey radiographic performance. This eliminates the need for repeated anesthetic procedures on the animal in a short period of time.

Animals with spinal trauma must be moved and positioned with caution to prevent further trauma to the spinal cord. A backboard is often employed in these animals to provide external spinal stability. If the animal is taped to a backboard that is not radiopaque, it should be carefully moved from the board onto the radiographic table. This can be accomplished by unfastening the tape and controlling the movement of the animal onto the radiographic table. More than one person should help during this movement, with at least one of these people supporting the unstable spinal area with two hands.

Changes in the alignment of the vertebrae or other vertebral and soft tissue inconsistencies may be subtle; therefore, the clinician must be familiar with the most appropriate radiographic views and techniques necessary to facilitate diagnosis of spinal trauma. Two or more radiographic views are indicated when investigating for evidence of spinal column injury, with the lateral and ventrodorsal (VD) radiographic views being the most commonly obtained. There have been many instances in which the spinal column appeared normally aligned in one radiographic view but obviously dislocated in another. For the lateral view, the spinal column should be kept parallel to the table with the use of positioning aids such as foam rubber cushions. If a ventrodorsal radiographic view is indicated, the radiographic tube should ideally be positioned in a cross-table orientation to collect the dorsoventral (DV) or VD radiographic view. If this is not possible, the animal should be carefully rolled onto its back, keeping the spinal column as straight and still as possible. Again, this is facilitated by having multiple individuals help in the moving of the animal. Rolling the animal into a foam V-shaped trough

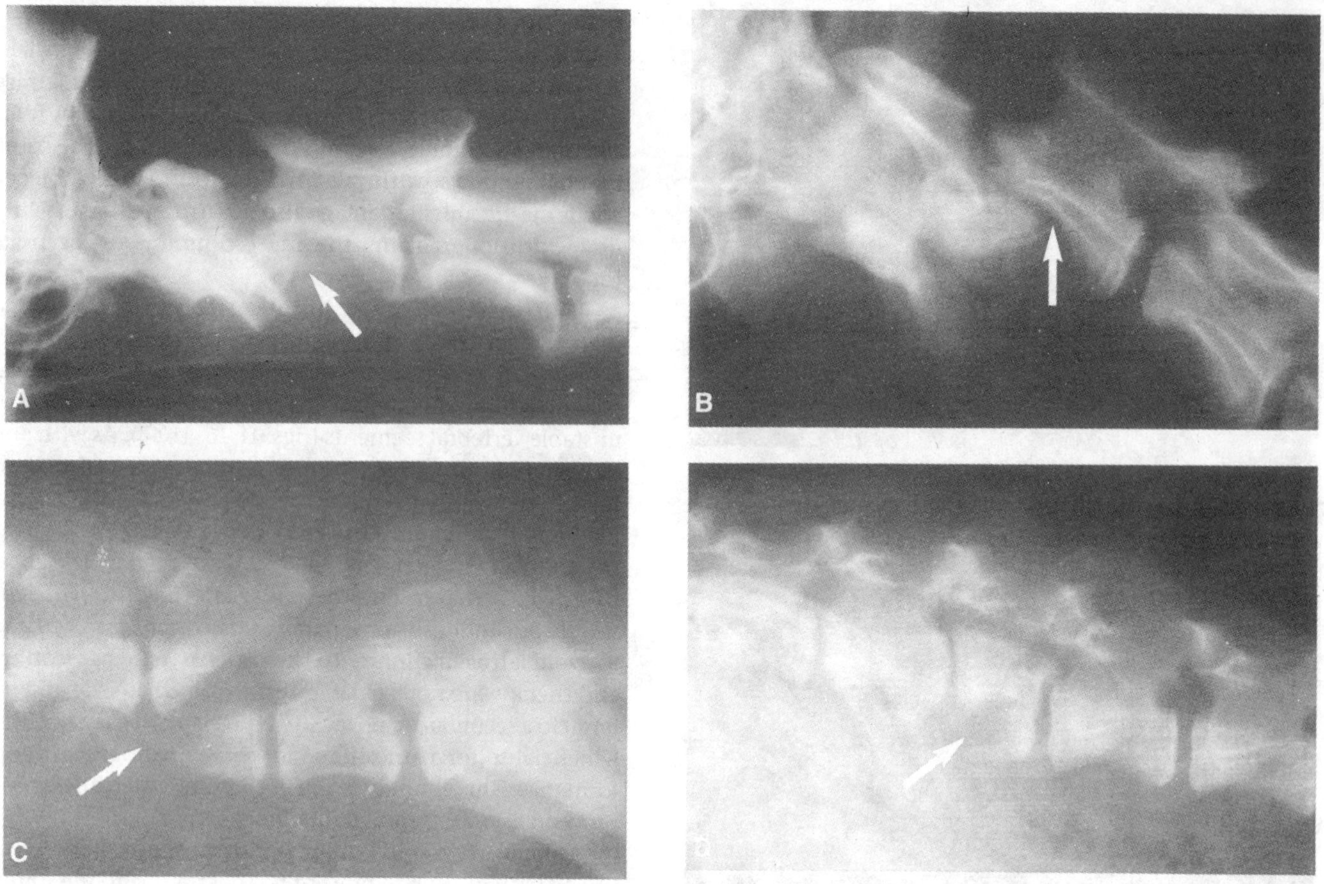

Fig. 11.46. (A,B) Lateral survey radiograph of two dogs with C2 fractures (*arrows*) and (C,D) two dogs with thoracolumbar fractures (*arrows*).

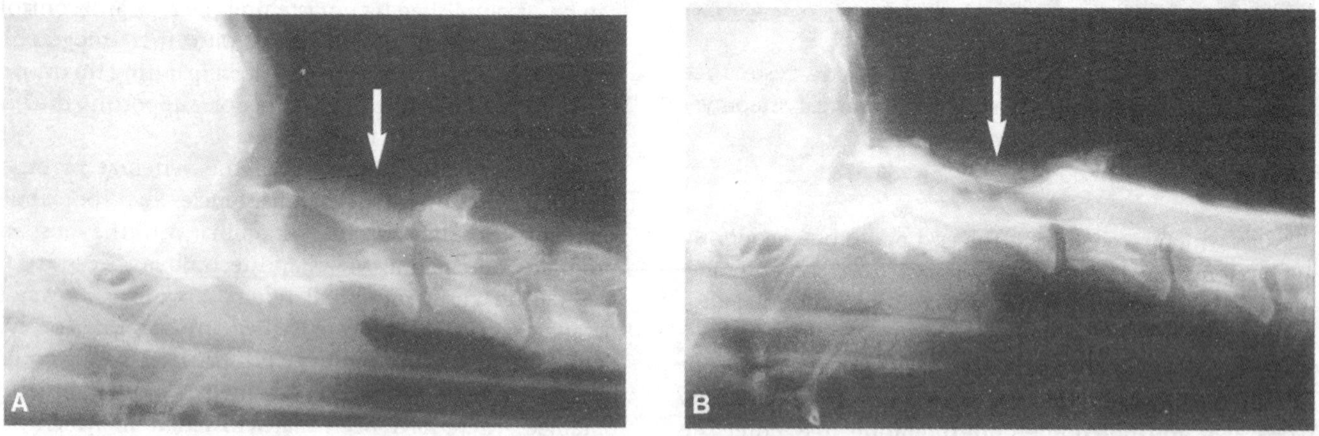

Fig. 11.47. (A) Lateral survey and (B) myelographic views of a dog with a fracture of the dorsal arch of C2 (*arrows*).

prior to movement is helpful in this regard. Specific radiographic positioning for each segment of spine is detailed in several veterinary radiology technique publications.

With spinal injury, it is important to remember that radiographs represent a static (single time) view of a lesion. The vertebral column may have suffered a significant amount of motion (luxation) during the traumatic event, but due to the effects of the strong musculature in the paraspinal region, the vertebrae may become ultimately positioned in a near normal-appearing alignment. In this situation, the clinical signs may be worse than the radiographic abnormalities would suggest. Disturbances to the adjacent soft tissue, such as paraspinal muscle disruption or hematoma, may also be an additional radi-

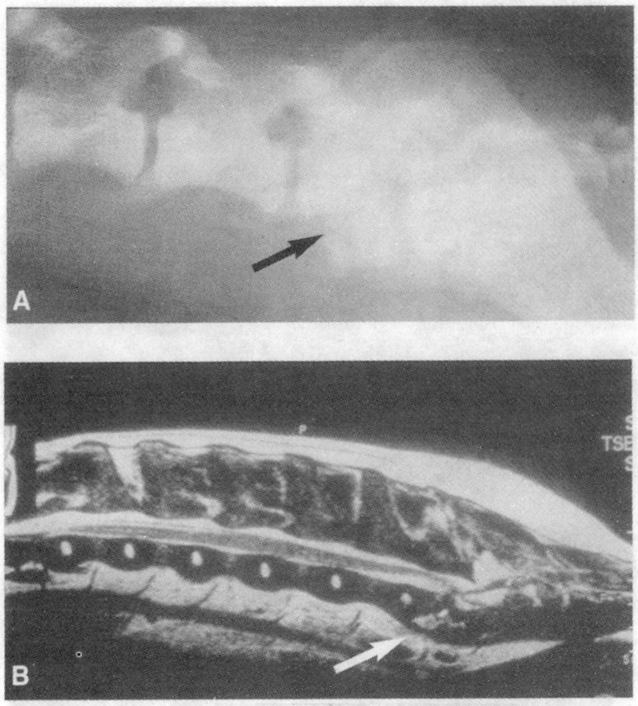

Fig. 11.48. (A) Lateral survey and (B) T2-weighted MR image of a dog with a fracture of the L7 vertebral body (*arrow*).

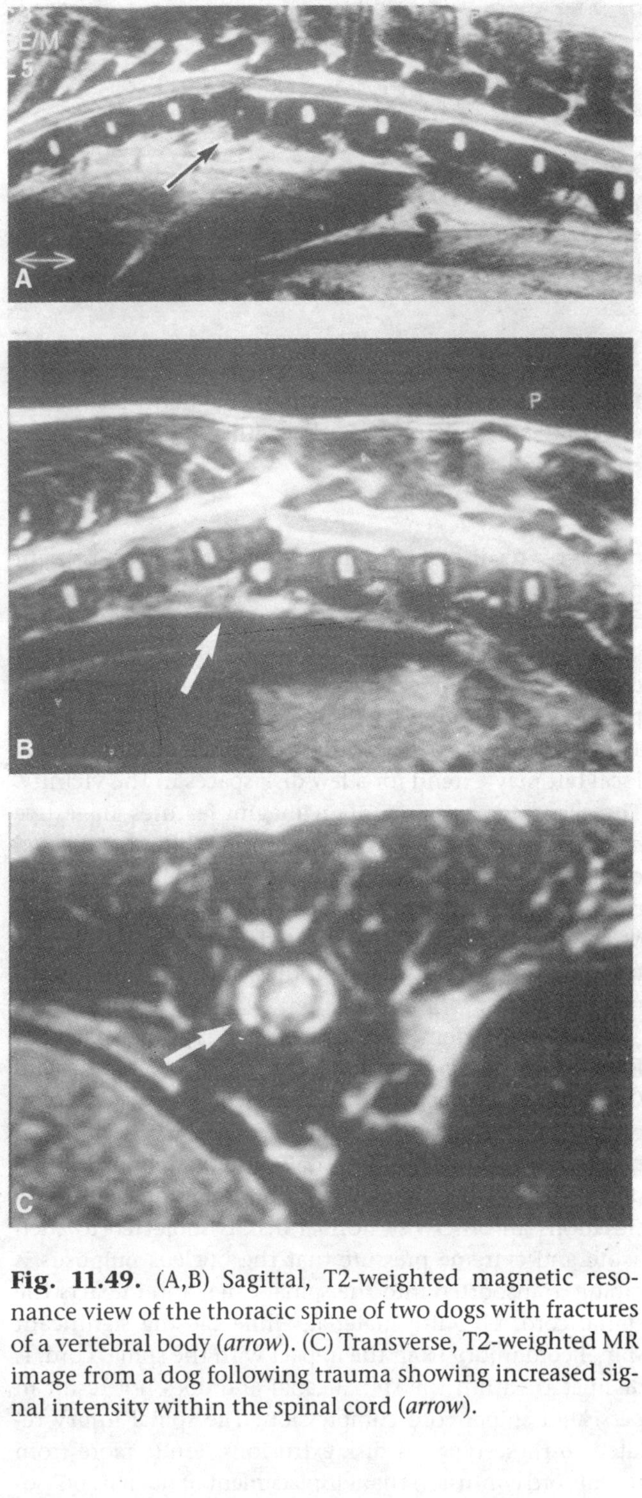

Fig. 11.49. (A,B) Sagittal, T2-weighted magnetic resonance view of the thoracic spine of two dogs with fractures of a vertebral body (*arrow*). (C) Transverse, T2-weighted MR image from a dog following trauma showing increased signal intensity within the spinal cord (*arrow*).

ographic clue to the site of injury. Conversely, in other instances the radiographic appearance of the vertebrae may show severe malalignment, however, the clinical signs may be minimal.

Computed tomography is an excellent study for detecting small fractures underappreciated on survey radiographs. Magnetic resonance clearly establishes the presence of associated acute spinal pathology (figs. 11.48, 11.49). When examination with MR is abnormal, the area affected may then be accessed by CT, if further clarification of vertebral involvement is necessary. Cerebrospinal fluid collected caudal to the lesion may show increases in red blood cells, xanthochromia, and erythrophagocytosis. Increases in nucleated cells and protein concentration may be present with concurrent spinal cord inflammation.

Fibrocartilaginous Emboli

Ischemic myelopathy, or *fibrocartilaginous emboli,* is a disease entity diagnosed with increasing frequency in dogs over the last 15 years (Cauzinille and Kornegay 1996; Hawthorne et al. 2001). This disease has been thought to result secondary to vascular thrombosis and infarction of the spinal cord with some pathologic evidence to support these conclusions. The speculated cause of the infarction centers around fibrocartilage material, similar to that found in intervertebral disks, entering the vascular system and resulting in the embolization of the spinal cord vasculature. How this fibrocartilage enters the vascular system is unclear. Theories include disk extrusion into the vascular system, either directly or through neovascularization of the IVD associated with disk degeneration. It has also been suggested that the fibrocartilage actually arises from within the vascular system and subsequently becomes dislodged. A reasonable pathophysiologic explanation for this disease has been elusive.

Diagnosis is supported by the appropriate clinical signs and exclusion of other disease processes. Definitive diagnosis can only be made at necropsy. Myelography is often normal or may show cord swelling during the acute

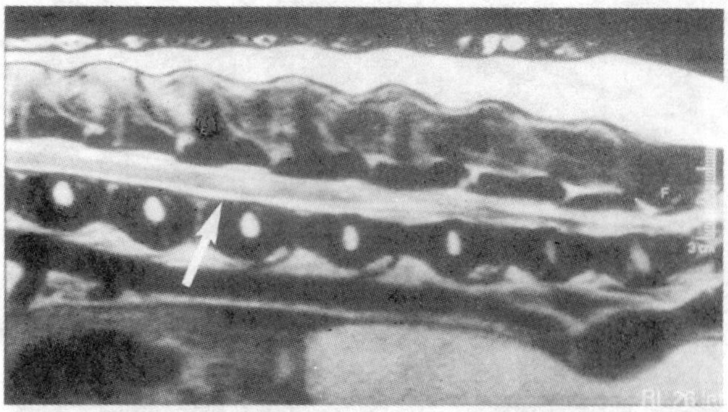

Fig. 11.50. Sagittal, T2-weighted magnetic resonance view of the lumbar spine of a dog with a fibrocartilaginous emboli (*arrow*).

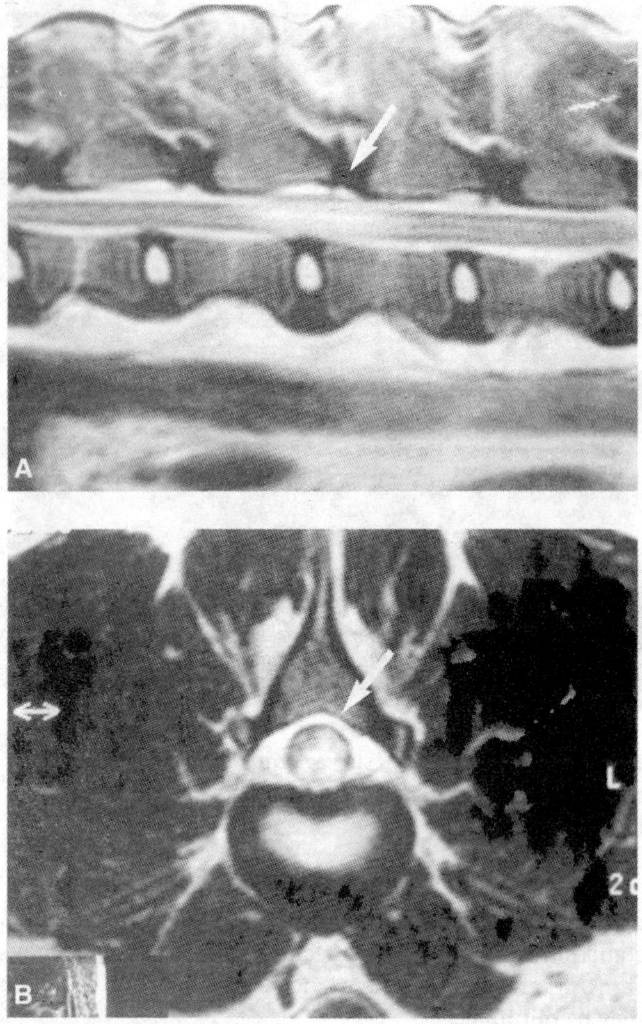

Fig. 11.51. (A) Sagittal and (B) transverse T2-weighted magnetic resonance view of the lumbar spine of a dog with a fibrocartilaginous emboli (*arrow*).

phases of the disease. Computed tomographic assessment may show similar changes as with myelography. An intramedullary spinal cord lesion is usually present on MR imaging of the affected spinal region. This abnormality usually has the appearance of edema or fluid (hyperintense or whiter signal on T2-weighted studies) (figs. 11.50, 11.51). The abnormality within the spinal cord is usually focal but may extend for a few disk spaces in the vicinity. These lesions may also contain imaging features suggestive of spinal cord hemorrhage. Cerebrospinal fluid, collected caudal to the lesion, may be normal or contain increases in nucleated cells and protein. A predisposition to formation of thrombi should be investigated with platelet counts, bleeding times, coagulation profiles, and antithrombin III measurements.

The antemortem diagnosis of FCE is somewhat confounded by the fact that similar clinical, myelographic, and CSF findings may occur in acute, noncompressive intervertebral disk herniation, vascular infarction, focal spinal hemorrhage, or myelitis (fig. 11.52). Intervertebral disk "explosions" have been previously reported in dogs. In these situations an otherwise normal disk is subjected to such acute and extreme pressure that the nucleus pulposus is rapidly transported into the spinal canal and impacts the spinal cord. The disk material, while causing significant spinal cord injury from the impact with the spinal cord, is dissipated within the spinal canal and does not result in persistent spinal cord compression. The spinal injury related to these types of disk extrusions results more from spinal cord contusion than displacement of nucleus pulposus into the spinal cord parenchyma. In these dogs, in addition to the focal spinal cord edema and injury evident on MR studies, the associated nucleus pulposus of the intervertebral disk space may be distorted and irregular compared to adjacent or normal disk spaces.

Clinical Clues to Fibrocartilaginous Emboli

- Appropriate clinical signs are present.
- Survey spinal radiographs are normal.
- Myelography, CT, or MR may show intramedullary spinal disease.
- CSF may contain alteration consistent with inflammation, hemorrhage, or spinal injury.

Spina Cord Hemorrhage or Hematoma

Spinal cord hemorrhage or hematoma may result in clinical signs of spinal cord dysfunction (Applewhite et al. 1999). Hemorrhage can occur at any level of the spinal cord. In most instances, extradural hematoma occurs from trauma, intervertebral disk extrusion, or underlying coagulopathies, platelet dysfunction, or vasculopathies. Extradural hematomas often appear as compressive spinal abnormalities. Intramedullary hematomas have also been reported.

Hemorrhagic CNS complications should be suspected in any animal with acute neurologic signs and associated signs of either thrombocytopenia or coagulopathy. In some instances, the nervous system signs will occur prior to any obvious systemic signs of a bleeding disorder. A thorough examination of the body for petechia is important, including the mucous membranes (especially of the penis, prepuce, and vulva) and the retina. Pallor, low-grade heart

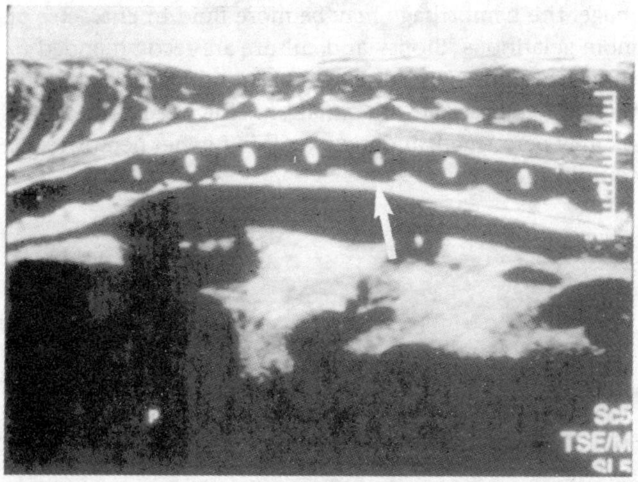

Fig. 11.52. Sagittal, T2-weighted magnetic resonance view of the thoracolumbar spine of a dog with a traumatic intervertebral disk extrusion (*arrow*).

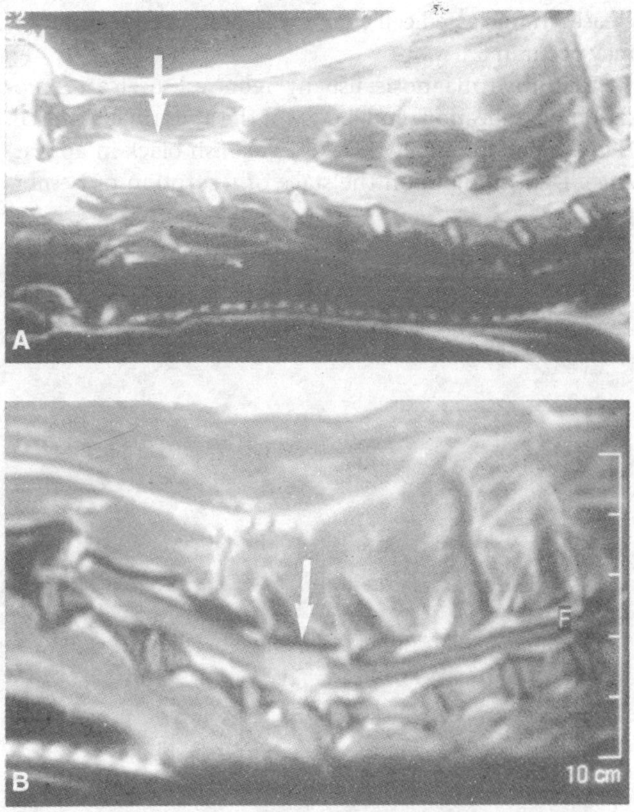

Fig. 11.53. (A) Sagittal, T2-weighted magnetic resonance view of the cervical spine of a dog with a spinal hemorrhage (*arrow*). (B) Sagittal, T1-weighted magnetic resonance view of the cervical spine of a dog with a focal spinal hematoma (*arrow*).

murmurs, weakness, and tachycardia are hallmark signs of coagulopathies with larger amounts of bleeding into body cavities. Thoracic auscultation for pleural fluid and abdominal palpation for hemoperitoneum is important. Radiographs and ultrasound may help when the physical examination is unrewarding but large amounts of internal bleeding are suspected. Remember that large amounts of blood can be lost through the gastrointestinal tract, and examination of the stool for hematochezia or melena is important.

Complete blood cell count, with special attention to red cell numbers and platelet counts, is important especially for the diagnosis of anemia and thrombocytopenia. Specific coagulation testing (bleeding time, PT, PTT, FDPs) are also commonly evaluated. Biochemical evidence of a predisposition to hypercoagulability such as proteinuria should be documented.

With most vascular diseases of the spinal cord survey spinal radiographs are normal. Myelography may reveal evidence of extradural or intramedullary abnormalities that distort the subarachnoid space. With extradural compression, the subarachnoid columns may be distorted inward toward the center of the spinal canal with myelographic evaluation. With intramedullary hematoma, the spinal cord appears focally enlarged.

Clarification of the cause of the clinical signs often requires advanced spinal imaging such as MR imaging (fig. 11.53). Computed tomography may aid in delineation of the compressive abnormality. With intraparenchymal hemorrhage, acute hemorrhage usually appears hyperdense within an hour as the clot retracts. This hyperdensity lasts a few days and then fades to isodensity and eventually hypodensity. On MR, hemorrhage less than 12 to 24 hours old may not be able to be differentiated from vasogenic edema. In the circulating blood, hemoglobin fluctuates between the oxyhemoglobin state and the deoxyhemoglobin state. The heme iron in both oxyhemoglobin and deoxyhemoglobin form is in the ferrous Fe^{2+} state. When hemoglobin is removed from the high-oxygen environment of the circulation, the heme iron undergoes oxidative denaturation to the ferric state (Fe^{3+}) forming methemoglobin. Continued oxidative denaturation forms ferric hemichromes (hemosiderin). As red blood cells break down, the various forms of hemoglobin have changing paramagnetic properties influencing the appearance of the clot on the various images (T1- and T2-weighted). Besides the form of hemoglobin present, the signal intensities of a blood clot may vary depending on the operating field strength, the type of signal the operator chooses, and the technique (T1- vs. T2-weighted). Hemorrhage may also vary in appearance depending on where the bleed occurred, for example in the subdural vs. intraparenchymal vs. subarachnoid regions.

Cerebrospinal fluid analysis may reveal red blood cells with subarachnoid hemorrhage. Xanthochromia and erythrophagocytosis are evidence of prior hemorrhage. As blood in the subarachnoid space may create an associated inflammatory response, CSF may contain increases in nucleated cells and protein concentrations. Neutrophils are often present in combination with subarachnoid hemorrhage. If an extradural hemorrhage or hematoma occurs and results in spinal cord compression, nonspecific increases in nucleated cell counts and protein concentration may occur in CSF.

Definitive diagnosis usually requires surgical exploration, visualization, and biopsy of the abnormal material. Hematomas are usually black or greenish black in appearance. Depending upon the stage of resorption of hemorrhage, the hemorrhage may be more fluid in character or more gelatinous. Biopsy and culture are recommended to eliminate underlying diseases that result in hemorrhage, such as neoplasia or inflammation. Fine needle aspiration is rarely performed, and may result in further hemorrhagic complications.

12 Diagnosis of Important and Common Diseases Involving the Peripheral Nervous System, Neuromuscular Junction, and Muscles of Dogs and Cats

The lower motor neuron (LMN) includes structures of the peripheral nerve, neuromuscular junction, and muscle. As with central nervous system diseases, the diagnosis of LMN diseases is often suspected based on breed associations and clinical features. Confirmation of diagnosis, however, usually still requires supportive evidence from diagnostic tests. With some diseases involving LMN structures reported historically, the definitive diagnosis has been made at necropsy without antemortem diagnostic testing performed. In other instances, the disease process has only been reported in a few individual animals and diagnostic testing results are inconsistently performed. Specific diagnostic testing results are, therefore, unavailable for comparison to those found in similarly affected animals in the current era. The available antemortem diagnostic testing information regarding disease of the LMN will be further discussed in this chapter. Pathologic alterations are described elsewhere (Summer et al. 1995).

In general, there are relatively few diagnostic tests that yield useful information regarding the integrity of the LMN structures. Many of these diagnostic tests are included in the diagnostic plan when evaluating animals with disease of the LMN.

Routine laboratory evaluations such as CBC and serum biochemical evaluations provide information regarding general health and organ function, but rarely yield information regarding the anatomical or functional integrity of LMN structures. Serum *creatine kinase (CK)* may be elevated by diseases causing muscle membrane damage. *Antiacetylcholine receptor antibodies* may be found in serum of animals with acquired myasthenia gravis (Shelton 1998). Diseases involving the *peripheral nerve* or *muscle* are often evaluated with *electromyography studies* (EMG, nerve conduction velocity). Other electrical studies such as the assessment of late potentials (F waves, H waves) are used to assess the integrity of the more proximal peripheral nerve and nerve roots (Sims 1981; Steiss 1984; Knecht 1985). Still other special electrical testing such as repetitive stimulation (Malik et al. 1989) and single fiber EMG (Hopkins et al. 1993) may be necessary when neuromuscular disease, and specifically myasthenia gravis, is suspected. Many electrodiagnostic evaluations have characteristic, but not pathognomonic, diagnostic features that aid in the determination of LMN disease. Cerebrospinal fluid analysis is usually normal in LMN disease, except in some instances where both the peripheral and central nervous system (CNS) structures are involved. In other situations such as polyradiculoneuritis where the proximal nerve roots in the subarachnoid space are involved with the disease process, CSF may be abnormal. *Muscle* and *nerve biopsy* provides objective morphological data as to the anatomical alterations in these structures (Braund 1991; Summers 1995). Specific disease etiologies, however, may not be determinable as end-stage nerve and muscle disease from a variety of diseases may appear similar pathologically. In other instances, biopsy of these structures is pathognomonic of a specific disease process. Importantly, biopsies of nerve and muscle should be evaluated by a pathologist experienced in LMN disease assessment (Braund et al. 1991). Studies, such as electron microscopy, of nerve samples are necessary to clarify pathological features.

DIAGNOSIS OF DISEASES OF THE LMN

Degenerative Neuropathies

There are numerous diseases that may be associated with primary degeneration of the peripheral nervous structures (see bibliography under Degenerative Neuropathies; Degenerative Myopathies). Degenerative peripheral neuropathies occur in a variety of age groups (both young and old) and are usually progressive diseases. Primary peripheral nerve degenerative processes which occur without apparent cause are sometimes classified as idiopathic neuropathies and are described under this section heading.

The presumptive diagnosis of primary degenerative neuropathies is based on a combination of the appropriate breed associations and clinical signs (see appendix 2 and chapter 7 for breed associations and clinical descriptions of disease processes, respectively). If denervation (loss of nerve influence over the muscle) is present, electromyographic studies may be abnormal. Spontaneous activity including fibrillation potentials and positive sharp waves may be found in diseases that involve or damage the axon or muscle-nerve interaction (fig. 12.1). Decreases in nerve conduction velocities may be found with diseases involving peripheral nerve myelin. Biopsy of peripheral nerve or muscle may confirm morphologic abnormalities in these tissues (fig. 12.2) (Braund et al. 1991). Pathognomonic features within nerve biopsy abnormalities may occasionally be apparent that allow for a specific or etiologic diagnosis. For example, with hypertrophic neuropathy of Tibetan mastiffs, a disorder of myelin is characterized by repeated demyelination and remyelination. Nerves from affected animals have a characteristic layering ("onion-bulb" formation) appearance of peripheral nerve samples. With many primary degenerative diseases, however, there are nonspecific pathologic alterations in affected nerves.

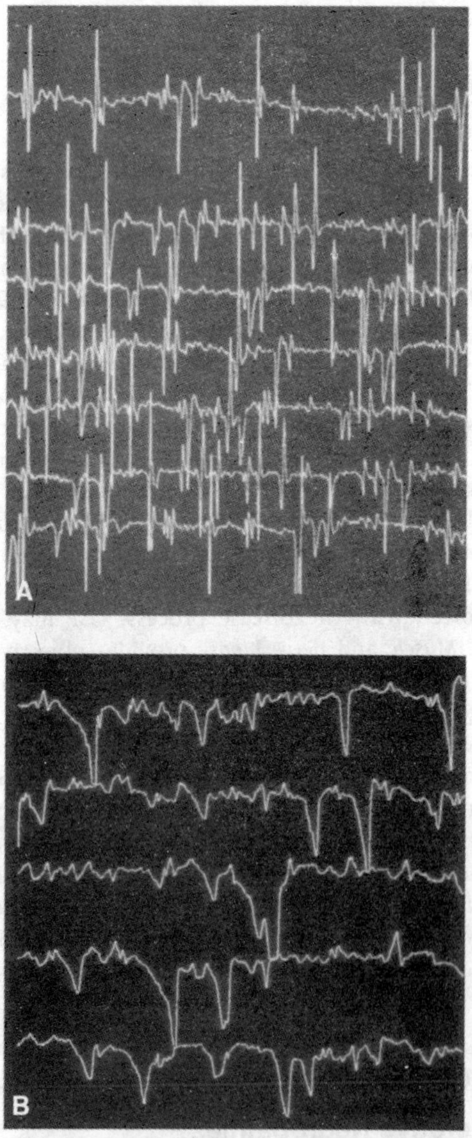

Fig. 12.1. Electromyographic abnormalities showing predominately (A) fibrillation potentials and (B) positive sharp waves.

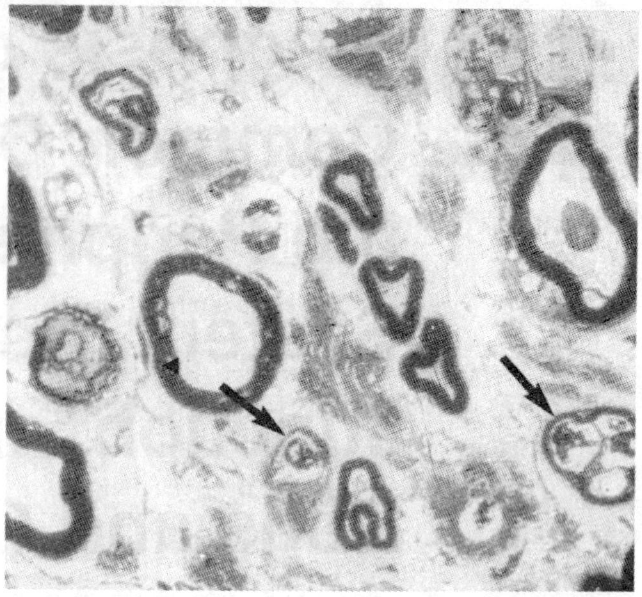

Fig. 12.2. Nerve biopsy from a dog showing axonal abnormalities (*arrows*).

Degenerative motorneuronopathies result from degeneration of neuronal cell bodies, which are located primarily in the central nervous system. Presumptive diagnosis is made based on the combination of appropriate breed associations and clinical signs (see chapter 7 and appendix 2). Degeneration of motor neuron cell bodies can result in denervation of limb and trunk muscles. Mild to moderate fibrillation potentials, consistent with denervation, can be found in the appendicular (limb) and paraspinal muscles with electromyography. Biopsy of peripheral nerves may show secondary alterations in axons and myelin. Muscle biopsy may show alterations consistent with denervation. Definitive diagnosis is usually confirmed definitively by necropsy examination of CNS tissues. Histologic lesions are most severe in the ventral spinal grey matter and consist of neuronal cell loss and gliosis.

Degenerative myopathies are presumptively diagnosed based on clinical signs and breed associations (see also chapter 7 and appendix 2). In some diseases, such as X-linked muscular dystrophy of golden retrievers and other breeds, serum CK may be elevated indicating underlying muscle disease. In these dogs, CK tends to increase early in life, with levels plateauing after 6 to 8 weeks. Electromyographic abnormalities with spontaneous muscle electrical activity (such as complex repetitive discharges) may be found with EMG evaluations. Biopsy of muscle and specialized microscopic evaluation may help to confirm the diagnosis. Abnormalities found with muscle biopsy include fiber hypertrophy, fiber splitting, myonecrosis, calcium deposition, internalized nuclei, and occasional fiber-type grouping.

In other primary myopathies, such as a hereditary myopathy of Devon rex cats and Labrador myopathy, serum CK levels are normal. Occasional fibrillation potentials and positive sharp waves are found with electromyographic examination in affected muscle groups. Muscle biopsies show variability in muscle fiber size, internal nuclei, myofiber necrosis, regeneration, and fibrosis. With nemaline rod myopathy, nemaline rods are a characteristic feature within muscle biopsies (see Summers et al. 1995).

Sudden death may occur in association with anesthesia in some myopathic conditions such as myotonia and muscular dystrophy, possibly due to spasm and contraction of the laryngeal muscles. Caution should be exercised when anesthetizing these animals for diagnostic testing procedures.

Metabolic Neuropathies and Myopathies

Metabolic Neuropathies. *Diabetic neuropathy* commonly affects cats, with clinical signs more obvious in the sciatic (tibial) nerve. Many diabetic cats are affected prior to initiation of treatment (untreated diabetes mellitus) or if they have poorly controlled (insulin resistant) diabetes mellitus. Many affected cats have a classic plantigrade stance in the pelvic limbs, suggesting sciatic (tibial) nerve dysfunction and tarsal extensor muscle weakness. This is the classic "dropped hock" appearance. This clinical feature is not pathognomonic, however, for diabetic neuropathy as other neuropathies and myopathic (tendon) processes may result in a similar clinical appearance. Clinical signs of polyuria, polydipsia, and weight loss, together with hyperglycemia (usually blood glucose is >250 to 300 mg/dl) and glucosuria found on serum biochemical analysis and urinalysis, respectively, are usually diagnostic for diabetes mellitus.

Additional diagnostic testing is needed to clarify clinical features of an associated peripheral neuropathy. Electromyographic abnormalities supporting a diagnosis of diabetic neuropathy include evidence of denervation (fibrillation potentials and positive sharp waves) and decreases in nerve conduction velocities. Nerve biopsies may show axonal degeneration and/or demyelination. These changes, however, are not specific for diabetic neuropathy as they may be found with other peripheral neuropathies.

Hypoglycemia can occur secondary to endocrine disorders such as hypoadrenocorticism, insulin overdose, lack of glucose production with liver failure, in association with some extrapancreatic neoplasia, and with insulinoma. In addition to the CNS signs, a *peripheral neuropathy* has been recognized in dogs with insulinoma fairly frequently. Diagnosis of hypoglycemia is based upon finding persistent hypoglycemia (blood glucose <60 mg/dl) on serum biochemical analysis in association with the appropriate clinical signs. Serum insulin concentration measured concurrently with serum glucose concentrations will help in determining the presence of an insulin-secreting tumor. An inappropriately elevated serum insulin concentration occurring in the face of hypoglycemia is often found in association with insulin-secreting tumors. Conversely, nonpancreatic tumors producing hypoglycemia are associated with concurrently low serum insulin concentrations. Abdominal ultrasound may be helpful when assessing the pancreas, liver, and lymph nodes for presence of tumor.

Electromyographic abnormalities supporting a diagnosis of neuropathy in instances of insulinoma include evidence of denervation (fibrillation potentials and positive sharp waves) and possibly decreases in nerve conduction velocities. Nerve biopsies usually show primarily axonal degeneration with secondary demyelination.

Hypothyroid neuropathy may involve the facial and limb muscles. Cranial nerve signs appear in some dogs. Head tilts are common. Other signs include facial paralysis, ventrolateral strabismus, nystagmus, hemiparesis, circling, and decreased corneal or facial sensation. The diagnosis is supported by decreases in certain thyroid hormone studies. Occasionally, EMG studies will show evidence of spontaneous muscle activity, however, the significance of these abnormalities is uncertain.

Hyperchylomicronemia is seen in cats due to a reduction in lipoprotein lipase activity (Jones et al. 1986). Clinical signs occur around 8 months of age. Xanthomata (lipid granulomas) may compress peripheral nerves. Clinical abnormalities include Horner's syndrome, facial paralysis, tibial nerve paralysis, femoral nerve paralysis, trigeminal nerve abnormalities, radial nerve (inability to extend digits) abnormalities, and recurrent laryngeal disease. A presumptive diagnosis is made when the appropriate clinical signs are present in combination with increases in serum lipid concentration. Electrodiagnostic and biopsy results are infrequently reported.

In cats with *hyperoxaluria (L-glyceric aciduria)* neuropathy, urine contains increased oxalate and L-glycerate levels (McKerrell et al. 1989). Positive sharp waves, milder fibrillation potentials, and occasional bizarre high-frequency discharges were found with electromyographic examination. Pathologically, neurons in the ventral grey matter of the spinal cord and their proximal axons were most affected. Swollen axons were present in the ventral nerve roots and dorsal root ganglion cells.

Metabolic Myopathies. *Hypokalemia myopathy* has been described in cats as a cause of muscle weakness (Dow et al. 1987). Affected cats may have increased serum CK and often have decreased serum potassium. *Burmese cats* have an inherited *hypokalemic myopathy* producing signs of periodic muscle weakness, with signs first evident before 12 months of age, usually between 4 and 12 weeks (Jones 2000). Hypokalemia may be exacerbated after fluid administration because of volume dilution and increased urinary potassium loss.

Diagnosis of hypokalemic myopathy is suggested by establishing decreased serum potassium concentrations (usually <3.5 mmol/L) in association with clinical signs. The severity of signs is variable in cats when serum potassium is 2.5–3.5 mmol/L. Below 2.5 mmol/L, and especially below 2.0 mmol/L, signs are life threatening, with death occurring from respiratory muscle failure. Serum CK may be elevated reflecting underlying muscle cell membrane damage. Electrodiagnostic evaluation abnormalities reported include increased insertional activity, fibrillation potentials and positive sharp waves, and occasionally bizarre high-frequency discharges. Muscle biopsies often have minimal change present however mild myonecrosis may be found.

Hyperkalemia and *hypernatremia* are possible, but less commonly recognized causes of myopathy in dogs and cats. Diagnosis is supported by the appropriate clinical signs in the presence of increases in serum potassium and sodium, respectively, when serum electrolyte concentrations are evaluated. In animals with hypernatremic myopathy, serum CK may be increased. Electrodiagnostic and muscle biopsy alterations are not well established for these metabolic myopathic processes.

Decreases in calcium lower the threshold for neuronal and muscle depolarization. The diagnosis of hypocalcemia is confirmed by finding decreased (usually less than 6 mg/dl) serum calcium on serum biochemical analysis.

Hyperadrenocortical myopathy most commonly occurs in dogs. Affected dogs often have a stiff, stilted gait. In some instances, there are increases in muscle mass and the muscles of the body will be well defined similar to the muscle appearance of myotonia. This myopathy is most commonly found in dogs with chronic, untreated hyperadrenocorticism. This disease may reflect a positive affect on muscle growth from a steroid (possibly with more anabolic effects) secreted in association with this disease.

Electromyographic studies may show myotonic or pseudomyotonic (complex repetitive discharges) potentials. Hyperadrenocortical myopathy is associated microscopically with mild degeneration changes associated with fiber size variation, presence of subsarcolemmal mass, focal necrosis, and splitting, fiber atrophy especially of the type II fibers.

Cats with *hyperthyroidism* may have a variety of associated clinical signs including LMN or muscle abnormalities. Diagnosis is readily established by demonstrating elevated serum total thyroxine (T_4) concentrations or evidence of the present excessive thyroid hormone production or secretion. When total T_4 concentration is at the high end of normal but signs are consistent with hyperthyroidism, measurement of free T_4 or a T_3 suppression test may help to confirm the diagnosis. In some cats, electromyography shows evidence of denervation, however, these studies are infrequently reported.

Hypothyroid myopathy is usually subclinical in dogs. The diagnosis is supported by decreases in certain thyroid hormone studies.

Mitochondrial myopathy has been reported in dogs such as Clumber and Sussex spaniels and Old English sheepdogs (Breitschwerdt et al. 1992; Shelton 1995; Shelton et al. 1998). Affected animals usually have elevated levels of serum lactate and pyruvate, which are greatly increased with muscle activity. More definitive diagnosis is obtained with muscle biopsy, which contains characteristic abnormalities (such as ragged red fibers) pathognomonic for this disease process.

Neoplastic Neuropathies and Myopathies

Lymphoma commonly occurs extradurally in cats and can involve nerve roots (see bibliography under Neoplasia). Rarely, only peripheral nerve involvement is seen (Presthus et al. 1986). Cranial nerves (V, VII) may be involved with hematogenous neoplasia (leukemias) due to direct involvement with the tumor cells (Carpenter et al. 1987). Hematological neoplasia such as leukemia may be present on CBC or bone marrow assessments. In cats, assessment of FeLV status may provide clues to a possible association between this virus infection and an underlying lymphoid neoplastic disease. The majority of cats with spinal lymphoma are FeLV positive. Cytologic evaluation of CSF may reveal the presence of neoplastic cells. In some instances, nonspecific increases in CSF protein concentration and nucleated cell counts may occur in association with neoplastic disease. With MR imaging, enlargement and enhancement of cranial or peripheral nerves may be evident in instances of peripheral nerve neoplasia. Biopsy of the affected nerve may be necessary for definitive diagnosis if a cytologic diagnosis cannot be rendered in another way (i.e., on CSF cytologic evaluations).

Nerve sheath tumors (Schwannoma, neurofibroma, neurofibrosarcoma) commonly involve the peripheral nerves of the thoracic limb in older dogs and occasionally, cats. Affected dogs often present for a lameness that, in some instances, may have been present for a year or more prior to presentation. Often dogs are initially diagnosed with arthritis or another orthopedic disease. Clinical clues include atrophy of selected thoracic limb muscles and pain upon local palpation of the nerve. In some instances, a discrete mass can be palpated in the nerve. Animals that are extremely painful may require general anesthesia for adequate palpation.

If the tumor damages the nerve, EMG may reveal denervation in muscles innervated by the affected nerves. If a peripheral nerve near the intervertebral foramen is involved, enlargement of the foramen may be found with survey radiographic evaluation of the spine (see figure 11.39 A). Computed tomography scanning or MR imaging may show enlargements of peripheral nerve elements and associated muscle atrophy (figs. 12.3, 12.4). Biopsy of the affected nerve is necessary for definitive diagnosis.

Nutritional Myopathies

Nutritional myopathies are infrequently reported in dogs and cats (deLahunta 1983). Selenium deficiency has been suspected in some of these disorders. Dogs may have stiff

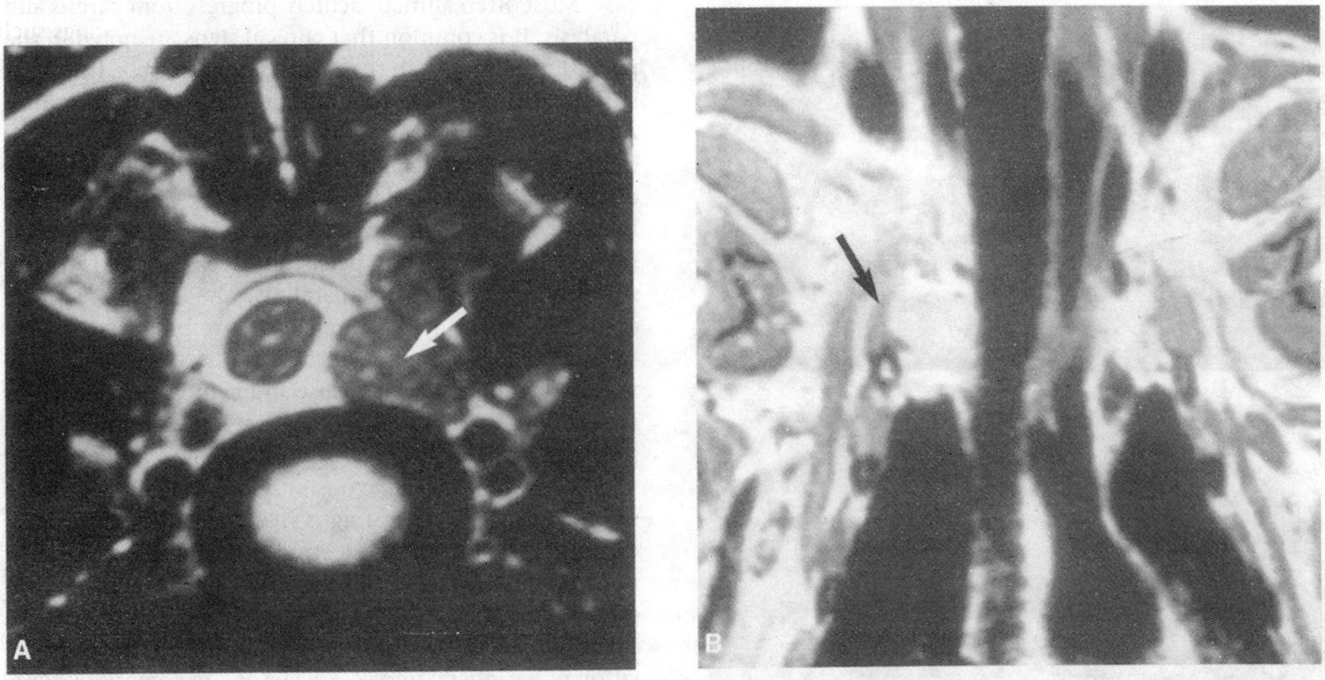

Fig. 12.3. (A) Transverse, T2-weighted MR image from a dog showing a tumor of the peripheral nerve (*arrow*). (B) Dorsal, T1-weighted MR image following intravenous contrast administration showing a peripheral nerve sheath tumor in the brachial plexus area (*arrow*).

movements of the limbs and take short steps. Exercise may exacerbate muscle weakness. Serum CK may be elevated, and electromyography may show evidence of myotonic potentials. Definitive diagnostic testing is infrequently reported.

Infectious and Inflammatory Neuropathies and Myopathies

Infectious Neuritis. *Toxoplasma gondii* and *Neospora caninum* are protozoal organisms that can affect any area of the nervous system resulting in encephalitis, myelitis, peripheral neuropathy or myositis (see bibliography under Protozoal Neuritis). Clinical signs may include peripheral nerve or muscle dysfunction. Diagnosis is presumptively made based upon the presence of IgM or increasing IgG serum or CSF titers indicative of an antibody response to the presence of the organism (toxoplasmosis). Serum antibody titers to *Neospora caninum* may also be determined.

Electromyographic studies may show nonspecific abnormalities associated with denervation in affected muscles and help in localization of the abnormalities in muscle or associated peripheral nerves. If these organisms involve the proximal nerve roots or the spinal cord structures, evidence of inflammation with increases in nucleated cells (primarily mononuclear cells) and protein concentrations may be found with CSF evaluations. Titers for these organisms can also be performed on CSF samples.

Ideally, visualization of the protozoan organism is found in biopsy specimens (both organisms) of either peripheral nerve or, more commonly, muscle. Clinical distinction between the two organisms is not always possible, but increased awareness of the latter protozoal organism as a disease entity and special staining and EM characteristics have increased the identification of this disease process.

Noninfectious Neuritis. A number of animals have been reported with suspected acute polyneuritis without evidence of a specific infectious cause. Diagnostic testing may reveal alterations in electrodiagnostic studies similar to those found with other peripheral neuropathies (i.e., alterations in spontaneous muscle activity—fibrillation potentials and positive sharp waves—or in nerve conduction velocities). Nerve biopsies can contain a variety of pathologic alterations including axonal degeneration, fragmentation, and loss of axons, as well as demyelination and accumulation of macrophages. In chronic, relapsing polyneuropathy of cats, for example, electrodiagnostic evaluation showed fibrillation potentials and positive sharp waves in the limb and paraspinal muscles as well as decreased nerve conduction velocities. Demyelination and remyelination were present in nerve biopsies. In one cat with the acute, severe polyneuritis, pathologically there was extensive destruction of myelin associated with macrophages.

Coonhound paralysis or *polyradiculoneuritis* is a disease of dogs similar to Guillain-Barré disease in human beings. A suspected antigen (possibly in raccoon saliva in the instance of coonhound paralysis) results in an immunologic-mediated inflammation directed primarily toward the nerve root and proximal nerves of the peripheral nervous system (see chapter 7). Other antigens may also initiate this disease, as raccoon exposure in not found in all animals. Clinical signs are of an acutely evolving, diffuse LMN dis-

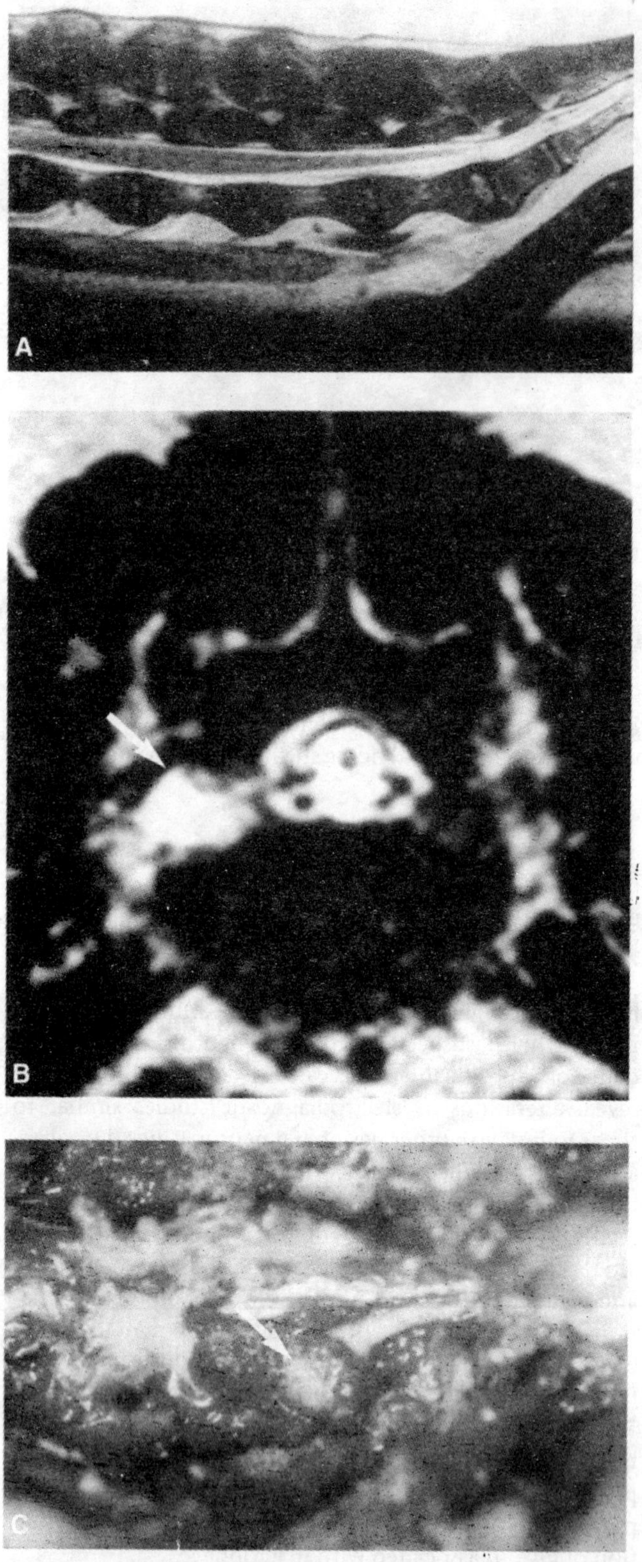

Fig. 12.4. (A) Sagittal and (B) transverse, T2-weighted MR image from a dog with a pelvic limb lameness showing a tumor of the peripheral nerve (*arrow*). The sagittal view is normal, however, the transverse view shows the tumor. (C) Appearance of the tumor at surgery (*arrow*). Histologic diagnosis was a neurofibroma.

ease. Most often animals acutely progress from paresis and paralysis. It is common that clinical signs are noted in the pelvic limbs initially. If the animals can still walk, the gait is stiff and stilted due to resultant decreases in step distance. Animals seem hyperesthetic to minimal pressure such as minimal pressure toe pinching as a clinical hallmark of this disease. Cranial nerve functions usually remain normal, however some dogs may have decreases in their palpebral reflex. Clinical signs can persist for weeks. Death is the result of respiratory muscle paralysis. Abdominal breathing and a "whispering" bark are clues to respiratory compromise. Muscle atrophy may occur and become severe. This may be a combination of disuse and neurogenic atrophy as some affected animals have evidence of denervation electrophysiologically.

The presumptive diagnosis of polyradiculoneuritis is supported by the clinical signs (see discussion of polyradiculoneuritis, chapter 7). Electrodiagnostic testing is often normal early (hours to first few days) in the course of the disease. In some instances, alterations occur in the electrical potentials evoked in muscle following electrical stimulation of peripheral nerves. F-wave or late potential recordings often are abnormal suggesting proximal nerve disease. As inflammation is present proximally in the nerves within the subarachnoid space, CSF collected in the lumbar area often contains increases in protein concentration and, rarely, nucleated cells. Nerve and muscle biopsies are usually normal initially. If muscles and nerves are biopsied more chronically, some evidence of muscle denervation and axonal alterations may be found.

Brachial plexus neuritis is suspected to be an immune-mediated neuritis that preferentially affects the thoracic limbs. Diagnosis is usually based on appropriate clinical signs. Cerebrospinal fluid collected in the lumbar area is usually normal, but may contain increases in protein concentration and/or nucleated cells if the proximal nerve roots are involved. Electrodiagnostic studies are infrequently reported but may show evidence of spontaneous muscle activity suggestive of denervation. Biopsy of an affected nerve may show inflammatory alterations in peripheral nerve.

Cauda equina polyradiculoneuritis has been rarely described in dogs. Affected animals present for signs of lumbosacral nerve dysfunction including bladder and bowel abnormalities, pain, and LMN paresis. Cerebrospinal fluid collection from the lumbar region may reveal increases in nucleated cell counts (usually lymphocytes or mononuclear cells) and/or protein concentration. Electrodiagnostic studies are uncommonly reported. Histologically, there is interstitial and periventricular infiltration of mononuclear cells (lymphocytes, plasma cells, and macrophages).

Infectious Myositis. Infectious myositis is uncommon in animals. Organisms such as protozoa including *Toxoplasma gondii* and *Neospora caninum* are the most common etiologies associated with infectious myositis. Occasionally, other infectious myopathies, such as from viral infections, may result in muscle inflammation. A subclinical myopathy has been shown to occur in experimentally infected FIV cats. Primary bacterial and fungal myositis is extremely rare in small animals. Cats with leptospirosis surprisingly will often present with muscle pain as a primary clinical problem. Infectious myositis has also been associated with *Leptospira australis* in a 10-year-old greyhound. *Trichinella* has also resulted in muscle inflammation in a dog. In some instances, muscle damage and associated inflammation may result from excessive use (exercise) or muscle trauma.

Serum CK may be elevated in these diseases. Similarly, serum titers to these infectious etiologies may provide clinical clues to the presence of these organisms. Fecal examination may sometimes uncover parasitic organisms that may migrate through muscle. Electrodiagnostic evaluations may show alterations in muscle function such as spontaneous activity. Biopsy of affected muscle may sometimes disclose a specific infectious organism.

Noninfectious Myositis. Clinical signs of *polymyositis* include muscle pain, muscle atrophy, and generalized muscle weakness. In cats, neck ventroflexion is common. Some animals have elevated serum CK levels suggestive of muscle disease. Megaesophagus may occur with polymyositis and be evident on thoracic radiographic evaluation. Abnormal spontaneous muscle electrical activity consistent with myocyte inflammation, and abnormal membrane electrical activity such as fibrillation potentials, positive sharp waves, and complex repetitive discharges may be present on electromyography. Muscle biopsies may show inflammatory changes including perivascular and pericapillary lymphocytic infiltration and myofiber necrosis, phagocytosis, and regeneration of muscle fibers.

Myositis may also affect only selected muscle groups or regions of the body. Muscle inflammation primarily of the *masticatory muscles (masticatory myositis)* is common. This disease is thought to result as an immune-mediated destruction of the type-2 M fibers found selectively in these muscles (Gilmour et al. 1992). Clinical signs can occur acutely with animals presenting for enlarged, painful temporalis and masseter muscles. Animals may be reluctant or unable to open the mandible. Muscle groups are most commonly bilaterally affected. As the disease progresses, the muscles of the head may become atrophic and fibrotic with increasing definition of the bony landmark of the skull. Muscle fibrosis at this stage also often results in an inability to open the jaw. Similar clinical findings may be present in dogs with trauma to the head and jaw.

Serum CK may be elevated, but this finding is inconsistent and may not occur. Historically, some affected dogs had a peripheral eosinophilia, but this is also inconsistent. A serum test detecting antibodies to the type-2 M muscle fibers is available. Electromyographic studies of the muscles of mastication may show spontaneous electrical potentials. Inflammatory abnormalities can be found on muscle biopsy of affected muscles.

Extraocular polymyositis has been reported primarily in young dogs between 6 and 18 months of age. Golden retrievers have been the most common breed affected, however, other breeds including Doberman pinschers, German shepherds, and mixed breeds may also have this problem. Bilateral exophthalmos is the most common clinical sign present, along with inability to move the globe through the various phases of gaze. If the extraocular muscle enlarges significantly, compression of the optic nerve may result, subsequently affecting vision and causing blindness. Evidence of spontaneous muscle activity may be present on EMG evaluations of the extraocular muscles. Similarly, spontaneous EMG activity may be found in other muscle groups affected with myopathic processes (laryngeal muscles).

Myositis ossificans is a disease reported primarily in cats. Muscle alterations include fibrosis, muscle necrosis, dystrophic mineralization, and ossification. Clinically affected animals may show weakness and swollen, painful muscles. Radiographic evaluation of affected body regions may disclose calcification of muscle regions.

Neuromuscular Junction Disease. *Myasthenia gravis* has two major clinical forms of the disease: a *congenital form* that is associated with congenital abnormalities, or a reduction in number, of acetylcholine receptors, and an *acquired form* that is associated with antibodies being produced against the acetylcholine receptor (see discussion of myasthenia gravis, chapter 7). The clinical consequence of either of these forms is neuromuscular junction (NMJ) dysfunction and muscle weakness.

An edrophonium (Tensilon) or similar product response test may suggest the disease if a positive response (significant increase in muscle strength) is found following administration of the drug (fig. 12.5). Edrophonium is an anticholinesterase that potentiates acetylcholine (ACH) at the NMJ. This drug, when given intravenously (0.1 to 0.2 mg/kg for a dog or 0.25 to 0.5 mg/cat), can improve the clinical weakness seen with myasthenia gravis for a short period of time. Unfortunately, a positive clinical response to this drug is not pathognomonic for myasthenia as occasionally signs of other diseases of the LMN will be improved following edrophonium administration. In animals that have associated systemic illness, such as concurrent aspiration pneumonia from megaesophagus, a positive clinical response to this drug may be masked by overall debility.

Complications of edrophonium administration consist primarily of muscarinic receptor stimulation (similar to organophosphate toxicity) and exacerbation of clinical weakness. Edrophonium may cause increases in salivation, urination, and defecation. Some clinicians treat animals with atropine prior to edrophonium administration to prevent these side effects. The duration of clinical effects of edrophonium are usually short (minutes). If exacerbation of muscle weakness occurs with this drug, animals may be unable to breathe from associated respiratory muscle weakness. As animals could potentially stop breathing following administration of this drug, it is a good practice to have an

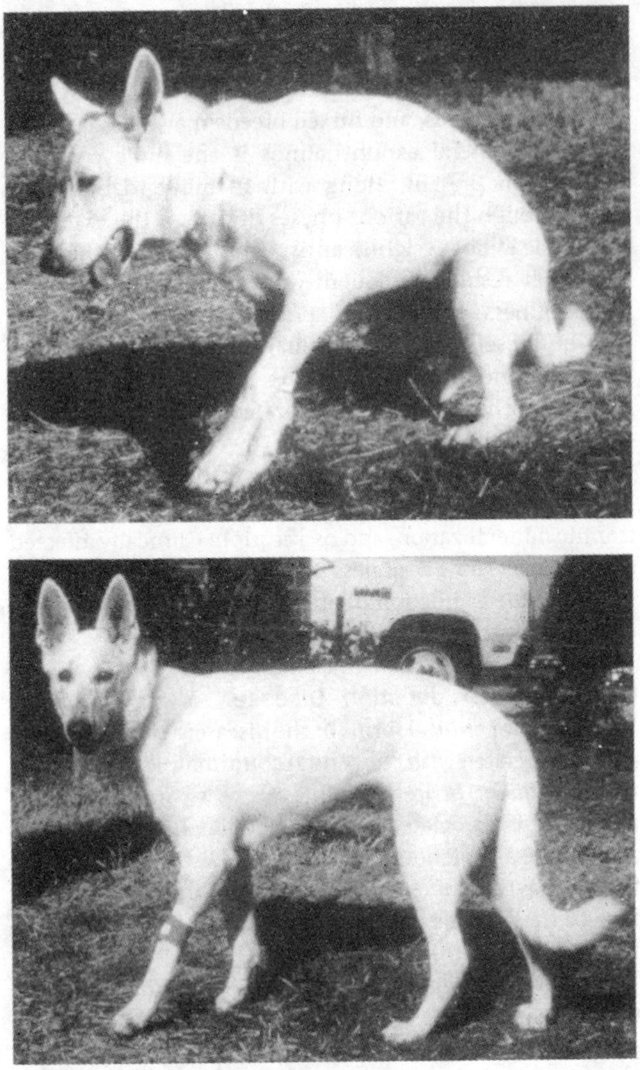

Fig. 12.5. (A) Dog with myasthenia gravis showing kyphotic posture and drooping of the facial muscles. (B) Normal appearance of the dog following the administration of edrophonium.

endotracheal tube and a self-inflating resuscitation (ambu) bag or similar means of acute ventilatory support readily available.

Thoracic radiographic studies may establish the presence of megaesophagus and aspiration pneumonia (figs. 12.6, 12.7). Routine electromyography and NCV studies will usually be normal in animals with myasthenia gravis. A decremental response of muscle activity may be seen during repeated stimulation of a peripheral nerve in some, but not all, cases of myasthenia gravis. Single fiber EMG is a relatively new technique that may be an aid to diagnosis of this disease in the future but requires special electrodiagnostic equipment and expertise for performance and interpretation (Hopkins et al. 1993). This electrodiagnostic technique is a more specific test of NMJ function.

Documentation of antibodies to the acetylcholine receptor in serum appears to be the most definitive diagnostic test for the acquired form of MG (antiacetylcholine re-

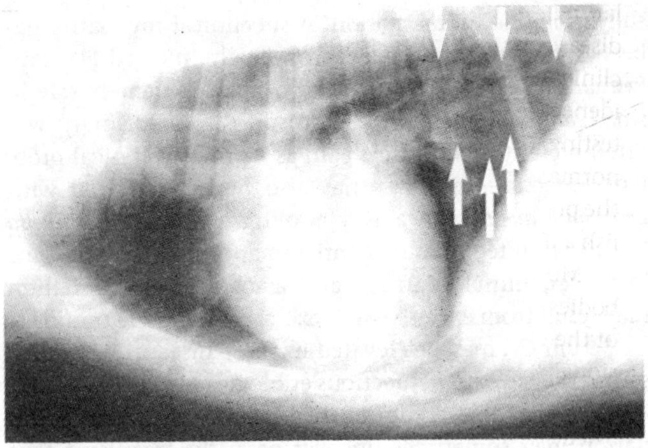

Fig. 12.6. Dog with a myasthenia gravis and megaesophagus (*arrows*).

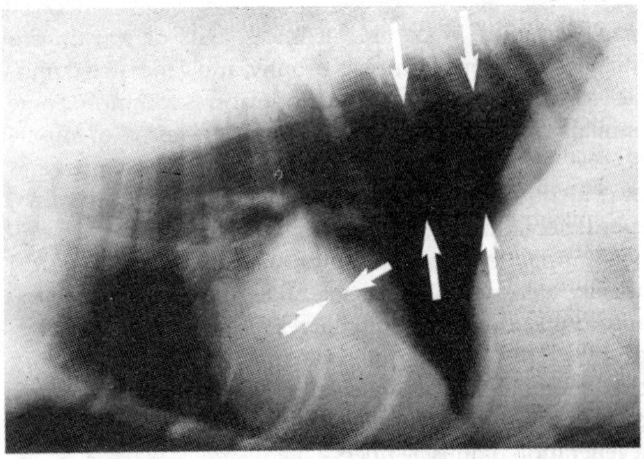

Fig. 12.7. Dog with megaesophagus (*large arrows*) and aspiration pneumonia. Note the air bronchogram (*small arrows*).

ceptor antibody testing). False negative results for this test are apparently rare with acquired MG. In congenital disease, however, these antibodies will not be present. Rarely, intercostal muscle biopsy with microscopic evaluation of the NMJ may be necessary for diagnosis.

Neuropathies and Myopathies without an Obvious Cause

The numerous neuropathies and myopathies of dogs and cats are still being recognized and clarified clinically (see bibliography under Neuropathies and Myopathies Without Known Cause). Many different clinical entities have been reported, however, the etiologic cause of these diseases is not always determined. The clinical features of many of these disease entities are discussed in the degenerative section of chapter 7. Examples include distal denervating disease, distal symmetrical polyneuropathy, Rottweiler distal sensorimotor polyneuropathy, hypomyelination of peripheral nervous system in Golden retrievers, Walker hound mononeuropathy, laryngeal paralysis, and Dalmatians with laryngeal-polyneuropathy complex. The diagnosis of these diseases is suspected based on the combination of breed and clinical signs (see chapter 7 and appendix 2). Supportive evidence of these diseases is provided with electrodiagnostic testing as well as nerve and muscle biopsy morphologic abnormalities. Oftentimes results of EMG and biopsy confirm the presence of a neuropathy or myopathy but do not establish a definitive etiologic diagnosis.

Motor neuronopathies are diseases that affect the cell bodies of the lower motor neuron leading to degeneration of the cell in the ventral horn of the spinal cord and, occasionally, the cranial nerve nuclei. Examples include diseases such as spinal muscular atrophy in Brittany spaniels, Swedish Lapland dogs, English pointers, German shepherds, and Rottweilers. A presumptive diagnosis is suggested with appropriate breed and clinical signs association. Electromyographic alterations consistent with denervation may be present in paraspinal or limb muscles. Peripheral nerve biopsies may show some evidence of secondary axonal loss. Definitive diagnosis is often made only at necropsy evaluation of the spinal cord.

Familial myoclonus (reflex myoclonus) of Labrador retrievers is a disease of marked, intermittent muscular hypertonicity that occurs in young dogs (usually around 3 weeks of age; Fox et al. 1984). Extensor muscle rigidity is usually initially episodic, but can progress to become more frequent. Muscle contractions are worsened by stimulation and handling. Other breeds are occasionally affected. The cause is unknown but it is suspected to be an inhibitory neurotransmitter abnormality of neurons in the spinal cord, possibly similar to spastic paresis of cattle. The presumptive diagnosis is made primarily on clinical features. Electrodiagnostic studies may be normal or disclose evidence of periodic excessive muscle activity. Muscle biopsy is often normal.

Dancing Doberman syndrome is a disease characterized by alternating pelvic limb flexion when the animal is standing (Chrisman 1990). Dobermans between 6 months and 7 years may be affected. Flexion of one or both pelvic limbs when standing is characteristic. This is usually associated with atrophy of pelvic limb muscles, especially the gastrocnemius. Abnormal spontaneous activity (fibrillation potentials and positive sharp waves) may be found on EMG evaluation of affected muscles. Microscopic evaluation of muscle biopsy may show atrophy and hypertrophy, internal nuclei, focal necrosis, endomysial-perimysial fibrosis, and fiber type grouping. Occasionally there are associated mild nerve alterations including demyelination and axonal necrosis.

Dysautonomia is an idiopathic autonomic nervous system disease seen sporadically and regionally in both cats and dogs (see bibliography under Dysautonomia). Clinical signs reflect autonomic system dysfunction. This disease is regional in the United States in dogs, with primary concentrations of disease in Kansas and Missouri (the Midwest). Dogs are often presented for vomiting and other gastrointestinal abnormalities. Other clinical signs include poor gastrointestinal motility, megacolon, dilated pupils, xerostomia, and keratoconjunctivitis sicca. Affected dogs may have a dilated anal sphincter. Dogs may also have LMN signs suggestive of a peripheral neuropathy affecting the limb muscles. A common environmental toxin or bacteria such as *Clostridium* is suspected.

In cats, dysautonomia has historically been primarily a disease entity in the United Kingdom and Europe, or found in cats imported from these regions. The prevalence has decreased markedly and it is now uncommon. Younger cats (<3 years) were more often affected. Clinical signs were often acute in onset over 48 hours with all cats showing depression and anorexia. Other signs reflect autonomic system dysfunction and included ocular signs such as fixed, dilated pupils without blindness, prolapsed third eyelids, and dry eyes (keratoconjunctivitis sicca). Gastrointestinal signs included regurgitation, megaesophagus, constipation and megacolon, loss of the anal reflexes, dry mouth (xerostomia), bradycardia (90–120 beats/minute), dysuria and/or distended bladder or incontinence with an easily expressive bladder, and generalized weakness.

Diagnosis is based primarily on clinical signs and evidence of autonomic dysfunction. Thoracic and abdominal radiographs and associated intraluminal contrast studies (barium swallow or GI series) may identify gastrointestinal motility abnormalities. The indirect-acting parasympathomimetic, physostigmine (0.02 mg/kg IV) produces no ocular response, but direct-acting pilocarpine (topically) results in immediate miosis, demonstrating postganglionic denervation hypersensitivity. Normal animals usually do not demonstrate these responses.

Neuropathies have been seen that only involve the *sensory nerves*. Breeds affected include the dachshund, boxer, border collie, English pointer, Siberian husky, Brittany spaniel, Welsh corgi, Doberman pinscher, whippet, Scottish terrier, golden retriever, Scotch collie, and other breed dogs. Clinical signs may include proprioceptive deficits, apparent ataxia, decreased or absent spinal reflexes, facial hypalgesia or paresthesia, megaesophagus, head tilt, loss of hearing and voice, anisocoria, dysphagia, a stiff gait, and self-mutilation. Dogs often have a characteristic paddling gait wherein the distal palmar and plantar aspects of the feet are flipped forward to impact the ground. Dogs may also sink on these limbs during impact. This may also be associated with a jerky movement from side to side that may be misidentified as ataxia.

Electromyographic assessments may be normal due to the predominant sensory nerve abnormalities. Sensory nerve conduction velocities may be abnormally slowed. Biopsy of sensory nerves may reveal pathologic changes involving axons or myelin.

Idiopathic Myopathies

Some of the important idiopathic myopathies of dogs and cats have previously been discussed under the degenerative myopathy section of this chapter (also see chapter 7 for clinical features). Diagnosis of these idiopathic myopathic processes may be supported by abnormalities of serum CK, electrodiagnostic testing, and muscle biopsy. Abnormalities of these diagnostic tests, however, are inconsistently present among the various myopathic diseases. Some of these diseases such as X-linked muscular dystrophy, Labrador retriever myopathy, nemaline rod myopathy, and mitochondrial myopathies have characteristic abnormalities on muscle biopsies. Other diseases such as idiopathic cramping syndromes are more functional abnormalities and rather show morphological abnormalities on histologic muscle assessments.

In golden retriever muscular dystrophy, serum CK is often (marked) elevated. Electrodiagnostic studies may show some spontaneous muscle activity (complex repetitive discharges). In Labrador retriever myopathy, serum CK is often normal. With Bouvier des Flandres myopathy, serum CK may be elevated and electrodiagnostic testing may show complex repetitive discharges in muscle. Exertional myopathy may be associated with myoglobinuria by 48 hours following exercise, however, the serum CK is variable.

Scotty cramp is characterized by paroxysms of muscular hypertonicity, usually precipitated by excitement or exercise. The disease is believed to be inherited as a recessive trait. The underlying mechanism for these episodes is thought to be the result of decreased central serotonin effects. During movement, initially there is abduction of the thoracic limbs. Arching of the back, pelvic limb stiffness, jumping into the air, falling, and curling into a ball may follow. Respirations may cease and facial muscles may be contracted. A similar syndrome is seen in Dalmatian and Norwich terriers. Diagnosis is presumptive based on clinical signs. Diagnostic testing is invariable normal.

Episodic falling of Cavalier King Charles is seen mostly in animals from the UK. Dogs are affected by 3 to 4 months of age. During exercise, dogs develop a bounding pelvic limb gait with stiff pelvic limbs, falling, and extensor rigidity of the limbs. The episodes are usually life-long in duration. Similar to Scotty cramp, diagnosis is based primarily on breed-associated clinical features as diagnostic tests are usually otherwise normal.

Myotonia occurs as a congenital problem in various dog breeds including the Chow Chow and cats. The excessive muscle contraction is thought to be due to an abnormal muscle cell membrane that supports persistent depolarization. Electromyography demonstrates the characteristic myotonic potentials, sounding similar to a motorcycle engine revving. In cats this same EMG activity may sound like bees buzzing. Muscle biopsies are often normal. In instances where myotonia is acquired due to herbicide exposure, the presence of the herbicide may be found in urine samples.

"*Cold tail*" may be the same as "limber tail" or "Limp tail," and has been described as a myopathy of the tail muscles. This syndrome is usually an acute onset of the flaccid tail in certain, primarily working breeds of dogs such as Labrador retrievers and pointers. Clinical diagnostic features include mild elevation of creatine kinase acutely, with evidence of EMG abnormalities in the coccygeal muscles several days after onset. Biopsy of the coccygeal muscles shows evidence of muscle fiber damage. Specific muscle groups, such as the intertransversarius ventralis caudalis muscles, were affected most severely.

Some animals will have problems from *self-mutilation* without apparent cause. Breeds affected are often described as "high strung" including Siamese, Burmese, Himalayan, and Abyssinian cats, and Doberman pinschers, German shepherds, Great Danes, Irish setters, and spitzs. Animals usually self-mutilate the tail, limbs, or flank. It is unknown if this is a behavior abnormally (obsessive compulsive disorder) or whether these animals are reacting to pain or other abnormal sensations. With the latter, peripheral neuropathies with paraesthesia have been suggested. Many of these dogs should be evaluated for a behavior component to their problem. Diagnostic testing in many of these animals reveals no obvious abnormalities.

Traumatic Neuropathies and Myopathies

Trauma can occur to a single nerve (misplaced injection into the sciatic nerve) or multiple nerves (brachial plexus avulsion) (see bibliography under Trauma; Brachial Plexus Trauma). The diagnosis is presumptive based on a history of a traumatic episode and the appropriate clinical signs. If the injury is acute, no electrodiagnostic abnormalities may be found. Denervation may be detectable as spontaneous muscle activity approximately 5 days following a peripheral nerve injury. In instances of brachial plexus avulsion, abnormalities suggestive of nerve rootlet trauma (edema, hemorrhage, nerve root enlargement) may be present on spinal MR imaging performed in the cervicothoracic intumescence region.

The severity of involvement clinically will determine prognosis. A neuropraxia (least severe injury) is an interruption in function and conduction in the nerve, usually associated with a lesion of the myelin without severe axonal involvement. Axonotmesis suggests separation and damage of axons, where neurotmesis (most severe injury) is complete severance of all structures of the nerve. The likelihood of regeneration is less with neurotmesis as compared to neuropraxia.

Toxic Neuropathies and Myopathies

Botulism is due to the exotoxin of *Clostridium botulinum*. Many toxin types have been described, however, type C toxin appears to cause the disease most readily in dogs (see bibliography under Botulism). This exotoxin blocks the presynaptic release of acetylcholine from the neuromuscular junction.

Presumptive diagnosis of botulism is based on characteristic clinical features. Diagnosis is supported by isolation of the toxin in serum or vomitus. Electromyography and NCV studies may show decreased amplitude of the compound muscle action potential, normal to decreased nerve conduction velocity, and occasionally fibrillation potentials or positive sharp waves consistent with denervation. Nerve and muscle biopsies are normal.

Tetanus is due to a neurotoxin (tetanospasmin) secreted by the organism *Clostridium tetani*. This toxin binds to interneurons and inhibits the release of inhibitory neurotransmitter (glycine) in inhibitory interneurons (Renshaw cells). The organism gains access to the body through a wound. Dogs and cat are inherently resistant to this disease, with cats being more resistant than dogs. Therefore, as the wound on a dog may be undetectable, the wound on a cat is usually obvious.

The diagnosis of tetanus is primarily based upon characteristic clinical signs. Electrocardiography may reveal disturbances of the cardiac rhythm (Panciera et al. 1988). Thoracic radiography may reveal hiatal hernia or megaesophagus associated with tetanus (Dieringer and Wolf 1991). If an abscess is suspected in a body cavity, ultrasound, CT, or MR imaging may be useful in establishing the location of the infection. Anaerobic culturing of a wound may reveal the organism. Biopsy and culture at the time of wound debridement of infected tissue may reveal inflammation or the organism. A serum test for antibodies has occasionally been useful, but is not readily available (Baker et al. 1988).

Tick paralysis is due to infestation with ticks. In North America, *Dermacentor andersoni, Dermacentor variabilis*, and *Argas (Persicargas) radiatus* are the species of ticks most commonly associated with paralysis. In Australia, the paralysis tick is *Ixodes holocyclus*, which is found along the eastern coast of Australia. Ticks secret a toxin that prevents release of ACH from the neuromuscular junction. In the United States, clinical signs are those of a diffuse LMN disease. Diagnosis is made presumptively based on the appropriate clinical signs in combination with tick infestation. The diagnosis is supported if removal of the tick results in reversal of clinical signs in 12 to 72 hours. In Australia, the disease is often life-threatening (see chapter 7).

Organophosphate intoxication potentiates the effect of acetylcholine at the neuromuscular junction and other synapses, by binding with and inactivating acetylcholinesterase. This leads to increased acetylcholine concentrations at the neuromuscular junction, increased receptor stimulation, and fatigue. Chronic exposure can result in peripheral neuropathies, and cats are one of the species most prone to delayed neurotoxicosis. Organophosphate and carbamate toxicity can result in a multitude of clinical signs including muscle weakness. Muscarinic signs classically include salivation, lacrimation, bradycardia, and pupillary constriction. Nicotinic signs include muscle fasciculations, tremors, and twitching. Chronic organophosphate toxicity can result in weakness, primarily in cats (Jaggy et al. 1990). A delayed neurotoxicity in cats is reported associated with the use of chlorpyrifos spray for household application against fleas.

A presumptive diagnosis of organophosphate toxicity is made when the appropriate clinical signs are found in an animal with a history of organophosphate exposure. The concentration of serum cholinesterase activity may lend support to the diagnosis. Depending upon the laboratory, values less than 500 IU/L (normal 900–1200 IU/L) are considered consistent with organophosphate toxicity. Cats with polyneuropathy from chronic OP toxicity may have normal serum cholinesterase activity. Electromyographic changes are occasionally present and include fibrillation potentials, positive sharp waves, and bizarre high-frequency discharges. A decremental response to repetitive nerve stimulation may be present. An edrophonium (used to test for myasthenia gravis) response test in these animals may produce an acute worsening of signs.

Envenomation can result in a variety of signs of nervous system dysfunction. Bites from brown snakes (*Pseudonaja* sp.), coral snakes (*Micrurus fulvius*), tiger snakes (*Notechis scutatus*), and death adders (*Acanthophis antarcticus*) can cause ataxia, paralysis, and dilated pupils. Additionally, bites from the red-backed spider (*Latrodectus* sp.) and ingestion of the tetrodotoxin from toadfish (*Sphaeroides hamiltoni*) may also result in weakness. Red-backed spider venom results in depletion of acetylcholine reserves at the motor end plate. A presumptive diagnosis is based on appropriate clinical signs and a history of a snake bite or access.

Vascular Neuropathies and Myopathies

Ischemic neuropathy is most often associated with aortic thromboembolism (see bibliography under Vascular Neuropathies and Myopathies). In cats, aortic thrombosis is the consequence of cardiomyopathy (hypertrophic). Occasionally, these thrombi can lodge in vessels supplying a thoracic limb. In dogs, aortic thrombus is associated with diseases of hypercoagulability such as protein-losing nephropathies (glomerular disease) and hyperadrenocorticism.

Clinical signs include acute onset paraplegia, with firm, hard painful muscles in the affected limb(s) (Griffiths et al. 1979). Spinal reflexes will usually be decreased or absent. Cats invariably show apparent distress usually with associated vocalizing. Absent femoral pulses, cold cyanotic extremities, and absent bleeding when a toenail is cut are also found. Serum CK is usually significantly elevated in affected animals and can be an important diagnostic clue. Aortic angiography is rarely used for diagnosis.

13 Treatment of Important and Common Diseases Involving the Intracranial Nervous System of Dogs and Cats

Once a diagnosis is established, appropriate treatment decisions can be formulated that we hope will enhance animal comfort and survival. The most appropriate treatment decisions can be made only when a *definitive diagnosis* is established. In some instances, a definitive diagnosis cannot be obtained due to patient influences, disease characteristics, or owner financial considerations. Treatments are initiated in these animals based on the *presumptive* (or most likely), or in other instances, a possible *diagnosis*.

When considering treatment of intracranial disease, both medical and surgical therapies may be necessary. Medical therapies primarily include antiseizure (anticonvulsant), antiedema, antimicrobial, and anti-inflammatory drug therapies. The influence of the blood-brain barrier (BBB) is an important consideration when medically treating for intracranial disease, as this barrier may effectively prevent drugs from penetrating into the central nervous system (CNS). The lack of ability of some drug therapies to actually be presented to the CNS limit the therapeutic concentrations of these drugs that can be achieved in intracranial structures.

The spectrum of therapies for animals with intracranial disease varies from routine to sophisticated. As animals with intracranial disease may be unable, in some instances, to perform activities necessary for basic systemic functions such as eating and drinking, treatments that support basic essential life processes, such as fluid therapy for maintenance of vascular volume and nutrition, are often a necessary aspect of treatment for animals with intracranial disease. Maintaining animals comfortable, hydrated, and clean is an important aspect of what is commonly referred to as "supportive care." In addition to support of basic life functions, another important aspect of treatment of animals with intracranial disease is the treatment of basic pathophysiologic abnormalities resulting secondary to the primary disease process. Principal secondary pathophysiologic abnormalities include seizures, decreased cerebral perfusion, and increases in intracranial pressure (ICP). Finally, treatment of the primary intracranial disease process is necessary to bring about resolution of clinical signs.

In the initial portions of this chapter, general treatments for intracranial disease will be discussed including basic aspects of medical and surgical treatment. The latter portions of this chapter will focus on treatment options in specific disease situations where these treatments have been utilized.

TREATMENT OF PATHOPHYSIOLOGIC ALTERATIONS OF INTRACRANIAL DISEASE: SEIZURES AND INCREASED INTRACRANIAL PRESSURE

Of the important pathophysiologic alterations secondary to intracranial disease, seizures and increases in intracranial pressure often require acute treatment. Seizures are treated most commonly with anticonvulsants, whereas there is a variety of methods for treating increased intracranial pressure.

Anticonvulsants

Seizures are one of the most common clinical problems associated with disease of the CNS. Seizures often require treatment independent of the primary disease process. As there are numerous intracranial diseases that may result in seizures, the ultimate treatment of a seizure disorder will depend upon the appropriate treatment of the primary cause. Seizures are such an important clinical problem that an in-depth discussion of seizure disorders is found in chapter 17 and appendix 3.

Seizures often need to be treated both short-term in emergency situations, and long-term through repeated administration of anticonvulsant medications (maintenance therapy). If it is necessary to terminate seizures acutely in an emergency situation, diazepam or a similar product (such as midazolam) is often helpful (see chapter 17 for dosages and treatment protocols). Diazepam is an effective anticonvulsant, but is rapidly metabolized in dogs and therefore its duration of efficacy is relatively short (seconds to minutes). This often necessitates using repeated or increasing dosages of diazepam to acutely terminate seizure activity. Diazepam may be administered in a variety of routes (orally, intravenously, intramuscularly, rectally), however, the intravenous route of administration is preferred. Repeated intravenous bolus dosages or constant rate infusions of diazepam are often needed to terminate severe seizure activity. If intravascular access is not available, diazepam may be admininstered rectally to achieve the desired effect. Diazepam is also an appropriate anticonvulsant for termination of acute seizure activity in cats, but is occasionally associated (idiosyncratic) with liver failure.

Maintenance anticonvulsants are administered in an attempt to decrease the overall frequency and severity of seizures (see chapter 17). While there are several maintenance anticonvulsants currently available for use in animals, the two most commonly used in the contemporary era are phenobarbital and potassium bromide. Both of these drugs seem reasonably effective as anticonvulsants in dogs. They do, however, have different metabolism, toxicities, and methods of administration and monitoring. The most appropriate choice of an anticonvulsant for one animal may not be the most appropriate choice for another. Specific information about anticonvulsants is found in chapter 17 and in appendix 3. As a general rule, maintenance anticonvulsants are helpful in approximately 70% of animals with recurrent seizures. Conversely, this leaves approximately 30% of animals with seizure disorders that do not receive significant benefit from these drugs for control of their seizures.

Phenobarbital. Phenobarbital is a barbiturate that has been used for a number of years as a monotherapy for seizures in dogs and cats(also see chapter 17 and appendix 3). This drug is initiated at 3 mg/kg orally every 12 hours. Serum phenobarbital levels should be assessed at 2 weeks after beginning therapy to determine whether the actual serum concentration of phenobarbital has been obtained. Trough therapeutic concentration (within 1 hour of the next dose) seems to correlate best with clinical seizure control but levels taken at various times during the day may yield similar information. The suggested therapeutic range for serum phenobarbital concentration is between 20 and 40 μg/ml. It is important to remember that this therapeutic range is based on a general population of dogs. Individual dogs may be controlled at various levels within, and sometimes outside, the therapeutic range. As serum phenobarbital levels become 35 μg/ml or greater, the potential for associated toxicity (primarily liver complications) is significantly increased.

There is no established mg/kg dose of phenobarbital that is efficacious or for that matter toxic for an individual animal. The actual mg/kg dose of phenobarbital an animal is administered is clinically inconsequential compared to the actual serum phenobarbital level that is achieved in the patient. Oral dosages in the range of 11 to 13 mg/kg given on a repeated basis often result in serum phenobarbital levels near or greater than 35 μg/ml. The correlation between orally administered dose and serum concentration of phenobarbital, however, is variable in individual dogs. Phenobarbital administration actually increases liver metabolism of phenobarbital itself, leading to decreasing serum phenobarbital levels following repeated or chronic phenobarbital administration. Serum phenobarbital concentrations, in consideration of the drug's effect on seizure frequency and severity, should be assessed before deciding that an animal is getting too little or too much phenobarbital. If toxic levels of phenobarbital are obtained, or if seizure control is not adequate, then an additional anticonvulsant is added to the treatment regime. If the serum phenobarbital concentrations are found to be in the toxic range, then phenobarbital dosages should be decreased, and possibly (cautiously) discontinued.

Side effects of phenobarbital administration include polyuria, polydipsia, polyphagia, and sedation. Sedation is most profound after the initial administration (first days to weeks) of the drug in animals that have never been administered phenobarbital previously. Occasionally, animals will become agitated, persistently vocalize, and become hyperactive when this drug is first administered (during or within the first 3 to 5 days). This reaction appears to be the result of the animal receiving too little medication. It has been likened to stage 2 or the excitement phase of anesthesia. In these animals, increasing the dose rapidly, including loading the dog on phenobarbital, will help to relieve this hyperactive reaction.

The most concerning side effect of phenobarbital is its liver-damaging effects. This side effect is more likely when relatively higher dosages of the drug are administered (i.e., drug levels are >35 μg/ml), if other medications that alter the metabolism of phenobarbital are used concurrently, or if administration of phenobarbital is chronic. Liver damage from phenobarbital therapy can be severe and potentially irreversible. Importantly, even appropriate phenobarbital administration will result in increases in commonly measured liver enzymes such as ALT and SAP. It is difficult, therefore, to determine if serum biochemical liver enzyme elevations reflect underlying liver damage or not. Conversely, severe liver failure can occur and liver enzyme concentrations can be normal (such as in the instance of cirrhosis). This underscores the point that, in an animal receiving phenobarbital, routine liver biochemical enzymes measurements do not always provide clinically helpful information regarding underlying liver dysfunction. A periodic test of liver function, therefore, is imperative in animals receiving phenobarbital as seizure therapy.

In an individual patient, if seizures are controlled and the dosage of phenobarbital remains consistent, serum bile acids or some similar liver function test should be assessed at regular intervals and at least every 6 months. If systemic abnormalities occur, or if seizure control is less than adequate, serum bile acids should be assessed more frequently. An animal that becomes excessively sedate on a seemingly appropriate oral dosage of phenobarbital should have an assessment of both serum phenobarbital concentrations and liver function to determine if an alteration of phenobarbital metabolism is occurring.

Routine administration and appropriate doses of phenobarbital should not result in increases in serum bile acids unless there is underlying liver pathology. Phenobarbital administration, however, may affect the results of some other commonly evaluated serum tests such as thyroid hormone concentrations. Measured serum T4 levels will decrease when an animal is receiving phenobarbital, without the animal having clinical evidence or affects of hypothyroidism.

Phenobarbital can affect the metabolism of certain drugs that are metabolized similarly. Additionally, other drugs may alter the metabolism of phenobarbital leading to either increased metabolism with resultant decreased efficacy or decreased metabolism with resultant toxicity. Protein-bound drugs such as nonsteroidal analgesics can displace phenobarbital from binding sites and increase the metabolism of phenobarbital, effectively lowering therapeutic concentrations. Other drugs, most notably chloramphenicol, but also possibly cimetidine, prevent the metabolism of phenobarbital leading to excessive serum concentrations. Excessive concentrations of phenobarbital can then result in a coma, respiratory depression, and eventual death.

Potassium Bromide. Potassium bromide (KBr) has become an important anticonvulsant for control of seizures in dogs and, occasionally, cats (see chapter 17). This product is actually produced as a chemical, not a drug formulation. Its use as an anticonvulsant has shown reasonable efficacy for treatment of seizures in dogs. The normal maintenance dose of bromide is 20 to 60 mg/kg/day. Potassium bromide has a relatively long half-life (~24 days) and, therefore, requires a significant period of time to reach steady state (up to 4 months) concentrations of the drug in dogs. In an effort to increase the therapeutic drug levels of potassium bromide more rapidly, a loading dose of potassium bromide can be administered at the initiation of treatment. For loading, a total dose of 400–600 mg/kg can be administered at the onset of therapy in an attempt to acutely increase KBr serum concentrations. Potassium bromide, when given in increased concentrations in a single dose, however, is often irritating to the stomach and results in vomiting. To avoid this complication, the total loading dose is divided in multiple, smaller doses over a 2- to 4-day period. During the loading period, the total loading dose is given over 48 to 96 hours by giving multiple doses of the maintenance dose of the medication. For example, the loading dose of potassium bromide for a 20 kg dog would be calculated as follows:

- 20 kg dog × 400 mg/kg (loading dose) = 8000 mg needed for loading.
- Maintenance dose of KBr for 20 kg dog is 20 kg × 30 mg/kg = 600 mg.
- To decrease the chance of gastric irritation with the maintenance medication, the 600 mg daily dose can be divided into two 300 mg dosages, which will ultimately be the maintenance dosage of KBr.

For loading, a 300 mg capsule is administered every 2 hours until a final dose of 8000 mg is achieved. This would require approximately 26 dosages over a period of approximately 52 hours. Some modifications of dosing schedule can be made to accommodate ease of medication administration. Depending upon the patient, the animal may be able to handle increased amounts of KBr at a single dosing interval without vomiting. This would decrease the number of individual dosages used during the loading phase. Conversely, administering smaller dosages at any single dosing interval would increase the number of dosages (and time) of the loading period. After loading is completed, the animal is begun on the maintenance dosage the following day.

Potassium bromide is reasonably safe but has some side effects. The bromide component is toxic to humans, who can get headaches, skin rashes, tremors, and gastrointestinal disturbances if exposed to this chemical in sufficient quantities. Owners should be careful in handling the chemical and not expose themselves either through ingestion, inhalation, or skin contact to this chemical. Avoiding exposure may require placing the medication in the animal's food rather than direct pilling, wearing gloves when pilling or handling the chemical, not opening previously compounded capsulated forms of the chemical, and washing hands after touching of the capsule.

The main side effects of KBr in dogs include sedation, ataxia (usually with increased dosages), and vomiting due to the local irritant effects of the chemical on the stomach. Diets with differing levels of sodium chloride, alterations in fluid intake, or dehydration may alter the therapeutic levels in the blood of KBr. Rarely, skin irritation, itchiness, or rashes may be noted in dogs. An association of KBr administration and pancreatitis and possibly renal insufficiency has been suggested. Importantly, in cats, KBr can result in a fatal asthmatic condition. Caution should be exercised when using this drug in cats, and if any respiratory signs are noted, the drug should be discontinued immediately.

If an animal becomes toxic from bromide administration, forced diuresis is used to eliminate the chemical from the body. Intravenous administration of NaCl-containing fluids is used for this purpose. Similar to phenobarbital, serum concentration of KBr can be measured. Suggested therapeutic levels for KBr range from 1 to 3 mg/ml. This range, however, is a less-reliable indicator of efficacy and toxicity compared with serum phenobarbital concentrations. As with other anticonvulsants, achievement of the desired effect (reduction or elimination of seizures) is balanced with side effects and toxicity of the medication.

Treatment of Elevated Intracranial Pressure

Increases in intracranial pressure (ICP)are often the most important consequence of structural intracranial disease (see bibliography under Intracranial Pressure). In many instances, appropriate treatment of increases in ICP will have a more profound effect on acute patient survival than primary treatment of the actual disease. Treatment of increases in ICP can bring about short-term stabilization of the severely impaired animal allowing time for additional, more specific disease treatments to have an affect.

Maintenance of Systemic Function. Basic life support measures may be necessary including blood or isotonic fluid administration. Of all of the reported treatments for increases in ICP, appropriate fluid resuscitation may, in fact, provide the greatest benefits. By maintaining appropriate intravascular fluid volumes, cerebral perfusion can be maintained. Improved cerebral perfusion will result in decreases in ICP. The difficulty becomes clinically determining what "appropriate" vascular volume is. Common clinical parameters of adequate fluid volumes such as skin turgor and mucous membrane dryness are often insensitive. Blood pressure measurements may be the best objective and most clinically practical measure to provide some indication of intravascular volume and subsequent perfusion.

Fluid administration should be critically monitored, however, as overhydration with isotonic fluids may perpetuate brain edema. Again, monitoring of systemic blood pressure and central venous pressure may aid in reestablishment of normovolemia. The goal is to provide or maintain appropriate fluid balance.

Diuretics

Mannitol. As cerebral edema contributes to intracranial volume and, subsequently, increases in ICP, treatments that decrease cerebral edema are often used to lower ICP. Mannitol is the most commonly used diuretic in clinical practice to decrease cerebral edema and ICP. Mannitol has been thought to decrease ICP primarily through its associated osmotic effects, although other effects such as concurrent decreases in blood viscosity and free-radical scavenging are, in fact, more beneficial. By decreasing blood viscosity, cerebral perfusion will be increased at the same level of systemic blood pressure. Vasoconstriction will result, lowering cerebral blood volume and concurrently lowering ICP.

Mannitol is administered intravenously at 0.25 up to 1 gm/kg over 5 to 10 minutes. Maximal lowering of ICP most often occurs in 10 to 20 minutes. In both humans and dogs with normal ICP, mannitol infusion is associated with an initial, short-lived increase in ICP. If ICP is elevated prior to treatment, ICP decreases consistently. Therefore, mannitol appears more effective in patients who have increased ICP, wherein precipitous decreases in ICP are seen. In patients where ICP is normal, the effect of mannitol on lowering ICP is less dramatic.

Contraindications to mannitol use include hypovolemia and ongoing intracranial hemorrhage. Mannitol has also been shown to induce histamine release from basophils, which may result in hypotension and a shocklike state. Additionally, after the initial decrease in ICP from mannitol administration, ICP may increase (rebound) back to similar or even higher levels than even before its administration. A decrease in fluid intake and subsequently an increase in vascular viscosity may be responsible. Sludging of cerebral blood flow then results in vasodilation of cerebral vessels, increases cerebral blood volume, and, subsequently, increases ICP. Preventing dehydration in the post-mannitol administration period may decrease this potential secondary complication.

Furosemide. Furosemide (0.7 mg/kg IV) is a loop diuretic that may help to lower ICP primarily or may potentiate the effects of mannitol. Furosemide given as a preoperative diuretic in humans lowered ICP comparably to mannitol. Additionally, furosemide did not result in an initial increase in ICP as with mannitol. Furosemide given minutes after mannitol administration potentiates the intracranial pressure-lowering effects of the latter.

Other hypertonic solutions such as dextrose and albumin appear less effective at lowering ICP as compared to mannitol and furosemide. This may be the result of these latter solutions being more freely diffusible across cell membranes with a resultant inability to establish a quantitatively significant osmotic gradient for fluid movement.

Hypertonic Saline. Treatment with hypertonic saline has been used to maintain intravascular volumes, arterial blood pressure, and cerebral perfusion. In some instances, hypertonic saline is equal to mannitol in decreasing ICP experimentally (see chapter 22) (Qureshi 1999, 2000, 2002).

Head Elevation. Head elevation to 30°above heart level will decrease ICP primarily by facilitating venous drainage. There is debate concerning this therapy with opponents suggesting that head elevation may decrease cerebral perfusion and, therefore, be detrimental to brain function. A study in humans, however, has shown that cerebral perfusion pressure and cerebral blood flow are maintained in the 30°head elevation position as ICP is concurrently decreased. Reduction of ICP with this relatively simple treatment may be beneficial in combination with other ICP decreasing measures.

Hyperventilation. Hyperventilation can decrease ICP due to the established effects of $PaCO_2$ concentrations on cerebral blood flow (see chapter 2). As cerebral vessels are directly responsive to $PaCO_2$ concentrations, if cerebrovascular autoregulation is intact, hyperventilation to decrease $PaCO_2$ will cause cerebral vasoconstriction, decreased cerebral blood volume, and subsequently decreased ICP. Hyperventilation in this instance should be used to maintain $PaCO_2$ between 28 and 32 mm Hg to avoid cerebral hypoxia from poor ventilation, which will also be detrimental to neuronal survival. Hyperventilation should not be used excessively to avoid hypoxemia. Endotracheal intubation and ventilator support can be performed under the influence of barbiturate anesthesia or neuromuscular blockade. Appropriate ventilator management, of course, is imperative.

Craniotomy. A major tenet of the Monro-Kellie doctrine is that intracranial contents are confined within the cranium. It would follow, therefore, that surgical removal of this structure would potentially relieve ICP elevations (see surgery below). Unilateral or bilateral craniectomy has been used as a treatment for ICP elevations that cannot be decreased by the more conventional methods stated above. While skull removal alone may be beneficial, subsequent dural incision appears significantly more effective in lowering ICP. This has been shown clinically in humans and experimentally in dogs as well as cats. Ultimate functional recovery remains dependent upon the underlying primary brain damage inflicted by the disease process. Because ICP may increase during wound closure and anesthetic recovery, the magnitude of ICP decrease subsequent to surgery, nevertheless, remains uncertain.

Craniectomy and durotomy have been shown to lower ICP by 15 and 65%, respectively, in dogs, cats, and humans. Intracranial pressures in normal dogs approached atmospheric pressure when a lateral rostrotentorial craniectomy and durotomy were performed. Adequate decompression of the brain in animals with structural disease would be suggested if intraoperative ICP approached similar levels.

Treatments with Possible but Uncertain Efficacy

Corticosteroids. Corticosteroids are often used as a treatment of intracranial disease and increased ICP. Beneficial effects of methylprednisolone in nervous system injury include inhibition of lipid peroxidation and its associated detrimental effects. The role of corticosteroids in the treatment of head injury, however, is unclear and the administration of corticosteroids in these instances is often discouraged (Procaccio et al. 2000). Potential detrimental effects of corticosteroids to the nervous system occur when neuronal ischemia is present. It is known that corticosteroids potentiate ischemic injury to neurons. It is not established whether this is due to direct toxic effects of corticosteroids or due to secondarily induced metabolic derangements. It is also established that humans that are hyperglycemic at the time of head injury have a worse overall prognosis than people who are normoglycemic. The increased concentrations of glucose in anaerobic brain tissue associated with ischemia may potentiate lactic acid accumulation and increase neuronal damage. Considering that severe head trauma is most likely associated with some degree of cerebral ischemia and that corticosteroids can result in a short-term increase in blood glucose, these same detrimental effects may apply when exogenous corticosteroids are used for treating brain injury secondary to increased ICP.

Cerebrospinal Fluid Aspiration. Cerebrospinal fluid aspiration is sometimes used as a means to decrease ICP in humans. This is most helpful in humans if a ventriculostomy is present and if ICP elevations do not exceed 30 mm Hg. The use of a CSF tap alone is not recommended in animals with suspected increased ICP, however, due to the increased risk of precipitating brain herniation. Similar to humans, however, removal of CSF from the ventricular system can be helpful in lowering increased ICP in animals.

Barbiturates. Barbiturates (pentobarbital 3 mg/kg IV to effect) were historically used to induce coma thereby decreasing cerebral metabolism, cerebral blood flow, and subsequently ICP in selected human patients. Barbiturates may benefit brain blood flow by causing vasoconstriction in normal tissue and shunting blood to ischemic areas. Other suggested benefits include decreases in vasogenic edema, oxygen metabolism, intracellular calcium, and increases in free radical scavenging. Pentobarbital is usually administered as a constant intravenous infusion in order to achieve and maintain a burst-suppression pattern on the electroencephalogram. Arterial blood pressure should be monitored closely, as barbiturates can result in hypotension, which may decrease cerebral blood flow and increase cerebral ischemia.

Beneficial effects from barbiturate coma in humans with intracranial pressure elevations have been variable. Similar to other treatments, success should be assessed based not only on the ability of the treatment to lower ICP, but also on the ultimate degree of functional recovery. Barbiturate therapy may, however, be more beneficial for patients with brain trauma who have preserved cerebrovascular reactivity to changes in $PaCO_2$ than those who do not.

Hypothermia. Hypothermia has been used experimentally in dogs and clinically in humans to decrease ICP when other treatments are less effective. Cooling of the body may prevent the ischemia-induced release of excitatory neurotransmitters such as glutamate. This decrease in extracellular levels of the excitatory neurotransmitters may prevent the rapid influx of extracellular calcium into the cell, which leads to free radical production and, eventually, cell death. Further studies, however, may support the use of hypothermia as an adjunct therapy for elevated ICP.

Miscellaneous Drugs. Other drugs have been suggested possibly as potential adjunctive therapies in brain injury, although clinical studies to support experimental information are less readily available. The antioxidant drug deferoxamine mesylate has been shown to reduce cold-induced brain edema in cats. Other drugs under investigation for use in brain injury include superoxide dismutase, allopurinol, opiate antagonists (naloxone), thyrotropin-releasing hormone, and calcium channel blockers. Future clinical trials in naturally occurring head injury are needed to determine the efficacy of these drugs.

ANTIMICROBIALS

Due to the presence of the blood-brain barrier (BBB), few antimicrobials normally penetrate the CNS adequately to achieve therapeutic concentrations. Trimethoprim sulfa products readily cross the BBB and are bactericidal. These drugs are often an initial choice for treating CNS bacterial infections and are also useful in treating toxoplasmosis and possibly neosporosis.

Ampicillin penetrates the CNS in adequate therapeutic concentrations only in the presence of inflammation and

BBB disruption. With resolution of the inflammation, therapeutic concentrations of this drug may subsequently not be achieved within the brain.

Clindamycin is a macrolide antimicrobial that is used in the treatment of toxoplasmosis and possibly neosporosis. Doxycycline and other tetracyclines are used in the treatment of rickettsial diseases and some bacterial diseases (*Brucella canis* infection). Metronidazole is often used for treatment of CNS anaerobic infections. Toxic effects associated with this latter drug primarily are neurologic abnormalities, such as vestibular signs in dogs, and central blindness and seizures in cats. Therefore, metronidazole should be used with caution in animals with underlying neurologic abnormalities, and animals should be diligently monitored for side effects. Other antibiotics, such as third-generation cephalosporin antimicrobials may be used in selected instances of bacterial encephalitis.

Chloramphenicol is a bacteriostatic antimicrobial that also readily crosses the BBB. It is useful for treating CNS infections due to rickettsial organisms and bacteria, but is rarely used in the modern era. This drug will inhibit the metabolism of other drugs (most notably phenobarbital) by decreasing drug metabolism (by inhibiting liver enzymes). Chloramphenicol should never be used with phenobarbital in combination as coma and respiratory arrest can occur even when using adequate dosages of each. Chloramphenicol also may result in hematologic abnormalities (bone marrow suppression) and aplastic anemia (in susceptible humans). The latter should be a concern for the veterinary team as well as owners.

Antimicrobials are often used in combination with corticosteroids for treatment of intracranial inflammatory conditions (see below, Inflammatory Disease). Antimicrobials also often have associated anti-inflammatory effects in addition to their effects on infectious organisms. As many CNS diseases, regardless of whether there is an infectious cause or not, result in CNS inflammation, antimicrobial therapy may result in improvements in clinical signs independent of any direct antimicrobial effects. This may result in a false presumption of the presence of an infectious agent if a positive therapeutic response is achieved following antimicrobial administration.

CORTICOSTEROIDS

Corticosteroids are commonly administered in animals with neurologic disease primarily for their anti-inflammatory and antiedema effects. Corticosteroids may greatly improve clinical signs in animals with neoplastic or inflammatory CNS disease and may even benefit animals with certain infectious diseases. Corticosteroids are used as the sole means of control of certain CNS inflammatory diseases. The role of corticosteroids in the treatment of spinal trauma is commonly, but not universally, accepted, however, the use of corticosteroids in instances of head trauma is debatable (see chapter 22) (Procaccio et al. 2000). While corticosteroids have shown benefit by reducing cerebral edema in brain tumor patients, caution has been suggested when using corticosteroids for other types of brain injury (Hall 1992, 1985). Corticosteroids are known to perpetuate neuronal damage if cerebral ischemia is present (Braakman 1983; Sapolsky 1985). Corticosteroid administration may increase blood glucose, a factor that may negatively influence outcome after brain injury (Lam et al. 1991).

Side effects associated with corticosteroid administration in animals with neurological disease include the propensity for gastrointestinal ulceration and pancreatitis. Dexamethasone appears to be more ulcerogenic than prednisolone in the gastrointestinal tract. This may be due in part to inappropriate dosing. Published doses of dexamethasone seem high considering pharmacologic properties and potency of this drug. Ulceration that leads to bowel perforation is often life-threatening. The most common site of intestinal perforation in animals receiving dexamethasone is at the antimesenteric side of the junction between the transverse and descending colon. Colonic perforation at this site has been uniformly fatal. Corticosteroid treatment may also predispose the animal to increased infection or superinfection processes via immunosuppressive effects of these drugs. Delayed wound healing, increased incidence of decubital ulceration, and urinary tract infection may result in recumbent patients.

SURGICAL TREATMENTS: INDICATIONS FOR INTRACRANIAL SURGERY

Intracranial surgery is most commonly employed for removal of intracranial masses, biopsy of intracranial lesions, placement of ventricular CSF shunting devices, decompression and debridement of intracranial tissues, and treatment of increased ICP. Surgery may include removal of sizable portions of the skull (craniotomy or craniectomy) or be limited to smaller burr holes for decompression and evacuation of hematoma or stereotactic biopsy. Other indications for intracranial surgery in humans include treatment for seizures, chronic pain, and movement disorders.

A craniotomy is the removal of a portion of the skull for access to the intracranial space, with subsequent replacement of bone. A craniectomy is the removal of a portion of the skull for access to the intracranial space, without subsequent replacement of bone (fig. 13.1). Maximum exposure of the lesion is a key aspect contributing to a successful intracranial surgical outcome. Limited approaches make lesion visualization difficult and increase the risk of iatrogenic brain disease from excessive brain manipulation. Often, when the intracranial nervous tissues are manipulated, brain swelling ensues. Adequate skull removal in the area of the swelling will provide a decompressive effect for this swollen brain (fig. 13.2) (Bagley 1996). Conversely, overzealous skull removal increases the risk of postoperative scarring (craniectomy membrane formation) and allows for significant shifts of brain parenchyma, which, in itself, may lead to further brain damage from vascular compromise. Multiple surgical approaches to intracranial structures have been used in dogs (table 13.1). Many of the basic

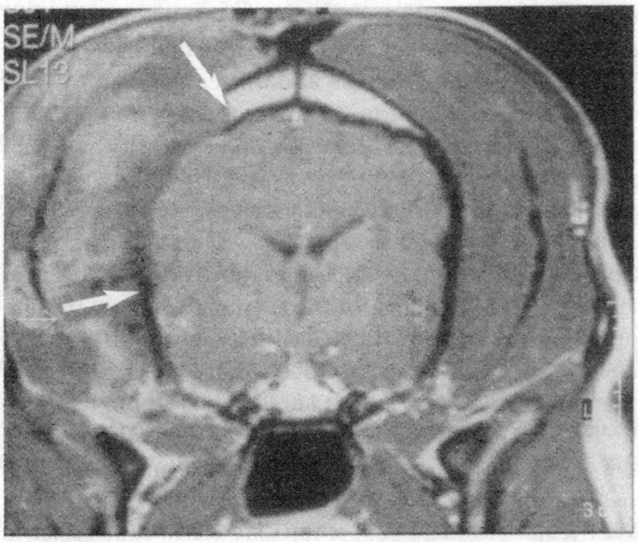

Fig. 13.1. Transverse T1-weighted magnetic resonance of a dog showing a craniectomy defect (*arrows*).

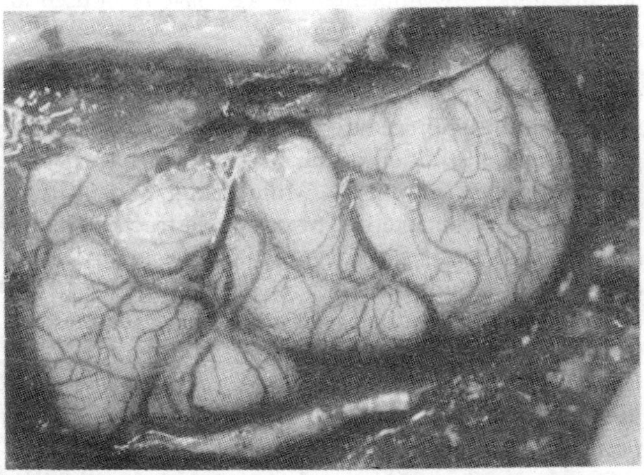

Fig. 13.2. Appearance of the dog cortex following a craniotomy.

Table 13.1. Surgical approaches to intracranial structures

- Lateral Rostrotentorial Craniotomy/craniectomy
  This approach is used for exposure of the lateral parietal, temporal, and occipital cortices.
- Radical Rostrotentorial Craniotomy/craniectomy
  An extension of the lateral rostrotentorial craniotomy/craniectomy has been described for access to more rostral and lateral cortical lesions.
- Suboccipital Craniotomy/craniectomy
  This approach is used for exposure of the caudal cerebellum, caudal medulla oblongata (obex), and cranial cervical spinal cord (foramen magnum area).
- Combined Rostrotentorial/suboccipital Craniectomy with Transverse Sinus Occlusion
  This approach is used for exposure of the dorsolateral cerebellopontine medullary angle and unilateral tentorial area.
- Bilateral Rostrotentorial (dorsal) Craniotomy/craniectomy
  This approach is used for exposure of the dorsal olfactory, frontal, parietal, temporal, and occipital cortices.
- Combination Dorsal, Bilateral Frontal, and Transfrontal Craniotomy/Craniectomy
  A more radical extension of the dorsal and transfrontal rostrotentorial craniotomy/craniectomy is used for exposure of the dorsal frontal cortices, olfactory bulbs, and ethmoidal areas.
- Pituitary Surgery
  Surgical approaches to the pituitary gland, primarily via a transsphenoidal approach, have been described.
- Approach to the Trigeminal Nerve
  In dogs, a lateral rostrotentorial craniectomy or a transzygomatic craniectomy has been used to access the ventral and ipsilateral floor of the skull in the area of the trigeminal nerve.

neurosurgical techniques have been described elsewhere (Bagley 2003).

Treatment of Specific Intracranial Diseases

Degenerative Diseases. Of the numerous primary degenerative intracranial diseases that have been described, many are found as only pathologic descriptions of the disease process identified at the time of necropsy. Treatments for many of these primary degenerative diseases either have not been attempted or no proven treatment is recognized. Some storage diseases are being treated experimentally with bone marrow transplantation, genetic transfer therapies, or parenteral enzyme replacement therapy. These treatments are not routinely available in the present era of clinical practice.

Primary age-related degenerative brain diseases are suspected in some older dogs. A suggested treatment for cognitive dysfunction of older dogs is L-deprenyl (selegiline). This drug is used to restore dopamine balance and may enhance catecholamine levels. Reported dosages are 0.5 to 1 mg/kg every 24 hours for dogs and 0.5 mg/kg every 24 hours for cats. Ideally, clinical signs should improve within the first month. Clinical improvement, however, is not pathognomonic for this disease process, as this drug may nonspecifically increase activity and alertness. Antioxidant-type diets are also available for use in older dogs. The lack of definitive diagnosis of these disorders, however, makes it difficult to accurately assess clinical treatment responses. Importantly, the spectrum of underlying diseases that may result in a more general description of "cognitive dysfunction" need to be identified and treated primarily, if present.

Anomalous Disease. As these are congenital anatomical abnormalities, primary treatment for the disease is not possible. Treatment of secondary pathophysiologic sequelae such as seizures may require, for example, anticonvulsant therapy.

Primary cystic structures may also be present in the intracranial region, usually in or around the caudal and dorsal third ventricle. These cystic structures are often referred to as arachnoid or subarachnoid cysts. In some instances, surgical fenestration through a craniotomy or craniectomy can produce improvement in clinical signs. Similarly, epidermoid or dermoid cysts may be surgically resectable (see figs. 5.7, 10.3). While there is no primary treatment for occipital dysplasia, the clinical consequences of Chiari malformation such as syringomyelia may be improved with a foramen magnum decompression via a suboccipital craniectomy with subsequent surgical reconstruction of this region.

Hydrocephalus. There are several medical and surgical treatment options that may be beneficial for animals with hydrocephalus (see bibliography under Hydrocephalus). The choice of treatments is generally dictated by degree of physical impairment, age of the animal, and cause of the hydrocephalus, if known. Medical treatment may include general supportive care and medications to limit CSF production and reduce intracranial pressure. Surgical treatment is designed to provide drainage of CSF from the brain to another site within the body for reabsorption.

Medical therapy may provide long-term control, or in some cases, resolution of the clinical signs in mildly affected animals. Medical therapies may also be used for perioperative stabilization of animals undergoing surgical treatment and for management of cases whose owners have limited financial resources. Medications used in the medical treatment of hydrocephalus include glucocorticoids, diuretics, or a combination of these drugs.

Glucocorticoids are often administered to animals with hydrocephalus in an attempt to decrease CSF production, intracranial edema, and inflammation. In some situations, corticosteroids may also help to limit increases in intracranial pressure. Prednisone given at 0.25–0.5 mg/kg orally twice daily is often used initially. If clinical signs improve, this dose is gradually reduced at weekly intervals to 0.1 mg/kg every other day. If clinical signs are controlled, the medication is eventually discontinued. It is more likely, however, that chronically administered dosages of corticosteroids are required daily or every other day to control clinical signs. Alternatively, dexamethasone may be given orally at 0.025 mg/kg every 6 to 8 hours, however, dexamethasone appears to be associated with more gastrointestinal ulceration compared to prednisolone or prednisone. The dose of dexamethasone is gradually reduced over 2 to 4 weeks, if possible. Some animals with congenital hydrocephalus can be adequately managed with long-term glucocorticoid administration at relatively low doses indefinitely. If no clinical benefits are observed within 2 weeks, or if side effects develop, other forms of therapy should be considered.

Acetazolamide, a carbonic anhydrase inhibitor, has been used in an attempt to reduce CSF pressure by decreasing CSF production. Therefore, this diuretic has been suggested to be especially useful for short-term management of animals with elevated intracranial pressure. A dose of 10 mg/kg is given orally every 6 to 8 hours. Electrolyte status should be monitored closely because acetazolamide, especially when used with corticosteroids, may cause potassium depletion. Some animals may have gastrointestinal abnormalities associated with this drug. The clinical efficacy of acetazolamide for treatment of hydrocephalus in animals is presently not established.

Mannitol is an osmotic diuretic that decreases CSF production and reduces ICP (see treatment of ICP above). A dose of 0.25 to 1 g/kg is given intravenously over 15 or 20 minutes and may be repeated two to four times over the following 48 hours. Animals administered mannitol and other diuretics should be monitored closely for dehydration, as dehydration can increase blood viscosity and, subsequently, decrease cerebral perfusion. This may, in fact, be associated with worsening clinical signs.

Surgical Shunting. Surgical treatment for hydrocephalus is generally required for those animals that do not improve within 2 weeks of medical therapy, or for those animals whose clinical signs deteriorate during medical therapy. Surgical procedures are designed to provide controlled CSF flow from the ventricles of the brain to either the peritoneal cavity or the right atrium. Shunt systems designed for use in humans seem to be adaptable for animals. Ventriculoperitoneal (VP) shunts are technically easier to install and are most commonly used in human neurosurgery (figs. 13.3, 13.4). Emergency placement of shorter-term CSF removal devices may be used in the management of secondary hydrocephalus. Vascular access ports or similar subcutaneously implanted devices have been used for this purpose.

Successful, long-term resolution of clinical signs of hydrocephalus has been achieved in dogs with these types of surgical shunting procedures. Experimental evidence suggests that reconstitution of the cerebral hemispheres after shunting occurs only in the white matter. Reconstituted white matter is characterized by myelin destruction, remyelination, and reactive astrocytosis. Because neuronal loss and cortical laminar destruction are irreversible, hydrocephalus should be treated aggressively as early as possible.

Shunting Complications. Regardless of the type of shunt used, strict aseptic technique and thorough hemostasis must be utilized to avoid shunt failure. The two most common complications of shunt placement in humans are infection and undershunting. Overshunting and seizures are less commonly encountered but possible. Undershunting (not removing enough CSF from the ventricle through the shunt) results from blockage, disconnection, or kinking of the catheter system.

Complications associated with overshunting have not been well described in the animals but mostly likely occur. In humans, overshunting results in formation of subdural hematomas and very small ventricular size (slit ventricle syndrome). Overshunting of CSF can cause collapse of the brain with tearing of vessels, which produces subdural hematoma formation.

Metabolic Encephalopathies

Treatment principles for metabolic encephalopathies include primary treatment of the specific underlying systemic condition and treatment of the secondary intracranial consequences (edema, hemorrhage, seizures) of the metabolic disturbance (see bibliography under Metabolic Diseases). Treatments for some metabolic disorders are listed in table 13.2. Current literature should be consulted

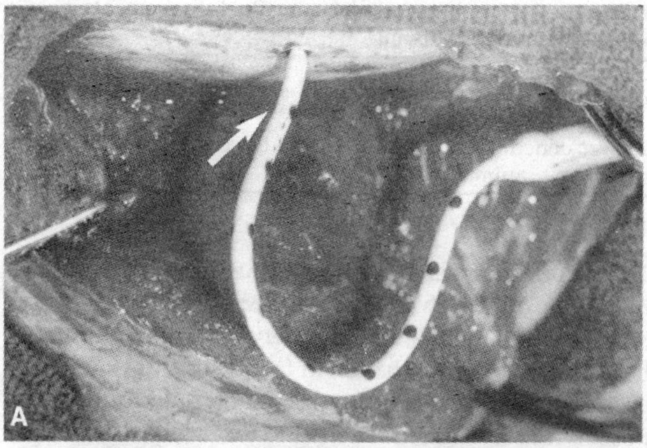

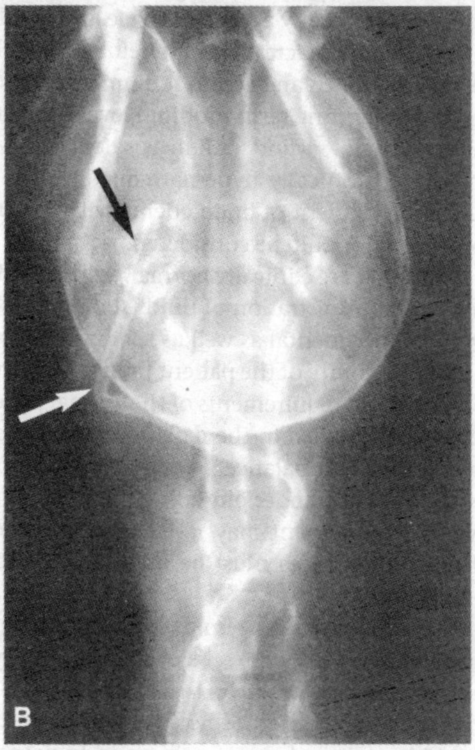

Fig. 13.3. (A) View at surgery of a ventriculoperitoneal shunt placed through a burr hole in the skull (*arrow*). (B) Ventrodorsal radiographic view of the VP shunt (*arrow*).

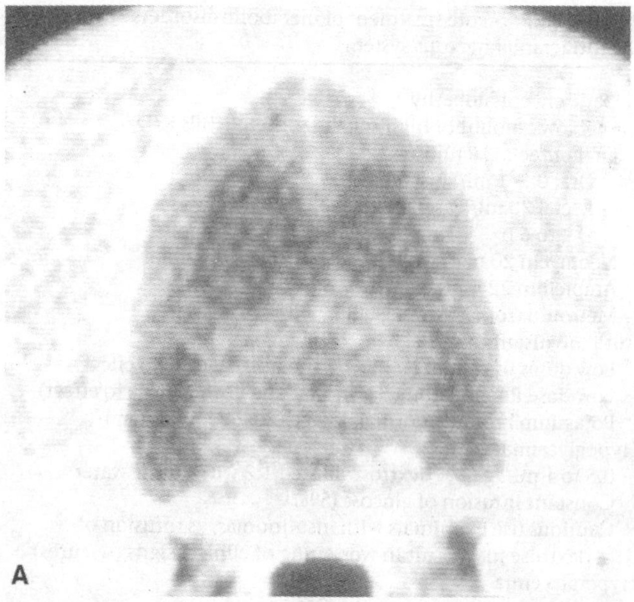

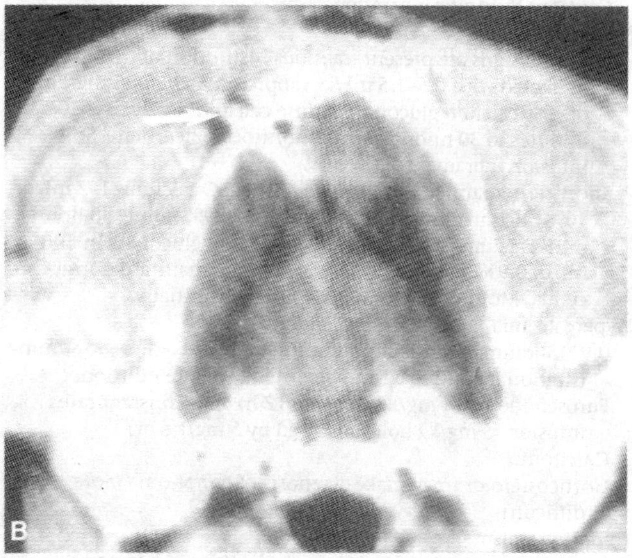

Fig. 13.4. Transverse CT image of a dog with hydrocephalus (A) before and (B) after implantation of a ventriculoperitoneal shunt (*arrow*).

regarding the most up-to-date treatment of specific metabolic conditions.

Cats with hyperglycemia from acromegaly most often have an associated pituitary tumor. These tumors may be treated with radiation therapy (see below, Neoplasia, Radiation Therapy).

Of the electrolyte disorder treatments, treatment of disorders of sodium have the potential to have significant influences on the CNS. Hypernatremia is most extreme in animals with abnormalities of thirst and drinking, which may also be associated with hypothalamic disease (Bagley 1994). Too rapid correction of hypernatremia with intravenous fluid administration can result in cerebral edema and severe alterations in mentation if not death. Acute hypernatremia can be treated by acute reduction of serum sodium concentrations. This can be accomplished by intravenous administration of relatively hypotonic fluids. Considering the elevation in serum sodium in many of these animals, even an isotonic fluid such as 0.9% sodium chloride is a relatively hypotonic fluid.

In established or chronic instances of sodium elevation, the brain compensates for a persistently hyperosmotic extracellular (EC) environment by the intracellular production of osmotically active products known as osmolytes (previous referred to as idiogenic osmoles). The composition of these osmolytes is unclear, but they may be glucose moieties or amino acids such as glutamate, aspartate, and GABA and other possible neurotransmitters.

Table 13.2. Acute treatment of metabolic disorders affecting the intracranial nervous system

- Hepatic encephalopathy
  - Diet low amount of high-quality protein (Hills K/D)
  - Oral or rectal lactulose
    - Oral 0.5–1 ml/kg Q 8 h
    - Rectal 20 ml/kg retained for 15 to 20 minutes Q 4 to 6 h
  - Neomycin 20 mg/kg q 8 h
  - Ampicillin 22 mg/kg q 8 h
  - Metronidazole 7.5 mg/kg q 8 h
- Anticonvulsants
  - Low doses of valium (1/4 to 1/2 the normal dose to effect)
  - Low dose Phenobarbital (1/4 to 1/2 the normal dose to effect)
  - Potassium bromide normal dosage (20–60 mg/kg/day)
- Hypoglycemia
  - 0.5 to 1 ml/kg 50% dextrose diluted 1:2 with sterile water
  - Constant infusion of glucose (5%)
  - Cautious use in animals with insulinomas, as infusion of dextrose may result in worsening of clinical signs (seizures)
- Hyperglycemia
  - Insulin
  - Cautious fluid administration
- Hypocalcemia
  - If clinical signs are present, cautious institution of treatment is indicated with 0.5–1.5 mL/kg (approximately 5–15 mg/kg) IV of 10% calcium gluconate. Infuse calcium slowly over 10 minutes to 30 minutes while monitoring heart rate. Stop infusion if bradycardia occurs.
  - Short-term maintenance involves either SC calcium (1–2 mL of 10% calcium gluconate diluted 1:1 in 0.9% saline q 8 hours) or IV calcium (10–20 mL of 10% calcium gluconate in 500 mL of 0.9% saline) with rate adjusted to maintain normocalcemia. Monitor calcium 2–3 times daily initially.
- Hypercalcemia
  - 0.9% Sodium chloride fluid administration at a diuretic administration level (2 to 3 times maintenance rate infusions)
  - Furosemide 1 to 4 mg/kg IV q 8 to 12 h) or as constant rate infusion (5 mg/kg bolus followed by 5 mg/kg/hr)
  - Calcitonin
  - Corticosteroids (may make diagnosis of lymphoma more difficult)
- Hypothyroidism
  - Myxedema coma (0.066–0.11 mg/kg IV thyroid hormone)
- Hypertriglyceridemia
  - Low fat diet
  - Gemfibrozil (7.5–10 mg/kg daily)
  - Marine (fish) oils rich in omega-3 fatty acids may help to decrease triglyceride concentrations.

Osmolytes are produced beginning between 1 and 4 hours after persistent ECF hyperosmolality, and are maximally effective at stabilizing brain water content by 7 days. While these osmolytes may be produced quickly in the hyperosomotic environment, they are broken down and removed much slower. If the serum sodium (and osmolality) is reduced acutely by too rapid administration or by a relatively hypotonic fluid, these osmolytes will serve to maintain intracellular hyperosmolality, and water will shift from the ECF intracellularly resulting in intracellular edema and potentially cell death.

Established hypernatremia (duration greater than 1 week) should be treated by *slowly* decreasing the serum sodium levels over *at least 48 hours* to prevent brain edema.

Table 13.3. Formulas for calculating fluid requirements in animals with hypernatremia

Water deficit (L) = 0.6 × lean body weight (kg) × animals sodium/normal sodium – 1
Sodium deficit (mEq/l) = 0.6 × lean body weight (kg) × (normal sodium – animal's sodium)

This can be performed by intravenous administration of a hypotonic fluid such as dextrose in water, but this may predispose to too rapid lowering of serum sodium and should be avoided. It is often better, in fact, to use an isotonic, or even a slightly hypertonic resuscitation fluid for this purpose. While recommendations and formulas exist as to the preferred rate of lowering of serum sodium (table 13.3), no specific rate is universally accepted as safe and is subject to individual patient characteristics. Therefore, clinical monitoring of patient status and serum sodium levels should be performed to determine serum sodium levels. In general, a slower reduction in serum sodium is safer. If neurologic signs occur in chronically hypernatremic animals during fluid therapy, treatment of brain edema with mannitol or hypertonic saline should be considered.

In animals that are clinically normal, adipsic and hypernatremic, oral administration of fluids should be a safe alternative. In experimental as well as spontaneously occurring adipsia, the ability of the patient to eat is not impaired. Therefore, the fluid requirements of the animal per day can be calculated and mixed in the daily food intake to maintain water intake and balance. Because this type of water administration is not under physiologic control, the anticipated water requirement may not always equal maintenance levels. Allowances must be made for situations of greater water loss.

In a chronically hyponatremia (hypoosmotic) environment, intracranial cells will translocate osmotically active particles such as potassium to the extracellular environment. In this compensated osmotic environment, similar to too rapid lowering of serum sodium in hypernatremia, too rapid correction of an established *hyponatremia* can result in intracranial lesions. In humans, these abnormalities tend to occur in the brain stem, hence the name for this syndrome is osmotic or central pontine myelinolysis. In dogs, bilaterally symmetrical lesions are common in the thalamus or may occur elsewhere in the brain (Churcher et al. 1999; O'Brien et al. 1994). These abnormalities are thought to result secondary to axonal shrinkage and associated demyelination.

For other primary intracellular metabolic abnormalities such as *mitochondrial encephalopathy,* there is no established treatment. Most affected animals have been euthanized due to deteriorating clinical signs.

Neoplasia

The most appropriate treatment for dogs with brain tumors has yet to be defined. Survival for dogs with brain tumors that are not treated is reportedly dismal (see bibliography under Brain Tumor). In one study, median survival for dogs with varying tumor types that did not have treatment was 6 days (Heidner et al. 1991). There are, however, anecdotal reports of dogs with brain tumors living for months to years without definitive treatment. The natural course and overall survival times of animals with brain tumors are not well established. This makes determination of treatment effects difficult.

Corticosteroids (beginning at 0.5 to 1 mg/kg every 12 hours orally) are often administered for sympathomatic treatment of the secondary pathophysiologic alterations of the tumor. In some instances, dramatic treatment responses are seen within hours or days following corticosteroid treatment. Usually, however, clinical improvement is finite. If the animal is rapidly deteriorating, intravenous corticosteroids (methylprednisolone sodium succinate or prednisone sodium succinate at 30 mg/kg IV administered over 10 to 15 minutes) can be administered.

Surgical Treatment. Surgical removal is ideal for superficially located, encapsulated, relatively small, benign tumors of which meningiomas would be the most common (figs. 13.5, 13.6, 13.7). Surgery also affords the possibility of

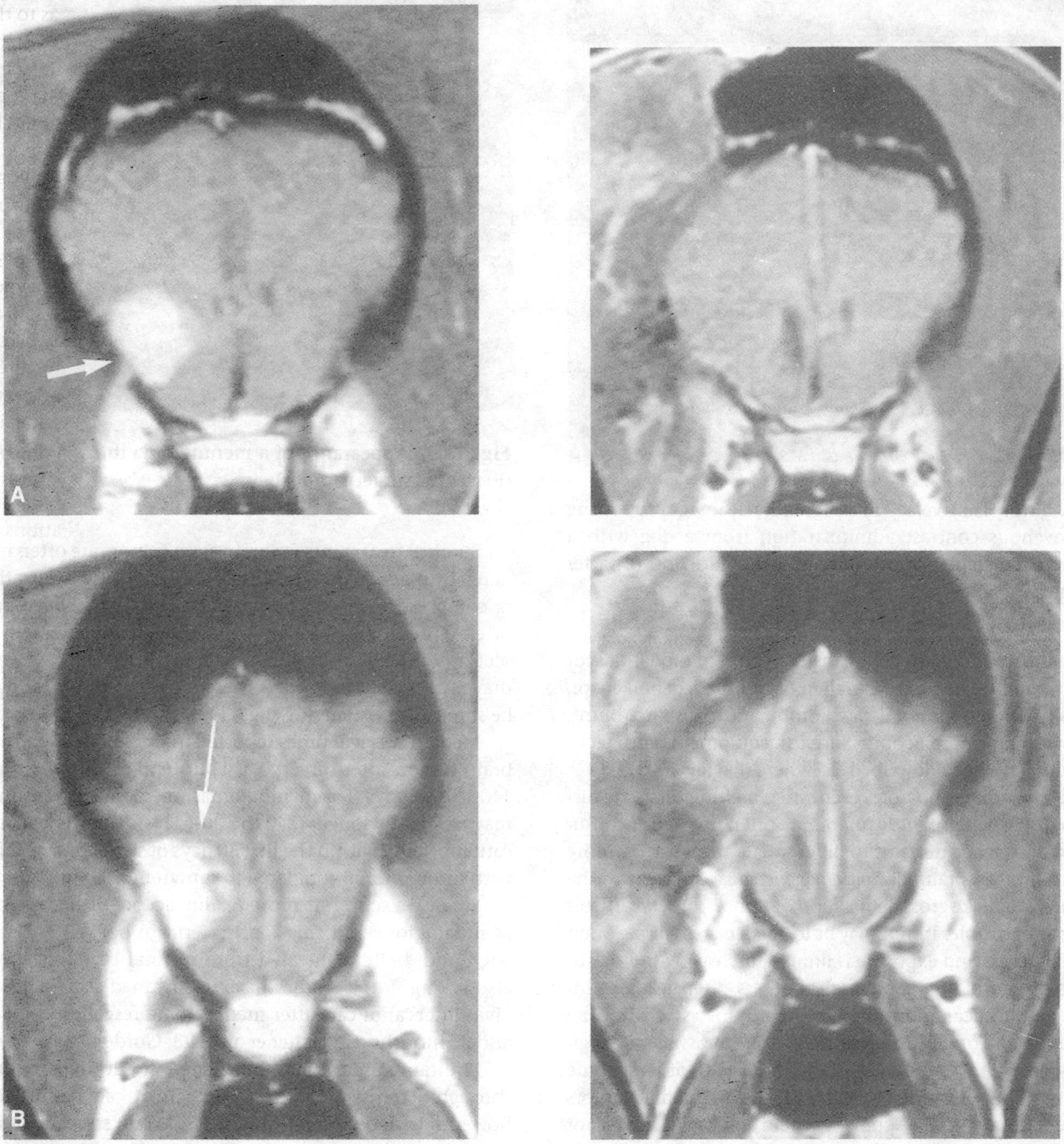

Fig. 13.5. (A,B) Transverse, T1-weighted MR images following intravenous contrast administration of dogs with meningioma (left) before and (right) after surgical removal.

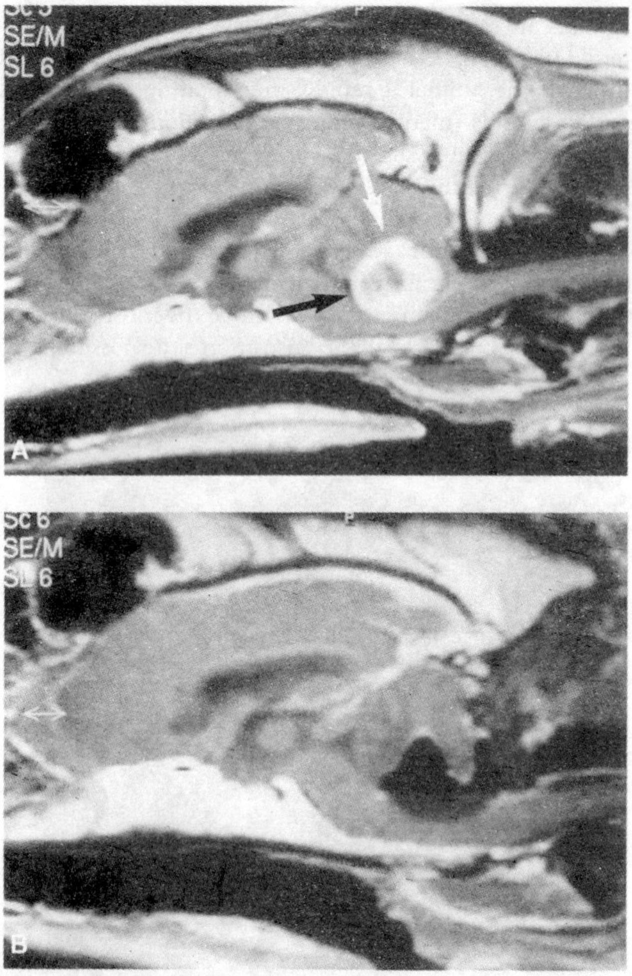

Fig. 13.6. Transverse, T1-weighted MR images following intravenous contrast administration from a dog with a fourth ventricular tumor (*arrows*) (A) before and (B) after surgical removal.

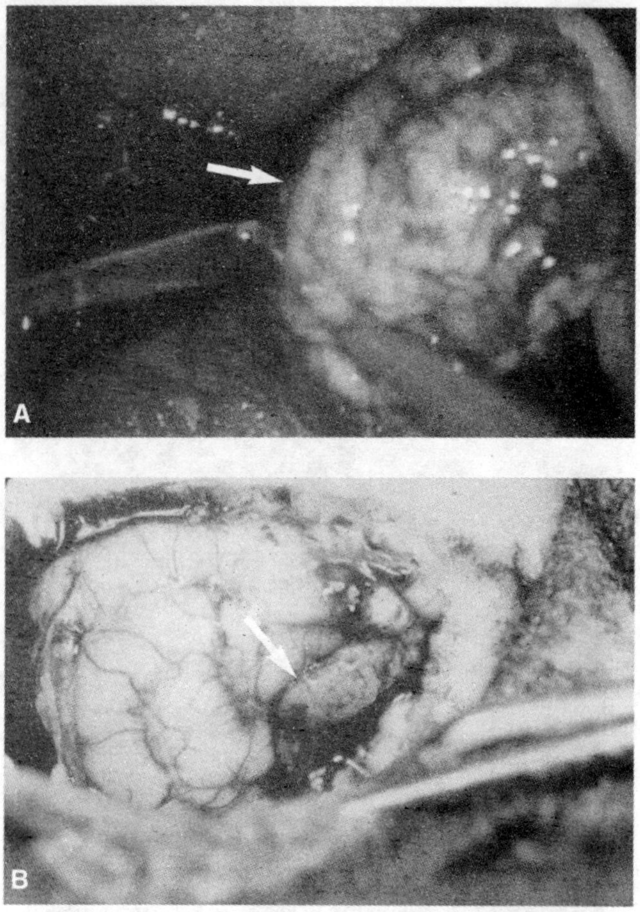

Fig. 13.7. Appearance of a meningioma in (A) a dog and (B) a cat at surgery (*arrow*).

cure that is uncommon with other treatment modalities for brain tumor. The tumor can then be biopsied, debulked, or, ideally, removed in total via a combination of sharp, blunt, and aspiration resection. Surgical equipment and techniques have been described elsewhere (Bagley 2003).

Unfortunately in dogs, even when meningiomas are histologically benign, these tumors are often not well encapsulated and hence difficult to differentiate from surrounding nontumorous brain. Brain damage in areas adjacent to the tumor can make gross delineation of tumor borders difficult if not impossible. Tumor may be located in areas of the brain where access and exposure is limited, increasing the risk of surgical morbidity. Poor surgical access often leads to increased surgical mortality. If the tumor is within the parenchyma or within a ventricle, it is impossible to surgically access these lesions without damage to at least some surrounding or overlying brain. Many intracranial tumors have multiple vessels supplying them lending to the risk of hemorrhage during resection. Possibly from these factors and others, dogs have historically had less than encouraging results with surgical treatment of brain tumors.

Surgical treatments for brain stem tumors are often hindered by inadequate exposure of the lesion and infiltration or compression of vital brain structures. Cranial nerves are often entwined within these masses making complete resection difficult. Tumors of the cranial nerves themselves may also occur. Removal of these types of tumors tends to be surgically challenging (figs. 13.8, 13.9).

Median survival times reported in dogs with all types of brain tumors after surgery vary but tend to cluster around 140 to 150 days. For meningiomas, median survival times may be slightly longer (240 to 300+ days). There is a significant mortality within the first 30 days of surgery for animals with infratentorial compared to supratentorial tumors.

Surgical excision is more readily accomplished in cats, as meningiomas in this species tend to be well encapsulated and easily delineated from normal brain (fig. 13.7; also see fig. 5.11). Studies have determined a median survival interval of cats after meningioma resection to be 22 and 27 months (Gallagher et al. 1993; Gordon et al. 1994).

Pituitary tumors may be treated surgically primarily through a transsphenoidal approach. It can be difficult, however, to access larger tumors (>1.0 cm) surgically leading to incomplete removal and increased surgical morbidity. While these tumors are generally radiation responsive, the associated endocrine abnormalities may require longer

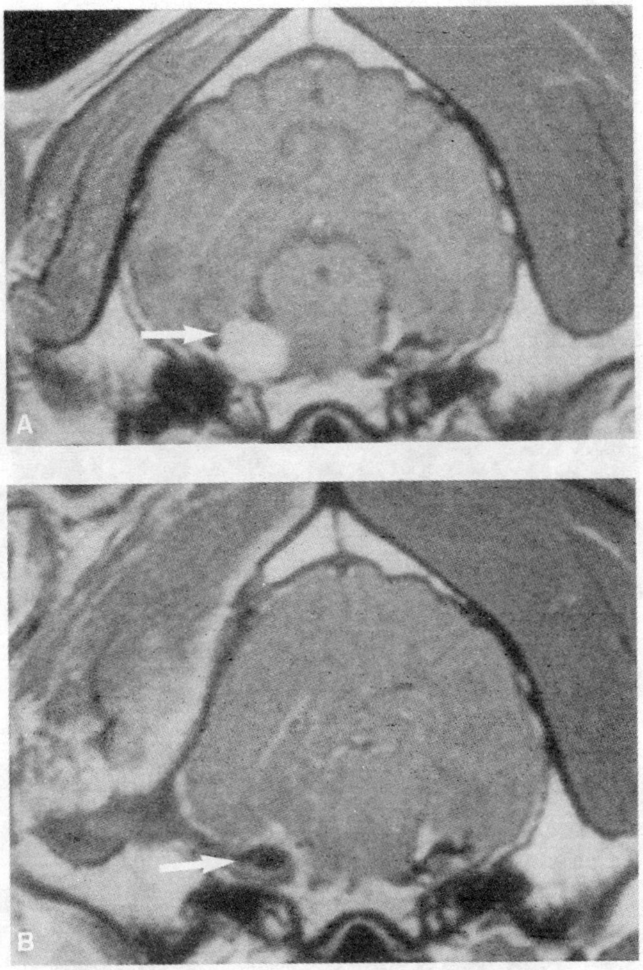

Fig. 13.8. Transverse, T1-weighted MR images following intravenous contrast administration from a dog with a trigeminal nerve tumor (*arrow*) (A) before and (B) after surgical removal.

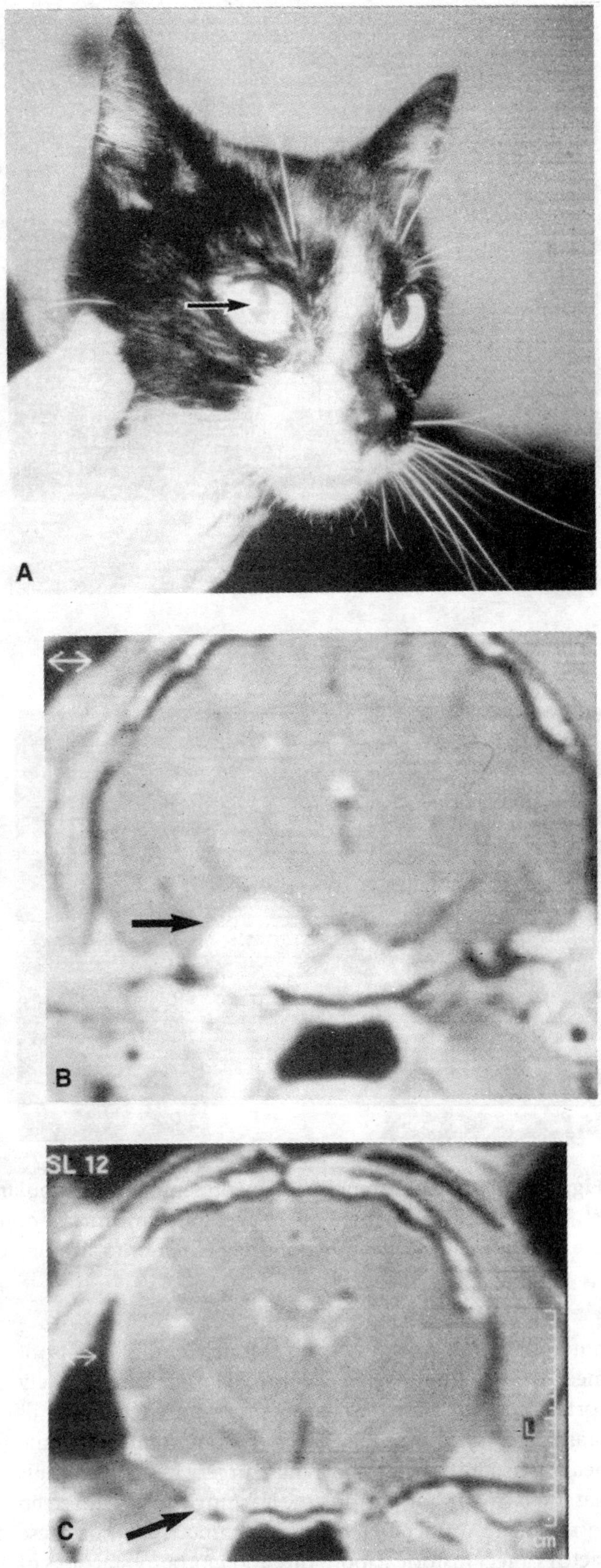

Fig. 13.9. (A) Corneal ulcer in a cat with a trigeminal nerve tumor. Transverse, T1-weighted MR images following intravenous contrast administration from the cat with a trigeminal nerve tumor (B) before and (C) after surgical removal.

periods of time (weeks to months) to resolve. In some instances, it is speculated that smaller pituitary tumors can enlarge rapidly after antiadrenal therapy (Nelson's syndrome) (Feldman et al. 1996). The resultant increased intracranial mass effect results in an acute onset of intracranial signs.

Treatment of metastatic tumor to the brain is rarely performed in animals. With humans, however, surgical removal of metastases often improves survival. Tumors invading the skull, such as multilobular chondrosarcoma or osteosarcoma, may also be surgically removable if treated early before significant skull involvement occurs (fig. 13.10).

Many factors may affect survival following brain surgery including neurologic and systemic abnormalities. In general, most dogs are probably diagnosed relatively late in the course of their disease and only when clinical signs become obvious. By this time, the tumors are relatively large, have caused significant associated brain injury, and are often infiltrative or tightly adherent to the nervous tissue. There may be an overall deterioration of systemic health prior to definitive treatment either from lack of adequate

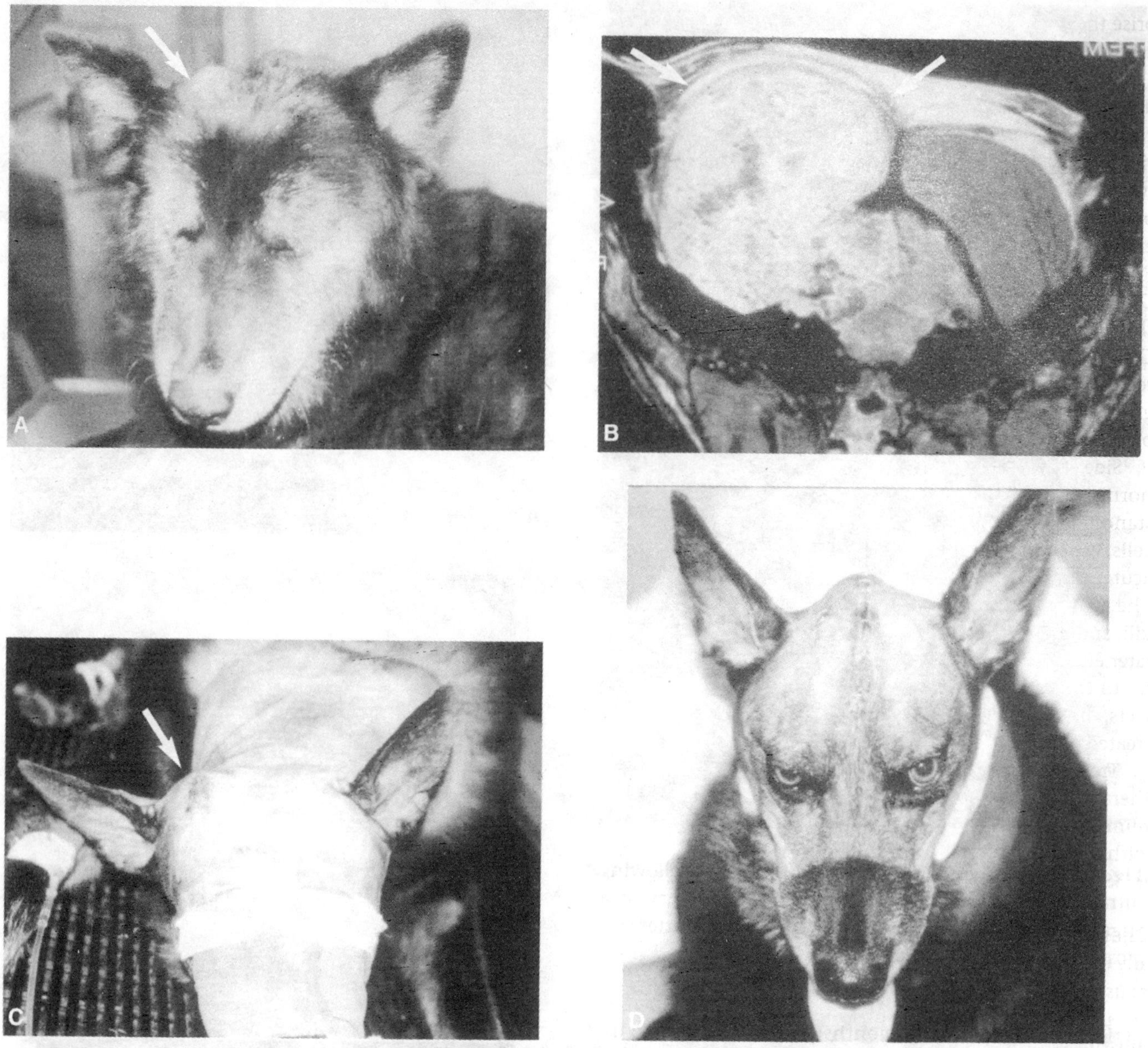

Fig. 13.10. (A) Appearance of a dog presented for vestibular signs and an enlargement of the right side of the head (*arrow*). (B) Transverse, T1-weighted MR images following intravenous contrast administration from the same dog showing a mass of the skull (*arrows*). Appearance of a dog (C) prior to and (D) following surgical resection of the tumor.

nutrition, chronic stress, pain, or deleterious effects of medications administered to control clinical signs, namely corticosteroids. Nonnervous system organ effects such as brain-heart syndrome may adversely compromise systemic health. In addition, as intracranial surgery in small animals has a relatively short history, the learning curve is still steep in regard to intracranial surgical techniques. All of these factors affect historical morbidity and mortality statistics of animals with brain tumors.

Surgical treatment of brain tumor should ideally not only cure the tumor but also improve or resolve the clinical signs associated with the tumor. Surgical resection of tumors, for example, may increase the likelihood of seizure control or help in the control of effects of increased ICP.

Radiation Therapy. As a primary therapy for brain tumors, conventional radiation therapy has been shown reasonably effective for brain tumor in dogs. Radiation therapy is more apt to control tumor progression, and, in some instances, it may eradicate the tumor completely. The main goal of the radiation treatment is to administer to the tumor the highest possible radiation dose while minimizing the dose to the surrounding normal tissue. Conventional radiation therapy techniques vary and are beyond the scope of this chapter. Mass localization can only be approximated from CT or MR imaging studies. It is generally accepted to treat a 2–4 cm size margin around the contrast enhancing mass seen on the imaging studies. When using CT or MR planning, the portal should comprise the contrast enhancing mass, peritumor edema, and a 1 cm margin.

Fractional dosing schemes (administering smaller doses of radiation more frequently) have been used to decrease the acute toxicity of the radiation. A coarse (higher single dose) fractionation scheme is around 6 Gy fractions twice weekly over 3 weeks. The majority of dogs treated for brain masses have been treated with 10–12 fractions, generally given three times weekly (Monday, Wednesday, and Friday) of approximately 4 Gy each, for a total dose of 48 Gy. These doses appeared to be generally well tolerated for the periods studied. It is suggested that a fraction size of 3 Gy will reduce the incidence of late responding tissue. It is recommended, therefore, that daily fractions of 3 Gy be given up to 4 weeks, with the total normal tissue dose below 50–55 Gy.

Side effects usually are the result of radiation damage to normal structures surrounding the tumor. In many instances, this damage involves blood vessel endothelial cells, with subsequent cerebrovascular complications. Both acute, early delayed, and late delayed affects can be seen. The acute effects may be the result of edema due to tumor kill, and may be reversed with antiedema medications. The later effects may not be reversible and may be as detrimental to the animals as the underlying disease. Late side effects, however, are relatively rare (<15% of all animals treated depending upon treatment protocols utilized).

Treatment protocols and survival analysis for radiation therapy of brain tumors has been reported in a limited number of studies in dogs. Median survival in dogs treated with conventional radiation therapy is usually between 150 to 350 days.

Chemotherapy. Chemotherapy is used as primary therapy or as an adjunct to surgery in selected instances in animals with brain tumors (Dimiski 1990). Chemotherapies are primarily used for treatment of gliomas. BCNU (carmustine) and CCNU (lomustine) are alkylating agents that have some effectiveness primarily against gliomas. These are given intravenously at 6-week intervals (depending on the protocol). Dosage is 50 to 60 mg/m^2. Side effects include bone marrow suppression (monitor CBC 1 week after administration). Hydroxyurea (20 mg/kg orally every 24 hours) is also being evaluated for treatment of meningiomas and other brain tumors. Other chemotherapeutic agents that have been used for CNS neoplasia such as primary lymphoma include cytosine arabinoside (crosses the BBB readily) and methotrexate.

Nutritional

Thiamine deficiency is most common in cats, but is occasionally recognized in dogs. Treatment for this vitamin deficiency is administration of thiamine dosed typically at 5–30 mg/cat/day orally. The maximum dose is usually up to 50 mg/cat/day. Dogs can be given 5–50 mg/day. Severely affected cats should receive at least 1 mg of thiamine parenterally. Change the diet to one with adequate thiamine and supplement with thiamine for at least a week following the change. Treatment of any primary disease that results in anorexia may also be important.

Inflammatory Diseases

Treatment of encephalitis and meningitis is ideally directed at a specific causative organism. Without a definable specific cause, the author has had the best treatment success using multiple drug therapies rather than single agent modalities, and by treating earlier rather than later in the disease course. Trimethoprim-sulfadiazine (30 mg/kg q 12 h), clindamycin (20–25 mg/kg q 12 h), and corticosteroids (prednisone 1–4 mg/kg q 12 h) are used in combination. While corticosteroids may seem contraindicated with infectious diseases, they are often beneficial in the acute treatment of brain inflammation and edema. These associated pathophysiological events are more often the cause of the neurologic deterioration than primary cell death from the organism itself. If rickettsial diseases are suspected, doxycycline (10–20 mg/kg q 12 h PO) or, less ideally, chloramphenicol (15–25 mg/kg q 8 h PO) can be substituted or added to the regime. If the animal is receiving phenobarbital, *do not* use chloramphenicol, as this drug will decrease the metabolism of the barbiturate and the animal will become comatose and possible die.

Bacteria. If possible, antimicrobial therapy for bacterial encephalitis should be based on the results of bacteria identification (culture) and subsequent antimicrobial sensitivity toward the organism. As identification of the organism may take a few days and the clinical signs are often rapidly progressive, treatment is commonly initiated prior to definitive culture results being established. As stated previously, prior to a specific cause being identified, the author uses trimethoprim sulfadiazine, clindamycin, doxycycline, and corticosteroids in combination for treatment of CNS inflammation/infection. Metronidazole (10 mg/kg IV slowly every 8 hours) may be used when anaerobic infections are suspected. Ampicillin (22 mg/kg every 6 to 12 hours), enrofloxacin (10 mg/kg IV every 12 hours), or cefotaxime (25 to 50 mg/kg IV every 8 hours) may also be used. If improvement is seen, antibiotic therapy should be continued at least 4 weeks or past resolution of all clinical signs.

Methylprednisolone sodium succinate (30 mg/kg) can be administered intravenously initially if the animal is severely impaired or rapidly deteriorating and if the animal is unable to swallow. If the animal is more mildly affected and can swallow effectively, oral prednisone/prednisolone (beginning at 1 to 2 mg/kg every 12 hours) can then be initiated at anti-inflammatory dosages. Low-dose dexamethasone (dexamethasone sodium phosphate at 0.1 to 0.15 mg/kg) may also be used. There appears to be an increased incidence of gastrointestinal ulceration in animals with severe neurologic impairment that are administered corticosteroids (primarily dexamethasone). Daily assessment for GI bleeding (such as examination of feces) should be performed. Prophylactic antiulcer medications (Carafate, ranitidine, omeprazole) may be used concurrently, and certainly in the presence of obvious GI ulceration. Assessment for associated GI disease (i.e., parasites) is also prudent.

In some instances, intracranial bacterial infection will coalesce to form a discrete abscess. As an abscess and its associated inflammation can rapidly increase intracranial pressure, surgical drainage/decompression of a focal abscess should occur as soon as possible after detection. Similarly, penetrating intracranial wounds may require debridement to avoid infectious complications.

Virus. Treatment of viral encephalitis is rarely reported. Antiviral agents such as acyclovir or zidovudine (AZT) have been alluded to, but clinical reports are scarce. Corticosteroids, while seemingly contraindicated, may decrease inflammation and improve clinical signs in some dogs. For feline infectious peritonitis (FIP) immunosuppressive therapy (usually with corticosteroids) may result in short-term improvement of clinical signs.

Protozoan. *Toxoplasma gondii* and *Neospora caninum* are protozoal organisms that often affect the nervous system. These organisms can result in encephalitis, myelitis, and occasionally a peripheral neuropathy, or myositis in dogs. Of the CNS infectious diseases, treatment of toxoplasmosis is usually the most successful.

Treatment recommendations for toxoplasmosis currently include administering clindamycin, however, this drug is often used in combination with a potentiated sulfa drug in immunosuppressed humans with CNS toxoplasmosis. Treatment for toxoplasmosis currently is clindamycin (8–25 mg/kg, q 8–12 hours; do not exceed 50 mg/kg q 24 hours) for 14–28 days, however, the addition of trimethoprim sulfa drugs PO, IM, or SC may provide a better clinical response. Trimethoprim sulfa antibiotics alone have also been used successfully to treat CNS toxoplasmosis. A similar treatment is used for neosporosis, however, few cases with definitive treatment success have been reported. Treatment courses of antibiotics usually are 4 weeks or more in duration. If clinical signs resolve within this time, antimicrobial therapy may be discontinued after 4 weeks and the animal monitored for clinical deterioration. Some animals with toxoplasmosis will have periodic relapses (recrudescence?) of clinical signs that require additional courses of therapy. In still other animals, continual (chronic) treatment with antimicrobials is necessary to control clinical signs. Newer drugs, such as azithromycin and clarithromycin (macrolides), are being evaluated for treatment of toxoplasmosis.

Rickettsia. Infection with rickettsial organisms associated with Rocky Mountain spotted fever (RMSF) and *Ehrlichia* commonly involve the brain stem, particularly the vestibular system. Dogs with clinical features of vestibular disease after a systemic febrile illness associated with thrombocytopenia should be treated with tetracycline or doxycycline (10 mg/kg every 12 to 24 hours) prior to establishing a definitive diagnosis with titers. For RMSF, treatment usually is only necessary for 7 to 14 days. Chloramphenicol may also be effective for RMSF but is rarely used in the modern era. For ehrlichiosis, treatment may need to be prolonged (weeks to months).

Fungal. Of the fungal diseases that can affect the nervous system, cryptococcus, blastomycosis, coccidiomycosis, candidiasis, and aspergillosis are most common. Immunodeficiency may play a role in these uncommon nervous system infections. Definitive diagnosis is made through viewing the organism in CSF or biopsy samples and fungal culture of infected nervous tissues. Treatment can be attempted with antifungal agents, however, the presence of an intact blood-brain barrier may hinder the ability of the drug to reach therapeutic concentration in CNS tissues. Fluconazole and itraconazole hold the most promise for treating fungal encephalitis/meningitis. These drugs have historically been comparatively expensive and owner financial constrains often limit long-term therapy with these drugs. Additionally, treatment for these fungal infections is often prolonged, if not lifelong, to control clinical signs.

Parasites. Ivermectin (400 µg/kg single dose administered subcutaneously) has been suggested as a treatment for CNS parasites, but its efficacy is unknown. It is recommended to pretreat with diphenhydramine (1 to 4 mg/kg IV) and corticosteroids (dexamethasone 0.1 mg/kg) prior to administration of ivermectin to avoid systemic anaphylactic-type reactions. Decreases in the secondary inflammatory responses to parasitic migration may be achieved with corticosteroids. Ivermectin has increased toxicity in collies, some shelties, and possibly other dogs due to cellular transport abnormalities (deficient P-glycoprotein).

Noninfectious Diseases

Of the spectrum of inflammatory diseases that can affect the CNS, more often the cause of the inflammation is either undetermined or not associated with an established infectious agent. For many of these conditions, effective treatment does not exist. Corticosteroids are often a mainstay of therapy for many animals with inflammatory intracranial diseases. For some diseases, such as pug, Yorkshire terrier, and Maltese encephalitis, corticosteroid therapy is inconsistently helpful. In other instances, such as with "corticosteroid responsive meningitis," eosinophilic meningoencephalitis, and some spinal cord vasculitis syndromes, corticosteroid therapy may be beneficial. Prednisolone beginning at 1–2 mg/kg every 12 hours is used. If clinical signs improve in 3 to 5 days, this treatment should be continued for at least 2 weeks. If, after this time the animal's clinical signs resolve, the dosage of corticosteroid can be slowly decreased over weeks to months to avoid recurrence.

If corticosteroid therapy provides beneficial, it is often necessary to administer these medications for prolonged periods of time, if not for the life span of the animal. Discontinuation of the therapy should be performed slowly over weeks if not months to prevent recurrence of clinical signs.

Table 13.4. Suggested medical treatments for GME

Prednisolone or prednisone
- 1–4 mg/kg every 12 to 24 hours

Cyclophosphamide
- 50 mg/m^2/day (orally) 4 days/week

Azathioprine
- 2 mg/kg orally initially, then 0.5–1 mg/kg every 48 hours

Cytosine arabinoside
- 50 mg/m^2 (SC) every 12 hours for 2 days, repeat every 3 weeks

Procarbazine
- 25–50 mg/m^2 (orally) daily, try to reduce to every other day after first month

Leflunomide
- 4 mg/kg every 24 hours

Cyclosporin A
- 5–10 mg/kg/day divided

Granulomatous meningoencephalitis can occur as a disseminated disease, as a focal mass-lesion, or as a primary ocular disease. Treatment options include immunosuppression (corticosteroids, cyclophosphamide, azathioprine), other immunomodulators (leflunomide), chemotherapeutics such as lomustine, surgery (if a focal mass), or radiation therapy (table 13.4). The latter has shown the most promise recently for definitive treatment of this disease. Newer medical treatments under investigation that show promise in treatment of GME include cytosine arabinoside and procarbazine (Cuddon 1998). Many of these treatments, however, are based on presumptive diagnosis of GME and anecdotal treatment responses. The efficacy of any of these treatments, therefore, is uncertain. As these drug therapies may affect bone marrow cellular production, monitoring of CBC for cytopenias is important.

There is a unique clinical syndrome (generalized tremor syndrome; white shaker dog syndrome) associated with generalized tremoring, which is usually associated with CNS inflammation. Generalized tremor secondary to nervous system inflammation usually improves with administration of glucocorticoids at immunosuppressive dosages. The tremor usually lessens or resolves within 1 to 3 weeks with this therapy. The dosage of corticosteroid can then be slowly decreased. If the drug is decreased too rapidly, tremor may recur. If recurrence is seen, a prolonged tapering of corticosteroid over 4 to 6 months may be necessary. Occasionally, a dog may require corticosteroid treatment indefinitely to control the tremor.

Idiopathic

Treatment of *idiopathic epilepsy* with anticonvulsants is discussed in chapter 17, which deals with seizures (see also appendix 3). *Narcolepsy* can be treated with sympathomimetics or other CNS stimulants (Thomas 2003). Sympathomimetics include methylphenidate (0.25 mg/kg orally every 8 to 12 hours) and dextroamphetamine (5–10 mg orally every 8 to 12 hours). Selegiline or L-deprenyl (1 mg/kg orally daily) has been suggested to increase activity, primarily in older dogs with potential cognitive dysfunction. Cataplexy often accompanies narcolepsy. Treatment recommendations for cataplexy include tricylic antidepressants to block reuptake of norepinephrine and imipramine to block serotonin reuptake. Suggested dosage for these drugs are: amitriptyline (1–2 mg/kg orally every 12 hours), fluoxetine (1 mg/kg orally every 24 hours), protryptiline (5–10) mg orally every 24 hours), and imipramine (0.4–1.0 mg/kg orally every 8 to 12 hours). Imipramine has also been suggested as a diagnostic test for narcolepsy and may increase, in certain dosages, narcoleptic activity.

Treatment for *feline hyperesthesia syndrome* usually includes initial anti-inflammatory drugs. Corticosteroid therapy (prednisolone) may help if a flea allergy or other inflammatory stimulus is suspected. Strict flea control may improve clinical signs. Behavior modifying drugs such as the tricyclic antidepressants amitriptyline (2 mg/kg or 5–10 mg/cat PO q 24 h), clomipramine (1–5mg/cat PO q 12-24 h) or the selective serotonin uptake inhibitors fluoxetine (Prozac 0.5–4 mg/cat PO q 24 h) or paroxetine (Paxil, 0.5 mg/kg PO q 24 h) may be helpful in some cats. Anticonvulsants (phenobarbital beginning at 3 mg/kg PO q 12 h with dose adjustments to maintain trough serum levels at 20–35 mcg/ml) may help if anti-inflammatories and behavior modifying drugs are unsuccessful. Feeding food without preservatives has been suggested as helpful. Carnitine/coenzyme Q_{12} may help cats with vacuolar myopathy. Also antioxidants and omega-3 fatty acids may be useful. Decreases in environmental stress may also be helpful.

Trauma

Treatment recommendations for traumatic brain injury is controversial and oftentimes confusing. For a more in-depth discussion see chapter 22. Much of the confusion arises because anecdotal information from noncontrolled observations becomes accepted into management strategies, and experimental studies usually focus on a single aspect of traumatic brain injury while intracranial and systemic pathophysiological events associated with brain trauma are complex and interdependent. Many issues regarding management of traumatic brain disease remain controversial in humans as well and a consensus on the most appropriate management of these injuries still does not exist.

Treatment for the primary injury associated with the traumatic incident is obviously not possible. Treatment is directed, therefore, toward the secondary pathological effects of the trauma, such as edema, impairment of vascular supply to normal tissue (ischemia), impairment of cerebrovascular autoregulation, hemorrhage (intraparenchymal, intraventricular, extradural or subdural), irritation (seizure generation), obstruction of the ventricular system, production of physiologically active products, and finally, increased intracranial pressure (ICP).

Fluid resuscitation is critical to maintain cerebral perfusion and aid in stabilizing intracranial pressure. Other treatments mainly center around stabilization of cerebral blood flow and reversal of increased intracranial pressure (see treatment of ICP in this chapter). Surgical decompres-

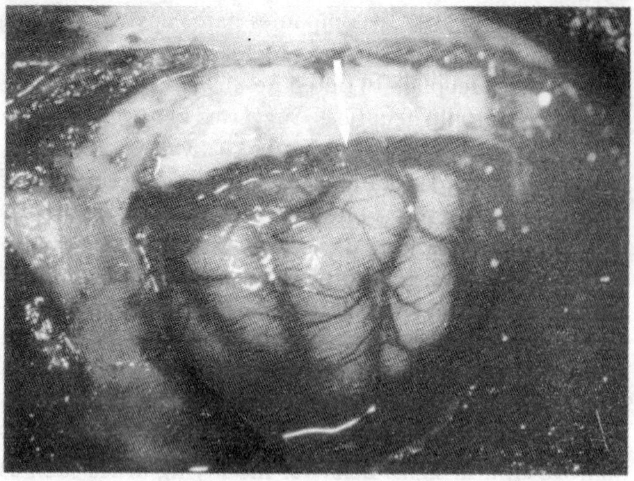

Fig. 13.11. Appearance of a cat brain swelling beyond the limits of a craniectomy *(arrow)*.

Table 13.5. Treatment of head trauma

Therapies with established efficacy
- Fluid resuscitation
  Isotonic fluids
- Diuretics
- Mannitol

Therapies with possible but currently unknown efficacy
- Hypertonic saline
- Head elevation
- Furosemide
- Hyperventilation
- Cerebrospinal fluid aspiration
- Miscellaneous drugs
  Deferoxamine mesylate
  Superoxide dismutase
  Allopurinol
  Opiate antagonists (naloxone)
  Thyrotropin-releasing hormone and calcium channel blockers
- Craniotomy

Therapies with unknown efficacy and potential detrimental effects
- Corticosteroids
- Cerebrospinal fluid aspiration

sion may be indicated to remove hemorrhage or debris. Craniectomy also allows for primary intracranial decompression (fig. 13.11). A list of apparently helpful and questionable efficacy treatments is found in table 13.5.

Toxicity

Treatment for CNS toxicities vary with the toxin agent (Dorman 2003). Current poison control treatment guidelines should be consulted for up-to-date treatment options. Lead toxicity can be treated with chelation therapy with calcium EDTA (25 mg/kg SC, IM, or IV q 6 h for 2 to 5 days) or penicillamine (10–15 mg/kg PO q 12 h) may be necessary to improve clinical signs. Treatment of strychnine poisoning and metaldehyde toxicity includes control of seizure activity and muscle rigidity with barbiturates and, possibly, muscle relaxants. Treatment of metronidazole toxicity is primarily supportive following discontinuation of the medication. Diazepam administration appears helpful for this toxicity (Evans et al. 2003).

Cerebrovascular Diseases

Primary treatment for cerebrovascular disease is not possible once the thrombosis or embolus has occurred. Intracranial treatments are directed at the secondary pathophysiological events such as edema, hemorrhage, ischemia, and increases in ICP. Cerebral edema can be treated primarily with diuretics but will be benefited by control of increased ICP. As cerebral edema contributes to intracranial volume and, subsequently, increases in ICP, treatments that decrease cerebral edema are often used to lower ICP. Caution should be exercised in some instances, as rapid decreases in ICP can actually result in intracranial hemorrhage (Coulter and Gooch 1993).

Treatment for CNS bleeding includes treatment of any underlying bleeding disorder and stopping or resolving the local effects of any accumulated hemorrhage. Various treatments exist for individual coagulopathies and for thrombocytopenia. Current recommendations for treatment of these bleeding disorders should be reviewed.

Treatment for a localized hematoma within the CNS is focused on evacuation of the hematoma usually via a craniotomy or craniectomy. If the underlying bleeding disorder is still active, a dilemma exists between the need for surgical hematoma drainage and the risk of causing increasing amounts of hemorrhage. Short-term hemostatic support with blood products or platelets may provide a window of patient stability for a surgical procedure to be performed. Ultimately, if the accumulation of bleeding in the central nervous system is becoming life-threatening, surgical drainage is a necessity, which is undertaken in view of the increased risk of hemorrhagic complications. While it is impossible to reverse all of the effects of the hemorrhage, decreasing the size of an expanding hematoma with the resultant decrease in nervous tissue pressure may improve clinical signs. There are two caveats to consider. One is that by decreasing intraparenchymal pressure, blood flow to the area may be restored, and a rebound hemorrhage may occur. Second, along the same lines, if the original cause of the bleeding was a ruptured vessel (aneurysm or arteriovenous malformation), hematoma removal may result in rebleeding. In both of these situations, however, hemostasis can hopefully be employed intraoperatively to decrease this possibility.

In chronic hematomas, especially if the initial bleeding tendency has subsided, surgical drainage is reasonably straightforward if the extent of the hematoma can be localized. Usually, a black, sometimes greenish, soft lesion consistent with an established hematoma is found. This can be removed with suction aspiration. The edges of the hematoma tend to be more organized requiring blunt dissection for removal.

Treatment for hypertensive encephalopathy includes treatment to lower blood pressure, with concurrent treatment of intracranial mass effect (e.g., hemorrhage), or increased intracranial pressure. Treatment of hypertensive crisis often includes administration of angiotensin-converting enzyme inhibitors (e.g., enalapril), calcium channel blockers (e.g., amlodipine), and sometimes cardioselective beta blockers (e.g., atenolol) (Littman 2002; Blumenfeld 2001).

Diuretic administration may have significant advantages in patients with both hypertension and associated intracranial disease to lower total vascular volume and decrease blood viscosity (to lower resistance and improve cerebral blood flow). One of the most important factors in treating brain injury, however, is to maintain cerebral blood flow, primarily through maintenance of systemic blood pressure. Caution should be exercised in the hypertensive animal that has concurrent intracranial disease to prevent rebound hypotension during treatment for hypertension (Goldstein 2000). This relative decrease in blood pressure may ultimately result in more significant intracranial injury due to cerebral ischemia and hypoxia.

In some instances, metabolic diseases such as hypothyroidism and hyperadrenocorticism may result in cerebrovascular abnormalities. Treatment for these and other underlying conditions is also necessary current with any specific intracranial treatments. Prophylactic treatment of animals with a propensity for thrombosis or emboli formation is important to avoid cerebrovascular complications of underlying systemic disease.

Treatment for Diseases of Cranial Nerves

Cranial nerves can occasionally be affected with disease independent of the intracranial nervous structures. In some instances, specific treatments exist for these abnormalities.

Optic neuritis not associated with a specific etiology is often treated with corticosteroids (prednisolone or prednisone at 1 to 4 mg/kg orally every 12 hours) usually administered for at least 1 to 2 weeks, depending upon return of vision. Often, corticosteroid treatments are maintained for 2 to 4 weeks in duration. In some instances, intravenous corticosteroids (methylprednisolone sodium succinate at 30 mg/kg IV slowly over 10 to 15 minutes) are given for a more rapid clinical response. If optic neuritis is associated with another disease process, such as a fungal infection, appropriate treatment for this underlying disease should also be initiated.

Dysautonomia is a disease characterized by dysfunction of the autonomic system. In addition to other clinical signs, such as vomiting and constipation, dilated, poorly to unresponsive pupils may be seen. Treatment for this disease is usually directed at supporting bodily functions including fluid and nutritional support.

Trigeminal neuritis is a poorly characterized but surprising common disease of the mandibular branches of cranial nerve V bilaterally. Most dogs should improve within the first 4 weeks following clinical signs. Corticosteroid therapy has been suggested, however, no treatment has shown benefit. Most complications from this disease are associated with the animal's inability to close the mouth when eating or drinking. In some instances, providing the animal a large, raised water bowl may provide the dog with an easier method of lapping water. Soft food may be manually placed in the caudal mouth so that it can be swallowed. Caution should be exercised in doing so, however, to avoid aspiration of food material. In other instances, esophagostomy or gastrostomy tube placement will allow for administration of food and water until the clinical signs improve.

Tumors may arise on or around the trigeminal nerve. Trigeminal nerve abnormalities can occur with infiltrating neoplasia (*lymphosarcomas*) that involve a branch or the entire nerve. *Myelomonocytic leukemias* and other hematocellular neoplasia may affect this nerve. Chemotherapies for lymphoma and leukemias may be used as treatment if these etiologies are identified. Cytosine arabinoside is often added to chemotherapeutic treatment protocols due to the relatively good CSF penetration with this drug.

Tumors of the coverings of the nerve (*nerve sheath tumors*) may arise on or around the trigeminal nerve. Surgical removal of these tumors has been performed but can result in cosmetic consequences due to complete trigeminal denervation of head muscles (figs. 13.8, 13.9). Radiation therapy has been used in a limited number of cases with apparently encouraging results.

Facial Nerve. Facial paralysis is the most common abnormality seen with facial nerve disease. This can occur as an idiopathic condition (especially in cocker spaniels) as a result of otitis media/interna, with trauma, and with tumor of the middle ear canal. Speculation in humans centers around a chronic herpes virus infection as a cause of idiopathic facial nerve (Bell's) palsy. Acyclovir may be attempted as therapy, however, therapeutic responses are poorly described. Hypothyroidism is a possible associated cause in some dogs. Treatment of hypothyroidism with thyroid hormone replacement therapy may bring about resolution of clinical signs in some instances. Occult or obvious middle ear or inner ear infection may also result in facial paralysis. Treatment for otitis interna such as systemic antibiotics (clavulanic acid) or surgical debridement (bulla osteotomy) may be necessary.

Vestibulocochlear Nerve. Diagnosis and treatment of vestibular disease is also discussed in chapter 18. Treatment of any primary disease process is necessary to bring about resolution of clinical signs.

Hypothyroidism is an infrequently associated cause in some dogs. Treatment of hypothyroidism with thyroid hormone replacement therapy may bring about resolution of clinical signs in some instances. Tumors of the ear more often occur in older animals. Squamous cell carcinoma and adenocarcinoma are most common. Treatment may include surgical resection or radiation therapy. Inflammatory polyps occur in cats. These may be seen on otoscopic evaluation or with oral examination. Surgical removal of these polyps is often helpful. As vestibular complications may occur with some drug therapies, discontinuation of such drugs may bring about improvement in clinical signs.

Otitis media/interna is a common cause of vestibular dysfunction. Treatment for otitis interna such as systemic antibiotics (clavulanic acid) or surgical debridement (bulla osteotomy) may be necessary.

Idiopathic peripheral vestibular disease occurs in both dogs and cats. Older dogs (*canine geriatric vestibular disease*) and young to middle-aged cats are most commonly affected. Treatment with diphenhydramine (1 mg/kg IV or orally every 8 to 12 hours), diazepam (5 to 10 mg PO q 6 to 8 hours) or meclizine may provide some relief. Similarly, valium administration may decrease anxiety and allow for some relaxation.

Clinical signs of idiopathic vestibular disease usually improve dramatically in 1 to 2 weeks. The nystagmus usually resolves quickly (within the first few days). Improvements in posture and walking occur within 5 to 7 days, whereas a mild head tilt may remain persistent. While most animals compensate well, some may have episodic ataxia when performing tasks such as jumping up on furniture. No primary treatment has proved beneficial and recurrence is possible.

Toxicity with *metronidazole* may result in central vestibular signs in both dogs and cats (Dow et al. 1989; Saxon and Magne 1993). There is no definitive treatment for this toxicity. Discontinuation of the drug and supportive care may be helpful if clinical signs are not severe. Diazepam may be helpful in some instances (Evans et al. 2003). Clinical signs will usually resolve in 1 to 2 weeks following discontinuation of the drug. Some severely affected animals may die, and others may have residual clinical abnormalities.

Aminoglycosides, administered either systemically or topically, may cause deafness and vestibular signs. Immediate discontinuation of these treatments should occur if clinical signs result.

Tumor of the infratentorial space such as meningiomas and choroid plexus tumors may cause vestibular signs due to infiltration or compression of the vestibular nerve. Surgical debulking or resection of these tumors is ideal, but it is often hindered by lack of surgical exposure and intimate association with vital brain structures. Irradiation may provide some benefit by slowing tumor growth. Choroid plexus tumors, however, are relatively radiation resistant.

Inflammatory disease can affect the vestibular nuclei in the brain stem. Specifically, the rickettsia associated with *Rocky Mountain spotted fever* commonly involve the brain stem, particularly the vestibular system (Greene et al. 1985). Dogs with clinical features of vestibular disease after a systemic febrile illness associated with thrombocytopenia should be treated with tetracycline or doxycycline (10 mg/kg every 12 to 24 hours) prior to establishing a definitive diagnosis with titers. For RMSF, treatment usually is only necessary for 7 to 14 days. Chloramphenicol may also be effective for RMSF but is rarely used in the modern era. For ehrlichiosis, treatment may need to be prolonged.

REHABILITATION OF THE BRAIN INJURED ANIMAL

As important as any primary treatment, rehabilitation from brain injury requires patience, attention to system complications such as pneumonia, and physical therapy or activity. In general, lesions of supratentorial structures or the cerebellum have a better overall prognosis for recovery than lesions involving the brain stem. After the acute effects of brain injury are controlled (usually within 7 days), the goal is to allow time for brain healing and recovery of function to occur. Smaller animals are often better candidates for prolonged nursing care in comparison to larger animals due to the relative ease of physical manipulation. Good nursing care includes the prevention of decubital ulcers in the recumbent animal and monitoring for secondary infections primarily of the pulmonary and urogenital systems. Pneumonia is a common complication of brain-injured animals. Oral feeding should be reserved for animals that are alert. Prolonged alterations of consciousness and awareness may require feeding tube or intravenous nutrition. This, however, is not a guarantee against aspiration pneumonia.

Recumbent animals should be placed on clean, soft bedding and turned frequently (ideally every hour, but at least every 4 hours). Physical therapy can begin as soon as possible if there are no unstable vertebral injuries. Physical therapy is individualized to the animal's needs, but may include supported or nonsupported walking, passive flexion and extension of the limbs, massage, or swimming. Cats may be more reluctant than dogs to perform the latter physiotherapy but may respond to swimming. A daily record of physical therapy will ensure that this therapy is not overlooked, and allows for multiple individuals, including the owner, to become involved in the healing process.

In general, clinical signs of unilateral supratentorial injury improve within the first 2 weeks following trauma. Usually the animal is ambulatory by 4 weeks postinjury, although, residual paresis and blindness may continue. A tendency to circle may also persist, being especially prominent when the animal is distressed or excited.

Recovery from brain stem injury may be less complete, and residual signs commonly remain. Recovery from cerebellar injury often occurs in a similar time frame as for supratentorial injury. If the secondary effects of brain injury are controlled, many animals can recover from the primary brain insult associated with trauma.

14 Basics of Treatment of Important Spinal Cord Diseases of Dogs and Cats

Once a spinal cord abnormality has been diagnosed, treatment options can be considered. Some spinal neurologic diseases, such as many of the spinal degenerative disorders, either are not treatable or have no treatment. Treatments for spinal cord disease can be divided into either medical (nonsurgical) or surgical types. In many instances these general categories of treatments are combined. Rehabilitation, physical therapy, and pain management are also important aspects in the treatment of spinal diseases. In this chapter, basic aspects of spinal treatment will be discussed, followed by recommendations for treatment of individual diseases.

BASIC MEDICAL (NONSURGICAL) TREATMENTS FOR SPINAL DISEASES

Cage Confinement and Restricted Activity

Restricted activity or cage confinement is often necessary for animals with a variety of spinal injury, especially those associated with vertebral instability. Restricted activity is also an important treatment aspect in animals with intervertebral disk disease (IVDD). Animals should be restricted to an area (cage) just large enough so that the animal can get up and move around but not walk or run. Cage confinement is the veterinary equivalent of bed rest for human beings with spinal injury. The area should be comfortable, warm, clean, and have stable footing so that the animal will not slip and fall. Food and water should be provided in the cage environment. Animals may be cautiously assisted out of doors for urination and defecation, but should not be allowed to move without being controlled by the owner.

Depending on the size of animal, animals should be confined to a comfortable space but one no larger than 3 feet by 3 feet in dimension with the sides usually 3 feet or greater. Smaller areas may be necessary for smaller animals, and slightly larger areas necessary for larger animals. Commercially available animal crates, carriers, or cages are manufactured in various sizes and are made for this purpose. A baby playpen is an alternative. The confinement area should be a place where there is as direct access as possible to outdoors without intervening steps or stairs if the animal is to be taken outdoors for urination and defecation. The confinement area should have level, nonslip flooring so the animal has an area of good footing. The animal should remain in this area at all times except when cautiously carried or assisted outside to urinate or defecate. The animal should never be left to walk freely in larger areas as this may create excessive strain on the back and subsequently the IVD.

Outside areas should also be level and have good footing. Smaller animals may be picked up and carried from the cage to an outside area for urination and defection. Larger animals should be supported and controlled with harness or support device outside of the cage. If the animal has a cervical problem, a chest-type harness should be used instead of a collar to avoid pressure on the cervical area from the leash.

The animals should remain confined for at least the initial 2 weeks following injury. Weekly veterinary assessments are ideal, but will depend on the clinical circumstances. The animal should not be allowed from confinement until a veterinary assessment deems that cage confinement is no longer necessary (i.e., the clinical signs have resolved). If the clinical signs are improved but not resolved within the initial 2 weeks, cage confinement is continued in weekly intervals with continual clinical reassessment until the clinical signs are resolved.

The duration of cage confinement necessary is arbitrary. Generally, the animal's clinical progress should be critically assessed in at least 2-week intervals. If clinical signs are no better after the initial 2-week confinement period, a more complete diagnosis (if not already rendered), prolonged confinement, and/or additional therapies should be considered. If the animal is improving but not normal, confinement is continued, and improvement monitored weekly. If the animal's clinical status deteriorates at any time during the confinement period, reassessment by a veterinarian should be performed as soon as possible.

Nonsteroidal Anti-inflammatory Medications

Nonsteroidal anti-inflammatory medications are used in a variety of musculoskeletal diseases for their anti-inflammatory and pain-relief benefits. Data regarding efficacy of nonsteroidal drug effects in animals with spinal disease are usually based on anecdotal observations in clinical practice. Commonly prescribed nonsteroidal medications for dogs include carprofen (2.2 mg/kg orally every 12 hours or 4.4 mg/kg orally daily) and etodolac (10–15 mg/kg orally every 24 hours). Nonsteroid anti-inflammatory medications such as aspirin and phenylbutazone are usually avoided in the current era due to the increased risk of gastrointestinal (ulceration) and renal adverse effects. These latter drugs should especially not be used in combination with corticosteroids, as the incidence of life-threatening gastrointestinal complications appears increased when nonsteroidal and steroidal medications are used concurrently. Idiosyncratic hepatic toxicity occurs in some animals with carprofen (MacPhail 1998). The efficacy of chondroprotective agents such as glucosamine and chondroitin sulfate for spinal disease is not known.

Corticosteroids

Corticosteroids are commonly prescribed in animals with spinal disease due to the anti-inflammatory and antiedema effects of this class of drugs. Corticosteroids may greatly improve clinical signs in animals with neoplastic or inflammatory disease and may even benefit animals with some infectious diseases. The role of corticosteroids in the treatment of spinal trauma is commonly, but not universally, accepted. The use of corticosteroids in instances of intervertebral disk disease also is debatable.

Corticosteroid therapy has been thought to be an important adjunctive therapy for humans and animals suffering acute spinal trauma, and hence is administered in many instances of spinal injury in animals. The dogma of administering methylprednisolone sodium succinate to humans with spinal injury, however, is currently being questioned in human medicine. Questions regarding this treatment include those surrounding treatment efficacy and number and severity of side effects. Therefore, the recommendations for using this drug in treatment of spinal injury in humans may change in the future.

Ideally, in both humans and animals methylprednisolone sodium succinate is administered as soon as possible after a spinal injury, prior to or during radiographic evaluation. Multicenter studies in human beings with spinal injury suggested that methylprednisolone sodium succinate given up to 8 hours after a spinal trauma was beneficial. Experimental studies in small animals, however, have suggested that only soluble corticosteroids (methylprednisolone sodium succinate) given within 1 hour of the trauma are beneficial at mitigating secondary pathophysiologic events associated with spinal trauma. This information suggests that there may be a significant difference in time of treatment and recognized benefit for these medications between small animals and humans, with the time frame following spinal injury of benefit being shorter in small animals. It is also important to recognize that other corticosteroids such as dexamethasone have not been proven effective for treatment of experimental spinal trauma in animals and have been associated with significant complications in clinically affected animals with spinal disease. For these reasons, the author does not use dexamethasone treatment for spinal injury.

In studies in humans following spinal trauma, a 30 mg/kg intravenous (IV) bolus of methylprednisolone sodium succinate was administered initially followed by 5.4 mg/kg/hour IV for the next 23 hours as a constant infusion. This protocol was an attempt to maintain increased concentrations of the corticosteroid in the injured cord for a longer duration of time following a spinal injury. An alternative protocol used in small animals (however experimentally and scientifically unproved) is to administer methylprednisolone sodium succinate as an initial bolus (time 0) at a dose of 30 mg/kg IV, with subsequent doses of 15 mg/kg IV given at 2 and 6 hours after the initial dose as an attempt to avoid the additional labor and expense of administering the medication as a constant infusion. The efficacy of this protocol, however, has not been scientifically established.

If methylprednisolone sodium succinate is administered IV too rapidly in an awake animal, vomiting often occurs. If the medication is given too rapidly with the animal under general anesthesia, hypotension often is noted. For these reasons, it is advisable to administer the methylprednisolone sodium succinate IV over approximately 5–10 minutes. Acute death has been also reported (rarely) experimentally in dogs following bolus injections of methylprednisolone. Acute death following IV methylprednisolone administration in clinically affected dogs and cats is extremely rare in clinical practice.

Corticosteroid administration in animals with spinal disease is also associated with an increased incidence of gastrointestinal ulceration and possibly pancreatitis. This complication is more likely when animals are given larger dosages of corticosteroids, or when the medication is given over a prolonged duration of time. If severe, gastrointestinal ulceration can be a life-threatening complication of corticosteroid administration in animals with spinal injury. The most common site of intestinal perforation in animals with spinal disease administered dexamethasone is at the antimesenteric surface of the border between the transverse and descending colon. Colonic perforation at this site has been uniformly fatal in dogs. Dexamethasone appears to be more ulcerogenic than prednisolone. This may be due in part to inappropriate dosing. Published doses of dexamethasone seem high considering the drug's pharmacologic properties.

Recommendations for prolonged corticosteroid administration for animals with spinal disease vary as they are based primarily on anecdotal experiences. Generally, oral prednisolone or prednisone is preferred, beginning with anti-inflammatory dosages of corticosteroids followed by decreasing doses as soon as a clinical response is achieved. In some instances, oral dexamethasone is used, however, the incidence of gastrointestinal ulceration may be higher in animals with spinal disease when this drug is administered. Importantly, oral corticosteroids should be used only if the animals can be confined to avoid further deterioration in clinical status due to improvements in activity and pain relief following corticosteroid administration.

Corticosteroid treatment may also predispose the animal to increased infection or superinfection processes via immunosuppressive effects of these drugs. Delayed wound healing or increased incidence of decubital ulceration and urinary tract infection may result in surgical or recumbent patients.

MANAGEMENT OF SPINAL PAIN

Pain is an unfortunate consequence of many neurologic diseases, especially those diseases that involve the spinal cord or exiting peripheral nerves (see chapter 21 for further information regarding management of spinal pain). In very few instances is pain a "good thing," and therefore it requires appropriate diagnosis and effective, aggressive treatment to improve patient welfare and comfort.

Pain is most effectively managed when the stimulus for pain is removed or exhausted. If a mechanical cause of the pain (e.g., intervertebral disk material compressing a spinal nerve) is causative, surgical removal of that material may be necessary to bring about long-term pain relief. If a surgically correctable abnormality is not found, modulation of the experience of pain by altering either its transmission or integration is necessary. Additionally, pain may be managed by evoking the body's own endogenous pain-modulating systems.

Pharmacological Modulation of Pain

Opiates. Opiates are often the most common pharmacological means of treating pain in animals. A variety of opiate drugs exists for this purpose, with morphine being the gold standard by which other opiates are judged (table 14.1). Opiates work through activation of descending antinociceptive systems and/or through direct inhibition of pain projection at the spinal cord level.

Table 14.1. Types of Pain Medications

Morphine
- Natural opioid agonist
- After administration, may see initial excitement, panting, salivation, nausea, vomiting, urination, defecation or hypotension. These effects are attributed to stimulation of chemoreceptor trigger zone, vagal stimulation, and histamine release.
- Can be administered SC, IM, or IV, however, the IV route is used with caution to prevent hypotension associated with acute histamine release.
- Level of analgesia achieved is dose dependent.
- Major side effects include mental and central respiratory depression.

Oxymorphone
- Semisynthetic opioid agonist
- ~10 times the analgesic potency of morphine but less-pronounced effects on respiratory, cardiovascular, and gastrointestinal systems

Meperidine
- Synthetic opioid agonist
- One-eighth the analgesic potency of morphine

Pentazocine
- Synthetic opioid antagonist with some agonistic properties
- One-fourth the analgesic potency of morphine

Butorphanol
- Synthetic opioid agonist-antagonist
- Five times the analgesic potency of morphine

Codeine
- Oral opioid that is very effective in longer term management of pain

Corticosteroids. Commonly used as anti-inflammatory agents, corticosteroids will produce analgesia by inhibiting prostaglandin production. Corticosteroids inhibit the enzyme phospholipase, which catalyzes the conversion of phospholipids to the prostaglandin precursor arachidonic acid. These drugs may also reduce the effects of substance P, histamine, and bradykinin.

Nonsteroidal Anti-inflammatory Drugs. Analgesic effects of this group of drugs is also attributed mainly to their antiprostaglandin activity. These prevent the conversion of arachidonic acid to prostaglandins by inhibiting cyclooxygenase. Drugs in this class include carprofen and etodolac.

Local Anesthetics. Local anesthetics work peripherally as the name would suggest. Many alter sodium conductance into axons and subsequently inhibit depolarization and conduction of action potentials. Lidocaine would be a commonly used representative of this class of drugs. Anesthesia is usually short-lived. Bupivicaine may be more effective for longer duration analgesia via local instillation. This may be applied topically around nerve roots or paraspinal muscles as an addition to postoperative pain management in surgery patients.

Nonpharmacological Pain Relief. A multiple modality approach to pain control that incorporates an underlying attempt at patient well-being is more likely to be successful. This includes relatively simple efforts such as keeping the animal's environment quiet and dimly lit, providing appropriate water and nutrition, and having clean, comfortable bedding. In addition, activity to keep the patient engaged in other tasks seems helpful. For most patients, that may include physical therapy, massage, swimming, other hydrotherapy, ultrasound, or electrical stimulation.

TENS units and similar devices can be very helpful in providing analgesia. These devices are relatively inexpensive and are additive to other local and systemic pain control approaches. Some problems exist with patch application in haired animals, and with establishing a soothing yet nonpainful level of electrical stimulation, but usually these problems are not insurmountable. Electroacupuncture is an extension of this form of analgesia. Trigger point therapy may be beneficial for some animals.

Acupuncture has also gained acceptance as a pain relief treatment modality and can be used independently or sometimes concurrently with other treatment modalities. While the true effects of acupuncture are not always established, there is some reasonable Western scientific information to suggest its efficacy. Some of acupuncture's benefits may occur through physiologic endogenous pain modification. Following cutaneous stimulation, ascending pain information from the ascending reticular formation (possibly also through the spinothalamic tracts) projects to the periaqueductal grey of the brain stem to excite enkephalinergic neurons in the nucleus raphe magnus possibly through serotonergic mechanisms. Inhibitory synapses on pain responses are projected caudally in the spinal cord in the raphe spinal tract. Stimulation of these central nervous system areas, such as periaqueductal grey, nucleus reticularis paragigantocellularis, nucleus gigantocellularis pars alpha, prefrontal cortex, septal nuclei, caudate, amygdala, or the lateral hypothalamus, may result in pain relief. This is likely mediated through the release or alteration in concentrations of neurotransmitters such as endorphins, enkephalins, serotonin, norepinephrine, and others. Additionally, pain transmission may be blocked locally at the spinal cord level in the substantia gelatinosa (gating). These endogenous antinociception mechanisms may be a physiological explanation for why acupuncture and acupressure may be beneficial.

Current Pain Control Recommendations for Animals with Neurologic Pain

Spinal injury and disease are associated with a significant amount of postoperative pain. Opiate analgesics are commonly used to alleviate pain (table 14.2). Some prefer nonsteroidal anti-inflammatory drugs either alone or in conjunction with opiate analgesics. Nonsteroidal and corticosteroids administered concurrently, however, increase the risk of gastrointestinal ulceration. Fentanyl, a synthetic opioid, is available in a dermal patch (Duragesic, Fentanyl Transdermal System, Janssen Pharmaceutica, Titusville, NJ), allowing a more convenient way to manage postoperative pain for up to 72 hours. Adequate blood levels may take up to 24 hours to be reached in some animals. Initial pain management, therefore, should be supplemented with injectable agents such as morphine administered at 0.3 to 0.5 mg/kg IM q 4 hours for first 12 to 24 hours (at least). The patch is applied as soon as possible or, in some instances such as with planned surgery, prior to the painful episode. The patch is applied to the dorsal neck or rump area away from any possible surgical site. In some instances, placing the patch around the lower limb and paw can be used. In order for the drug delivery system to make adequate contact with the skin, an area 3 square inches should be shaved prior to adherence of the patch. An elevated body temperature may increase the amount of drug administered through the patch, so the animal should be checked for the presence of a fever on a daily basis. Occasionally an animal will develop dermatitis at the patch site necessitating removal of the patch and alternative pain therapy.

In our hospital, the most effective means of pain control for animals with neurologic and other painful conditions is by administering codeine. This narcotic has significant advantages as it can be administered orally, is titratable, is relatively safe, and is effective for severe forms

Table 14.2. Commonly prescribed narcotic analgesics and doses

Morphine	Dog	0.25–1.25 mg/kg q 4–6 h IM, SC
	Cat	0.1 mg/kg q 6–7 h IM, SC
Oxymorphone	Dog	0.05–0.2 mg/kg q 6 h IM, SC
	Cat	0.01 mg/kg q 6 h IM, SC
Meperidine	Dog	2–5 mg/kg q 1–2 h IM, SC
	Cat	Same
Pentazocine	Dog	1.5–3.0 mg/kg q 2–3 h IM, SC
	Cat	0.75–1.5 mg/kg q 2–4 h IM, SC
Butorphanol	Dog	0.1–0.2 mg/kg q 2–4 h IV or 0.2–0.4 mg/kg q 2–4 h SC, IM
	Cat	Same
Fentanyl patch		2–4 μg/kg
Codeine		1 mg/kg PO A 4–6 hours PRN

of pain. Disadvantages include its potential for human abuse, and therefore, its schedule II narcotic status requiring strict administration and dosing records. Gastrointestinal upset and constipation are rare but possible side effects. Regardless, this drug is extremely effecting in relieving most painful situations. Codeine is administered at 1 mg/kg q 6 hours PO PRN, and may be increased to Q 4 hours (or possibly more frequently) if necessary. Monitoring of the patient for overdose or underdosage of this medication is imperative, as with all pain medications.

PHYSICAL THERAPY AND REHABILITATION OF ANIMALS WITH NEUROLOGICAL DISEASE

Physical therapy is often an underutilized aspect of treatment in animals with spinal injury or disease. While the concept may seem somewhat daunting at first, in many instances, physical therapy is based upon common sense, a positive attitude, and persistence. Certainly, rehabilitation from any spinal or brain injury can be a long, tedious, difficult process. If the animals are large, physical therapy can be more physical for the therapist than the patient. While physical therapy often comes down to hard work, it may be some of the most important and rewarding medicine that can be offered.

Physical therapy attempts to improve physical strength, function, and mobility for the patient. Improvements in such a psychological boost may be more difficult to objectively assess but are likely. It is important, therefore, that those veterinary care individuals involved in physical therapy be positive and upbeat about the chances for recovery. The attitude of the therapist may, in fact, be more important than the attitude of the patient.

Accurate Neurological Assessment

Paramount to establishing an appropriate physical therapy plan is to have a thorough understanding of the disease process and other effective treatments. Neurologic status should be assessed by examination before beginning, and periodically during therapy to determine benefits and detriments of the therapy. A complete neurological examination should ideally be performed and recorded weekly during therapy.

General Medical Status

Many animals with neurologic disease have other complicating problems, some of which, if unrecognized may be more harmful to the animal than the neurological disease itself. As examples, urinary tract infection is common in animals that are not emptying their bladder effectively. If unrecognized, this infection can ascend to involve the kidney, with pyelonephritis and renal damage as consequences. Often, pneumonia occurs in recumbent animals, especially those with swallowing problems or megaesophagus.

If animals are recumbent for long periods of time, decubital ulcers over bony prominences become more likely. This is especially true in parts of the body where pain sensation is diminished. Soft bedding (i.e., water beds), frequent turning, frequent bathing (to remove debris, urine and feces), good nutrition, and focal padding may be helpful in this regard.

If muscles are not being used normally, muscle atrophy is commonly seen. If the lower motor neuron to the muscle is damaged with the disease, muscle atrophy may be severe (neurogenic atrophy).

Functional Ability

Before beginning therapy, an assessment should be made of the ability of the animal to perform normal functions. This will help in determining which therapies can be safely utilized. It is important that the animal not be forced to do something that will result in further physical damage, compounding the rehabilitation period.

Psychological

As stated previously, one of the most important aspects of rehabilitation is to encourage a positive mental attitude in the patient. Verbal encouragement is often most useful in animals. Instilling a feeling of confidence in the therapist's ability is also important.

Pain Control

Pain control is a very important component of the rehabilitation and recovery process from injury. Pain therapy is discussed previously in this chapter and in chapter 21.

Types of Physical Therapy

There are differing types of physical therapies that may be used in individual instances (table 14.3). Realistic decisions based on resources available and degree of patient incapacitation are used to individualize a physical therapy program for each animal.

Table 14.3. Types of physical therapy

Turning
Turning from one side to the other, or to sternal recumbency, should be performed every 2 hours. This is primarily to prevent decubital ulcers and static lung and bladder complications. Atelectasis is common if dependent lungs are not allowed to expand. This can lead to pneumonia, hypoxemia, and hypercapnia (increased $PaCO_2$).
Walking
Walking with or without support is used to stimulate the musculoskeletal and nervous mechanism used in purposeful movement. A sling supported on a wheeled cart is useful in animals that are unable to use both thoracic and pelvic limbs. Various devices are available or can be made if only the pelvic limbs need support. If some but not a significant amount of support is needed, the base of the tail may be held to direct movement of the pelvic limbs.
Passive Flexion and Extension
Passive flexion and extension of the limbs and other body areas are performed by the therapist. This is primarily to prevent stiffness and contractual joint and muscle complications. Each affected limb should be manipulated for 5 to 10 minutes, three to four times/day.
Massage
Massage can be performed by stroking (effleurage)—running the hands lightly over the surface of the skin; compression (pétrissage)—kneading, squeezing, and friction (a circular motion performed by placing a small part of the hand on the area). Reflex benefits of massage include sensations of pleasure and relaxation produced by skin stimulation of peripheral receptors, which are then transmitted through the spinal cord to the brain. Mechanical effects include improving circulation of blood and lymph, and producing intramuscular motion to stretch adhesions between muscle fibers and mobilize accumulations of intramuscular fluid.

Physical Therapy after Spinal Injury

There are several simple, effective methods of performing physical therapy on recumbent postsurgical spinal trauma animals, which do not require the purchase of expensive equipment. As previously mentioned, massage can be an effective way of preventing or treating limb edema as well as increasing general circulation to the limb. The touching sensation may also result in decreased apprehension and an overall feeling of well-being. Passive range of motion exercises can help prevent joint stiffness, edema, and muscle atrophy. This includes extending and flexing each joint in the thoracic and pelvic limbs. It can also be helpful to simply mimic an exaggerated walking motion with the limb, moving it in a circular fashion and utilizing each of the joints. These exercises may be performed for 10–20 minute periods at least twice daily.

It is important to encourage the recumbent animal to begin walking again. To prevent slipping, a textured nonslip surface such as concrete or soil is helpful for this exercise. When the dog has deficits in its rear limbs only (paraparesis), it can be supported by a number of simple methods. The dog can be grasped by the base of the tail or supported by a towel under the abdomen and assisted to walk. Commercially made supports, such as the Walkabout (Santa Cruz, CA), can be helpful and are available in a wide variety of sizes. These devices can be used on both the thoracic and pelvic limbs to provide a sling effect. Due to possible binding in the axial and groin areas, Walkabouts should not be used for extended walking exercises. For the animal that is reluctant to walk or has deficits in all four limbs (tetraparesis), a supportive sling, preferably on wheels, may be necessary.

The use of specially made carts to support the pelvic limbs and rump of an animal recovering from spinal trauma is not encouraged unless the prognosis is hopeless. Any effort made by the animal to move from one area to another is a form of physical therapy and may aid in the return of function to the legs. If the animal is confined to a cart, it becomes less motivated to exercise the pelvic limbs. In circumstances when sufficient time (at least a month) has passed and the ability of the paraplegic dog to regain limb function is in serious doubt, a custom-sized cart such as those provided by K-9 Carts (Big Sky, MT) may benefit the animal's quality of life and extend its life span.

Although not practical in all hospital settings, hydrotherapy can also be an effective method of physical therapy. Swimming provides a buoyant environment for the animal to attempt movement of its limbs without having to support its full weight. The warm water also promotes adequate circulation and muscle relaxation. A nonslip surface such as a cage mat should be placed on the bottom of the tub or deep sink. Sterile petrolatum ointment should be applied over the surgical incision. Rarely are wound complications such as infection noted if clean water is used at each therapy. The water can be filled to a depth that provides enough support for the animal to attempt to stand on its own and encourages the animal to swim. An animal should never be left unattended in water. Therapists should keep their hands on the animal at all times to prevent slipping or attempts at jumping out. A variety of children's floatation devices can be helpful in supporting the animal in the water. These range from simple inflatable toys from a local discount or department store to specially adapted canine life vests, which can be purchased from water ski or dive equipment stores. Another popular swim toy that can be found near pool accessories are long, foam-rubber tubes. These can be useful as a support under the abdomen of a swimming dog and can also be assembled into a raftlike device to support a heavy or tetraparetic animal.

A more elaborate device that combines the positive effects of hydrotherapy and walking is an underwater treadmill. The walking motions may stimulate neural circuits where as the buoyant effects of the water help in supporting the body against gravity.

Management of Animals with Neurogenic Abnormalities of Bladder Function

Urination is an important function of the body which requires significant nervous system input. Urination requires both local spinal and central reflex mechanisms as well as central nervous system coordination. Abnormalities of urination may occur with both upper motor neuron (UMN) and lower motor neuron (LMN) disease. Lesions in the UMN result in clinical features referred to as an UMN bladder. Lesions in the LMN result in LMN bladder clinical characteristics.

With ascending spinal cord sensory pathway involvement, the bladder may not be consciously recognized as full or distended. With descending UMN motor pathway involvement, coordinated bladder emptying may be interrupted. For these reasons, UMN disease can result in large bladder. Because the local peripheral nerves (S1–S3 spinal cord segments and associated nerves (pelvic, pudendal) to the bladder are not impaired, the bladder muscle has good tone (i.e., it feels turgid), and because of hyperreflexia of the bladder outflow region, the UMN bladder is difficult to manually express. This is the same concept as hyperreflexia of the patellar reflex seen with UMN lesions. After a period of time (usually around 2 weeks), reflex bladder expression may begin to occur.

Additionally with UMN lesions, poor coordination between the phases of urination may occur (i.e., poor synchrony between detrusor contraction and urethral sphincter relaxation). Affected animals may begin to urinate normally, but then the urine stream is stopped abruptly before the bladder is completely emptied. This abnormal urinary pattern is referred to as reflex dysynergia.

With LMN lesions affecting the sacral spinal segments or associated peripheral nerves, the bladder may also be large because the ascending and descending information cannot project through the damaged peripheral nerves. Bladder tone is decreased, and the bladder feels flaccid (jelly-like). If the bladder is maximally distended, however, bladder tone (based on palpation) can seem adequate. Additionally, the bladder is often easily manually expressed because the local tonic reflex to maintain tone in the bladder outflow tract is not diminished or absent.

The animal's ability to urinate following spinal injury or disease is an important factor in determining prognosis for recovery and quality of life. With the availability of custom-made carts, even paralyzed dogs can lead a long and happy life. An incontinent dog, however, presents sometimes overwhelming nursing care demands for owners. The inability to control bladder function, therefore, can have greater influence on the dog's quality of life than the return of its leg function. Assessing the animal's bladder function both prior to and following spinal surgery is crucial. The presence or absence of urine on the animal's bedding or in the cage, witnessed voluntary urination, and the ease or difficulty with which the bladder is expressed are important observations. Animals with no voluntary urinary control may leak urine (overflow incontinence) from a maximally distended bladder in a cage. Therefore, the presence of urine in a cage is not indicative that an animal can voluntarily urinate. The bladder should be gently palpated regularly (at least every 6 hours; more frequently in animals that are polyuric) to determine the volume of urine it contains and to establish whether or not the animal is fully emptying its bladder each time it urinates. Urine retained in the bladder due to inadequate bladder emptying can lead to cystitis. Manual expression may be necessary every 6 hours if the animal is not able to urinate on its own. The bladder should be gently manually expressed if indicated. Gentle (nontraumatic) manual bladder expression avoids additional injury to the bladder wall and other abdominal structures, including the muscular abdominal wall.

The color and smell of the urine collected or expressed should be evaluated at each voiding. A daily urinalysis using a urine dipstick and sediment evaluation is performed to determine if an infection is occurring. Appropriate aerobic or anaerobic bacterial cultures are submitted if pyuria, bacteriuria, or hematuria is noted.

If expression is difficult, the bladder should be drained by introduction of a sterile urinary catheter on an as needed basis, but at least every 6 to 8 hours if the animal is not polyuric. Indwelling urinary catheters are avoided if at all possible as they increase the risk of introducing a bladder infection. If an animal is constantly leaking urine and soiling its skin, an indwelling urinary catheter may be necessary. In female dogs where intermittent urinary catheterization is difficult, an indwelling urinary catheter may also be used.

Depending on the nature of the neurologic lesion and the cause of the abnormal bladder function, a number of pharmacological agents are routinely used to assist in bladder management (tables 14.4, 14.5).

Phenoxybenzamine is administered in an attempt to reduce tone in the internal urethral sphincter. Increased tone of the external urethral sphincter is treated with diazepam or dantrolene. Detrusor contractility is enhanced with bethanechol. Each of these agents is used for a highly specific action and strict attention must be paid to contraindications which can cause more harm than good.

The inability to voluntarily urinate often requires the animal to be hospitalized. Some owners, however, feel comfortable with home-bladder management, and the animals may then be discharged from the hospital for the recovery period. Appropriate client communication as to the important aspects of posttrauma or postoperative care is critical for an overall successful outcome of the animal with spinal trauma.

Neurogenic bladder abnormalities are frequently managed incorrectly, with potentially devastating consequences. The two most frequent complications of poor bladder management are urinary tract infection (due to incomplete expression) and detrusor atony (stretched bladder wall due to overdistention). Detrusor atony usually results from a prolonged overdistended bladder. As the bladder muscle cells are not innervated by a single nerve fiber, a single nerve fiber may only innervate one out of every three or more muscle fibers. For the muscle fibers that are not directly innervated to be excited to contract, they must rely upon depolarization waves that are projected from adjacent and directly innervated muscle cells. These depolarization waves spread between cells via connections in tight junctions. With bladder wall distention, muscle cells are pulled apart and these tight junctions are disrupted. Therefore, with nervous stimulation, complete bladder wall depolarization is not achieved. Chronic or severe detrusor atony is often irreversible.

Table 14.4. Types of drugs used for neurogenic bladder and urination abnormalities

- Bladder Outflow Relaxation Agents

  Inhibits the internal urethral sphincter. The representative drug in this class is *phenoxybenzamine*. This drug blocks the alpha adrenergic innervation to the bladder neck resulting in increased ease of expression.

- Skeletal Muscle Relaxation

  Two representative drugs fall in this class: diazepam and dantrolene. *Diazepam* is a benzodiazepine most commonly used as a short-acting anticonvulsant. *Dantrolene* may be more efficacious in cats, whereas diazepam may not be effective for urethral skeletal muscle relaxation in this species.

- Parasympathomimetic Agents

  Bethanecol is the most commonly used parasympathomimetic agent used in clinical practice. It is beneficial in increasing the strength of contraction of the detrusor muscle.

Table 14.5. Dosages of drugs used in the pharmacological management of urination disorders

Urethra Sphincter Incompetence (Decreased Sphincter Tone)		
Phenylpropanolamine	Dog	75 mg/40 lb q 12h; alpha agonist
Ephedrine	Dog	4–10 mg PO q 8–12 h; alpha agonist
Propranolol	Dog	5–40 mg PO q 8–12 h; beta blocker
	Cat	2.5–5 mg PO q 8–12 h
Increased urethral tone, smooth muscle relaxation		
Phenoxybenzamine	Dog	2.5–15 mg POq 8 h; alpha blocker
	Cat	2.5–5 mg PO q 8 - 24 h
Skeletal Muscle Relaxation		
Diazepam	Dog	2–10 mg PO q 8 h
	Cat	2–5 mg PO q 8 h
Dantrolene	Dog	1.0 mg/kg to 5 mg/kg PO q 8 to 12 h
Detrusor Atony		
Bethanechol	Dog	5–20 mg PO q 8–12 h
	Cat	2.5–5 mg PO q 8–12 h
Detrusor Atony with Increased Urethral Resistance (Reflex Dysynergia)		
Bethanechol + phenoxybenzamine		
Bethanechol + diazepam		

Management of the Recumbent Animal

In some situations, owners elect to pursue nonsurgical management for animals with severe neurologic impairment that prevents the animal from standing or even moving. In this situation, the animal may be recumbent for prolonged periods of time and require more extensive care in addition to confinement and pain medications.

Recumbent animals should be kept in a comfortable environment that prevents them from moving freely and further injuring themselves. Animals that are recumbent may be confined similarly to those that can still walk. The recumbent animal should be turned at least every 1–4 hours to prevent decubital ulcers from developing on bony protuberances such as hips or shoulders. Extra padding under the animals with foam rubber or thick fleece material is necessary. Small soft-sided waterbeds are helpful in preventing bed sores. Frequent turning is also important in preventing atelectasis, which may lead to pneumonia. Ideally, the animal should be kept in a sternal or sternal oblique position to allow for chest expansion.

Urine and feces may contaminate the animal or the area, and should be removed as rapidly as possible to avoid skin irritation from contact with these substances. The recumbent animal is often unable to move itself from an area it has soiled. Absorbent, waterproof pads, such as Val-U-Sorb Underpad (Professional Medical Products, Greenwood, SC), can be useful in soaking up urine and preventing the saturation of bedding material with urine or feces. Absorbent pads that can be changed frequently are often helpful in keeping animals clean and dry. Strategic placement of cage padding and absorbent materials in relation to the animal is necessary so that body fluids will be directed away from the recumbent position. Frequent bathing may be necessary to prevent urine scald. This may be accomplished during hydrotherapy. Long-term recumbency can lead to limb edema, and muscle atrophy. Massage to the effected limb and other forms of physical therapy can prevent or help treat these complications.

Animals that are recumbent may not be able to move to food and, most important, water. In these animals, water and food must be placed within the range of access for the animal. If the animal is laterally recumbent, a caregiver will often have to hold the animal in a sternal position and offer food and water by hand.

SURGICAL TREATMENTS FOR SPINAL CORD DISEASE

The indications for spinal surgery include but are not limited to decompression of the spinal cord or nerve roots, stabilization or realignment of vertebral structures, diagnosis of spinal disease (biopsy), resection of spinal tumors, and preventative treatments such as for intervertebral disk disease. General aspects of spinal surgery are discussed further in this section. The specific utility of spinal surgery in the treatment of spinal disease is discussed under the treatment of specific spinal disease processes.

Spinal Cord Decompressive Procedures

If the spinal cord is compressed by disease, access to the spinal cord and removal of the compressive abnormality is necessary. There are two basic decompressive surgical procedures; the *hemilaminectomy* and the *dorsal laminectomy.* In addition, for ventral cervical decompression, a specialized partial spondylectomy referred to commonly as a *ventral slot* is useful.

As the term "laminectomy" implies, these procedures involve removal of bone (i.e., the lamina) from various areas around the spinal cord to provide access to the epidural space and dural tube. A hemilaminectomy is used in most cases due to the increased incidence of ventral and unilateral spinal compression (figs. 14.1-14.4). The thoracolumbar area can be accessed for decompression via a dorsal approach for either a hemilaminectomy or a dorsal laminectomy. With localized lesions on one side and centered exclusively around the nerve root, a *foraminotomy* (surgically enlarging the intervertebral foramen) may be the procedure of choice.

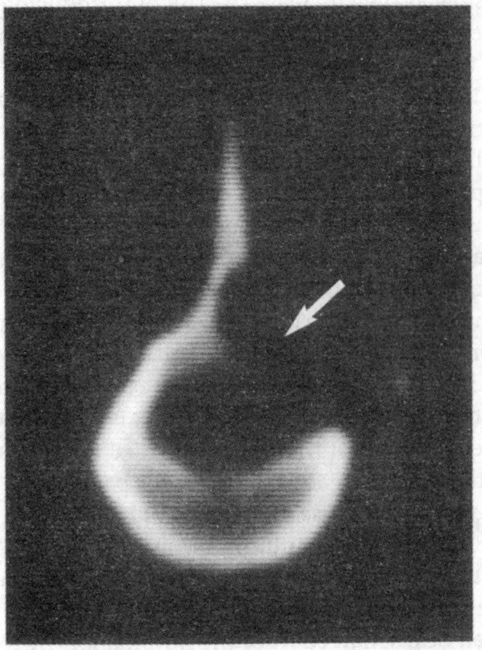

Fig. 14.1. Transverse CT image of a vertebra with a hemilaminectomy (*arrow*).

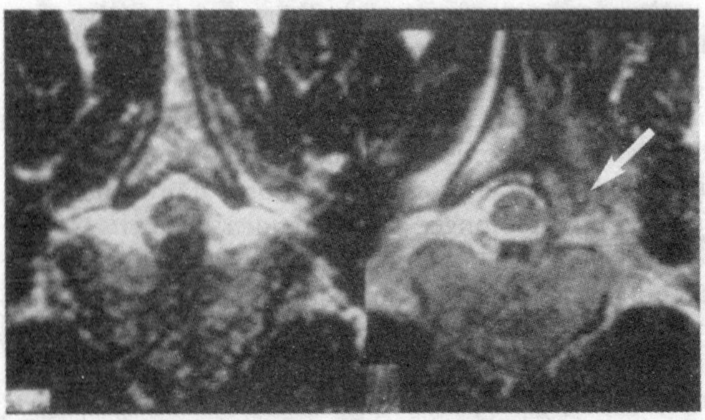

Fig. 14.2. Transverse T2-weighted MR images from a dog (A) before and (B) after a hemilaminectomy (*arrow*).

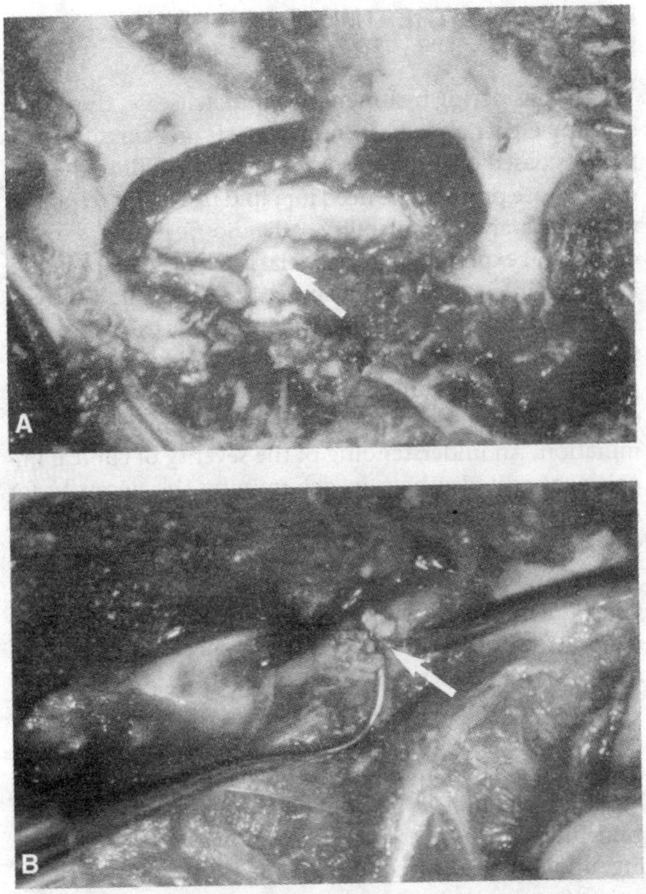

Fig. 14.3. (A,B) Appearance of acutely herniated intervertebral disk material at the time of a hemilaminectomy in two dogs (*arrow*).

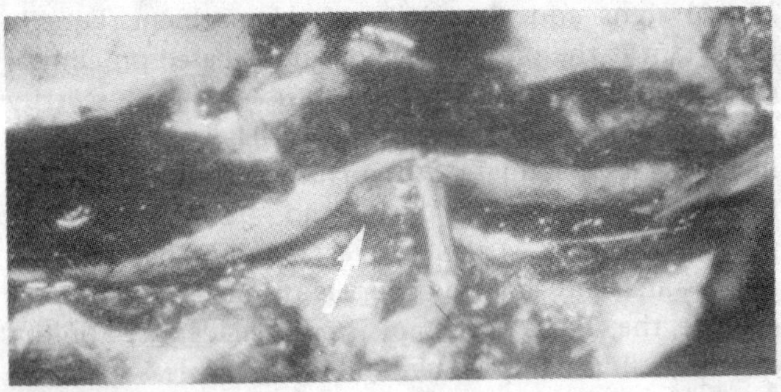

Fig. 14.4. Appearance of chronically protruded intervertebral disk material at the time of a hemilaminectomy (*arrow*).

Advantages and Disadvantages. The major advantage of the hemilaminectomy is that this procedure provides for adequate exposure of the dorsal, lateral, and ventral spinal cord and unilateral nerve root (table 14.6). This degree of exposure is beneficial in most instances of IVDD as the herniated disk material is found usually ventrally or laterally. Problems with the hemilaminectomy include the need for accurate localization of the side of the lesion and the potential for hemorrhage from the vertebral sinuses in the vertebral canal.

Table 14.6. Comparison of hemilaminectomy and dorsal laminectomy

Hemilaminectomy
Advantages
• Allows for access to the dorsal, lateral, and ventral aspects of the spinal cord
• Results in the least amount of instability of the vertebral segments
• Allows for adequate exposure of the nerve root
Disadvantages
• Increases risk for rupturing the ventral vertebral sinus (usually not a major problem, however, in some instances, hemorrhage can be significant)
• Allows access to only one side of the spinal cord (i.e., need accurate side localization to perform)
Dorsal Laminectomy
Advantages
• Allows for access to the dorsal aspect of the spinal cord
• Allows for access to both lateral aspects of the spinal cord as compared to the hemilaminectomy
Disadvantages
• Difficult to expose ventrally located lesions
• Cannot be performed continuously over as many disk spaces as a hemilaminectomy

The dorsal laminectomy is useful for lesions located exclusively in the dorsal aspect of the spinal cord or canal. This technique results in a greater degree of instability of the spine than does the hemilaminectomy. Surgeons experienced with this technique find it useful even for ventrally situated lesions, however, an increased amount of spinal cord manipulation may result.

Three basic types of dorsal laminectomy exist: Funkquist types A and B, and the modified dorsal laminectomy. Problems with laminectomy membrane formation (postoperative scarring resulting in spinal cord compression) occurred commonly with the Funkquist type A laminectomy and this procedure is almost never performed in the modern era. The Funkquist type B laminectomy was developed to decrease this postoperative scarring complication, but it results in limited ventral exposure to the spinal cord. The modified dorsal laminectomy was developed to allow for better exposure to the ventral spinal cord while decreasing the risk of laminectomy membrane formation. This procedure is most adequate for dorsal compressive lesions in the thoracolumbar area, however, it may be less ideal for ventrolateral compression. In general, the dorsal laminectomy is less commonly used in the current era.

The cervical area can be accessed for decompression via a ventral, lateral, or dorsal approach. A ventral slot is the common phrase used to describe a ventral decompressive spinal surgical procedure used exclusively in the cervical region (fig. 14.5). This procedure is usually adequate for access to ventral compressive lesions associated with IVDD in the cervical region from C2–3 through C6–7 and possibly C7–T1. This approach allows limited access to the ventral

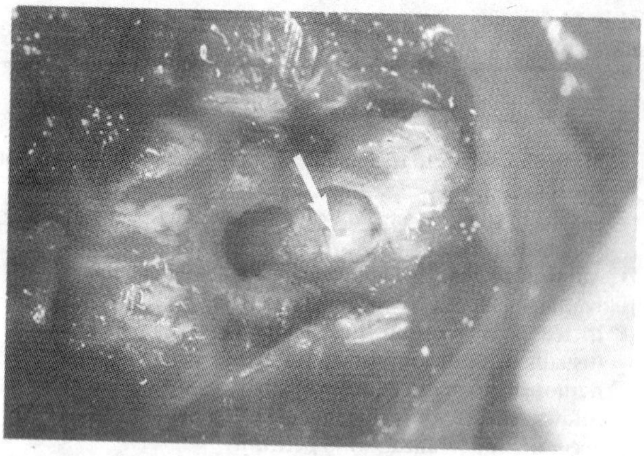

Fig. 14.5. Appearance of acutely herniated intervertebral disk material at the time of a ventral slot (*arrow*).

aspect of the spinal cord overlying the disk space. Access is limited due to the normal course of the ventral vertebral sinuses. Additionally, removal of excessive amounts of the vertebral body results in significant spinal instability. A ventral slot is often inadequate for spinal cord lesions other than those associated with IVDD.

Cervical hemilaminectomy or dorsal laminectomy is most useful for surgical decompression of dorsal, lateral, and ventral compressive lesions in the cervical region from C2–3 through C6–7 and possibly C7–T1. A specific *lateral cervical approach* may be used to access the lateral aspect of the caudal cervical area. If necessary, a hemilaminectomy of the caudal cervical and cranial thoracic vertebrae can be performed through this approach. The major disadvantage of the lateral cervical approach is that only C3–4 to C5–6 can be accessed easily. An approach similar to the craniolateral approach to the brachial plexus may allow access to the more caudal cervical area if desired.

Brachial Plexus Procedures

The brachial plexus is most often surgically accessed for nerve sheath tumor arises from these nerves. Biopsy of affected nerves, as in the case of brachial plexus neuritis, can also be performed through this approach. If necessary, a hemilaminectomy of the caudal cervical and cranial thoracic vertebrae can be performed concurrently . Also, this surgical approach can be adapted for limb amputation if necessary (as in the case of brachial plexus tumor).

Nondecompressive Procedures

Fenestration is a prophylactic procedure wherein portions of the intervertebral disk is removed prior to this material extruding. The vertebral canal is not entered during a fenestration. The annulus fibrosis of the intervertebral disk (IVD) space is incised and the nucleus pulposus is removed. This may prevent further extrusion of nucleus pulposus and may result in fibrosis of the IVD. Success with this procedure varies primarily with the severity of the clinical signs. Fenestration alone, however, is not a spinal decompressive procedure.

CHOOSING A TREATMENT FOR SPINAL DISEASE

When considering treatments for spinal disease, the choice of using either a medical (nonsurgical) or a surgical treatment is based on a multitude of factors including the specific disease process, the need for rapid treatment responses to avoid paralysis, availability of diagnostic testing, surgical or medical expertise, and financial aspects. A major factor, however, in choosing a nonsurgical versus a surgical treatment is often the degree of impairment or the severity of the clinical signs and the potential for rapid reversal or improvement in the clinical signs (table 14.7). The severity of clinical signs is often ranked or graded to help in this determination. An understanding of the severity of clinical impairment will also help in determining the necessity for rapid diagnosis and treatment (i.e., the need for emergency surgery).

Ideally, scientific data would be available to be used as a guide in making decisions regarding when surgical (or medical) treatment of spinal disease is necessary. Unfortunately, clinical decisions are often based on individual opinion from anecdotal experiences. The following are guidelines for surgical management of animals with spinal cord disease. These should serve only as general guidelines. Modification of the recommendations based on these guidelines may be necessary in individual animals depending upon special circumstances (e.g., systemic health, owner finances).

When Is Surgery on the Spine Necessary?

Decisions regarding when and if surgical versus nonsurgical treatment for spinal cord disease is indicated are primarily made based on two main factors: the severity of neurological signs and chronicity of the problem. Equally important is the presumptive diagnosis based on clinical evaluation. The ranked scale can be used to assess severity of spinal injury (table 14.7). Animals that are presumed to have diseases that might result in further clinical deterioration should always be evaluated and treated as rapidly as possible. If a disease (such as an acute injury) has occurred to the spinal cord and this injury is assumed to be nonprogressive, the choice of therapy is often made based on the degree of clinical impairment (table 14.7). Diseases such as intervertebral disk extrusion or protrusion and exogenous spinal injury usually fall into this category. In some instances, an acute spinal injury will result in progressive clinical signs over the ensuing hours or days. If a nonsurgical treatment option is initially chosen, however the clinical signs continue to worsen, a surgical treatment should be considered as rapidly as possible prior to significant clinical impairment.

Therefore, a dog with a signalment, history, and clinical features that suggest an acute intervertebral disk problem or exogenous spinal injury can be managed generally via these guidelines. Approximately 60–70% of dogs with acute intervertebral disk disease that are grade 6 (walking) or higher at initial presentation improve or completely re-

Table 14.7. Clinical status

Least Severe	
10	Normal
8	Pain only
6	Paresis (walking)
5	Paresis (not walking)
4	Plegia (urination, deep pain intact)
3	Plegia (urination absent, deep pain intact)
2	Plegia (deep pain absent <48 hours)
1	Plegia (deep pain absent >48 hours)
0	Myelomalacia
Most Severe	

solve this problem without surgical intervention. If clinical signs worsen during strict confinement, a more thorough evaluation should be pursued.

Generally, animals who are a grade 6 or higher who have had clinical signs for less than two weeks in duration and have a presumptive diagnosis of a spinal injury, either from an intervertebral disk problem or exogenous injury, are candidates for nonsurgical management of their spinal problem. Nonsurgical management primarily includes strict cage confinement for at least a 2-week period of time, acute anti-inflammatory medications (for the first day, possibly more), and treatment for spinal pain (as necessary) with subsequent reevaluation and reassessments performed as necessary. Clinical assessments are made at least daily if not more frequently until clinical signs are nonprogressive for at least a 48-hour period of time. These assessments are often performed with the animal hospitalized for the first 24 to 48 hours following a spinal injury. At home or in the hospital, cage confinement and restricted activity need to be continued for 4 to 8 weeks depending upon the rapidity and completeness of recovery. Corticosteroids can be administered acutely (methylprednisolone sodium succinate 30 mg/kg IV slowly), however, should be continued cautiously after the first 24 hours as the risk of gastrointestinal complications (gastric and colonic ulceration) significantly increases with a longer duration of therapy.

Animals who are grades 5 through grade 1 (unable to stand and walk) tend to be considered as candidates for surgical treatment. Animals with acute intervertebral disk disease that are judged to be within grades 5–2 who have surgery performed within a reasonable time frame (48 hours) have approximately an 80+% recovery rate of useful function. Animals that lose deep pain sensation and are operated on within 48 hours have conservatively a 50% chance of recovery and, in some instances, as high as a 70% or better recovery rate. Animals who have lost deep pain sensation for greater than 48–72 hours have a much poorer (5% or less?) chance of recovery of useful function with or without surgery. A dog with obvious signs of myelomalacia will recover no useful spinal cord function. Animals with extensive myelomalacia often appear systemically ill and have fevers. If myelomalacia ascends to involve the nerves responsible for respiration (i.e., the cervical area), the prognosis is grave and it is best to euthanize the animal to relieve further suffering.

An exception to aforementioned rules is the animal who has suffered a traumatic (hit by car, gunshot injury) spinal problem and has no deep pain at presentation. The rate of return of useful function in this group of animal is far less than 50% even if the animal is treated rapidly following the injury.

If the diagnosis is uncertain, or if the clinical signs are periodically recurrent, performance of diagnostic tests to establish a definitive diagnosis and determination of the need for surgical intervention should be considered as soon as possible. If the clinical signs are not responding to nonsurgical treatment in a reasonable amount of time (2 to 4 weeks depending), reassessment, rediagnosis, and surgical assessment are warranted.

While the above discussion provides general guidelines, this clinical classification system has been shown useful in management of most animals with spinal cord injury. If a question arises, a neurologist or neurosurgeon should be consulted to offer further opinions. Not only should these guidelines be useful for clinical management of animals with spinal compressive disease, they should also allow for communication with the owner of realistic expectations of recovery potential in the animal with spinal injury. All guidelines, however, are modified based on individual patient and disease characteristics. Definitive treatment judgments need to be made by the primary clinician responsible for the care of the animal.

TREATMENTS OF SPINAL CORD DISEASES

Treatments of individual diseases affecting the spinal cord or surrounding structures vary. As new treatments may be developed, the current literature should be consulted for the newest treatment options. Additionally, drug dosages and other therapeutic modalities may vary depending upon individual clinician's experience, the unique clinical manifestations of any individual animal's disease, and the animal's overall systemic health. The following treatments are suggested as guidelines and may have to be altered or modified in individual clinical situations.

Degenerative Diseases

Many of the primary degenerative spinal diseases are not currently treatable. *Degenerative myelopathy* is a degenerative spinal cord disease that results in paraparesis in adult animals. No curative treatment is known for this disease. One author has claimed success in stopping or slowing the progression of the disease using epsilon aminocaproic acid (500 mg/dog three times daily) (Clemmons 1989). Other treatments, as yet unproved, include forced exercise, vitamin supplementations, acetylcystiene, and other alternative nutrient supplementation. A slowly (weeks to months) worsening paraparesis progressing to paraplegia is unfortunately the norm in many instances, regardless of treatment.

Intervertebral Disk Disease

Similar to other spinal conditions, treatment options for intervertebral disk disease usually involve either medical (nonsurgical) treatment or surgery (see bibliography under Intervertebral Disk Disease). When and if surgical compared to nonsurgical treatment for intervertebral disk disease is utilized is primarily based on three main clinical features of the disease process: (1) the severity of neurological signs (tables 14.7, 14.8), (2) the chronicity of the clinical signs, and (3) the recurrence or repeatability of the clinical signs.

It can be helpful to think of an acute intervertebral disk extrusion (rupture) in the same way that one would think of a healing skin wound. With both injuries, there is the healing process occuring in stages that require a certain time period. A skin wound that is constantly manipulated and stretched will be less likely to heal or, at least, will require a longer period to heal. Similarly, a rupture in the annulus fibrosis of an intervertebral disk requires a staged, time-dependent healing process. Continuous or excessive force on the disk structure will prevent such healing from occurring in a timely manner, and may also affect the quality of the healing process. As an added concern, the longer a persistent defect remains in the annulus, the longer there remains the potential for additional amounts of nucleus pulposus to be extruded and result in a worsening of clinical signs. Therefore, time and quiescence are important factors in the healing process for intervertebral disk disease.

Treatment decisions may differ depending upon whether the problem is acute, chronic, or recurrent. Treatment of acute IVDD will be discussed first. Generally, animals who are a grade 6 or higher (walking with impairment or painful only) who have clinical signs for less than 2 weeks in duration and have a presumptive diagnosis of a spinal injury from an intervertebral disk problem are candidates for medical (nonsurgical) management of their spinal problem (table 14.8). Animals with intervertebral disk disease that are unable to stand and support their own weight when walking are more likely to be considered for surgical treatment of their intervertebral disk problem.

Medical (Nonsurgical) Management of Intervertebral Disk Disease

Animals presented for evaluation of acute intervertebral disk disease that are mildly affected clinically are often managed without surgical treatment. When animals are presented to the hospital, an examination and survey spinal radiographs are often performed, however, a more extensive diagnostic evaluation may not always be performed for a variety of reasons. Therefore, the diagnosis of IVDD is often a presumptive diagnosis, and treatment is initiated based on this presumption. The animal is ideally hospitalized for the first 12 to 24 hours to assess for further clinical deterioration and initial treatment responses unless the animal is minimally affected. As animals with acute intervertebral disk disease are often painful, this first 24 hours of hospitalization also allows for an assessment and acute treatment of pain.

Table 14.8. Nonsurgical treatment of acute intervertebral disk disease

- Cage confinement
- Pain medication
- Monitoring of urination and defecation
- Keep the animal clean
- Nonimpact physical therapy
- Provide access to food and water
- +/- corticosteroid or nonsteroidal anti-inflammatory medications

Medical therapy for intervertebral disk disease may include:

- Cage confinement
- Corticosteroids
- Analgesic therapy
- Low-impact physical therapy
- Management of the recumbent animal as needed
- Management of bladder and bowel abnormalities

Prognosis with Nonsurgical Treatments for Intervertebral Disk Disease. Approximately 60–70% (and possibly up to 90%) of dogs with acute intervertebral disk disease that are grade 6 or higher at initial presentation improve or completely resolve this problem without surgical intervention within the first 1 to 3 months. Nonsurgical treatments, therefore, are often successful in treatment of these dogs (table 14.8). If clinical signs worsen and confinement has been performed appropriately, a more thorough diagnostic evaluation should be pursued. If nonsurgical treatments are not effective, a surgical consultation should occur as soon as possible to avoid prolonged delays or incomplete recoveries.

Surgical Treatment of Intervertebral Disk Disease

Animals with acute intervertebral disk disease that are unable to stand and walk, are paralyzed, or have abnormalities of deep pain sensation are often considered for surgical treatment. Ideally, animals that are more severely affected with IVDD should be treated as soon as possible following the occurrence of their disease. For animals that still have voluntary movement, this is often within 24 to 48 hours following onset of clinical signs.

Surgical treatment for intervertebral disk disease is most successful if performed following an appropriate anatomical diagnosis regarding the location and extent of the intervertebral disk abnormality. Surgical experience with the numerous varieties and locations of intervertebral disk disease will influence the surgical procedure and outcome. It is recommended that only those individuals with experience in spinal surgery attempt surgical treatment of animals with intervertebral disk disease. While these procedures are often helpful in resolving clinical signs if performed correctly, removal of part of the vertebra may increase the risk of vertebral instability in some instances (fig.

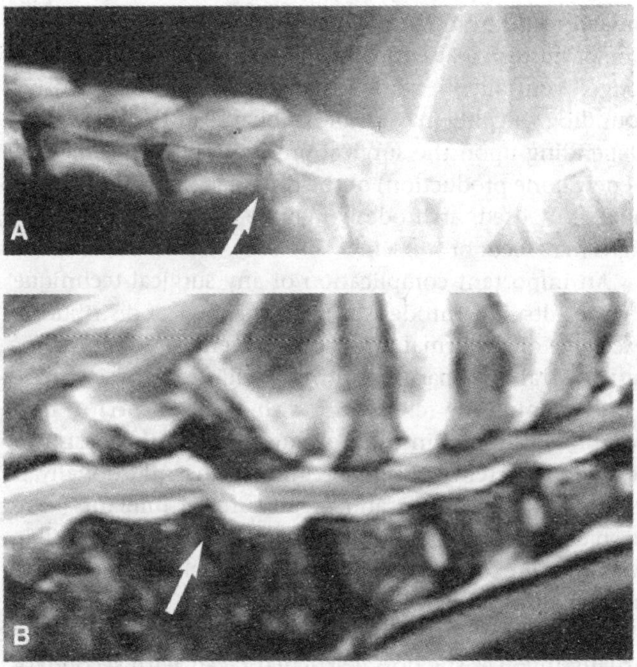

Fig. 14.6. (A) Lateral myelographic view of a dog with collapse of the cervical vertebrae and subsequent spinal cord compression (*arrow*) following a ventral slot. (B) Sagittal, T2-weighted MR image from a dog with collapse of the cervical vertebrae following cervical surgery (*arrow*).

14.6). Obviously, an important goal of surgical treatment is to not make the animal worse from the surgery itself.

Prognosis for Animals with Surgical Treatment of Intervertebral Disk Disease. Animals with intervertebral disk disease within grades 5–2 who have appropriate surgery performed within 48 hours of injury have approximately an 80 to 90+% recovery rate of useful function (walking without assistance). Animals that lose deep pain sensation due to their injury and have surgery within 48 hours have, conservatively, a 50% and possibly as high as a 70% chance of recovery to walking. Animals who have lost deep pain sensation for greater than 48 to 72 hours by the time of definitive treatment have a much poorer (5% or less ?) chance of recovery of useful function with or without surgery. A small percentage of dogs with intervertebral disk disease and prolonged loss of deep pain sensation may improve following surgery. A dog with obvious signs of myelomalacia will recover no useful spinal cord function. If myelomalacia ascends to involve the nerves responsible for respiration (i.e., the cervical area), the prognosis is grave, and it is best to euthanize the animal to relieve further suffering.

Management of the Animal Following Spinal Surgery for Intervertebral Disk Disease. In the immediate hours following surgery for IVDD, animals are usually monitored in a critical care or intensive care environment for abnormalities of vital functions such as respiration and cardiovascular health. Until the body temperature is normal, keeping the animal warm is necessary. Rarely, animals will emerge from surgery and be hyperthermic, requiring cooling procedures. Intravenous fluid therapy is continued until the animal is alert enough to drink effectively. Urine is evacuated from the bladder either by manual expression or catheterization until the animal is able to urinate normally. Obviously, bladder management may need to be continued following the immediate postoperative period if the animal cannot voluntarily urinate. If the animal is not too hypothermic, a cold or iced compress can be applied to the surgical wound in an attempt to reduce wound swelling and inflammation.

Management and treatment of the animal in the days following spinal surgery include many of the aforementioned nonsurgical treatments. Appropriate assessments are made of the surgical wound, looking for abnormalities such as excessive redness, swelling, heat, pain, or abnormal discharge from the wound. If a seroma occurs, hot packing or drainage may be necessary.

Spinal surgery can be associated with a significant amount of postoperative pain. Opiate analgesics are commonly used to alleviate pain. Fentanyl, a synthetic opioid, is available in a dermal patch (Duragesic, Fentanyl Transdermal System, Janssen Pharmaceutica, Titusville, NJ), allowing a convenient way to manage postoperative pain for up to 72 hours. Adequate blood levels may take up to 24 hours to be obtained in some animals, therefore initial pain management should be supplemented with injectable agents such as morphine administered at 0.3 to 0.5 mg/kg IM q 4 hours for the first 12 to 24 hours (at least). The patch is applied as soon as possible or, in some instances such as a previously planned surgery, prior to surgery. The patch is applied to the dorsal neck, rump area, or lower limb area away from any possible surgical site. In order for the drug delivery system to make adequate contact with the skin, an area 3 square inches should be shaved prior to adherence of the patch. An elevated body temperature may increase the amount of drug administered through the patch, so the animal should be checked for the presence of a fever on a daily basis. Occasionally, an animal will develop dermatitis at the patch site necessitating removal of the patch and alternative pain therapy.

In our hospital, the most helpful pain medication for use in the days following surgery is codeine (1–4 mg/kg orally every 6 hours PRN). This narcotic has significant advantages as it can be administered orally, is titratable, has few side effects, and is reasonably effective even for severe pain. This drug can be used either concurrently or independently of a fentanyl patch. Codeine is initially administered at 1 mg/kg q 6 hours PO PRN, and may be increased to Q 4 hours (or possibly more frequently) if necessary. Disadvantages include its potential for human abuse, and, therefore, its schedule II narcotic status requiring strict administration records. Gastrointestinal upset and constipation are rare but are possible side effects. Monitoring the patient for overdose or underdosage of this medication is imperative, as with all pain medications.

Follow-up Assessments. When the animal no longer requires in-hospital care and evaluation, it can be discharged from the hospital to its owner or other caregiver. The animal that has had IVD spinal surgery should be periodically assessed by a veterinarian. The frequency and intensity of this assessment will depend upon the individual animal's recovery and complications. In most instances, veterinary assessments should be performed no later than 10 to 14 days after surgery, if for no other reason than to remove sutures or staples. Most animals will require 1 to 3 months to fully recover from spinal surgery, and periodic assessments throughout this time are often helpful.

Wobbler Syndrome

Both medical (nonsurgical) and surgical treatments have been historically used for this disease (see bibliography under Wobbler Syndrome). Medical treatments including confinement or exercise restriction, analgesics, and sometimes short-term corticosteroid or nonsteroidal anti-inflammatory medications are used. Using a harness instead of a collar may help to avoid trauma to the neck region during leash walking. If clinical signs are poorly or minimally responsive to these nonsurgical treatments, if clinical signs are severe, or if clinical signs are worsening, an appropriate diagnosis and assessment for surgical treatment should be performed.

A number of surgical techniques for the disease have been described, suggesting that no one technique is adequate. Surgery may be performed with a primary goal of decompressing the spinal cord, or it can be used to internally fuse the affected spinal segments. Both dorsal and ventral decompressive techniques have been described depending upon the location of the spinal compression.

Multiple techniques to internally stabilize the caudal cervical area have been employed. The flexion force that occurs in this area in the awake animal often leads to dislocation of the apparatus and return of instability unless the construct is well attached to the underlying bone and stable. If the dorsal annulus fibrosis and dorsal longitudinal ligaments have not been surgically removed, further collapse of the disk space leads to recurrent spinal cord compression if distraction of the IVD is not maintained with the apparatus. Therefore, it is often necessary to combine internal stabilization with ventral decompression to ensure the best postoperative result (fig. 14.7).

The ultimate goal of any surgical treatment for this disease is to result in arthrodesis and bony fusion of the vertebrae adjacent to the affected disk space. If arthrodesis can be achieved, resolution of ligamentous hypertrophy and osteophyte production can occur with time. Another current utilized surgical technique for this disease involves "plugging" of the affected IVD spaces with polymethyl methacrylate alone. After the IVD space is distracted, a small amount of PMMA is placed into the disk space and allowed to harden and maintain distraction of the IVD. An external support brace is sometimes placed on the animal during the weeks following surgery to help maintain stability of the cervical region. Complications from this approach result from failure of the plug to maintain distraction of the disk space, usually due to the plug becoming dislodged ventrally. In some instances, bone resorption surrounding the plug may result in collapse of the IVD space. Depending upon the surgical preparation (for promotion of new bone production) of the disk space and the amount of PMMA used, arthrodesis may be delayed and clinical signs may recur or worsen.

An important complication of any surgical technique that results in arthrodesis is the possibility of distributing excessive or abnormal forces on adjacent or adjoining intervertebral disk spaces resulting in failure of these spaces. This is commonly referred to as the *domino effect.* A new compressive lesion in the area adjacent to arthrodesis can result in recurrence of similar clinical signs. Additionally, if clinical signs do recur and metal surgical implants have been used, imaging of the surgical area may not be possible with MR due to the artifact created by such metal precluding visualization of the area.

In younger dogs with wobbler syndrome, the pathology usually involves the dorsal articular facets with secondary hypertrophy of the associated joint capsules and ligaments (see chapter 6 discussion of wobbler syndrome). As dorsal instability and joint failure most likely contribute to the pathophysiology of the disease, surgical treatment involves removal of abnormal tissues to result in spinal cord decompression. A dorsal laminectomy is performed, and abnormal soft tissues, synovial cysts, and associated bony stenosis are removed (fig. 14.8). As instability of the dorsal articular joint spaces contributes to the progression of the disease, internal stabilization dorsally may decrease the progression of the disease. This may be achieved by removal of the articular cartilage of the affected articular joint spaces, placement of bone grafting material in these spaces, and stabilization of these spaces using transarticular cortical bone screws (fig. 14.9). In some instances, ventral surgical techniques to result in arthrodesis of these joints via the production of ventral bony fusion have been attempted.

In general, clinical signs in approximately 75% of affected dogs that are walking prior to surgery will either stop progressing or improve after surgery. Recovery percentages fall to approximately 50% in dogs that are not walking prior to surgery. Although worsening paralysis after surgery occurs less frequently, it is important to inform owners of this risk. As always, appropriate nursing care and physical therapy often significantly contribute to a successful outcome.

Lumbosacral Disease

Lumbosacral (LS) disease can occur as a congenital stenosis of the lumbosacral region or be acquired due to malarticulation, malformation, occult osteochondritis dessicans (OCD) lesions, or, most commonly, IVD degeneration and protrusion (see chapter 6 and bibliography under Lumbosacral Disease). If the disease is mild, clinical signs may be improved with confinement and restricted activity (for 4 to 8 weeks) and analgesics. Any jumping or activity

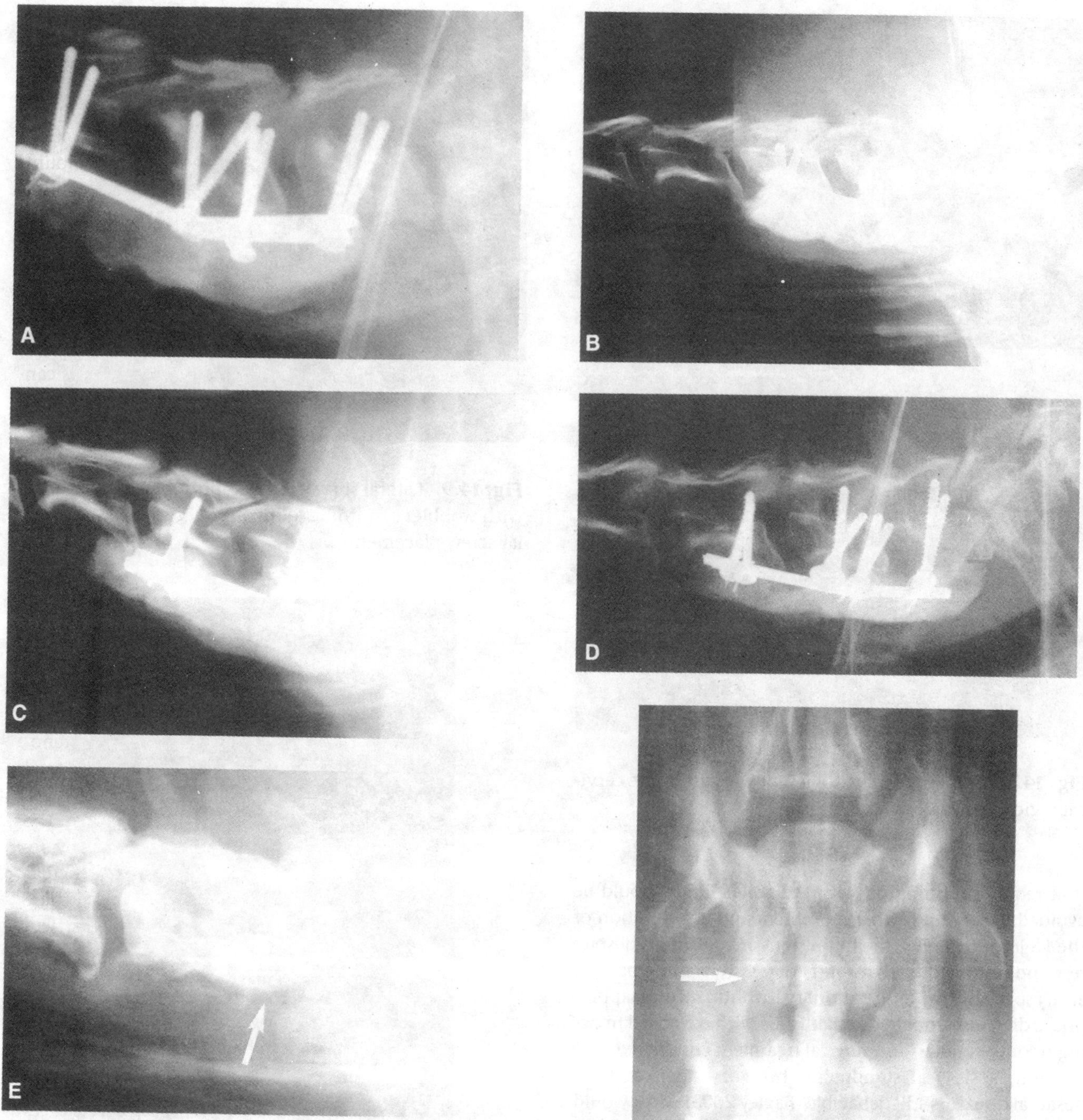

Fig. 14.7. (A,B,C,D) Lateral survey radiographic view of dogs with wobbler syndrome following surgical stabilization. (E) Lateral survey radiographic view of a dog with a PMMA plug (*arrow*). (F) Ventrodorsal survey radiographic view of a dog with a PMMA plug (*arrow*).

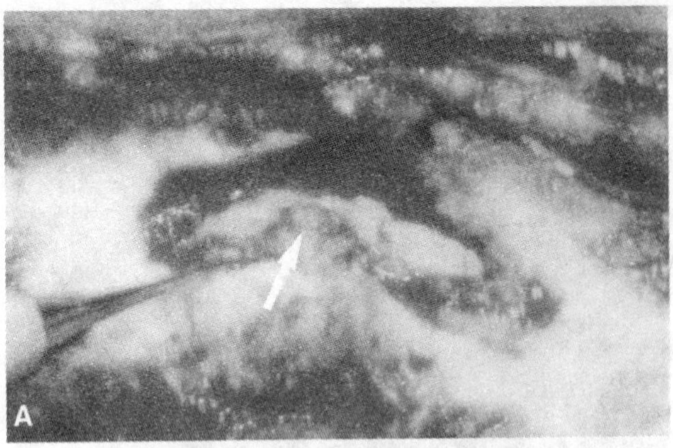

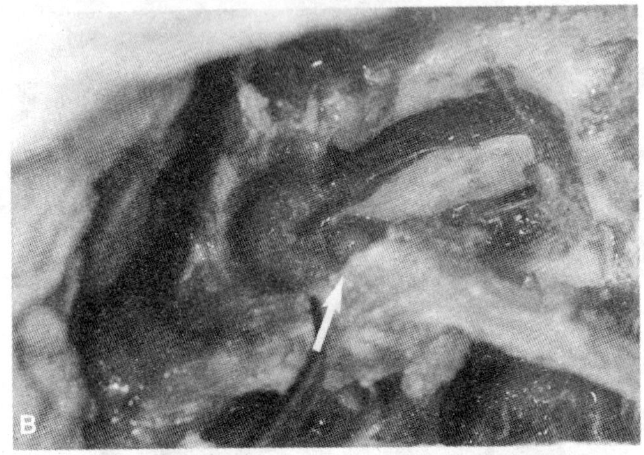

Fig. 14.8. (A,B) Appearance of a synovial cyst in the cervical region of two dogs (*arrow*).

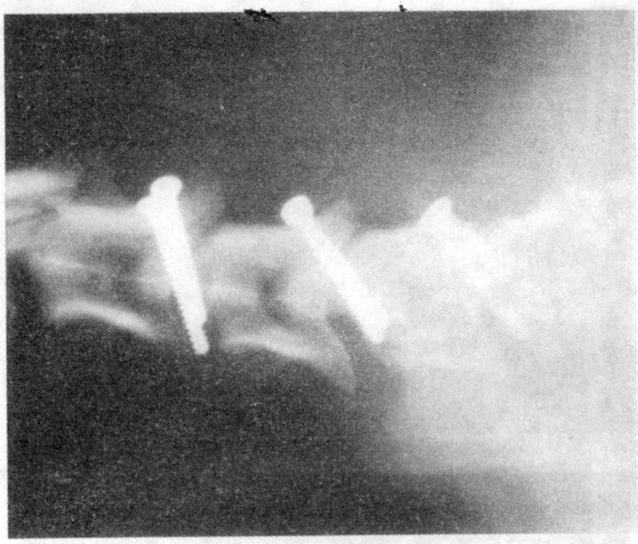

Fig. 14.9. Lateral survey radiographic view of a young dog with wobbler syndrome following surgery and transarticular screw placement.

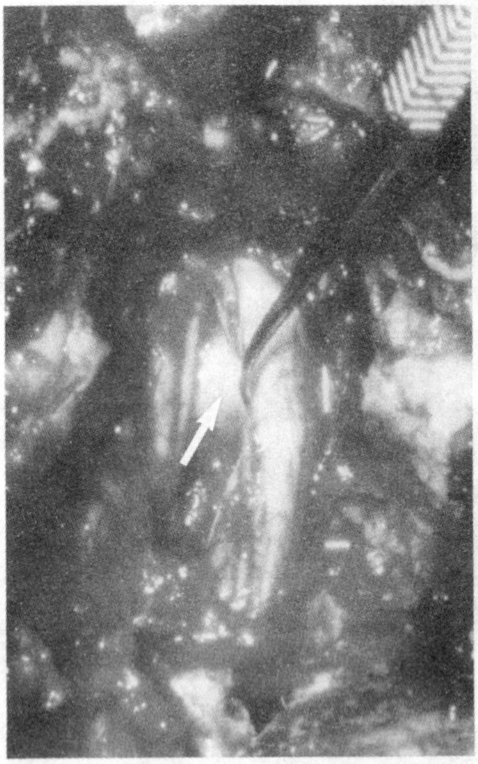

Fig. 14.10. Appearance of a lumbosacral disk protrusion following a dorsal laminectomy in a dog (*arrow*).

that requires pushing off with the pelvic limbs should be avoided to prevent further movement and deterioration of the LS joint complex. If clinical signs are persistent despite rest and restricted activity, or if there is worsening paresis, and, especially, any fecal or urinary incontinence, an appropriate diagnosis should be established with advanced imaging or other studies, and surgical treatment considered.

From a surgical standpoint, how best to treat lumbosacral disease is still debatable (Bagley 2003). Most would agree that decompression via laminectomy is often helpful, however not always successful, and failure to improve or recurrence of clinical signs may be attributable to instability. Generally, dogs with milder signs are more likely to respond to laminectomy alone (fig. 14.10). Dorsal laminectomy is almost exclusively chosen for decompression of the lumbosacral space. The nerve roots in this area can be pulled gently to the side to afford ventral exposure. Decompression itself via laminectomy and diskectomy may also facilitate spontaneous fusion of the LS joint, which may contribute to the overall success of this procedure.

There is clinical and radiological evidence that there is instability in instances of LS disease. Because of these factors, we have opted to surgically treat LS disease using a combination of decompression via laminectomy and internal stabilization (fig. 14.11). While objective comparative data are lacking, clinical outcomes with this approach have been very favorable, additional surgical time for the stabilization procedure is acceptable, and recurrence of the disease is minimal. Comparative studies still need to be performed to determine if either approach is better than the other to bring about return to normal function and activity and, importantly, long-term resolution of clinical signs.

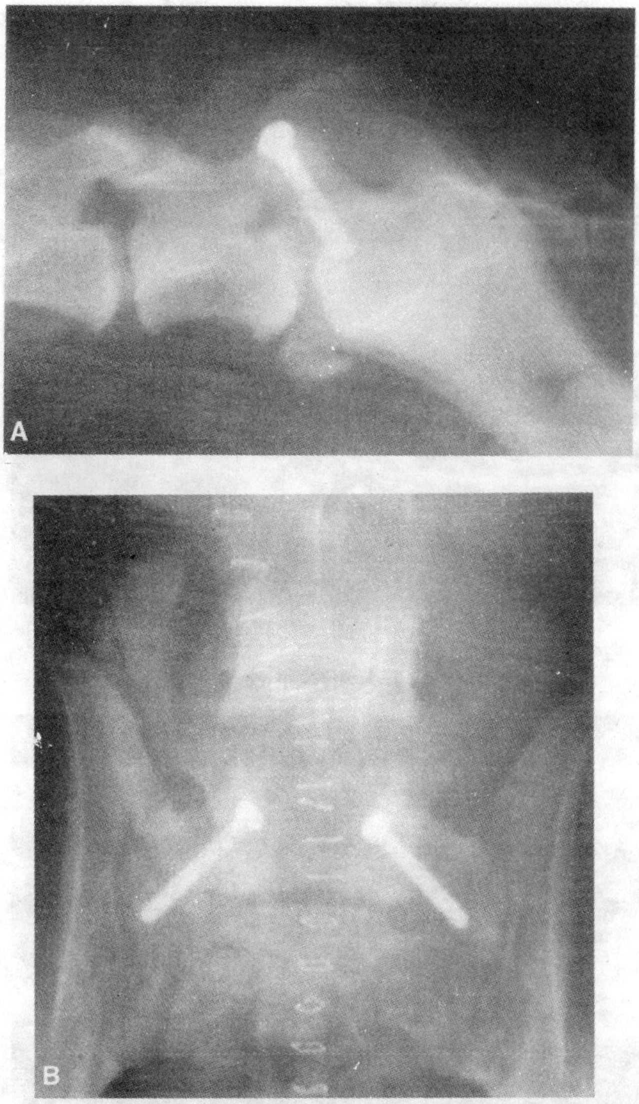

Fig. 14.11. (A) Lateral and (B) ventrodorsal survey radiographic view following transarticular screw placement at the lumbosacral junction.

Complications of stabilization are few and are comparable to those of laminectomy and diskectomy alone. Potential complications associated with internal fixation include increased surgical time, breakage or migration of the implants, fracture of the articular facets, infection, and failure at adjacent sites in the spine secondary to increased strain resulting from fusion of the LS junction. Currently, these complications have been rarely encountered. Additionally, if clinical signs do recur and metal surgical implants have been used, imaging of the surgical area may not be possible with MR due to the artifact created by such metal precluding visualization of the LS area.

Rest and analgesics are used following surgical decompression. Dogs should be confined with exercise restriction for at least 4 and preferably 8 weeks following surgery. If no major complications occur, physical therapy consisting of leash walking and/or swimming is used for 4–6 weeks with a gradual return to normal activity over 2 to 3 months. Milder clinical signs are more likely to respond to medical therapies. Once incontinence occurs, improvement in clinical signs, even with surgical decompression, is less likely.

Spondylosis Deformans/Ventral Bridging Spondylosis

Spondylosis deformans or ventral bridging spondylosis is a commonly encountered, assumably degenerative vertebral and paravertebral abnormality (see Bagley and Tucker 1996). If nerve impingement is found, surgical removal through laminectomy or foraminotomy may bring about improvement in clinical signs. Pain management may also be helpful.

Anomalous Diseases

A variety of spinal cord congenital abnormalities may involve the vertebrae, the meninges, or the spinal cord proper. These defects may be associated with protrusion or adhesion of the meninges (meningocele) or meninges and spinal cord (meningomyelocele). The spinal cord may be tethered to the skin resulting in traction on the spinal cord and cauda equina nerves. In these situations, surgical removal of this meningocele and associated structures may untether the underlying associated spinal cord and result in improvement or resolution of clinical signs.

Rhodesian ridgeback dogs and, occasionally, other breeds of dogs, such as Shih tzus and boxers, have a congenital connection from the spinal cord to the skin referred to as a dermoid sinus. Surgical removal of this tissue may resolve or improve clinical signs. This requires dissection of these abnormal tissues from the spinal cord and dura (fig. 14.12).

Abnormalities of the vertebral structures may sometimes be associated with clinical signs of spinal cord dysfunction. If clinical signs are mild, nonsurgical treatments with confinement, restricted activity, corticosteroids, or pain medication may provide symptomatic relief. If no response is achieved with nonsurgical therapies, spinal cord decompression, stabilization, or realignment may be attempted surgically. Depending on the type, severity, and location of the vertebral defect, surgery may be variably successful.

Atlantoaxial Subluxation

Atlantoaxial instability occurs in numerous, usually small but occasionally large, dog breeds (see bibliography under Atlantoaxial Subluxation). If clinical signs are mild, nonsurgical treatments with confinement, restricted activity, corticosteroids, or pain medication may provide symptomatic relief. External support splints or bandages are occasionally helpful, but are difficult to apply properly to reduce motion in the AA joint.

Surgical treatment for AA instability is used to eliminate spinal instability at this articulation and realign the vertebral column (Thomas et al. 1991). Dorsal fixation techniques using wires were originally developed but had a

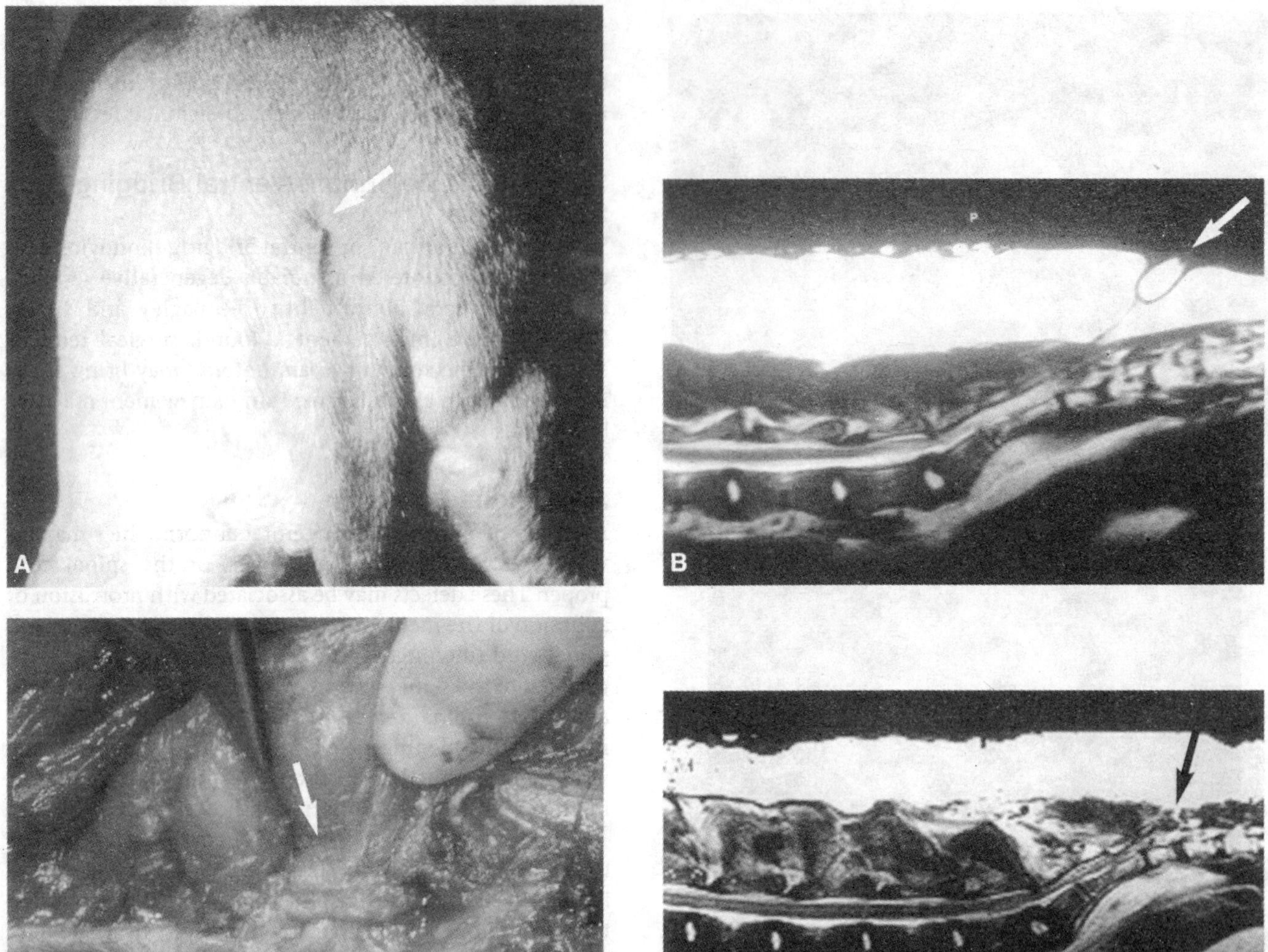

Fig. 14.12. (A) Appearance and (B) sagittal T2-weighted MR image of a dog with a dermoid sinus (*arrow*). (C) Appearance of the tract extending into the spinal canal at surgery (*arrow*). (D) Sagittal, T2-weighted MR image from the same dog following surgery (*arrow*). (E) Appearance of the dog following surgery.

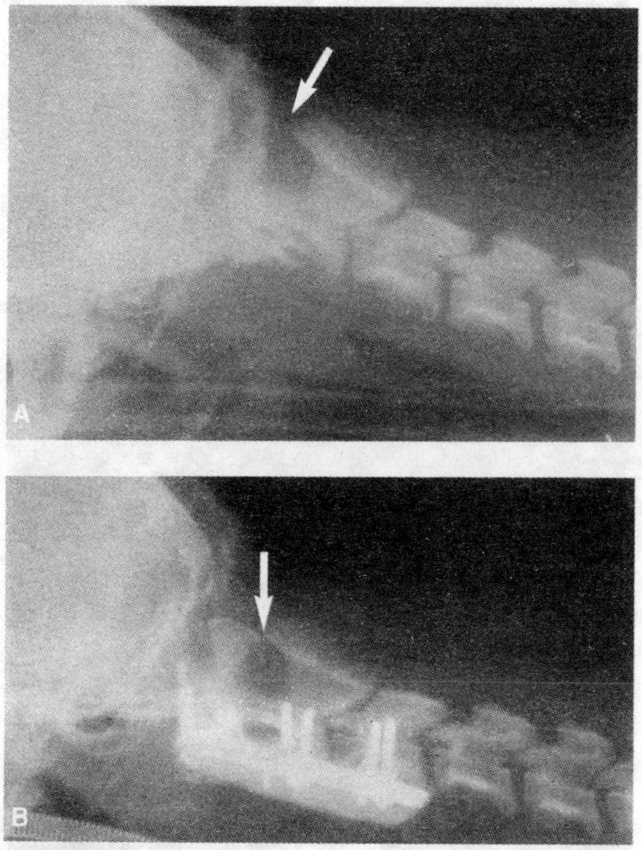

Fig. 14.13. Lateral survey radiographic view of a dog with atlantoaxial instability (A) before and (B) after surgery stabilization of the articulation.

high incidence of failure. Conventional surgical recommendation is stabilizing this joint via a ventral approach and lag screwing of C2 to C1. Complications include acute death and trachea necrosis due to retraction of soft tissues for ventral surgical exposure to this articulation.

In our hospital, a technique wherein screws (1.5–2 mm) are placed into the C1, C2, and C3 vertebrae and then anchored together using a combination of Steinmann pins or Kirschner wires, wire, and polymethyl methacrylate has been used successfully (fig. 14.13). This technique affords maximum stabilization of the AA joint. The pins are placed to prevent dorsal movement of C2 in relation to C1. Caution should be exercised, as always, during soft tissue manipulation in this area to avoid iatrogenic damage to the larynx or esophagus. Laryngeal paralysis may be an associated complication from excessive soft tissue manipulation.

Syringomyelia and Hydromyelia

Syringomyelia and hydromyelia are increasingly diagnosed as a cause of spinal cord dysfunction in dogs, and rarely, in cats (see Bagley et al. 1996; Bagley et al. 2000). If clinical signs are mild, nonsurgical treatments with confinement, restricted activity, corticosteroids, or pain medication may provide symptomatic relief. Medical management of this condition may improve clinical signs in some dogs, and is often attempted prior to, or concurrent with, surgical treatments. Corticosteroids (prednisone) are most often used at anti-inflammatory dosages (0.5–1 mg/kg every 12 to 24 hours). If medical treatment is the sole treatment to be used (i.e., in an owner not wishing to pursue surgical treatment), corticosteroid dosages are adjusted (increased) if clinical signs are not improved, and the animal is monitored closely for side effects. If improvement or resolution of clinical signs occurs within the first 1 to 2 weeks following corticosteroid therapy, this medication can be used in decreasing doses to provide the lowest dose necessary to achieve remission of clinical signs.

If the clinical signs are the result of a Chiari or other foramen magnum or infratentorial abnormality, surgical removal of any stenosis and decompression of the brain stem, cerebellum, and cranial spinal cord may benefit clinical signs (fig. 14.14). Decompressive surgery of the foramen magnum usually includes a suboccipital craniectomy and durotomy. After portions of the occipital bone and associated fibrous tissues are removed, a dura graft, such a temporalis fascia graft, is placed over the foramen magnum area in an attempt to prevent further scarring of tissues in this area.

In other situations where syringomyelia is associated with hydrocephalus, ventriculoperitoneal shunting may improve clinical signs. In still other instances, if the syringomyelia is associated with local spinal cord disease such as focal arachnoid scarring, surgical removal of abnormal tissues through laminectomy may be necessary.

Scoliosis

Scoliosis is a lateral deviation of the spine that is often associated with underlying spinal cord abnormalities such as syringomyelia and myelodysplasia in dogs (see Bagley et al.

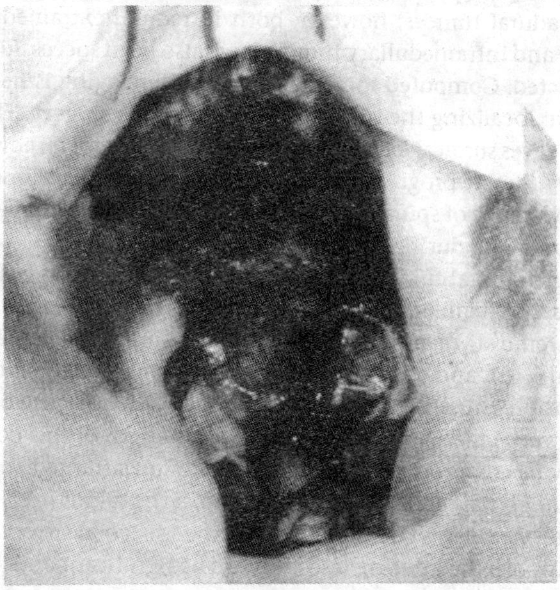

Fig. 14.14. Appearance of the foramen magnum area in a dog with a dilated fourth ventricle and syringomyelia following a suboccipital craniotomy.

1997). Medical therapy may include treatment of associated spinal pain (analgesics) and anti-inflammatory medications (steroid or nonsteroid). If clinical signs are progressive, surgical treatment may be considered. Surgical treatment should only be attempted after underlying spinal cord defects have been determined. Depending upon the type and extent of any spinal defects, surgical treatment may include spinal cord decompression, drainage of abnormal intraspinal fluid accumulations, and realignment of the vertebral frame with surgical stabilization may be attempted.

Arachnoid Cysts

Spinal arachnoid cysts have been reported with increasing frequency in dogs. A similar lesion is also seen in humans (see bibliography under Arachnoid Cysts). Clinical signs associated with arachnoid cysts may be treated medically with anti-inflammatory (corticosteroid) medication. If clinical signs are progressive, surgical removal of the cystic cavity associated scar tissue is performed through a laminectomy (fig. 14.15). The abnormal tissue is usually sharply dissected from the spinal cord and the overlying dura is removed. Surgical treatments for this disease are often successful if the abnormal tissue is removed completely and pial adhesions are released.

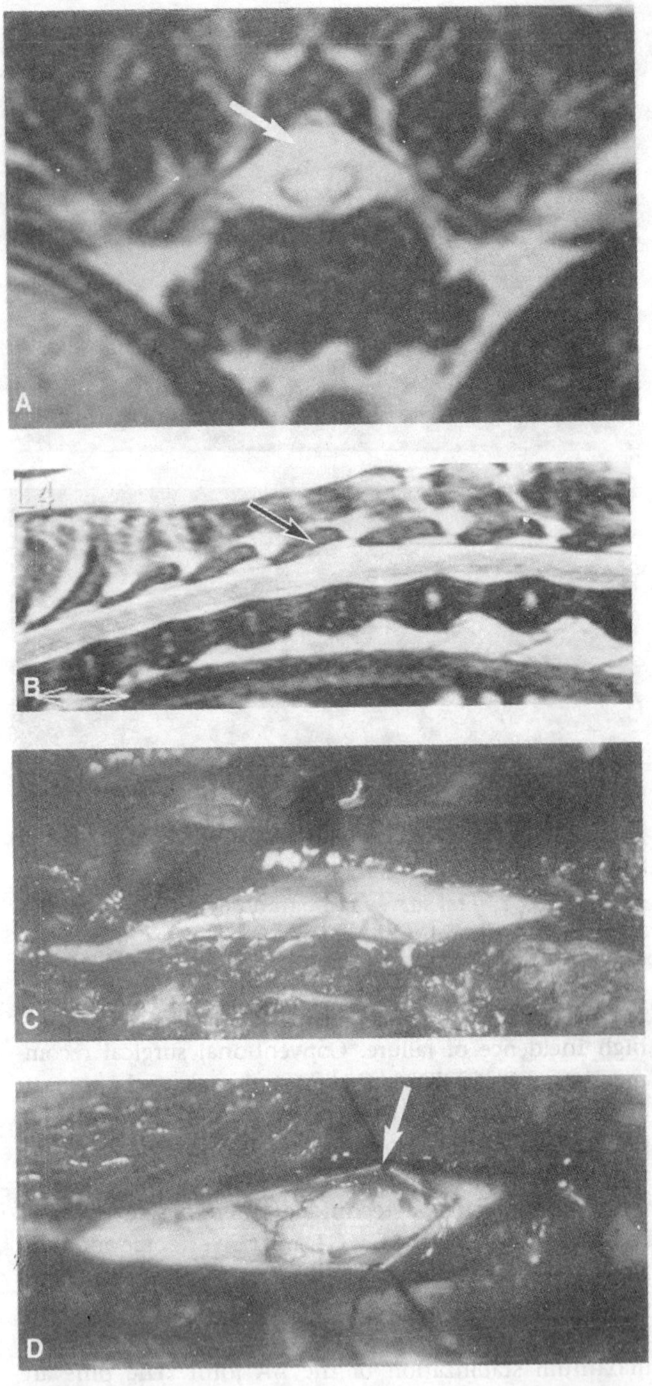

Fig. 14.15. (A) Transverse and (B) sagittal, T2-weighted magnetic resonance views of a dog with a subarachnoid cyst (*arrow*). Appearance of the cyst at surgery (C) before and (D) after incision of the cyst.

Neoplasia

Spinal neoplasms are often categorized initially based upon the anatomical area, in relation to the dura and spinal cord, of spinal involvement (see bibliography under Spinal Tumor). Determining the tumor type and extent is important when choosing appropriate therapies.

Palliative treatments include confinement, restricted activity, corticosteroids, and pain medication as needed to provide symptomatic relief. Definitive treatment options for spinal tumors include surgical removal and, possibly, radiation therapy. Surgical removal is most often reserved for extradural tumors, however, both intradural/extramedullary and intramedullary tumors have also been successfully resected. Computed tomography and MR imaging is helpful in localizing the tumor extension prior to surgery. This improves surgical exposure and subsequent tumor removal. The ultimate prognosis depends upon degree of local resection, degree of spinal infiltration, associated spinal damage prior to and during surgery, and tumor type.

Extradural tumors are removed by laminectomy, either dorsal or hemilaminectomy. Ventral slotting is inadequate for removal of most cervical tumors. Abnormal tissue is identified and removed via blunt or sharp dissection. Caution is used during drilling with lesions that involve the vertebrae, as the consistency and strength of this bone may be compromised. This may lead to unwarranted entry of the spinal canal with the drill. Also, if the tumor involves large vascular structures such as the vertebral artery or sinus, bleeding during resection can be significant and life-threatening.

Wide surgical margins are a main tenet of surgical oncology, however, this is often an unrealized goal when dealing with neoplasia in the vertebrae or spinal cord due to the obvious vital nature of the surrounding nervous system. With vertebral neoplasia, a significant portion if not all of a vertebral body, lamina, or pedicles may be involved requiring extensive surgical resection. Often, while total vertebrectomy is possible, tumor margins extend to the edge and beyond reasonable limits of vertebral resection. If the amount of bone removal is excessive, surgical stabilization of the involved spinal segments may be necessary (fig.

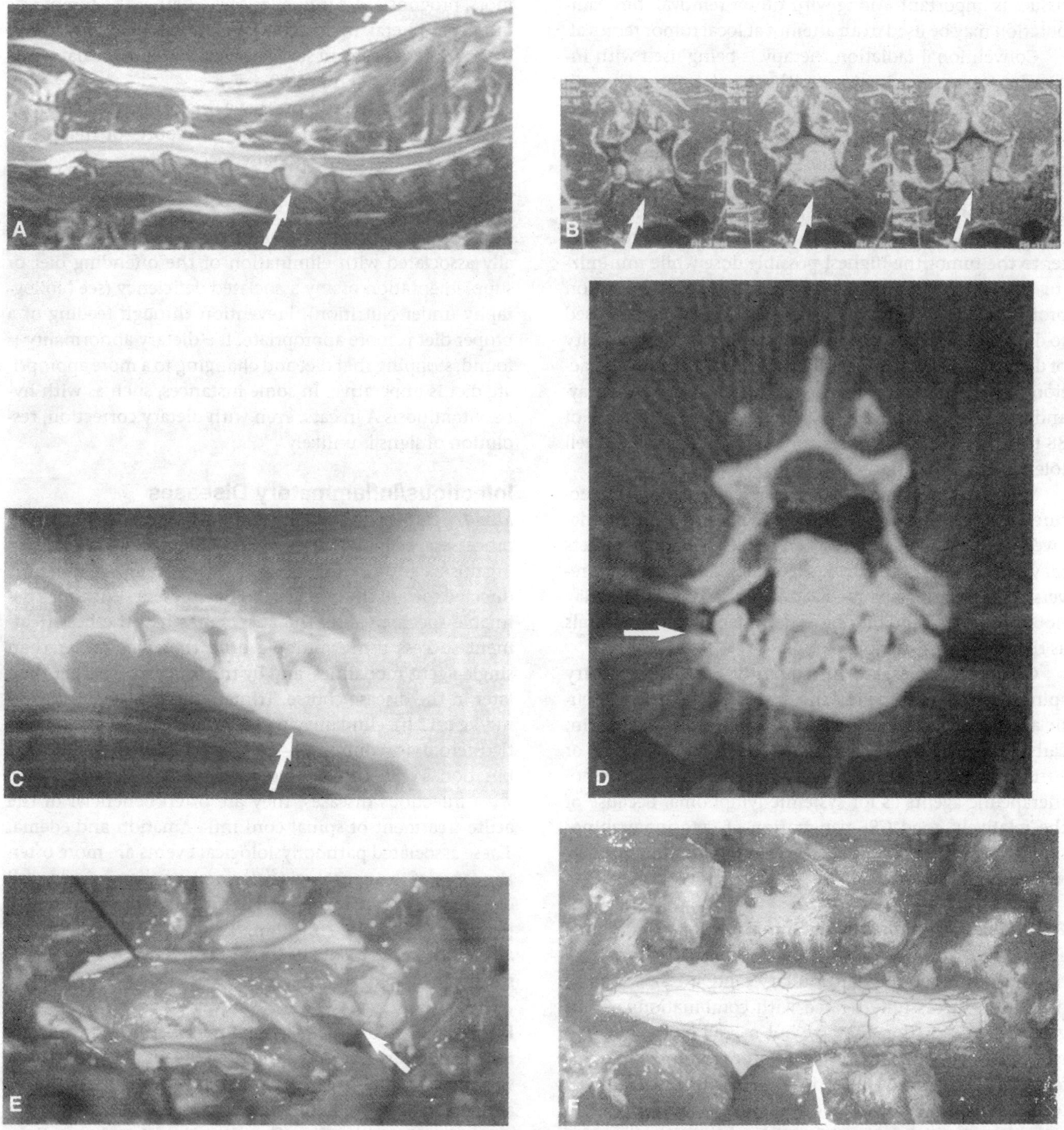

Fig. 14.16. (A) Sagittal T2-weighted, and (B) transverse T1-weighted following intravenous contrast administration magnetic resonance images of a dog with a vertebral body tumor (*arrows*). (C) Lateral, survey radiography from the same dog following surgical resection and internal stabilization. (D) Transverse CT image from the same dog showing the implanted construct. (E) Appearance at laminectomy of a meningioma (*arrow*). (F) Appearance at laminectomy of an intraspinal tumor (*arrow*).

14.16). This can be accomplished as with spinal fractures using a combination of bone screws, Steinmann pins, K-wires, and polymethyl methacrylate.

If the tumor is located within the nerves that contribute to the brachial plexus, an approach to this area may be necessary concurrently with an approach that will afford lateral access to the cervical spinal cord. A hemilaminectomy can be performed with the animal in lateral recumbency, if necessary, for spinal cord decompression if the tumor extends proximally into the spinal cord. Tumors that arise from within peripheral nerve structures are usually locally invasive, therefore, aggressive surgical removal of affected tissues is important. Along with tumor removal, limb amputation may be used in an attempt at local tumor removal.

Conventional radiation therapy is being used with increasing frequency in dogs with spinal tumor. Overall, small numbers of animals with spinal tumors have been treated. Radiation therapy is more apt to control tumor progression, however, in some instances it may eradicate the tumor completely. Significant and rapid reduction in spinal lymphoma, for example, may occur following radiation therapy. The main goal of the treatment is to administer to the tumor the highest possible dose while minimizing the dose to the surrounding normal tissue. Radiation protocols vary. Fractional dosing schemes have been used to decrease the acute toxicity of the radiation. The majority of dogs treated for spinal tumors have had, with 10–12 fractions, generally given 3 times weekly (Monday, Wednesday, and Friday) of approximately 4 Gy each, for a total dose of 38 to 48 Gy. All of the doses appeared to be generally well tolerated for the periods studied.

Side effects include radiation damage to normal structures surrounding the abnormality. Both acute, early delayed, and late delayed affects can be seen. The acute affects may be the result of edema due to tumor kill, and may be reversed with antiedema medications. The later effects may not be reversible and may be as detrimental to the animals as the underlying disease.

Chemotherapies are infrequently used for primary spinal tumors. In some instances, similar chemotherapeutic agents used for appendicular osteosarcoma (cisplantin, carboplatin) are used for vertebral osteosarcoma. Spinal or perispinal lymphoma may be responsive to similar chemotherapeutic agents as for systemic lymphoma. Because of the relatively good CSF penetration of cytosine arabinoside, this drug is often added to spinal lymphoma treatment regimens.

Prognosis of Animals with Spinal Tumor. Individual animals with tumor in each of the three locations (extradural, intradural/extramedullary, and intramedullary) have been successfully treated with combinations of surgery and/or radiation therapy, but overall efficacy of specific treatments in statistically significant numbers of affected animals is not known. Advances in microsurgical techniques have afforded the ability to successful operate on tumors involving the spinal cord, however, reports of larger numbers of similarly affected animals will be required to make objective outcome conclusions. In one report on 37 dogs with a variety of spinal tumors, median survival of all dogs that survived 20 days following diagnosis was 240 days. Forty percent of these dogs, however, were euthanized or died within the first 20 days following diagnosis. These dogs were not figured into the overall survival statistics. Tumors primarily involving the vertebrae may be associated with shorter survival times.

Median survival in dogs with peripheral nerve sheath tumors who had surgery varied depending upon whether the tumor was benign (median survival 1410 days) or malignant (median survival 180 days). For nerve sheath tumors, prognosis was influenced by whether the tumor was more peripheral in location versus involving the nerve plexus or root (median survival plexus group 360 days, median survival root group 150 days).

Intramedullary tumors have historically been diagnosed at necropsy with infrequent reports of treatment. Surgical removal is occasionally successful.

Nutrition

Primary treatments for nutritional spinal diseases are usually associated with elimination of the offending diet or supplementation of any associated deficiency (see bibliography under Nutrition). Prevention through feeding of a proper diet is more appropriate. If a dietary abnormality is found, stopping that diet and changing to a more appropriate diet is imperative. In some instances, such as with hypervitaminosis A in cats, even with dietary correction, resolution of signs is unlikely.

Infectious/Inflammatory Diseases

Myelitis can be the result of a variety of inflammatory processes (see bibliography under Myelitis). Both *infectious* organisms and noninfectious diseases occur. Treatment is directed toward the specific etiology present. Without a definable specific cause, the author has had the best treatment success using multiple drug therapies rather than single-agent modalities, and by treating earlier rather than later in the disease course. Trimethoprim sulfadiazine (30 mg/kg q 12 h), clindamycin (20–25 mg/kg q 12 h), and corticosteroids (prednisone 1–4 mg/kg q 12 h) are used in combination. While corticosteroids may seem contraindicated with infectious diseases, they are often beneficial in the acute treatment of spinal cord inflammation and edema. These associated pathophysiological events are more often the cause of the neurologic deterioration than primary cell death from the organism itself. If rickettsial diseases are suspected, doxycycline (10–20 mg/kg q 12 h PO) or, less ideally, chloramphenicol (15–25 mg/kg q 8 h PO) can be substituted or added to the regime.

Bacterial Diseases. Bacterial meningitis or myelitis is rare in dogs and cats. Treatment is ideally directed at the specific causative bacteria based on culture identification and sensitivity results collected from the infected area or, in some situations, the CSF. If a culture is not available, then the choice of antimicrobial is directed toward the suspected organism. Combinations of trimethoprim sulfadiazine (30 mg/kg q 12 h), clindamycin (20–25 mg/kg q 12 h), cephalosporins, or ampicillin may be used. If an anaerobic infection is suspected, then metronidazole may be added. If the infection or abscess results in a mass effect and spinal cord compression, surgical decompression of empyema through a laminectomy may be necessary.

Viral Diseases. *Viral myelitis* may result from systemic viral infections. *Canine distemper* remains a surprisingly common cause of spinal cord dysfunction in dogs. Specific treatment for distemper virus infection is rarely reported.

Corticosteroids may decrease associated spinal cord inflammation, however, may allow for further viral proliferation.

Feline infectious peritonitis (*FIP*) results from a coronavirus-induced vasculitis in cats. As with distemper virus infection in dogs, no specific antiviral treatment currently exists for this disease. Immunosuppression with corticosteroids may improve clinical signs, but this is usually only for a short duration. In other instances, corticosteroids will not improve clinical signs.

Feline leukemia virus may result in lymphoma that can affect the spinal cord. Treatment for lymphoma may include various chemotherapeutics or radiation therapy. Cytosine arabinoside is often added to these protocols due the improved CSF penetration with this drug. Direct effects of the virus on the spinal cord are unclear. Feline leukemia virus, however, has been associated with a myelopathy independent of the presence of lymphoma. No treatment recommendations exist for this disease.

Protozoal Disease. *Toxoplasma gondii* and *Neospora caninum* are protozoal organisms that can affect any area of the nervous system resulting in myelitis, peripheral neuropathy, or myositis in dogs. Treatment for toxoplasmosis currently is clindamycin (8–25 mg/kg, q 8–12 hours; do not exceed 50 mg/kg q 24 hours) for 14–28 days, however the addition of trimethoprim sulfa drugs PO, IM, or SC may provide a better clinical response. The most appropriate treatment of neospora is not established. Treatment as for toxoplasmosis with clindamycin and trimethoprim sulfa drugs has been used successfully for spinal cord *Neospora* infection.

Rickettsia. Infection with rickettsial organisms associated with Rocky Mountain spotted fever (RMSF) and *Ehrlichia* rarely involve the spinal cord. Dogs with clinical features of spinal cord disease thought to be associated with rickettsial organisms can be treated with tetracycline or doxycycline prior to establishing a definitive diagnosis with titers. For RMSF, treatment usually is only necessary for 7 to 14 days. For ehrlichiosis, treatment may need to be prolonged.

Fungal Disease. Of the fungal diseases that can affect the nervous system, cryptococcus, blastomycosis, coccidiomycosis, candidiasis, and aspergillosis are most common. Fungal infection involving the spine is usually associated with diskospondylitis. Treatment can be attempted with antifungal agents, however, the ability of these drugs to reach therapeutic concentration in central nervous system tissue is questionable. Fluconazole and itraconazole hold the most promise for treating fungal encephalitis/meningitis in the future. These drugs have historically been rather expensive and owner financial constraints often limit the ability to use long-term therapy.

Parasites. Parasitic disease involving the spinal cord is uncommon. Ivermectin (400 ug/kg single sq dose) has been suggested as a medical treatment for CNS parasites, but its efficacy is unknown. It is recommended to pretreat with diphenhydramine (1 to 4 mg/kg IV) and corticosteroids (dexamethasone 0.1 mg/kg) prior to administration of ivermectin. Decreases in the secondary inflammatory responses may be achieved with corticosteroids. If the parasitic infection results in a focus of inflammation, surgical removal or debridement may be possible. Cuterebra infection and migrating heartworm larvae may be treated in this way.

Noninfectious Diseases

Of the spectrum of inflammatory diseases that can affect the CNS, more often the cause of the inflammation is either undetermined or not associated with an established infectious agent. These diseases are primary inflammatory CNS diseases without a clinically recognized cause.

A *steroid-responsive meningitis* is found primarily in young (<2 years of age), large-breed dogs such as Labrador retrievers. Usually this disease responds to corticosteroid administration (prednisolone or prednisone 1–4 mg/kg q 12 h). Treatment is continued at higher dosages for 1 to 2 weeks or until clinical signs resolve or improve significantly. If clinical signs are controlled, the dosage of corticosteroid can slowly be decreased over weeks to months so as to achieve the lowest dosage of medication that will control clinical signs. Corticosteroid dosage should be tapered slowly to avoid iatrogenic hypoadrenocorticism and, most importantly to avoid recurrence of clinical signs due to subtherapeutic concentrations of the medication. *Spinal cord vasculitis syndromes* (Beagle—Beagle pain syndrome—German short-haired pointer, Bernese Mountain dog, and other breeds) are treated similarly with corticosteroid administration (prednisolone or prednisone 1–4 mg/kg q 12 h).

Granulomatous meningoencephalitis can result in clinical signs of spinal cord disease. Corticosteroid administration (prednisolone or prednisone 1–4 mg/kg q 12 h) is often used in the treatment of this disease, similar to other noninfectious myelitis syndromes. If corticosteroid therapy is beneficial, it is often necessary for prolonged periods of time, if not lifelong therapy. Discontinuation of the therapy should be performed slowly over weeks if not months to prevent recurrence of clinical signs.

If corticosteroids are not effective, other treatment options include immunosuppression (cyclophosphamide, azathioprine), other immunomodulators (leflunomide), chemotherapeutics such as lomustine, surgery (if a focal mass), or radiation therapy. The latter has shown the most promise recently for definitive treatment of this disease. Newer medical treatments under investigation in treatment of GME include cytosine arabinoside and procarbazine (Cuddon 1998). Many of these treatments are based on presumptive diagnosis of GME and anecdotal treatment responses. The efficacy of any of these treatments, therefore, is uncertain.

There is a unique clinical syndrome (generalized tremor syndrome; white shaker dog syndrome) associated with generalized tremoring. This disease is usually associated with CNS inflammation, which may involve spinal cord structures. Generalized tremor secondary to nervous system inflammation usually improves with administration of glucocorticoids at immunosuppressive dosages (1–4 mg/kg orally every 12 hours). The tremor usually lessens or resolves within 1 to 3 weeks with this therapy. The dosage of corticosteroid can then be slowly decreased. If the drug is decreased too rapidly, tremor may recur. If recurrence is seen, a prolonged tapering of corticosteroid over 4 to 6 months may be necessary. Occasionally, a dog may require corticosteroid treatment indefinitely to control the tremor.

Diskospondylitis

Diskospondylitis is infection in the IVD space and surrounding vertebral bodies (see bibliography under Diskospondylitis). Treatment is initiated with antimicrobial administration specific for the organism present. The choice of antimicrobial depends on the sensitivity spectrum of the organism cultured. Prior to definitive culture results, or when cultures are negative in association with radiographic signs suggestive of this disease, a first-generation cephalosporin such as cephalothin (22 mg/kg orally every 8 hours) is prescribed. If the organism is susceptible, clinical signs will usually improve in 3 to 7 days. If no improvement is noted, reassessment of the diagnosis should be performed. Ensure that fungal causes of diskospondylitis have been excluded. A different antimicrobial can then be used. If antimicrobial drugs bring about improvement in clinical signs, these medications should be administered for at least 6 weeks. In some instances, medications will need to be given for longer than 6 weeks to eliminate the infection. If brucellosis is present, treatment with minocycline or other tetracycline products has been historically successful. Brucellosis can also be persistent in the face of treatment, so prolonged duration of treatment is often necessary.

If blood and urine cultures remain negative, and a clinical improvement is not seen on antimicrobials, direct disk space culture should be performed. This can be performed percutaneously with needle aspiration, but it usually requires fluoroscopic imaging to ensure accuracy of needle penetration. For access to the affected intervertebral disk space, a open surgical approach (as for a laminectomy) and disk space fenestration are most often performed. Often the infected disk space is fibrous in character and does not contain an obvious abscessation. In some situations, if diskospondylitis is associated with vertebral instability, surgical stabilization of the affected adjacent vertebrae may be necessary. In some instances of diskospondylitis, the infectious process may extend from the disk into the perispinal tissues and fat.

Vertebral body osteomyelitis is uncommon in dogs and cats but can result from hematogenous infection or local penetrating trauma. Grass awn and porcupine quill migration may enter the spinal canal and result in focal infection. *Actinomyces* and *Nocardia* may be present in these locations. Fungal granulomas have also occurred in the spinal canal. Surgical exploration, debridement, and culture may be necessary to remove the offending foreign body or abscess accumulation.

Idiopathic Disease

Calcinosis circumscripta is a primarily a disease of German shepherds but has been reported in other breeds. Surgical resection and spinal cord decompression may improve clinical signs. Treatment for *Feline hyperesthesia syndrome,* which may mimic signs of spinal painful disease, is discussed in chapter 13.

CLINICAL MANAGEMENT OF ANIMALS WITH SUSPECTED SPINAL TRAUMA

Animals may have spinal injury from exogenous trauma such as being hit by an automobile, falling, and getting impacted with objects and missile projectiles. Treatment of animals with spinal injury is discussed in chapter 22. The animal should be carefully placed on a rigid, movable surface such as a spinal board (fig. 14.17).

Once spinal injury is established, it is important to assess the severity of injury in order to develop a management strategy and a realistic prognosis for the owner. Severity of a spinal cord injury is usually graded based on clinical findings (table 14.7). Animals that are less-severely affected (painful only; mildly paretic) are more often managed without surgical intervention. Animals that are more severely neurologically impaired (nonambulatory paretic or paralyzed) are often considered for possible surgical treatment (stabilization). It is important to recognize, however, that scientific data to support many of the current treatment recommendations for animals with spinal trauma are lacking. Individual clinical experience with the various treatments is often the overriding factor in decision making. These anecdotal experiences, however, are difficult to prove without case-controlled studies. Unfortunately, until this information is available, individual assessments based on clinical experience and owner wishes are the guiding forces behind management decisions in animals with spinal trauma.

Animals that lose deep pain sensation concurrent with their spinal injury have a worse chance for return to function. Loss of deep pain sensation in an animal with a verte-

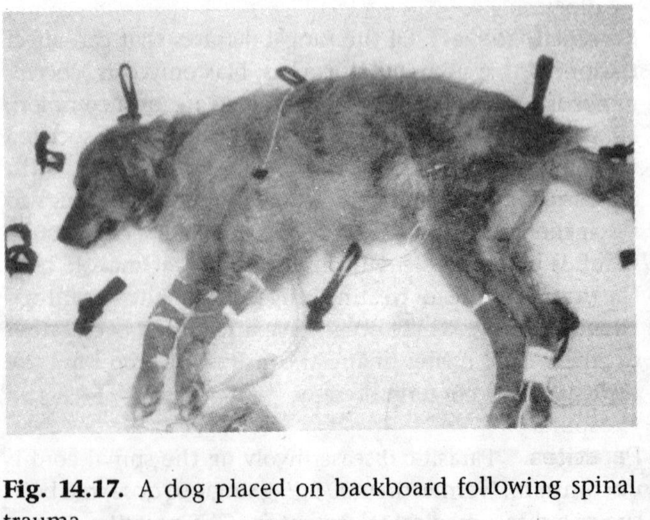

Fig. 14.17. A dog placed on backboard following spinal trauma.

bral fracture or luxation is a very poor prognostic indicator. Additionally, if deep pain sensation is absent in an animal with 100% or greater displacement of the vertebral canal on radiographic assessment, the prognosis for walking is exceedingly poor.

NONSURGICAL TREATMENTS FOR SPINAL TRAUMA

Corticosteroid Therapy

Corticosteroid therapy has been shown to be an important adjunctive therapy for humans and animals suffering spinal trauma. Methylprednisolone sodium succinate administration was established as the standard of care for humans suffering spinal trauma in the early 1990s. Since that time, controversy has arisen as to the efficacy and the degree of side effects associated with administration of methylprednisolone in this group of patients. The dogma of administering methylprednisolone sodium succinate to humans with spinal injury is currently being questioned in human medicine. Questions regarding this treatment include those of treatment efficacy and number and severity of side effects. Therefore, the recommendations for using this drug in treatment of spinal injury in humans may change in the future.

As a controlled, blinded clinical study has not been performed to determine the efficacy of methylprednisolone therapy in animals with acute spinal injury, many of the recommendations for use of this steroid have been based on information from studies in animals of experimentally induced spinal injury. Until a definitive study is available in animals, clinicians will have to make individual determinations as to whether or not to administer methylprednisolone sodium succinate to animals with spontaneously occurring spinal injury.

Ideally, corticosteroids are administered as soon as possible after a spinal injury, prior to, or during radiographic evaluation. Experimental studies in small animals have suggested that only soluble corticosteroids (methylprednisolone sodium succinate) given within 1 hour of the trauma are beneficial at mitigating secondary pathophysiologic events associated with spinal trauma. Many of these experimental studies have been performed in cats. Less information is available in dogs.

In human beings, it has been suggested that methylprednisolone sodium succinate given up to 8 hours after a spinal trauma was beneficial. This dichotomy between time of administration and benefit in humans versus animals suggests that the time frame of benefit following injury is shorter in small animals. It is also important to recognize that other corticosteroids such as dexamethasone have generally not been proven effective for treatment of experimental spinal trauma and have been associated with significant complications in clinically affected animals with spinal disease. For these reasons, the author does not use dexamethasone treatment for spinal injury.

In studies in humans, a 30 mg/kg intravenous (IV) bolus of methylprednisolone sodium succinate was administered initially followed by 5.4 mg/kg/hour IV for the next 23 hours as a constant infusion. This was in an attempt to keep a high level of this corticosteroid in the injured cord for a longer period. An abstracted report of the use of this same treatment regime in dogs with intervertebral disk disease suggested a benefit, however was poorly controlled. An alternative protocol used in small animals (however, experimentally unproved) is to give methylprednisolone sodium succinate as an initial bolus (time 0) at a dose of 30 mg/kg IV, with additional doses of 15 mg/kg IV given at 2 and 6 hours after the initial dose as an attempt to avoid the additional labor and expense of administering the medication as a constant infusion. The efficacy of this protocol, however, is not established.

If the methylprednisolone sodium succinate is given too quickly in an awake animal, vomiting often occurs. If the medication is given too rapidly with the animal under general anesthesia, hypotension often is noted. Acute death has been also noted experimentally with bolus injections of methylprednisolone, however, this is extremely rare in normal clinical practice. For these reasons, it is advisable to administer the methylprednisolone sodium succinate IV over approximately 5–10 minutes.

Corticosteroid administration in animals with spinal disease is also associated with an increased incidence of gastrointestinal ulceration and possibly pancreatitis. This complication is more likely when animals are given larger dosages of corticosteroids, or when the medication is given over a prolonged duration of time. If severe, gastrointestinal ulceration can be a life-threatening complication of corticosteroid administration in animals with spinal injury. The most common site of intestinal perforation in animals with spinal disease administered dexamethasone is at the antimesenteric surface of the border between the transverse and descending colon. Colonic perforation at this site has been uniformly fatal in dogs. Dexamethasone appears to be more ulcerogenic than prednisolone. This may be due in part to inappropriate dosing as published doses of dexamethasone seem high considering its pharmacologic properties.

Confinement and External Support Bandages

Cage confinement may be necessary for 4 to 6 weeks in animals with nonsurgically managed spinal fracture. In some instances, confinement may be as beneficial for recovery as surgical treatment.

External support bandages or casts have also been used successfully in nonsurgical treatment animals (see chapter 22). The goals of external support should be immobilization of the vertebral segments above and below the damaged area. This support should be as rigid as possible to ensure that minimal, and ideally no, motion of the vertebral column occurs around the affected area. External supports are ideally left on the animal for 4 to 6 weeks or until healing is complete. The bandage associated with the external support is changed as needed during this time and especially if skin irritation occurs. A bandage that becomes loose fitting or soiled needs to be removed and replaced.

Follow-up evaluations can be scheduled as necessary based upon clinical course. It is ideal to evaluate the animal at 3 and 6 weeks after injury to critically assess neurologic progress. If an external support bandage has been applied, more frequent evaluations may be performed to change soiled bandages. Radiographic assessment of fracture healing may also be used to determine when cage confinement or external support can be terminated. If healing is suspected to be complete, a gradual return to exercise should be initiated. Short leash-controlled walks are begun (10–15 minutes; one to three times per day for the first 1–2 weeks) on flat surfaces with good footing, and the animal is monitored for any pain or decline in neurologic status. If leash walks are tolerated, the duration and number of walks during the day can be increased over the next 2–4 weeks. If the animal tolerates this exercise, it may have free activity after this time, provided that the activity area is enclosed (e.g., fenced backyard), and there is good footing.

SURGICAL TREATMENTS

Indications for surgical treatment of spinal trauma are numerous and often controversial. Some authors suggest that similar results are obtained with both surgical and nonsurgical treatments for spinal fracture, irrespective of severity of clinical signs. Intuitively, however, surgical stabilization of spinal instability seems reasonable when the chance of increasing instability is likely.

If instability is documented, spinal stabilization should be considered (fig. 14.18). External fixation with splints and bandages may be helpful if applied correctly. Internal fixation and stabilization, however, is often necessary. A variety of techniques have been used and have been previously reviewed. Each technique has advantages and disadvantages, which may be utilized in different situations.

In our hospital, internal fixation using a combination of bone screws, Kirschner wires, Steinmann pins, and polymethyl methacrylate (PMMA) cement is most often chosen for stabilization (figs. 14.18, 14.19). These methods of fixation are modifications of previously described techniques. Screws and pins are used to anchor the PMMA to the bone. Similar fixation devices have been shown to provide adequate protection against excessive spinal rotation in canine cadaver spine preparations. Rigid spinal fixation increases the chance of fracture healing in dog spines.

Follow-up Management

The animal that has had surgical spinal fixation is treated in the same manner as animals recovering from other types of spinal surgery (see above, Intervertebral Disk Disease). Important management areas include attention to systemic health, confinement in an appropriate area, pain control, bladder assessments, and physical therapy. Appropriate wound management is used until skin healing is complete. If clinical improvement in limb function is noted, the aforementioned exercise scheme can be followed. Radiographs should be taken at least 6 weeks after surgery to assess the alignment, surgical implants, and fracture healing. Postoperative infection of implants can result in systemic illness or draining tracts in the area of the surgery. If infection is present but localized, appropriate antibiotics are prescribed until fracture healing is thought to be complete.

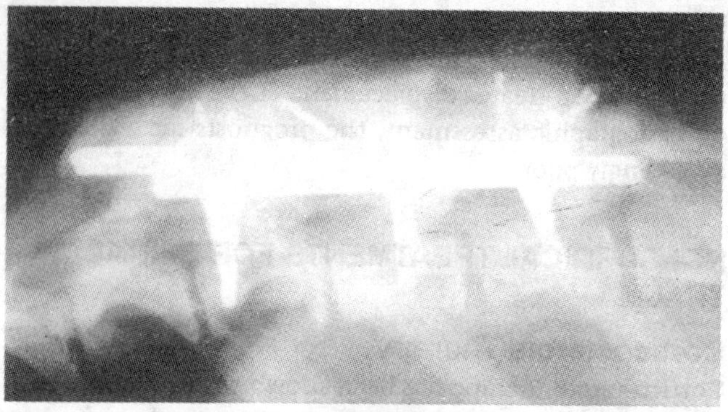

Fig. 14.18. Lateral survey radiographic image from a dog with a spinal fracture following surgical stabilization.

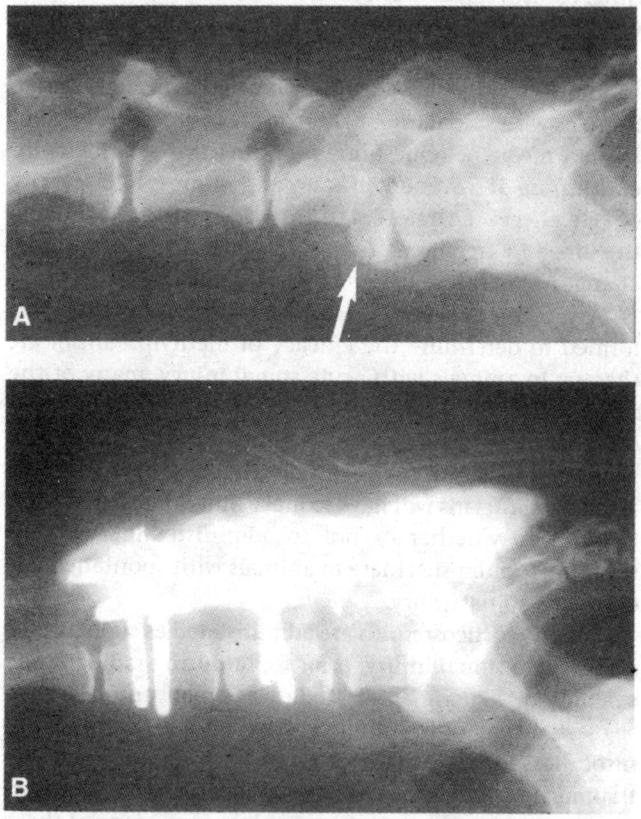

Fig. 14.19. Lateral survey radiograph (A) before and (B) following surgical stabilization of an L6 vertebral body fracture (*arrow*).

FIBROCARTILAGINOUS EMBOLI

Ischemic myelopathy or fibrocartilaginous emboli is a spinal cord vascular disease (infarction) that results in a noncompressive myelopathy. Other diseases such as noncompressive intervertebral disk extrusion and spinal contusion may present similarly.

There is no specific treatment for this condition. Corticosteroids are sometimes used acutely following the onset of clinical signs, but the benefit of their administration is unknown. The prognosis of dogs with fibrocartilaginous emboli depends primarily on the severity of clinical signs. Loss of deep pain sensation is a poor prognostic sign for return to function. If deep pain sensation remains, even if the animals are paralyzed initially from the disease, many animals will recover useful spinal function. Basic management guidelines for the animal recovering from spinal injury or intervertebral disk disease should be followed.

SPINAL CORD HEMORRHAGE AND HEMATOMA

Treatment for CNS bleeding includes treatment of any underlying bleeding disorder and stopping or resolving the local effects of any accumulated hemorrhage. Various treatments exist for individual coagulopathies and for thrombocytopenia. Current recommendations for treatment of these bleeding disorders can be found in other sources. If a hematoma compresses the spinal cord in an extradural location, laminectomy and evacuation concurrent with treatment of any underlying bleeding disorder should be performed. As focal neoplasia and infectious diseases may predispose to bleeding, it is always prudent to biopsy and culture the hematoma or associated abnormal tissue to ensure that these diseases are not concurrently present. If the hematoma is in the intradural but extramedullary area, a durotomy is performed to access the hemorrhage.

Treatment for a localized hematoma within the spinal cord centers is directed toward evacuation of the hematoma through a laminectomy and myelotomy (incision into the spinal cord). If the underlying bleeding disorder is still active, a dilemma exists between the need for surgical hematoma drainage and the risk of causing increasing amounts of hemorrhage. Short-term hemostatic support with blood products or platelets may provide a window of patient stability for a surgical procedure to be performed. Ultimately, if the accumulation of bleeding in the central nervous system is becoming life-threatening, surgical drainage is a necessity that is undertaken in view of the increased risk of hemorrhagic complications. While it is impossible to reverse all of the effects of the hemorrhage, decreasing the size of an expanding hematoma with the resultant decrease in nervous tissue pressure may improve clinical signs. There are two caveats to consider. One is that by decreasing intraparenchymal pressure, blood flow to the area may be restored, and a rebound hemorrhage may occur. Second, if the original cause of the bleeding was a ruptured vessel (aneurysm or arteriovenous malformation), hematoma removal may result in rebleeding. In both of these situations, however, hemostasis can, hopefully, be employed intraoperatively to decrease this possibility.

In chronic hematomas, especially if the initial bleeding tendency has subsided, surgical drainage is reasonably straightforward if the extent of the hematoma can be localized. Usually, a black, sometimes greenish, soft lesion consistent with an established hematoma is found. This can be removed with suction aspiration. The edges of the hematoma tend to be more organized requiring blunt dissection for removal.

15 Treatment of Diseases Involving the Peripheral Nervous System, Neuromuscular Junction, and Muscle of Dogs and Cats

DEGENERATIVE NEUROPATHIES

The vast majority of these degenerative neuropathic diseases either have no known effective treatment, or treatment of these diseases has not been attempted (table 15.1) (Braund 1996a, 1996b, 1996c). In some instances, experimental treatments are currently being investigated but are not practically available for widespread use. Many degenerative diseases are progressive and will eventually result in significant incapacitation of the animal.

METABOLIC NEUROPATHIES AND MYOPATHIES

Primary treatment for the neuropathy is not possible, however, treatment of the associated diabetes mellitus in order to achieve good systemic glycemic control may result in improvements in clinical signs providing substantial peripheral nerve damage has not occurred prior to diagnosis and therapy (Kramek et al. 1984; Munana 1995). Treatments for diabetes mellitus often include exogenous insulin therapy and dietary modifications.

As with diabetic neuropathy, there is no primary treatment for insulinoma neuropathy. Clinical hypoglycemia can be treated with intravenous dextrose (20–50%) 1–5 ml to effect. In some instances of insulinoma, however, intravenous dextrose therapy may result in an exacerbation or worsening of clinical signs, particularly seizure activity. As these tumors retain some responsiveness to serum glucose concentrations, dextrose administration may result in further increases in insulin secretion by the tumor. Surgical removal of an insulinoma may normalize serum glucose concentrations if the tumor can be removed in total and if there are no metastases.

Medical management of insulinoma is primarily palliative and consists of frequent small meals low in carbohydrate, diazoxide (12.5 mg bid PO), and corticosteroids (0.5–6 mg/kg/day in divided doses, beginning at lower dose) to increase blood glucose. The somatostatin analogue octreotide has also been used in some instances. Definitive treatment for insulinoma such as surgical resection of the pancreatic tumor may result in improvements of the clinical neuropathic signs if the pathological changes in peripheral nerves are not severe.

Table 15.1. Degenerative and idiopathic neuropathies and myopathies without known or currently available treatment

Neuropathies
Alaskan malamute neuropathy
Boxer axonopathy
Birman cat polyneuropathy
Dancing Doberman syndrome
Distal denervating disease
Distal symmetric polyneuropathy
Giant axonal neuropathy
Golden retriever hypomyelination
Hypertrophic neuropathy of Tibetan mastiffs
Laryngeal paralysis/polyneuropathy complex
Lysosomal storage diseases (some of these have experimental treatments available)
Neuronopathies
Rottweiler neuropathy
Sensory neuropathies
Spinal muscle atrophy
Myopathies
Hereditary myopathy of Devon Rex cats
Labrador retriever myopathy
Muscular dystrophy (some of these have experimental treatment options)
Nemaline rod myopathy

For treatment of *hypokalemic myopathy*, supplementation with potassium is essential (Dow et al. 1987). Oral supplementation is more effective and is associated with fewer complications than intravenous administration. Intravenous administration should be reserved for cats with severe, life-threatening muscle weakness. Administering potassium intravenously in fluids should be performed cautiously, as further decreases in serum potassium concentration may occur as a result of dilution of plasma and enhanced loss of potassium in urine. If IV fluids are indicated because of dehydration, the rate of administration should not induce diuresis, as catastrophic decreases in potassium can occur. Increased urinary potassium loss occurs secondary to renal sodium and water loss, when fluids are administered in excess of maintenance to induce diuresis. In severely weak cats, administering a lower volume of fluid with a higher potassium concentration, such as 160 mEq/L, might be a reasonable choice. It is recommended to not exceed an administration rate of 0.5 mEq/kg/hr as cardiac arrest may occur. Until serum potassium reaches >3.5 mEq/L, maintenance fluid rates such as 10 ml/cat/h are recommended with potassium supplementation together with oral potassium supplementation (5–8 mg/cat PO q 12–24 h). Endotracheal intubation and ventilatory support are required if the cat is in respiratory muscle failure, and this type of respiratory support may be required for 1 to 2 days. Do not give corticosteroids as these increase urinary potassium excretion. Oral supplementation (potassium gluconate) is used for long-term management. An empirical dose of 2–6 mEq/cat/day is usually effective. Regular monitoring of serum potassium is required to determine the effective maintenance dose for individual cats.

The prognosis for cats with hypokalemic myopathy is usually favorable provided respiratory paralysis does not occur. Signs resolve usually in 24 hours to 3 days following appropriate treatment. If respiratory paralysis occurs, intensive care and ventilatory support are required for survival. As many older cats may have underlying renal disease, periodic evaluation of renal function and serum potassium concentration is suggested.

Treatment of *hyperkalemic myopathy* with acetazolamide 2 mg/kg orally every 12 hours has been recommended in idiopathic instances of hyperkalemia. In instances of hypoadrenocorticism, fluid therapy, mineralocorticoid, and glucocorticoid therapy may result in improvement in muscle strength.

Hypernatremic myopathy has been reported in young domestic cats (<1 year). Established hypernatremia (duration greater than 1 week) should be treated by slowly decreasing the serum sodium levels over at least 48 hours to prevent brain edema (also see chapter 13 treatment of hypernatremia). This is most often performed by intravenous administration of an isotonic fluid, or in some instances, a slightly hypertonic fluid (see also chapter 13). Therefore, clinical monitoring of patient status and serum sodium levels should be performed to determine serum sodium levels. In general, a more gradual reduction (occurring over days) in serum sodium is safer.

Treatment of *hypocalcemia* involves calcium supplementation and vitamin D therapy. If clinical signs are severe and life-threatening, rapid institution of treatment is indicated with 0.5–1.5 mL/kg IV of 10% calcium gluconate. Infuse IV calcium slowly over 10 minutes while monitoring heart rate and stop the infusion if bradycardia occurs. Short-term maintenance therapy with calcium involves either subcutaneously administered calcium (1–2.5 mL of 10% calcium gluconate diluted 1:1 in 0.9% saline q 8 hours) or intravenously administered calcium (10–20 mL of 10% calcium gluconate in 500 mL of 0.9% saline) with administration rates adjusted to maintain normocalcemia. Calcium concentrations need to be monitored frequently (in some cases up to two to three times daily) during initiation of calcium therapies.

Longer-term maintenance therapy of hypocalcemia includes supplementation with oral calcium (25 mg/kg q 8–12 hours) and vitamin D. Serum calcium should be monitored carefully, as hypercalcemia is nephrotoxic. Adjustments to doses should be made every 1–3 days based on calcium concentrations. If hypocalcemia is the result of thyroidectomy, calcium and vitamin D therapy can be reduced gradually over 2 to 3 weeks, and stopped if calcium remains in the normal range.

Cats with *hyperthyroidism* may have a variety of nervous system signs. The weakness may improve with treatment for hyperthyroidism (medical, surgical, and radiation) and correction of any hypokalemia.

Hypothyroidism has been suggested to cause both a neuropathy and myopathy. Clinical signs of hypothyroid in both of these abnormalities may improve with oral thyroid hormone supplementation.

Hyperadrenocortical myopathy most commonly occurs in dogs. Definitive treatment for hyperadrenocorticism may bring about improvements in mobility, but clinical signs often remain persistent once established.

Hyperchylomicronemia is seen in cats due to a reduction in lipoprotein lipase activity (Jones et al. 1986). Feeding a low fat diet resulted in resolution of the neuropathy in 2 to 3 months in a few cats with peripheral neuropathy. Gemfibrozil (7.5–10 mg/kg daily) is indicated if dietary therapy does not normalize triglyceride concentrations. Marine (fish) oils rich in omega-3 fatty acids may help to decrease triglyceride concentrations.

Hyperoxaluria (L-glyceric aciduria) is thought to be inherited as an autosomal recessive disease in cats. No treatment was attempted for these cats.

Mitochondrial myopathy has been reported in Clumber and Sussex spaniels and Old English Sheepdogs. No definitive treatment has been described. Supplementation with L-carnitine (50 mg/kg orally every 12 hours), coenzyme Q (4 mg/kg/day), and B vitamins, may help some instances of mitochondrial and other myopathies.

NEOPLASTIC NEUROPATHIES AND MYOPATHIES

Lymphoma commonly occurs extradurally in cats and can involve nerve roots. Rarely, only peripheral nerve involvement is seen. Systemic treatments for lymphoma and leukemia may result in resolution of clinical signs and remission. Cytosine arabinoside may be added to chemotherapeutic protocols as this drug achieves good drug concentrations in the CSF.

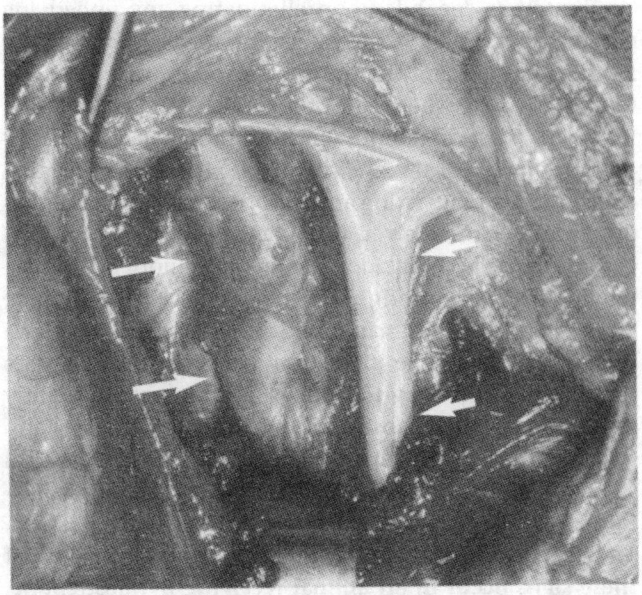

Fig. 15.1. Appearance of a peripheral nerve tumor in the brachial plexus at exploratory surgery. The abnormal nerve (*large arrows*) is compared to the normal nerve (*small arrows*).

Nerve sheath tumors (Schwannoma, neurofibroma, neurofibrosarcoma) commonly involve the peripheral nerves of the limbs or cranial nerves and in some instances are surgically resectable. Prognosis is poor when the tumor invades in and around the spinal cord or brain. Local recurrence is common, and extensive resection and amputation (of a limb) is recommended (fig. 15.1). Some cranial nerve sheath tumors may be surgically resectable. Radiation therapy has also been used, however, too few cases have been reported to determine efficacy. Preliminary results with postoperative radiation therapy to the tumor bed have been encouraging, but too few cases have been evaluated to make firm recommendations.

Paraneoplastic neuropathy without tumor infiltrate into peripheral nerves is occasionally recognized in dogs (Braund 1990; Mariani et al. 1999). Treatment of the underlying neoplastic condition may improve clinical signs.

INFECTIOUS AND INFLAMMATORY NEUROPATHIES AND MYOPATHIES

Botulism is the result of the effects of an exotoxin of *Clostridium botulinum.* Treatments for botulism include administration of polyvalent antitoxin and supportive care for the recumbent animal (see also chapter 14). As botulism in dogs is usually associated with ingestion of preformed toxin, antimicrobials such as penicillin products are not necessary, however, are usually administered regardless.

Tetanus is due to a neurotoxin (tetanospasmin) secreted by the organism *Clostridium tetani.* Treatment includes wound debridement, administration of tetanus antitoxin (administered once IV), penicillin or similar antimicrobials, muscle relaxants, enteral or parenteral nutrition support, a quiet environment, and good supportive care. Anticonvulsants are given if seizures occur.

Neuritis

Toxoplasma gondii and *Neospora caninum* are protozoal organisms that can affect any area of the nervous system resulting in encephalitis, myelitis, peripheral neuropathy, or myositis. Current recommendations for treatment for toxoplasmosis is *clindamycin* (8–25 mg/kg, q 8–12 hours; do not exceed 50 mg/kg q 24 hours) for 14–28 days, however, the *addition of trimethoprim sulfa drugs* PO, IM, or SC may provide a better clinical response. Treatment of neospora infection is less established. Clindamycin and trimethoprim sulfa drugs as for the treatment of toxoplasmosis are often used in the treatment of neospora.

Coonhound paralysis or polyradiculoneuritis is suspected to be an immune-mediated or autoimmune radiculoneuritis. There is no definitive treatment for polyradiculoneuritis. Corticosteroid administration does not appear to influence clinical signs. With this disease, the animal may be recumbent for prolonged periods of time and require additional care in conjunction with confinement and pain medications. Management of recumbent animals is discussed in chapter 14.

With a similar disease in cats (chronic, relapsing polyneuropathy), improvement, if not resolution of clinical signs, may occur in some cats after corticosteroid therapy. In one cat reported with acute, severe polyneuritis, no treatment was attempted.

Respiratory complications, due to paralysis of respiratory muscles, are the most life-threatening consequences of polyradiculoneuritis. In some instances, an animal may need to be placed on a respirator (fig. 15.2). If clinical signs become this severe, the animal is usually unable to breath spontaneously for a number of days. A tracheostomy is necessary to avoid prolonged sedation for intubation.

Plasmapheresis and immunoglobulin therapy are often used as a treatment for a similar disease (Guillain-Barré syndrome) in human beings. In essence, this is a way to filter antibodies causing the neuritis from the serum and ulti-

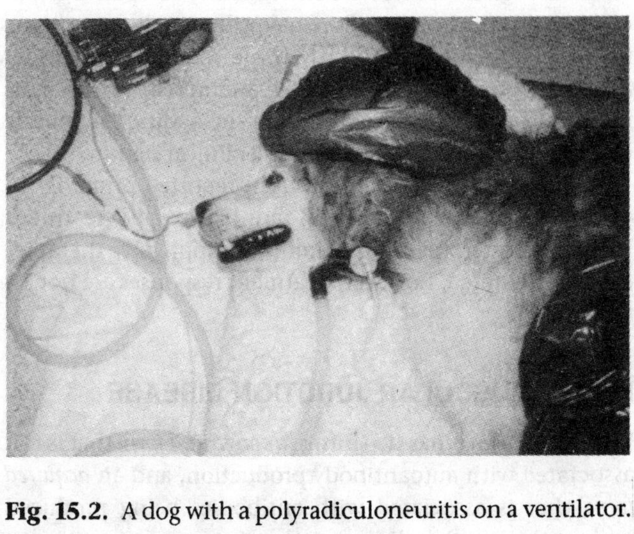

Fig. 15.2. A dog with a polyradiculoneuritis on a ventilator.

mately, reduce the severity of the disease. Plasmapheresis has infrequently been used in dogs for treatment of other immune-mediated diseases such as myasthenia gravis, but the efficacy of plasmapheresis in dogs is not established. Immunoglobulin administration has been used as treatment for other immune-mediated diseases in animals, such as hemolytic anemias, but its use for polyradiculoneuritis is also not established.

Brachial plexus neuritis is suspected to be an immune-mediated neuritis that preferentially affects the thoracic limbs. Treatment may be attempted with immunosuppression, usually by using corticosteroid therapy (1–4 mg/kg every 12–24 hours). If improvement in clinical signs is seen in 1 to 2 weeks, a slow reduction in the corticosteroid medication over weeks should be performed to avoid recurrence of clinical signs.

Cauda equina polyradiculoneuritis has been reported rarely in dogs. Immunosuppressive therapy may be attempted with corticosteroids but few reports of treatment exist.

Myositis

Infectious polyradiculoneuritis or *myositis* can also result from toxoplasmosis (dogs and cats) or *Neospora* (dogs). Current recommendations for treatment for toxoplasmosis is clindamycin (8–25 mg/kg, q 8–12 hours; do not exceed 50 mg/kg q 24 hours) for 14–28 days, however, the addition of trimethoprim sulfa drugs PO, IM, or SC may provide a better clinical response.

Polymyositis may be idiopathic or immune-mediated, or may result from infections with protozoa such as *Toxoplasma gondii*, some viral infections, bacteria such as *Leptospira australis*, fungi, and some parasites (*Trichinella*). If a specific infectious etiology is identified, therapy is directed toward this organism. If an immune-mediated polymyositis is suspected, immunosuppression with corticosteroids is indicated as with other immune-mediated diseases.

Myositis may also affect only selected muscle groups or regions of the body such as the masticatory muscles (masticatory myositis)(Gilmour et al. 1992). Treatment is primarily focused on systemic immunosuppression using corticosteroids or other immunosuppressive therapies. Even in animals with severe fibrosis and inability to open the jaw, corticosteroid administration may still provide some benefit. Manually opening the jaw while the animal is under anesthesia has been historically attempted, however, is rarely effective and usually results in additional muscle damage and recurrent or worsening clinical signs.

Extraocular polymyositis has been reported primarily in young dogs between 6 and 18 months of age. Treatment with corticosteroids or other immunosuppressive therapies can be attempted, however, treatment responses are not established.

NEUROMUSCULAR JUNCTION DISEASE

Myasthenia gravis has two forms: a *congenital form* that is not associated with autoantibody production, and an *acquired form* that is associated with antibodies being produced against the acetylcholine receptor.

Treatment depends upon eliminating any underlying etiology, potentiating the affects of acetylcholine at the NMJ, or modulating the immune response with corticosteroids. If MG is the result of a paraneoplastic effect of a thymoma, surgical removal of this tumor may result in resolution of clinical signs. If the disease is either congenital or acquired, a long-acting anticholinesterase product (pyridostigmine) can be given to enhance the effect of acetylcholine at the NMJ. Pyridostigmine (Mestinon) is administered to effect beginning at 0.5–3 mg/kg PO q 8–12 hours). Start at the lower doses and increase as required to achieve the clinically desirable effect. Cats may be more sensitive to the effect of this drug than dogs, and, therefore, slightly lower dosages than those used in dogs should be used initially. Toxicity from this drug is associated with clinical signs similar to organophosphate toxicity including salivation, excessive urination and defecation, and weakness. These signs are also similar to naturally occurring MG. If these signs occur in an animal receiving pyridostigmine, signs could be the result of either too little or too much pyridostigmine. In this situation, an edrophonium response test is cautiously performed. If the clinical signs are improved following edrophonium, the animal most likely needs an increased dose of pyridostigmine. If clinical signs are exacerbated with edrophonium, the animal is most likely showing toxicity from the pyridostigmine, and doses need to be decreased.

Additionally, immunosuppressive therapy with corticosteroid (1–2mg/kg PO q 12 hours) or plasmapheresis may be needed to control clinical signs in the acquired form. Corticosteroids are administered as for other immune-mediated diseases. Lower doses may be used initially to avoid worsening of clinical signs acutely. Initial doses are used for 1 to 3 weeks depending upon clinical response. If significant improvements are seen, the corticosteroid dosage can be successively decreased over the following weeks to months to determine the lowest dosage needed to control clinical signs. In some instances, clinical signs of MG will remit, and corticosteroids can be discontinued.

Standard treatment for megaesophagus and aspiration pneumonia is often necessary in animals with these complications from MG. Treatments for megaesophagus include elevated feedings and possible administration of drugs such as metaclopromide to potentially enhance esophageal motility. If regurgitation is a severe problem, precluding oral administration of medications such as pyridostigmine, injectable neostigmine can be used to provide some NMJ transmission benefits.

Aspiration pneumonia is a life-threatening complication of megaesophagus and MG. Fever can be an important clue to this problem. Maintaining the animal's hydration, usually with intravenous fluid therapy, is an important component of treatment for AP. Antibiotics are administered ideally based on culture and sensitivity results of organisms cultured through tracheal washings or bronchoalveolar lavage. Nasal oxygen administration, nebulization, and coupage may also be helpful. Bronchodilators and expectorants may also provide some benefit, but are debatable.

Prognosis for some animals with MG is good, with occasional spontaneous cures or remission within 6 months to 1 year. Recurrences are possible. Treatment responses may not be as dramatic in cats compared to dogs. Complicating factors include severe weakness with respiratory compromise, aspiration pneumonia secondary to megaesophagus, and laryngeal paralysis, which may make recovery difficult.

NEUROPATHIES AND MYOPATHIES WITHOUT AN OBVIOUS CAUSE

The numerous neuropathies and myopathies of dogs and cats are increasingly being recognized and clarified. Many different disease types have been reported, however, many of these diseases are without specific etiologic cause and either have no known treatment, or treatments have not been attempted.

Motor neuronopathies are diseases that affect the cell bodies of the lower motor neuron. There is no current effective therapy for these diseases.

Familial myoclonus (reflex myoclonus) of Labrador retrievers is a disease of marked, intermittent muscular hypertonicity that occurs in young dogs (usually around 3 weeks of age). Treatment with diazepam or clonazepam is occasionally helpful.

Dancing Doberman syndrome is a disease characterized by alternating pelvic limb flexion when the animal is standing (Chrisman 1990). No definitive treatment is known.

Dysautonomia is an idiopathic autonomic nervous system disease primarily seen in cats and, occasionally, dogs. No specific treatment is available, but supportive care is important. Nutritional support may involve syringe or tube feeding and watering. Parasympathomimetic agents may improve some clinical signs. Pilocarpine ophthalmic drops (1%/1 drop q 6 h) may result in pupillary contraction and increase salivation. Bethanechol (1.25–5 mg, PO, q 8–12 h) may benefit constipation and urinary retention. Metaclopromide (0.2–0.5 mg/kg, PO, SC, q 8 h) may improve gastric motility. A mortality rate of up to 70% has been reported.

Neuropathies have been seen that only involve the *sensory nerves*. These include sensory neuropathy of boxers, long-haired dachshunds, and other breeds. Treatment is sometimes attempted with corticosteroids, however, responses are usually poor.

Laryngeal paralysis may be part of more diffuse polyneuropathy or myopathy. Surgical treatment, such as laryngeal tieback procedures, may be necessary in severe cases of inspiratory dyspnea.

MYOPATHIES

Many of the myopathies of dogs and cats are not treatable or treatments are not currently available in the clinical setting. In some of these conditions, clinical signs may stabilize after a period of progression and animals may be able to survive with this disability. In some instances, L-carnitine (50 mg/kg every 12 hours), coenzyme Q_{10} (4 mg/kg/day), and B vitamin supplements have been suggested as possible treatments for some myopathies (Shelton 2002).

Fibrotic myopathy occurs primarily in German shepherds between 2 and 7 years of age. Surgical transection of the fibrotic muscle has been attempted, but is usually ineffective as clinical signs often return following surgery. *Infraspinatous muscle* contraction usually occurs in hunting breeds. Surgical transaction of the infraspinatous tendon is often helpful for this abnormality.

Scotty cramp is characterized by paroxysms of muscular hypertonicity, usually precipitated by excitement or exercise. A similar syndrome is seen in Dalmatians and Norwich terriers. Treatment has been attempted with diazepam and promazine tranquilizers with variable benefits.

Episodic falling of Cavalier King Charles spaniels may be a disease similar to Scotty cramping. The episodes are usually life-long in duration. Slight improvements in clinical signs have been noted with diazepam.

Myotonia most often occurs as a congenital problem, and, rarely, can be acquired due to toxicity with some herbicides or with hyperadrenocorticism. Treatment with procainamide has been used with limited improvement in clinical signs. In some instances, long-acting diazepam derivatives such as clorazepate or clonazepam may be helpful. If myotonia is acquired due to toxicity, clinical signs can resolve following excretion or metabolism of the toxin. If animals have hyperadrenocorticism, definitive treatment for this disease may bring about some improvement in clinical signs. No treatment has been described in cats with congenital myotonia.

Cold tail may be the same as *limber tail* or *limp tail*, and has been described as a myopathy of the tail muscles. No specific treatment exists for this problem, however, clinical improvement with time is often seen.

Some animals will have problems from self-mutilation without apparent cause. It is unknown if this is a behavior abnormality (obsessive compulsive disorder) or if these animals are reacting to pain or other abnormal sensations. If organic disease is eliminated, behavior modification and drug therapies for obsessive compulsive disorders may be helpful.

TRAUMATIC NEUROPATHIES AND MYOPATHIES

Trauma can occur to a single nerve (misplaced injection into the sciatic nerve) or multiple nerves (brachial plexus avulsion). If the level of the nerve injury can be identified, decompression or neurolysis (surgically freeing the nerve) may be helpful. If nerve transaction occurs, surgical reapposition may allow for some improvements in regeneration.

Brachial plexus avulsion occurs as a result of a trauma. No treatment for the primary avulsion is currently available, however, experimental surgical treatments are being developed and tested for future use.

TOXIC NEUROPATHIES AND MYOPATHIES

Tick paralysis is due to infestation with ticks. In North America, *Dermacentor andersoni, Dermacentor variabilis,* and *Argas (Persicargas) radiatus* are the species of ticks most commonly associated with paralysis. In Australia, the paralysis tick is *Ixodes holocyclus*, which is found along the eastern coast. In general, these ticks secrete a toxin that prevents release of ACH from the neuromuscular junction. Clinical signs are those of a diffuse LMN disease.

Treatment of tick paralysis in the United States is focused on removing or killing of the tick(s). The tick can be removed manually using curved forceps or a pair of partially opened scissors to lever out the tick while avoiding any pressure on the tick's body. Administration of a tick dip may help in killing the ticks if one is not visually apparent. In some instances, the ticks may be in hard to find places such as the ear canals, under heavy coats, in between toes, and even in the anus.

In Australia where tick paralysis is more life threatening, an antitoxin is often necessary (table 15.2). Tick antitoxin serum (TAS) is manufactured from canine serum and can be given to dogs.

Heavy metals, such as mercury, arsenic, and lead, toxicity have been associated with peripheral neuropathies. While there is no specific treatment for the neuropathy, removal of the source of toxicity may allow for resolution over time.

Organophosphate (OP) intoxication potentiates the effect of acetylcholine at the neuromuscular junction and other synapses by binding with and inactivating acetylcholinesterase. For acute organophosphate toxicity, treatment includes protopam chloride 2-PAM (20 mg/kg q 12 h IV), which reactivates cholinesterase, and diphenhydramine (1–2 mg/kg PO q 81–12 h), which reduces muscle fasciculation. Atropine (0.2–0.4 mg/kg) can be given with acute toxicity to decrease autonomic signs. Current recommendations are that it only be used if marked bradycardia is present, because it may precipitate respiratory arrest. Salivation and defecation are not life threatening and generally do not require atropine.

For chronic OP toxicity, diphenhydramine (1–2 mg/kg PO q 8–12 h) can be administered to improve muscle strength. If diphenhydramine is administered IV to these cats, there may initially be some exacerbation of weakness. Diazepam should be avoided in these cats as it may result in generalized muscle tremor, hypersalivation, miotic pupils, and vomiting similar to acute muscarinic signs of organophosphate toxicosis.

Envenomation can result in a variety of signs of nervous system dysfunction. For snake bite, identification of the snake is often helpful when planning treatment as both monovalent and polyvalent antivenins are available. Dosages are often standardized and dispensed as one dose. Anaphylactic reactions are possible, so caution should be used when administering these products. For red-back spider venom, an antivenin exists as possible treatment.

VASCULAR NEUROPATHIES AND MYOPATHIES

Ischemia neuromyopathy is most often associated with aortic thromboembolism. Various treatments have been tried. Low-dose aspirin or heparin has been used to reduce the incidence of perpetuation of thrombosis. Tissue plasminogen activator (TPA) administration may be the most effective but carries the risk of significant mortality (50%). Supportive care to maintain systemic health and management of the recumbent animal is necessary. Some animals can recover useful function with ischemic neuromyopathy. In cats, treatment of underlying cardiac disease is often necessary. Prognosis is usually poor for long-term recovery because of the underlying heart disease. In dogs, treatment for underlying diseases such as hyperadrenocorticism or hypercoagulability with glomerular disease can help to prevent repeated episodes.

Table 15.2. Treatment of tick paralysis in Australia

Tick Antitoxin Serum (TAS)

TAS (0.5–1 mL/kg) diluted 50:50 with 0.9% NaCl and warmed to room temperature

Administer TAS—either give slowly IV (over 20–30 minutes) or give IP. TAS can also produce a vagally mediated systemic reaction seen clinically as bradycardia, hypotension, and circulatory shock (B-J reaction). To minimize these risks give:

- Acepromazine (0.03 mg/kg SC or IM) to relieve anxiety and respiratory distress. Wait 20–30 minutes before giving TAS.
- Atropine (0.04–0.1 mg/kg SC) to reduce salivation and produce bronchodilation. Wait 20–30 minutes before giving TAS.
- Prednisolone sodium succinate (5–10 mg/kg IV) to reduce the likelihood and severity of anaphylaxis. Wait 10–30 minutes before giving TAS.
- Epinephrine 1: 10,000 (3 mL SC) about 5 minutes prior to administration of TAS to reduce the likelihood of anaphylaxis.

Supportive Care

- Oxygen therapy (oxygen cage, flow-by, nasal catheter, or positive pressure ventilation) is indicated for severe dyspnea.
- Furosemide (2–5 mg/ kg IV) should be given to reduce pulmonary edema in dyspneic animals and repeated as necessary.
- Metaclopromide (0.5 mg/ kg IM or IV) is indicated in vomiting animals to reduce the risk of aspiration.
- Eye ointment should be applied to prevent corneal desiccation.
- Nothing per os is essential until the gag reflex returns. Then introduce oral fluids slowly.
- Parenteral fluids are not routinely indicated and must be used with care due to the potential worsening of pulmonary edema. Colloid or heta/penta starch fluids may be used to maintain circulating fluid volume if the hematocrit is significantly elevated. Crystalloids may be given after 24 hours at submaintenance rates if the slow return of the gag reflex delays introduction of oral fluids.
- If possible animals should be positioned sternally to minimize pulmonary ventilation-perfusion mismatching. Laterally recumbent animal should be positioned with the shoulders elevated to aid pharyngeal drainage and turned every 2 hours to reduce ventilation-perfusion mismatching.
- Urine retention often occurs and manual expression of the bladder may be needed during recovery.
- Stress must be minimized.
- Provision of a cool environment alleviates signs.

II Common Clinical Problems

16 Assessment and Management of Animals with Stupor or Coma

Animals admitted with severe alterations of consciousness and awareness present some of the most challenging of clinical evaluation problems. A rapid, complete neurologic assessment is imperative, but it is hindered by the fact that these animals are poorly responsive or unresponsive to external stimuli used for assessment of neurologic function. Clinical examinations that rely on the animal's being conscious of the stimulus, such as menace response testing (vision), sensation assessments (pain), and conscious proprioception testing, will be, invariably, abnormal. The following provides a clinical approach used when evaluating animals with acute and severe alterations of consciousness.

CLINICAL ASSESSMENT OF ANIMALS WITH STUPOR AND COMA

Clinical signs of alterations in consciousness and behavior are described under examination of animals with nervous system disease in chapter 3. Once dysfunction of consciousness or awareness is established, it is important to determine if the primary problem lies within the intracranial nervous system or is the result of dysfunction within a nonneural body system (tables 16.1 and 16.2). It is taken for granted that any disease process that results in life-threatening changes in systemic metabolic or cardiovascular dysfunction will ultimately affect consciousness in the terminal stages of the disease. Intracranial dysfunction may result from a primary lesion, from secondary intracranial pathophysiologic sequelae to a focal lesion (such as increases in ICP), or from global CNS dysfunction as a consequence of extracranial systemic disease (see chapter 2).

Diagnostic Evaluation

The owner should be questioned as to circumstances surrounding the animal prior to admission to the hospital, any known trauma, or exposure to toxic products.

- Perform a complete systemic examination to determine clinical abnormalities that might suggest an underlying metabolic disease.
- Perform a complete neurological evaluation to determine evidence of a primary intracranial abnormality.

Important assessments on the physical examination include the following:

- Body temperature
- Mucous membrane (color and CRT), limb temperature, and other assessments of perfusion
- Heart rate and rhythm including heart auscultation
- Respiratory rate and character including auscultation of the lung sounds
- Abdominal palpation for organomegaly, fluid or gas distention, and pain
- Rectal examination and assessment of stool for blood or melena, foreign material, toxic products
- Retinal examination for evidence of hypertension, bleeding, or inflammatory disease
- Skin for evidence of lacerations, bite wounds, burns, exposure to foreign substances, ticks, and other arthropods and insects
- Neurologic assessments including pupil size and reactivity, muscle tone, proprioceptive testing (if the animal is not comatose), cranial nerve and spinal reflex assessments, and palpation for pain

Once physical assessments and have been completed and differential diagnoses have been considered, assessment of diagnostic tests that can be performed as quickly as possible and provide the broadest assessment of systemic health should be considered. Routine blood work and urinalysis will often provide clues to underlying metabolic diseases. CBC, serum chemistry, and urinalysis are standard assessments. Other assessments to be considered include:

- Blood pressure
- Blood gas determination
- Urine or blood assessment for ethylene glycol
- Buccal mucosal bleeding time
- Coagulation panel (PT, PTT, FDP, platelet determination)
- Fecal examination for parasites
- ECG
- Thoracic radiograph
- Abdominal radiograph

Table 16.1. Primary diseases that affect the intracranial nervous system and result in coma

Anomalous	Hydrocephalus
Neoplastic	Primary brain tumor Metastatic tumors Local Extension
Nutritional	Thiamine deficiency
Inflammatory brain diseases	Infectious Distemper (dog) Herpes virus Parvovirus Parainfluenza virus (hydrocephalus) Feline infectious peritonitis (cat) Fungal disease Toxoplasmosis Neosporosis Rickettsial Rocky Mountain spotted fever (vestibular) Ehrlichia Bacteria Protothecosis Parasite migration
Trauma	Head trauma Intracranial hemorrhage Subdural hematoma
Toxicity	Metronidazole Lead Strychnine CNS depressants
Vascular	Arteriovenous malformation Infarction Feline ischemic encephalopathy Primary hemorrhage Coagulopathy Platelet disorder DIC Hypertension

Table 16.2. Common systemic disease: processes that secondarily result in coma

Liver disease (hepatic encephalopathy)
Renal failure
Pancreatic disease
Hyperglycemia
Diabetic ketoacidosis
Nonketotic diabetic coma
Hypoglycemia
Hyper or hyponatremia
Hyper or hypokalemia
Acidosis and alkalosis
Hypo or hyperthyroidism
Hypo or hyperadrenocortism
Cardiac disease
Cardiac arrhythmias
Pulmonary disease
Abdominal organ rupture
Gastrointestinal
Liver
Spleen
Kidney
Bladder
Uterus
Diseases associated with poor peripheral delivery of oxygen
Anemia
Toxicity
Cyanide
Acetaminophen
Diseases associated with poor perfusion
Blood loss
Hypovolemia
Shock
Thromboemboli disease
Glomerular disease
Hyperadrenocorticism
Bacterial endocarditis
Pyometra
DIC

- Ultrasound (abdomen for fluid or gas, heart for pericardial effusion)
- If ultrasound is not available, and fluid or air is suspected in the abdomen or thoracic cavity, abdominal or thoracocentesis

If the results of these tests are normal or nondiagnostic, consideration should be directed toward primary CNS diseases.

- Ideally, the animal should undergo an advanced imaging study such as a CT or MR to determine the anatomical integrity of the intracranial structures.
- If such testing is not feasible or available, consideration should be given to performing a CSF analysis. Abnormal CSF results can indicate intracranial involvement with a disease process. Collection of CSF does present a risk to the animal that may have increased ICP. The risks of CSF collection need to be considered compared to the potential diagnostic benefits (see chapter 9). If there is a strong clinical suspicion of primary inflammatory intracranial disease, the potential diagnostic benefits of CSF collection may outweigh the risks to the patient.

TREATMENT

Treatment of the animal with stupor or coma is directed toward the underlying cause.

- Systemic disease processes and known toxicities are treated as per current treatment recommendations.
- Treatment for CNS disease is also directed toward the primary cause (see chapter 13 for treatment of specific intracranial diseases).
- Unfortunately, in the emergency situation, a primary diagnosis is not always established. If a primary cause is not determined or is unobtainable in a timely manner, and the animal's abnormality is considered life threatening, treatment is directed toward the "best guess" or presumptive diagnosis.

Table 16.3. Treatment of increased intracranial pressure

Fluid resuscitation to maintain cerebral perfusion
- Isotonic fluids, hypertonic saline

Diuretics
- Mannitol (0.25–1.0 gm/kg IV bolus)
- Furosemide (0.07 to 1 mg/kg IV)
- Hypertonic saline (3%) (5.3 ml/kg IV)

Head elevation

Hyperventilation (if the animal is intubated)
- Monitor blood gas on end-tidal CO_2 concentration to maintain CO_2 approximately 28 to 30
- Corticosteroids (methylprednisolone sodium succinate or prednisone sodium succinate at 30 mg/kg IV slowly over 15 minutes, repeat at 15 mg/kg IV slowly at 2 and 6 hours after initial dose. Alternative, dexamethasone sodium phosphate at 0.01–0.025 mg/kg IV every 6 hours)

Surgical decompression (craniotomy)

- Concurrent treatments for increased ICP are also useful (table 16.3).

If a structural intracranial disease is suspected, every attempt should be made to obtain an advanced imaging study (CT or, ideally, MR) as soon as possible.

- In some instances such as intracranial bleeding, tumor, or abscess, surgical decompression is the best treatment option.
- If intracranial imaging is not immediately available or feasible, and systemic metabolic disease has been excluded, treatment is initiated for the presumptive structural disease.
- If hydrocephalus or a brain tumor is very likely, treatment for ICP and corticosteroids should be administered (table 16.3).
- If intracranial hemorrhage from a bleeding disorder is suspected, treatment for coagulation abnormalities (plasma or whole blood, vitamin K administration) or platelet disorders (platelet-rich plasma, corticosteroids, other immunosuppressive drugs) should be performed.
- If thiamine deficiency is suspected, treatment with thiamine is initiated (table 16.4).
- If encephalitis is suspected, treatment with a broad combination of antimicrobial and anti-inflammatory therapies may be helpful (table 16.4).

PROGNOSIS OF ANIMALS WITH COMA

The prognosis of animals with coma is dependent upon the prognosis associated with the underlying disease process and the potential for response to definitive treatment. Primary intracranial diseases that are nonprogressive offer the best chance of recovery if clinical signs are not severe. After the acute pathophysiological effects of brain disease are controlled (usually up to 7 days following the acute brain injury), the goal is to allow time for brain healing and recovery of function to occur.

Generally, clinical signs of unilateral supratentorial injury improve within the first 2 weeks following trauma. Usually the animal is ambulatory by 4 weeks postinjury, although, residual paresis and blindness may continue. A tendency to circle may also persist, being especially prominent when the animal is distressed or excited.

Recovery from brain stem injury may be less complete, and residual signs commonly remain. Recovery from cerebellar injury often occurs in a similar time frame as for supratentorial injury. If the secondary effects of brain injury are controlled, many animals can recover from the primary brain insult associated with trauma.

Table 16.4. Nonsurgical Emergency Treatments for Specific Intracranial Diseases

Hydrocephalus
- Treatment for ICP
- Corticosteroids (methylprednisolone sodium succinate or prednisone sodium succinate at 30 mg/kg IV slowly over 15 minutes, repeat at 15 mg/kg IV slowly at 2 and 6 hours after initial dose. Alternative, dexamethasone sodium phosphate at 0.01–0.025 mg/kg IV every 6 hours)

Brain Tumor
- Treatment for ICP
- Corticosteroids (see above)

Thiamine Deficiency
- Thiamine (severely affected cats should receive at least 1 mg parenterally)
- 5–30 mg IV in isotonic fluids

Encephalitis and Meningitis
- Trimethoprim-sulfadiazine (30 mg/kg q 12 h)
- Clindamycin (20–25 mg/kg q 12 h)
- Doxycycline (10 mg/kg q 24 h PO)
- Corticosteroids (prednisone 1–4 mg/kg q 12 h or methylprednisolone sodium succinate or prednisone sodium succinate at 30 mg/kg IV slowly over 15 minutes, repeat at 15 mg/kg IV slowly at 2 and 6 hours after initial dose. Alternative, dexamethasone sodium phosphate at 0.01 to 0.025 mg/kg IV every 6 hours)
- If anaerobic infection, can use metronidazole (10 mg/kg IV slowly every 8 hours)
- Other antibiotics
  - Ampicillin (22 mg/kg every 6 to 12 hours)
  - Enrofloxacin (10 mg/kg IV every 12 hours)
  - Cefotaxime (25 to 50 mg/kg IV every 8 hours)

17 Clinical Evaluation and Management of Animals with Seizures

Seizures are among the most common admitting complaints of a neurologic nature in small animals. Due to the numerous causes, clinical ramifications, and treatments possible, a logical evaluation of affected animals is imperative. An initial but important determination is whether, in fact, the animal is having a seizure or another episodic abnormality mistakenly interpreted as a seizure. The diagnosis of a seizure disorder often requires assessments for potential structural and metabolic intracranial causes for the seizure. Finally, client communication regarding possible treatments and realistic future expectations for the animal affected with a seizure disorder is one of the most important aspects of effective management for the seizuring animal.

CLINICAL EVALUATION OF ANIMALS WITH SUSPECTED SEIZURES

Many owners use the word "seizure" to describe a variety of episodic abnormalities that occur with their animal. When an animal is presented for a possible seizure disorder, it is important to determine if, in fact, the animal has a seizure abnormality or some other episodic disorder that may be misinterpreted by the owner (or even the clinician) as a seizure. It may be helpful to record observations and assessments in some written descriptive form to ensure all information is collected and assessed (fig. 17.1). Video recordings of any potential seizure event are also very helpful in the determination of the possibility of a true seizure event occurring episodically.

IS THE ANIMAL HAVING A TRUE SEIZURE, OR SOMETHING ELSE?

What Is a Seizure?

A seizure is defined as a paroxysmal, transitory disturbance of brain function that has a sudden onset, ceases spontaneously, and has a tendency to recur. Seizures are usually associated with autonomic disturbances such as urination, salivation, and defecation. Epilepsy is a recurrent seizure disorder irrespective of cause.

Unfortunately, "seizure" is a common word that nonmedical individuals are familiar with and apply to episodic disturbances that affect their animals. This may lead to inappropriate diagnoses and treatments if the actual cause of the episodic disturbance is not appropriately identified and treated.

History and owner descriptions of the events in question are important aspects of clinical evaluation of animals with seizure disorders, as often the events are not witnessed by the clinician in the hospital. The owner should not be asked leading questions to avoid introducing bias that may affect later interpretations. One way to avoid this is to simply ask the owner to describe what happens to the animal when it is having its "seizure."

Seizures are of differing types and have differing stages (phases). The *prodome* is the period prior to a seizure. This phase may occur hours to minutes before seizure activity. Animals may have behavior abnormalities, restlessness, or changes in daily behavior patterns such as eating or sleeping. The *aura* is best defined in human beings with seizures as the sensation or feeling immediately prior to a seizure. Animals most commonly have behavior abnormalities during this phase of the seizure cycle. The *ictus* is the actual seizure event. This usually lasts less than a few minutes unless that animal has continual seizure activity termed *status epilepticus*. The period following ictus is the *postictal period*. This phase may last minutes to hours and, in some instances, days. Again, behavior abnormalities predominate this phase, with abnormalities ranging from somnolence to hiding to agitation and frenzied activity. Importantly, it is possible that animals have physical (and sometimes focal) neurologic examination abnormalities during this phase of the seizure cycle.

Animal identification

Seizure Evaluation

Clinician ____________________

Date: ____________________

Time: ____________________

History of seizures prior to this episode? ____ **Y** ____ **N**

Previous anticonvulsant treatment? ____ **Y** ____ **N**

Which Anticonvulsant Drug? Phenobarbital KBr Valium

Other

Dose ____________________

Previous anticonvulsant level when taken? _______ **days** _______ **weeks** _______ **months**

Last anticonvulsant level? Phenobarbital _______(20-40 ug/ml) KBr _______(1-3 mg/ml)

Side effects of the medication? (circle): none PU PD PP excitement sedation anorexia Ataxia vomiting skin irritation diarrhea other

Description of the Event: (circle)

Falls over (lateral) Falls down (sternal) Remains standing

Urination Defecation Salivation Conscious Unconscious

Paddling tremor shaking Vomiting

Other:

Duration of Episode(s): _______ **seconds** _______ **minutes**

Number of Episode(s): _______ **per hour** _______ **per day** _______ **per week** _______ **per month**

How long ago was the last episode? _______ **hour(s)** _______ **day(s)** _______ **week(s)** _______ **month(s)**

Multiple seizures/ day? ____ **Y** ____ **N** **Cluster seizures?** ____ **Y** ____ **N** **Status epilepticus** ____ **Y** ____ **N**

____ **Number**

Summary Neurologic examination findings (complete separate neurologic examination form)

Normal Interictal exam Focal deficits Symmetric deficits Multifocal

Fig. 17.1. Example of seizure evaluation form for the medical record.

Differential Diagnosis (prioritize 1, 2, 3)

Metabolic ____________ **Structural** ____________ **Idiopathic** ____________

(Extracranial) **(Intracranial)**

____

Etiologic Differential Diagnosis (circle if appropriate)

Degenerative
Storage diseases
Other degenerative processes
Anomalous
Hydrocephalus
Hydraencephaly
Lissencephaly
Metabolic
Liver (hepatic encephalopathy)
Renal Encephalopathy
Pancreatic disease
Glucose abnormalities
Thyroid
Adrenal (Hyper / hypo)
Cardiovascular
Neoplastic
Primary Brain tumor
Metastatic tumors
Local Extension

Nutritional
Thiamine deficiency
Idiopathic Epilepsy
Infectious
Viral -Distemper (Dog)
Herpes virus
Parvo Virus
Parainfluenza virus (hydrocephalus)
Feline Infectious Peritonitis (Cat)
Fungal disease
Toxoplasmosis
Rickettsial
Rocky Mountain spotted fever (Vestibular)
Ehlichia
Bacteria
Parasites

Trauma
Head trauma
Toxicity
Lead
unclassified
Vascular
Arteriovenous malformation
Infarction
Feline Ischemic Encephalopathy
Hemorrhage (coagulation abn)
Hypertension

Diagnostic Testing

Test	Order	Completed	Results
CBC/Chem/UA			
Bile acids			
Blood pressure			
MR/ CT			
CSF			
EEG			
Phenobarbital level			
KBr level			

Signature ____________

Comments

____

Diagnosis

____

Generalized, tonic clonic seizures have characteristic features in most dogs and cats allowing for their differentiation from other events. Important clues that a generalized seizure is occurring include falling over or becoming laterally recumbent, paddling or running movements of the limbs, urination, defecation, or salivation. It may be difficult to ascertain from the owner if an animal is conscious or aware of the event, but this is often an important aspect of determining that a seizure has occurred. Animals with generalized seizure often have their eyes open, which may confuse an owner into believing that the animal is conscious. If the animal is responsive to external stimuli, such as touching or talking, this may indicate that at least some consciousness is preserved. With focal seizures, however, consciousness may remain intact adding confusion to the clinical evaluation.

Generalized seizures often last a short period of time. Single, generalized (grand mal) seizure events often are only 30 to 90 seconds in duration. There may be a preictal phase of varying lengths. Often, during this period, the animals have behavioral abnormalities such as hiding or becoming apprehensive. Following a seizure, there is frequently a phase (postictal) when the animal may also behave abnormally, and, most importantly, have focal neurologic examination abnormalities. These postseizure features become important when interpreting the results of the clinical examination and in subsequently formulating a differential diagnosis for seizuring animals.

It is often observed that seizures occur in the middle of the night in dogs. One explanation suggests that during low levels of awareness, drowsiness, and dreamless sleep, decreased activity in the reticular formation allows for reverberating circuits between the thalamus and the cortex to synchronize. Additionally, groups of neurons that are only mildly hyperactive in the awake state become excitable and fire consistently during sleep.

Events that are often confused with true seizures include syncope, narcolepsy, cataplexy, behavior disorders, weakness episodes, vestibular disorders, cramping syndromes, cervical painful responses, tremors, and other episodic movement disorders (table 17.1). If the description of the event is not clear, and if the event occurs frequently at home, asking the owners to videotape the event for further review is often helpful in the clinical diagnosis.

Classification of Seizures

Once it has been determined that a seizure abnormality is present, characteristics of the seizure activity and patterns may be important clues to the underlying cause. Seizures can be classified in numerous ways depending upon where the seizure activity originates, which areas of the brain are affected, or the actual etiologic cause of the seizure. A simplistic yet realistic classification system initially categorizes seizures as having either a generalized or focal onset. An attempt to describe seizure disorders of dogs exactly as in human beings often adds confusion. The existence in animals of these various seizure types that occur in humans is not yet universally proven, but is likely. Obviously, the inability of animals to verbally communicate what they feel or experience during the events is problematic.

Generalized seizures affect the entire body simultaneously. The generalized tonic clonic or grand mal seizure is thought to be the most common seizure seen in animals. This may, however, only represent the fact that this type of seizure is more readily recognizable to veterinarians, while other, less commonly recognizable seizure phenomena are overlooked.

Focal seizures remain localized to one body region, but may progress to generalized seizure activity. Focal seizure activity may be of value in localization of the seizure focus to one side of the brain. Generally, a clinical abnormality on one side of the body is the result of a seizure focus in the contralateral supratentorial structures. Focal seizures are also more often associated with structural brain disease.

A "petit mal" seizure is a term commonly, and inappropriately, used to mean "small" or focal seizures in animals. The term is an older term for a generalized seizure disorder of humans wherein the individual experiences periods of absence. Hence, this type of seizure is now referred to as "absence" seizures with an associated characteristic EEG pattern. The term "petit mal," therefore, should not be used as a descriptive term for focal seizures in dogs and cats.

Bizarre behaviors may be manifestations of seizure disorders, possibly initiated in components of the limbic system. Fly biting is one example. Other behavior disorders such as flank sucking or tail biting may result from a seizure focus, but definitive evidence is lacking. These activities are more likely obsessive-compulsive types of behavioral disorders. Vomiting may be a manifestation of some types of unusual seizure activity. This is often referred to as visceral epilepsy in humans.

Seizures may also be classified based on the actual cause of the seizure disorder. Seizure types are those that occur without cause (idiopathic) compared to those with a specific cause (symptomatic). Cryptogenic seizures are those that presumably have a specific cause but the etiology is not identified.

DIFFERENTIAL DIAGNOSIS

After the clinician is convinced that a seizure disorder is present, a differential diagnosis list should be generated. A most important question to be answered is whether the seizure focus is the result of primary intracranial disease, the result of an extracranial disturbance, or is occurring without either a metabolic or structural derangement (idiopathic). Generally, the causes for seizures can be categorized into those secondary to an intracranial anatomical or structural cause (*structural*), an extracranial cause (*metabolic*), or idiopathic epilepsy (*idiopathic*). Some use the terms "intracranial" to indicate structural and "extracranial" to indicate metabolic etiologies for seizure activity.

Metabolic

Extracranial disease resulting in seizures can be divided into those causes arising within the animal itself (endoge-

Table 17.1. Clinical abnormalities commonly mistaken for seizure activity

- **Tremor**
  An involuntary, rhythmic, oscillatory movement of all or part of the body. It results from the alternate or synchronous contraction of reciprocally innervated, antagonistic muscles. True tremor ceases with sleep. Tremor can be localized to one body area or be generalized (whole body). Localized tremor usually involves the head or pelvic limbs.
- **Myoclonus**
  A shocklike contraction of a muscle or muscles. This most often occurs in a thoracic limb, however, a pelvic limb or the facial muscles may also be involved. Myoclonus in dogs is usually the result of distemper infection that establishes a pacemaker-like depolarization of local motor neurons.
- **Reflex myoclonus**
  Characterized by episodic, stimulation-evoked extensor rigidity of the body and is most commonly seen in Labrador retrievers. Other breeds (Dalmatian) are occasionally affected. As this is a congenital disorder, young (weeks to months of age) animals are affected.
- **Narcolepsy/cataplexy**
  Narcolepsy (excessive daytime sleepiness) and cataplexy (periods of acute muscular hypotonia); acute onset of REM sleep, usually occurring with stimulation such as eating, is characteristic of narcolepsy. Breeds of dogs predisposed to narcolepsy include Doberman pinschers, Labrador retrievers, miniature poodles, dachshunds, beagles, and Saint Bernards. Clinical signs usually begin at a young age, however, dogs as old as 7 years have been diagnosed with this disorder.
- **Scotty Cramp**
  Characterized by paroxysms of muscular hypertonicity, usually precipitated by excitement or exercise; during movement, initially there is abduction of the thoracic limbs. Arching of back, pelvic limb stiffness, jumping into the air, falling, curling into a ball may follow. Respirations may cease and facial muscles may be contracted. A similar syndrome is seen in Dalmatians and Norwich terriers.
- **Episodic falling of Cavalier King Charles**
  Seen mostly in animals from the UK; dogs are affected by 3 to 4 months of age. During exercise, dogs develop a bounding pelvic limb gait with stiff pelvic limbs, falling, and extensor rigidity of the limbs.
- **Myotonia**
  Sustained muscle contraction, which is initiated voluntarily or with stimulation, and sustained involuntarily. Myotonia most often occurs as a congenital problem, however, the disease can be acquired with some toxicities and secondary to hyperadrenocorticism. Occurs in dogs such as Chow Chows, Staffordshire terriers, Great Danes, Rhodesian ridgebacks, and cats. Animals with myotonia may have a short, stilted gait, possible bunny hopping, and apparent stiffness or extensor rigidity of the limbs. Affected animals may also have large, bulky muscles on palpation. Muscle dimpling may occur with direct muscle percussion.
- **Dyskinesias**
  Defined as impairment of the power of voluntary movements resulting in fragmented or incomplete movements. Involuntary movements are usually manifested through abnormal motion of the limbs, trunk, or head. Flexing movements of the limbs may occur. These types of episodes need to be differentiated from partial seizure activity and muscle disorders.
- **Syncope**
  Short, episodic loss of consciousness that results from transient cerebral hypoxia or anoxia. If the hypoxia is prolonged, actual seizure may result and confound the clinical interpretation. Syncope is most often the result of a cardiopulmonary disorder (usually a bradyarrhythmia) and, therefore, attention should be paid to the cardiopulmonary systems during the routine physical examination.
- **Pain**
  Acute and severe painful episodes, especially involving the neck, may cause animals to become rigid, vocalize, and fall over.
- **Vestibular disease**
  Acute vestibular episodes may result in animals falling, having extensor rigidity, appearing apprehensive, sometimes salivating, and having exaggerated or flailing movements of the limbs. Nystagmus, heading tilting, and ataxia may be other clues to an underlying vestibular disturbance.
- **Unclassified episodic abnormalities**
  Some episode disorders have features of seizure activity, but may also represent other types of involuntary movement disorders. One such example occurs in the Chinook breed of dog (see D. P. O'Brien at http://www.canine-epilepsy.nect/chinook/chinook.htm). Clinical abnormalities range from stopping and standing, to falling over, curling of the body, and flexing of the limbs. Similar to many dyskinesias, these types of clinical abnormalities await further clarification.

nous disease such as hepatic encephalopathy) and those causes arising external to the animal (exogenous diseases such as toxins). There are numerous metabolic diseases that can result in seizures. These include hypo- or hyperglycemia, liver disease, renal disease, electrolyte disturbances, many toxins, anemias, and cardiopulmonary diseases. In most instances, seizures with these diseases result from an abnormality of nerve cell metabolic function or neurotransmission. Multiple factors are required for effective nerve cell function including energy (oxygen, glucose), electrical current (electrolytes, electrolyte pumps), and synaptic transmission (neurotransmitters). More often, it may be a combination of metabolic derangements rather than a single factor that results in the seizure.

Structural

Structural intracranial diseases resulting in seizures include hydrocephalus, storage diseases, neoplasia (primary and secondary brain tumor), inflammatory diseases (infectious and noninfectious encephalitis), trauma (injury), and vascular-based diseases. Intracranial disease can alter normal physiological relationships through numerous mechanisms that result in seizures. These include, but are not limited to, physical invasion and/or destruction of neurons, metabolic alterations in neuronal or glial cells, impairment of vascular supply to normal tissue (ischemia or hypoxia), impairment of autoregulation, hemorrhage (intraparenchymal or intraventricular), irritation, obstruction of the ventricular system, edema formation, production of physiologically active substances, and increases in intracranial pressure (ICP). These processes may initiate and perpetuate each other.

Idiopathic

Idiopathic epilepsy is the primary disease in this category. There is a significant population of dogs (possibly >100,000 dogs in the United States) who have a seizure disorder without an obvious metabolic or structural cause. A diagnosis of idiopathic epilepsy is always presumptive, as there is no definitive diagnostic test that confirms this disease. Assuredly there are multiple causes for idiopathic seizures that are not identified and therefore obligate a diagnosis of idiopathic epilepsy. Possibly the initiating event is no longer present, however alterations in neuronal depolarization persist. Conversely, there likely are some dogs that have abnormal neuronal depolarizations as a genetically determined alteration of neuronal cell physiology.

CLINICAL DIAGNOSIS OF SEIZURE DISORDERS

The clinical diagnosis of a seizure disorder will be aided by both historical information gathered from the owner and physical examination clues found during neurologic assessments. Important aspects of evaluation of animals with seizure include how old the animal is (was) at the time of its first seizure, and whether there are any persistent interictal physical abnormalities found during neurologic examination.

What Is the Age of Onset of the First Seizure?

Seizures resulting from idiopathic epilepsy usually begin in animals between 1 year and 4 years of age. A dog, therefore, that begins having seizures at 5 years of age frequently has another cause for the seizure activity besides idiopathic epilepsy. Certain breeds of dogs are known or thought to have an increased incidence of idiopathic epilepsy, such as beagles, Belgian Tervurens, German shepherds, keeshonds, and collies. High-incidence breeds associated with idiopathic epilepsy include Saint Bernards, golden retrievers, Irish setters, American cocker spaniels, wire-haired fox terriers, Alaskan malamutes, Siberian huskies, and miniature poodles. An obvious question from owners is whether idiopathic epilepsy is inherited or genetic. Without extensive breeding studies, this question is impossible to definitively answer in individual animals. There is often a suspicion that idiopathic epilepsy has a genetic component.

History of systemic illness or toxin exposure may be important when establishing a differential diagnosis. Previous head trauma, oftentimes months or even years prior to the onset, may result in a seizure disorder (posttraumatic epilepsy).

In some animals, their first seizure is not witnessed and therefore is undocumented. If, for example, an animal is left alone for long periods of time (at night, or during the day when the owners are working), and the seizure occurs without causing damage to the animal or the environment, the existence of the seizure disorder may not be obvious to the owner. Another situation influencing accurate determination of the initial seizure event is where a new family adopts an animal in adulthood, and a history of previous seizure activity is not known. In these instances, when the seizure is witnessed for the first time (i.e., in adulthood or later age), the owners will assume that this is the onset of the seizure disorder. This percentage of animals with idiopathic epilepsy have seizures that escape detection in earlier life, and only come to be identified later in life with a seizure abnormality.

Are There Any Interictal Deficits Detected During the Neurologic Examination?

The *neurological examination* can be extremely informative in animals with seizures. Idiopathic seizures are usually not associated with interictal neurological deficits unless seizures are severe or persistent. A percentage of dogs, even with idiopathic epilepsy, may have neurological deficits in the minutes, hours, or sometimes days following a seizure. Knowledge of when the seizure(s) occurred in relationship to the clinical examination is important. Often, with severe seizures (multiple or cluster seizures, or status epilepticus), deficits will remain for extended periods of time following the seizure (hours to days).

Metabolic causes may result in persistent interictal neurological deficits, especially if the animal's mental status is altered. Physical deficits are usually symmetric but occasionally can be worse on one side of the body. While the initiating cause of the seizure activity may be an underlying systemic metabolic abnormality, a consequence of the seizure activity may result in a structural alteration in the brain, such as edema, hypoxia, infarction, ischemia, or neuronal cell body damage. These focal anatomical (structural) alterations may be reflected as deficits on the clinical neurologic examination.

What Is the Most Likely Cause of the Seizure?

Prioritizing these general categories of causes of seizures may help in the logical evaluation of affected animals and allow for reasonable communication with the owner about potential causes, reasons for diagnostic testing, and prognoses. The following are general guidelines for establishing likely categories of seizure-related disease entities by using information from age of onset of first seizure and clinical examination findings.

Based on the age of onset of first seizure, and evidence of any persistent neurologic abnormalities, likely causes of seizure activity can be considered. As with all generalizations, exceptions to each of these conclusions exist for individual animals.

The Young Animal with Seizures

- The animal is <6 months of age at the time of first seizure.
- The animal has no interictal neurologic examination deficits.

- Think:
  1. *Metabolic diseases*
  2. *Structural diseases*: Some animals with structural disease have disease in regions of the brain that do not result in abnormalities on the neurologic examination.
  3. *Idiopathic epilepsy*: Some animals with idiopathic epilepsy begin having seizures at a young age.

In the animal less than 6 months of age with seizures and persistent neurologic deficits, while metabolic causes should always be searched for, structural causes for seizure need to be excluded. In these animals, consideration should be given to performing a diagnostic test that will show anatomical structures within the brain (CT or MR imaging). Cerebrospinal fluid collection is important in determining the presence of brain inflammation.

- The animal is <6 months of age at the time of first seizure.
- The animal has focal interictal neurologic examination deficits.
- Think:
  1. *Structural diseases more likely*
  2. *Metabolic diseases*: In some animals, metabolic abnormalities secondarily result in structural disease and subsequently result in abnormalities on the neurologic examination.
  3. *Idiopathic epilepsy*

The Older Animal with Seizures

- The animal is >5 years of age at the time of first seizure.
- The animal has no interictal neurologic examination deficits.
- Think:
  1. *Metabolic diseases*
  2. *Structural diseases*: Some animals with structural disease have disease in areas of the brain that do not result in abnormalities on the neurologic examination.
  3. *Idiopathic epilepsy*: Some animals with idiopathic epilepsy begin having seizures at an older age, or, the initial seizure has been not documented.

In the older animal with seizures and no obvious persistent neurologic deficits, metabolic causes should be searched for by performing some routine blood and urine testing. Liver function or other specific organ testing may be necessary in individual animals. If obvious metabolic diseases are excluded, animal should have an anatomical imaging study to assess for clinically occult structural brain disease.

- The animal is >5 year of age at the time of first seizure.
- The animal has focal interictal neurologic examination deficits.
- Think:
  1. *Structural diseases*
  2. *Metabolic diseases*: In some animals, metabolic abnormalities secondarily result in structural intracranial disease and subsequently abnormalities on the neurologic examination.
  3. *Idiopathic epilepsy*: In some animals with idiopathic epilepsy, severe seizure activity can result in structural intracranial disease and subsequently abnormalities on the neurologic examination.

In animals older than 5 years of age that have an initial seizure and have persistent, associated neurologic examination abnormalities, structural intracranial causes need to be excluded from consideration by performing CT or MR imaging of the intracranial region.

The Most Common Presentation for Animals with Idiopathic Epilepsy

- The animal is between 1 and 5 years of age at the time of first seizure.
- The animal has no interictal neurologic examination deficits.
- Some animals with structural disease have disease in areas of the brain that do not result in abnormalities on the neurologic examination. Other animals between 1 and 5 years of age may have metabolic diseases resulting in seizures.

After establishing the likelihood of categories of seizure causes, specific etiologies pertinent to the individual patient should be considered (see chapter 5 for specific intracranial diseases).

Diagnostic Plan. Once the likely causes of seizures are considered, a reasonable diagnostic plan can be established. Evaluation for metabolic abnormalities include a complete physical examination, CBC, serum biochemical panel, urinalysis, fecal examination, thoracic and abdominal radiographs, heartworm (dog) or FeLV/FIV testing (cat), blood pressure measurements, and electrocardiography (ECG). As hepatic encephalopathy is a common cause of metabolic encephalopathy, bile acids testing or other liver function tests should also be evaluated. Other specific tests such as blood lead levels are assessed based on possible exposure and other individual patient characteristics.

Evaluations for a possible structural (anatomical) intracranial abnormality include performance of an anatomical imaging study (CT or MR imaging) and CSF evaluation for possible inflammatory/hemorrhagic and neoplastic causes. Electroencephalography (EEG) evaluations may be helpful in individual animals but are not universally available. As idiopathic epilepsy is a diagnosis made through exclusion of *all* other possible causes of seizures, to be most confident of this diagnosis, a complete evaluation for all metabolic abnormalities and structural intracranial diseases needs to be performed to be most assured of the diagnosis. Regardless of the extent of diagnostic testing, idiopathic epilepsy is always a *presumptive* diagnosis.

Treatment. Once an appropriate diagnosis is made, treatments can more realistically be considered. Treatment decisions are individualized to the needs of the particular animal and owner. An important dialogue should occur between the veterinarian and the owner prior to initiating treatment to establish treatment goals and to describe administration, side effects, and monitoring of anticonvulsant medication.

WHEN SHOULD SEIZURES BE TREATED?

When a seizure disorder requires treatment is not clearly defined. Guidelines have been established in the veterinary literature as to when to initiate anticonvulsant treatment based on the number and type of seizures occurring. Many of these guidelines, however, are based on anecdotal experiences and arbitrary time frames. Most clinicians would consider that more than one seizure per month probably requires treatment. There is some information to suggest that earlier and more aggressive treatment of seizures is justified. Evidence to support the phenomenon of kindling suggests that seizure activity can perpetuate or lead to further seizure activity. With time, kindled foci may become autonomous and form a new, independent seizure focus, which may compound the overall treatment of seizure disorders. Persistent seizure activity can also result in anatomical structural alterations in the brain, possibly the result of excitotoxins, cellular metabolic or membrane damage, cytotoxic edema, ischemia, and hypoxia. These alterations in neuronal cell populations may lead to potentially increased seizure activity, or seizures that are less responsive to treatment.

Prior to initiating treatment for animals with seizures, realistic goals for anticonvulsant therapeutic interventions should be established to avoid later frustrations for the owner and the veterinarian alike. *Seizure control* may be interpreted as stopping all seizure activity, or as simply decreasing the clinical severity or the frequency of the seizure. Animals that have idiopathic epilepsy will most often continue to have at least some seizures even when receiving appropriate anticonvulsant medications. The fact that some seizure activity may be expected should be discussed with owners to avoid unrealistic expectations on the part of the owner that all seizures will stop after anticonvulsant medication is initiated. If an associated underlying disease is resulting in the seizure activity, it should be communicated that, even with effective treatment of this underlying disease, seizure activity may intermittently continue in the future.

What is considered a *treatment response* should also be established. A response to anticonvulsant treatment may be reflected as termination of all seizure activity, or as a reduction in the severity and frequency of seizure activity. In many instances of anticonvulsant treatment for idiopathic seizures, only the latter is realistic. It is important for both the owner and the veterinarian to understand that even with "effective" treatment responses, some frequency of seizure activity is likely in the future.

The administration schedule and side effects of the medications should be clearly communicated and understood, as the administration of anticonvulsant medication will become the responsibility of the owner at home. Finally, how therapy will be monitored, management of at home seizures, and expected future financial expenses to be incurred with treatment should be discussed. Appropriate owner education and communication are as important to a successful treatment outcome in animals with seizures as any administered anticonvulsant drug.

WHAT SHOULD I BE TREATING WITH?

The treatment of a seizure disorder will depend upon appropriate treatment of any primary cause. If no cause can be found for the seizure activity, or if the seizures are a life-threatening problem regardless of cause, anticonvulsant medication should be initiated. Many dogs with intracranial structural diseases require anticonvulsant medication independent of additional treatments for the primary intracranial abnormality.

Generally, anticonvulsants may provide benefit either by altering (raising) the seizure threshold or by preventing the spread of the electrical activity within the brain. Differing anticonvulsants may have different mechanisms of seizure control as well as different metabolism, administration schedules, and side effects. As will most treatments, anticonvulsant medications that the clinician is most familiar with and have experience with in treating animal with seizures are more likely to be safe and effective.

Seizures are treated either short-term, in emergency situations, or chronically with repeated administration of medication (maintenance therapy). Anticonvulsant drugs are chosen for therapy of seizures based on their mechanism of seizure control, onset and duration of action, ease of administration and monitoring, and side effects of administration.

Persistent seizures often need to be terminated acutely to prevent life-threatening complications and intracranial injury. In these instances, diazepam (or sometimes other benzodiazepines such midazolam) is often used. Diazepam is an excellent anticonvulsant, but is rapidly metabolized in dogs. This often necessitates using repeated dosages or increased dosages of diazepam to terminate seizures acutely. Diazepam may be administered by a variety of routes, however, the intravenous route of administration is preferred to acutely terminate seizure activity. If intravascular access is not available, diazepam may be administered intrarectally to achieve the same desired effect. Diazepam is also an appropriate acute anticonvulsant for cats, but is occasionally (idiosyncratic reaction) associated with severe liver failure.

Maintenance anticonvulsants are administered chronically in an attempt to decrease the frequency and severity of seizure activity. While there are numerous maintenance anticonvulsants available, the two most commonly used in animals in the current era are phenobarbital and potassium bromide. Both of these drugs seem reasonably effective (65 to 75%) for dogs. They do, however, have different metabolism, toxicities, and methods of administration and monitoring. The most appropriate choice of an anticonvulsant for one animal may not be the best choice for another. Therefore, the best way to choose the most appropriate anticonvulsant drug is to become familiar with the efficacy and side effects of the anticonvulsant, to discuss these aspects of the therapy with the owner, and to come to a mutual decision on which drug to try first based on expectations and lifestyle.

Phenobarbital

Phenobarbital is a barbiturate that has been used for a number of years as a monotherapy for seizures in dogs and cats. This drug is initiated at 3 mg/kg orally every 12 hours. At this dosage, serum phenobarbital concentrations at steady state (10 to 14 days following initiation of the drug) will usually be between 15 and 22 µg/ml. Serum phenobarbital levels should be assessed at approximately 2 weeks after initiating or altering therapy to determine the current serum concentration. Trough therapeutic concentrations (within 1 hour of the next dose) seem to correlate best with clinical seizure control but levels taken at various times during the day may yield the similar information.

Serum phenobarbital concentrations can be measured to determine relative amount of the drug in circulation. When collecting serum for phenobarbital level determination, do not use serum separator tubes, as containers result in false concentrations of measured phenobarbital (falsely low due to silicone binding of phenobarbital). The commonly accepted serum therapeutic range for dogs receiving phenobarbital is between 20 and 40 µg/ml. This range is a general one based on a population of dogs and may not correlate with the efficacy of phenobarbital as an anticonvulsant in any particular dog. Individual dogs may be controlled at various levels within, and sometimes outside (lower), the therapeutic range. For example, one dog may receive significant benefit from phenobarbital when its serum phenobarbital level is at 23 µg/ml, while another dog may not receive anticonvulsant benefit until its level is at 35 µg/ml. If an animal has a serum phenobarbital level within, but not at the high end, of the general therapeutic range, and is not receiving anticonvulsant benefits at that concentration, the dosage of phenobarbital may be increased in an attempt to increase the serum phenobarbital levels. This animal may have improved anticonvulsant benefit at this new level. If the serum phenobarbital levels are increased toward 40 µg/ml, and the animal is receiving no therapeutic benefit from the medication, then further increases in phenobarbital dosage are unlikely to generate any additional therapeutic benefit. As serum phenobarbital levels increase beyond 35 µg/ml, the potential for toxicity becomes greater.

There is no exact mg/kg dose of phenobarbital that will benefit or will be toxic to an individual animal. The actual mg/kg dose of phenobarbital the animal receives is somewhat inconsequential compared to the actual serum phenobarbital level that is achieved. In general, animals receiving 11–13 mg/kg orally every 12 hours will have serum phenobarbital levels greater than 35 µg/ml. It is imperative, however, to determine the serum phenobarbital concentrations before deciding that an animal is getting too little or too much phenobarbital.

Side effects of phenobarbital include polyuria, polydipsia, polyphagia, and sedation. Sedation is most profound after the initiation of phenobarbital therapy, or subsequent to increases in dosages. Sedation usually lasts for 3 to 5 days following the initiation of phenobarbital, but is dose dependent. Animals that have been receiving phenobarbital chronically are less likely to become sedated following increases in phenobarbital, unless toxic concentrations are obtained. Occasionally, animals will become very agitated and hyperactive when phenobarbital is first initiated. These animals often pace compulsively and vocalize. This reaction appears to be the result of the animal receiving too little medication. It has been likened to stage 2 or the excitement phase of anesthesia. In these animals, increasing the dose rapidly, possibly by loading the dog on phenobarbital, will help to relieve this agitation.

The most concerning side effect of phenobarbital is its liver damaging effects (fig. 17.2). Liver damage can be severe and irreversible with phenobarbital treatment. Liver complications with phenobarbital treatment are more likely when relatively high dosages of the drug are used (i.e., drug levels are >35 µg/ml), if other medications are used concurrently, or with chronic drug administration. It is important that a liver function test (bile acids or equivalent) be monitored on a routine basis in animals receiving phenobarbital to establish the possibility of liver dysfunction. Even appropriate phenobarbital dosages and administration will result in increases in commonly measured liver enzymes such as ALT and SAP on a biochemical assessment. These enzyme elevations, therefore, cannot be used solely as a signal of underlying liver dysfunction. Conversely, severe liver fail-

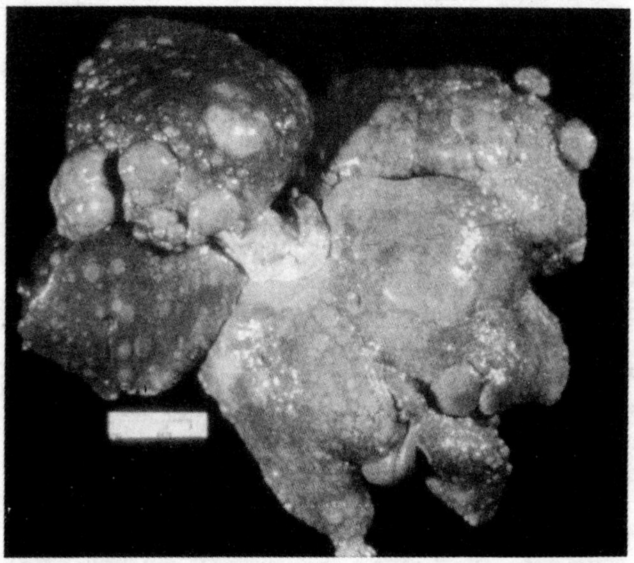

Fig. 17.2. Appearance of the liver at necropsy of a dog with cirrhosis following chronic phenobarbital administration.

ure can occur with liver enzymes measured normal, such as when little functioning liver tissue survives. This underscores the point that, in an animal receiving phenobarbital, routine liver enzymes measurements are less clinically useful during monitoring for underlying liver disease. A liver function such as bile acids assessments is required to make the most accurate determination of underlying liver disease in these animals. If the seizures are controlled on a stable level of phenobarbital, bile acids should be assessed at least every 6 months. If systemic complications arise, bile acids should be assessed sooner. Also, if an animal suddenly becomes sedate on what appears to be an adequate dosage of phenobarbital, assessments for underlying liver disease (and subsequent reduction in phenobarbital metabolism) should be performed.

Phenobarbital can affect the metabolism of other drugs that are metabolized similarly. Additionally, other drugs may alter the metabolism of phenobarbital leading to either increased metabolism with resultant decreased efficacy or decreased metabolism with resultant toxicity. Protein-bound drugs such as nonsteroidal analgesics can displace phenobarbital from binding sites and increase the metabolism of phenobarbital, effectively lowering therapeutic concentrations. Still other drugs, most notably chloramphenicol and possibly cimetidine, prevent the metabolism of phenobarbital leading to excessive serum concentrations. These excessive concentrations can then result in a comatose state, respiratory depression, and eventual death.

Routine administration of phenobarbital should not result in increases in bile acids unless there is underlying liver pathology. Phenobarbital administration, however, may affect the results of some other commonly evaluated serum tests such as thyroid level. Measured T4 levels will decrease when an animal is on phenobarbital, making the diagnosis of hypothyroidism in these dogs more difficult. The decrease in thyroid hormone concentrations with phenobarbital does not result in clinical manifestation of hypothyroidism.

If toxic levels of phenobarbital are attained, or if seizure control is not adequate, then an additional anticonvulsant is added. Potassium bromide is most often added in these dogs.

Potassium Bromide

Another reasonable option for maintenance anticonvulsant therapy, especially for younger animals that may require anticonvulsants, is potassium bromide (KBr). This medication is actually a chemical, not a drug formulation. Potassium bromide has reasonable efficacy for treatment of seizures in dogs. It was initially difficult to obtain in formulations for administration to dogs, but this is less of a problem currently as there are a number of veterinary compounding laboratories that provide therapeutic distribution of this drug.

Potassium bromide has a relatively long half-life (~24 days in dogs, 10 days in cats), and, therefore, requires significant amounts of time to reach steady state concentrations (up to 4 months in dogs, 6 weeks in cats) . In an effort to increase the therapeutic drug levels of potassium bromide sooner, a loading dose of potassium bromide can be given at the initiation of treatment. The normal maintenance dose of bromide is between 20 and 60 mg/kg/day. If sodium bromide is used, the dosage is slightly reduced (17 to 30 mg/kg/day). If more rapid seizure control is needed, an initial dose of 400–600 mg/kg, usually divided over a 2 to 3 day period, can be administered. Potassium bromide, when administered in increased concentrations in a single dosing period, is often irritating to the stomach and results in vomiting. To avoid this problem, this loading dose is administered in multiple, smaller doses over the 2 to 3 day period. It often helps when using the loading dose to calculate the maintenance dose expected first. This will most likely be the capsule size that can be formulated by a compounding laboratory. During the loading period, the total loading dose is given over 48 to 72 hours by giving multiple doses of the maintenance dose of the medication. For example, the loading dose of potassium bromide for a 20 kg dogs would be calculated as follows:

Maintenance dose of KBr for 20 kg dog is

20 kg × 30 mg/kg = 600 mg

To decrease the chance of gastric irritation with the maintenance medication, the 600 mg daily dose is divided into two, 300 mg dosages, which is how the medication will be compounded.

For loading,

20 kg (dog) × 400 mg/kg (loading dose) = 8000 mg (needed)

For loading, take the 300 mg capsules and administer this dose every 2 to 4 hours until a final dose of 8000 mg is attained. This requires approximately 27 dosages over a 2 to 4 day period. Some modifications of this method can be made to accommodate ease of medication administration. The animal may be able to handle increased amounts of KBr without vomiting, and this would decrease the number of individual dosages used during the loading phase. After loading is completed, the animal is started on the maintenance dosage the following day.

Potassium bromide is reasonably safe but has some side effects. The bromide component is toxic to humans who can get headaches, skin rashes, tremors, and gastrointestinal disturbances. Therefore, owners should be careful in handling the medication and not expose themselves to the chemical. This may require placing the medication in the food, wearing gloves when pilling, and washing hands after touching the capsule. Diets with relatively high chloride (sodium chloride) content may increase bromide elimination as bromide competes with chloride for elimination. Renal disease may decrease elimination of bromide, requiring decreases in dosage of bromide up to 50% of normal levels to avoid toxicity.

The most common side effects of potassium bromide

administration in dogs include sedation and ataxia. Pancreatitis is associated with the use of this drug, but the actual cause and effect relationship is not clear. With some dosages, vomiting may occur due to the local irritant effects on the stomach. Diets, alterations in fluid intake, or dehydration may alter the therapeutic levels in the blood of KBr. Rarely, skin irritation, itchiness, or rashes may be noted. Importantly, in cats, KBr can result in a fatal asthmatic condition. Caution should be exercised when using this drug in cats, and if any respiratory signs are noted, the drug should be stopped immediately. Rarely, dogs may become aggressive while receiving bromide therapy. When performing routine serum chemistry evaluations, measured serum chloride concentrations will be increased as the analysis methods measure the serum bromide as chloride.

If toxic levels of bromide are present, diuresis is used to eliminate the drug from the body. Intravenous administration of NaCl-containing fluids is used for this purpose.

Similar to phenobarbital, serum concentration of KBr can be measured to provide a more objective measure of circulating KBr concentrations. Levels range from 1 to 3 mg/ml. This range, however, is not correlated with efficacy or toxicity as reliably as serum phenobarbital concentrations. With KBR, toxic effects are usually evident clinically (primarily sedation and ataxia).

Diazepam

Oral or injectable diazepam is usually not appropriate for use as a maintenance anticonvulsant in dogs due to its relatively short half-life. Diazepam, however, does have utility in the home treatment of dogs with seizures for acute administration following or during seizure activity (see below, Status Epilepticus). Injectable diazepam can be administered rectally (at usually 1.5 times the normal intravenous dosage) to help in terminating a seizure or breaking a seizure cycle. The medication is given to the owner in a dark glass container (diazepam is degraded by light and plastic) in 3 to 5 dosing increments.

The owner should be instructed in how to administer the medication. The liquid drug should be removed from the bottle (usually with a needle and syringe) to the appropriate dosing amount. The needle is then removed from the syringe, and either a teat canula or similar nontraumatic device, or the unneedled syringe is inserted into the rectum and the medication is injected. For some seizuring animals, at-home administration of diazepam by owners may help with acute seizure control and avoid trips to the veterinary hospital.

Additional Medical Therapies for Seizures

Approximately 70% of idiopathic epileptic dogs will be controlled with currently available anticonvulsant medications. If monotherapy with these drugs is not effective, combining these drugs may be helpful in some animals. If phenobarbital or potassium bromide is not effective, there are a number of other anticonvulsants that have been tried in animals. Many of these either are not as effective as phenobarbital and potassium bromide, or they have not been used extensively enough in animals to assess efficacy. Additionally, new anticonvulsants are constantly being developed for human use, and often are similarly tried in animals (see appendix 3). Drugs such as felbamate and gabapentin have been used as additional drugs in difficult-to-control epileptic dogs. These drugs also have side effects that may be life-threatening and should be reviewed before administration in animals. As these drugs are available in the human market, oftentimes they are expensive as well (tables 17. 2, 17.3).

Table 17.2. Comparative cost per dose of anticonvulsants (costs may vary based on drug availability and generic forms)

Drug[1]	Wholesale price	Retail price	Price/dose[2]
Phenobarbital 30 mg	$5.58/1000	$7.99/100	$0.08
Phenobarbital 60 mg	$10.82/1000	$7.99/100	$0.08
Phenobarbital 90 mg	$17.97/1000	$8.95/100	$0.09
Potassium bromide 1000 mg	$20.00/30,000 mg		$0.75
Felbamate3 400 mg	$168.44/100	$156.01/90	$1.73
Felbamate 600 mg	$193.05/100	$188.76/90	$2.10
Gabapentin4 100 mg	$28.68/100	$34.99/90	$0.39
Gabapentin 300 mg	$53.67/100	$59.99/90	$0.67
Gabapentin 400 mg	$71.31/100	$74.99/90	$0.83
Gabapentin 600 mg	$99.70/100	$89.99/90	$1.00
Gabapentin 800 mg	$118.62/100	$89.99/90	$1.00
Clonazepam 0.5 mg	$2.00/100	$19.89/90	$0.22
Clonazepam 1.0 mg	$2.55/100	$21.87/90	$0.24
Clonazepam 2.0 mg	$4.58/100	$23.86/90	$0.27
Clorazepate 3.75 mg	$7.93/100	$67.69/90	$0.75
Clorazepate 7.5 mg	$11.55/100	$83.78/90	$0.93
Clorazepate 15 mg	$20.14/100	$113.02/90	$1.26
Diazepam 5 mg	$2.27/100	$13.95/90	$0.16
Diazepam 10 mg	$3.04/100	$11.63/90	$0.13

[1] Costs in the author's hospital in 2005.
[2] Exact costs may vary. Cost will also depend on amount of drug used.
[3,4] In the previous 2 years, for example, costs for Felbamate have increased, whereas costs for Gabapentin have decreased.

Table 17.3. Relative costs of common anticonvulsants

Drug	Relative expense
Phenobarbital	1
Potassium bromide	1.25
Felbamate	4.25
Gabapentin	4
Clonazepam	4 to 8
Clorazepate	8+
Levetiracetam	3
Zonisamide	4+
Topirmate	8+

Note: Relative cost per day for a 20 kg dog at standard dosages (cost may vary depending on tablet strength and on amount of drug needed for seizure control); scale is based on a dosage of phenobarbital = 1 (approximately $0.32/day)

Alternative Treatments for Seizures

Alternative therapies for seizure control include treatments with acupuncture and dietary modification. Implantation of vagal stimulation devices have been used in dogs for treatment of seizure activity. Also, dietary modification, such as using an all-natural diet or even a ketogenic diet, may help seizure control in some dogs.

FUTURE DIRECTIONS—SURGICAL TREATMENTS OF SEIZURES

Surgical treatments for seizure control are used for selected human patients with seizures that are not controlled adequately with medical therapies. Similar surgical treatments are rare in animals, but we hope will increase with a better understanding of seizure generation and location. This hopefully will occur through advances in intracranial imaging and electrophysiological monitoring for animals.

SEIZURES IN CATS

Seizure disorders in cats are less well defined compared to dogs. Cats have been suggested to uncommonly have true genetic or idiopathic epilepsy. Instead, it is commonly accepted that cats have cryptogenic epilepsy, possible resulting from previous vascular or infectious intracranial disease that results in a residual seizure focus. This may be one reason why cats appear to have more focal varieties of seizures compared to dogs. Focal seizures in cats may consist of movements of a part of the face or body, or involve only the facial muscles.

In general, the basic thought process for evaluation of seizures in dogs can be followed when evaluating cats with seizures. Assessments for underlying causes such as metabolic, infectious, and structural intracranial diseases (tumors, encephalitis, hydrocephalus, trauma, and vascular diseases) should be performed. If underlying disease is eliminated, persistent seizures, regardless of previous cause, may require treatment. Treatment options for cats with seizures are limited and less established compared to dogs. Phenobarbital is a commonly used option that is helpful in many cats. Dosages and monitoring of therapy is similar as for dogs. Potassium bromide may be helpful in some cats, however, cats can develop a potentially fatal asthmatic condition while receiving KBr. If this is not recognized and KBr promptly discontinued, this abnormality can result in death. Therefore, KBr should be used cautiously in cats, and if any respiratory abnormalities occur in a cat receiving KBR, this medication should be promptly discontinued.

Diazepam has historically been used as a supportive maintenance anticonvulsant, however, for cats this drug has been associated with potentially fatal liver disease. The risks of use of this drug compared to the anticonvulsant benefits for individuals cats need to be considered if this drug is to be used for seizure control. Other historically used anticonvulsants such as primidone and phenytoin may be toxic to cats and should be avoided.

Gabapentin has been used as an anticonvulsant in cats. Excessive sedation is possible, especially when this drug is initiated. Gradually increasing dosages are recommended to avoid this adverse effect. Initial doses of 5 to 10 mg/kg every 24 hours are increased to the same dose every 12 hours after 3 to 5 days of therapy.

STATUS EPILEPTICUS

Status epilepticus is a state of persistent seizure activity without a break in the seizure cycle. This type of seizure activity can rapidly have life-threatening consequences, and should be considered an emergency situation. The goal in management of animals with status epilepticus is to quickly terminate the seizure activity, to rapidly determine the cause of the seizure activity, and to treat any associated systemic or intracranial consequences of the seizure activity. An outline for treatment of status epilepticus is found in table 17.4.

Seizure activity is most often terminated with diazepam administered intravenously or rectally if diazepam is administered frequently enough and in adequate dosages. If an animal is suspected of having a portal systemic shunt or other type of liver dysfunction, be cautious in administering diazepam as these animals will have trouble metabolizing this medication and may become heavily sedated or comatose.

Administer an appropriate dosage of diazepam for the size of the animal being treated (general ranges include 5 mg for animals under 10 kg, 10 mg for animals 10–20 kg, and 15 or 20 mg for animals over 20 kg). Administer the initial dosage either intravenously or rectally. Concurrently, establish intravenous access with an intravenous catheter if possible. If the initial dosage of diazepam terminates the seizure activity, then begin the diagnostic process through examination and laboratory assessments while monitoring physical signs and seizure activity.

If the initial dosage of diazepam does not terminate the seizure activity, or if the seizure activity is only terminated for a short time (seconds to minutes), administer a second dosage of diazepam. If the seizure activity returns rapidly or is not terminated appropriately, administer additional

Table 17.4. Management of status epilepticus

1. Take your own pulse (calm down).
2. Give diazepam (Valium) IV or rectally—0.5–2 mg/kg. Average doses are listed below.

Small dogs	5 mg
Medium dogs	5–10 mg
Large dogs	10–20 mg

1.5–2 mg/kg rectally

Note: Do not be afraid to give significant amounts of diazepam, as long as you are not suspicious of a liver problem (portosystemic shunt). Wait 1 minute to assess effect. Keep giving single doses every minute until seizure stops.

3. If seizures stop, give phenobarbital IV and proceed with additional diagnostics.

If animal has not been on phenobarbital, give 12 mg/kg IV.
If animal is currently receiving phenobarbital, give up to 12 mg/kg.

4. If seizures return quickly, again give additional 0.5–2 mg/kg diazepam. If seizure stops, consider diazepam infusion. Give the amount of diazepam that stopped the seizure as a continuous infusion over 1 hour (approximately 5–20 mg/dog/hour; puppies, 5–10 mg/hour; large dog, 10–20 mg/hour). Mix dose in small volume of 0.9% NaCl or 5% dextrose in water in buretrol. Avoid light. Run 5 mg diazepam through line to saturate diazepam binding sites in plastic infusion line. Another option is to use infusion pump.
5. If seizures are unresponsive to diazepam, give

Propofol 1–2 mg/kg IV; constant infusion of 0.1–0.6 mg/kg/minute or 6 mg/kg/hour to effect

OR

Phenobarbital 3–6 mg/kg IV

OR

if the animal has not been on phenobarbital previously, 12–16 mg/kg IV or IM. *Wait 20 minutes for effect.*
Give 1 mg/kg phenobarbital to raise serum phenobarbital by 1 μg/ml. Can give up to 2–4 mg/kg/hourly phenobarbital IV. Monitor for respiratory depression and be prepared to ventilate. If seizures return, can use phenobarbital continuous infusion similar to valium infusion at 2–4 mg/kg/hour

(120 mg phenobarbital diluted to 20 ml total volume = 6 mg/ml)

If seizures stop, continue on BID phenobarbital at 3 mg/kg IV, IM or PO (or appropriate increased dose depending upon how much phenobarbital the animal was receiving previously).

6. If all else fails, plan to anesthetize the animal with isoflurane (less ideally, pentobarbital at 3 mg/kg IV to effect PRN). This stops the motor manifestations of the seizure but not the electrical seizure activity occurring intracranially.
7. Sodium bromide has been given intravenously and rectally.
8. Maintain blood pressure with appropriate intravenous fluid therapy.

May administer B vitamins (vitamin B_1 25–50 mg/animal IM).

If seizures have been prolonged, treat for possible increased ICP with

Mannitol (0.25–1 g/kg IV)
Furosemide (0.07 mg/kg IV)

OR

Hypertonic saline (3% solution, 5.3 ml/kg IV)

Many animals also benefit from administration of corticosteroids (methylprednisolone sodium succinate or prednisone sodium succinate at 30 mg/kg IV slowly).

Basic supportive critical care, maintain body temperature.

9. Other unproven or inconsistently effective options for termination of seizures:

Lidocaine at 1–2 mg/kg IV (Seizures are a side effect of lidocaine overdose.)

Phenytoin continuous infusion?

(Note: Constant infusions can be discontinued 2–4 hours following the last seizure event.)

dosages of diazepam while monitoring seizure activity and vital signs such as respiration. If the animal's seizures can be terminated, even for a short time, with repeated dosages of diazepam, consider using constant intravenous administration of diazepam.

Animals that present in status epilepticus often benefit from acute phenobarbital therapy. Depending upon whether the animal has previously been treated with phenobarbital, loading with between 10 and 12 mg/kg IV or IM of injectable phenobarbital is often used. As a general rule, administer 1 mg/kg of phenobarbital to raise the serum phenobarbital levels by 1 μg/ml. If, for example, an animal with a previous serum phenobarbital level of 26 μg/ml is presented in status epilepticus, a dosage of injectable phenobarbital of 10 mg/kg could be expected to acutely increase this level to 36 μg/ml.

Animals that present in status epilepticus often have associated cerebral edema or increases in intracranial pressure. These animals often benefit from treatments for increased intracranial pressure such as mannitol (0.25–1 g/kg IV) or hypertonic saline (3% at 5.3 ml/kg IV) administration concurrent with treatment for their seizure activity. Intravenous corticosteroid administration (methylprednisolone sodium succinate at 30 mg/kg intravenously slowly over 10 to 15 minutes) have been helpful for some of these animals. Appropriate intravenous fluid administration is also critical to maintain systemic blood pressure and, subsequently, cerebral perfusion pressure.

In some instances, a variety of other treatments is used for treatment of status epilepticus in animals. Pentobarbital has been used for a number of years. As this drug is primarily an anesthetic agent, it is used to terminate the external manifestations and movements of seizure activity. It is debatable if pentobarbital has an effect on the actual seizure activity within the brain, therefore, it may not help in quelling the intracranial damage secondary to seizures. Propofol administration has also been used for treatment of seizure activity, primarily in animals with associated liver disease. If seizure activity is severe and uncontrollable with diazepam and phenobarbital, consideration should be given to using isoflurane gas anesthesia for a short period (30 minutes to an hour). Isoflurane inhalant anesthesia has been associated anecdotally with termination of severe seizure activity in some dogs.

18 Evaluation of Dogs and Cats with Vestibular Disease

Disease of the vestibular system results in some of the most dramatic clinical presentations seen in clinical neurology. The vestibular system is largely responsible for keeping the animal oriented with respect to gravity. Disease process may affect the vestibular system either in the peripheral portions of the nerve or in the more central portions associated with vestibular nuclei in the brain stem.

CLINICAL SIGNS OF VESTIBULAR DISEASE

Clinical signs of vestibular dysfunction reflect abnormal orientation of the head, limbs, and eyes. Clues to vestibular or cerebellar disease include:

- Head tilt (usually toward the side of the lesion)
- Ataxia
- Nystagmus
- Falling
- Rolling
- Vomiting
- Lateral recumbency (prefer to lie on the side of a unilateral lesion)

NEUROANATOMICAL LOCALIZATION

Differentiation as to whether the lesion is central (within the brain stem) or peripheral (within CN VIII proper or its peripheral receptors) is important for selection of appropriate diagnostic tests (table 18.1).

Once the lesion has been localized, appropriate differential diagnoses can be formulated (tables 18.2, 18.3, 18.4).

Unfortunately, intracranial lesions occasionally result in signs indicative of a peripheral lesion. Conversely, animals with acute, severe peripheral vestibular dysfunction may be so incapacitated that accurate interpretation of neurologic examination findings may not be possible. Because of these nuances, if the examiner is unsure of the location of the lesion, an evaluation for central vestibular disease should occur concurrently with an evaluation for peripheral disease.

DIAGNOSTIC TESTING

1. If a lesion is suspected to involve the central vestibular structures (supratentorial, brain stem, or cerebellum), an advanced imaging study such as CT or MR imaging is used to assess the structural integrity of these areas.
    - These studies are noninvasive but do require anesthesia in all but the comatose animal.
    - One disadvantage of CT is the significant beam-hardening artifacts that often occur in the posterior fossa of animals hindering evaluation of the vestibular area.
2. Survey radiographs of the skull are useful in instances of skull fracture or middle ear (bulla) disease, however, do not allow for assessment of nervous system parenchyma.
3. If peripheral disease is suspected, a thorough otoscopic examination, preferably while the animal is anesthetized, is mandatory.
4. Cerebrospinal fluid (CSF) analysis is helpful primarily to determine the presence of inflammatory diseases.
    - In general, collection of spinal fluid caudal to the level of the lesion is most accurate for diagnosis. Fluid is analyzed for cellularity, protein content, and cell morphology.
    - While CSF analysis is often helpful in determining the presence of nervous system disease, used alone, it does not often lend a specific etiologic diagnosis.
    - Titers to specific infectious agents can be measured in CSF to assess for intrathecal production of antibody.
5. Recording the brain stem auditory potential (BSEP or BAER) may be helpful in determining the presence of intact hearing pathways and may also provide some information about the integrity of central (brain stem) projection pathways associated with hearing.
    - BSEP testing requires availability of the equipment and expertise in performing and evaluating the tests.
6. Surgical biopsy is often necessary for definitive antemortem diagnosis of structural intracranial disease.

Table 18.1. Signs of vestibular disease

Signs consistent with central vestibular disease
- Conscious proprioceptive deficits
- Vertical nystagmus
- Changing nystagmus with changing head positions
- Multiple cranial nerve deficits excluding CN VII

Signs consistent with either peripheral or central vestibular disease
- Head tilt
- Horizontal or rotatory nystagmus
- Ataxia
- Falling
- Rolling
- Positional strabismus
- Positional nystagmus (as long as the direction of the nystagmus does not change with changing head positions)

Table 18.2. Important and common diseases that affect the peripheral vestibular structures

Anomalous	Congenital peripheral vestibular disease: Akitas, beagles (bilateral), German shepherds, Dobermans, English cockers; Siamese and Burmese cats
Metabolic	Hypothyroidism (possibly)
Neoplastic	Middle/inner ear tumor: squamous cell tumor, adenocarcinoma
Idiopathic	Canine geriatric vestibular disease; feline idiopathic vestibular disease
Inflammatory/ infectious	Otitis media/interna
Inflammatory/ noninfectious	Idiopathic vestibulitis
Trauma	Trauma to internal ear structures,foreign material in ear
Toxicity	Ototoxic drugs (aminoglycosides, furosemide, chlorhexidine, cisplatin) Metronidazole (may initially have peripheral nerve signs)

Table 18.3. Central diseases commonly associated with vestibular signs

Anomalous	Arachnoid cysts Dermoid or epidermoid cysts Hydrocephalus Dandy-Walker syndrome
Metabolic	Hypothyroidism?
Neoplastic	Meningioma Choroid plexus tumor
Nutritional	Thiamine deficiency (cat and dog)
Inflammatory Brain Diseases	Infectious Viral *Distemper (dog)* *Herpes virus* *Parvovirus* *Parainfluenza virus* *Feline Infectious Peritonitis (cat)* Fungal Protozoal *Toxoplasmosis* Rickettsial *Rocky Mountain spotted fever* *Ehrlichia* Bacteria Parasites Noninfectious encephalitis GME Breed-specific meningitis Generalized tremor syndrome
Trauma	Head trauma Intracranial hemorrhage Subdural hematoma
Toxicity	Metronidazole
Vascular	Infarction Primary Hemorrhage (coagulopathies or platelet disorders) Hypertension

Note: Also see infratentorial diseases chapter 5.

- This is more difficult in the infratentorial space as surgical exposure, especially of ventrally located lesions, is often incomplete.

7. For lesions of the ear canal and bulla, lateral ear canal resection and bulla osteotomy, respectively or in combination, are useful for biopsy, lesion resection, and drainage of infected tissue.

TREATMENT

Specific treatments can be recommended best after a definitive diagnosis is made (table 18.5).

- Nonspecific treatments include protecting the eyes from damage, especially if there is an associated facial nerve deficit or if the animal is lateral recumbent and rolling into the ground.
- Antihistamines, such as diphenhydramine (1–2 mg/kg orally or IV), have been useful in decreasing anxiety and anorexia and, in some instances, the severity of the associated head tilt and nystagmus.
- Meclizine (dog: 25 mg orally every 24 hours; cat: 12.5 mg orally every 24 hours) has also been suggested to decrease nausea.
- Diazepam (5–10 mg/dog orally every 6 to 8 hours) may also help with anxiety and apprehension and may be useful in dogs with metronidazole toxicity.

Table 18.4. Important diseases that affect the cerebellum (or result in signs of cerebellar disease)

Degenerative	Abiotrophies (Channelopathies?) Spongiform encephalopathies Feline spongiform encephalopathy Neuroaxonal dystrophy Leukocephalomyelopathy Storage diseases
Anomalous	Arachnoid cysts Dermoid or epidermoid cysts Hydrocephalus Hypoplasia (panleukopenia infection in cats) Dandy-Walker syndrome
Neoplastic	Meningioma Choroid plexus tumor Medulloblastoma Glioma
Nutritional	Thiamine deficiency (dog)
Inflammatory brain diseases	Infectious Viral *Distemper (dog)* *Herpes virus* *Parvovirus* *Parainfluenza virus* *Feline infectious peritonitis (cat)* Fungal Protozoal *Toxoplasmosis* Rickettsial *Rocky Mountain spotted fever* *Ehrlichia* Bacteria Parasites Noninfectious encephalitis *GME* *Breed-specific meningitis* *Generalized tremor syndrome*
Trauma	Head trauma Intracranial hemorrhage Subdural hematoma
Toxicity	Metronidazole
Vascular	Infarction Primary Hemorrhage (coagulopathies or platelet disorders) Hypertension

Table 18.5. Treatment of Vestibular Disease

Nonspecific treatments

- Comfortable, safe environment
- Antihistamines, *diphenhydramine* (1–2 mg/kg orally or IV)
  Meclizine (dog 25 mg orally every 24 hours; cat 12.5 mg orally every 24 hours)
  Diazepam (5 to 10 mg/dog orally every 6 to 8 hours)
  Consider thyroid supplementation for hypothyroid

Treatment for suspected peripheral vestibular disease

- Otitis interna
  Systemic antibiotics: Amoxicillin/clavulanic acid (dog: 12.5–25 mg/kg orally every 12 hours; cat: 62.5 mg/cat orally every 12 hours)
  Remove aural foreign material
  Cleaning of ear
  Surgical debridement

Treatment of suspected central vestibular disease

- Stop administration of toxic medications such as metronidazole
- Diazepam
- Hydrocephalus
  Treatment for ICP
  1. Fluid resuscitation to maintain cerebral perfusion (Isotonic fluids, hypertonic saline)
  2. Diuretics
     a. Mannitol (0.25–1.0 gm/kg IV bolus)
     b. Furosemide (0.07 to 1 mg/kg IV)
     c. Hypertonic saline (3%) (5.3 ml/kg IV)
  3. Head elevation
  4. Hyperventilation (if the animal is intubated)
     a. Monitor blood gas on end-tidal CO_2 concentration to maintain CO_2 approximately 28 to 30
     b. Corticosteroids (methylprednisolone sodium succinate or prednisone sodium succinate at 30 mg/kg IV slowly over 15 minutes, repeat at 15 mg/kg IV slowly at 2 and 6 hours after initial dose. Alternative, dexamethasone sodium phosphate at 0.01–0.025 mg/kg IV every 6 hours)
  5. Surgical decompression (craniotomy)

  Corticosteroids (methylprednisolone sodium succinate or prednisone sodium succinate at 30 mg/kg IV slowly over 15 minutes, repeat at 15 mg/kg IV slowly at 2 and 6 hours after initial dose. Alternative, dexamethasone sodium phosphate at 0.01–0.025 mg/kg IV every 6 hours)

- Brain tumor
  Treatment for ICP (see above)
  Corticosteroids (see above)

- Thiamine deficiency
  Thiamine: Severely affected cats should receive at least 1 mg parenterally5–30 mg IV in isotonic fluids

- Encephalitis and meningitis
  Trimethoprim-sulfadiazine (30 mg/kg q 12 h)
  Clindamycin (20–25 mg/kg q 12 h)
  Doxycycline (10 mg/kg q 24 h PO)
  Corticosteroids (prednisone 1–4 mg/kg q 12 h or methylprednisolone sodium succinate or prednisone sodium succinate at 30 mg/kg IV slowly over 15 minutes, repeat at 15 mg/kg IV slowly at 2 and 6 hours after initial dose. Alternative, dexamethasone sodium phosphate at 0.01 to 0.025 mg/kg IV every 6 hours)
  Other antibiotics: ampicillin (22 mg/kg every 6 to 12 hours); enrofloxacin (10 mg/kg IV every 12 hours; cefotaxime (25 to 50 mg/kg IV every 8 hours)

19 Localization of Abnormalities of Vision and Pupils in Companion Animals

Animals may be presented for a variety of abnormalities of vision and pupils. These abnormalities may result from diseases primarily affecting the ocular structures, or the central and peripheral nervous pathways important for vision and pupillary functions. Primary abnormalities of ocular structures should be assessed through a thorough ophthalmologic examination. When evaluating, it is important to determine whether the animal is visual, the resting pupil size, and how the pupils react in both bright and dimly lighted environments.

ASSESSMENT OF VISION

- Vision is initially assessed subjectively in animals through observation of the animal's movements and behavior.
- Animals that have difficulty with vision often are apprehensive in unfamiliar environments, and tend to remain in areas that are "safe." In some cases, this is interpreted as the animal being less active or quieter than normal.
- Animals may appear startled more easily, or may even become apprehensive or aggressive when approached.
- If animals with visual deficits are forced to move, they may bump into walls or other objects in the examination area. When these animals do bump into objects, they tend to pull their heads backward and back away, suggesting that they "understand" that they impacted an unknown object or structure.
  - Animals with abnormalities of cognition and recognition of visual information may bump into walls and continue to walk or press forward.
- Assessments of vision can also be made by encouraging the animal to walk through an unfamiliar obstacle course. Animals with visual abnormalities may bump into objects that are placed in areas they are unfamiliar with.

THE MENACE RESPONSE

- An assessment of vision by performing a menace response test (see chapter 3).
- A menacing gesture is made to one eye as the other is covered (fig. 19.1).
- The menace response tests components of optic nerve and the central visual pathways (see chapter 3) (fig. 19.2).
- Visual-stimulated impulse is transferred in nerve fibers that project from the retina to the *optic nerve, optic chiasm, contralateral optic tract, lateral geniculate body* (in the thalamus, *optic radiations*) and, finally, to the *visual cortex (the occipital lobe)* where integration of visual information begins.
- Appropriate responses to visual stimulation are then mediated by areas within the CNS associated with visual integration (fig. 19.3).
  - These areas most likely include motor system excitation in the cerebral hemispheres, projection pathways in the brain stem, with additional influences provided by the cerebellum.
  - Animals with cerebellar disease can lack a normal menace response but have normal vision and normal CN VII function.
- The efferent response of the menace response test is mediated through *CN VII* (facial nerve) resulting in closure of the eyelid through activation of the orbicularis oculi muscle.

VISUAL FIELD DEFICITS

In some animals with visual deficits, it may be possible to discern a lesion in a single visual field or, more commonly, in one-half of the visual fields (fig. 19.4). A visual deficit affecting one-half of the visual fields is referred to as a hemianopia.

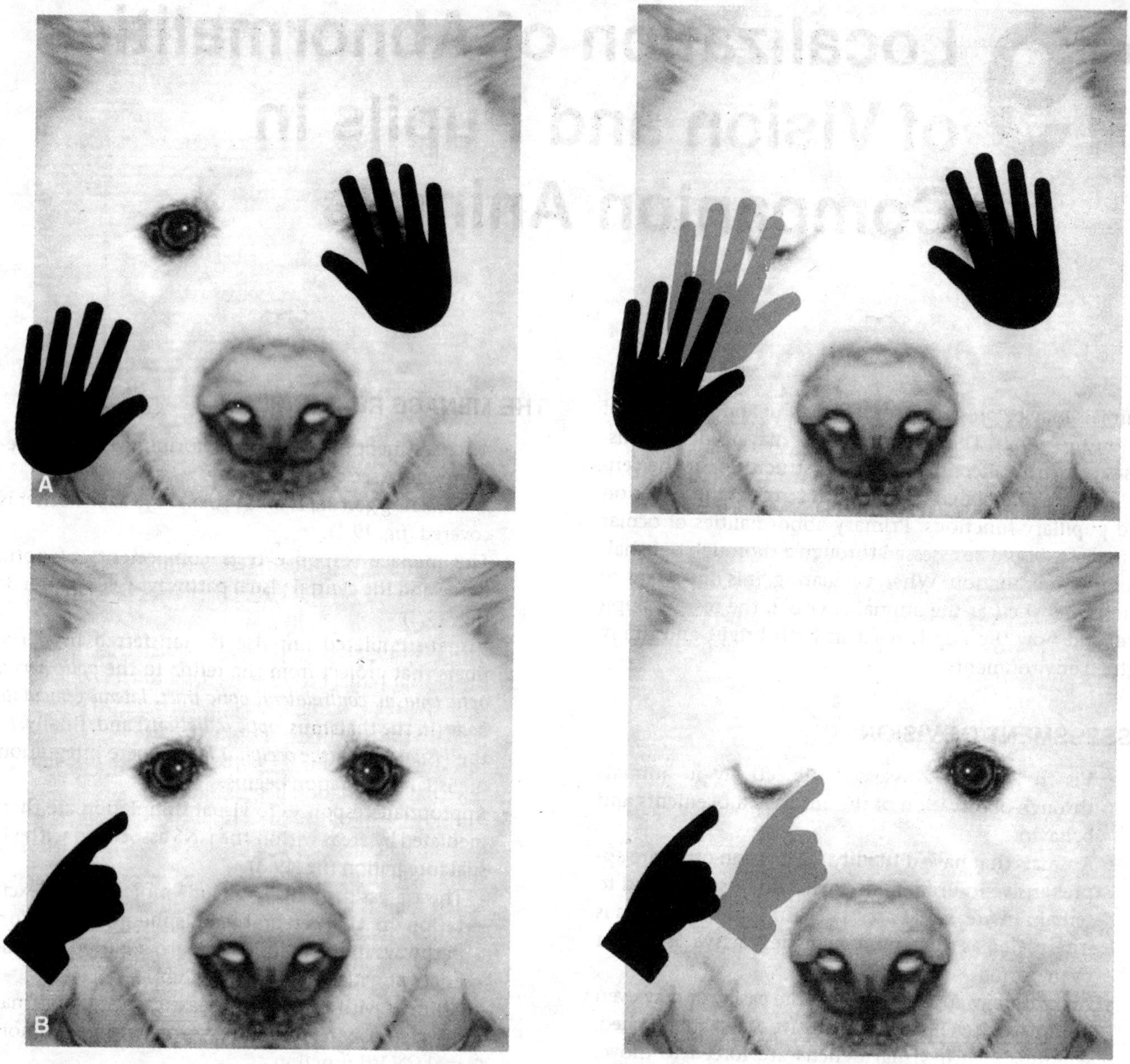

Fig. 19.1. Representation of the menace response (top figures) and the palpebral reflex (bottom figures).

- A visual deficit in corresponding visual fields is referred to as a homonymous hemianopia, such as a deficit in the nasal visual field in one eye and the temporal visual field of the opposite eye (fig. 19.5).
  - This is often present in animals with unilateral supratentorial lesions but is often difficult to detect clinically.
- A hemianopia in noncorresponding visual fields, such as in both temporal or both nasal fields, is described as a heteronymous.
  - This type of hemianopia is rarely recognized in animals.

DISEASES AFFECTING VISION

Diseases of the nervous system affecting vision may involve cranial II or the visual projection pathways associated with this nerve. Abnormalities of cranial nerve II include:

- Optic nerve hypoplasia
- Neoplastic diseases such as *meningiomas*
- Inflammatory diseases such as canine *distemper, granulomatous meningoencephalitis (GME),* and optic neuritis
  - In the ocular form of GME, animals are often presented for unilateral blindness with reduced or absent pupillary light reflexes. On fundic examina-

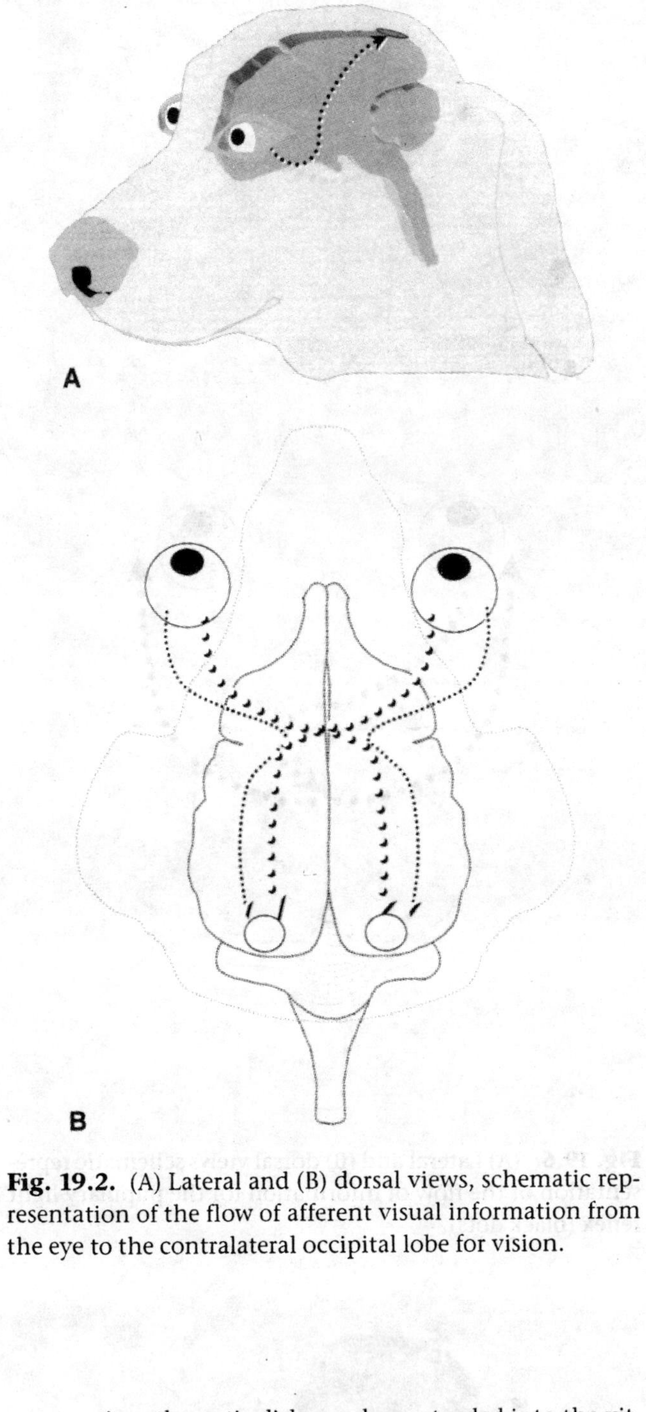

Fig. 19.2. (A) Lateral and (B) dorsal views, schematic representation of the flow of afferent visual information from the eye to the contralateral occipital lobe for vision.

tion, the optic disk may be protruded into the vitreous and be hyperemic and edematous. Retinal vessels may be dilated and focal retinal hemorrhages may be present.

- *Optic neuritis* is a primary inflammation of the optic nerves. Animals often present for blindness or visual difficulty, usually with associated absent or decreased pupillary light reflexes. Upon retinal examination, an edematous, elevated optic disk may be seen. Retinal vessels may be engorged and there may be associated focal retina hemorrhages.

- *Protothecosis* has been reported to cause central nervous system disease and also involve the eye. This may be primarily the result of an anterior uveitis.

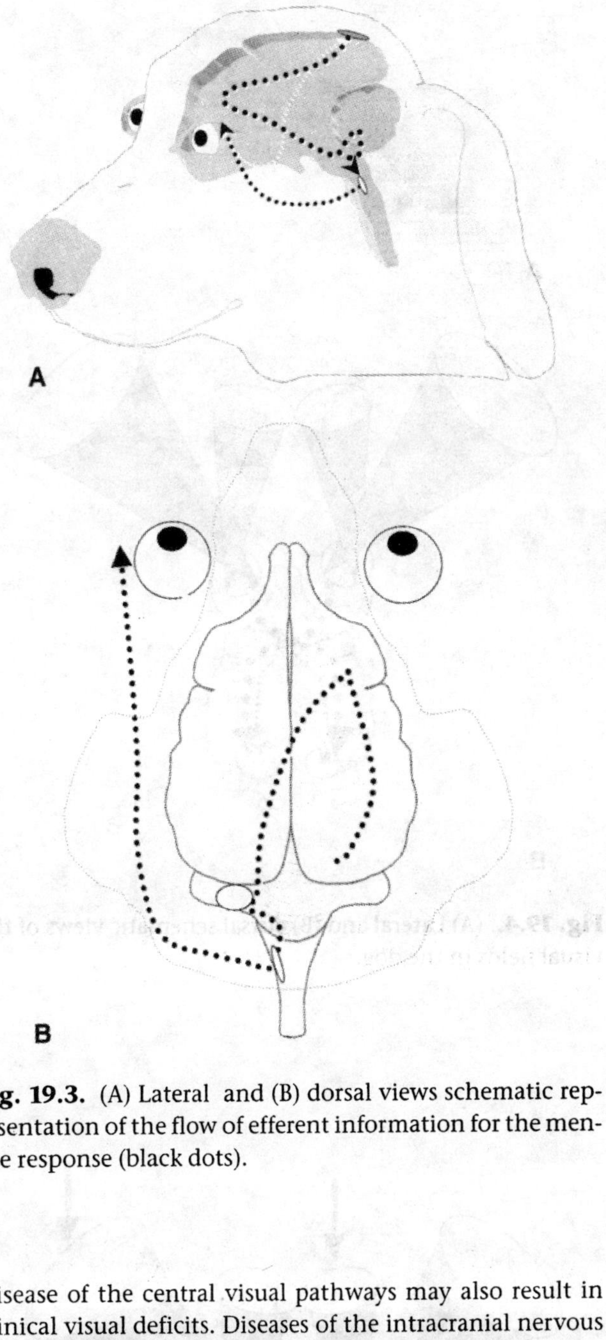

Fig. 19.3. (A) Lateral and (B) dorsal views schematic representation of the flow of efferent information for the menace response (black dots).

Disease of the central visual pathways may also result in clinical visual deficits. Diseases of the intracranial nervous structures are discussed in detail in chapter 5. The more common diseases affecting brain structure include *hydrocephalus, tumor, encephalitis, traumatic injury, and cerebrovascular disease.*

NEUROANATOMY OF PUPIL FUNCTION

The pupil is innervated by the two divisions of the autonomic nervous system, which are in turn controlled by many different areas within the nervous system. Pupil size and reactivity are controlled by both the parasympathetic and sympathetic systems. When stimulated, the parasympathetic system is responsible for constriction of the pupil and the *pupillary light reflex (PLR)* (fig. 19.6). Sympathetic system stimulation results in pupillary dilation (table 19.1, fig. 19.7).

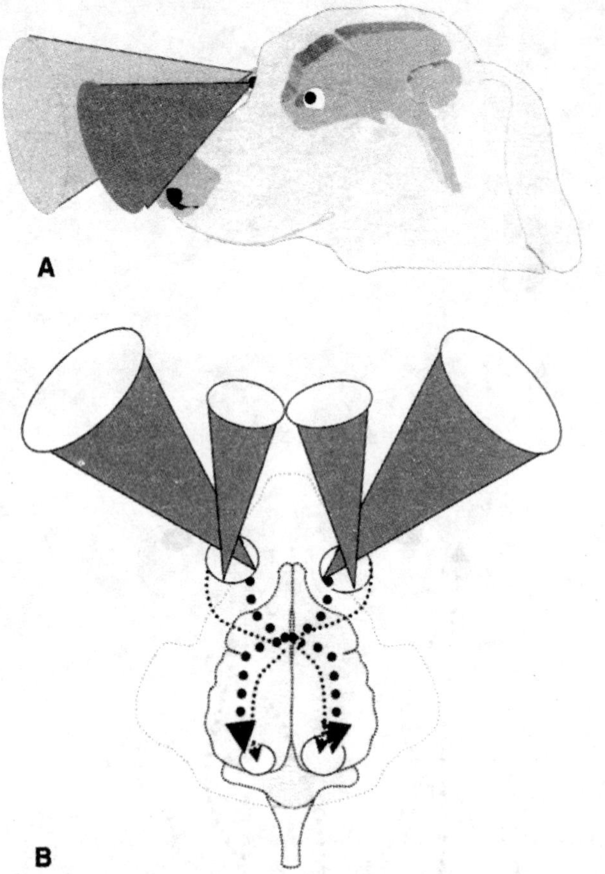

Fig. 19.4. (A) Lateral and (B) dorsal schematic views of the visual fields in the dog.

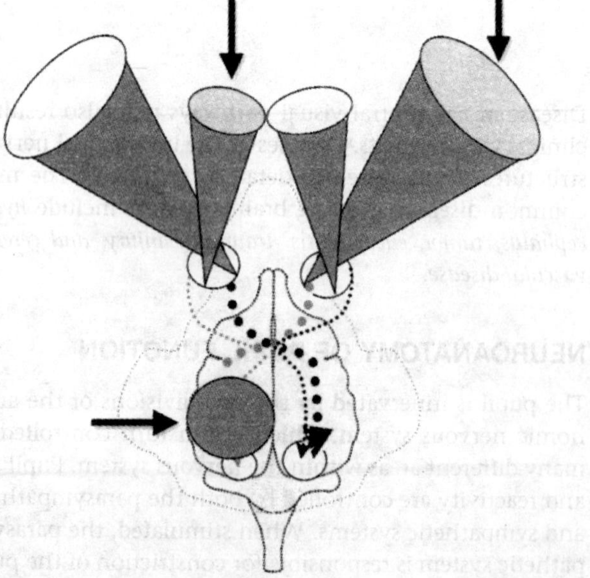

Fig. 19.5. Visual field deficits with a homonymous hemianopia (*arrows*) for a supratentorial lesion (*arrow*).

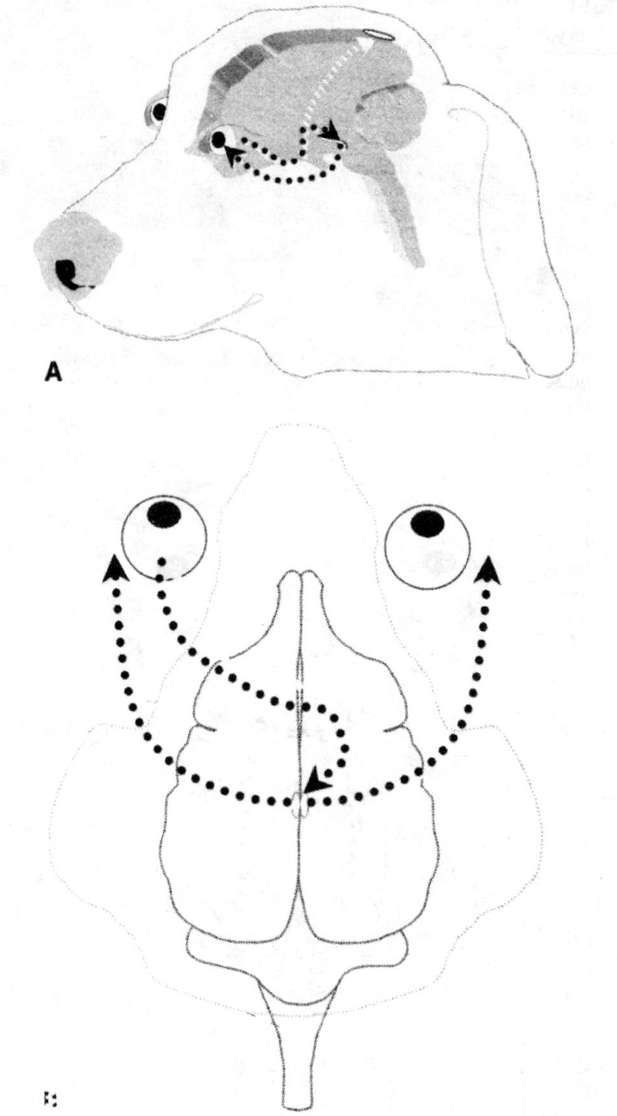

Fig. 19.6. (A) Lateral and (B) dorsal views schematic representation of the flow of information for the pupillary light reflex (black dots).

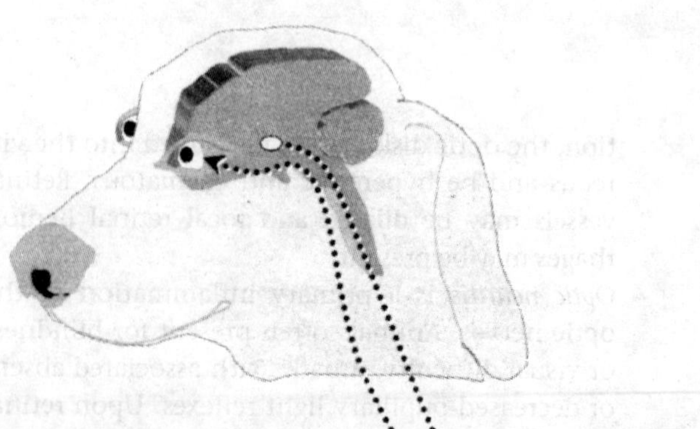

Fig. 19.7. Lateral view, schematic representation of the sympathetic innervation to the pupil.

Table 19.1. Anatomic pathway for sympathetic pupillomotor innervation (preganglionic and postganglionic)

- Cell bodies of preganglionic sympathetics in T1–3 intermediate grey matter (spinal cord) ventral root
- Segmental ramus communicans
- Thoracic sympathetic trunk (inside thorax ventrolateral to the vertebral column)
- Projects without synapse through the cervicothoracic ganglion and pass very close to the surface of the cranial lung lobe
- Continues in cervical sympathetic trunk (part of the vagosympathetic trunk)
- Synapses in the cranial cervical ganglion (medial to the origin of the digastric muscle and ventromedial to the tympanic bulla)
- Postganglionic fibers form a nerve plexus around the carotid artery
- Leaves plexus and enters the middle ear
- Joins the tympanic branch of CN IX to form the caroticotympanic nerves
- Exits middle ear and travels close to the cavernous sinus
- Joins the ophthalmic branch of CN V
- Exits skull through orbital fissure
- Aborizes into the nasociliary nerve
- Merges into the long ciliary nerve that enters eye
- Projects to ciliary body and iris dilator muscle

ABNORMALITIES OF PUPILS

The pupils are assessed as to their size in normal room light and under both light stimulated and dark adapted environments (fig. 19.8, 19.9, 19.10).

If an animal is blind in a single eye from a lesion of the prechiasmic ocular (retina) or optic nerve structures, when a light is shown in this abnormal eye, neither a direct nor consensual pupillary light reflex (pupillary constriction) will occur. If the light stimulus is directed in the normal eye, a normal direct and consensual reflex pupillary constriction should result. If, after causing constriction in both eyes by shining light in the normal eye, the light stimulus is moved quickly (swung) to the abnormal eye, the pupil in the abnormal eye may dilate as the light is projected into it. This is referred to as a positive swinging flashlight test and is indicative of a prechiasmic abnormality in the eye whose pupil dilates inappropriately.

ABNORMALITIES OF RESTING PUPIL SIZE

A constricted or miotic pupil that does not dilate in the dark may be present with the following abnormalities:

- The pupil may be small with anterior uveitis and sluggish to respond to light due to iridic vascular congestion and edema.
- Painful conditions of the cornea may cause a miosis.
- Instillation or administration of parasympathomimetic or sympatholytic drugs into the eye may cause miosis.
- The spastic pupil syndrome is a static anisocoria of cats that remains essentially unchanged during dark adaptation. Many of these cats are positive for the feline leukemia virus.
- Abnormality of sympathetic innervation to eye. This can result in a miotic pupil alone (Horner's pupil) or in signs of complete sympathetic denervation of the orbit—Horner's syndrome.
- Supratentorial disease affects the normal inhibition of these structures over CN III.

A dilated or mydriatic pupil that does not dilate in the dark may be present with the following abnormalities:

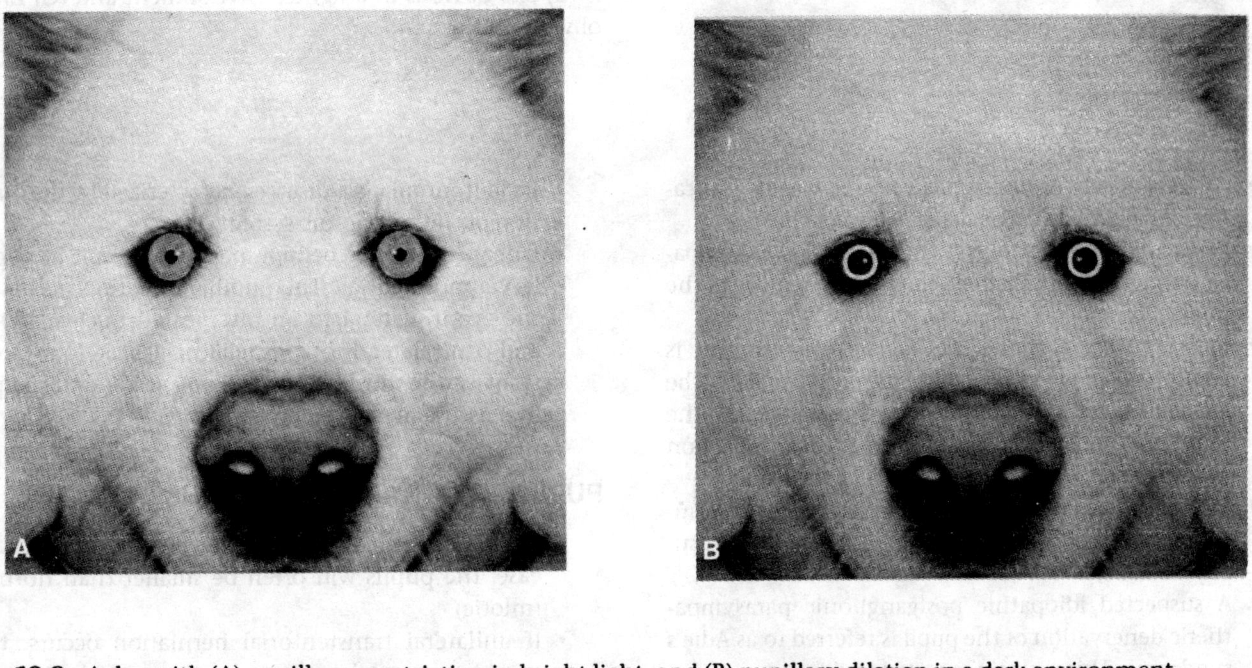

Fig. 19.8. A dog with (A) pupillary constriction in bright light, and (B) pupillary dilation in a dark environment.

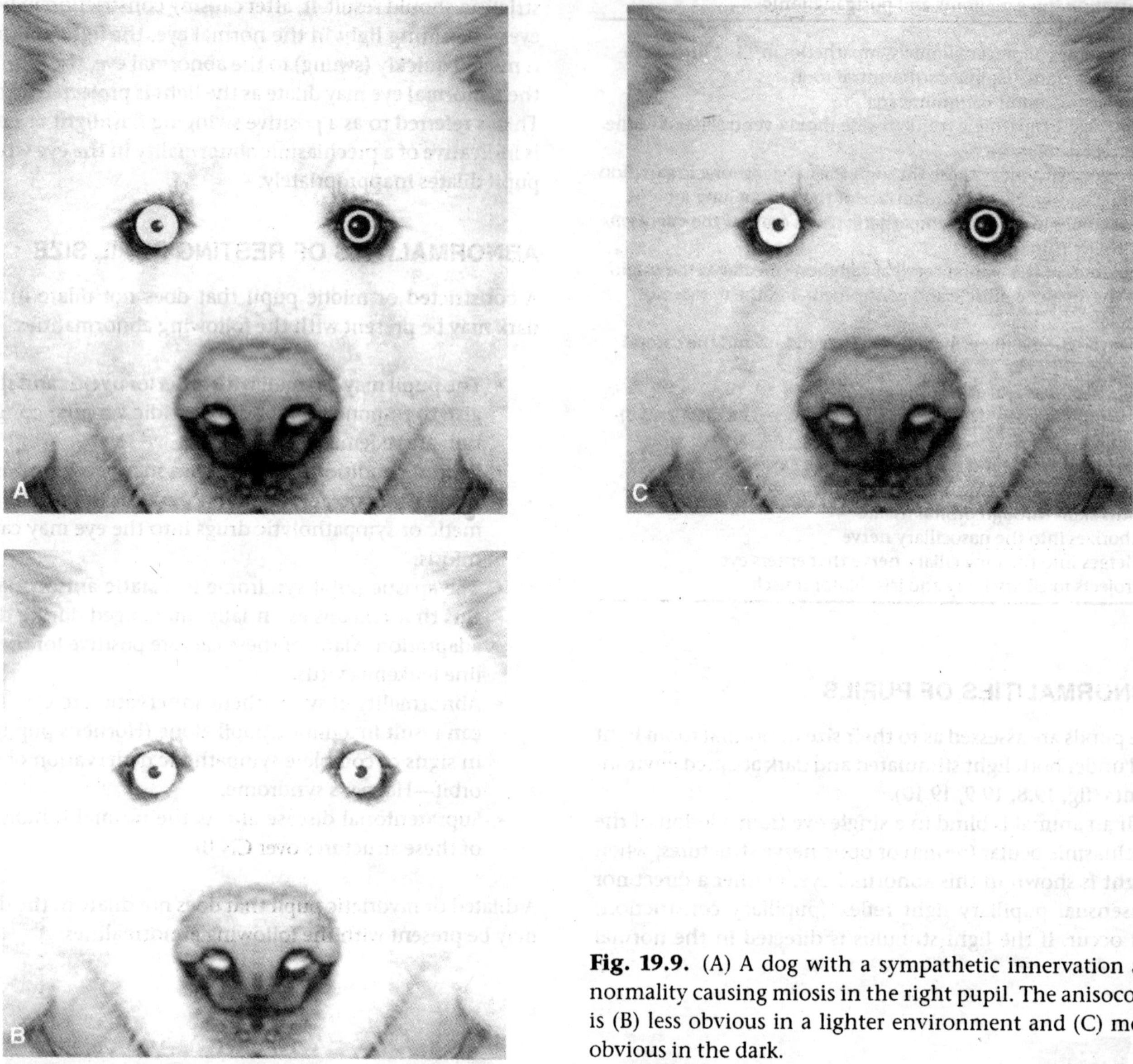

Fig. 19.9. (A) A dog with a sympathetic innervation abnormality causing miosis in the right pupil. The anisocoria is (B) less obvious in a lighter environment and (C) more obvious in the dark.

- A large, poorly or unresponsive pupil can be indicative of parasympathetic denervation of the iris.
- Parasympatholytic drugs, such as atropine, or sympathomimetic drugs instilled in the eye will dilate the pupil.
- Primary disease of the iris, such as iris atrophy, is common cause in older dogs. A dyscoric pupil may be a clue to underlying iris atrophy. The margins of the pupil are often irregular, and the tapedal reflection may be seen through some defects in the iris.
- Primary disease of the eye, such as synechia or glaucoma, can result in a dilated pupil. The animal is usually also blind.
- A suspected idiopathic postganglionic parasympathetic denervation of the pupil is referred to as Adie's syndrome. This is rarely reported in dogs.
- Dysautonomia is a disease characterized by dysfunction of the autonomic system.
- Disease of the cerebellum may rarely result in pupillary abnormalities. The pupillary dilation occurs in the eye ipsilateral to an interposital nuclear lesion and contralateral to a fastigial nuclear lesion. Occasionally, the third eyelid may protrude and the palpebral fissure may be enlarged.

PUPILLARY CHANGES WITH CNS DISEASE

- With bilateral, usually severe cerebrocortical disease, the pupils will often be smaller than normal (miotic).
- If unilateral transtentorial herniation occurs, the parahippocampal gyrus may compress the brain stem

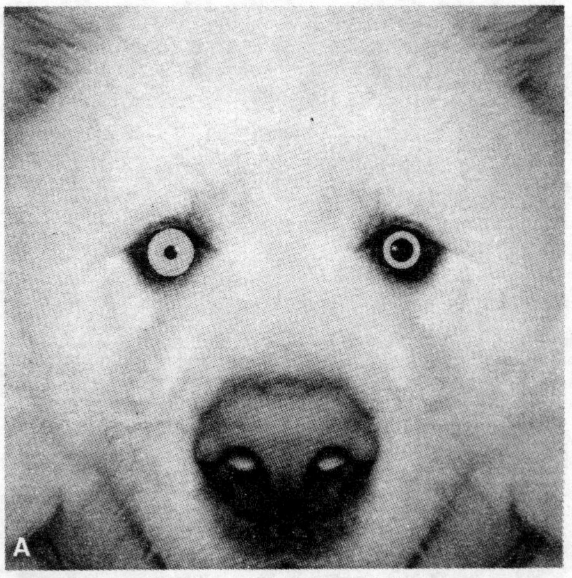

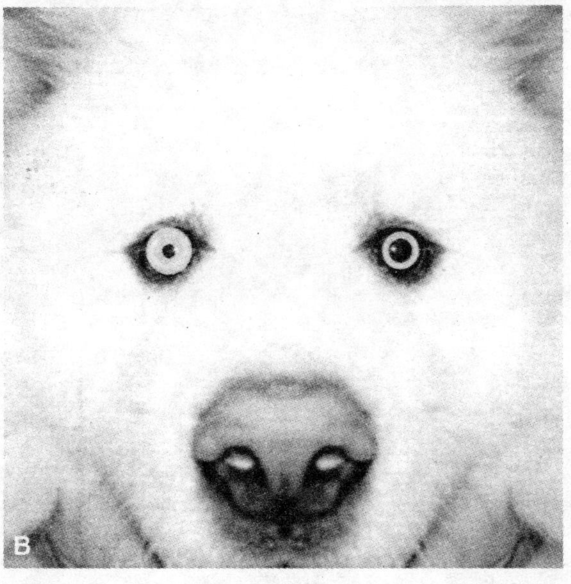

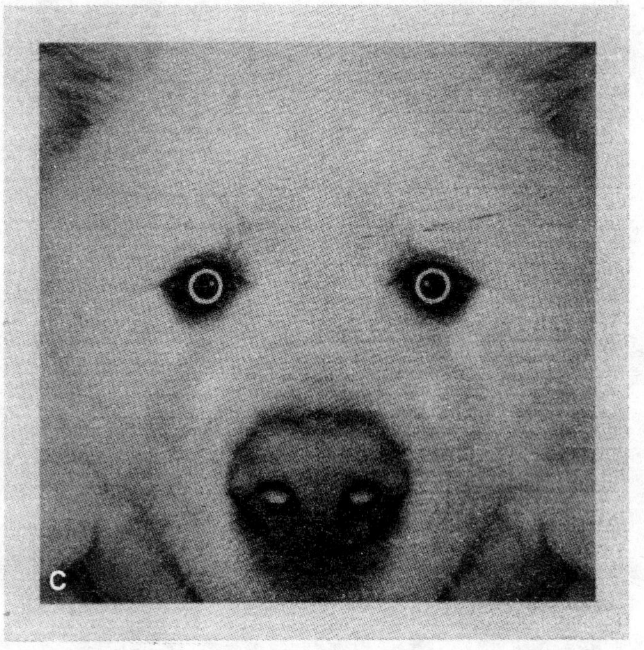

Fig. 19.10. (A) A dog with a parasympathetic innervation abnormality causing mydriasis in the left pupil. The anisocoria is (B) obvious in the lighter environment and (C) less obvious in a darker environment.

and CN III and result in unilateral mydriasis (fig. 19.11).

- As the midbrain is further compressed, fixed midrange pupils will occur.

PRACTICE CLINICAL CASE LOCALIZATIONS

Cases are presented in appendix 4 of animals with vision and pupillary abnormalities to illustrate localization of vision and pupillary abnormalities.

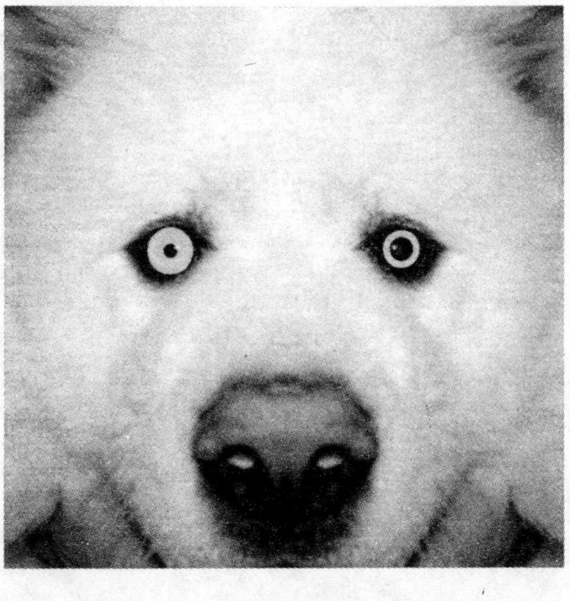

Fig. 19.11. A unilateral caudal transtentorial herniation can result in an ipsilateral dilated pupil due to cranial nerve III dysfunction.

20 Clinical Assessment of Gait and Voluntary Movement Abnormalities in Dogs and Cats

When presented with an animal that is unable to walk normally, it is important to first determine the pathophysiologic mechanism of the dysfunction (table 20.1).

CLINICAL ASSESSMENT OF THE ANIMAL WITH VOLUNTARY MOVEMENT ABNORMALITIES

Characteristics of Gait Abnormality

Abnormalities of numerous body components can affect gait. Some gait abnormalities are characteristic of a dysfunction of the nervous system, while others are characteristic of a musculoskeletal or other body system abnormality (tables 20.2 through 20.5).

- The step length is assessed as either normal, increased, or decreased relative to the step distance of a normal dog of the same breed (fig. 20.3).
- Step-length determination will often be helpful in determining whether a gait abnormality is more likely associated with dysfunction of the nervous system (table 20.6).
- Animals with UMN disease may appear irregular and uncoordinated in stepping, having a tendency to sway from side to side; some may fall to the side (table 20.6).
- Animals with neurologic disease may appear to have their feet contact the ground with increased force and potentially prior to when they expected the foot to contact the ground. Their subsequent step may be hypermetric.
- Many dogs with neurologic disease vary their step distance with subsequent steps. This results in some steps being longer and some steps being shorter in distance.
- Dogs with lower motor neuron (LMN) disease may hold the head low (possibly because of neck muscle weakness) and take short, choppy appearing steps.
    - The frequency of the steps is often increased.
    - Some have an associated kyphotic body posture.
    - Animals with LMN diseases may tire easily, may not be able to walk as far, and may eventually appear unwilling to perform. These animals may also sit and lie down.
- A consistent flexion of a limb may be associated with soft tissue injury of the limb, muscle fibrosis, and skeletal and joint abnormalities. When walking, this is commonly referred to as a (non-weight bearing) *lameness*.
- If the pain originates from a spinal or peripheral nerve abnormality, this is termed a *nerve root signature* (fig. 20.1). Nerve root signature may involve either the thoracic or pelvic limbs.
- Animals with musculoskeletal or orthopedic lameness may also stand in abnormal but characteristic postures (fig. 20.2).

Table 20.1. Anatomical structures required for movement

What does an animal require for movement?
- Nerves to signal muscle and sense joint position
- Muscles to move joints
- Bones, tendon, and ligaments for support
- Oxygen, via blood flow, to support muscle metabolism
- Nutrients and other metabolic building blocks of muscles

What components of the nervous system are required for movement?
- Supratentorial (forebrain) structures are important for voluntary control, especially of intricate movements.
- Brain stem structures are important for gait generation.
- The cerebellum, while not necessary for the initiation of movement, is important for coordination of movement. Cerebellar influences coordinate and smooth body movements by controlling rate, range, and force of limb motion. The cerebellum most likely is responsible for inhibition of the flexor component of gait.
- The spinal cord allows for information to be transferred to and from the intracranial structures to the limbs. The grey matter of the spinal cord is where the nerve cell bodies that give rise to the efferent peripheral nerves are found.
- The peripheral nerves carry efferent information to and afferent information from the muscles.
- The neuromuscular junction provides a mechanism for transfer of nervous information to the muscles.
- The muscles contract and provide the force for limb movement.

Table 20.2. Gait abnormalities characteristic of nervous system dysfunction

- *Ataxia*—Falling and swaying from side to side often associated with irregular step distances
- *Dysmetria*—Abnormal range and extent of movements
- *Hypermetria*—Overflexion, exaggerated movement, usually of a limb
- *Hypometria*—Decreased flexion of a limb; often appears as a stiff, stilted movement
- *Spasticity*—Extended, stiff appearance of the limb, however, step distances are usually normal to increased
- *Dragging of the limb*—Usually associated with conscious proprioceptive deficits
- *Nerve root signature*—Animals usually hold a limb upward in a flexed position; may be similar in appearance to lameness; often occurs in a single thoracic or pelvic limb. Often, the affected limb may appear painful upon manipulation, mimicking an orthopedic problem.

Table 20.3. Gait abnormalities associated with dysfunction of specific peripheral nerves

- *Femoral nerve*
  Inability to extend the stifle and support weight. The animal may have difficulty bringing the limbs forward and may bunny-hop or have shorter step distance in the affected limb. Bunny-hopping is the simultaneous advance of the pelvic limbs, and has classically been associated with UMN spinal cord disease (spinal dysraphism/myelodysplasia). Occasionally, animals with orthopedic disease (bilateral hip dysplasia or coxofemoral pain) will have the same gait abnormality. Animals with orthopedic disease (bilateral hip dysplasia or coxofemoral pain) may have the same gait abnormality.

- *Obturator nerve*
  Does not affect gait in dogs and cats. If an animal is placed on a slippery surface, however, the affected pelvic limb may slide laterally with weight bearing.

- *Sciatic nerve*
  Results in a characteristic gait wherein the distal foot is almost thrown forward by the movements of the more proximal muscles of the limb. When the animal is weight bearing, the hock joint may overflex resulting in the dropped-hock appearance. Atrophy associated with sciatic disease is often obvious in the cranial tibial muscle group. With lesions of the *cranial gluteal nerve,* the stifle may become abducted during the stance phase of gait.

- *Radial nerve*
  Affects the animal's ability to extend the carpus. If the lesion occurs proximally in the radial nerve, the elbow may be positioned more ventrally than normal. The limb may be carried off of the ground with the elbow flexed if the musculocutaneous nerve is intact.

- *Medial, ulnar, musculocutaneous, and suprascapular nerves*
  Gait is usually unaffected. The carpal joint may be overextended with medial and ulnar lesions. With musculocutaneous nerve paralysis, elbow flexion is poor and this joint may be held overextended.

Table 20.4. Gait Abnormalities Often Indicative of a Musculoskeletal Problem

- *Fibrotic Myopathy of the Semimembranous and Semitendinous Muscles*
  Results in an awkward jerking of the affected limb during the flight phase of limb movement. If the animal is observed from behind, as the affected pelvic limb begins to be lowered following the zenith of the flight phase of gait, the distal foot (from the hock level) is rapidly pulled in a medial direction due to the decreased elasticity of the fibrotic muscle.
- *Infraspinatous and Supraspinatous Muscle Fibrosis*
  The thoracic limb at the shoulder lever may be outwardly rotated, with the foot contacting the ground in a sideways position.
- *Rupture of the Gastrocnemius Tendon*
  Animals may sink at the hock joint when weight bearing. A similar phenomenon may occur with abnormal sciatic innervation to the gastrocnemius muscle. If, however, the gastrocnemius tendon ruptures and the superficial digital flexor tendon remains intact, as weight is placed on the limb and the hock sinks, the toes will be held in a flexed position. This characteristic toe position does not occur with neurologic weakness of the gastrocnemius muscle. Affected animals may have a leg-carrying lameness, and stand straight in the stifles when weight bearing. Animals often have associated muscle atrophy of the limb including the semimembranous, semitendinous, and gastrocnemius muscles. This may sometimes be confused with dancing Doberman syndrome.
- *Iliopsoas Muscle Disease*
  May result in pelvic limb lameness. Animals may position the hocks in an adducted way (cow-hocked).

Table 20.5. Gait abnormalities that may be associated with either neurologic or musculoskeletal disease

Stiffness and Decreased Step Length
Commonly seen with diseases of the peripheral neuromuscular apparatus (LMN cell body, nerve roots, peripheral nerve, neuromuscular junction and muscle), musculoskeletal disease, metabolic weakness, myotonia, or poor perfusion of the limb. Dogs with neuromuscular disease may also have a stiff, stilted, choppy gait due primarily to muscle weakness. These abnormalities may be episodic and occur, as in the case of myasthenia gravis, as the level of exercise increases.

Lameness
Decreased or non-weight bearing on a limb usually associated with pain in the limb from musculoskeletal disease. A similar clinical abnormality can also occur with nervous system dysfunction (and presumably pain) referred to as nerve root signature.

Nerve Root Signature
Animals usually hold a limb upward in a flexed position. May be similar in appearance to lameness. Often occurs in a single thoracic or pelvic limb. Often, the affected limb may appear painful upon manipulation, mimicking an orthopedic problem.

Bunny-hopping
Simultaneous advance of the pelvic limbs, has classically been associated with UMN spinal cord disease (spinal dysraphism/myelodysplasia). It can also occur with diseases that result in bilateral decreases in step distance. Occasionally, animals with orthopedic disease (bilateral hip dysplasia or coxofemoral pain) or poor perfusion to the limbs will have the same gait abnormality

Table 20.6. Gait abnormalities associated with UMN vs. LMN disease

Gait abnormalities suggesting UMN neurologic disease:
- Ataxia with either a normal or increased step distance
- Dysmetria (hypermetria) with either a normal or increased step distance
- Increased step distance
- Irregular step distances with varying steps

Gait abnormalities suggesting LMN neurologic disease:
- Decreased step distance
- Short and choppy appearance to limb movements

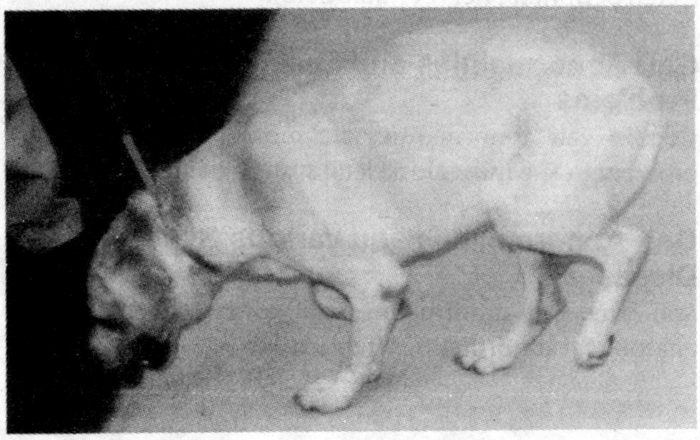

Fig. 20.1. Dog with a non-weight-bearing lameness of the left pelvic limb.

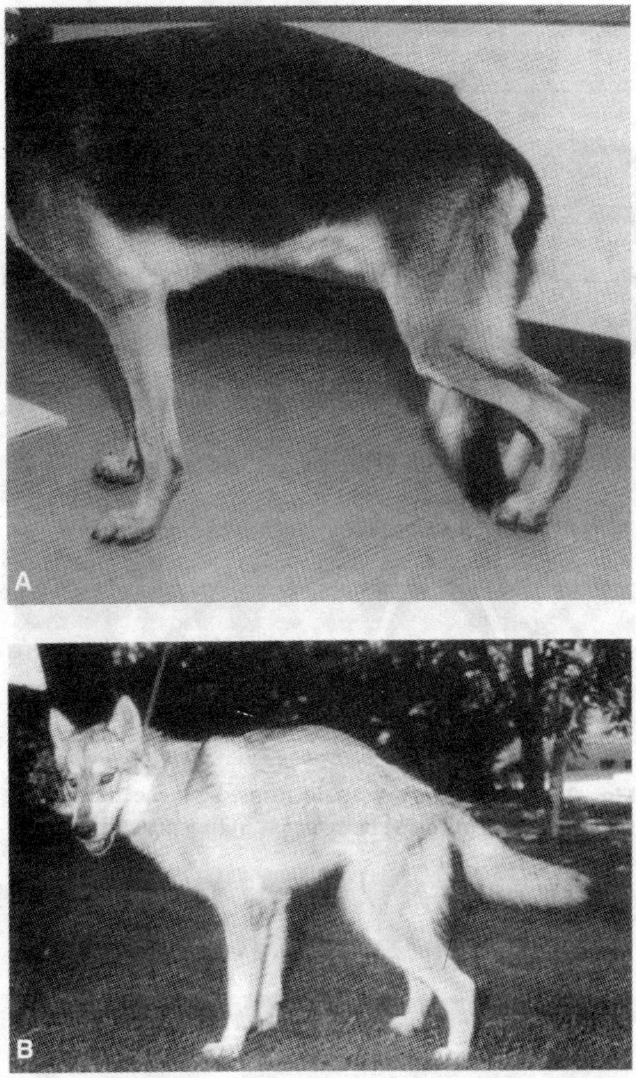

Fig. 20.2. Flexed stifle and sinking pelvic area appearance in (A, B) two dogs with bilateral cranial cruciate ligament ruptures.

- Animals with upper motor neuron (UMN) neurological abnormalities often have normal to increased step (or stride) lengths (fig. 20.3).
- Animals with orthopedic or lower motor neuron (LMN) and neuromuscular disease have shortened step or stride lengths.

LOCALIZATION OF NEUROLOGIC ABNORMALITIES RESULTING IN ABNORMAL GAIT

Intracranial Disease

- Supratentorial disease will often not affect the ability of the animal to walk, however, animals may wander, bump into walls and other objects, stumble, and circle.
- Animals with unilateral supratentorial disease usually circle in the direction of the lesion.
- Commonly, when circling, animals with supratentorial disease will "swing out" the thoracic limb on the side of the body opposite to the direction of the circling.
- Lesions of the brain stem often have dramatic effects on gait, frequently impairing the ability to stand and generate a gait. If the lesion occurs unilaterally, an ipsilateral hemiparesis may be present. If pathways are affected bilaterally, tetraparesis can be present. Spinal reflexes should reflect the UMN nature of the lesion.

Spinal Cord Abnormalities

Gait abnormalities in animals with spinal cord disease may be more UMN or LMN in character. The spinal cord can be functionally divided based upon the spinal segments and associated clinical signs of disease affecting these segments (table 20.7).

Lower Motor Neuron Disease

- The gait is usually short stepped and "choppy," if the animal is able to generate a gait.
- The limbs may appear flaccid and may tremor and buckle with weight bearing.
- With some diseases, weakness is exacerbated with exercise (e.g., myasthenia gravis).

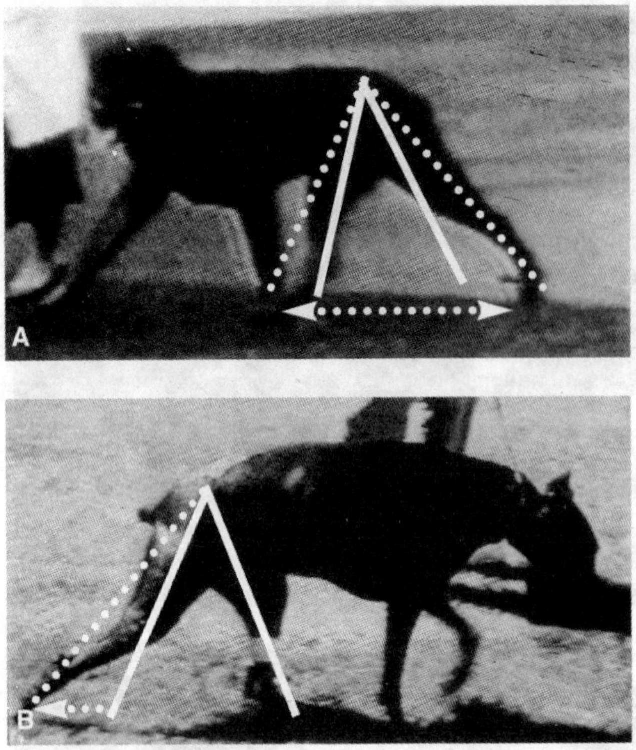

Fig. 20.3. Imaginary triangle formed by the limbs and their attachment to the body in (A, B) two dogs with UMN disease overstepping.

Table 20.7. Functional areas and associated clinical signs of the spinal cord

C1–C5	UMN tetraparesis/plegia, neck pain
C6–T2	UMN signs to pelvic limbs; LMN signs to thoracic limbs
T3–L3	UMN signs to pelvic limbs; thoracic limbs normal
L4–S3	LMN signs to pelvic limbs and/or bladder

Gait Abnormalities and Lesions of Selective Peripheral Nerves

Certain abnormalities of gait are seen with lesions of selected peripheral nerves (table 20.3).

Gait Abnormalities and Musculoskeletal Problems

Certain gait abnormalities are more characteristic of a problem in the musculoskeletal system (table 20.4).

Gait Abnormalities and Various System Diseases

Still other gait abnormalities may occur with a variety of anatomical abnormalities (table 20.5).

21 Clinical Assessment and Management of the Painful Dog and Cat

Animals that appear painful often prompt owners to seek veterinary attention. Numerous disease processes can result in neurologically generated or mediated pain. As with other disease processes, appropriate treatment of the painful animal is based on accurate diagnosis of the disease resulting in pain. Once a diagnosis is established, the most appropriate pain control strategy can be adopted for the individual animal. The following discussion provides some general guidelines for management of neuropathic pain in animals. Ultimately, treatment of pain is individualized to each animal's unique pathologic and physiologic characteristics.

CLINICAL ASSESSMENT OF THE PAINFUL ANIMAL

An assessment is made for both physiological and behavioral responses that are associated with pain (table 21.1 and 21.2).

PAIN ASSOCIATED WITH INTRACRANIAL DISEASE

Pain associated with intracranial disease can result from compression of the meninges, cranial nerves, and skull.

- Increases in intracranial pressure may result in meningeal stretching or cerebrovasospasm.
- Other animals with intracranial disease may appear oversensitive to touch, light, and sound.
- Importantly, animals with intracranial disease may exhibit signs of cervical pain and rigidity.

PAIN ASSOCIATED WITH SPINAL DISEASE

Pain associated with spinal cord disease can result from disease irritating or compressing bone (periosteum), ligament, cartilage, meninges, nerve rootlets, or exiting peripheral nerves. Diseases that involve these structures, consequently, are most likely to be associated with spinal pain (table 21.3).

Disease that is exclusively present within the spinal cord parenchyma (i.e., intramedullary tumor) may not be associated with clinical evidence of pain as there are no nociceptors within the neural parenchyma. Often, however, these intramedullary diseases result in some degree of expansion of the spinal cord, which then secondarily stretches the meninges or the nerve roots and/or exiting peripheral nerve and results in a painful process.

Focal diseases of the spinal cord often result in focal areas of spinal pain. Diffuse pain along the spinal axis may be associated with diffuse meningeal or spinal diseases such as inflammation (meningitis or myelitis) or diffuse neoplastic disease (e.g., lymphoma). Diffuse spinal pain may also be associated with polyarthritis of the articular facet joints, or much less commonly, paraspinal muscle disease or inflammation.

Paraspinal pain associated with paraspinal muscle atrophy may be associated with paraspinal or sublumbar muscle abscess or diskospondylitis. Of course, multiple areas of spinal pain may also be associated with multiple disease processes in differing spinal areas.

PAIN ASSOCIATED WITH PERIPHERAL NERVE DISEASE

When peripheral nerves are compressed, damaged, or irritated, pain can result.

- Trauma and injury to peripheral nerves, such as with brachial plexus avulsion, usually result in nonpainful nerve dysfunction.
- With coonhound paralysis or polyradiculoneuritis, animals frequently seem hyperesthetic even to minimal manipulation or palpation.

DIAGNOSIS OF ANIMALS WITH PAIN

The diagnosis of animals with pain begins with an appropriate physical, neurologic, and orthopedic evaluation for localization of the painful process. Diagnostic testing in animals with spinal pain should include anatomical assessments of these structures including spinal radiographs and advanced imaging studies (myelography, computed tomography [CT], or magnetic resonance [MR] imaging) (see also chapter 11 discussion of diagnosis of spinal disease).

Table 21.1. Clinical features associated with pain in animals

Abnormal Activities
- Varying from reclusive to restless and agitated
- Disruption of sleep-wake cycle
- Orienting toward the painful area
- Aggression

Abnormal Gaiting or Walking
- Shortened step distance
- Reluctance to move
- Take weight off limbs when sitting down

Abnormalities of Body Posture
- Rigid, tense muscles
- Abnormal use or guarding of a painful region (e.g., limb)
- Lameness

Vocalization
- Independent of apparent stimulation
- With direct pressure on a body region

Systemic Physiological Abnormalities
- Increased temperature
- Tachycardia
- Tachypnea
- Increased blood pressure
- Salivating

Table 21.2. Clinical features associated with neurologic pain in animals

Cervical Pain
- Holds head downward and lower to ground
- Neck muscle rigid
- Decreased range of motion in neck
- Kyphotic posture
- Neck straight in relation to the back
- Shortened step distance in thoracic limbs
- Thoracic limb flexion or lameness (root signature)

Thoracolumbar Pain
- Kyphotic or lordotic posture
- Sitting posture
- Head extended caudally
- Pelvic limb lameness (root signature)
- Pain on abdominal palpation
- Sphinxlike posture (cranial thoracic area pain)

Lumbar Pain
- Pelvic limb flexion or lameness (root signature)
- Kyphotic posture of the thoracolumbar spine
- Holds head lower to ground
- Reluctant to urinate, defecate
- Pain on rectal palpation

- Cerebrospinal fluid assessments should be helpful in instances of myelitis.
- Electromyographic studies of the limb or paraspinal muscles may be helpful in instances where peripheral nerves or muscles are involved.

For assessment of intracranial abnormalities associated with pain, advanced imaging studies (MR and CT) and cerebrospinal fluid analysis are often necessary for clarification of the disease process (see discussion in chapter 10 of diagnosis of intracranial diseases).

Table 21.3. Spinal diseases most often associated with pain

- Intervertebral disk disease
- Diskospondylitis/vertebral osteomyelitis
- Tumor (usually extradural, or intradural and extramedullary tumors)
- Trauma (fracture or luxation)
- Myelitis
- Atlantoaxial instability
- Lumbosacral instability

HOW IS PAIN MANAGED?

Pain is most effectively managed when the stimulus for pain is removed or exhausted. If a mechanical cause of the pain (e.g., intervertebral disk material compressing a spinal nerve) is causative, surgical removal of that material may be necessary to bring about long-term pain relief. If a surgically correctable abnormality is not found, modulation of the experience of pain by altering either its transmission or integration is necessary.

TREATMENT STRATEGIES FOR ANIMALS WITH SPINAL PAIN

Cage confinement is indicated in animals with suspected spinal injury, anomalies, and instability, and in animals with intervertebral disk disease (also see discussion in chapter 14 of treatment of spinal disease). *Opiates* are often the most effective pharmacological means of treating pain in animals (tables 21.4, 21.5).

Nonsteroidal anti-inflammatory medications are used in a variety of musculoskeletal diseases for their anti-inflammatory and pain relief benefits. Data on nonsteroidal effects in animals with spinal disease are usually based on anecdotal observations. Commonly used nonsteroidal medications prescribed include carprofen (2.2 mg/kg orally every 12 hours or 4.4 mg/kg orally daily) and etodolac (10–15 mg/kg orally every 24 hours).

Corticosteroids will produce analgesia by inhibiting prostaglandin production. In general, corticosteroids should be used for their pain and anti-inflammatory effects when a definitive diagnosis is established and that disease is known to be benefited by corticosteroid administration. Side effects of corticosteroid administration including gastrointestinal ulceration seem common in animals with neurologic abnormalities.

Nonpharmacological Pain Relief

Nonpharmacological pain relief includes the following:

1. Keeping the animal's environment quiet and dimly lit, providing appropriate water and nutrition, and having clean, comfortable bedding.

Table 21.4. Medications Used for Treatment of Pain

- Morphine
  Natural opioid agonist. After administration, may see initial excitement, panting, salivation, nausea, vomiting, urination, defecation, or hypotension. These effects are attributed to stimulation of chemoreceptor trigger zone, vagal stimulation, and histamine release.

  Can be administered SC, IM, or IV, however, the IV route is used with caution to prevent hypotension associated with acute histamine release.

  Level of analgesia achieved is dose dependent.

  Major side effects include mental and central respiratory depression.
- Oxymorphone
  Semisynthetic opioid agonist with ~10 times the analgesic potency of morphine but less pronounced effects on respiratory, cardiovascular, and gastrointestinal systems.
- Meperidine
  Synthetic opioid agonist; one-eighth the analgesic potency of morphine.
- Pentazocine
  Synthetic opioid antagonist with some agonistic properties; one-fourth the analgesic potency of morphine.
- Butorphanol
  Synthetic opioid agonist-antagonist; five times the analgesic potency of morphine.
- Codeine
  Oral opioid that is very effective in long-term management of pain.

2. Activity to keep the patient engaged in activities and tasks seems helpful. This may include physical therapy, massage, swimming, other hydrotherapy, ultrasound, or electrical stimulation.
   - Tens units and similar electrical stimulation devices can be very helpful in providing analgesia as well as in certain instances maintaining muscle mass and strength.

Table 21.5. Commonly prescribed narcotic analgesics and doses

Morphine	Dog	0.25–1.25 mg/kg q 4–6 h IM, SC
	Cat	0.1 mg/kg q 6–7 h IM, SC
Oxymorphone	Dog	0.05–0.2 mg/kg q 6 h IM, SC
	Cat	0.01 mg/kg q 6 h IM, SC
Meperidine	Dog	2–5 mg/kg q 1–2 h IM, SC
	Cat	Same
Pentazocine	Dog	1.5–3.0 mg/kg q 2–3 h IM, SC
	Cat	0.75–1.5 mg/kg q 2–4 h IM, SC
Butorphanol	Dog	0.1–0.2 mg/kg q 2–4 h IV Or 0.2–0.4 mg/kg q 2–4 h SC, IM
	Cat	Same
Fentanyl patch		2–4 µg/kg
Codeine		1–4 mg/kg PO A 4–6 hours PRN

   - Electroacupuncture is an extension of this form of analgesia.
   - Trigger point therapy may be beneficial for some animals.
   - Ultrasound therapy may also be helpful in selected instances.
3. Acupuncture has also gained acceptance of the pain relief treatment modality and can be used independently or sometimes concurrently with other treatment modalities.
4. Other alternative therapies such as herbal remedies are also gaining in popularity for treatment of painful conditions.

22 Management of Neurologic Trauma

Trauma to the nervous system may have devastating consequences for the animal resulting in emergency evaluation and treatment by veterinarians. In many instances, traumatic injury affects multiple body systems making clinical assessments and management challenging. This chapter provides an overview of assessment and management of animals with neurotrauma.

CLINICAL ASSESSMENT AND MANAGEMENT OF ANIMALS WITH INTRACRANIAL TRAUMA

After the animal is initially admitted to the hospital, life-threatening systemic abnormalities should be identified and treated. Important assessments on the physical examination include the following:

- Body temperature
- Mucous membrane (color and CRT), limb temperature, and other assessments of perfusion
- Heart rate and rhythm including heart auscultation
- Respiratory rate and character including auscultation of the lung sounds
- Abdominal palpation for organomegaly, fluid or gas distention, and pain
- Rectal examination and assessment of stool for blood or melena, foreign material, toxic products
- Retinal examination for evidence of hypertension, bleeding, or inflammatory disease
- Skin for evidence of lacerations, bite wounds, burns, exposure to foreign substances, ticks, and other arthropods and insects

Once critical care concerns are addressed, a neurological evaluation as complete as possible should be performed, and the results should be recorded for comparison with subsequent future examinations. Neurologic assessments include pupil size and reactivity, muscle tone, proprioceptive testing (if the animal is not comatose), cranial nerve and spinal reflex assessments, and palpation for pain.

DIAGNOSTIC PROCEDURES

Procedures include the following:

- *Survey radiographs* of the skull may aid in determining whether fractures are present.
- *Advanced imaging studies*, such as computed tomography (CT) or magnetic resonance (MR) imaging, are useful in determining the location and extent of intracranial injury. The results of these studies are also helpful in determining the need for surgical treatment of intracranial injury such as evacuation of subdural hematomas, removal of depressed skull fractures, or debridement of damaged tissue and foreign material.
- Routine *cerebrospinal fluid collection* is rarely necessary, and may, in fact, be contraindicated and detrimental, especially in animals with intracranial injury and elevated ICP.

IN-HOSPITAL MANAGEMENT

From a practical standpoint, monitoring for, and treatment of, the secondary effects of craniocerebral trauma may be the most important aspects of management of animals with head trauma in clinical practice. Recognition, understanding, and treatment of the secondary pathophysiological sequelae of brain injury often impact more on prognosis than does the initial injury.

- Fluid resuscitation with appropriate crystalloids or colloids is commonly administered to stabilize blood pressure and maintain cerebral perfusion.
- Monitoring of systemic blood pressure and central venous pressure may aid in reestablishment of normovolemia.
- After the initial neurological assessment, a decision should be made as to whether an advanced imaging study (CT or MR) is indicated to determine if addi-

tional treatments (such as surgery) are necessary. If these studies are unavailable or otherwise not feasible to perform, or if the clinical signs are mild, the animal should be frequently monitored for deteriorating neurological function. Deterioration in clinical status usually indicates the need for treatment of increased ICP.

TREATMENT

Treatments for head injury will depend on the clinical status of the animal (table 22.1). Deteriorating clinical signs may indicate cerebral ischemia, edema, intracranial hemorrhage, or increased ICP.

Treatments for Head Injury in Animals

- Maintenance of systemic blood pressure through basic life support measures includes blood or isotonic fluid administration.
- Nasal oxygen administration following trauma may help in overall inspiratory oxygenation.
- Mannitol administered at 0.25 up to 1 g/kg IV as a bolus. Contraindications to mannitol use include hypovolemia and possibly ongoing intracranial hemorrhage.

or

- Hypertonic saline (3%) administered at 5.3 ml/kg
- If seizure activity ensues, a constant infusion of diazepam or propofol may be needed for acute seizure control. If seizures are persistent, loading with phenobarbital (11–13 mg/kg IV) may be necessary to prevent further brain injury from the seizure activity.
- Head elevation to 30 degrees above the heart level
- Maintenance of respiration and possibly hyperventilation
- Craniectomy and durotomy may be necessary to decompress the intracranial region and aid in control of ICP.
- Corticosteroids are currently not recommended for treatment of humans with head injury.

Table 22.1. Treatment of head trauma

Therapies with established efficacy
- Fluid resuscitation
  - Isotonic fluids
- Diuretics
- Mannitol (0.25–1 g/kg IV)

Therapies with possible but currently unknown efficacy
- Hypertonic saline (3% solution, 5.3 ml/kg IV, 23.4% solution, 0.7 mg/kg)
- Head elevation
- Furosemide (0.07–1 mg/kg IV)
- Hyperventilation
- Cerebrospinal fluid aspiration
- Miscellaneous drugs
  - Deferoxamine mesylate
  - Superoxide dismutase
  - Allopurinol
  - Opiate antagonists (naloxone)
  - Thyrotropin-releasing hormone and calcium channel blockers
- Craniotomy

Therapies with unknown efficacy and potential detrimental effects
- Corticosteroids
- Cerebrospinal fluid aspiration

MANAGEMENT FOLLOWING HEAD INJURY

- If animals are alert following trauma, hospitalization for the first 24 hours is appropriate to monitor for clinical deterioration.
- Animals that are severely impaired are usually monitored in a critical care or intensive care area for signs of neurologic deterioration for at least 48 hours after injury.
- Animals should be kept in a comfortable, well-padded, and quiet environment with minimal light stimulation. Recumbent animals are positioned in a head-neutral or head-elevated position.
- Clinical parameters monitored include heart rate and rhythm, respiratory rate and pattern, blood pressure, urine production, and pain.
- Neurologic parameters monitored include pupil size and responsiveness to light, level of consciousness, behavior, and the ability to move and walk.
- Oral food and water are withheld until the animal is fully alert. Intravenous fluid therapy is given to maintain normal hydration and perfusion.
- Lacerations or wounds are managed as for other body areas.
- Exposure to sound and light following intracranial injury should be kept to a minimum to avoid further stimulation.
- Stools are monitored consistently for evidence of melena that might indicate gastrointestinal ulceration. If noted, an antiulcer medication (ranitidine) is administered concurrently due to the apparent increase in gastrointestinal ulcers in neurologic patients.
- Pain control is instituted with narcotics as needed.
- Massage and passive range of motion of the limbs are reasonable even in stuporous or comatose animals.
- Of the nonneurologic complications following intracranial injury, pneumonia is the most common. A fever is usually the first sign of pneumonia in animals with aspiration pneumonia. Any dog with a fever in the postinjury period should be evaluated with a thoracic radiograph to determine the presence of aspiration pneumonia. Radiographic changes, however, may not be present in the acute stages of the disease. Once established, pneumonia should be treated aggressively with appropriate pneumonia management.

REHABILITATION OF THE BRAIN INJURED ANIMAL

Good nursing care includes the prevention of decubital ulcers in the recumbent animal and monitoring for secondary infections primarily of the pulmonary and urogenital systems. Recumbent animals should be placed on clean, soft bedding and turned frequently (ideally every hour, but at least every 4 hours). Physical therapy can begin as soon as possible if there are no unstable vertebral injuries.

CLINICAL MANAGEMENT OF ANIMALS WITH SUSPECTED SPINAL CORD TRAUMA

Upon admission to the hospital, the animal with suspected spinal trauma should be physically or mechanically immobilized as soon as possible.

- Life-threatening injuries are identified and treated.
- Overt hemorrhage is controlled.
- A complete history of the current problem is obtained. Information that may be significant includes whether or not the owner witnessed the traumatic event and the relevant circumstances regarding the accident itself. Important questions to ask include:
  1. How long ago did the accident occur?
  2. What movement was the animal capable of immediately after the trauma and in the time since?
  3. Is the animal worse or better than immediately after the trauma?
  4. Did the animal attempt to walk and has it been able to urinate on its own?

At the initial admission to the hospital, the animal should be assumed to have an unstable spinal injury until proven otherwise. The animal should be expeditiously clinically evaluated and treated for systemic abnormalities using standard emergency and critical care procedures. A critical care physical diagnosis checklist or some similar format may be useful in these situations (table 22.2).

The animal is immobilized or secured in the position in which it is presented. This is usually a sternal or lateral recumbent position. If physical immobilization is impractical, or if the animal is not conscious (comatose), extreme caution should be exercised when physically evaluating the animal to avoid iatrogenic trauma to the spinal cord. Chemical restraint or sedation should be avoided until a thorough clinical evaluation has been performed.

For physical immobilization, any rigid surface that is freely movable can be used to support the spine during manipulations and movement. A board 8–10 feet wide, 4–5 feet long, and 3/4 to 1 inch thick can be useful. Strong, nonflexible tape, such as 2-inch white porous tape, is applied in a banding fashion extending over the point of the shoulder and fastened on both ends of the board. The tape is applied cranial and caudal to the shoulder, forming a crisscross pattern across the shoulder (fig. 22.1). Handles attached to the board make it easier to move the board/animal combination from flat surfaces such as floors. It is also helpful to record the weight of the board directly on all sides.

Table 22.2. Checklist for management of the animal with suspected spinal trauma

- Assess for immediately life-threatening abnormalities
- Immobilize the animal (reduce spinal motion)
- Assess for physical abnormalities
- Assess for neurological abnormalities

If neurological injury is strongly suspected:

- Administer methylprednisolone sodium succinate (30 mg/kg IV slowly)
- Radiograph affected areas of spine
- Determine severity of injury
- Determine need for medical versus surgical therapy

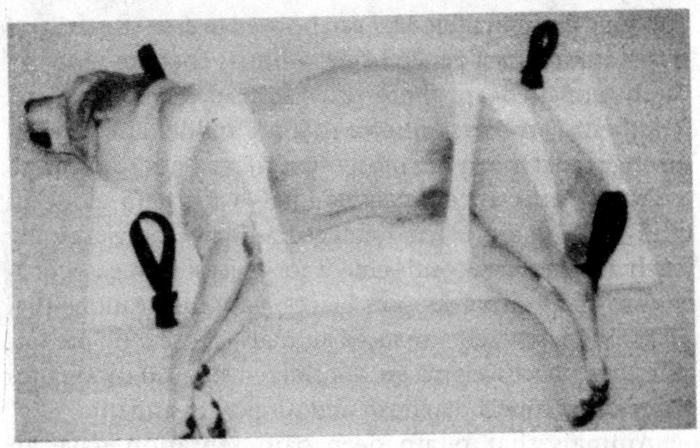

Fig. 22.1. A dog placed on a backboard following spinal trauma.

Neurologic Examination

Once the animal has been immobilized and systemic abnormalities identified (and treated as necessary), a more complete physical and neurologic exam should be performed. If the animal is physically or mechanically immobilized, the examination process may need to be modified to accommodate for this immobilization.

- The animal will most often be immobilized in a laterally recumbent position.
- While this position will not lend itself to evaluation of conscious proprioception and gait evaluation, much of the neurological examination can be performed and interpreted with the animal restrained.
- Mental status, cranial nerves, spinal reflexes, cutaneous trunci, anal tone, and deep pain sensation can be evaluated.
- Most importantly, the animal's spine can be palpated for areas of hyperesthesia.
- Any voluntary movement of the limbs is also important to ascertain. Voluntary movement is determined by observing for signs of purposeful movements.

- The presence or absence of deep pain is the most important factor in determining severity of a spinal cord lesion. When assessing for the presence of deep pain sensation, it is important not to confuse the withdrawing of a limb when pinching a digit with the actual presence of conscious pain perception and voluntary limb withdrawal.

When to Consider Nonsurgical (Medical) and Surgical Treatment

In animals with spinal trauma, an important decision is whether nonsurgical (medical) treatments are indicated, or whether surgical intervention is necessary. The need for surgical intervention will usually also determine the need for additional diagnostic testing such as advanced spinal imaging.

Decisions regarding when and if surgical versus nonsurgical treatment for spinal cord disease is indicated are primarily made based on the severity of neurological signs. The scale given in table 14.7 can be used to assess severity of spinal injury. As a general rule, animals that are more severely impaired are more often considered for surgical treatments, whereas animals that are mildly affected following spinal injury are most often treated nonsurgically.

Mildly affected animals (animals with pain alone or mild paresis) are often managed initially nonsurgically (such as with cage confinement for at least 6 weeks, corticosteroids, external support braces, pain medications)(fig. 22.2). More severely impaired animals (those who are unable to support weight) are considered surgical candidates and require timely diagnosis and surgical treatment.

Animals that retain deep pain sensation have an 80–90% chance of being able to walk at some time after injury. When deep pain is absent and an animal has suffered an exogenous spinal injury, the prognosis for walking falls to well below 50%.

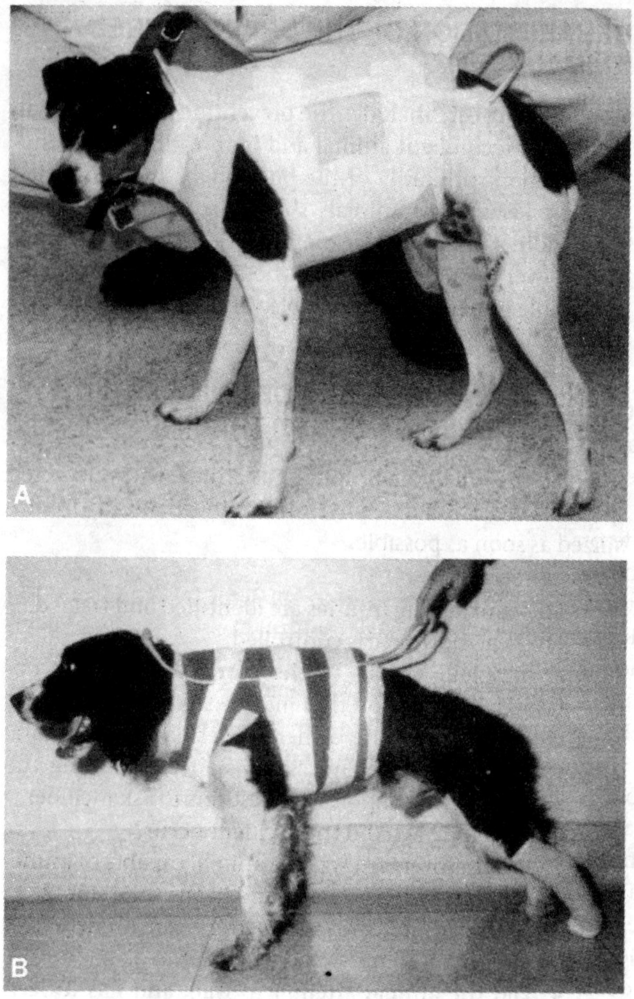

Fig. 22.2. (A, B) Two dogs with back braces.

Initial Diagnostic Testing

If, based upon initial physical and neurologic examinations, a vertebral injury is suspected, it is reasonable to perform survey radiographs of the affected area prior to performing additional physical manipulations. As with any radiographic procedure, proper positioning and radiographic technique are of utmost importance to avoid misinterpretation of the radiographic findings. Animals with spinal trauma and associated unstable vertebral segments must be moved and positioned with caution during radiographic procedures to avoid further and iatrogenic traumatic injury to the spinal cord.

Initial Treatment: Corticosteroids

A multicenter study in human beings reported in 1990 suggested that methylprednisolone given within the first 8 hours after a spinal trauma was beneficial for human patients with acute spinal injury. In this study, methylprednisolone was given at 30 mg/kg IV as a slow bolus, then 5.4 mg/kg/hour IV for the next 23 hours as a constant infusion. The use of methylprednisolone sodium succinate therapy as a standard of care for humans with spinal traumatic injury is currently being questioned and debated. Concerns regarding use of methylprednisolone sodium succinate in humans include both lack of significant benefit and increased amount of side effects.

Unfortunately, no scientifically valid randomized, controlled clinical trials exist regarding the use of methylprednisolone sodium succinate in animals. In the current era, clinicians are forced to make the decision as to whether to use this corticosteroid for treatment of spinal injury in animals based on experimental studies in animals.

If methylprednisolone therapy is to be used, dosing and administration schemes are debatable.

- One commonly used (but not necessarily scientifically supported) dosing regimen is to administer methylprednisolone sodium succinate at 30 mg/kg intravenously slowly for animals suffering spinal injury.
- There is experimental evidence to suggest that this medication is only effective if administered within a short time (1 hour) following experimental injury.

- As constant infusion administration and monitoring can be labor intensive in veterinary medicine, a subsequent dosing scheme of giving two additional bolus doses of the methylprednisolone at 15 mg/kg IV at 2 and 6 hours after the initial 30 mg/kg bolus dose has been used in place of the 23-hour constant infusion.
- Dexamethasone appears to be associated with increased side effects in animals with spinal disease. This may be a reflection of the relatively large dosages of dexamethasone that are currently recommended in many veterinary publications.

Nonsurgical Management

Cage confinement may be necessary for a minimum of 2 weeks and possibly up to 6 weeks (also see in chapter 14).

If walking, dogs should only be cautiously allowed outside on short leash walks only and should be prohibited from using stairs, running, or jumping. The animal should always be kept on surfaces with good footing to decrease slippage and further trauma. Additionally, the animal should always be controlled by the handler or care giver. This is usually accomplished with the use of slings and other support devices.

In some situations of traumatic spinal instability, a supportive spinal brace may be necessary. Although commercial varieties are available, an effective and economical version can be assembled at the veterinary hospital using bandage material and aluminum rods or casting material. Beginning cranial to the shoulders and ending cranial to the pelvis, several layers of cast padding or similar material are rolled around the animal's body, followed by two layers of stretch gauze. The bandage material should follow a "figure-eight" pattern around the animal's thoracic limbs and thorax. A layer of Vetrap (3-M Animal Care Products, St. Paul, MN) is then applied over the stretch gauze. As with any bandage application, care must be taken to avoid wrapping the bandage material too tightly. Following bandage placement, it is important to ensure that the animal can expand its ribcage and breathe comfortably with the bandage in place.

The rigid portion of the brace can be achieved with casting material or aluminum bars. Casting material is applied over the dorsal spinal (abnormal) area to form a rigid cover. Once the material has hardened, it can be attached to the underlying bandage material with tape or a similar product.

Aluminum bars offer the ability to mold the brace to the dimension of the animal while still providing strength. The aluminum rod is bent into an oblong, oval shape. The center portion of the oval should be straight and flat, positioned directly along the animal's spine. The two ends are positioned caudal to the occipital crest and cranial to the pelvis, but bent at approximately a 45-degree angle away from the animal's body. This allows for comfortable movement of the animal's head and neck and also provides handles to aid the owner or hospital staff in walking or physical therapy. This brace is then taped in place with 2-inch white porous tape. Modifications of this type of spinal brace are made for animals with traumatic injury in the cervical area.

Surgical Management

If surgical treatment is indicated, and surgery will not occur at the admitting hospital, preparation for referral to a facility for possible surgical evaluation is necessary. Prior to transport, systemic functions should be assessed and treated. The animal should be physically immobilized to avoid further iatrogenic damage to the vertebral column and spinal cord during transport. The appropriate contacts should be made so that the referring facility is prepared to receive the animal upon arrival to the referral hospital.

In preparation for surgery, survey radiographs may be followed by myelography to determine if compression of the spinal cord is present. In veterinary referral centers, computed tomography (CT) scans and magnetic resonance (MR) imaging are increasingly used in the diagnosis of spinal trauma.

Various types of surgical procedure are used for spinal stabilization, but they are beyond the scope of this chapter. Most commonly, the spine is realigned using cortical bone screws, Kirschner wires, Steinmann pins, and polymethyl methacrylate. The goal of surgery is to (1) realign the abnormal vertebrae, (2) decompress the spinal cord, and (3) stabilize the vertebrae to allow for fracture healing (fig. 22.3).

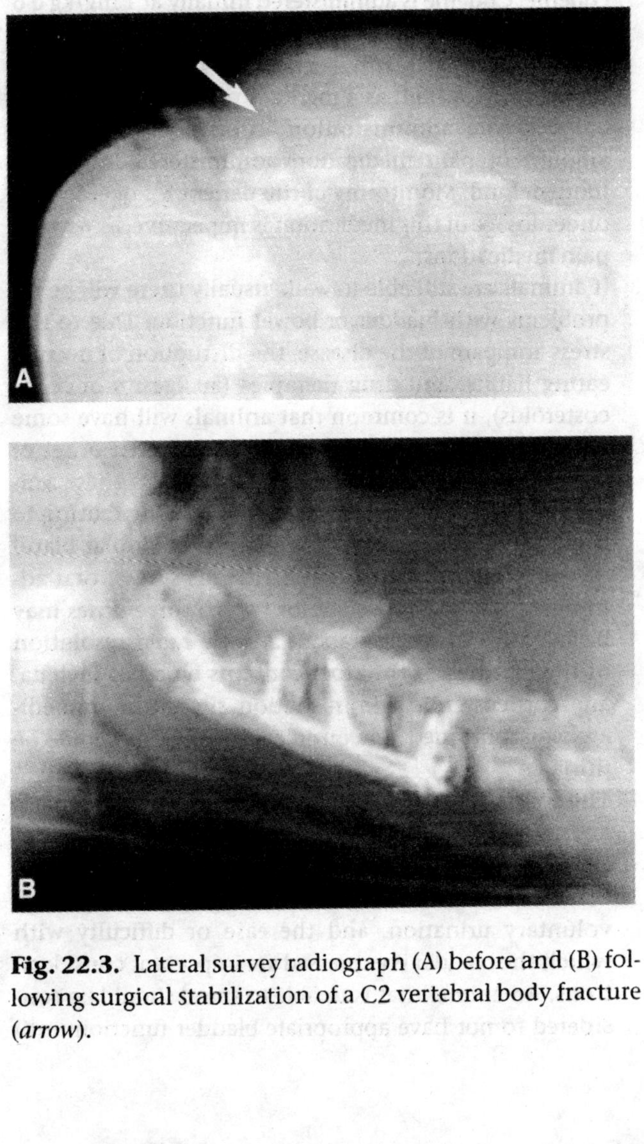

Fig. 22.3. Lateral survey radiograph (A) before and (B) following surgical stabilization of a C2 vertebral body fracture (*arrow*).

Postinjury or Postsurgery Management of the Animal with Spinal Injury

Postinjury or postsurgery management is detailed below. Additional information regarding care of the animal with spinal disease is found in chapter 14.

1. Confinement and restricted activity (rest). Depending on the size of animal (i.e., smaller areas for smaller animals), animals should be confined to a comfortable space no larger than 3 feet (width) by 3 feet (length) by 3 feet (height) in dimension. The animals should be kept confined for at least 4 to 6 weeks following a spinal injury. Weekly veterinary assessments are ideal, but will depend on the clinical circumstances, with evaluation possible more or less frequently. The animal should not be freed from confinement until a veterinary assessment deems that cage confinement is no longer necessary (i.e., the clinical signs have resolved). If the clinical signs are improved but not resolved, cage confinement is continued in weekly intervals with continual clinical reassessment until the clinical signs are resolved.
2. Opiate analgesics are commonly used to alleviate pain (table 14.2). In our hospital, the most effective means of pain control for animals with neurologic and other painful conditions is achieved by administering oral codeine. Codeine is administered initially at 1 mg/kg q 6 hours PO PRN, and may be increased to Q 4 hours (or possibly more frequently) if necessary. Dosages may be increased to as high as 4 mg/kg if needed, however, decreasing the administration interval to titrate the amount of pain medication administered is usually more helpful. Monitoring of the patient for overdose or underdosage of this medication is imperative, as with all pain medications.
3. If animals are still able to walk, usually there will be no problems with bladder or bowel function. Due to the stress and pain of the disease, the disruption of normal eating habits, and drug therapies (analgesics or corticosteroids), it is common that animals will have some diarrhea during the initial days following the onset of their disease. It is always prudent to assess these animals for internal parasites that may be contributing to the diarrhea. Providing a commercial or similar bland diet is often helpful. If the diarrhea is severe, oral administration of Kaopectate for two to three doses may be helpful in bringing about a more rapid resolution of the diarrhea. If the stool contains blood or melena, any corticosteroid administration should be immediately discontinued, and antiulcer mediations should be initiated.
4. The animal's ability to urinate following spinal trauma is an important factor in determining prognosis for recovery and quality of life. The presence or absence of urine on the animal's bedding or in the cage, voluntary or involuntary urination, and the ease or difficulty with which the bladder is expressed are important considerations. An animal that is unable to stand should be considered to not have appropriate bladder function until voluntary urination is proven. The bladder should be gently palpated regularly (at least every 6 hours; more frequently in animals that are polyuric) to determine the volume of urine it contains and to establish whether or not the animal is fully emptying its bladder each time it urinates. Urine left in the bladder due to inadequate bladder emptying can lead to cystitis. Manual expression may be necessary every 6 hours if the animal is not able to urinate on its own. The color and smell of the urine collected or expressed should be monitored. A daily urinalysis using a urine dipstick and sediment evaluation is performed to determine if an infection is beginning. Appropriate cultures are submitted if pyuria, bacteriuria, or hematuria is noted.

   If expression is difficult, the bladder should be drained by introduction of a sterile urinary catheter. Indwelling urinary catheters are not recommended as they increase the risk of introducing a bladder infection. Indwelling urinary catheters may be necessary in animals that are difficult to intermittently catheterize (small, female animals) or in animals that have urinary incontinence who are persistently dribbling urine and soiling themselves.

   Depending on the nature of the neurologic lesion and the cause of the abnormal bladder function, a number of pharmacological agents are routinely used to assist in bladder management (table 14.5).
5. Physical therapy is often an important aspect of recovery and rehabilitation from spinal injury. The amount and degree of physical therapy will vary with the experience of the veterinary hospital and owner. In animals with spinal injury that may have an unstable spinal segment, the degree and amount of physical therapy should be balanced to avoid further iatrogenic spinal injury. If used cautiously and appropriately, however, physical therapy can provide significant benefits in animals with spinal injury.

   Light massage of the back and limb often appears comforting. The touching sensation may also result in decreased apprehension and an overall feeling of well-being. Passive range of motion exercises can help prevent joint stiffness, edema, and muscle atrophy. With the animal in lateral recumbency, the therapist can extend and flex each joint in the thoracic and pelvic limbs. It can also be helpful to simply mimic an exaggerated walking motion with the limb, moving it in a circular fashion and utilizing each of the joints. These exercises may be performed for 10–20 minute periods at least twice daily. Electrical muscle stimulation is also gaining in popularity. More aggressive physical therapy (swimming, treadmill) is usually reserved for animals that have improved significantly from their disease or, at least, have been given sufficient time to allow healing of any spinal segment disruption.

Manangement of the Recumbent Animal. Recumbent animals should be kept in a comfortable environment that prevents them from moving freely and further injuring themselves. Animals that are recumbent are confined similarly to those that can still walk. If the animal is recumbent, padding the animal and frequent cautious turning (ideally every 1 to 2 hours) should be performed to avoid decubital ulcers. Urine and feces may contaminate the animal or the area and should be removed as rapidly as possible to avoid skin irritation. Absorbent pads that can be changed frequently are often helpful in keeping animals clean and dry. Strategic placement of the padding, the absorbent material, and the animal is necessary so that body fluids will be directed away from the recumbent animal.

Animals that are recumbent may not be able to move to have access to food and, most importantly, water. It is imperative to place water and food within the range of access for the animal. If the animal is laterally recumbent, someone will often have to hold the animal in a sternal position and offer food and water by hand. If the animal is tetraplegic, this may mean having to hand-feed and water the animal every 2 hours to maintain hydration. It is vital to avoid forcing food into the animal to prevent aspiration and subsequent pneumonia.

Extra padding under the dog with foam rubber or thick fleece material is necessary. Small, soft-sided waterbeds are helpful in preventing bed sores. Frequent turning is also important in preventing atelectasis, which may lead to pneumonia. Ideally, the animal should be kept in a sternal or sternal oblique position to allow for chest expansion.

The recumbent animal is often unable to move itself from an area it has soiled. Absorbent, waterproof pads, such as Val-U-Sorb Underpad (Professional Medical Products, Greenwood, SC), can be useful in soaking up urine and preventing the saturation of bedding material with urine or feces. Frequent bathing may be necessary to prevent urine scald. This may be accomplished during hydrotherapy. Although not practical in all hospital settings, hydrotherapy can be an effective method of physical therapy. Swimming provides a buoyant environment for the animal to attempt movement of its limbs without having to support its full weight. The warm water also promotes adequate circulation and muscle relaxation.

III Appendixes

1. Magnetic Resonance Imaging Brain Atlas for Dogs
2. Breed-Associated Neurologic Disease
3. Anticonvulsants in Dogs and Cats
4. Abnormalities of Vision and Pupils
5. Practice Clinical Cases

1 Magnetic Resonance Imaging Brain Atlas for Dogs

Magnetic resonance (MR) imaging has changed the clinical practice of neurology by allowing for exceptional anatomical imaging of the intracranial nervous system. Prior to interpretation of intracranial MR studies, the examiner must possess a thorough knowledge of intracranial sectional anatomy and the neurophysiologic correlations of these anatomic structures. The following is a sectional guide to intracranial neuroanatomy and the correlative appearance of these structures on MR images for dogs.

With all MR studies, the anatomical appearance of the brain may vary somewhat from individual to individual due to alterations in animal positioning during imaging, location of individual image acquisitions, anatomical differences among individual animals, and image acquisition parameters. Additionally, some distortion of the gross anatomical image is due to fixation of the brain prior to sectioning and lack of normal cerebral blood flow. CSF surrounding the intracranial structures is present in the antemortem MR images, but not in the postmortem anatomical images. Therefore, this atlas should be interpreted as a guide rather than an absolute depiction of the MR anatomy of the dog brain.

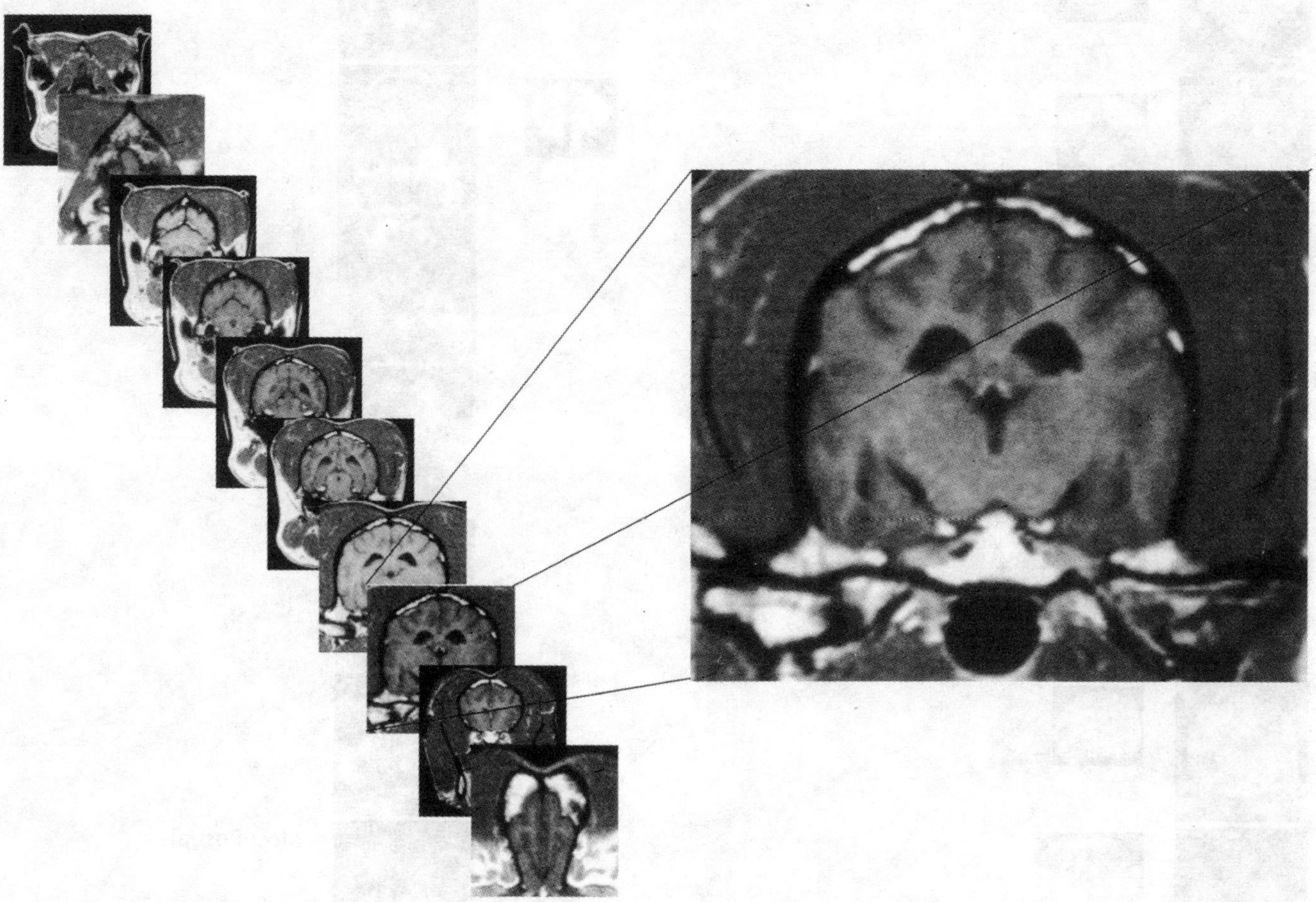

Fig. A1.1. Representation of transverse MR "slices" or images of a dog brain.

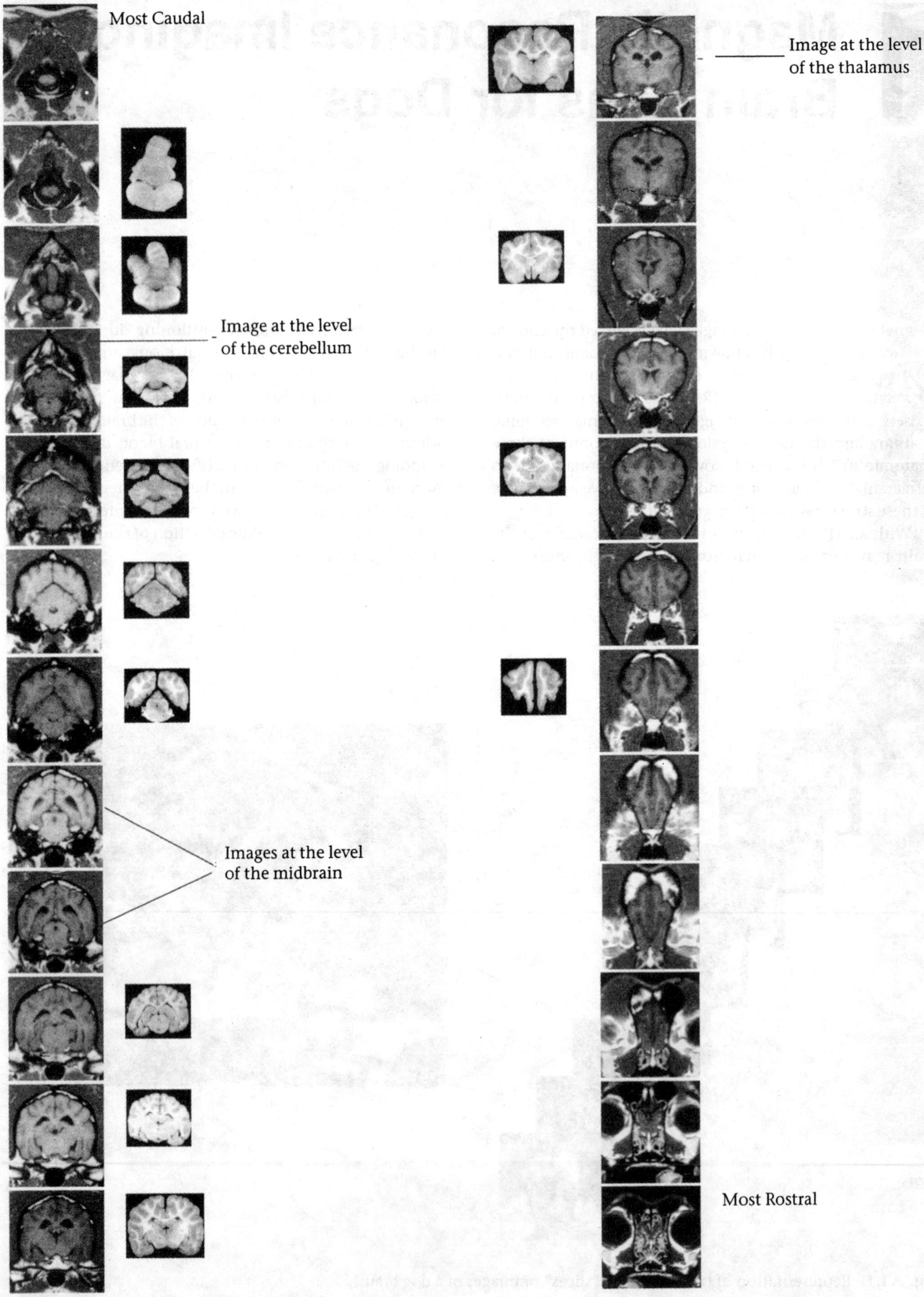

A1.2a. T1-weighted MR images of the brain from caudal to rostral, with associated gross anatomical images from a dog.

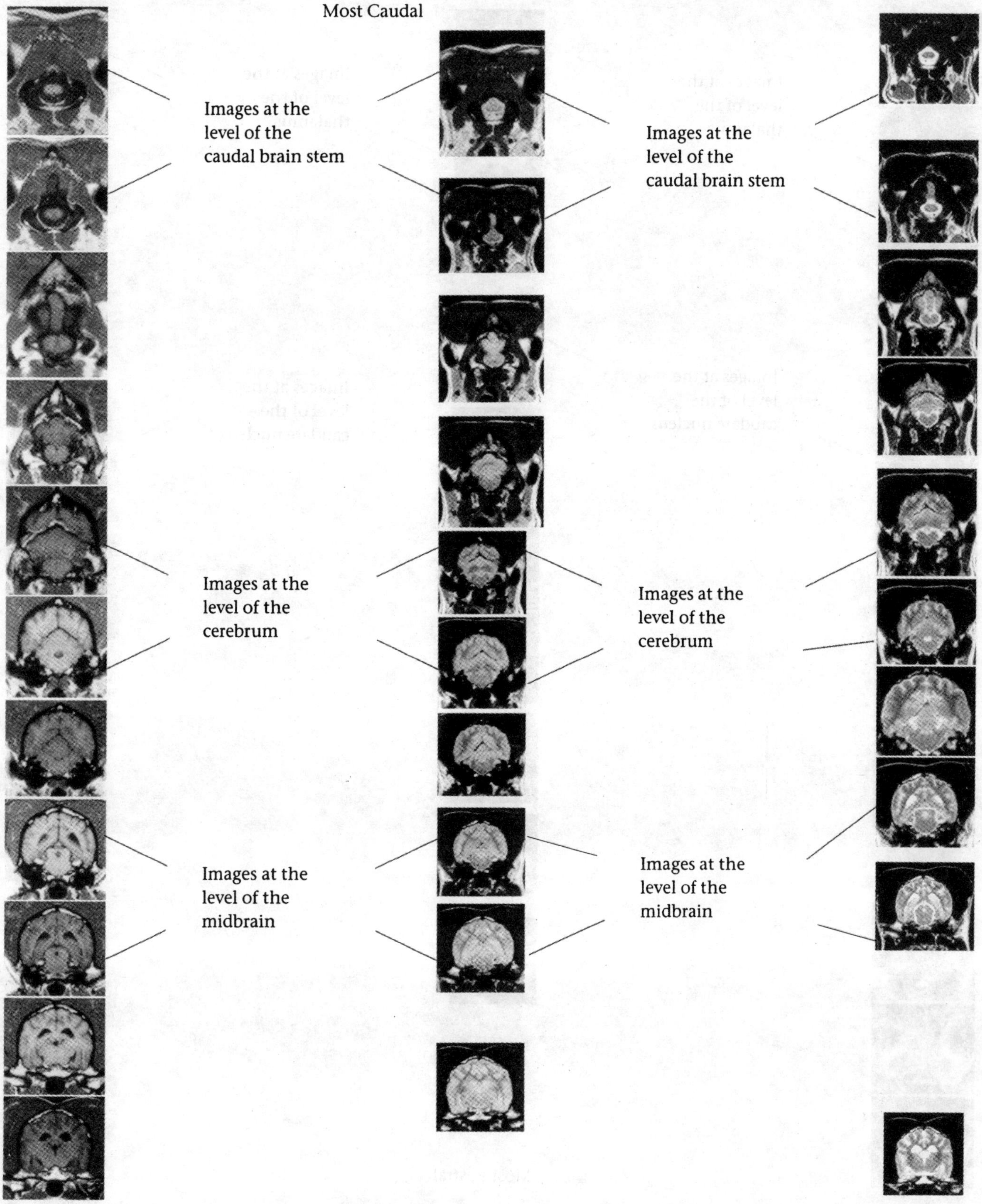

A1.2b. T1-weighted (left), proton density (center), and T2-weighted (right) MR images of a dog's brain, viewing from caudal to rostral. *(continues)*

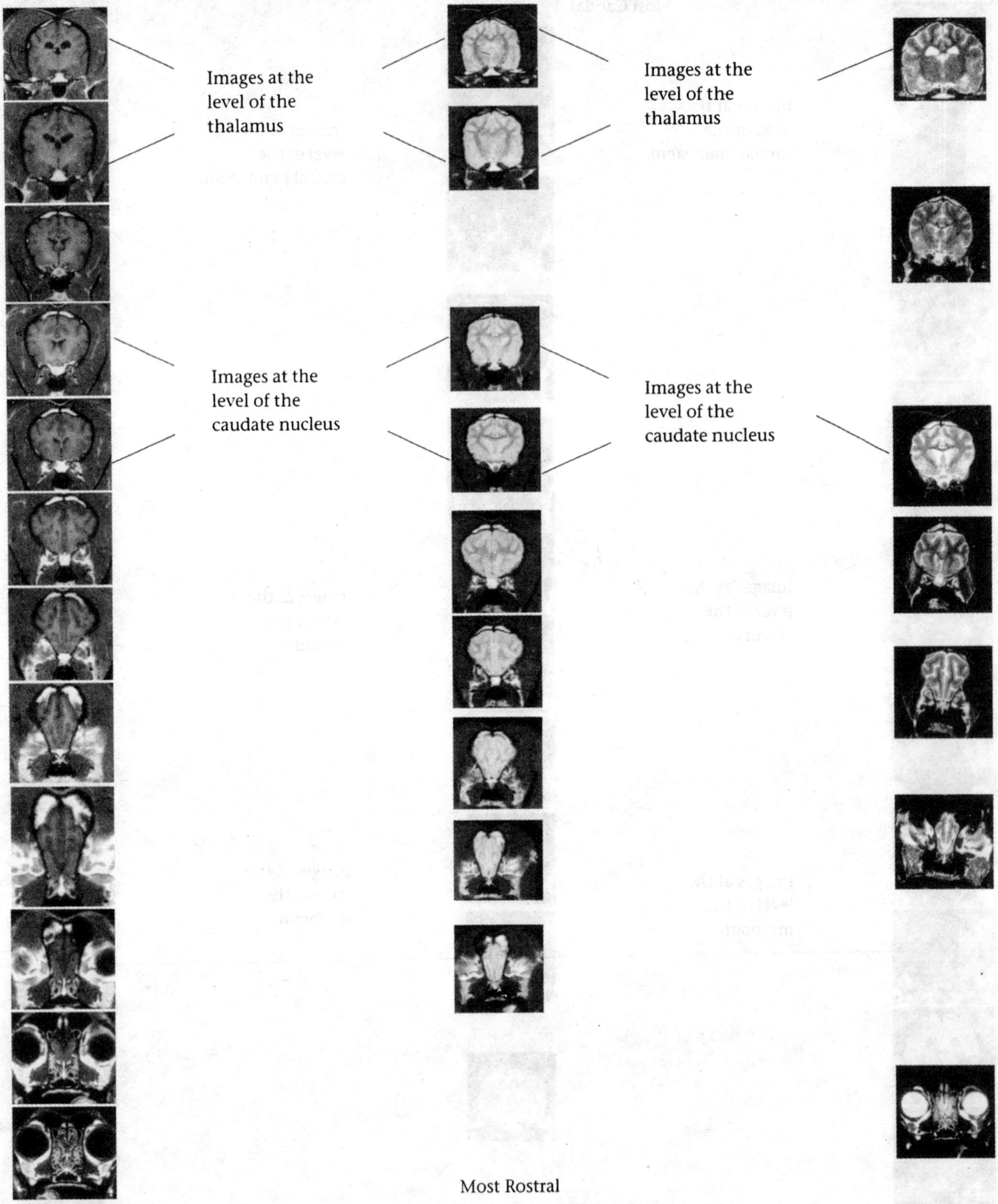

A1.2b. *Continued.*

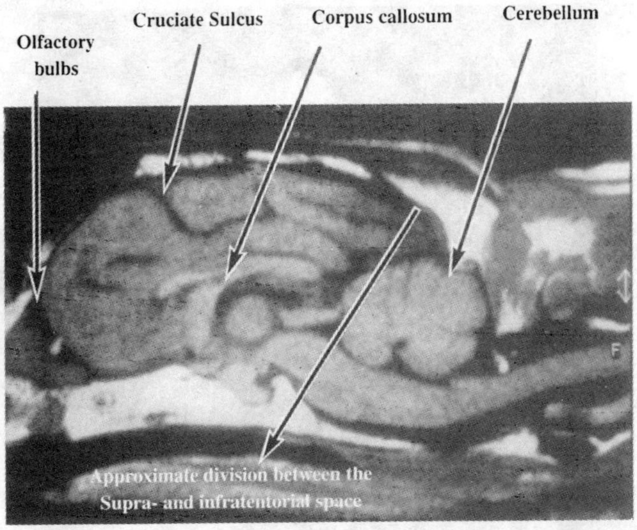

Fig. A1.3. Sagittal T1-weighted MR image of a dog brain.

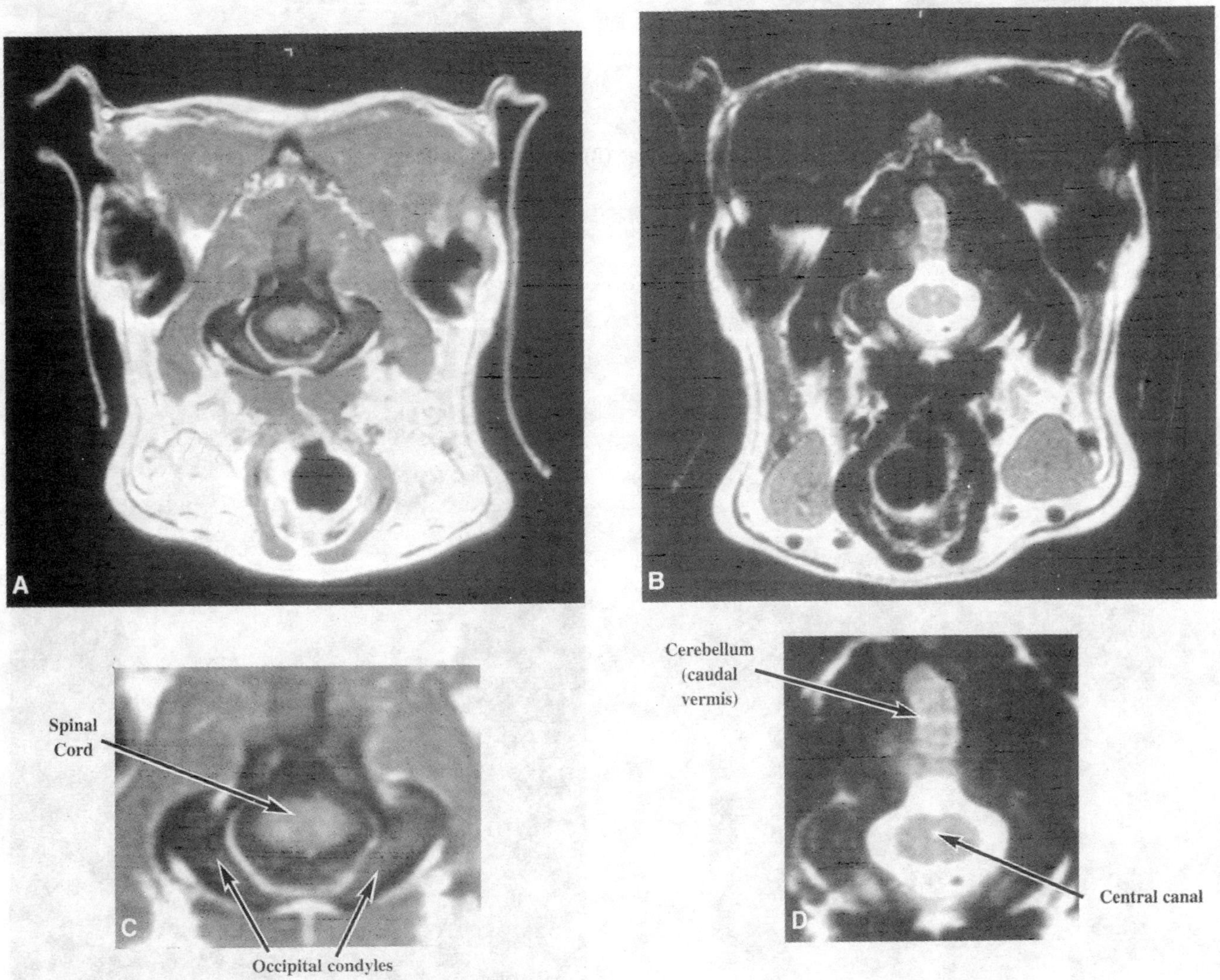

Fig. A1.4. T1-weighted (A, C) and T2-weighted (B, D) MR images at the level of the foramen magnum.

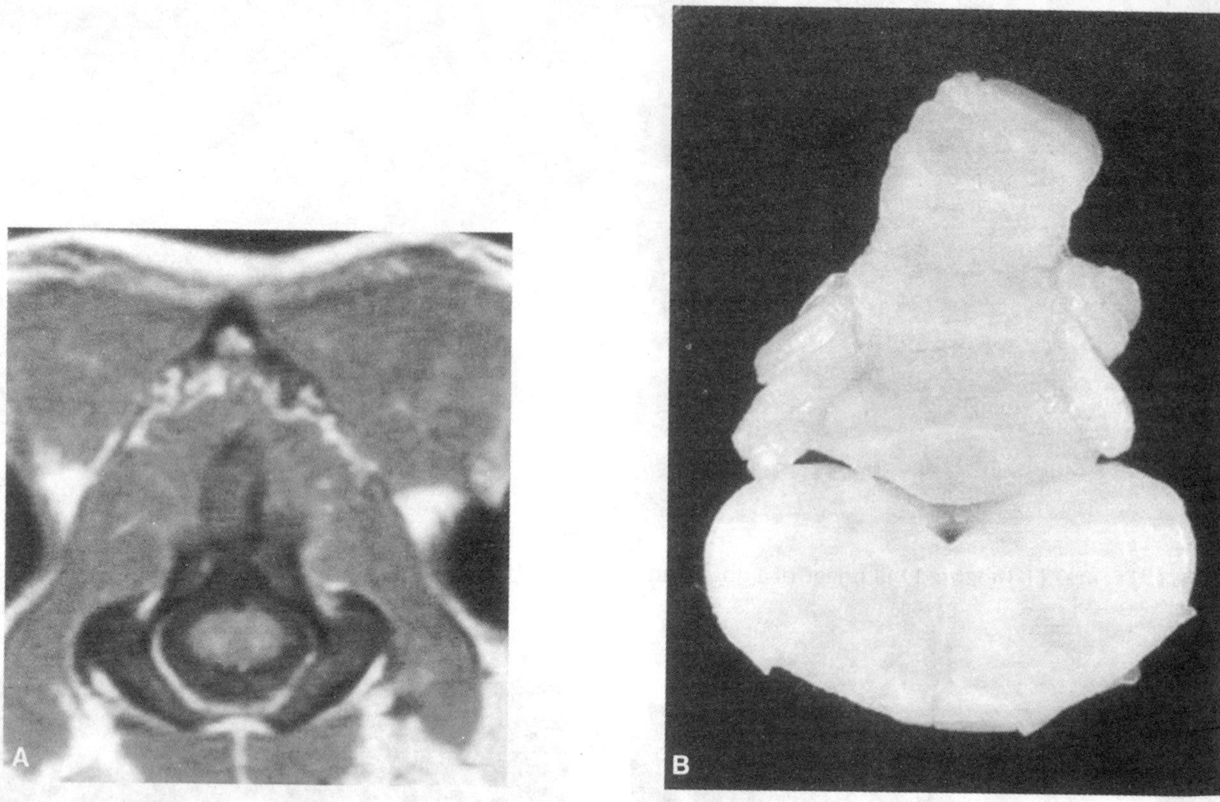

Fig. A1.5. T1-weighted MR image (A) and anatomical image (B) at the level of the caudal cerebellum and brain stem.

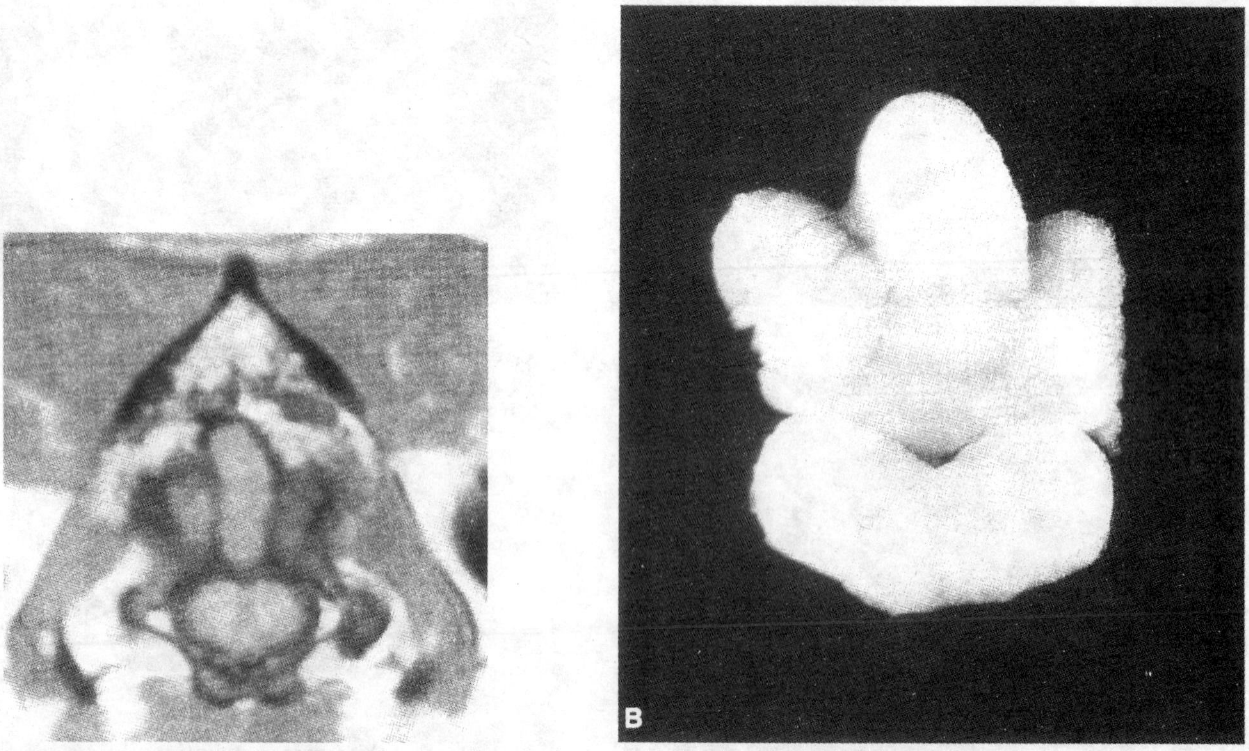

Fig. A1.6. T1-weighted MR image (A) and anatomical image (B) at the level slightly rostral to Fig. A1.5.

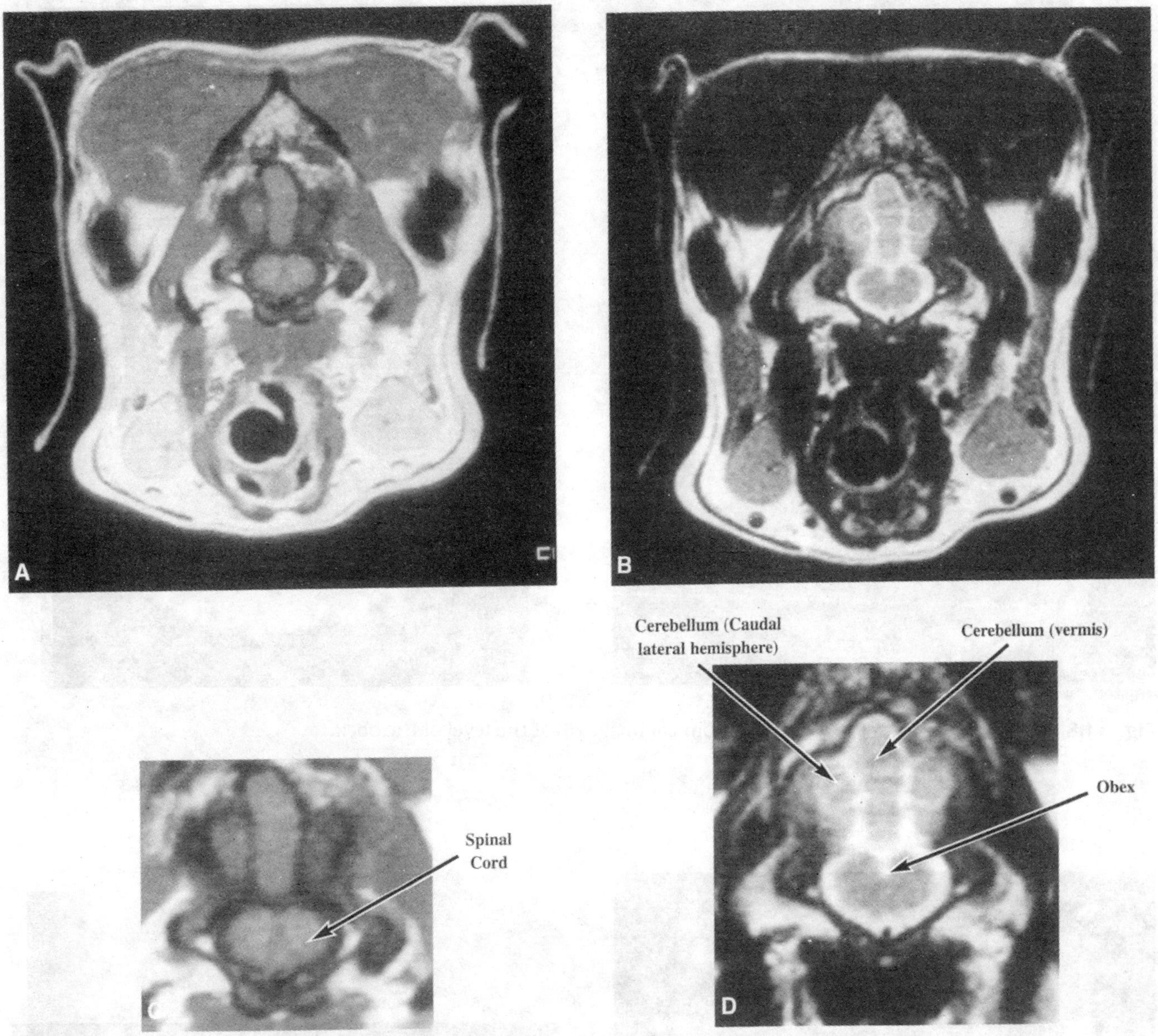

Fig. A1.7. T1-weighted (A, C) and T2-weighted (B, D) MR images at the level just rostral to the foramen magnum.

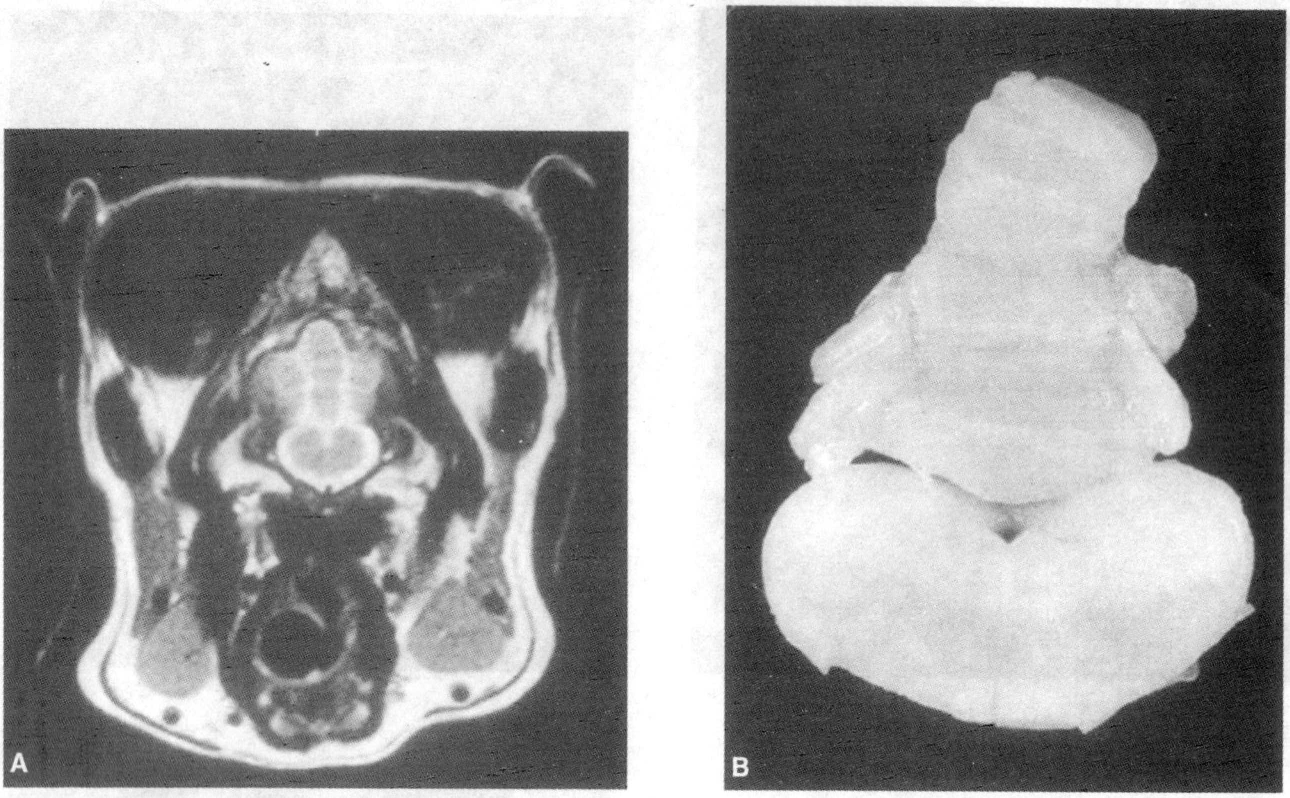

Fig. A1.8. T2-weighted MR image (A) and anatomical image (B) at the level of the obex.

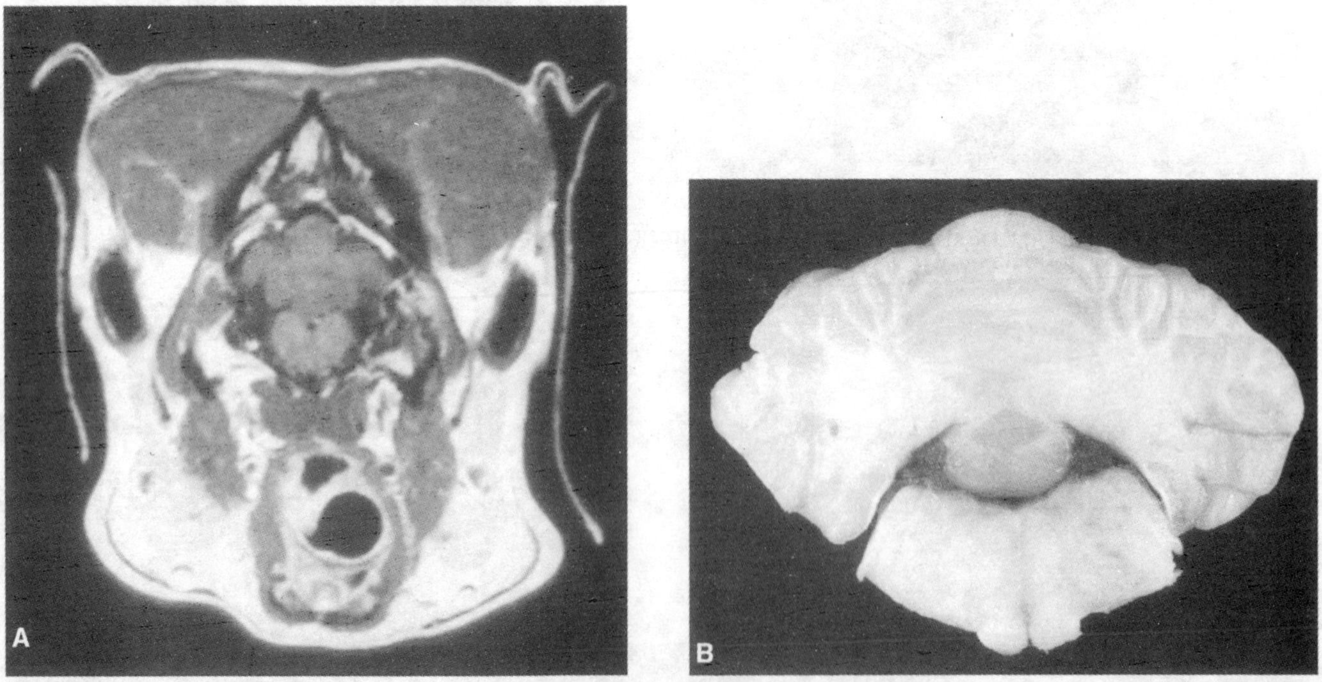

Fig. A1.9. T1-weighted MR image (A) and anatomical image (B) at the level of the pyramids.

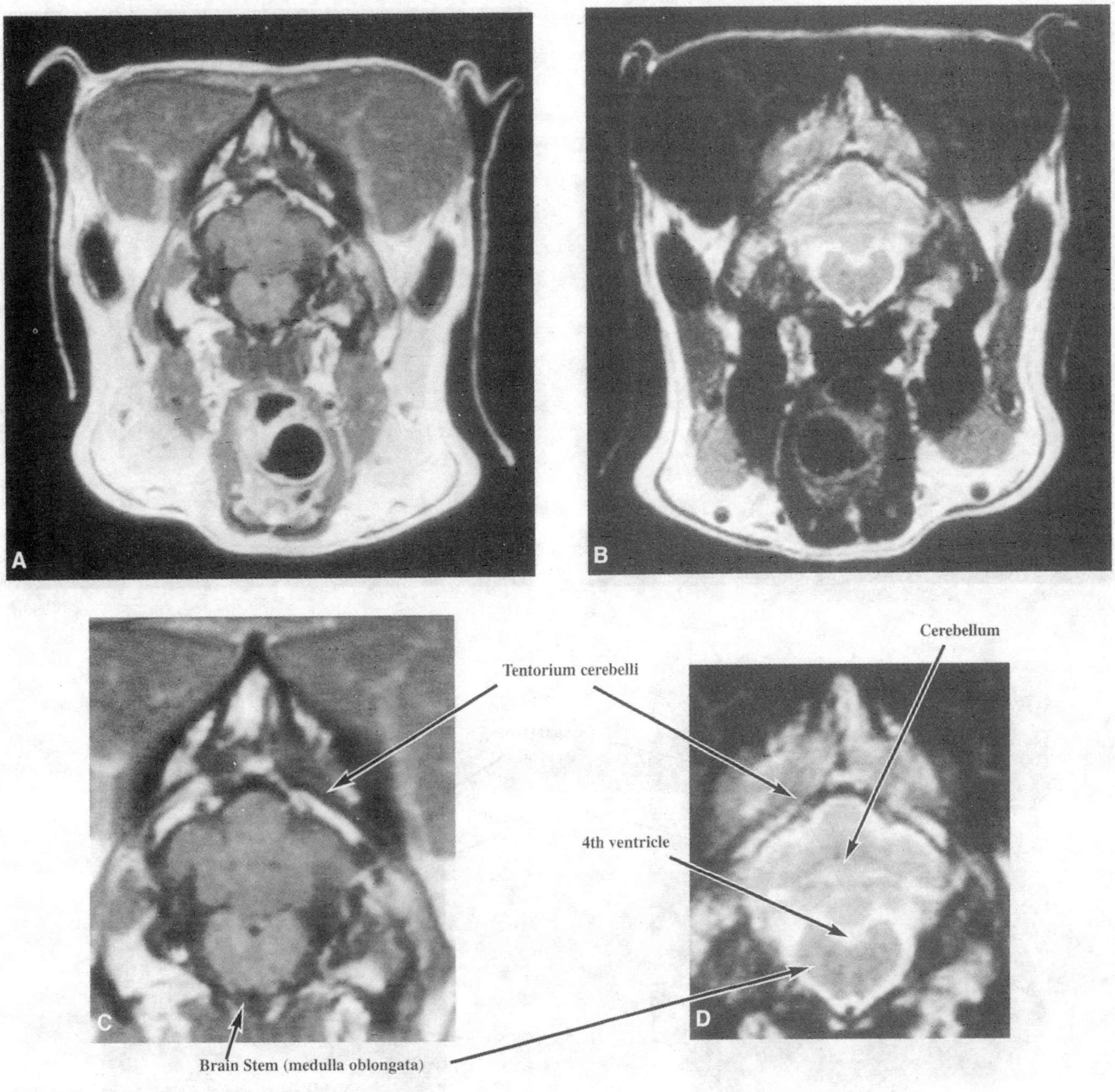

Fig. A1.10. T1-weighted (A, C) and T2-weighted (B, D) MR images at the level of the cerebellum.

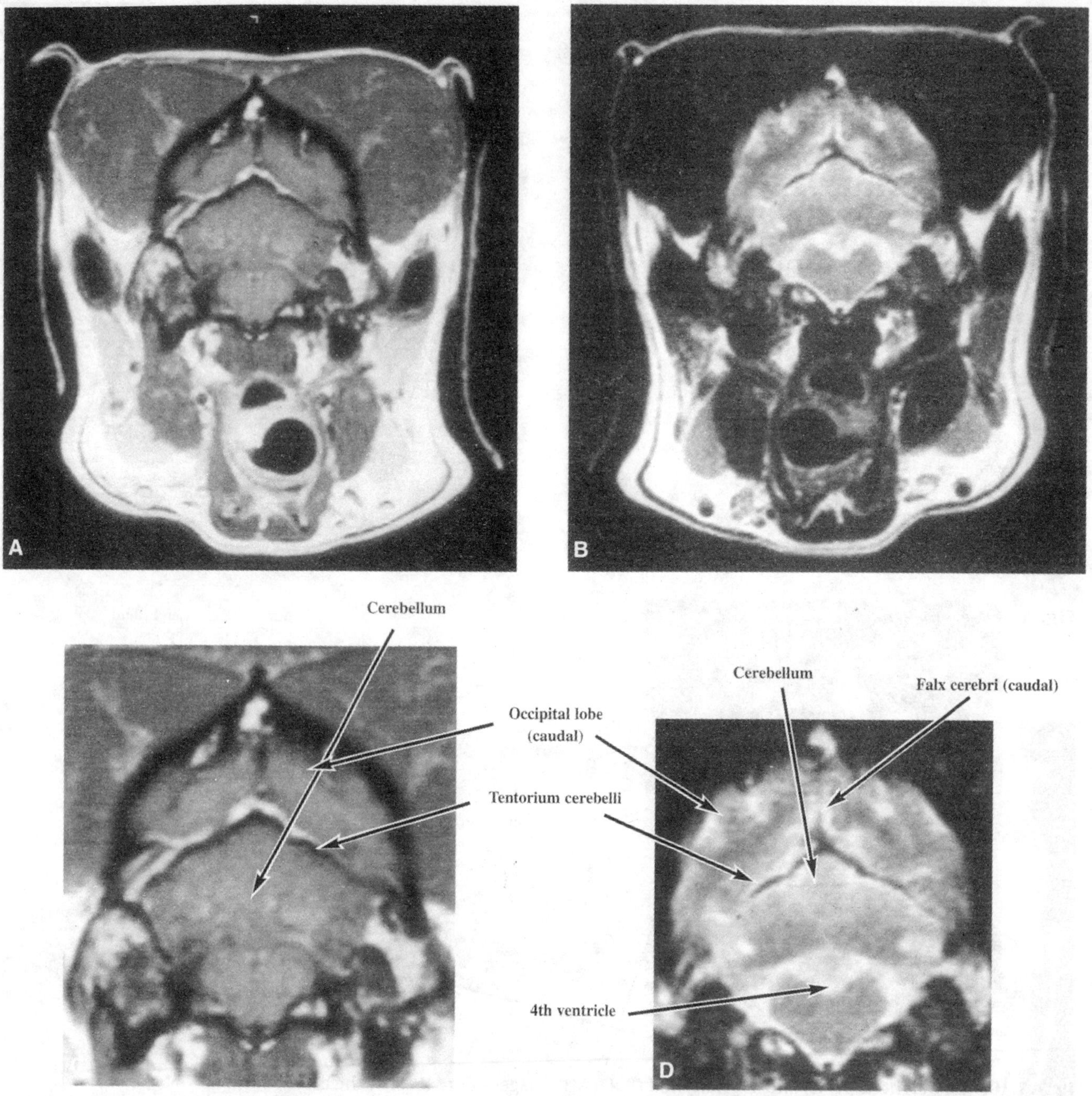

Fig. A1.11. T1-weighted (A, C) and T2-weighted (B, D) MR images at the level of the cerebellum and brain stem.

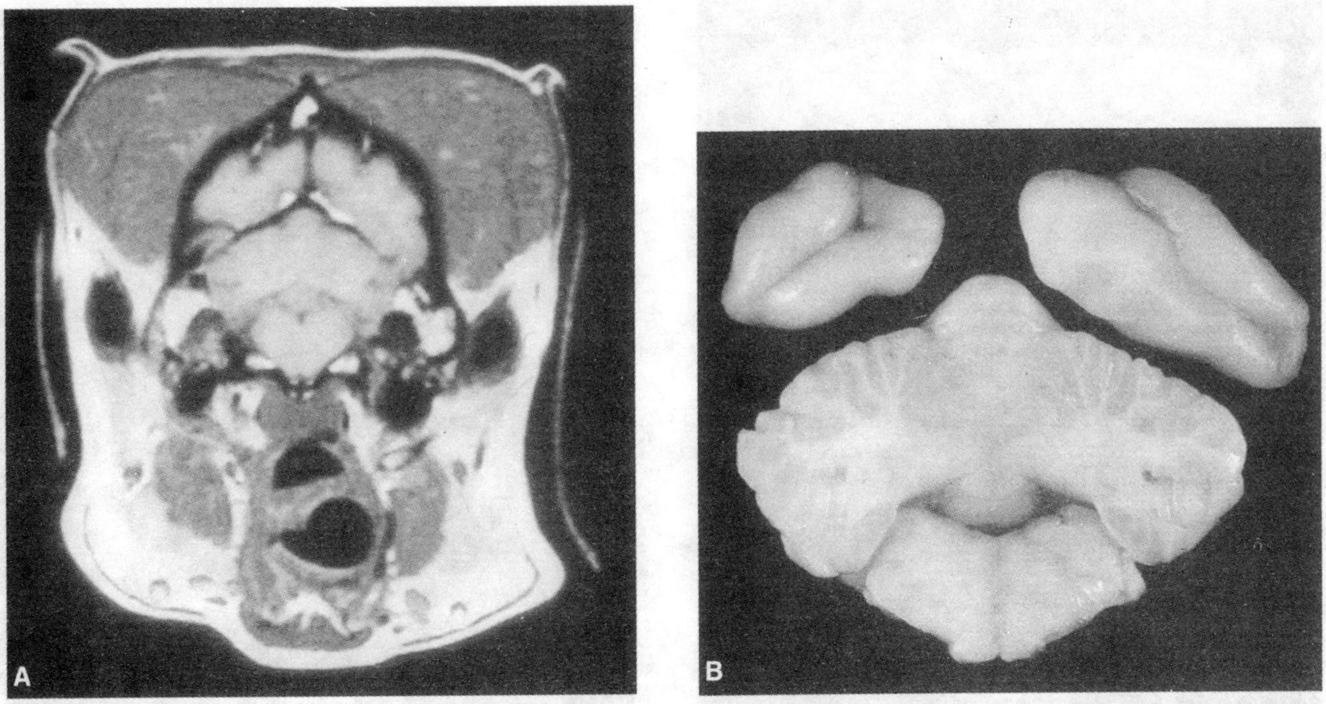

Fig. A1.12. T1-weighted MR image (A) and anatomical images (B) at the level of the caudal fourth ventricle.

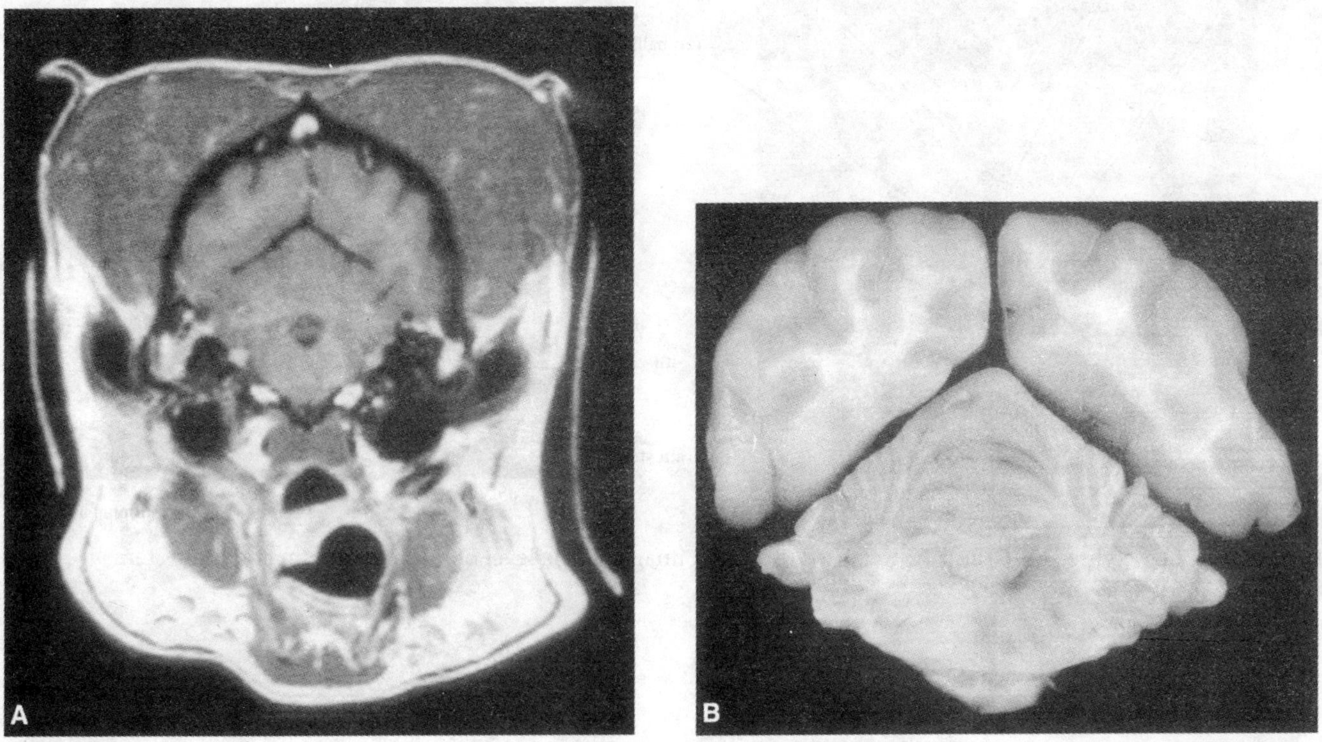

Fig. A1.13. T1-weighted MR image (A) and anatomical images (B) at the level of the caudal occipital lobes, brain stem, and cerebellum.

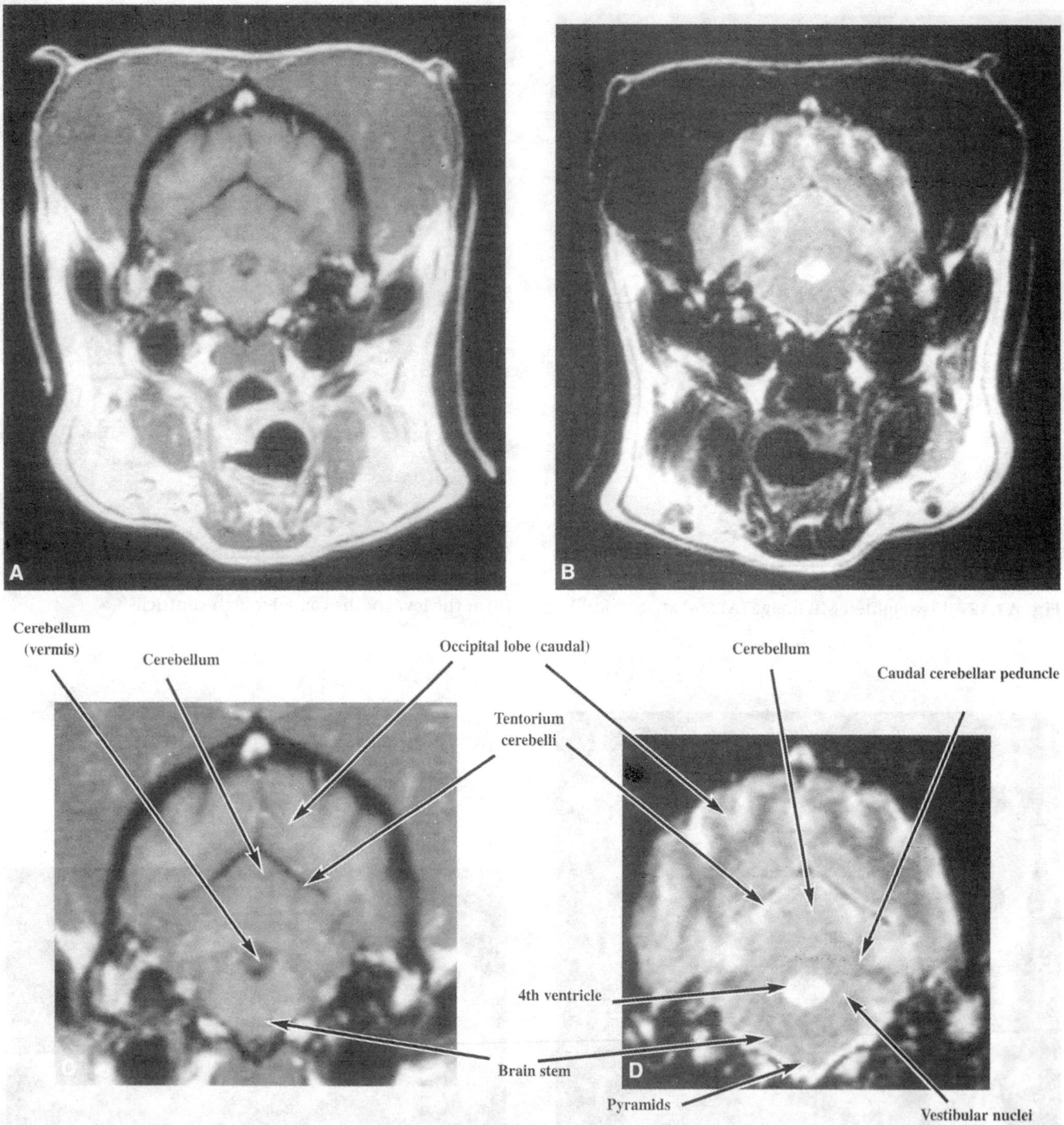

Fig. A1.14. T1-weighted (A, C) and T2-weighted (B, D) MR images at the level of mid-cerebellum and brain stem.

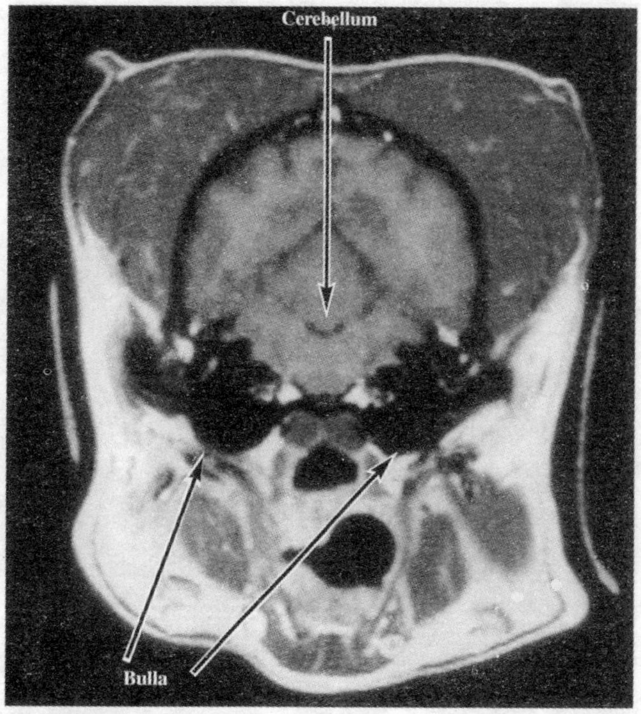

Fig. A1.15. T1-weighted MR image at the level of the bulla.

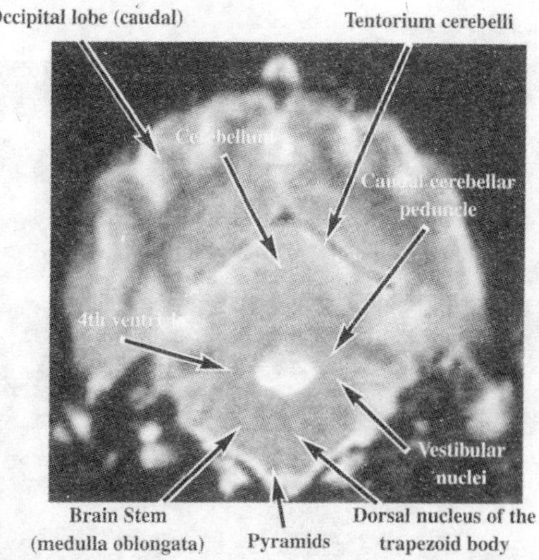

Fig. A1.16. T2-weighted MR image at the level of the caudal fourth ventricle.

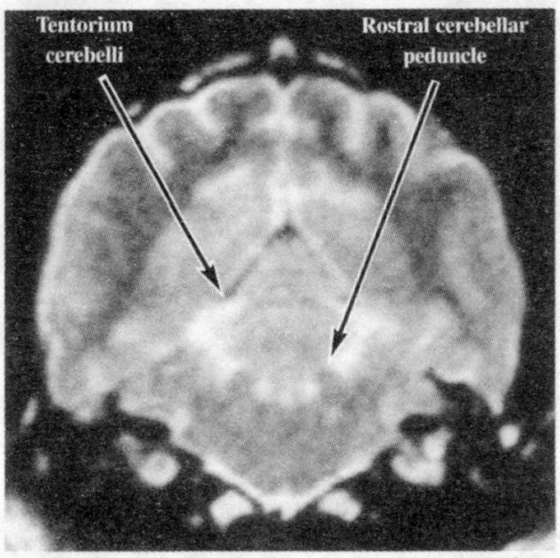

Fig. A1.17. T2-weighted MR image at the level of the rostral fourth ventricle.

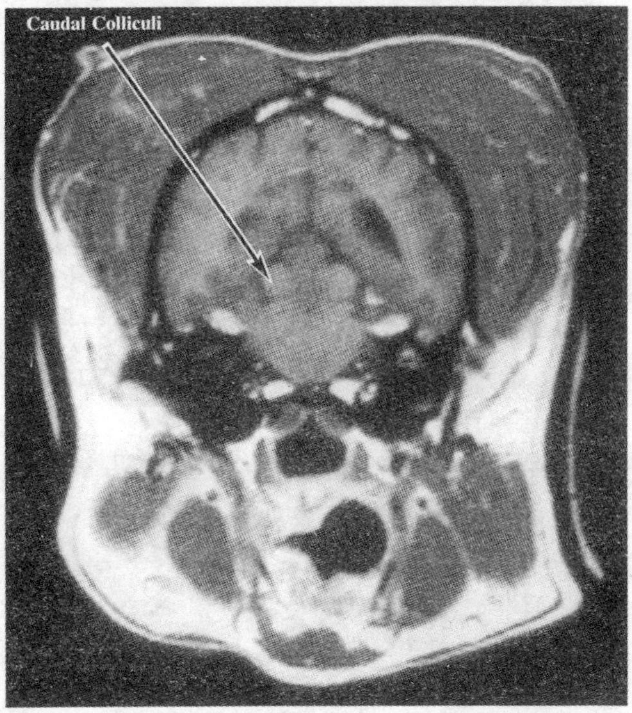

Fig. A1.18. T1-weighted MR image at the level of the caudal colliculi.

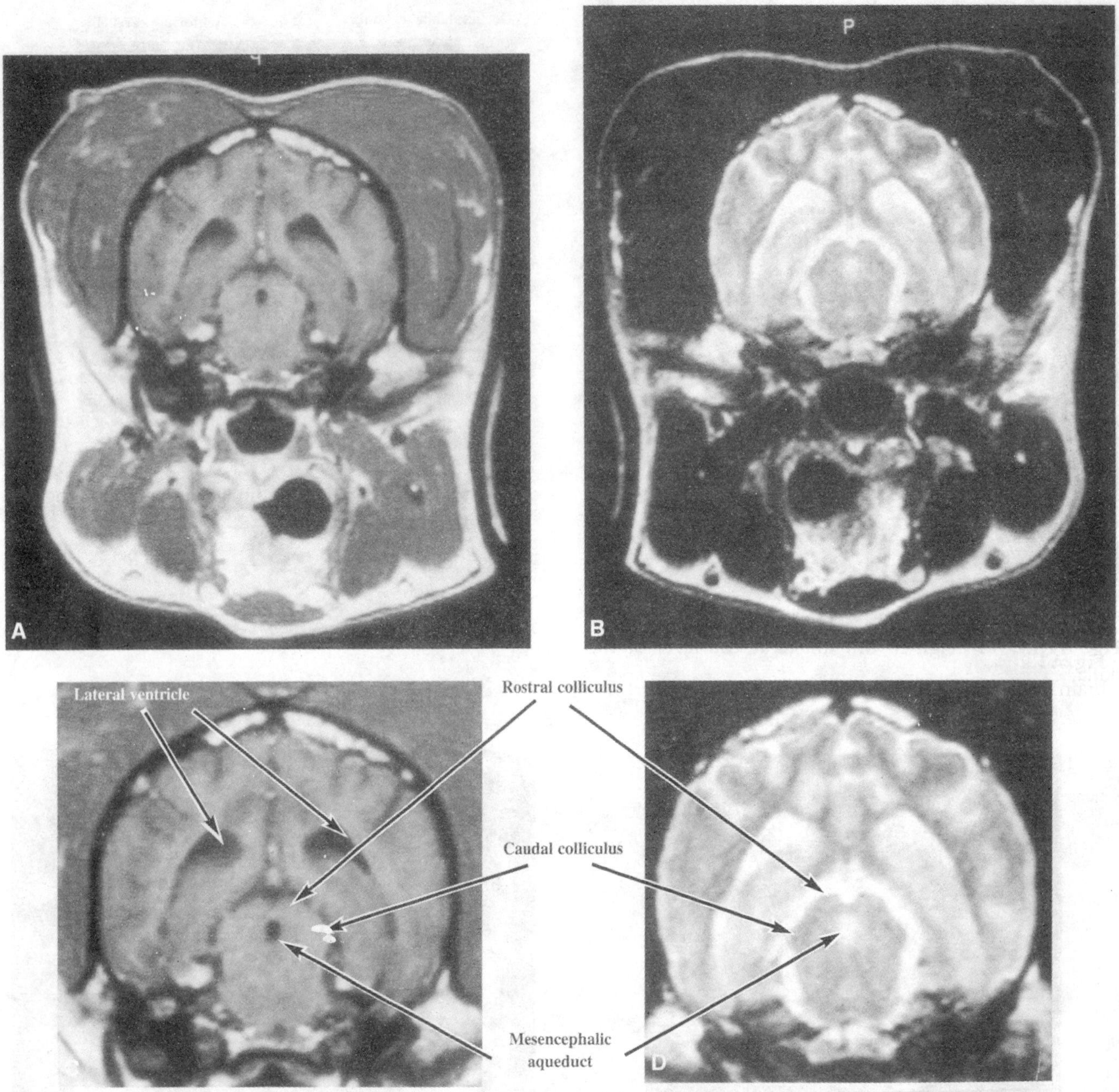

Fig. A1.19. T1-weighted (A, C) and T2-weighted (B, D) MR images at the level of the midbrain.

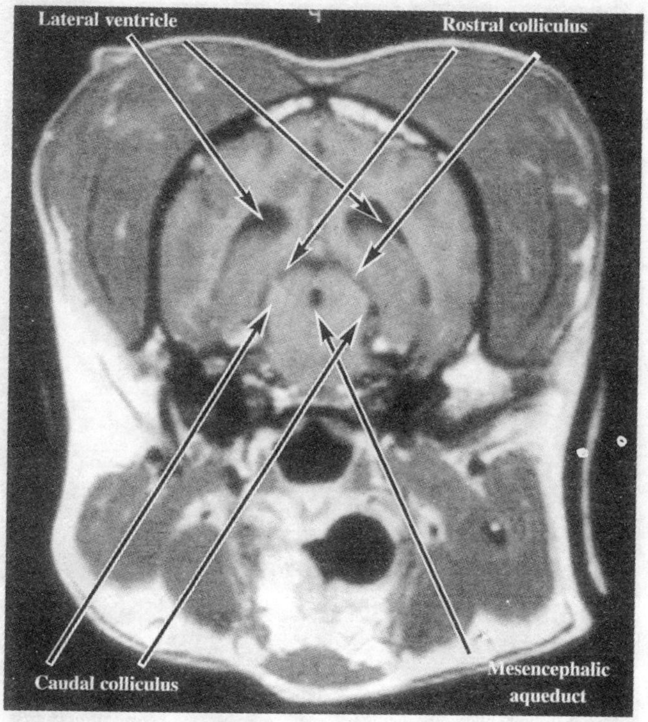

Fig. A1.20. T1-weighted MR image at the level of the midbrain.

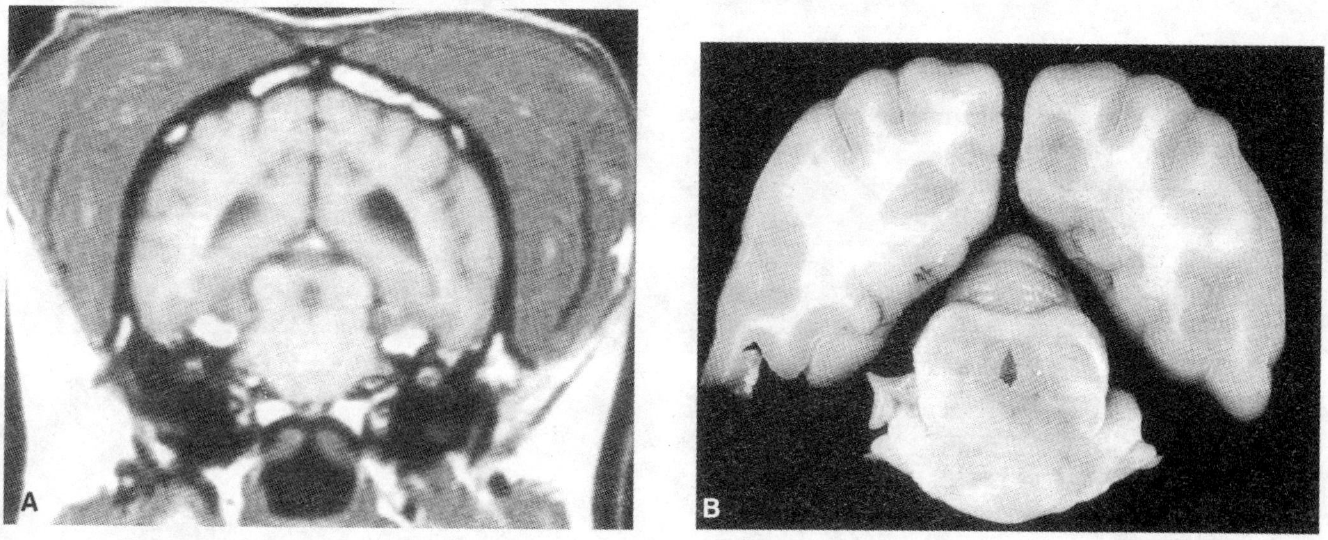

Fig. A1.21. T1-weighted MR image (A) and anatomical images (B) at the level of the midbrain.

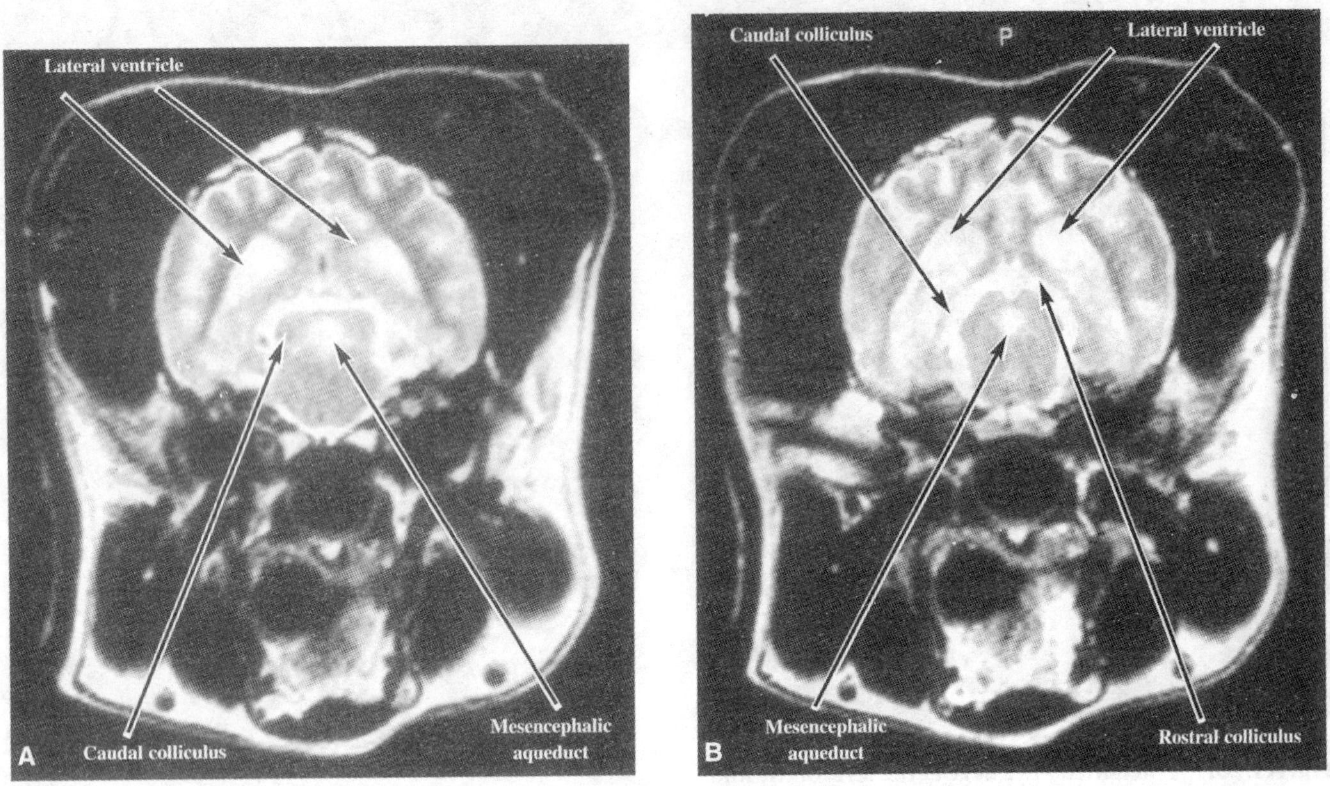

Fig. A1.22. T2-weighted MR images at the level of the midbrain.

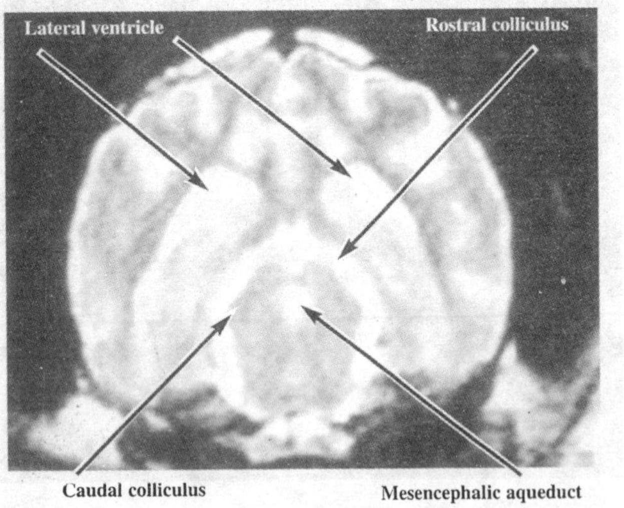

Fig. A1.23. T2-weighted MR image at the level of the midbrain.

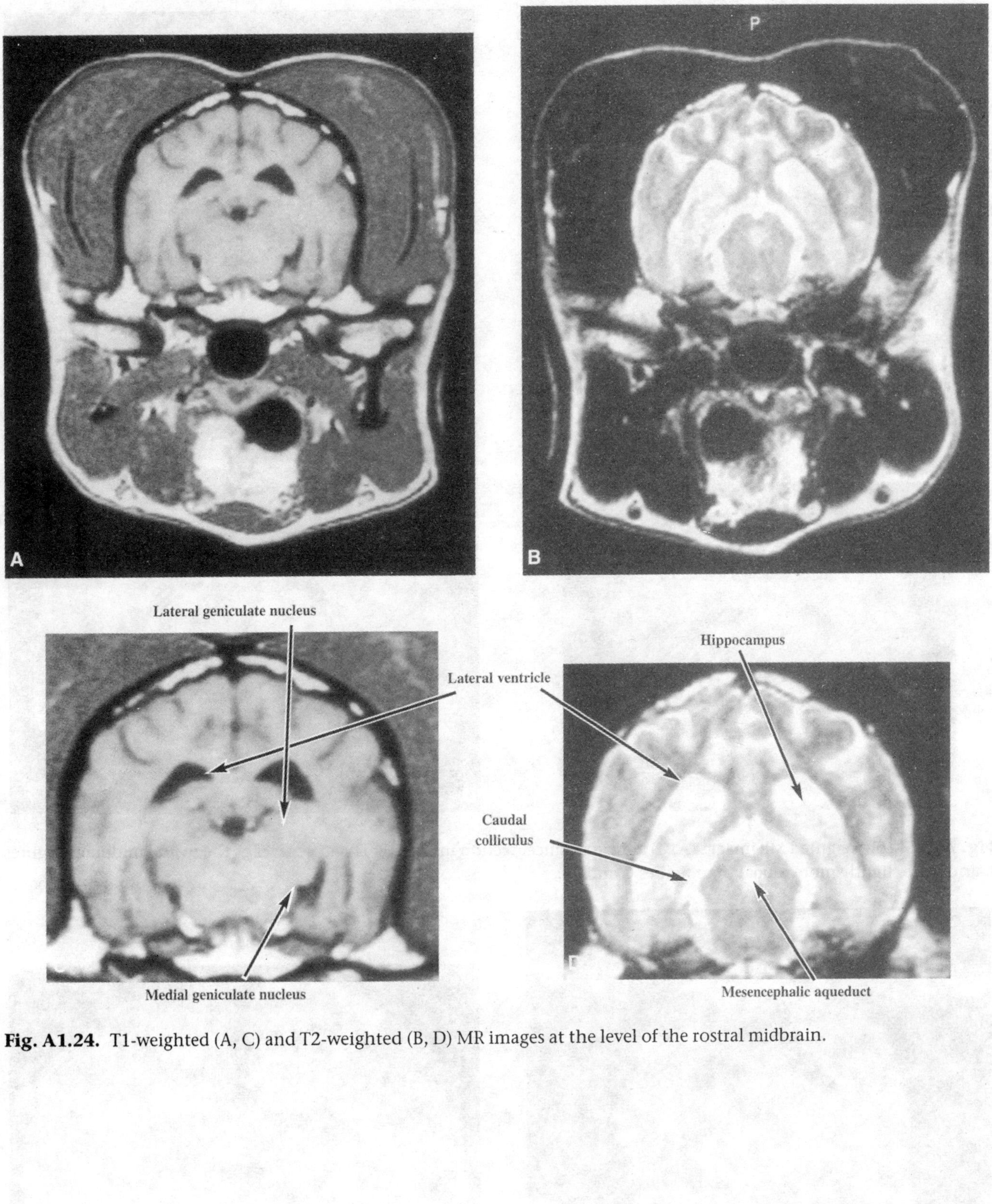

Fig. A1.24. T1-weighted (A, C) and T2-weighted (B, D) MR images at the level of the rostral midbrain.

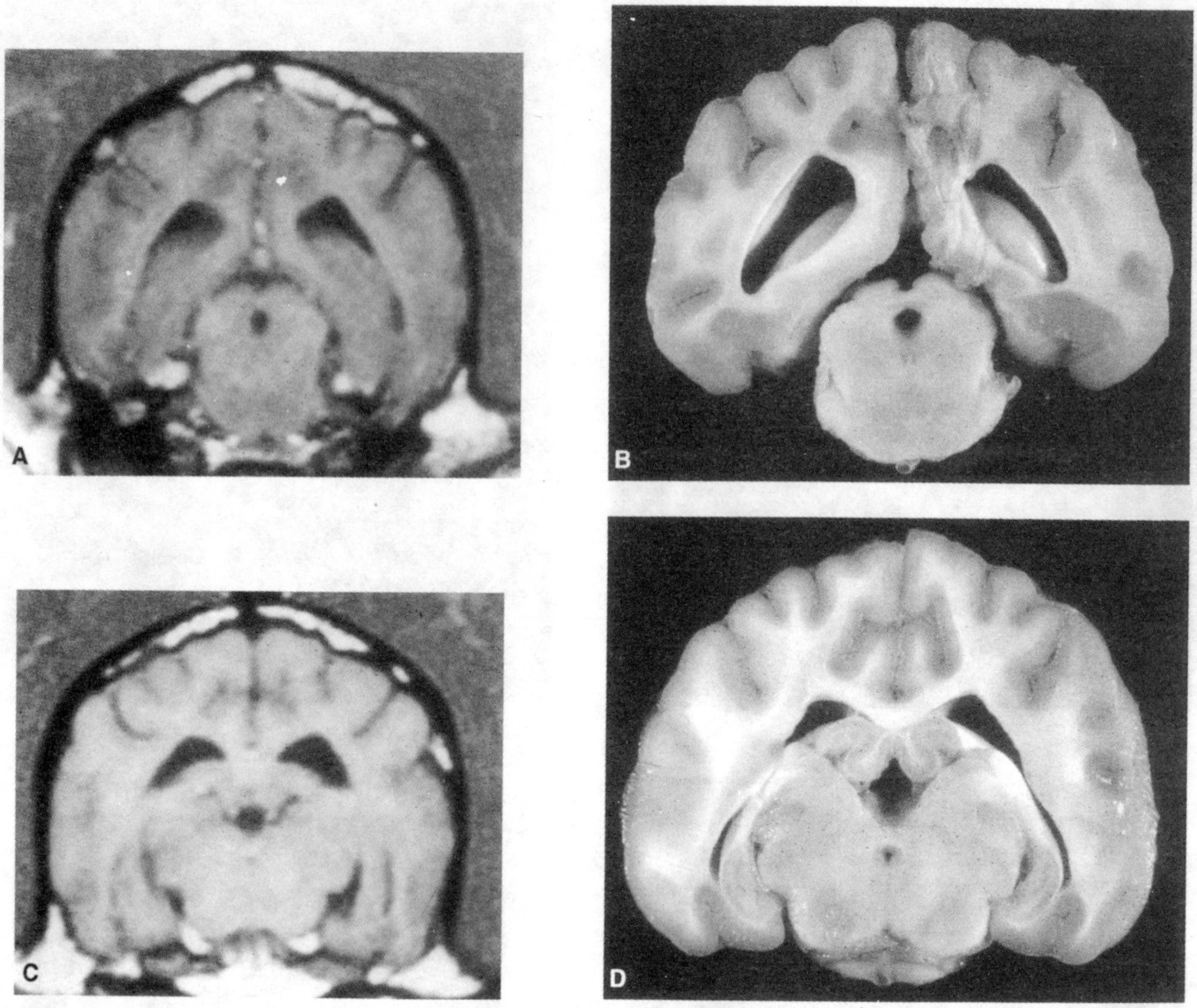

Fig. A1.25. T1-weighted MR images (A, C) and anatomical section images (B, D) at the level of the rostral midbrain (figures A and B are slightly more caudal than figures C and D).

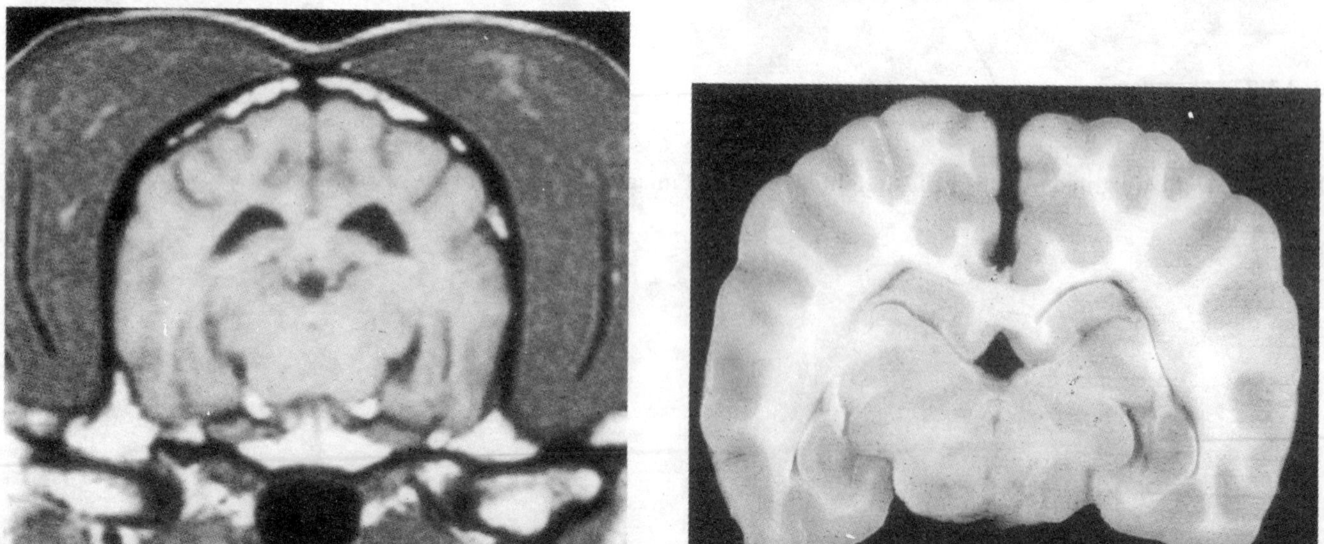

Fig. A1.26. T1-weighted MR image (A) and anatomical section (B) at the level of the caudal thalamus.

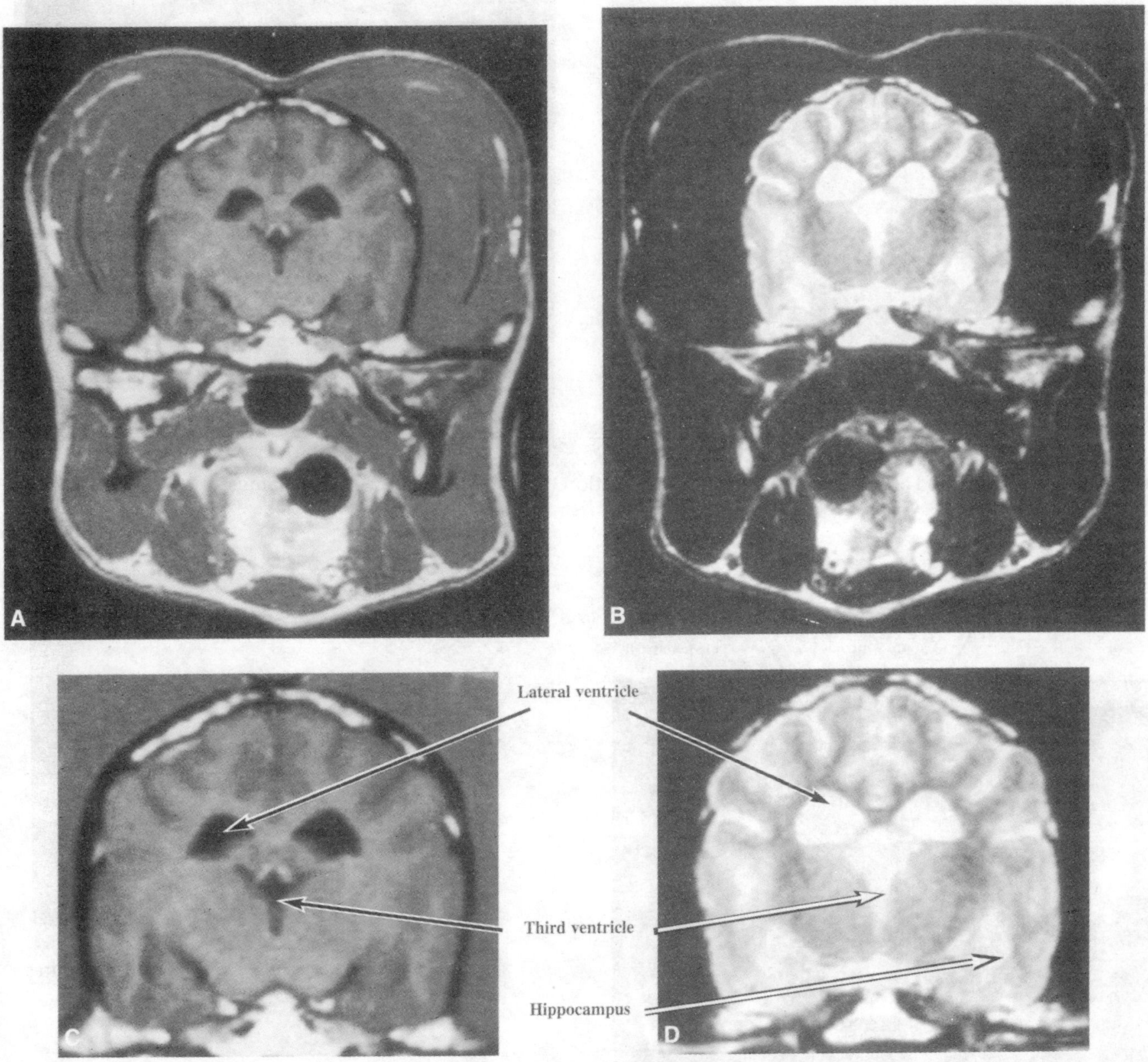

Fig. A1.27. T1-weighted (A, C) and T2-weighted (B, D) MR images at the level of the thalamus.

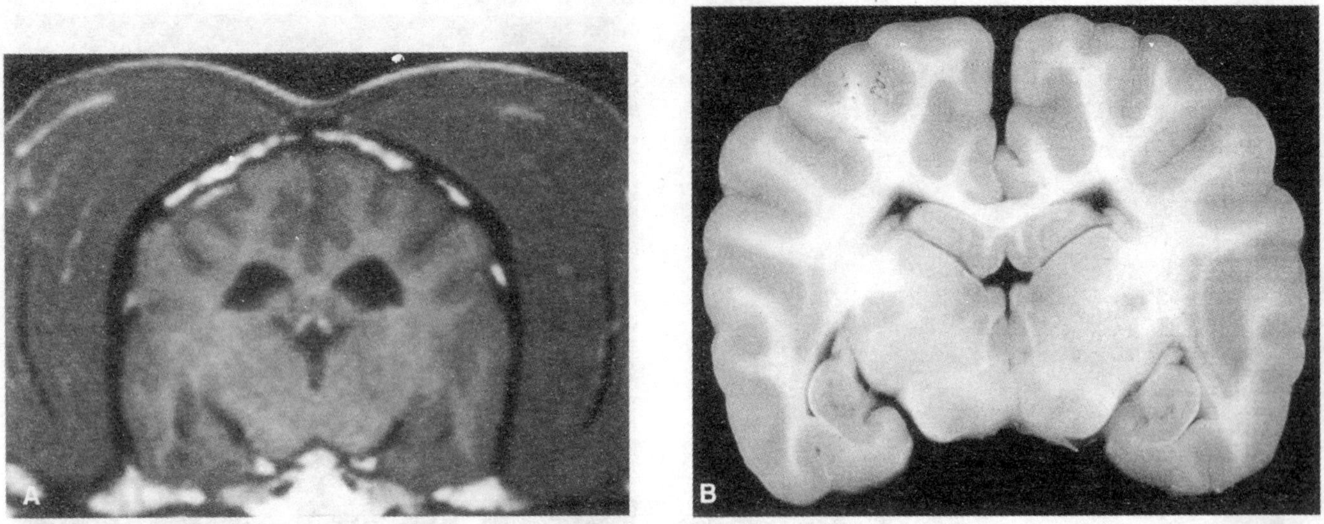

Fig. A1.28. T1-weighted MR image (A) and anatomical section (B) at the level of the mid thalamus.

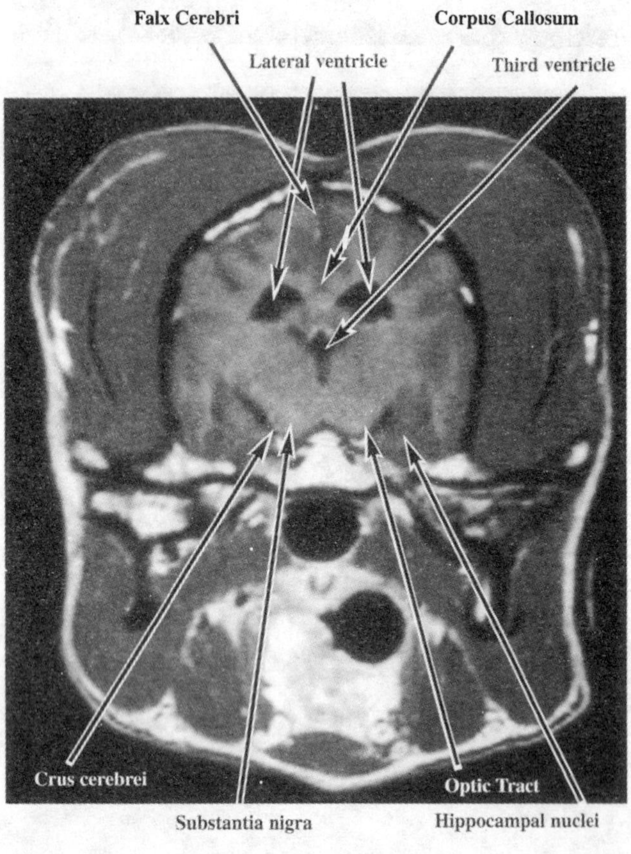

Fig. A1.29. T1-weighted MR image at the level of the thalamus.

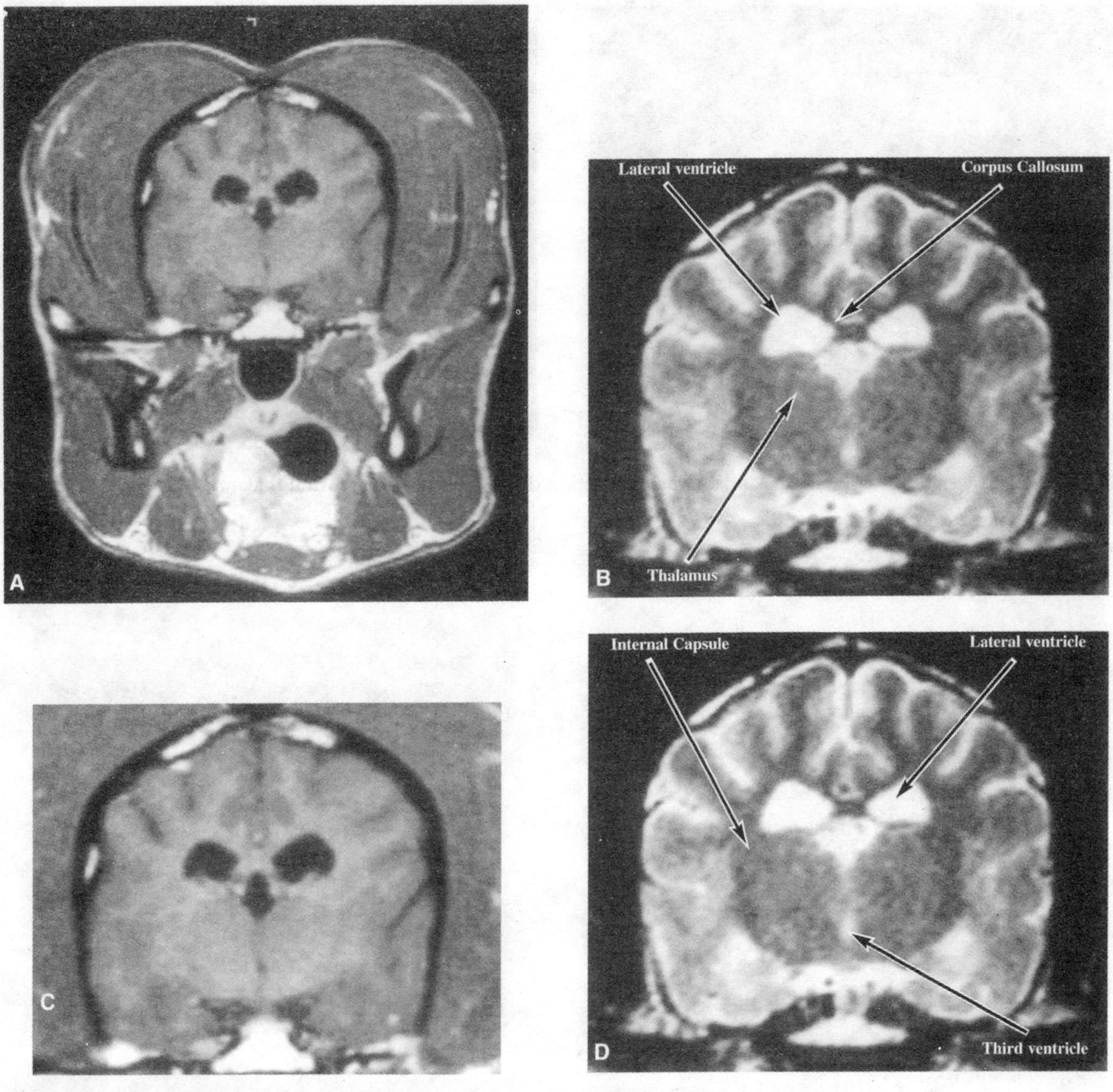

Fig. A1.30. T1-weighted (A, C) and T2-weighted (B, D) MR images at the level of the thalamus.

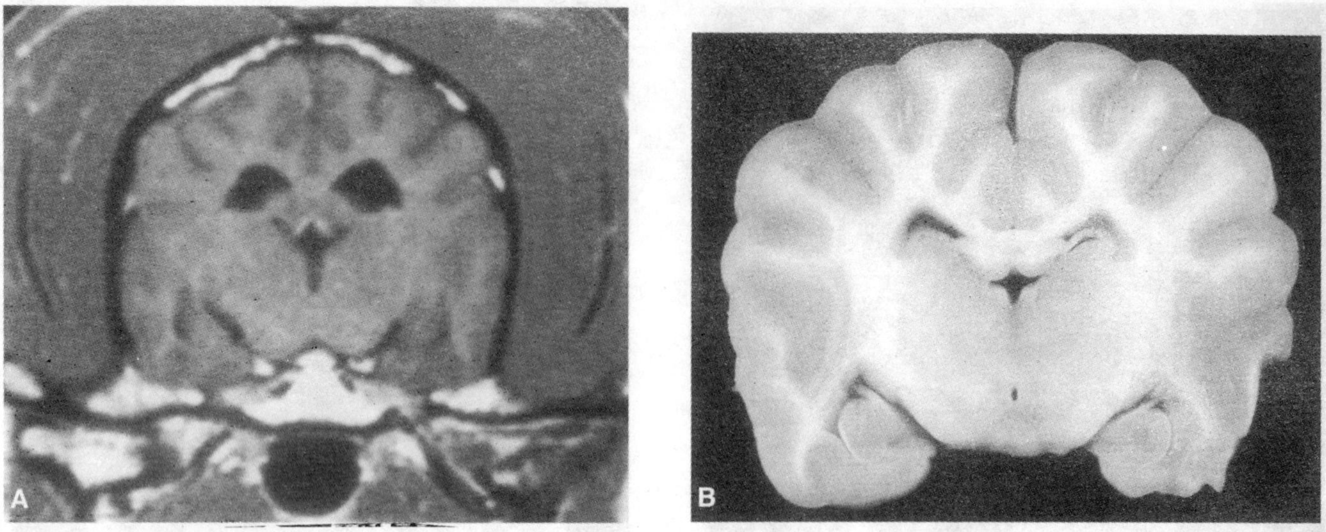

Fig. A1.31. T1-weighted MR image (A) and anatomical section (B) at the level of the rostral thalamus.

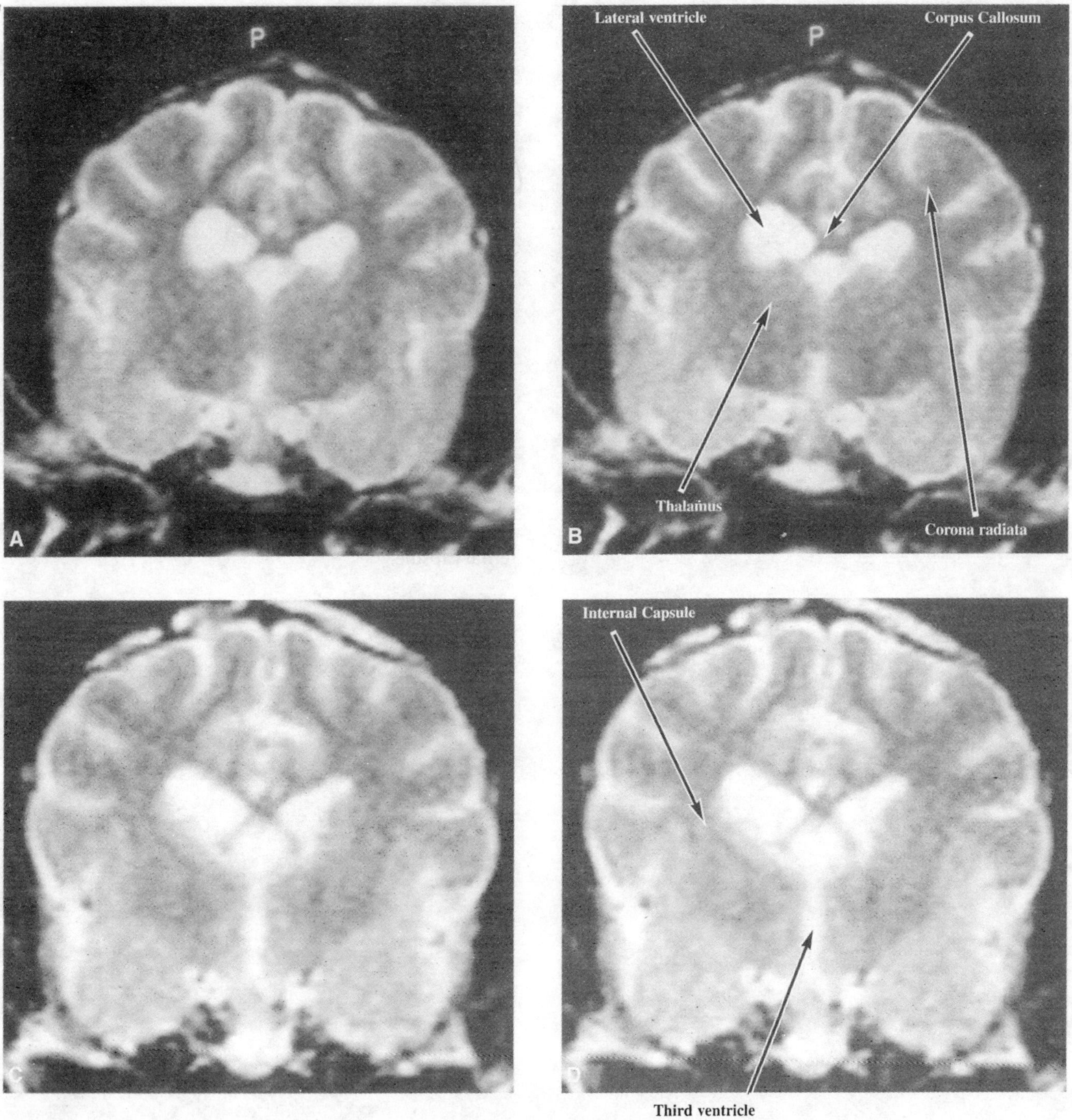

Fig. A1.32. T2-weighted (A–D) MR images at the level of the internal capsule.

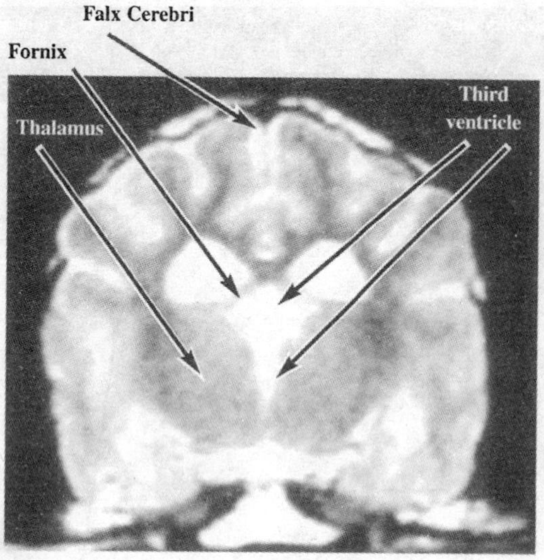

Fig. A1.33. T2-weighted MR image at the level of the thalamus.

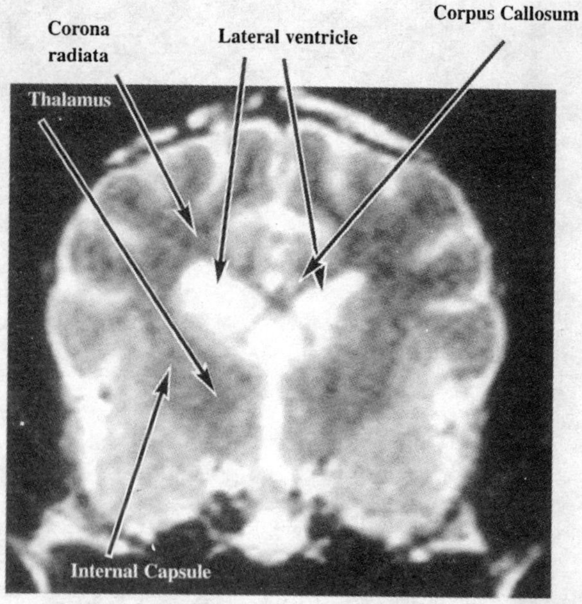

Fig. A1.34. T2-weighted MR image at the level of the internal capsule.

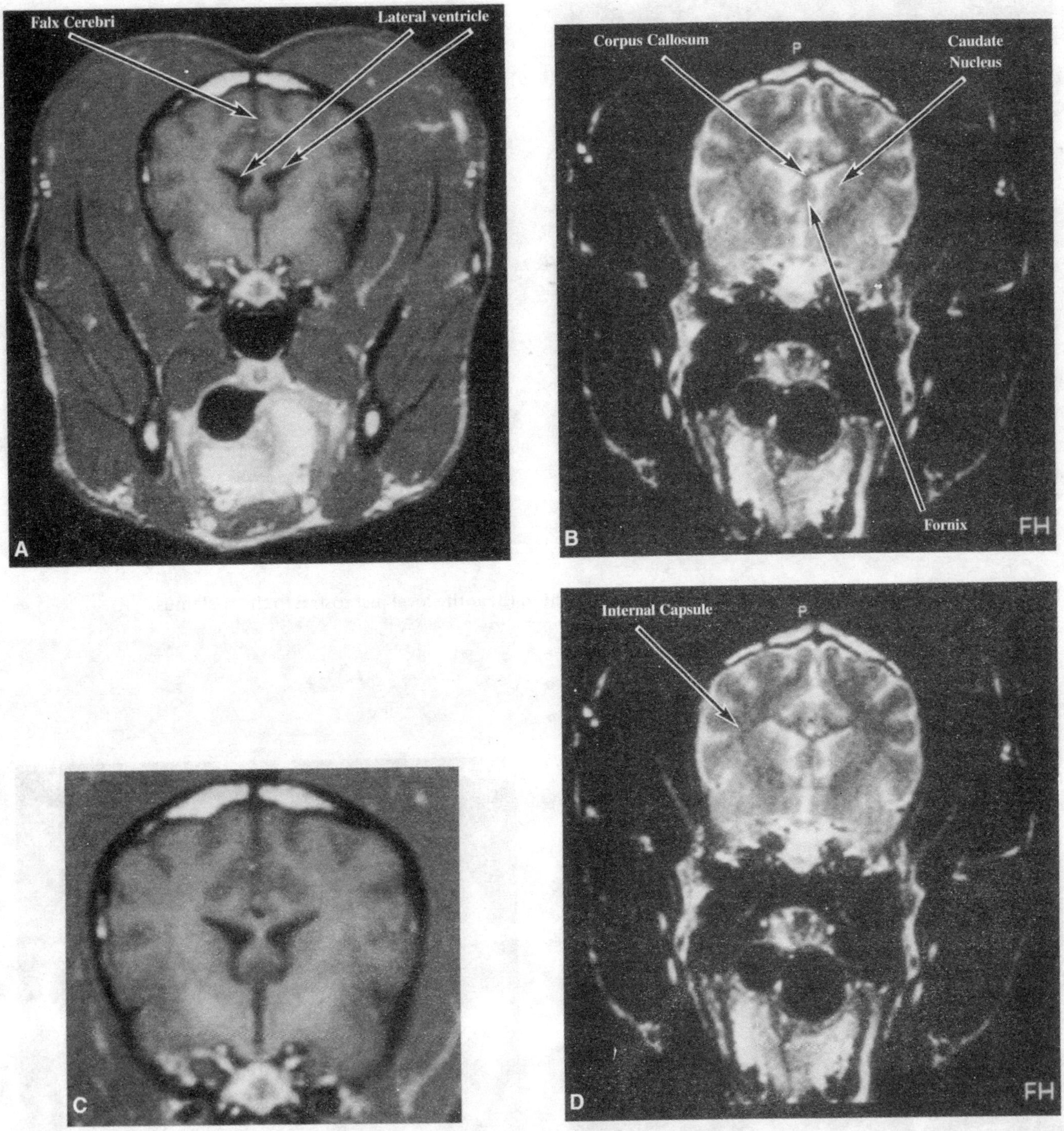

Fig. A1.35. T1-weighted (A, C) and T2-weighted (B, D) MR images at the level just rostral to the thalamus.

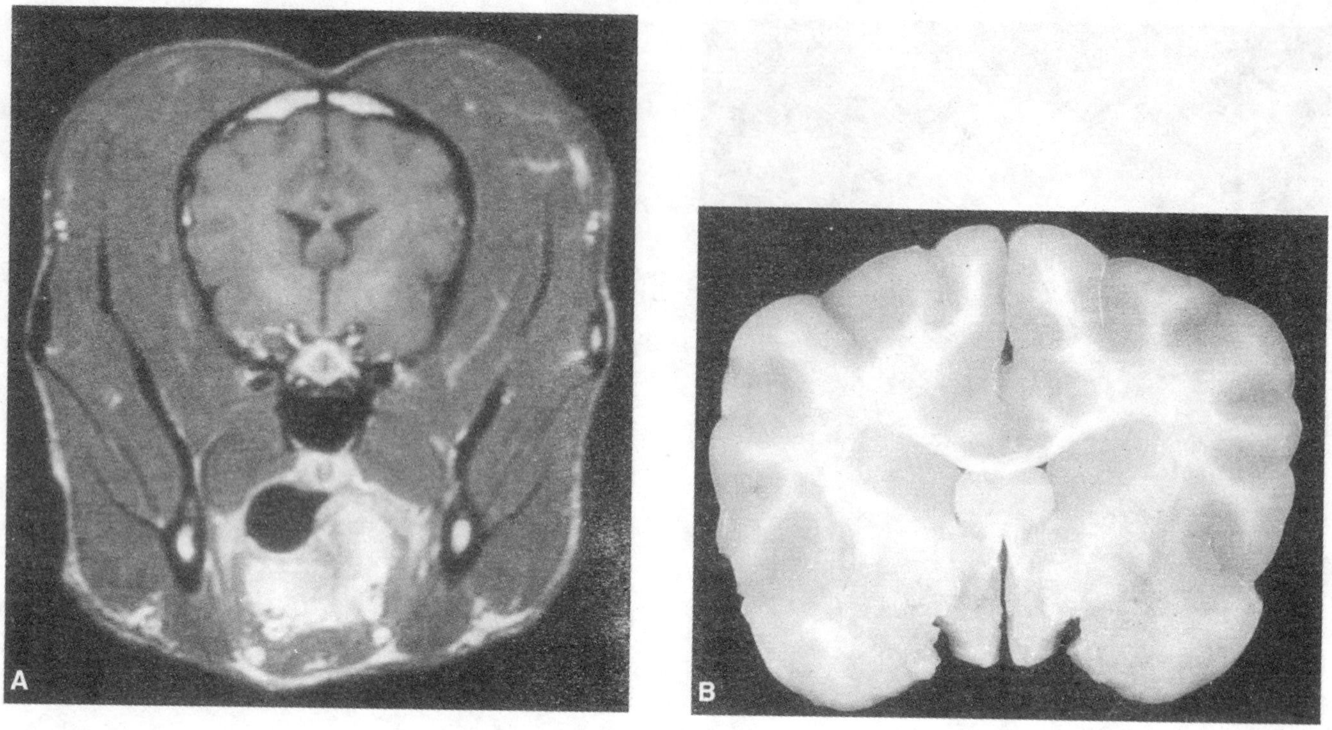

Fig. A1.36. T1-weighted MR image (A) and anatomical section (B) at the level just rostral to the thalamus.

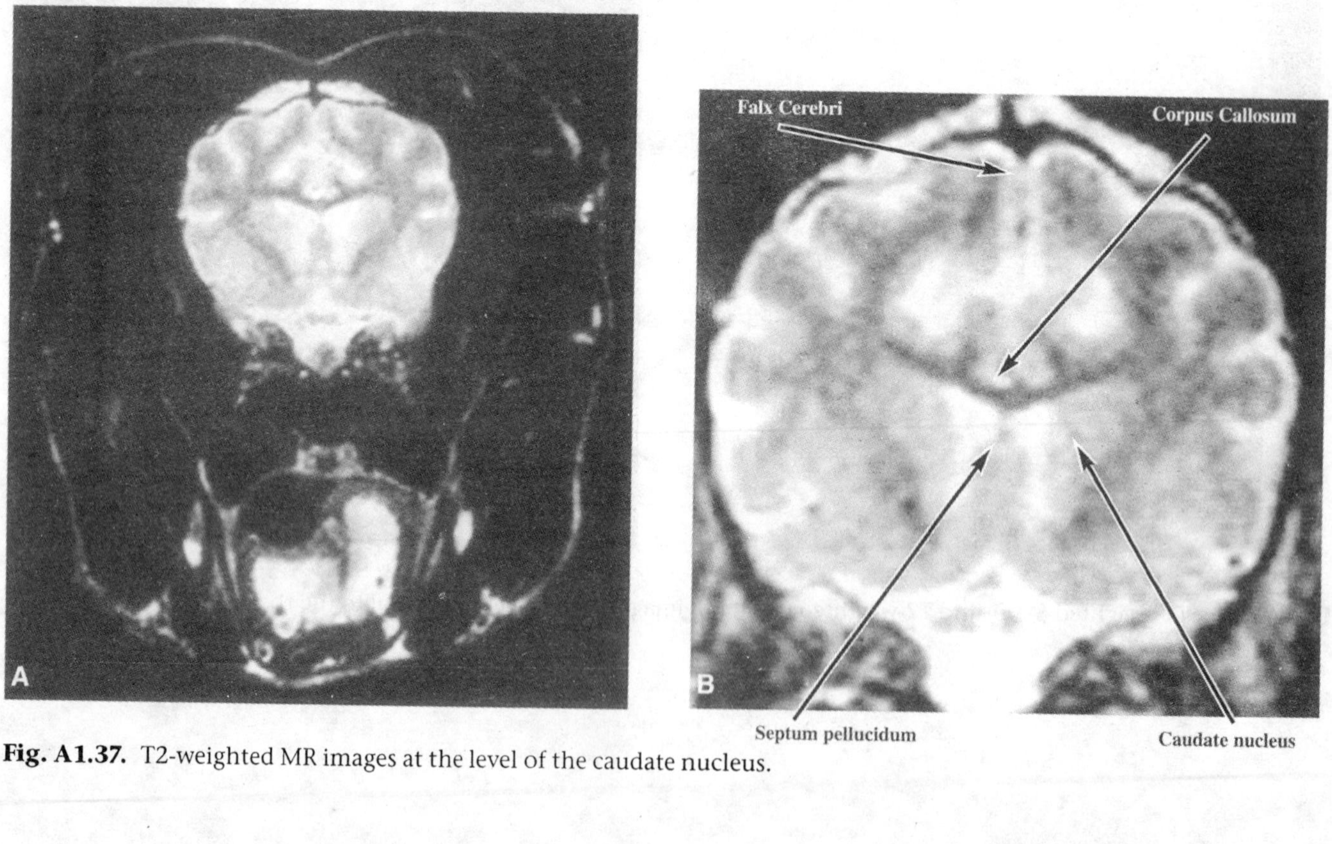

Fig. A1.37. T2-weighted MR images at the level of the caudate nucleus.

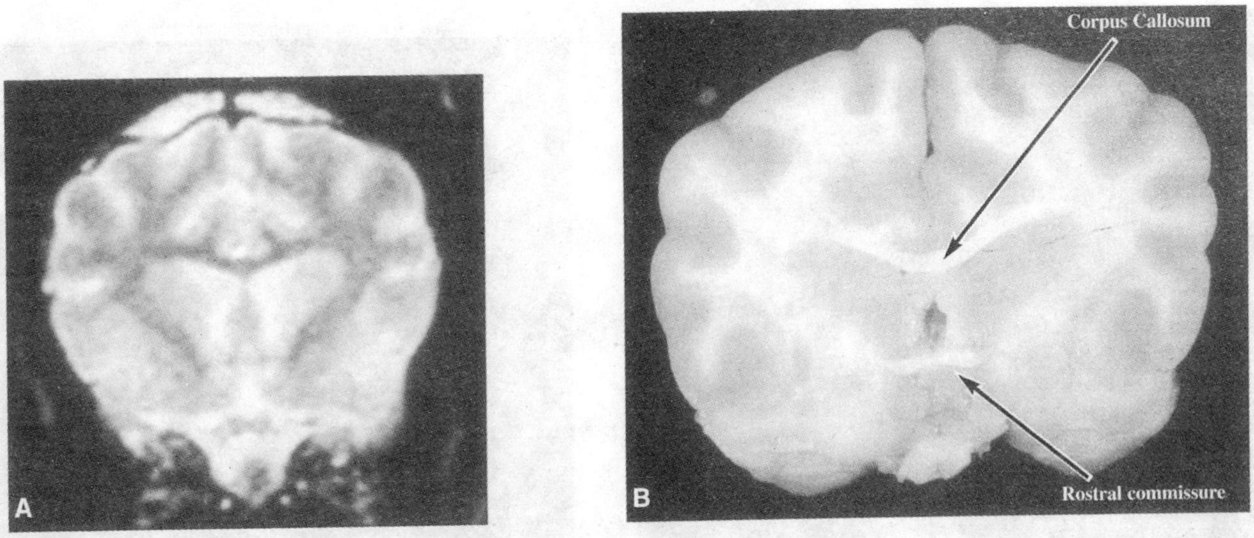

Fig. A1.38. T2-weighted MR image (A) and anatomical image (B) at the level of the rostral commissure.

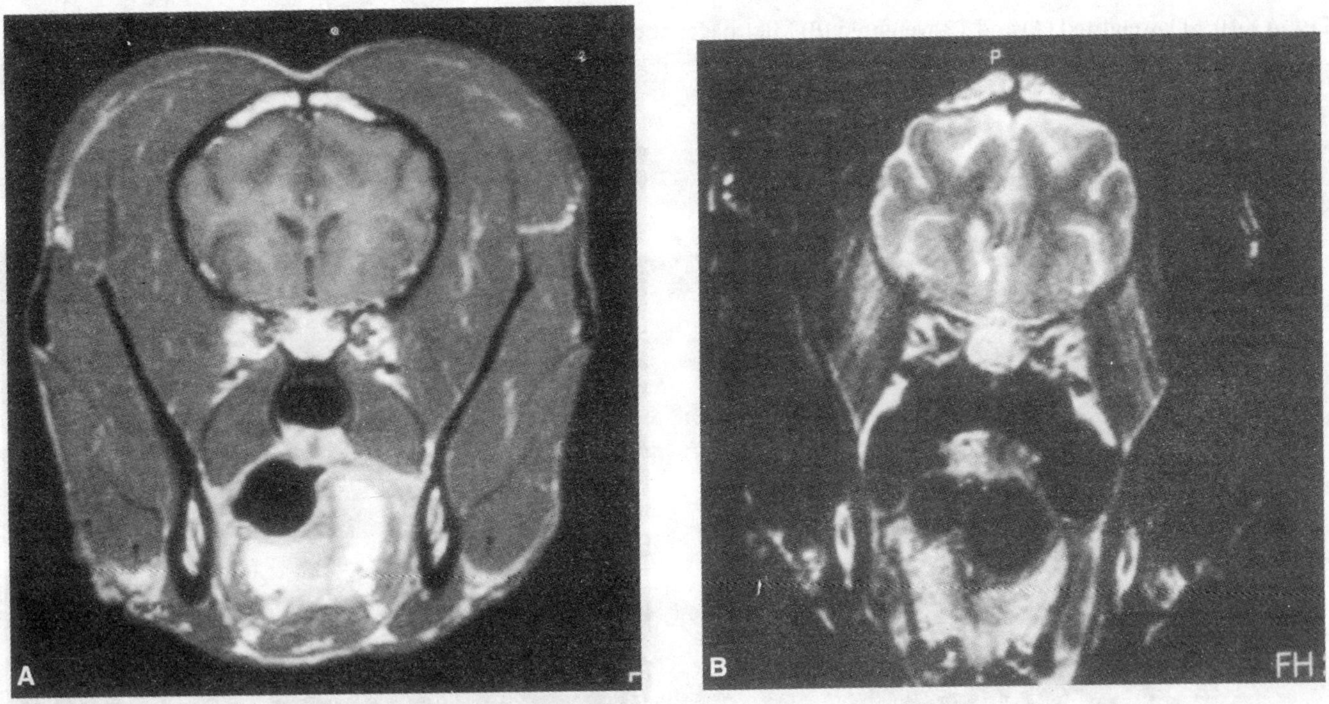

Fig. A1.39. T1-weighted (A) and T2-weighted (B) MR images at the level just rostral to the rostral commissure.

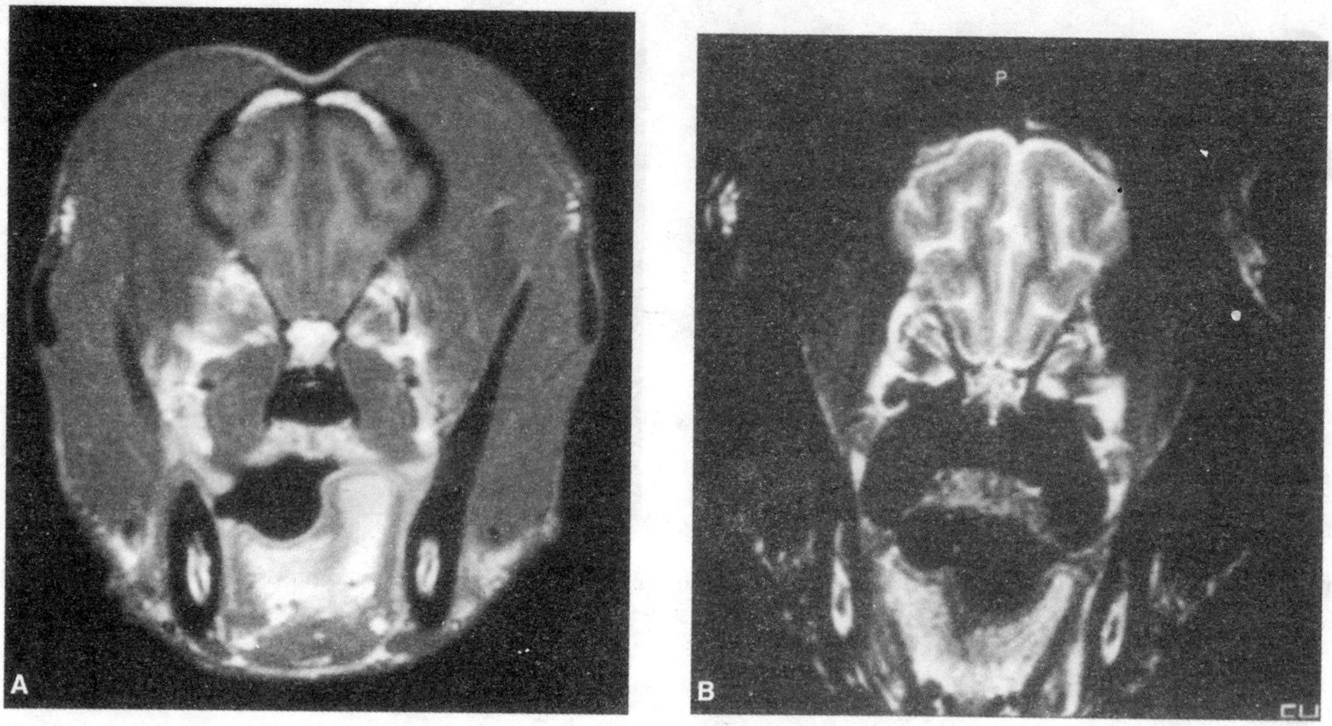

Fig. A1.40. T1-weighted (A) and T2-weighted (B) MR images at the level just rostral to A1.39.

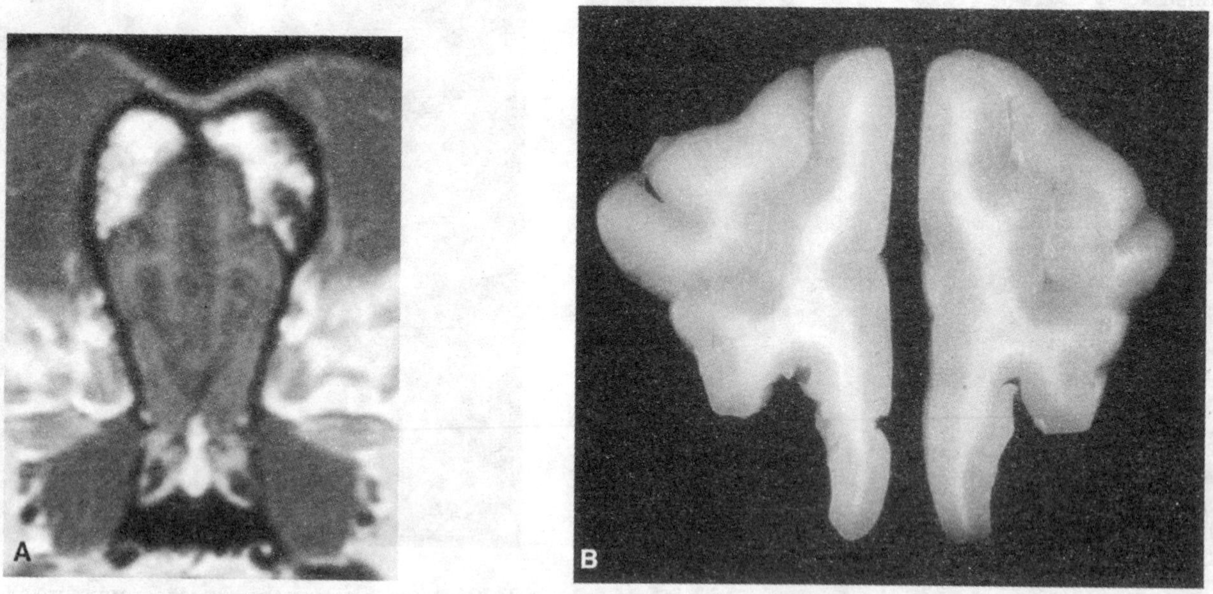

Fig. A1.41. T1-weighted anatomical images (A) and anatomical section (B) of the olfactory region.

2 Breed-Associated Neurologic Disease

Table A2.1. Common breed-associated neurological abnormalities of dogs

Breed	Abnormality
Afghan hound	Myelomalacia
	Narcolepsy/cataplexy
Airedale	Cerebellar degeneration
	Cerebellar hypoplasia
	Granulomatous meningoencephalomyelitis?
	Lumbosacral disease
Alaskan husky	Subacute necrotizing encephalopathy
Alaskan malamute	Mitochondrial encephalopathy
	Myelodysplasia
	Peripheral neuropathy
Australian cattle dogs	Ceroid lipofuscinosis
	Polioencephalomyelopathy
Australian kelpies	Cerebellar degeneration
Australian shepherd	Deafness
Basset hound	Cervical vertebral malformation
	Globoid cell leukodystrophy
	Glycoproteinosis
	Intervertebral disk disease
Bernese mountain Dog	Histiocytosis
	Hypomyelinogenesis
	Spinal cord vasculitis
Beagle	Bilateral peripheral vestibular disease
	Cerebellar cortical degeneration
	Globoid cell leukodystrophy
	Glycoproteinosis
	Idiopathic epilepsy
	Intervertebral disk disease (cervical)
	Narcolepsy
	Spinal cord vasculitis (Beagle pain syndrome)
Beagle mixed	Gangliosidosis GM_1
Belgian sheepdog	Congenital nystagmus
Belgian Tervuren	Idiopathic epilepsy
Belgian Malinois	Degenerative myelopathy
	Lumbosacral disease
	Neuronal degeneration
Bern running dog	Cerebellar degeneration
Bichon frise	Atlantoaxial subluxation
	Generalized tremors
Blue heeler	Ceroid lipofuscinosis
Blue tick hound	Globoid cell leukodystrophy
Border collie	Cerebellar degeneration
	Ceroid lipofuscinosis
	Deafness
Borzoi	Cervical vertebral malformation/Malarticulation
Boston terrier	Arachnoid cyst
	Cerebellar hypoplasia
	Hydrocephalus
	Vertebral anomalies
Bouvier des Flandres	Degenerative myopathy
	Laryngeal paralysis
Boxer	Dermoid sinus
	Primary brain tumor (glioma)
	Progressive axonopathy
Brittany spaniel	Cerebellar degeneration (late onset)
	Dystrophy-like myopathy
	Sensory ganglioradiculitis
	Spinal muscle atrophy
Bullmastiff	Cerebellar degeneration
	Cervical vertebral articular facet disease
Bull terrier	Cerebellar degeneration
	Deafness
	Laryngeal paralysis
Cairn terrier	Globoid cell leukodystrophy
	Multisystem neuronal degeneration
	Spinal muscle atrophy
Catahoula	Deafness
Cavalier King Charles spaniel	Fly-biting
	Episodic falling
	Chiari malformation
	Syringomyelia
Chesapeake Bay retriever	Distal polyneuropathy
	Laryngeal paralysis
Chihuahua	Atlantoaxial subluxation
	Ceroid lipofuscinosis
	Hydrocephalus
Chow chow	Arachnoid cyst
	Cerebellar hypoplasia
	Hypomyelination
	Myotonia
Clumber spaniel	Mitochondrial myopathy
Cocker spaniel	Ceroid lipofuscinosis
	Deafness
	Idiopathic facial nerve paralysis
	Intervertebral disk disease
	Multisystem neuronal degeneration
Collie (rough-coated)	Cerebellar abiotrophy
	Optic nerve hypoplasia
	Sensory trigeminal neuropathy
Collie (Scotch)	Deafness
	Dermatomyositis
	Distal polyneuropathy

(continued)

Table A2.1. Common breed-associated neurological abnormalities of dogs (*continued*)

Breed	Abnormality
Collie (sheepdog)	Neuroaxonal dystrophy
	Spinal muscle atrophy
Corgi	Degenerative myelopathy
	Intervertebral disk disease
Coton de Tulear dogs	Cerebellar disease
Dachshund	Ceroid lipofuscinosis
	Intervertebral disk disease
	Narcolepsy/cataplexy
	Myasthenia gravis
	Sensory neuropathy
Dachshund (dapple)	Deafness
Dachshund (long-haired)	Sensory neuropathy
Dalmatian	Cavitating leukodystrophy
	Ceroid lipofuscinosis
	Cramping syndrome
	Deafness
	Hypomyelination
	Laryngeal paralysis-polyneuropathy
	Wobbler syndrome
Doberman	Cervicalvertebral malformation/malarticulation
	Congenital vestibular disease
	Dancing Doberman syndrome
	Deafness
	Idiopathic head tremor
	Narcolepsy/cataplexy
	Sensory neuropathy
English bulldog	Head tremor
	Hemivertebra
	Spina bifida
	Sacrococcygeal malformation
English Cocker spaniel	Congenital peripheral vestibular abnormality
English pointer	Sensory neuropathy (self-mutilation)
	Motorneuron degeneration
English setter	Ceroid lipofuscinosis
	Deafness
English Springer spaniel	Muscular dystrophy
Finnish harrier	Cerebellar degeneration
Foxhound (English)	Hound ataxia
Fox terrier	Congenital vestibular disease
	Deafness
	Hereditary ataxia
Gammel Dansk honsehund	Myasthenia gravis
German shepherd	Calcinosis circumscripta
	Congenital vestibular disease
	Deafness
	Degenerative myelopathy
	Fibrotic myopathy
	Giant axonal neuropathy
	Intervertebral disk disease
	Lumbosacral instability/stenosis
	Masticatory myositis
	Motorneuron degeneration
	Multiple cartilaginous exostosis
	Spinal cord blastoma (neuroepithelioma)
German short-haired pointer	Hemivertebrae
	Gangliosidosis GM_2
	Pyogranulomatous meningoencephalomyelitis
Golden retriever	Eosinophilic meningitis(?)
	Extraocular polymyositis
	Hypomyelination polyneuropathy
	Muscular dystrophy
	Primary brain tumor (meningioma)
Gordon setter	Cerebellar degeneration
Great Dane	Corelike myopathy
	Distal symmetrical polyneuropathy
	Fibrocartilaginous emboli
	Disseminated idiopathic skeletal hyperostosis
	Myotonia
	Optic nerve hypoplasia
	Exertional myopathy
Harriers	Myelopathy
Hounds	Polyradiculoneuritis
	Hound ataxia (United Kingdom)
Ibizan hound	Deafness
Irish setter	Cerebellar hypoplasia
	Hereditary quadriplegia and amblyopia
	Idiopathic epilepsy
	Laryngeal paralysis
	Lissencephaly
Irish terrier	Muscular dystrophy
Irish wolfhound	Cervicalvertebral malformation/malarticulation
Jack Russell terrier	Congenital myasthenia gravis
	Hereditary ataxia
	Sensory neuropathy
Japanese Akita	Deafness
	Congenital vestibular disease (bilateral)
Japanese chin	Atlantoaxial subluxation
Keeshond	Idiopathic epilepsy
Kerry blue terrier	Cerebellar abiotrophy
Kooiker dogs (Dutch)	Hereditary necrotizing myelopathy
Kuvasz	Deafness
Labrador retriever	Central axonopathy
	Cerebellar degeneration
	Distal polyneuropathy
	Fibrinoid encephalomyelopathy
	Hereditary myopathy
	Myotonia
	Narcolepsy/cataplexy
	Reflex myoclonus
	Spongiform degeneration
Lapland dogs	Glycogenesis type II
Leonberger dogs	Polyneuropathy and laryngeal paralysis
Lhasa Apso	Hydrocephalus
	Lissencephaly
Lurcher hound	Hypomyelination
Malinois shepherd	Spongiform encephalopathy
Maltese terrier	Generalized tremor syndrome
	Hydrocephalus
	Necrotizing meningoencephalitis
Malamute	Multiple cartilaginous exostosis
	Neuropathy
Mastiff	Cerebellar disease
	Cervical stenosis
	Neuronal degeneration
Miniature pinscher	Generalized tremors
	Mucopolysaccharidosis
Mongrel	Myasthenia-like syndrome
Norwich terrier	Cramping syndrome
Nova Scotia duck trolling retrievers	Meningitis syndrome
Old English sheepdog	Cerebellar degeneration
	Deafness
	Mitochondrial myopathy
Papillon	Deafness
	Neuroaxonal dystrophy
Pekingese	Atlantoaxial Subluxation
	Hydrocephalus

Table A2.1. Common breed-associated neurological abnormalities of dogs (*continued*)

Breed	Abnormality
	Intervertebral disk disease
	Optic nerve hypoplasia
Plott hound	Mucopolysaccharidosis
Poodle (miniature)	Atlantoaxial subluxation
	Cerebellar and cerebral cortical degeneration
	Demyelinating myelopathy
	Fibrinoid encephalomyelopathy
	Glycoproteinosis
	Intervertebral disk disease
	Narcolepsy/cataplexy
	Optic nerve hypoplasia
	Sacrococcygeal dysgenesis
	Sphingomyelinosis
Poodle (Toy)	Atlantoaxial subluxation
	Hydrocephalus
Pomeranian	Atlantoaxial subluxation
	Globoid cell leukodystrophy
	Hydrocephalus
Portuguese water dogs	Gangliosidosis GM_1
Pug	Arachnoid cysts
	Pug encephalitis
	Spinal scarring
Rhodesian ridgeback	Dermoid sinus
	Myotonia-like syndrome
Rottweiler	Aplasia of the dens
	Arachnoid cysts
	Deafness
	Distal sensorimotor polyneuropathy
	Laryngeal paralysis-polyneuropathy
	Leukoencephalomyelopathy
	Motorneuron degeneration
	Neuroaxonal Dystrophy
	Neuronal Vacuolation
Russian wolfhound	Optic nerve hypoplasia
Saluki	Ceroid lipofuscinosis
	Spinal muscle atrophy
Samoyed	Cerebellar atrophy
	Hypomyelination
	Lissencephaly
	Myopathy
	Myotonia
	Spongiform degeneration
Saint Bernard	Idiopathic epilepsy
	Narcolepsy/cataplexy
Schnauzer (giant)	Narcolepsy/cataplexy
Schnauzer (miniature)	Fibrocartilaginous emboli
	Hyperlipidemia (seizures)
	Idiopathic adipsia
	Idiopathic epilepsy
	Intervertebral disk disease
	Muscular dystrophy
	Myotonia
Scottish terrier	Cerebellar degeneration
	Fibrinoid encephalomyelopathy
	Scotty cramp
Sealyham terrier	Deafness
Shar pei	Megaesophagus
Sheltie	Dermatomyositis
	Hyperlipidemia (seizures)
Shetland Sheepdog	Leukodystrophy
Shih Tzu	Atlantoaxial subluxation
	Dermoid sinus
	Intervertebral disk disease
Shropshire terrier	Deafness
Siberian husky	Cerebellar agenesis
	Degenerative myelopathy
	Laryngeal paralysis
	Sensory neuropathy
Silky terrier	Myopathy
	Spongiform degeneration
Spitz	Generalized tremor
Smooth coated fox terrier	Congenital myasthenia gravis
	Hereditary Ataxia
Springer spaniel	Congenital myasthenia gravis
	Fucosidosis
	Hypomyelination
Staffordshire terrier	Myotonia
	Cerebellar degeneration
Standard poodle	Polymicrogyria and Hydrocephalus
Sussex spaniel	Mitochondrial myopathy
Swedish Lapland	Glycogenesis type II
	Motorneuron degeneration
Sydney Silky terrier	Glucocerebrosidosis
Tibetan mastiff	Hypertrophic neuropathy
Walker hound	Mononeuropathy
Weimaraner	Hypomyelination
	Spinal dysraphism
Welsh Pembroke corgi	Intervertebral disk disease
	Muscular dystrophy
	Narcolepsy/cataplexy
West highland white terrier	Globoid cell leukodystrophy
Whippet	Sensory ganglioradiculitis
Wire-haired fox terrier	Cerebellar hypoplasia
	Deafness
	Lissencephaly
Wire-haired griffon	Narcolepsy/cataplexy
Yorkshire terrier	Atlantoaxial subluxation
	Hepatic encephalopathy (portosystemic shunt)
	Hydrocephalus
	Intervertebral disk disease
	Microvascular dysplasia (liver)
	Multiple cartilaginous exostosis
	Necrotizing encephalitis
Yugoslavian sheepdog	Ceroid lipofuscinosis

Note: Also see storage diseases discussed in chapter 5.

Table A2.2. Breed-associated neurological abnormalities of cats

Breed	Abnormality	Breed	Abnormality
Abyssinian	Myasthenia gravis	Egyptian Mau	Spongiform encephalopathy
Balinese	Sphingomyelinosis	Himalayan	Fibrotic myopathy
Birman	Distal polyneuropathy	Korat	Gangliosidosis GM1
	Spongiform encephalopathy	Manx	Sacrococcygeal dysgenesis
Burmese	Congenital vestibular disease	Norwegian Forest cats	Glycogenosis type IV
	Deafness	Persian	Mannosidosis
Domestic short-haired	Ceroid lipofuscinosis	Rex	Myopathy
	Gangliosidosis GM1	Siamese	Ceroid lipofuscinosis
	Gangliosidosis GM_2		Congenital strabismus/nystagmus
	Globoid cell leukodystrophy		Congenital visual pathway abnormal
	Glycogenesis type II		Deafness
	Hyperoxaluria		Gangliosidosis GM_1
	Mannosidosis		Hyperchylomicronemia
	Metachromatic leukodystrophy		Mucopolysaccharidosis
	Mucopolysaccharidosis		Myasthenia gravis
	Muscular dystrophy		Peripheral vestibular disease
	Myasthenia gravis		Sphingomyelinosis
	Spinal muscle atrophy		Spinal muscular atrophy
Domestic tricolor	Neuroaxonal dystrophy	Somali	Myasthenia gravis

Note: Also see storage diseases discussed in chapter 5.

3 Anticonvulsants in Dogs and Cats

See chapter 17. See also Bibliography under Intracranial Diseases, Idiopathic Diseases, Seizures.

STANDARD ANTICONVULSANTS

Phenobarbital

- Barbiturate-derivative
- Most commonly used anticonvulsant

Pharmacokinetics

- T 1/2 = 47–74 hours in most mongrel dogs. The T 1/2 in beagles is 25–38 hours (elimination proceeds at almost double the rate of other dogs); T 1/2 = 34–43 hours in cat.
- Bioavailability of oral phenobarbital is 88–95% (GI disease may interfere).
- Human beings: 70–90% absorbed after oral dose.
- 45% is protein bound in serum, slightly less than in humans.
  When given for longer periods of time, half-lives will decline.
- Maximum concentrations are observed 4 to 8 hours after oral administration, although food delays peak concentrations by an additional 2–4 hours.
- Ratio of CSF:plasma phenobarbital concentrations is 0.53; ratio of CSF:saliva is 0.39 (salivary concentration indicates unbound drug).
- Rate of entry from blood into CSF is 0.042/min.

Metabolism

- Metabolized to parahydroxyphenobarbital, which is renally excreted.
- Primarily through metabolism of hepatic microsomal enzymes, although up to 25% of the drug is eliminated by pH-dependent renal excretion of unchanged drug.
- Glucuronidation is not an important mechanism of elimination, and therefore cats do not appear to metabolize this drug differently than dogs.
- Metabolism increased with use due to hepatic enzyme induction (cytochrome P_{450}; occurs primarily in periportal regions rather than perivenous regions in liver.

Mechanism of Action

- Shortens the duration of electrically induced afterdischarges and increases the threshold of normal brain structures to afterdischarges.
- Increases responsiveness to inhibitory postsynaptic GABA-ergic interneurons by increasing Cl^- conductance into the cell and by reducing glutamate-induced depolarization of excitatory neurons.
- Blocks presynaptic entry of Ca^{+2} into nerve terminals, which results in diminished Ca^{+2}-induced neurotransmitter release into the synapse (inhibits calmodulin-dependent protein kinase).
- May have antiglutamate effects.
- Decreases cerebral blood flow and cerebral metabolism.
- With local acidosis, more phenobarbital becomes unionized and concentrates at the site of discharge.
- Summary: Suppresses epileptogenic foci discharges and inhibits kindling; decreases neuronal excitability and increases the action potential threshold to electrical stimulus.

Dosage and Monitoring

- Dosages vary depending on author; 2–4 mg/kg orally every 12 hours, initial dose.
- Serum concentrations more closely correlated with therapeutic benefit than administered dose. Therapeutic levels of 20–40 μg/ml have been suggested to maximize seizure control while minimizing side effects. Trough levels historically correlated better with therapeutic outcome than peak levels, however, this may not be as significant as initially thought.
- When changing from primidone to phenobarbital, give 65 mg phenobarbital/250 mg primidone.

Interactions, Side Effects, and Toxicity

- Toxicity signs: drowsiness/sedation, ataxia, PU/PD/PP, nystagmus, restlessness or hyperexcitability, drug rash, hyperprothrombinemia, blood dyscrasias, and osteomalacia.
- PU is thought to be due to central inhibition of ADH release.

- PP is believed to result from suppression of the satiety center in the ventromedial hypothalamus.
- Phenobarbital has been shown to induce coagulation defects in cats by reducing vitamin K-dependent clotting factors (II, VII, IX, X).
- Phenobarbital is displaced by sulfonamides and salicylates, and may increase the metabolism of many drugs. Does not alter digoxin levels.
- Chloramphenicol decreases metabolism of phenobarbital and can cause severe depression, sedation, and coma.
- Decreases T_4 (due to increased biliary excretion and possibly an increase in deiodination of T_4).
- Liver enzyme elevations may take 5 weeks up to 7 months to return to normal after D/Cing this drug.

Emergency Situations: Status Epilepticus

- Phenobarbital at 12–16 mg/kg IV (loading) in dog that has never been on phenobarbital prior.
- 2–4 mg/kg phenobarbital q 20 minutes IM or IV (requires 20 minutes to see full effect of the given dose).

Potassium Bromide

Metabolism

- Rapidly absorbed from small intestine.
- Not protein bound or metabolized.
- Slowly excreted in urine.
- Due to its lack of metabolism, ideal anticonvulsant for dogs with hepatotoxicity.

Mechanism of Action

- Not known; neuronal hyperpolarization and Cl^- channel alterations probable.
- Br actively transported across the choroid plexus.

Dosage and Monitoring

- Optimal dose not known.
- Dosage of 20–60 mg/kg PO q 24 hours (divided BID).
- If sodium bromide is used, the dosage is slightly reduced at 17 to 30 mg/kg/day.
- Achieve a therapeutic blood level of 1–3 mg/ml.
- Requires 2–3 weeks before bromide blood levels will enter the therapeutic range and 9 weeks before steady state concentrations are approximated.
- T 1/2 of bromide is 25 days, takes 4 months to reach full steady state.
- If seizure control is needed more rapidly, can give loading dose of 400–600 mg/kg orally, which will achieve serum bromide levels of 1–1.5 mg/ml. Give this dose over a 2 to 4 day period to avoid vomiting due to high osmolarity and potassium content.

Interactions, Side Effects, and Toxicity

- Acute toxicity includes vomiting, anorexia, constipation, sedation, and incoordination.
- Sedation likely with levels 1.5 mg/ml or higher.
- Chronic toxicity in human manifested by skin rash, neurological disturbances, and GI signs.
- Sodium losing states, i.e., dehydration and diarrhea reduce the therapeutic index.
- Fatal asthma possible in cats.

Diazepam

- Benzodiazepine
- Crosses the BBB faster than any anticonvulsant.

Metabolism

- Primarily demethylation to nordiazepam (desmethyldiazepam) and oxazepam.
- Metabolites have 25–33% of diazepam's anticonvulsant activity.
- Due to extensive first pass effect, oral systemic availability is only 1–3%.
- Serum T 1/2 is 3.2 hours.
- Serum protein binding is 96%.
- Tachyphylaxis is noted with repeated doses of benzodiazepines probably due to a feedback- regulated increase in benzodiazepine receptors or a decreased production of GABA.

Mechanism of Action

- Bind to benzodiazepine receptors causing allosteric changes that facilitate binding of GABA to its receptor.
- This opens Cl^- channel, allowing for Cl^- influx and enhanced inhibition of the postsynaptic neuron.

Dosages and Monitoring

- 1–2 mg/kg IV for acute seizure.
- In cats, as a PO anticonvulsant, 1–2 mg TID.
- Tolerance occurs within one week of dosing.
- Can be used as a continuous infusion at 5–20 mg/hour IV.
- May be associated with liver dysfunction in cats.
- Cautious use in animals with liver dysfunction.

Interactions, Side Effects, and Toxicity

- Acute toxicity includes drowsiness, lethargy, and CNS depression.
- T 1/2 of diazepam and nordiazepam are prolonged by drugs such as cimetidine that inhibit hepatic microsomal enzymes.

HISTORICAL ANTICONVULSANTS

Primidone

- 2-deoxybarbiturate

Metabolism

- Rapidly oxidized to phenobarbital and phenylethylmalonamide (PEMA) by microsomal enzymes in liver.

- Phenobarbital contributes 85% of the anticonvulsant activity due to its prolonged T 1/2.
- Relative percentages of metabolites at steady state concentrations are: phenobarbital, 64.6%; PEMA, 33.6%; primidone, 1.8%.

Mechanism of Action

- Effectiveness of primidone correlates better with serum phenobarbital concentration (correlation with primidone or PEMA and primidone dose is poor) T 1/2 of PEMA and primidone is 10–14 hours.
- Only 1 in 15 dogs in one study that were refractory to phenobarbital benefited from primidone.

Dosage and Monitoring

- 30–55 mg/kg/day divided TID. Others have recommended somewhat lower dosages of 10–15 mg/kg/d and 15/30 mg/kg/d divided B to TID.
- Adjustments in dose made on basis of serum phenobarbital levels.
- Cats: Has not been approved, and one initial study suggested it is toxic to cats.
- Recent work suggests that cats metabolize the drug differently than dogs (unmetabolized primidone attained higher serum concentrations than phenobarbital and had a T 1/2 of 7 H, at a dose of 40 mg/kg/day).

Interactions, Side Effects, and Toxicity

- Acute toxicity includes sedation, ataxia, PU/PD, nystagmus, profound tachycardia, episodic hyperventilation, and anorexia.
- Hepatotoxicity associated with the duration rather than daily dose.
- Histopathological changes after 6 months of therapy include hepatocellular hypertrophy and necrosis, lipidosis, and extramedullary hematopoiesis. If medication is discontinued after this time, these changes will result in hepatic fibrosis with some permanent loss of function.
- Primidone intoxication is associated with concurrent use of chloramphenicol.
- Dermatitis associated with the use of primidone in a dog and excessive licking of paws.
  - Alopecia, pruritus, scaling, pigmentation, and ulceration over back, elbows, hocks, face, and ears.
  - Biopsy: severe diffuse parakeratotic hyperkeratosis of epidermis and hair follicles, frequently associated with epidermal hyperplasia, dyskeratosis, and intracellular vacuolation; hint of anti-IgG staining.

Phenytoin

Metabolism

- In human beings, degraded to parahydroxy metabolites that have a T 1/2 of 22 hours. In dogs, metabolized primarily to a metahydroxy metabolite that has a T 1/2 of 4 hours.
- Biotransformation takes place in microsomal enzymes in liver.
- Stimulates its own degradation.
- Oral bioavailability is 40% in dogs.
- Phenytoin eliminated very slowly in cats. T 1/2 is 41 hours in adults and kittens following IV administration, 24–108 hours after oral administration.
- Smaller volume of distribution and shorter elimination half-life in puppies as compared to adults, therefore, higher peak serum concentrations in puppies.
- Protein binding is 77.5%, less than that noted in human beings.

Mechanism of Action

- Interferes with Na^{+2} conductance.
- Stabilizes neuronal membranes and restricts the spread of electrical discharge.
- Brain concentrations similar to serum concentrations.

Dosage and Monitoring

- Dosages up to 35–50 mg/kg TID may be required to maintain serum concentrations.
- Therapeutic range for serum concentrations in human beings is 10–20 μg/ml.

Interactions, Side Effects, and Toxicity

- Acute toxicity results in sedation, ataxia, and anorexia in dogs. In human beings, nystagmus becomes evident at concentration greater than 20 μg/ml; greater than 30 μg/ml → ataxia; greater than 40 μg/ml → mental changes and confusion.
- Hepatopathy: with chronic administration, results in hepatocellular hypertrophy and necrosis, lipidosis, and extramedullary hematopoiesis.
- Coagulation defects → vitamin K dependent.
- Reversible dermal atrophy in cats.
- Gingival hyperplasia.
- Chloramphenicol increases phenytoin toxicity.
- Decreases T_4 due to decreased plasma protein binding.
- Toxic to cats (due to inability to hydroxylate phenolic compounds). With chronic treatment, trough concentrations may rise. Can result in sialosis, frequent vomiting, and moderate weight loss.

OTHER ANTICONVULSANTS

Clonazepam

- Klonopin
- Extremely potent benzodiazepine.
- Used for simple absence seizure, atonic seizures, and bilateral massive epileptic myoclonus.
- Generalized EEG abnormalities are better suppressed than focal abnormalities, possibly because clonazepam limits the spread of epileptogenic discharge rather than suppressing the focus.

Metabolism

- Nearly 100% bioavailable as an oral solution.
- Peak concentrations 1–3 hours after PO dose.
- 82% protein bound.
- Hepatic clearance 10 times as efficient in dogs as compared to humans.
- Metabolism becomes somewhat saturated to therapeutic doses in 10–25% of dogs.
- Elimination T 1/2 increased from 1.4 hours at start of therapy to 1.6–2.9 hours after 1 week of treatment.
- Elimination of clonazepam is increased by phenobarbital, an effect due to hepatic enzyme induction rather than an alteration in hepatic blood flow.

Dosage and Monitoring

- 0.5 mg/kg PO BID to TID achieves peak serum concentrations of 130–179 ng/ml and trough concentrations of 22–77 ng/ml; These concentrations are near the therapeutic range in human beings.

Interactions, Side Effects, and Toxicity

- Sedation
- After prolonged treatment, abrupt cessation of therapy causes acute withdrawal signs including "wet dog shakes," listlessness, weight loss, increased body temperature, and dorsal recumbency. Signs are most severe 2 days after cessation, and will subside within 1 week of withdrawal. Therefore, gradually taper off of this medication.

Clorazepate

- Tranxene
- 15 times less potent than clonazepam.

Metabolism

- Rapidly and completely hydrolyzed in the stomach to nordiazepam.
- T 1/2 in human is 41 +/- 10 hours after oral clorazepate.

Dosage and Monitoring

- Preliminary evidence indicates the dosages of 2 mg/kg BID produce peak nordiazepam concentrations near 1 μg/ml with maximum concentrations from 1 to 2 hours after oral administration. Additional dosage recommendations at 0.5–1 mg/kg orally every 8 hours.
- Optimum seizure control in human beings is noted when serum nordiazepam concentrations are greater than 1 μg/ml.

Interactions, Side Effects, and Toxicity

- Clorazepate crosses the placenta slowly, but nordiazepam crosses very rapidly, and has been found in breast milk and the blood of nurslings.
- May increase concentrations of concurrently administered phenobarbital.

Carbamazepine

- Causes much less CNS depression in humans.
- Iminostilbene derivative.
- Used as an anticonvulsant and also for relief of pain in trigeminal neuralgia.
- Structurally related to tricyclic antidepressants.

Mechanism of Action

- Limits seizure propagation by reduction of posttetanic potentiation of synaptic transmission.
- Sedative, anticholinergic, antidepressant, muscle relaxant, antiarrhythmic, antidiuretic, and neuromuscular transmission-inhibitory actions.

Metabolism

- Metabolized to carbamazepine 10,11-epoxide (liver).
- Further metabolism to inactive metabolites is self-induced during multiple dosing.
- When dogs have been switched to this drug from standard regimes, they have lapsed into status epilepticus, possibly due to the rapid elimination of carbamazepine.
- Concentration in CSF of humans is 15% serum concentration.

Vigabatrin

- gamma-vinyl-gamma aminobutyric acid (see Speciale et al. 1991).

Metabolism

- Absorbed from GI tract, peak plasma concentration in 2 hours; bioavailability may be less in children as compared to adults.
- Little protein-binding.
- Minimal metabolism in humans; eliminated primarily by renal excretion.
- Does not induce hepatic enzymes.
- Elimination T 1/2 = 4–6 hours in humans.
- Steady state in 2 days.

Mechanism of Action

- A structural analogue of GABA is a selective and irreversible inhibitor of GABA- aminotransferase (GABA-T); takes 4–6 days to make new enzyme.
- Designed to prevent the breakdown of GABA.

Dosage and Monitoring

- Optimal dose not known
- People: 250–500 mg q 12–24 h increasing every 1–2 weeks until seizure control. Average maintenance in humans is 1000–1500 mg q 12 h.
- Children: starting dose 40 mg/kg/day; average maintenance dose is 80–100 mg/kg/day.
- Clinically, dogs have been given between 35 and 125 mg/kg/day (divided q 8 to 12 hours).
- In Speciale et al. (1991), this drug was often given concurrently with phenobarbital.

Interactions, Side Effects, and Toxicity

- One dog developed immune-mediated anemia.
- Intramyelinic edema in experimental dogs; not seen with clinical use in people.
- Sedation, dizziness, and headache in people.
- Increases in body weight.

NEWER ANTICONVULSANTS

Felbamate (Felbatol)

- 2-phenyl-1,3-propanediol dicarbamate

Metabolism

- Extensively metabolized by the liver via hydroxylation and conjugation.
- Half-life in dogs 5 to 6 hours.
- Well absorbed after oral administration.

Mechanism of Action

- Not known; works on the N-methyl-D-aspartate (NMDA) receptor.
- Appears to increase seizure threshold and prevent seizure spread.

Dosage and Monitoring

- Optimal dose not known.
- For dogs less than 10 kg, start at 200 mg PO q 8 h with a 200 mg per week increase up to a maximum dose of 600 mg PO q 8 h or until seizure control in obtained. For dogs greater than 10 kg, start at 400 mg PO q 8 h with a 400 mg per week increase up to a maximum dose of 1200 mg PO q 8 h or until seizures are controlled (Podell 1997).
- Other dosing recommendations at initial dose of 15 mg/kg every 8 to 12 hours orally. Increase in 15 mg/kg increments every 2 weeks until seizure control.
- Doses of 60–70 mg/kg given in dogs for metabolism studies without toxicity. Toxic dose of felbamate appears to be 300 mg/kg.

Interactions, Side Effects, and Toxicity

- Aplastic anemia and hepatic failure in humans.
- Severe hepatic disease in some dogs with this drug alone, or in combination with phenobarbital.
- Side effects in humans include anorexia, insomnia, weight loss, nausea, dizziness, fatigue, ataxia, and lethargy.

Gabapentin

- Neurontin
- Developed to be structurally similar to GABA; does not, however, work at the GABA receptor.

Metabolism

- Elimination T1/2 is 5–9 hours in humans.
- 30% undergoes hepatic metabolism in dogs.
- Peak serum levels in 2–4 hours.
- Steady state concentrations at 2–4 days.
- Not bound to plasma protein.
- Excreted unchanged, i.e., no liver metabolism.

Mechanism of Action

- Not known

Dosage and Monitoring

- Optimal dose not known.
- For dogs begin at 100 mg orally q 8 h with a gradual increase up to 900 mg PO q 8 h over the next 4 weeks or until seizures are controlled (Podell 1997).
- Other recommendations: Start at 100–300 mg/dog every 8 hours orally. Increase the dose upward every 1 to 2 weeks until seizures are controlled or maximum dose of 1200 mg/dog orally every 8 hours.
- Other recommendations: 25–60 mg/kg/day divided every 6 to 8 hours.

Interactions, Side Effects, and Toxicity

- Drowsiness, tiredness, fatigue, somnolence, dizziness, ataxia, nystagmus, headache, tremor, nausea, vomiting in humans.
- Side effects in dogs at higher doses: sedation and GI upset.
- Little effect on severe seizures in humans.
- Dogs commonly may appear sedated when receiving this drug. Other side effects and toxicity associated with this drug are currently unknown.
- This drug may be helpful for seizure control in animals with hepatic disease.
- Gabapentin has been used as an anticonvulsant in cats.
- Excessive sedation is possible, especially when this drug is initiated. Gradually increasing dosages are recommended to avoid this adverse effect. Initial doses of 5 to 10 mg/kg every 24 hours are increased to the same dose every 12 hours after 3 to 5 days of therapy.

Lamotrigine

- Lamictal
- 3,5-diamino-6-(2,3-dichlorophenyl-1,2,4-triazine)

Metabolism

- Well absorbed after oral administration.
- Peak concentration 1–3 hours after dosing in humans.
- 55% bound to plasma proteins.
- Drug undergoes extensive metabolism in the liver largely to an inert glucuronide conjugate.
- Does not induce or inhibit hepatic microsomal enzymes.

Mechanism of Action

- Believed to stabilize presynaptic neuronal membranes by blocking voltage-dependent sodium channels, thereby preventing the release of excitatory neurotransmitters such as glutamate and aspartate.

Dosage and Monitoring

- Dose not known for dogs.
- For children: begin at 2 mg/kg/day, increasing after 2 weeks to 5 mg/kg, and thereafter to a maintenance dose of 5–15 mg/kg/day.

Interactions, Side Effects, and Toxicity

- Rash, headache, ataxia, diplopia, nausea, dizziness, vomiting, somnolence in humans.
- Side effects in humans include anorexia, insomnia, weight loss, nausea, dizziness, fatigue, ataxia, and lethargy.

Zonisamide

- Zonegran
- Sulfonamide-based anticonvulsant

Metabolism

- Half-life appears to be 15 hours
- Hepatic metabolism

Mechanism of Action

May:

- Block T-type calcium and voltage-gated sodium channels in brain
- Modulate CNS dopaminergic metabolism
- Scavenge free radicals
- Enhance CNS GABA release
- Inhibit carbonic anhydrase

Dosage and Monitoring

- Efficacy dose not known for dogs
- Suggested 10 mg/kg orally every 12 hours
- Also 4–8 mg/kg/day
- Therapeutic levels in humans suggested at 10–40 mg/L.
- Dogs may be 18–24 μg/ml.

Interactions, Side Effects, and Toxicity

- Minimal side effects in beagles treated with 75/mg/kg/day
- Ataxia, drowsiness, gastrointestinal
- If phenobarbital administration is used concurrently, dosages of phenobarbital should be reduced by approximately 50%.

Levetiracetam

- Keppra
- Pyrrolidine-based anticonvulsant

Metabolism

- No hepatic metabolism
- 70% of drug eliminated in urine, remaining portions hydrolyzed in serum and other others.
- Half-life appears to be 4 hours.

Mechanism of Action

Unknown; may:

- Inhibit voltage-gated calcium channels.
- Ameliorate allosteric inhibition of GABA and glycine channels.

Dosage and Monitoring

- Efficacy dose not known for dogs.
- Suggested 20 mg/kg orally every 8 hours
- Also 3 to 30 mg/kg every 8 to 12 hours, and 500–4000 mg/day.

Interactions, Side Effects, and Toxicity

- Minimal side effects in beagles treated with less than 400/mg/kg/day.
- Salivation, restlessness, vomiting, ataxia.
- Signs resolved within 24 hours of discontinuation of the drug.

Others: Topiramate

- Topamax
- Dosage 10–25 mg/kg/day
- Very expensive drug currently

MANAGEMENT OF STATUS EPILEPTICUS

1. Take your own pulse (calm down).
2. Give diazepam (Valium) IV or rectally—0.5–2 mg/kg. Average doses are listed below.

Small dogs	5 mg
Medium dogs	5–10 mg
Large dogs	10–20 mg
2 mg/kg rectally	

   Note: Do not be afraid to give significant amounts of diazepam, as long as you are not suspicious of a liver problem (portosystemic shunt). Wait 1 minute to assess effect. Keep giving single doses every minute until seizure stops.
3. If seizures stop, give phenobarbital IV and proceed with additional diagnostics.

   If animal has not been on phenobarbital, give 12 mg/kg IV.

   If animal is currently receiving phenobarbital, give up to 12 mg/kg.
4. If seizures return quickly, give additional 0.5–2 mg/kg diazepam. If seizure stops, consider diazepam infusion. Give the amount of diazepam that stopped the seizure as a continuous infusion over 1 hour (approximately 5–20 mg/dog/hour; puppies, 5–10 mg/hour; large dog, 10–20 mg/hour). Mix dose in small volume of 0.9% NaCl or 5% dextrose in water or buretrol. Avoid light. Run 5 mg diazepam through line to saturate diazepam binding sites in plastic infusion line.
   Another option is to use infusion pump.

5. If seizures are unresponsive to diazepam, give

   Propofol 1–2 mg/kg IV; constant infusion of 0.1–0.6 mg/kg/minute or 6 mg/kg/hour to effect

   OR

   Phenobarbital 3–6 mg/kg IV

   OR

   if the animal has not been on phenobarbital previously, 12–16 mg/kg IV or IM. *Wait 20 minutes for effect.*
   Give 1 mg/kg phenobarbital to raise serum phenobarbital by 1 μg/ml.
   Can give up to 2–4 mg/kg/hourly phenobarbital IV. Monitor for respiratory depression and be prepared to ventilate. If seizures return, can use phenobarbital continuous infusion similar to Valium infusion at 2–4 mg/kg/hour.

   (120 mg phenobarbital diluted to 20 ml total volume = 6 mg/ml).

   If seizures stop, continue on BID phenobarbital at 3 mg/kg IV, IM or PO.

   OR

   Intrarectal bromide 100/mg/kg every 4 hours for 6 dosages (up to 600 mg/kg); may cause irritation and rectal prolapse.

   OR (less ideally)

   Pentobarbital 2–6 mg/kg IV TO EFFECT
   0.5–4.0 mg/kg/hour
6. If all else fails, plan to anesthetize the animal with isoflurane (less ideally, pentobarbital at 3 mg/kg IV to effect PRN). This stops the motor manifestations of the seizure but not the electrical seizure activity occurring intracranially.
7. Sodium bromide has been given intravenously and rectally.
8. Maintain blood pressure with appropriate intravenous fluid therapy.

   May administer B vitamins (vitamin B_1 25–50 mg/animal IM).

   If seizures have been prolonged, treat for possible increased ICP with

   Mannitol (0.25–1 g/kg IV)
   Furosemide (0.07 mg/kg IV)

   OR

   Hypertonic saline (3% solution, 5.3 ml/kg IV)

   Many animals also benefit from administration of corticosteroids (methylprednisolone sodium succinate or prednisone sodium succinate at 30 mg/kg IV slowly).

   Basic supportive critical care, maintain body temperature.
9. Other unproven or inconsistently effective options for termination of seizures:

   Lidocaine at 1–2 mg/kg IV (Seizures are a side effect of lidocaine overdose.)

   Phenytoin continuous infusion?

   (Constant infusions can be discontinued 2–4 hours following the last seizure event.)

4 Abnormalities of Vision and Pupils

PRACTICE CLINICAL CASE LOCALIZATIONS

The following cases are used to illustrate localization of vision and pupillary abnormalities.

Case 4.1

The dog has equal pupil size in examination room light (fig. A4.1.1). The dog has absent menace in the left eye (fig. A4.1.2). Palpebral reflex is normal bilateral (fig. A4.1.3). The pupillary light reflex is as shown, with both pupils responding to light stimulation by constriction (fig. A4.1.4). The dog is avisual in the left eye. Where is the lesion?

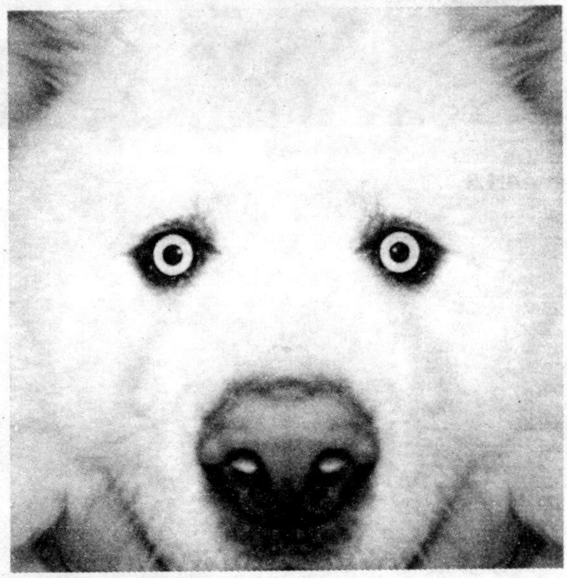

Fig. A4.1.1.

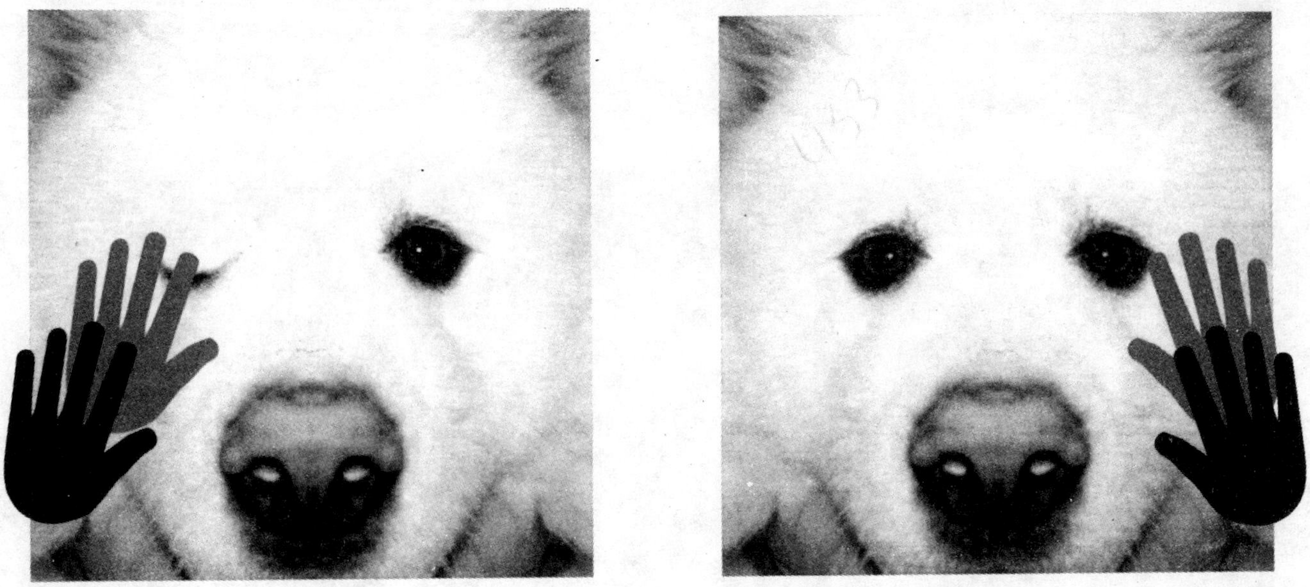

Fig. A4.1.2.

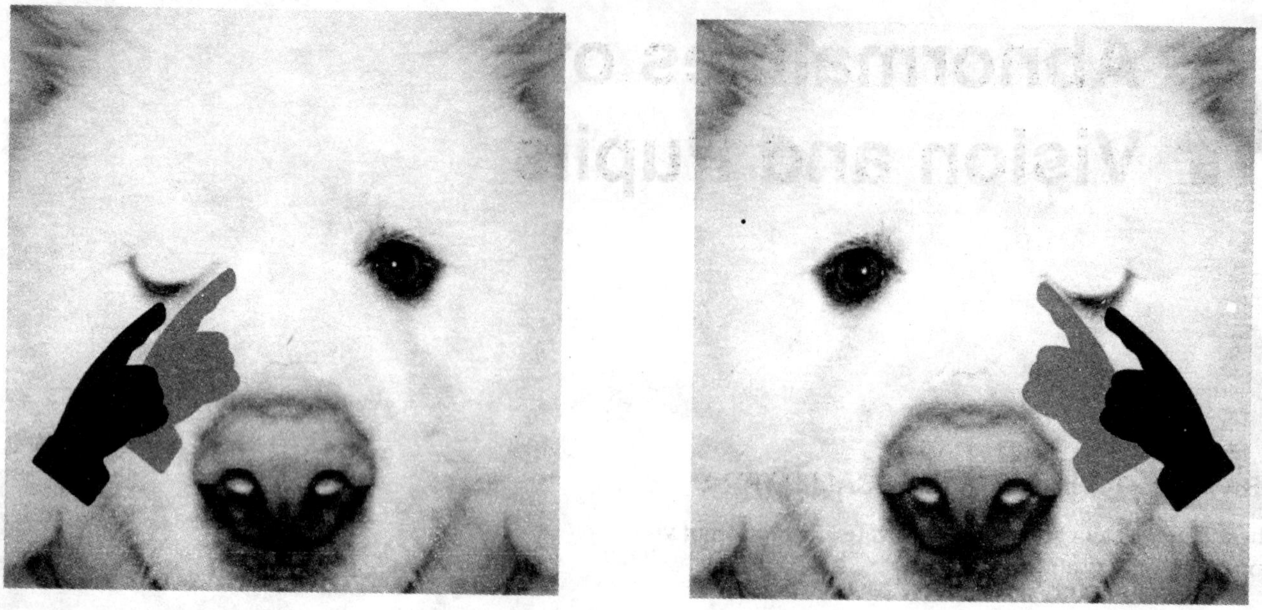

Fig. A4.1.3.

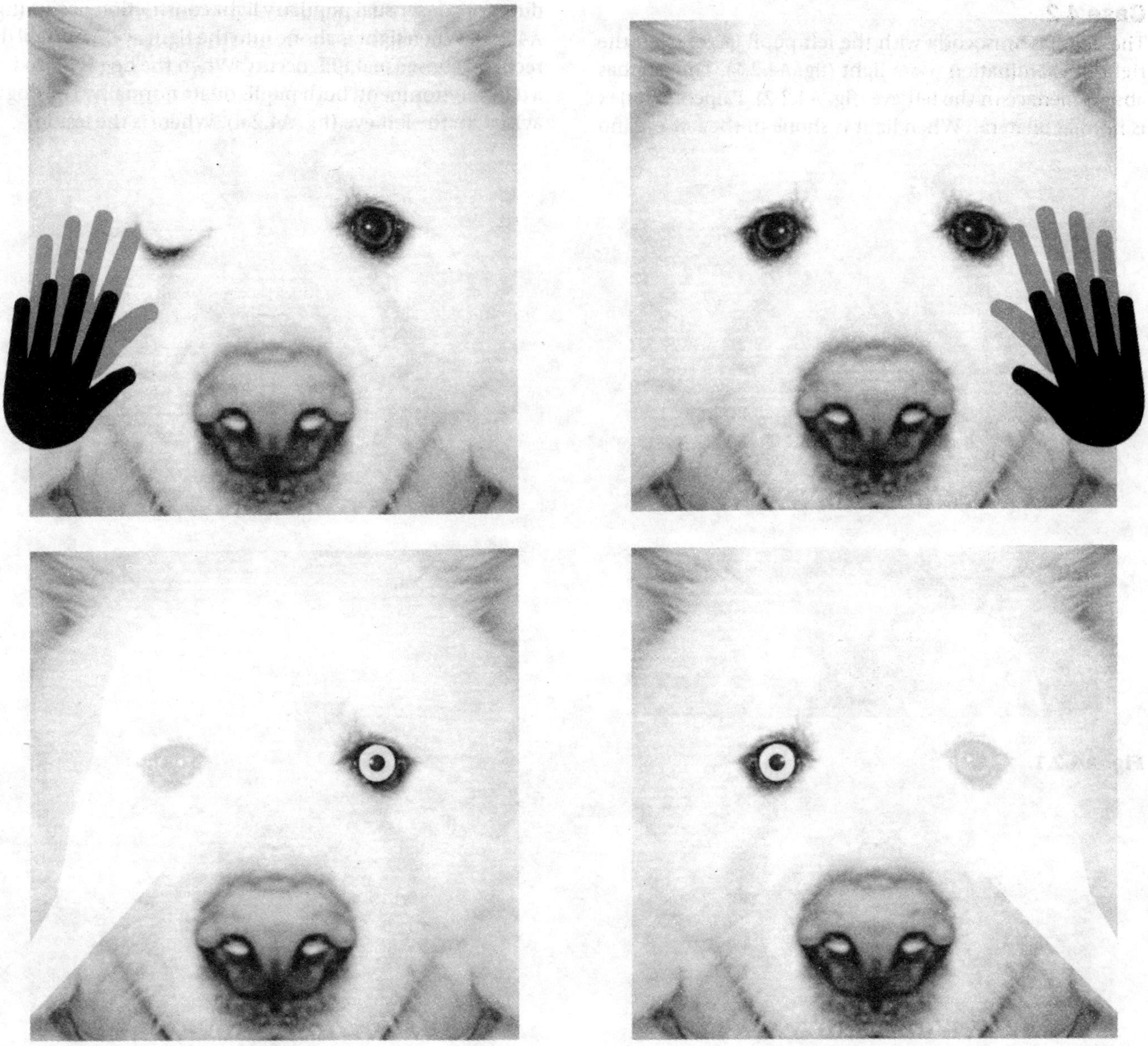

Fig. A4.1.4

Case 4.2

The dog has anisocoria with the left pupil larger than the right in examination room light (fig. A4.2.1). The dog has absent menace in the left eye (fig. A4.2.2). Palpebral reflex is normal bilateral. When light is shone in the left eye, no direct or consensual pupillary light constriction occurs (fig. A4.2.3). When light is shone into the right eye, a normal direct and consensual PLR occurs. When the dog is placed in a dark environment, both pupils dilate normally. The dog is avisual in the left eye (fig. A4.2.4). Where is the lesion?

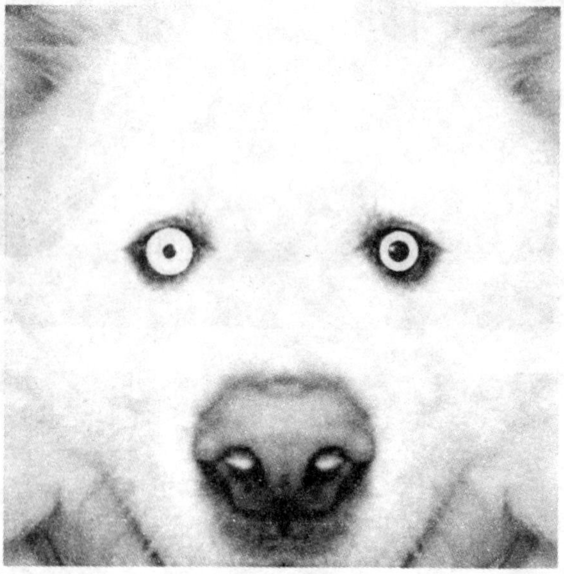

Fig. A4.2.1.

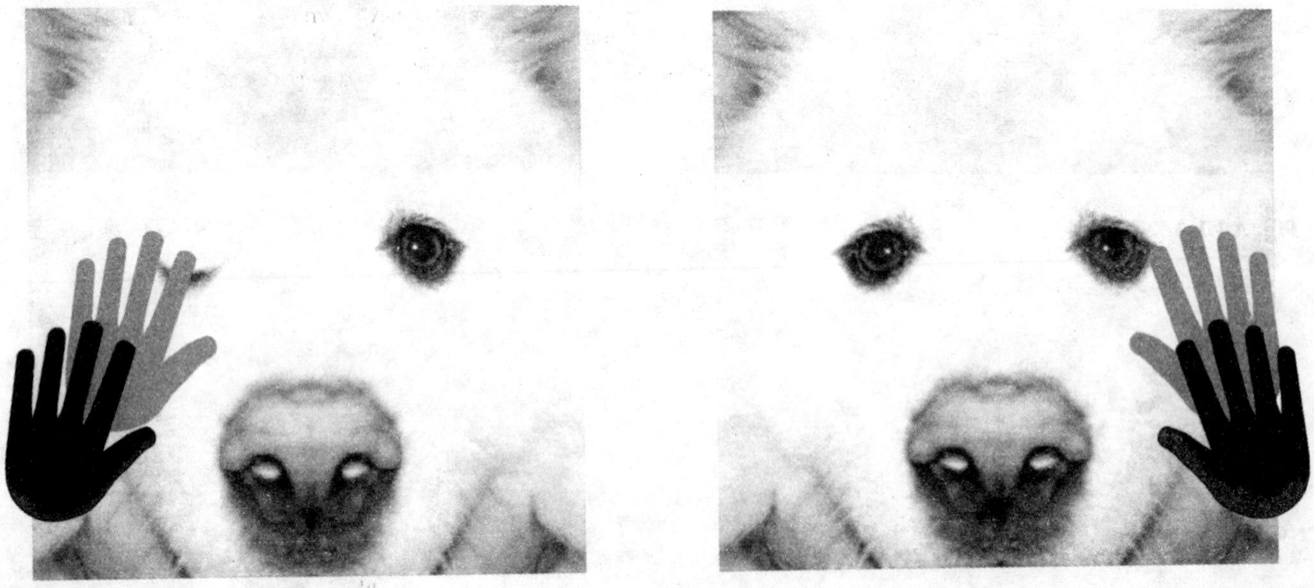

Fig. A4.2.2.

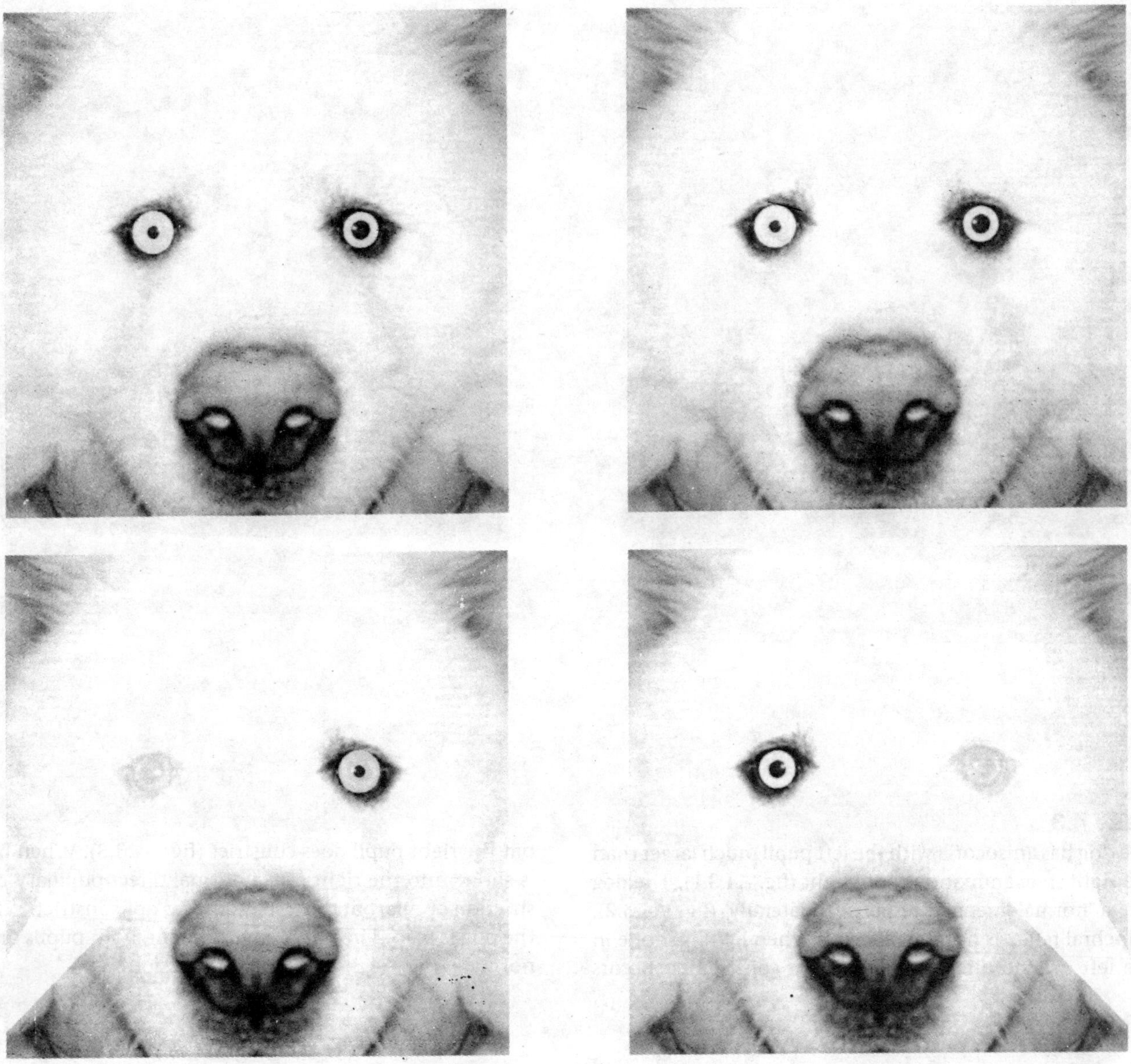

Fig. A4.2.3.

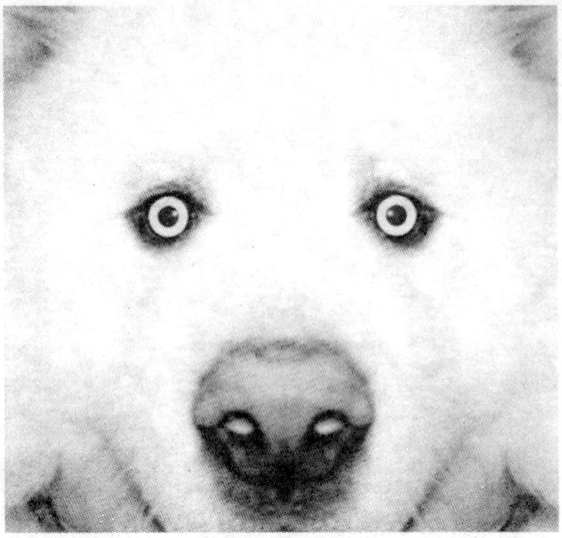

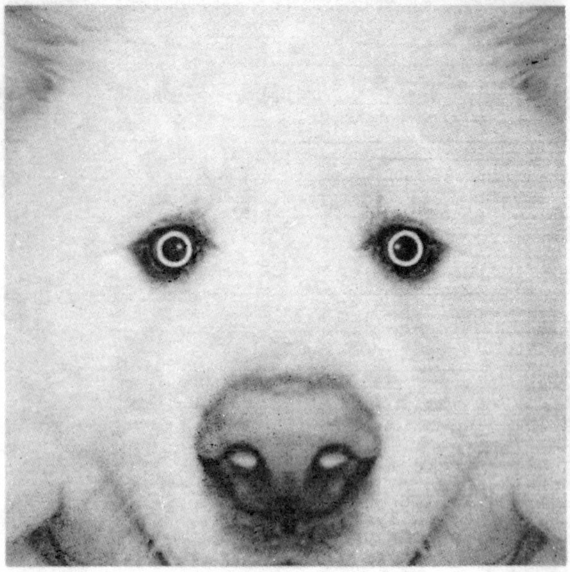

Fig. A4.2.4.

Case 4.3

The dog has anisocoria with the left pupil much larger than the right in examination room light (fig. A4.3.1). The dog has a normal menace response bilaterally (fig. A4.3.2). Palpebral reflex is normal bilateral. When light is shone in the left eye, no direct pupillary light constriction occurs but the right pupil does constrict (fig. A4.3.3). When light is shone into the right eye, a normal direct pupillary constriction occurs, but the left pupil does not constrict. When the dog is placed in a dark environment, both pupils dilate normally (fig. A4.3.4). Where is the lesion?

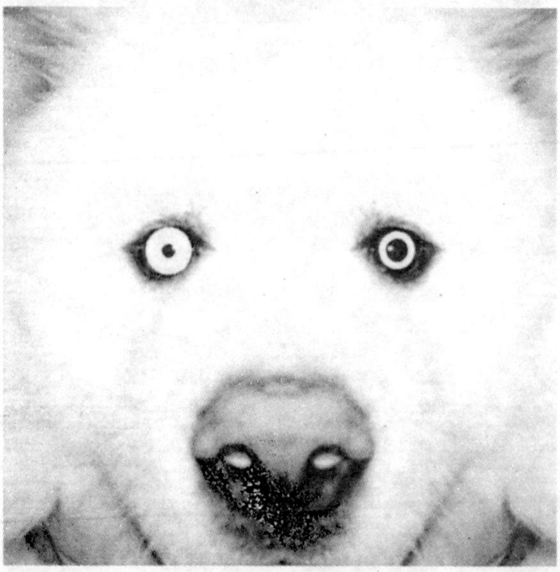

Fig. A4.3.1.

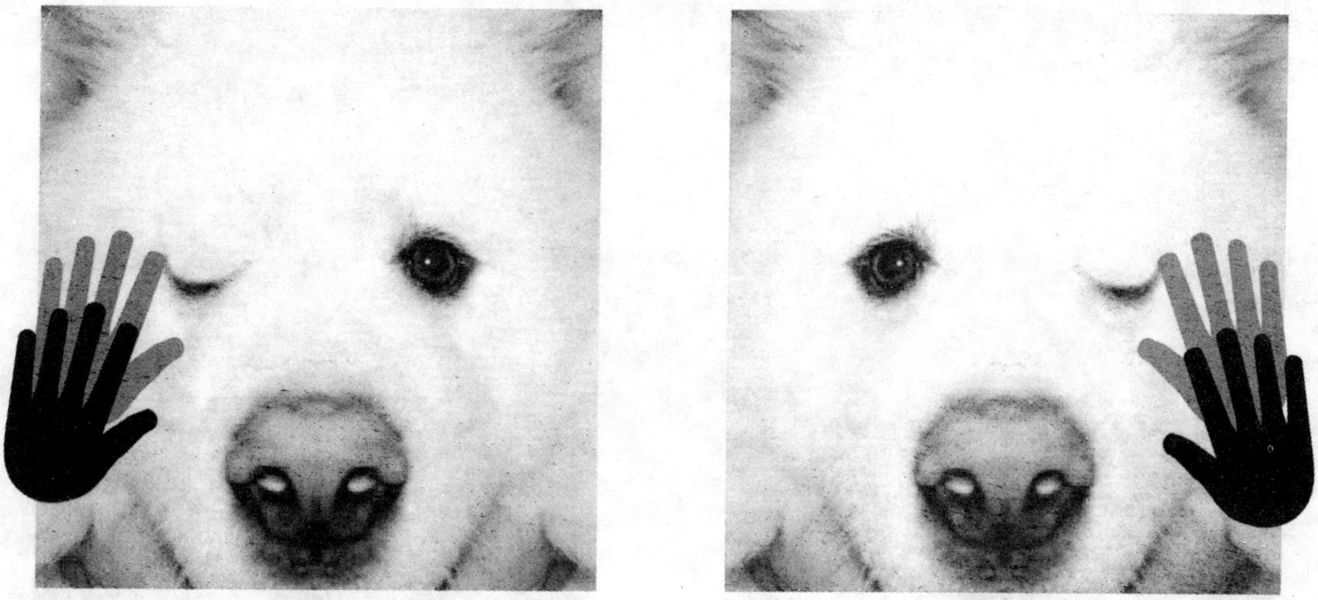

Fig. A4.3.2.

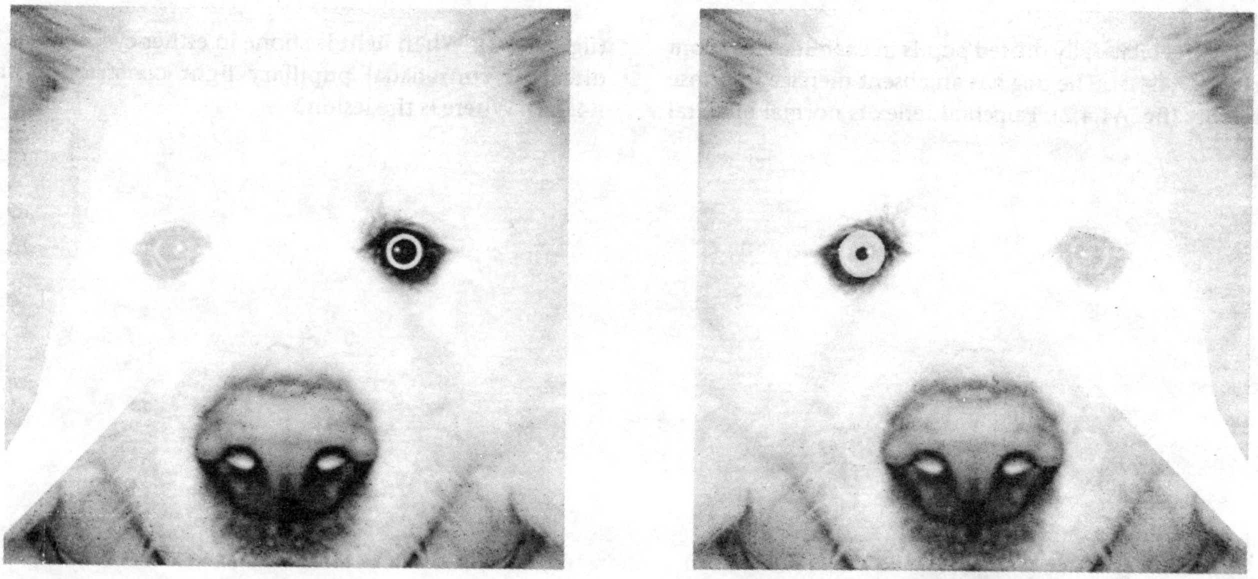

Fig. A4.3.3.

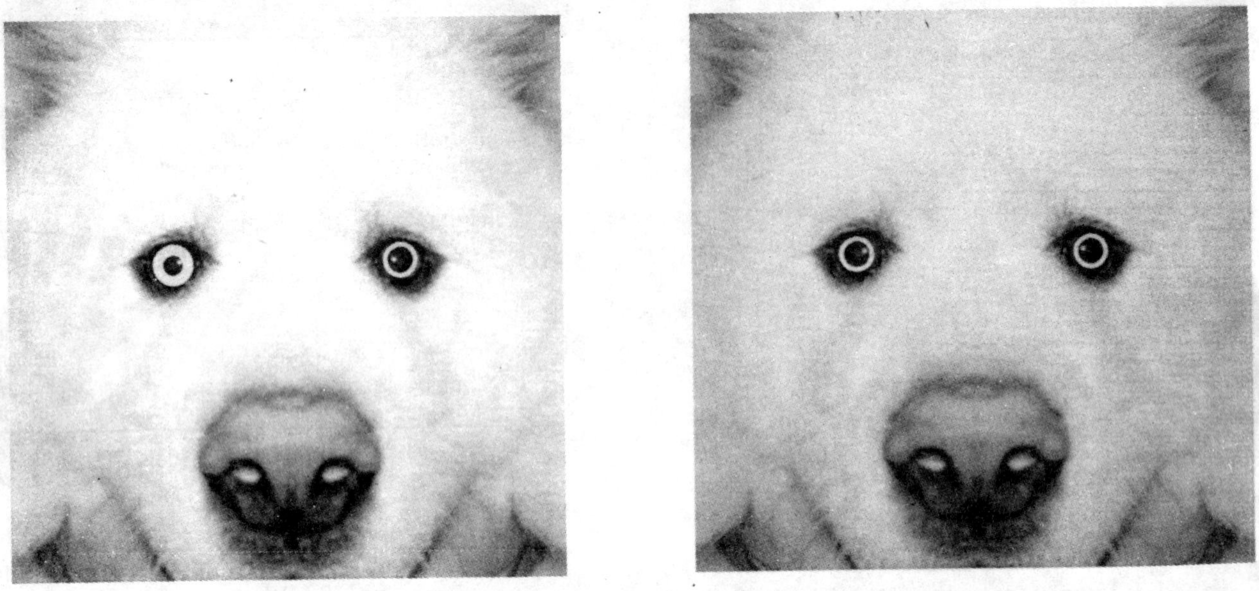

Fig. A4.3.4.

Case 4.4

The dog has bilaterally dilated pupils in examination room light (fig. A4.4.1). The dog has an absent menace response bilaterally (fig. A4.4.2). Palpebral reflex is normal bilateral (fig. A4.4.3). When light is shone in either eye, there is no direct or consensual pupillary light constriction (fig. A4.4.4). Where is the lesion?

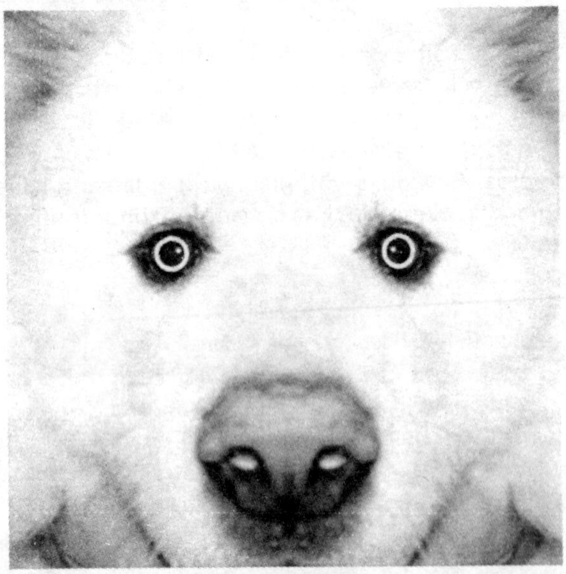

Fig. A4.4.1.

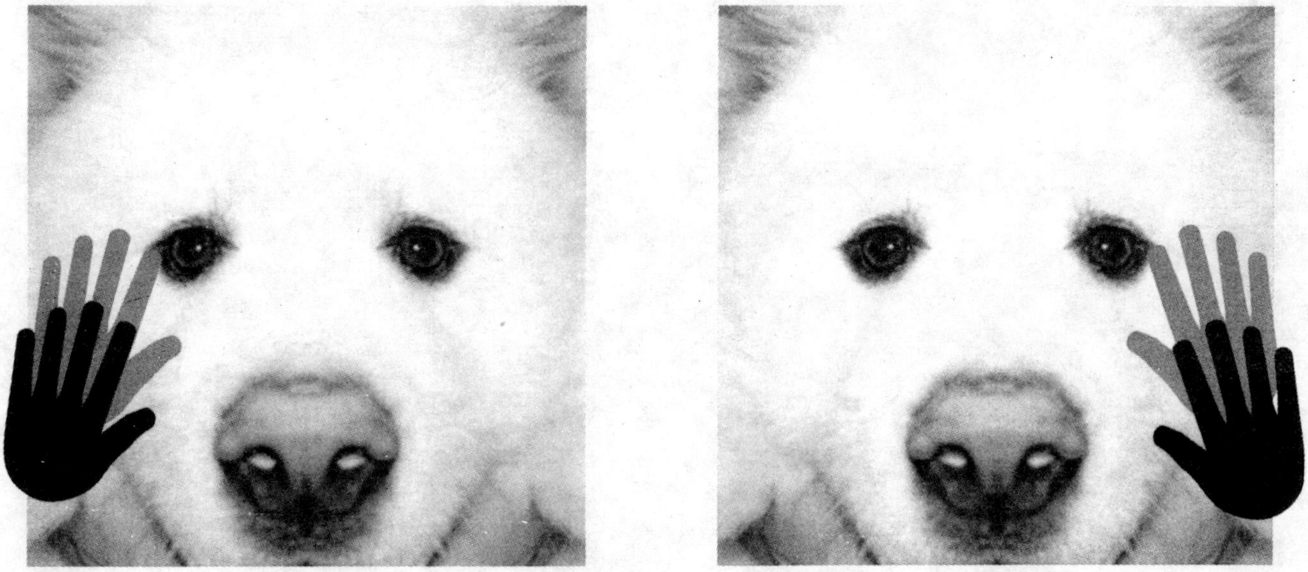

Fig. A4.4.2.

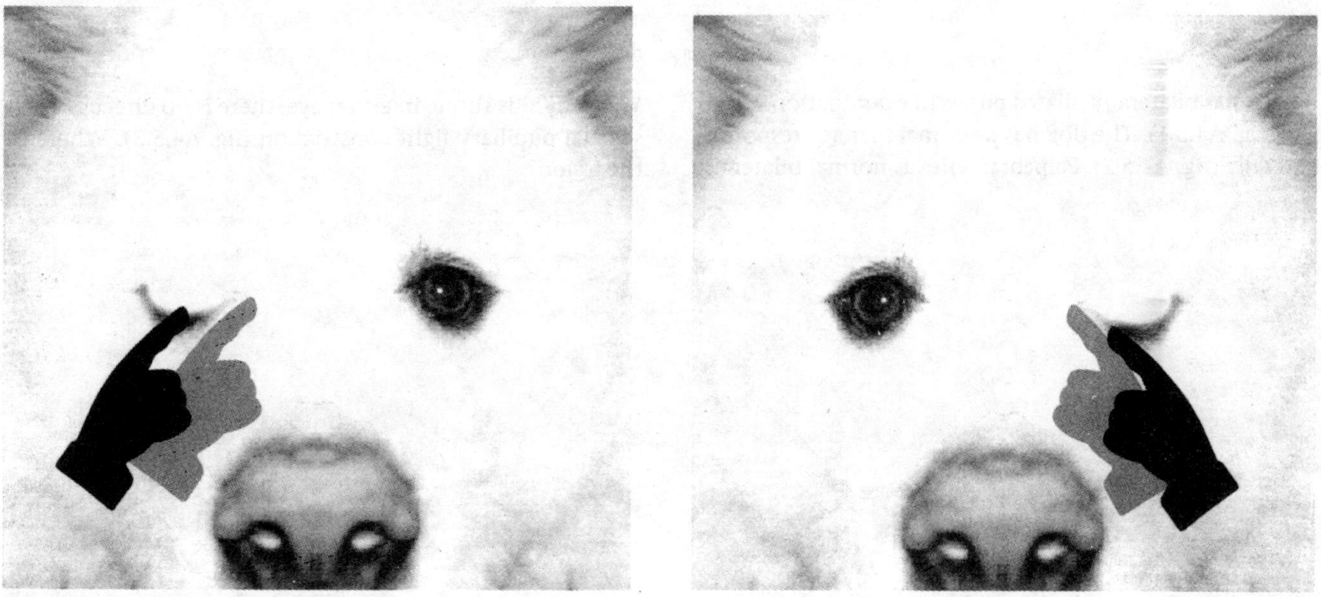

Fig. A4.4.3.

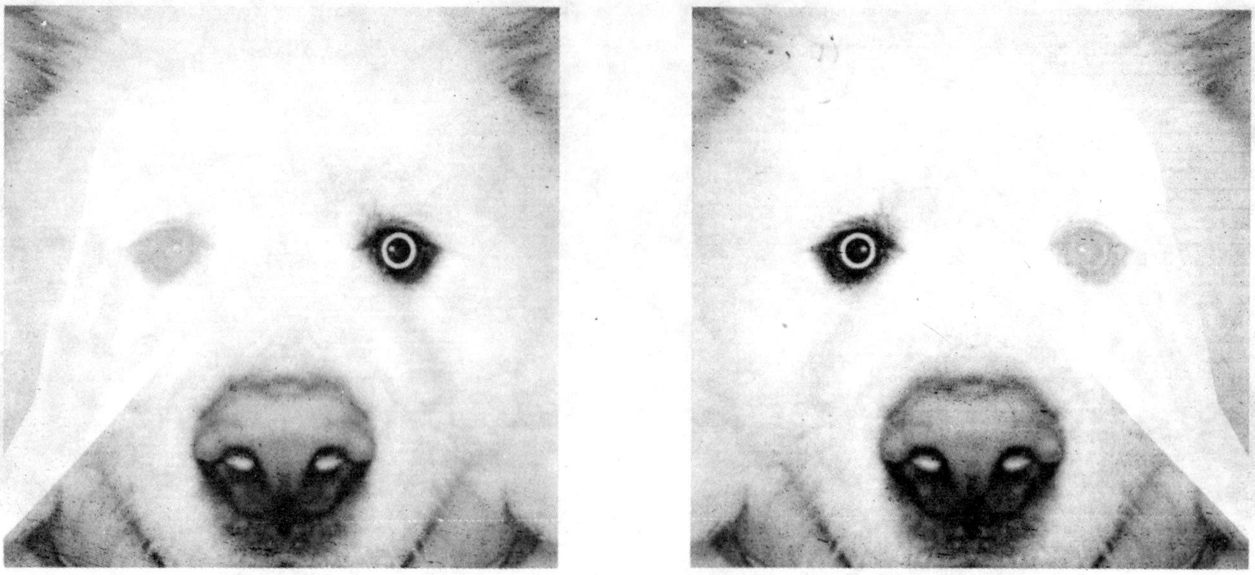

Fig. A4.4.4.

Case 4.5

The dog has bilaterally dilated pupils in examination room light (fig. A4.5.1). The dog has a normal menace response bilaterally (fig. A4.5.2). Palpebral reflex is normal bilateral. When light is shone in either eye, there is no direct or consensual pupillary light constriction (fig. A4.5.3). Where is the lesion?

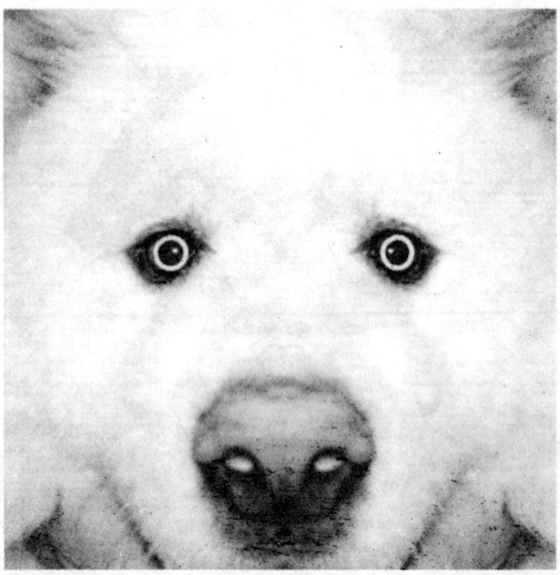

Fig. A4.5.1.

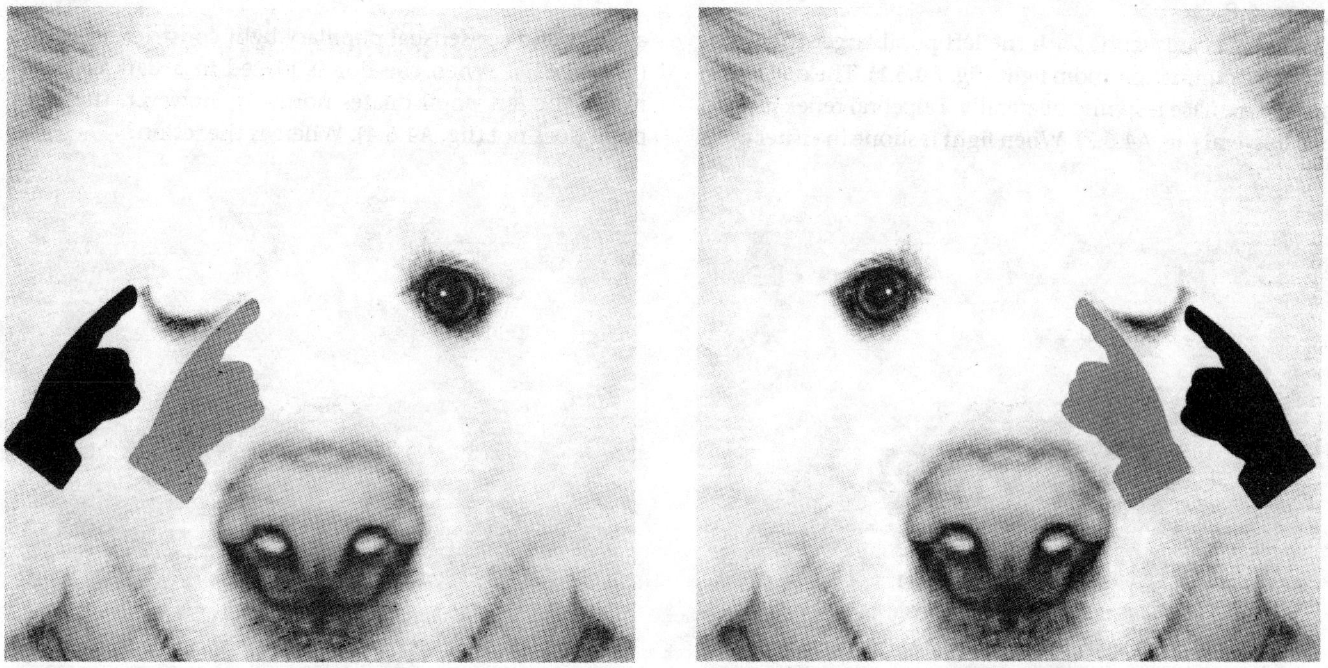

Fig. A4.5.2.

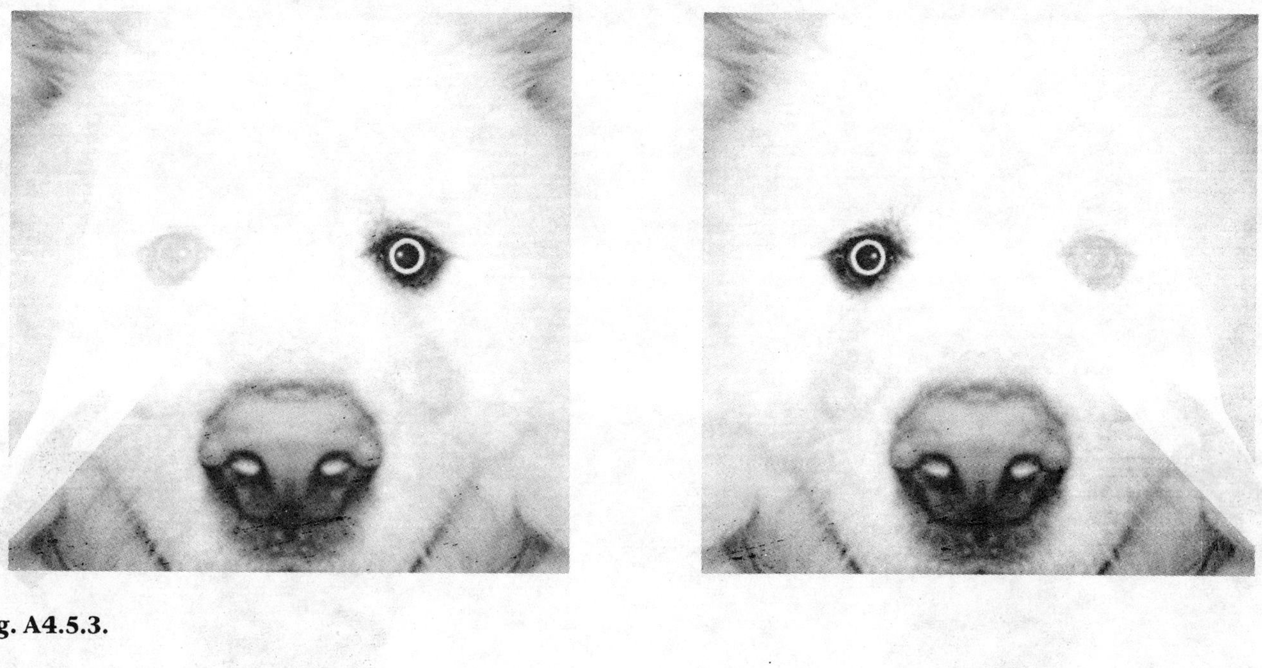

Fig. A4.5.3.

Case 4.6

The dog has anisocoria with the left pupil larger than the right in examination room light (fig. A4.6.1). The dog has a normal menace response bilaterally. Palpebral reflex is normal bilateral (fig. A4.6.2). When light is shone in either eye, a direct and consensual pupillary light constriction occurs (fig. A4.6.3). When the dog is placed in a dark environment, the left pupil dilates normally, however, the right pupil does not (fig. A4.6.4). Where is the lesion?

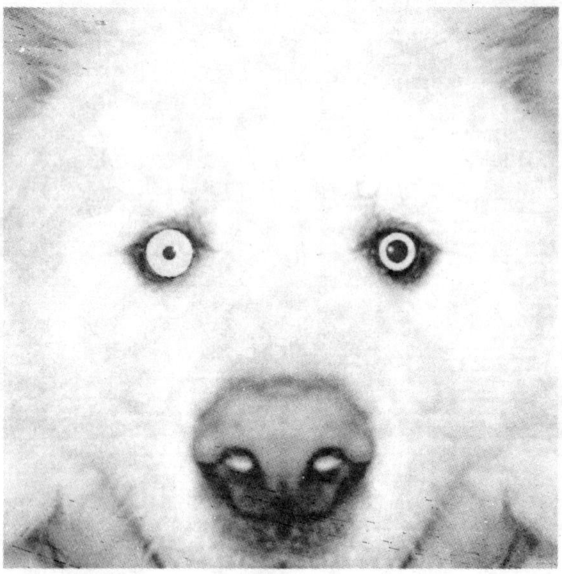

Fig. A4.6.1.

Fig. A4.6.2.

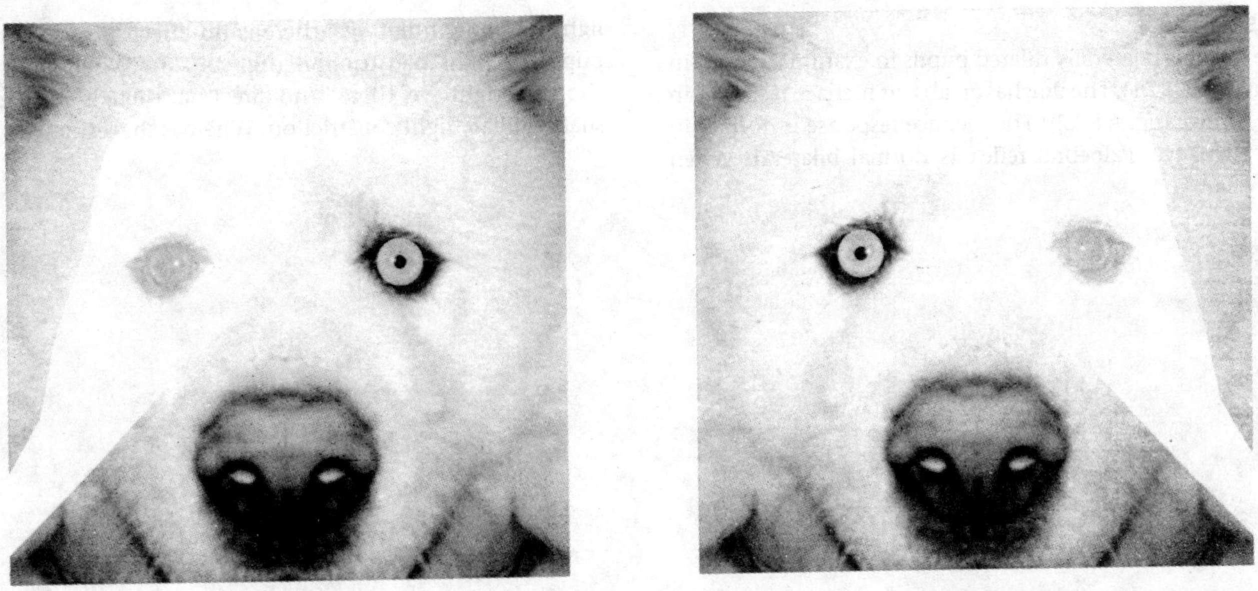

Fig. A4.6.3.

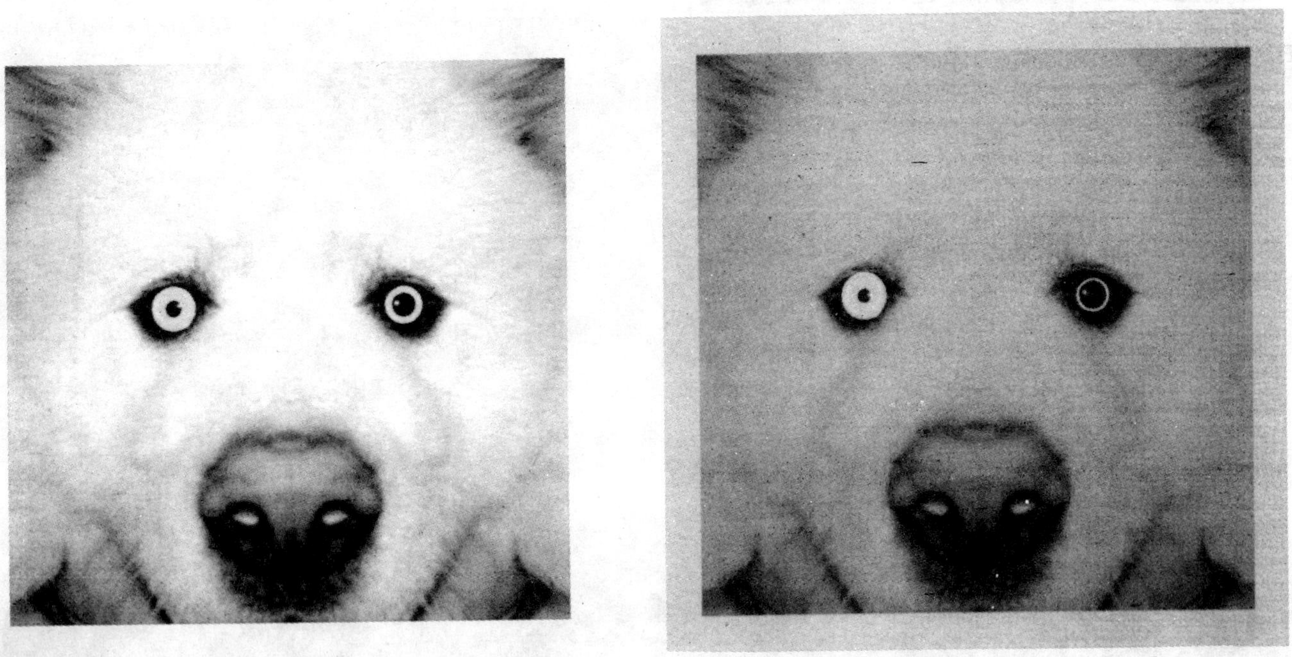

Fig. A4.6.4.

Case 4.7

The dog has bilaterally dilated pupils in examination room light (fig. A4.7.1). The dog has an absent menace response in the left eye (fig. A4.7.2). The menace response is normal in the right eye. Palpebral reflex is normal bilateral. When light is shone in left eye, there is no direct or consensual pupillary light constriction (fig. A4.7.3). When light is shone in right eye, there is no direct but there is a consensual pupillary light constriction. Where is the lesion?

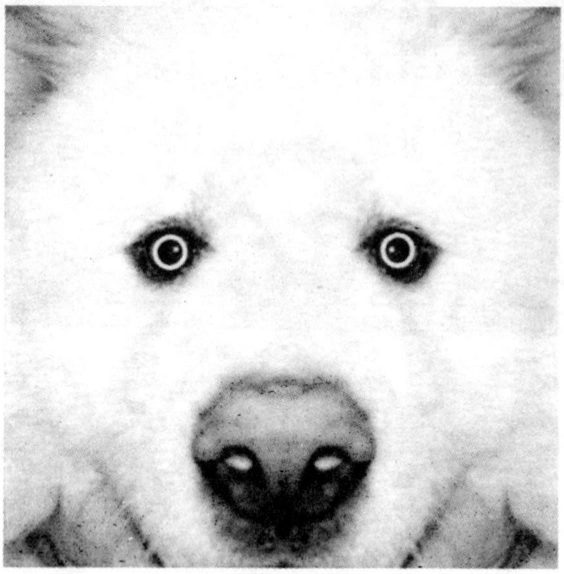

Fig. A4.7.1.

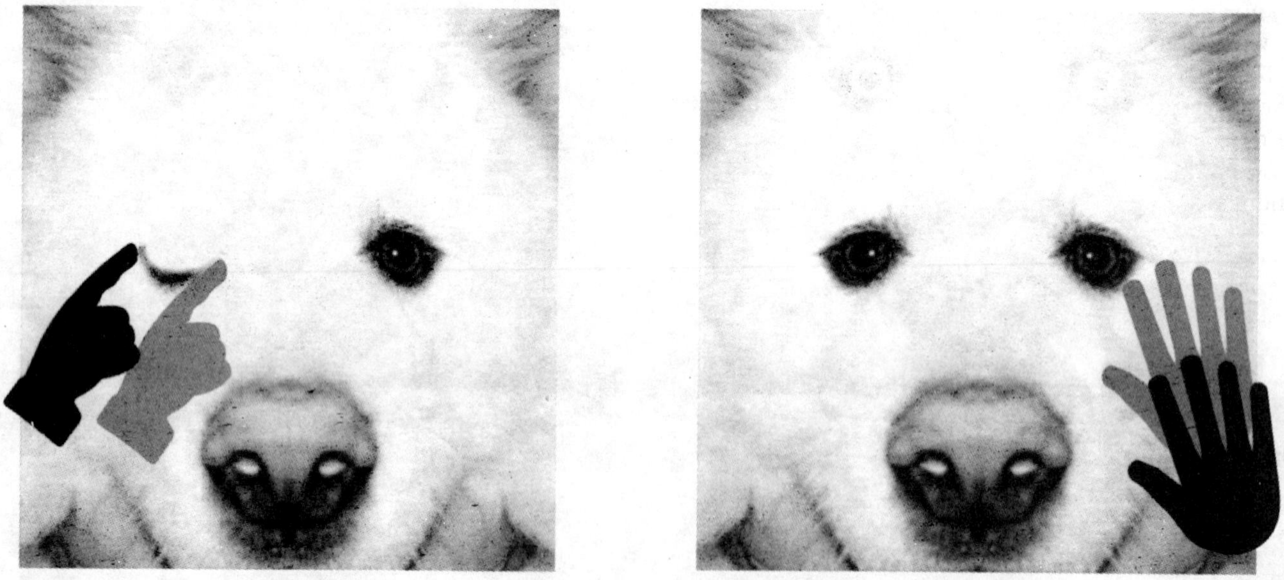

Fig. A4.7.2.

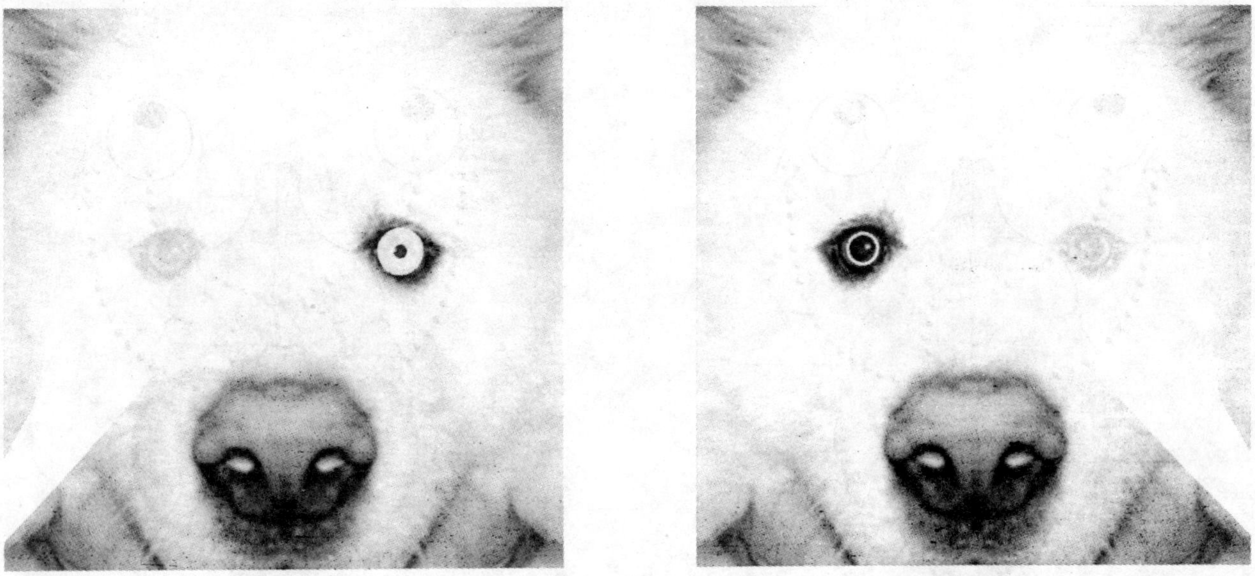

Fig. A4.7.3.

PRACTICE CLINICAL CASE LOCALIZATIONS EXPLANATIONS

Case 4.1 Explanation

First, we know that the menace is normal in the right eye, so the pathways shown in figure A4.1.5 must be intact. The palpebral reflex is normal bilaterally excluding a facial nerve abnormality as a cause for the lack of menace. Next we know that the PLR is normal both direct and consensually when light is directed into the left eye (fig. A4.1.6).

Therefore, the lesion must be caudal to where the fibers leave the right optic tract to result in the PLR. This leaves the right supratentorial region as abnormal (fig. A4.1.7). These clinical features would be an example of central blindness.

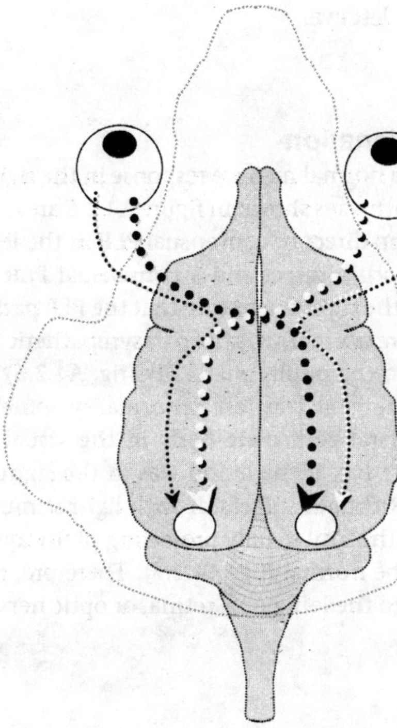

Fig. A4.1.5. Visual pathways from right eye (lighter dots) should be intact.

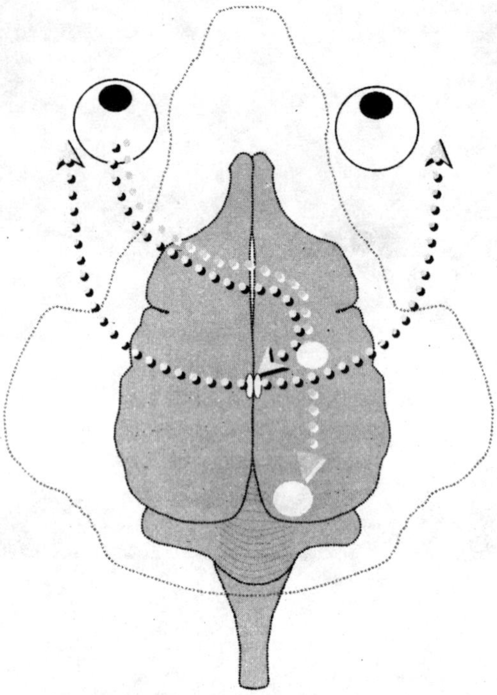

Fig. A4.1.6. Pathway for the PLR (darker dots) with light directed into the left eye.

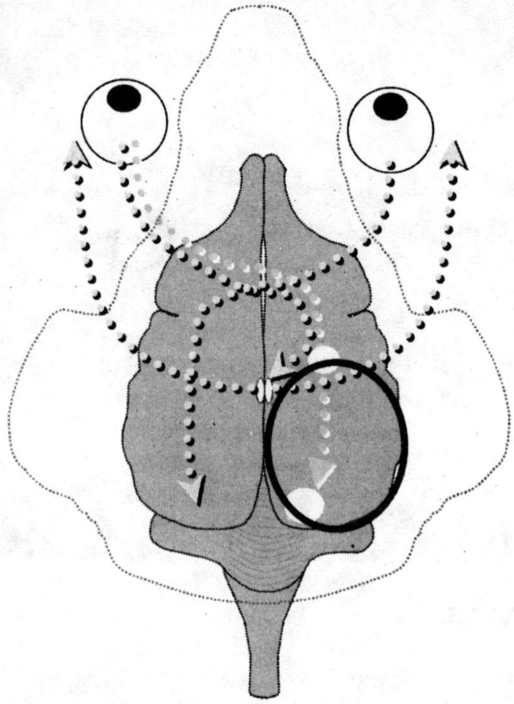

Fig. A4.1.7. Lesion most likely in the right supratentorial region.

Case 4.2 Explanation

This animal has a normal menace response in the right eye. Therefore, the pathways shown in figure A4.2.5 are normal. The animal has no direct or consensual PLR in the left eye, but does have both a direct and a consensual PLR when light is shone in the right suggesting that the PLR pathways in the right eye are normal, as is the parasympathetic innervation (CN III) to the pupils bilaterally (fig. A4.2.6) These suggest that there is at least an abnormality somewhere rostral to the lateral geniculate body in the visual pathway from the left eye. If the lesion was in the right-sided optic tract, a PLR should still result with light stimulation of the left eye as the ipsilaterally projecting pathways from this eye should be normal (fig. A4.2.7). Therefore, the lesion is localized to the left globe, retina, or optic nerve (fig. A4.2.8).

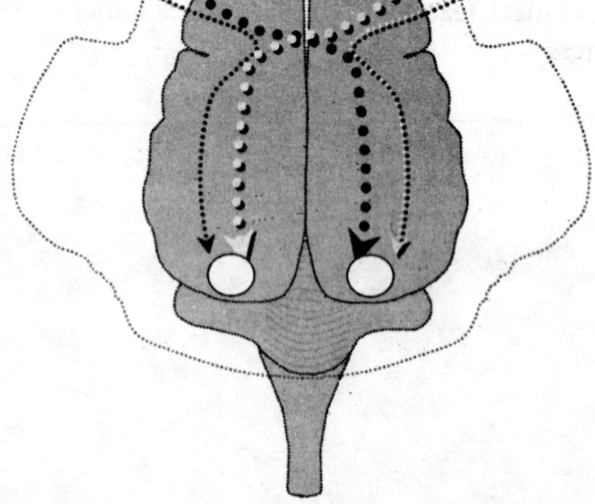

Fig. A4.2.5. Pathways for menace response from the right eye (light dots) should be intact.

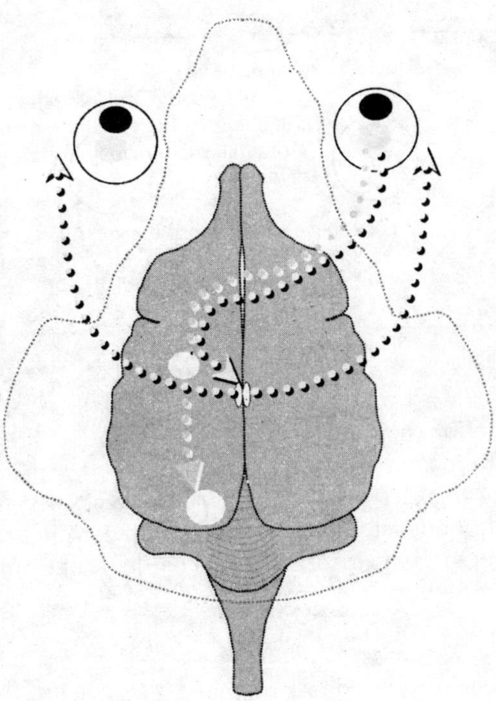

Fig. A4.2.6. Pathways for the PLR from the right eye appear normal.

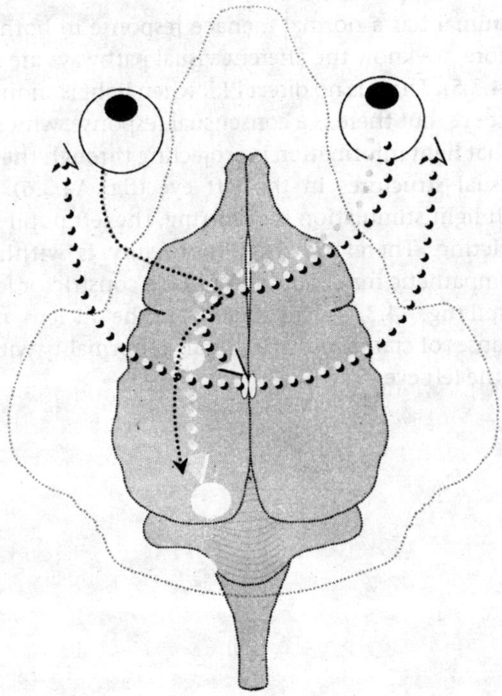

Fig. A4.2.7. Ipsilateral pathway for the PLR (small black dots) intact from the left eye.

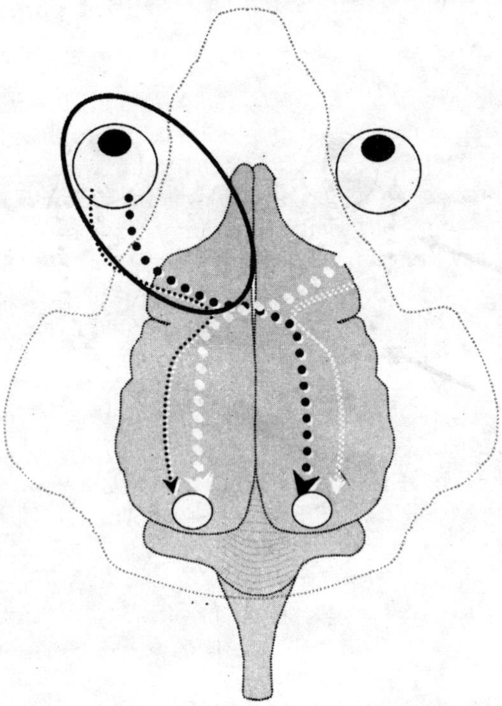

Fig. A4.2.8. Lesion should be prior to the chiasm in the left eye or optic nerve.

Case 4.3 Explanation

This animal has a normal menace response in both eyes. Therefore, we know the afferent visual pathways are intact (fig. A4.3.5). There is no direct PLR when light is shone into the left eye, but there is a consensual response, which suggests that light information is projecting through the afferent visual structures in the left eye (fig. A4.3.6). Even though light stimulation is occurring, the left pupil is not constricting. Therefore, the abnormality is within the parasympathetic innervation or muscle constrictor for the left pupil (fig. A4.3.7). This could be in the nucleus, nerve, or synapses of cranial nerve III, or an abnormality with the iris in the left eye.

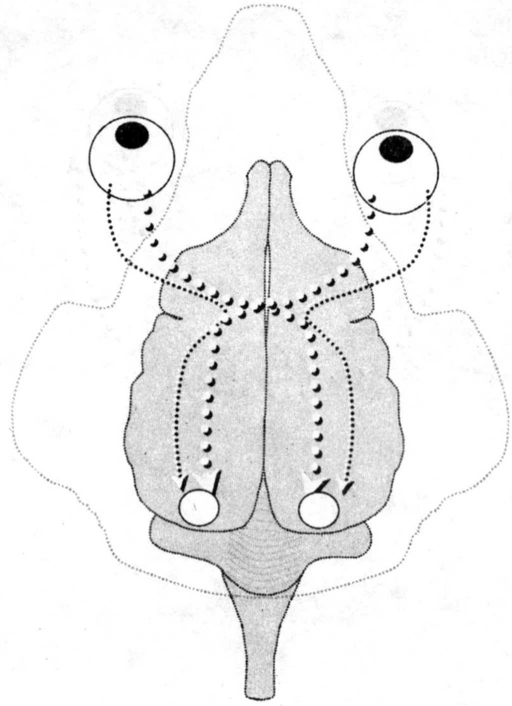

Fig. A4.3.5. Normal afferent visual pathways.

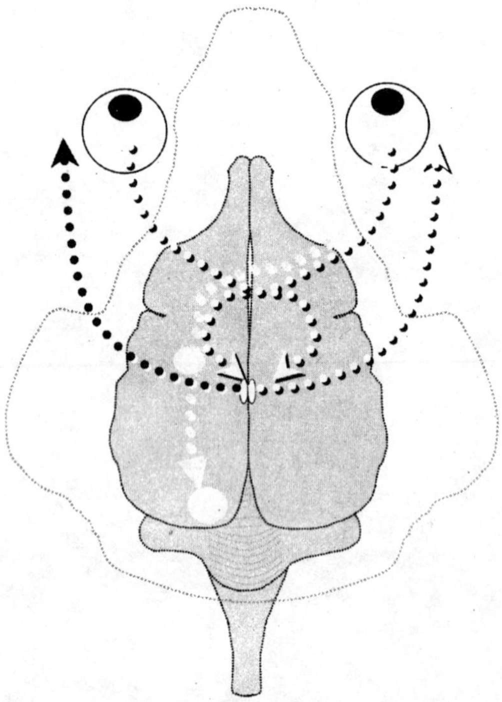

Fig. A4.3.6. Normal pupillary constriction of the right eye with light stimulation of the left eye.

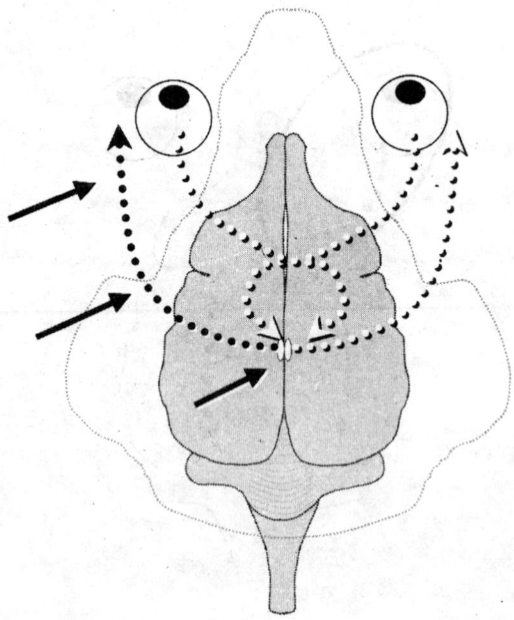

Fig. A4.3.7. Lesion most likely in the parasympathetic innervation to the iris or in the iris muscle of the left eye.

Case 4.4 Explanation

This animal has an absent menace response in both eyes. Therefore, we know the abnormality should be in the afferent visual pathways. There is no direct or consensual PLR in either eye suggesting the light information is not projecting along the initial portions of the visual pathways bilaterally (fig. A4.4.5). Therefore, the abnormality is either with the eye structure, including the retinas bilaterally, the optic nerves bilaterally, or within the optic chiasm (fig. A4.4.6).

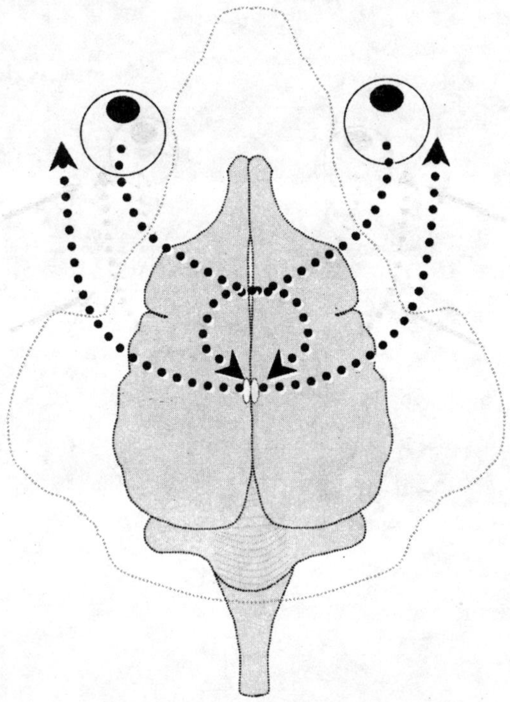

Fig. A4.4.5. Pathway for the PLR.

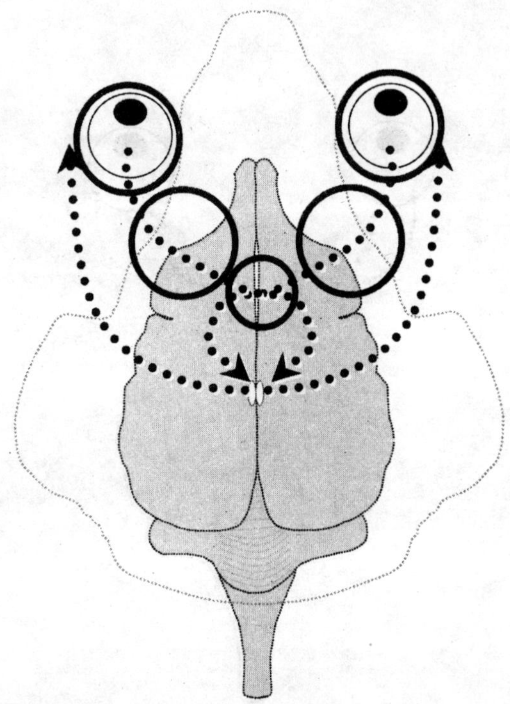

Fig. A4.4.6. Lesions may be in the eye structures (bilateral), optic nerves (bilateral), or optic chiasm.

Case 4.5 Explanation

This animal has a normal menace in both eyes. Therefore, we know the afferent visual pathways are intact (fig. A4.5.4). There is no direct or consensual PLR in either eye. As we know from the menace response that the afferent visual pathways are normal, an abnormality must exist within the parasympathetic innervation to the pupils bilaterally (fig. A4.5.5). This could be in the parasympathetic nuclei of cranial nerve III bilaterally, cranial nerve III or its synapses bilaterally, or an abnormality of the iris constrictor muscle bilaterally.

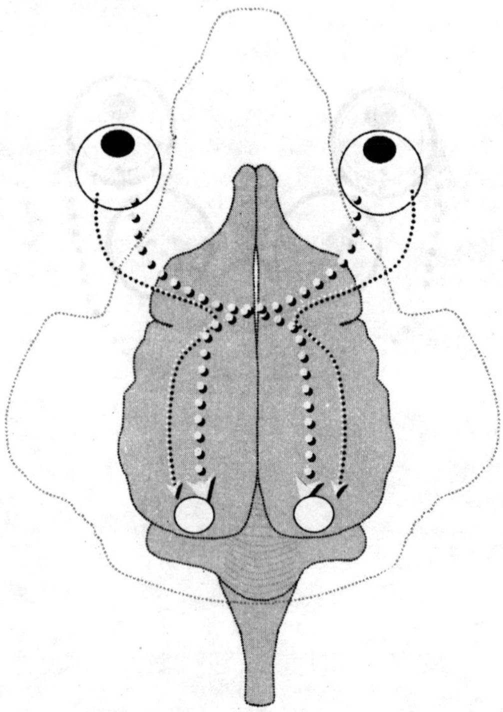

Fig. A4.5.4. Afferent visual pathways.

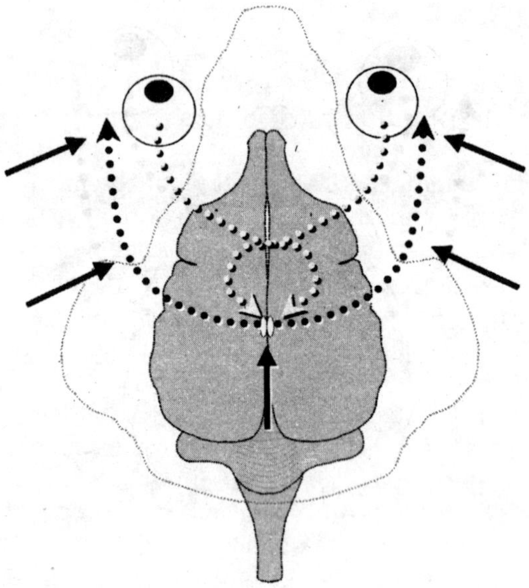

Fig. A4.5.5. Lesion of the parasympathetic innervation to the iris (bilateral) or in the iris muscle (bilateral).

Case 4.6 Explanation

This animal has a normal menace response and PLR in both eyes. Therefore, we know the afferent visual pathways and the PLR pathways are intact (fig. A4.6.5). When the animal is placed in a dark environment, the right pupil cannot dilate. This could indicate an abnormality with the iris dilator muscle, such as a synechia, or an abnormality in the sympathetic innervation to the right eye (fig. A4.6.6).

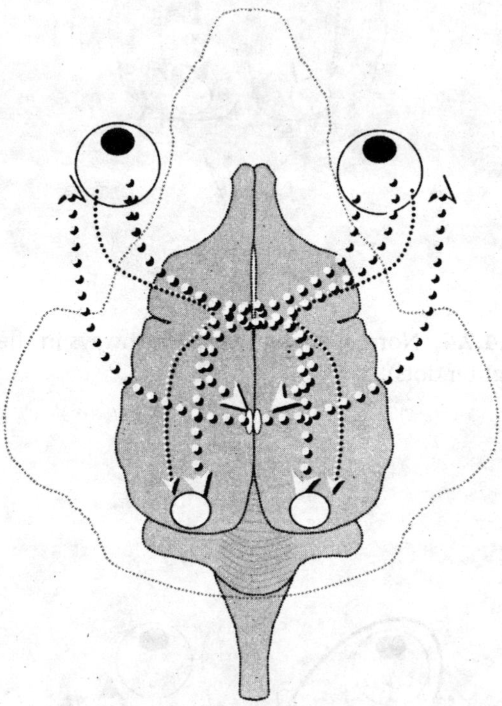

Fig. A4.6.5. Afferent visual pathways and the PLR pathways intact.

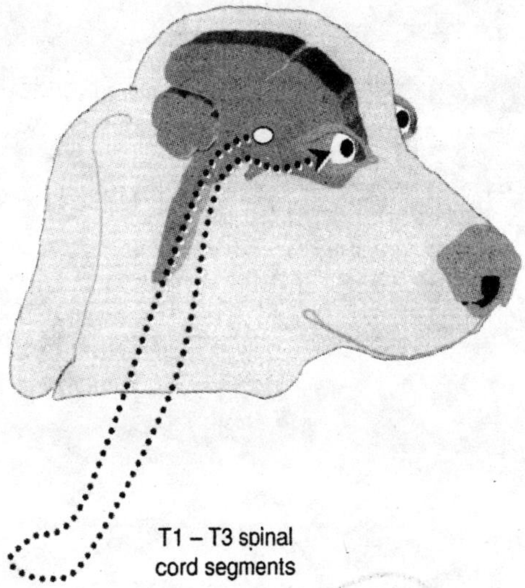

Fig. A4.6.6. Pathway for sympathetic innervation to the eye.

Case 4.7 Explanation

This animal has a normal menace response in the right eye. Therefore, the pathways are normal shown in figure A4.7.4. The animal has no direct or consensual PLR in the left eye suggesting a prechiasm abnormality in the left eye (fig. A4.7.5). The lesion may be localized to the left globe, retina, or optic nerve. If this were the only abnormality, both pupils should constrict when light is shone in the right eye. However, only the left pupil constricts when light is shone in right eye suggesting an abnormality of the constrictor system in the right eye (fig. A4.7.6). Therefore, this animal has multiple lesions in the visual and pupillary systems; in the left prechiasmic region and the right papillary constrictor system.

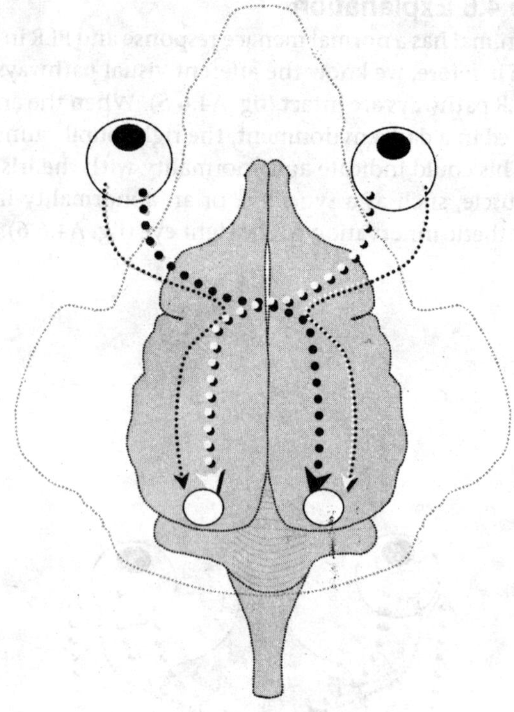

Fig. A4.7.4. Normal afferent visual pathways in the right eye (lighter dots).

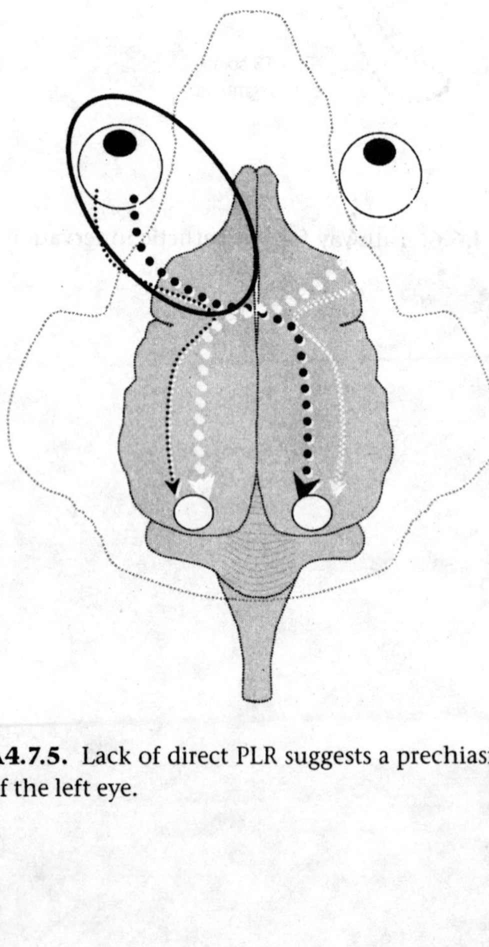

Fig. A4.7.5. Lack of direct PLR suggests a prechiasmic lesion of the left eye.

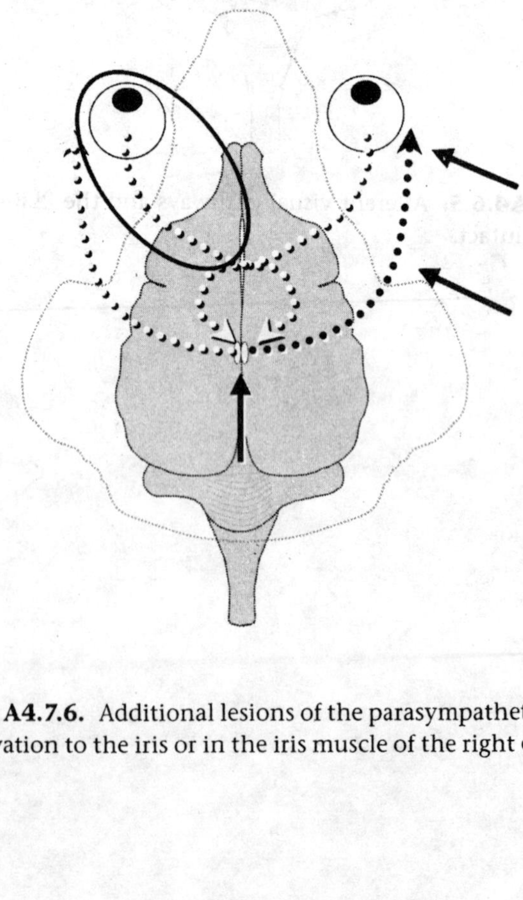

Fig. A4.7.6. Additional lesions of the parasympathetic innervation to the iris or in the iris muscle of the right eye.

5 Practice Clinical Cases

CASE 5.1

Signalment: *4-year-old Golden retriever*

Chief Complaint (CC): *Abnormal gait for 2 weeks, acute onset, nonprogressive signs*

Physical Examination: *Normal*

Neurologic Examination
Mental status: *Normal*
Posture: *Normal*
Gait: *Pelvic limb ataxia*
Conscious proprioception: *Decreased in both pelvic limbs; normal in the thoracic limbs*
Spinal reflexes: *Normal in all limbs*
Cranial nerves: *Normal*
Urination/defecation: *Normal*
Cutaneous trunci: *Normal*
Spinal pain: *None*
Deep pain: *Present*

Questions
What is the neuroanatomical explanation for ataxia?

Neuroanatomical Diagnosis
Where is the lesion?
What are the differential diagnoses?
What is the diagnostic plan?

CASE 5.2

Signalment: *5-year-old dachshund*

Chief Complaint: *Acute onset inability to stand 12 hours ago*

Physical examination: *Normal*

Neurologic Examination
Mental status: *Normal*
Posture: *Normal*
Gait: *Unable to stand*
Conscious proprioception: *Decreased in all limbs; conscious proprioception is worse in the right thoracic and pelvic limbs compared to the left thoracic and pelvic limbs*
Spinal reflexes: *Normal in all limbs*
Cranial nerves: *Normal*
Urination/defecation: *Normal*
Cutaneous trunci: *Normal*
Spinal pain: *None*
Deep pain: *Present*

Neuroanatomical Diagnosis
Where is the lesion?
What are the differential diagnoses?
What is the diagnostic plan?

CASE 5.3

Signalment: *10-year-old Rhodesian ridgeback*

Chief Complaint: *Acute onset of a behavioral change*

Physical Examination: *Some dental tartar*

Neurologic Examination
Mental status: *Dull*
Posture: *Normal*
Gait: *Normal, but tends to walk toward walls on the left side*
Conscious proprioception: *Decreased in left thoracic and pelvic limbs, Normal on the right thoracic and pelvic limbs*
Spinal reflexes: *Normal in all limbs*
Cranial nerves: *Decreased menace response in left eye with normal palpebral and pupillary light reflexes; decreased facial sensation in the left nostril; other cranial nerves normal*
Urination/defecation: *Normal*
Cutaneous trunci: *Normal*
Spinal pain: *None*
Deep pain: *Present*

Neuroanatomical Diagnosis
Where is the lesion?
What are the differential diagnoses?
What is the diagnostic plan?

CASE 5.4

Signalment: *7-year-old German shepherd dog*

Chief Complaint: *Progressive abnormality of facial expression occurring over the last 5 days*

Physical Examination: *Normal*

Neurologic Examination

Mental status: *Normal*
Posture: *Normal*
Gait: *Normal*
Conscious proprioception: *Normal*
Spinal reflexes: *Normal in all limbs*
Cranial nerves: *Decreased menace response (right); decreased palpebral reflex (right), otherwise, cranial nerves are normal. Note: During the menace response testing the dog tries to retract his eye in the orbit, but cannot completely close the palpebral fissure.*
Urination/defecation: *Normal*
Cutaneous trunci: *Normal*
Spinal pain: *None*
Deep pain: *Present*

Neuroanatomical Diagnosis

Where is the lesion?
What are the differential diagnoses?
What is the diagnostic plan?

CASE 5.5

Signalment: *3-year-old mixed-breed dog*

Chief Complaint: *Acute onset of inability to stand and falling*

Physical Examination: *Normal*

Neurologic Examination

Mental status: *Dull*
Posture: *Normal*
Gait: *Cannot stand, tends to fall*
Conscious proprioception: *Decreased in all limbs, worse on the right side*
Spinal reflexes: *Normal in all limbs*
Cranial nerves: *Spontaneous nystagmus, vertical direction*
Urination/defecation: *Normal*
Cutaneous trunci: *Normal*
Spinal pain: *None*
Deep pain: *Present*

Neuroanatomical Diagnosis

Where is the lesion?
What are the differential diagnoses?
What is the diagnostic plan?

CASE 5.6

Signalment: *5-year-old German shepherd*

Chief Complaint: *Abnormal gait for 2 weeks, progressive worsening of function during this time*

Physical Examination: *Normal*

Neurologic Examination

Mental status: *Normal*
Posture: *Normal*
Gait: *Pelvic limb dysfunction with dragging of the pelvic limbs*
Conscious proprioception: *Decreased in both pelvic limbs; normal in the thoracic limbs*
Spinal reflexes: *Normal in all limbs*
Cranial nerves: *Normal*
Urination/defecation: *Normal*
Cutaneous trunci: *Normal*
Spinal pain: *None*
Deep pain: *Present*

Neuroanatomical Diagnosis

Where is the lesion?
What are the differential diagnoses?
What is the diagnostic plan?

CASE 5.7

Signalment: *5-year-old German shepherd*

Chief Complaint: *Problems rising from a sitting position for 6 months*

Physical Examination: *Normal*

Neurologic Examination

Mental status: *Normal*
Posture: *Normal*
Gait: *Normal*
Conscious proprioception: *Normal*
Spinal reflexes: *Normal in all limbs*
Cranial nerves: *Normal*
Urination/defecation: *Normal*
Cutaneous trunci: *Normal*
Spinal pain: *Pain upon manipulating the tail base and on palpation over the LS area; also, the tail tone is poor.*
Deep pain: *Present*

Neuroanatomical Diagnosis

Where is the lesion?
What are the differential diagnoses?
What is the diagnostic plan?

CASE 5.8

Signalment: *7-year-old Labrador retriever*

Chief Complaint: *Gait abnormality for 6 weeks, progressive*

Physical Examination: *Normal*

Neurologic Examination
Mental status: *Normal*
Posture: *Normal*
Gait: *Right pelvic limb cannot be normally flexed at the hock during the flight phase of pelvic limb gait.*
Conscious proprioception: *Normal in thoracic limbs; decreased in right pelvic limb*
Spinal reflexes: *Normal in thoracic limbs; normal patellar reflex in the pelvic limbs; decreased withdrawal in the right pelvic limbs.*
Cranial nerves: *Normal*
Urination/defecation: *Normal*
Cutaneous trunci: *Normal*
Spinal pain: *Pain upon palpation over the caudal lumbar area*
Deep pain: *Present*

Neuroanatomical Diagnosis
Where is the lesion?
What are the differential diagnoses?
What is the diagnostic plan?

CASE 5.9

Signalment: *4-year-old Labrador retriever dog*

Chief Complaint: *Acute onset of facial asymmetry over the last 5 days*

Physical Examination: *Normal*

Neurologic Examination
Mental status: *Normal*
Posture: *Normal*
Gait: *Normal*
Conscious proprioception: *Normal*
Spinal reflexes: *Normal in all limbs*
Cranial nerves: *Temporalis muscle atrophy on the left side. The dog has decreased facial sensation in the left nostril, and a decreased palpebral reflex in the left eye coupled with a normal menace response in the left eye.*
Urination/defecation: *Normal*
Cutaneous trunci: *Normal*
Spinal pain: *None*
Deep pain: *Present*

Question
What are the three general causes of muscle atrophy?

Neuroanatomical Diagnosis
Where is the lesion?
What are the differential diagnoses?
What is the diagnostic plan?

CASE 5.10

Signalment: *6-year-old mixed-breed dog*

Chief Complaint: *Progressive gait problem for 1 month*

Physical Examination: *Normal*

Neurologic Examination
Mental status: *Alert*
Posture: *Head tilt to right*
Gait: *Hypermetric left thoracic limb*
Conscious proprioception: *Decreased in left thoracic and pelvic limbs; normal in the right thoracic and pelvic limbs*
Spinal reflexes: *Normal in all limbs*
Cranial nerves: *Head tilt to right*
Urination/defecation: *Normal*
Cutaneous trunci: *Normal*
Spinal pain: *None*
Deep pain: *Present*

Neuroanatomical Diagnosis
Where is the lesion?
What are the differential diagnoses?
What is the diagnostic plan?

CASE 5.11

Signalment: *9-month-old Labrador retriever dog*

Chief Complaint: *Clinical signs began with a left thoracic limb lameness, which progressed over the ensuing 5 days to a more significant impairment of gait.*

Physical Examination: *Normal*

Neurologic Examination
Mental status: *Normal*
Posture: *Normal*
Gait: *Dragging of left pelvic and left thoracic limbs*
Conscious proprioception: *Decreased in left thoracic and pelvic limbs; decreased in the right thoracic and pelvic limbs but less so than on the left side.*
Spinal reflexes: *Normal in pelvic limbs; decreased withdrawal in the thoracic limbs bilaterally*
Cranial nerves: *Normal*
Urination/defecation: *Normal*
Cutaneous trunci: *Normal*
Spinal pain: *None*
Deep pain: *Present*

Neuroanatomical Diagnosis
Where is the lesion?
What are the differential diagnoses?
What is the diagnostic plan?

CASE 5.12

Signalment: *10-year-old cat*

Chief Complaint: *Acute onset of a behavioral change 3 weeks prior to admission*

Physical Examination: *Normal*

Neurologic Examination
Mental status: *Alert*
Posture: *Normal*
Gait: *Normal, but tends to circle to the left side*
Conscious proprioception: *Decreased in right thoracic and pelvic limbs*
Spinal reflexes: *Normal in all limbs*
Cranial nerves: *Decreased menace response in right eye with normal palpebral and pupillary light reflexes; other cranial nerves normal*
Urination/defecation: *Normal*
Cutaneous trunci: *Normal*
Spinal pain: *None*
Deep pain: *Present*

CASE 5.13

Signalment: *10-month-old German shepherd dog*

Chief Complaint: *Abnormal gait for 2 weeks, gradual onset, progressive signs*

Physical Examination: *Normal*

Neurologic Examination
Mental status: *Normal*
Posture: *Normal*
Gait: *Step distance is progressively shorter with exercise.*
Conscious proprioception: *Decreased in all limbs when the animal supports its own body weight; conscious proprioception is normal, however, when the examiner supports all of the animal's weight.*
Spinal reflexes: *Normal in all limbs*
Cranial nerves: *Mild decrease in the menace and palpebral reflexes bilaterally. Otherwise normal*
Urination/defecation: *Normal*
Cutaneous trunci: *Normal*
Spinal pain: *None*
Deep pain: *Present*

Neuroanatomical Diagnosis
Where is the lesion?
What are the differential diagnoses?
What is the diagnostic plan?

CASE 5.14

Signalment: *5-year-old cat*

Chief Complaint: *Gait abnormality for 6 weeks, progressive*

Physical Examination: *Normal*

Neurologic Examination
Mental status: *Normal*
Posture: *Normal*
Gait: *Decreased ability to extend the hock. "Dropped hock" appearance or plantigrade stand; normal in thoracic limbs*
Conscious proprioception: *Decreased in pelvic limbs*
Spinal reflexes: *Normal in thoracic limbs; decreased in both pelvic limbs; normal patellar reflex in the pelvic limbs; decreased withdrawal reflex in the pelvic limbs*
Cranial nerves: *Normal*
Urination/defecation: *Normal*
Cutaneous trunci: *Normal*
Spinal pain: *None*
Deep pain: *Present*

Neuroanatomical Diagnosis
Where is the lesion?
What are the differential diagnoses?
What is the diagnostic plan?

CASE 5.15

Signalment: *5-year-old Akita dog*

Chief Complaint: *Progressive gait abnormality over 6 months*

Physical Examination: *Normal*

Neurologic Examination
Mental status: *Normal*
Posture: *Normal*
Gait: *Short steps in pelvic limbs, with longer, more irregular steps in the pelvic limbs*
Conscious proprioception: *Decreased in all limbs*
Spinal reflexes: *Normal in pelvic limbs; decreased withdrawal in the thoracic limbs*
Cranial nerves: *Normal*
Urination/defecation: *Normal*
Cutaneous trunci: *Normal*
Spinal pain: *None*
Deep pain: *Present*

Neuroanatomical Diagnosis
Where is the lesion?
What are the differential diagnoses?
What is the diagnostic plan?

CASE 5.16

Signalment: *1.5-year-old mastiff dog*

Chief Complaint: *Progressive gait abnormality over 6 months*

Physical Examination: *Normal*

Neurologic Examination
Mental status: *Normal*
Posture: *Normal*
Gait: *Dragging of the thoracic limbs*
Conscious proprioception: *Decreased in thoracic limbs; normal in the pelvic limbs*
Spinal reflexes: *Normal in all limbs*
Cranial nerves: *Normal*

Urination/defecation: *Normal*
Cutaneous trunci: *Normal*
Spinal pain: *None*
Deep pain: *Present*

Neuroanatomical Diagnosis
Where is the lesion?
What are the differential diagnoses?
What is the diagnostic plan?

CASE 5.17

Signalment: *5-year-old German shepherd*

Chief Complaint: *Gait abnormality for 4 weeks, progressive*

Physical Examination: *Normal*

Neurologic Examination
Mental status: *Normal*
Posture: *Normal*
Gait: *Drags right pelvic limb*
Conscious proprioception: *Normal in thoracic limbs; decreased in right pelvic limb*
Spinal reflexes: *Normal in thoracic limbs and in the left pelvic limb; exaggerated patellar reflex in right pelvic limb; decreased withdrawal reflex in the right pelvic limb*
Cranial nerves: *Normal*
Urination/defecation: *Normal*
Cutaneous trunci: *Normal*
Spinal pain: *Pain upon palpation over the caudal lumbar area*
Deep pain: *Present*

Neuroanatomical Diagnosis
Where is the lesion?
What are the differential diagnoses?
What is the diagnostic plan?

CASE 5.18

Signalment: *12-year-old mixed-breed dog*

Chief Complaint: *Clinical signs began with a right thoracic limb lameness, which progressed over the ensuing 5 months to a more significant impairment of gait.*

Physical Examination: *Normal*

Neurologic Examination
Mental status: *Normal*
Posture: *Normal*
Gait: *Lameness of the right thoracic limb*
Conscious proprioception: *Decreased in right thoracic and pelvic limbs*
Spinal reflexes: *Normal in pelvic limbs; decreased withdrawal in the right thoracic limb*
Cranial nerves: *Normal*
Urination/defecation: *Normal*
Cutaneous trunci: *Regardless of which side of the body is stimulated, only the left cutaneous trunci muscle contracts*
Spinal pain: *Pain upon palpation of the right axillary region*
Deep pain: *Present*

Neuroanatomical Diagnosis
Where is the lesion?
What are the differential diagnoses?
What is the diagnostic plan?

CASE 5.19

Signalment: *2-year-old Labrador retriever dog*

Chief Complaint: *Acute onset inability to stand on pelvic limbs 3 days prior to admission*

Physical Examination: *Normal*

Neurologic Examination
Mental status: *Normal*
Posture: *Normal*
Gait: *Cannot stand in pelvic limbs*
Conscious proprioception: *Normal in thoracic limbs; absent in both pelvic limbs*
Spinal reflexes: *Normal in thoracic limbs; absent in the left pelvic limb; decreased patellar and withdrawal in the right pelvic limb*
Cranial nerves: *Normal*
Urination/defecation: *No voluntary urination or defecation; anal tone is absent; bladder is large, flaccid, and easy to express.*
Cutaneous trunci: *Normal*
Spinal pain: *Mild pain upon palpation over the caudal lumbar area*
Deep pain: *Absent in the left pelvic limb; present in the right pelvic limb*

Neuroanatomical Diagnosis
Where is the lesion?
What are the differential diagnoses?
What is the diagnostic plan?

CASE 5.20

Signalment: *5-year-old beagle*

Chief Complaint: *Acute onset of pain 4 days ago; no improvement noted on anti-inflammatory drugs.*

Physical Examination: *Normal*

Neurologic Examination
Mental status: *Normal*
Posture: *Normal*
Gait: *Unable to stand*
Conscious proprioception: *Decreased in all limbs, worse on right side*

Spinal reflexes: *Normal in all limbs*
Cranial nerves: *Normal*
Urination/defecation: *Normal*
Cutaneous trunci: *Normal*
Spinal pain: *Pain in the cervical area*
Deep pain: *Present*

Neuroanatomical Diagnosis
Where is the lesion?
What are the differential diagnoses?
What is the diagnostic plan?

CASE 5.21

Signalment: *5-year-old cat*

Chief Complaint: *Acute onset abnormal posture 5 days ago; no change in clinical signs over the last 5 days*

Physical Examination: *Normal*

Neurologic Examination
Mental status: *Normal*
Posture: *Head tilt to the right*
Gait: *Ataxia and falling*
Conscious proprioception: *Normal in all limbs*
Spinal reflexes: *Normal in all limbs*
Cranial nerves: *Right head tilt; spontaneous rotatory nystagmus, does not change character with changing head positions.*
Other cranial nerves: *Normal*
Urination/defecation: *Normal*
Cutaneous trunci: *Normal*
Spinal pain: *None*
Deep pain: *Present*

Neuroanatomical Diagnosis
Where is the lesion?
What are the differential diagnoses?
What is the diagnostic plan?

CASE 5.22

Signalment: *9-month-old malamute dog*

Chief Complaint: *Abnormal gait for 1 month, slow onset, signs getting worse*

Physical Examination: *Normal*

Neurologic Examination
Mental status: *Normal*
Posture: *Normal*
Gait: *Step distance is progressively shorter with exercise, some bunny hopping*
Conscious proprioception: *Decreased in all limbs*
Spinal reflexes: *Decreased in all limbs*
Cranial nerves: *Normal*
Urination/defecation: *Normal*
Cutaneous trunci: *Normal*
Spinal pain: *None*
Deep pain: *Present*

Neuroanatomical Diagnosis
Where is the lesion?
What are the differential diagnoses?
What is the diagnostic plan?

CASE 5.23

Signalment: *3-year-old mixed-breed dog*

Chief Complaint: *Acutely unable to stand*

Physical Examination: *Normal*

Neurologic Examination
Mental status: *Alert*
Posture: *Laterally recumbent*
Gait: *Cannot stand to walk*
Conscious proprioception: *Absent in all limbs*
Spinal reflexes: *Absent in all limbs*
Cranial nerves: *Normal*
Urination/defecation: *Normal*
Cutaneous trunci: *Normal*
Spinal pain: *None*
Deep pain: *Present; The animal appears hyperesthetic to minimal touch of the limbs.*

Neuroanatomical Diagnosis
Where is the lesion?
What are the differential diagnoses?
What is the diagnostic plan?

CASE 5.24

Signalment: *7-month-old Samoyed*

Chief Complaint: *Involuntary movements for 3 days*

Physical Examination: *Normal*

Neurologic Examination
Mental status: *Alert*
Posture: *Wide-based stance at times*
Gait: *Ataxia, hypermetria, tremoring*
Conscious proprioception: *Normal*
Spinal reflexes: *Normal in all limbs*
Cranial nerves: *Decreased menace response in both eyes with normal palpebral and pupillary light reflexes; dog is visual, other cranial nerves normal.*
Urination/defecation: *Normal*
Cutaneous trunci: *Normal*
Spinal pain: *None*
Deep pain: *Present*

Neuroanatomical Diagnosis

Where is the lesion?
What are the differential diagnoses?
What is the diagnostic plan?

CASE STUDIES ANSWERS

Case 5.1 Discussion

Ataxia is a failure of muscular coordination or an irregularity of muscle action. It is associated with a variety of anatomic lesions within the nervous system, most commonly of the cerebellum, vestibular system, and spinal cord sensory pathways. Ataxia, without motor involvement or paresis, usually implies cerebellar or cerebellar pathway disease.

The dog has ataxia and conscious proprioceptive deficits in the pelvic limbs suggesting a neurologic problem.

The thoracic limbs are normal suggesting a problem caudal to the cervical intumescence (T2).

The spinal reflexes are normal, suggesting that the local reflex arcs beginning at the lumbar intumescence (L4–S1–3) are normal. These findings are consistent with a lesion between the T3 and L3 spinal segments.

Therefore, the neuroanatomical diagnosis is a lesion from *T3–L3 spinal segments.*

The *differential diagnosis* would include:

- Intervertebral disk disease
- Tumor
- Spinal trauma
- Myelitis/meningitis
- Diskospondylitis/osteomyelitis
- Fibrocartilaginous emboli (a nonpainful and nonprogressive disease)
- Other spinal defects, such as syringomyelia or hydromyelia

The *diagnostic plan* would include:

- Survey spinal radiographs to determine an anatomical spinal cord abnormality, advanced spinal imaging such as MR, CT, or myelography
- CSF analysis to rule out myelitis

Final Diagnosis. A MR image of the thoracic spine (fig. A5.1, arrow) showed an intramedullary tumor in the thoracic area.

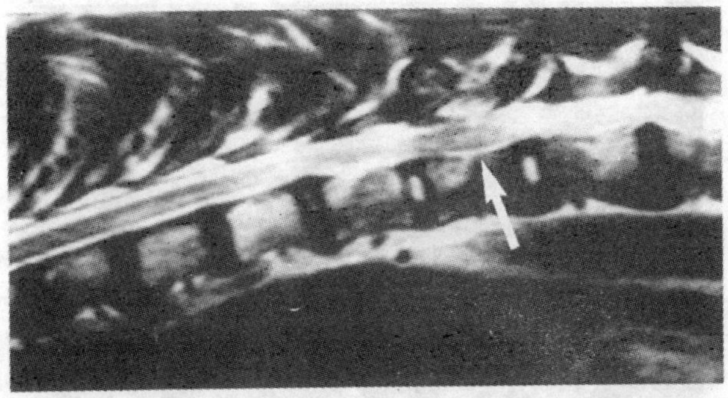

Fig. A5.1.

Case 5.2 Discussion

The dog has conscious proprioceptive deficits in all limbs suggesting a neurologic problem.

The dog has asymmetric signs and is worse on the right side.

The spinal reflexes are normal, suggesting that the local reflex arcs in the cervical intumescence (C6–T2) and the lumbar intumescence (L4–S1–3) are normal. These findings are consistent with a lesion cranial to the C5 spinal segment.

The cranial nerves are normal, suggesting a problem caudal to the foramen magnum.

Therefore, the neuroanatomical diagnosis is a lesion from *C1 to C5 spinal segments.* The dog is *worse on the right side* suggesting an *asymmetric lesion* more on *the right side.*

The *differential diagnosis* would include:

- Intervertebral disk disease
- Tumor
- Spinal trauma
- Myelitis/meningitis
- Diskospondylitis/osteomyelitis
- Fibrocartilaginous emboli (a nonpainful and nonprogressive disease; this is, however, very uncommon in chondrodystrophoid breeds of dogs, such as dachshunds.)
- Other spinal defects, such as syringomyelia or hydromyelia

The *diagnostic plan* would include:

- Survey spinal radiographs
- To determine an anatomical spinal cord abnormality, advanced spinal imaging such as MR, CT, or myelography
- CSF analysis to rule out myelitis

Final Diagnosis. An MR image of the cervical spine (fig. A5.2, arrow) showed an intervertebral disk extrusion at C2–3.

Case 5.3 Discussion

The dog is mentally dull.

The dog has conscious proprioceptive deficits in the left thoracic and pelvic limbs suggesting a neurologic problem. This is a left hemiparesis.

The dog has asymmetric signs and is worse on the left side.

The spinal reflexes are normal, suggesting that the local reflex arcs in the cervical intumescence (C6–T2) and the lumbar intumescence (L4–S1–3) are normal. These findings are consistent with a lesion cranial to the C5 spinal segments.

The menace response is abnormal in the left eye.

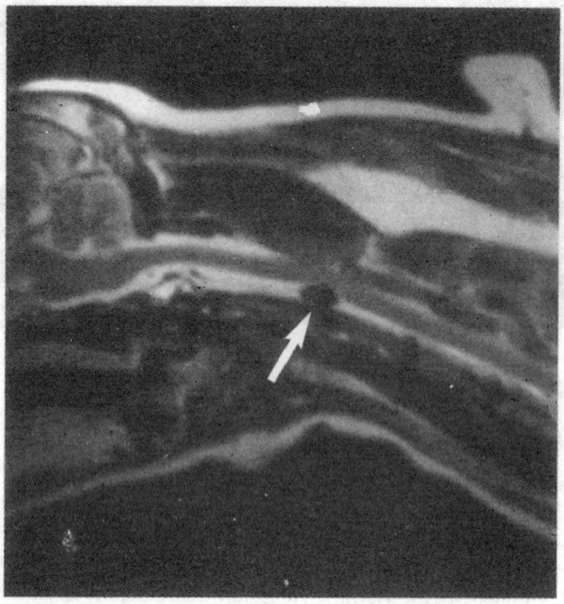

Fig. A5.2.

Considering the normal palpebral reflex and the normal pupillary reflex, this suggests a lesion within the opposite (i.e., right) supratentorial area (see vision and pupils case 4.1, appendix 4).

Therefore the neuroanatomical diagnosis is a lesion in the *supratentorial area.* The dog is *worse on the left side* suggesting an *asymmetric lesion* more on *the right side.*

The *differential diagnosis* would include:

- Brain tumor
- Head trauma
- Acquired Hydrocephalus
- Encephalitis
- Cerebrovascular disease

The *diagnostic plan* would include:

- Assessment of systemic health with CBC, Chem, UA, blood pressure
- Advanced intracranial imaging such as MR
- CSF analysis to rule out encephalitis

Final Diagnosis. An MR image of the brain (fig. A5.3, arrow) showed a tumor of the right supratentorial area. Histologic diagnosis was a glioma.

Case 5.4 Discussion

The dog is otherwise normal except for the function of CN VII (facial nerve).

Note that during the menace response testing the dog tries to retract his eye in the orbit, but cannot completely close the palpebral fissure.

These abnormalities are suggestive of a facial nerve abnormality. The lack of additional neurologic signs suggests a peripheral nerve problem.

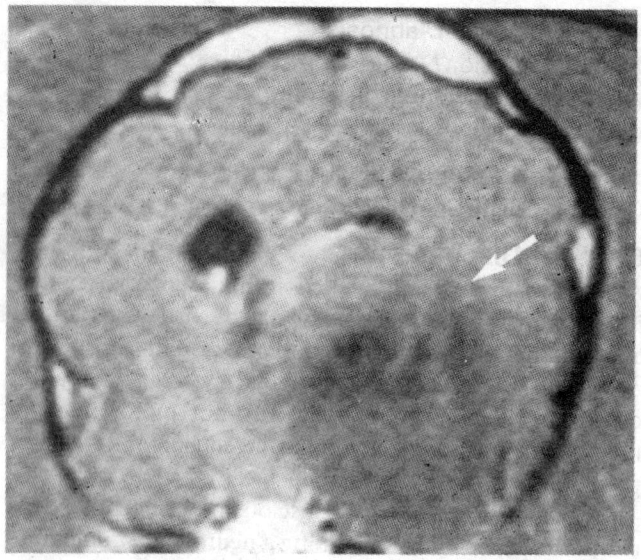

Fig. A5.3.

The *differential diagnosis* would include:

- Idiopathic facial paralysis
- Otitis interna
- Peripheral nerve tumor
- There is a weak association with facial nerve paralysis and hypothyroidism.
- Occult central nervous system problem (brain stem lesion) from tumor, trauma, encephalitis, hydrocephalus, or cerebrovascular disease

The *diagnostic plan* would include:

- Schirmer tear test for KCS
- Check systemic health with CBC, Chem, UA
- Probably assess thyroid status
- Otoscopic exam of ear
- If middle/inner ear disease suspicious, could perform skull radiographs looking for bulla disease. CT and MR imaging can also assess the bulla.
- Advantage of MR imaging is that it can assess the peripheral structure of the middle/inner ear concurrently with the brain stem and other central nervous system structures.
- CSF to rule out encephalitis if other tests are negative

Final Diagnosis. The dog had idiopathic facial nerve palsy.

Facial paralysis is the most common abnormality seen with facial nerve disease. This can occur as an idiopathic condition (especially in cocker spaniels), as a result of otitis media/interna, with trauma, and with tumor of the middle ear canal. Hypothyroidism is a loosely associated cause in some dogs. Hyperinsulinism (islet cell tumor) and other metabolic abnormalities also loosely associated. Rarely, primary tumor of CN VII (nerve sheath tumor, LSA, or meningioma) is seen. Trauma may affect only one branch of this nerve.

Case 5.5 Discussion

The dog has conscious proprioceptive deficits in all limbs suggesting a neurologic problem. This is referred to as a tetraparesis.

The spinal reflexes are normal, suggesting that the local reflex arcs in the cervical intumescence (C6–T2) and the lumbar intumescence (L4–S1–3) are normal. These findings are consistent with a lesion cranial to the C5 spinal segment.

The dog also has vertical nystagmus. Coupled with the conscious proprioceptive deficits, this suggests vestibular disease. Neuroanatomical localization would be a central vestibular lesion, most likely on the right side.

The *differential diagnosis* would include:

- Brain tumor
- Head trauma
- Acquired hydrocephalus
- Encephalitis
- Cerebrovascular disease
- Metronidazole toxicity (In a dog with vestibular disease, always ask about administration of this drug.)

The *diagnostic plan* would include:

- Assessment of systemic health with CBC, Chem, UA, blood pressure
- Advanced intracranial imaging such as MR
- CSF analysis to rule out encephalitis

Final Diagnosis. An MR image of the brain (fig. A5.5), showed a tumor in the right central vestibular area (arrow).

Case 5.6 Discussion

The dog has conscious proprioceptive deficits in the pelvic limbs suggesting a neurologic problem.

The thoracic limbs are normal suggesting a problem caudal to the cervical intumescence (T2).

The spinal reflexes are normal, suggesting that the local reflex arcs beginning at the lumbar intumescence (L4–S1–3) are normal. These findings are consistent with a lesion between the T3 and L3 spinal segments.

Therefore, the neuroanatomical diagnosis is a lesion from *T3 to L3 spinal segments.*

The *differential diagnosis* would include:

- Chronic intervertebral disk disease
- Degenerative myelopathy
- Tumor
- Spinal trauma
- Myelitis/meningitis
- Diskospondylitis/osteomyelitis
- Other spinal defect such as syringomyelia or hydromyelia

The *diagnostic plan* would include:

- Survey spinal radiographs to determine an anatomical spinal cord abnormality, advanced spinal imaging such as MR, CT, or myelography
- CSF analysis to rule out myelitis

Final Diagnosis. An MR image of the thoracolumbar spine (fig. A5.6A) showed multiple chronic intervertebral disk protrusions (arrows). Figure A5.6B shows the appearance of the chronic disk at surgery (arrow).

Case 5.7 Discussion

The dog has pain primarily in the LS area. Coupled with poor tail function, this suggests a lesion of the caudal spinal cord segments or exiting peripheral nerves.

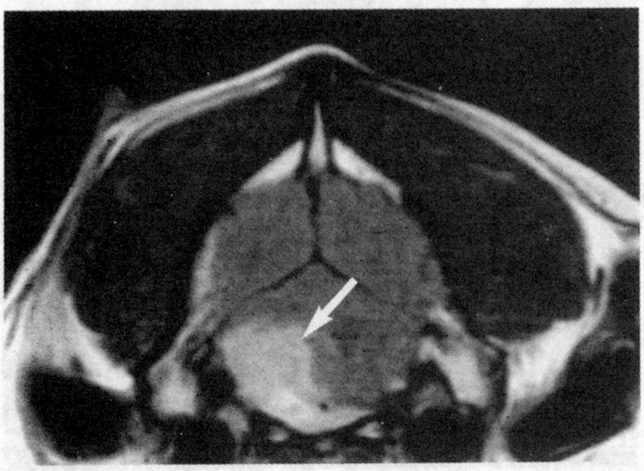

Fig. A5.5.

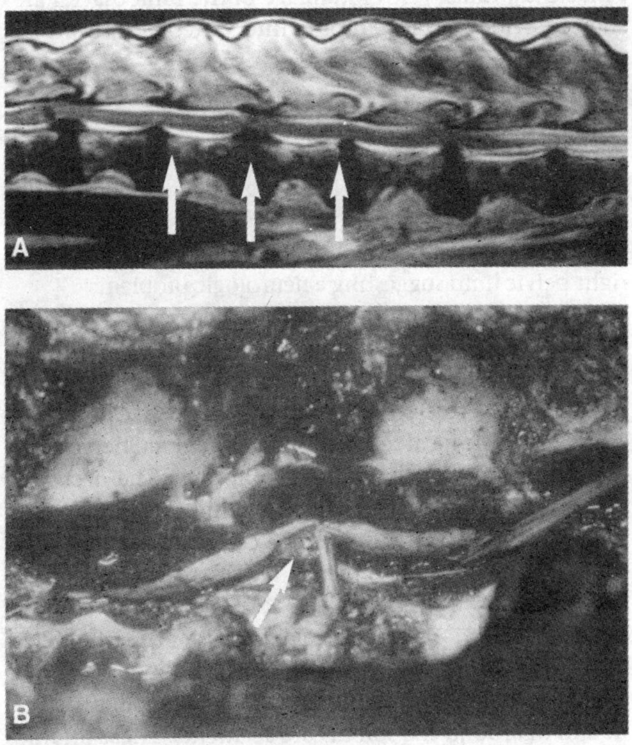

Fig. A5.6.

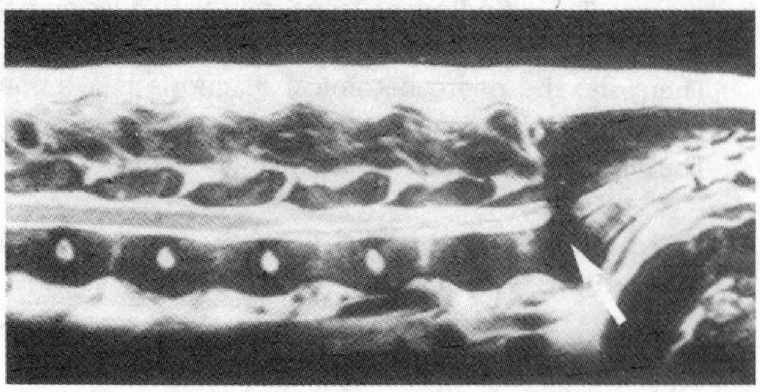

Fig. A5.7.

The *differential diagnosis* would include:

- Chronic intervertebral disk disease
- Lumbosacral stenosis
- Tumor
- Spinal trauma
- Myelitis/meningitis
- Diskospondylitis/osteomyelitis

The *diagnostic plan* would include:

- Survey spinal radiographs of LS area to evaluate for diskospondylitis, tumor, and fracture
- For definitive diagnosis, advanced spinal imaging such as MR, CT
- EMG may help in determination of local denervation
- CSF analysis to rule out myelitis

Final Diagnosis. An MR image of the lumbosacral area showed evidence of a chronic intervertebral disk protrusion at the L7–S1 intervertebral disk space (fig. A5.7, arrow).

Case 5.8 Discussion

The dog has an abnormal gait wherein the distal pelvic limb is "thrown" forward. This suggests poor ability to flex the hock joint.

The dog has a conscious proprioceptive deficit in the right pelvic limb suggesting a neurologic problem.

The thoracic limbs are normal suggesting a problem caudal to the cervical intumescence (T2).

The spinal reflexes are normal in the thoracic limbs.

The patella reflexes are normal in the pelvic limbs suggesting that the local reflex arcs for the femoral nerve at the lumbar intumescence (L4–L6) are normal. The decreased withdrawal reflex in the right pelvic limb suggests a lesion in the sciatic nerves, either in the cell bodies at the spinal cord (L6–S1-3 spinal segments), in the exiting peripheral nerves, or in the peripheral sciatic nerves distal the spinal canal. The L6–S1-3 spinal segments lie over the L4–5 vertebral segments.

The spinal pain in the caudal lumbar area suggests a lesion in or around the spinal cord segments. These findings are consistent with a lesion between the *L6 and the S1-3 spinal segments*, more on the right side.

The *differential diagnosis* would include:

- Intervertebral disk disease
- Tumor
- Spinal trauma
- Myelitis/meningitis
- Diskospondylitis/osteomyelitis

The *diagnostic plan* would include:

- Survey spinal radiographs of lumbar area to evaluate for diskospondylitis, tumor, and fracture
- For definitive diagnosis, advanced spinal imaging such as MR, CT
- EMG helpful in determination of local denervation
- CSF analysis to rule out myelitis

Final Diagnosis. An MR image of the lumbar spine showed a spinal tumor at the L5–6 intervertebral disk space.

Figure A5.8A is a sagittal T-2 weighted MR image of the lumbar spine showing an abnormality over the L5–6 intervetebral disk space (arrow). Figure A5.8B is a transverse T-2 weighted MR image over the same region showing a hypointense mass (arrow) displacing the spinal cord.

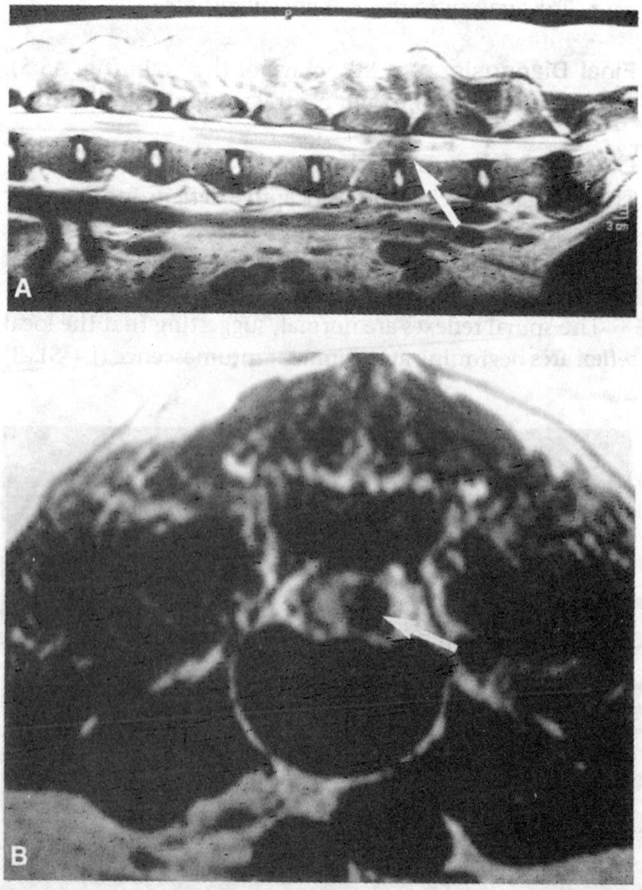

Fig. A5.8.

Case 5.9 Discussion

The three general causes of muscle atrophy are neurogenic (due to peripheral nerve injury or disease), disuse (atrophy due to lack of muscle use, most often seen with UMN diseases or musculoskeletal diseases), and primary myopathic atrophy (seen with disease of the muscle).

The dog has an acute onset of muscle atrophy, which is consistent with primary muscle disease or neurogenic atrophy.

The dog has a decreased palpebral reflex in the left eye suggesting a problem with either CN V for sensation or CN VII for the motor portion of this reflex. Since the menace response is normal, this suggests that the sensory portion of this reflex is abnormal. This sensory portion of this reflex is innervated through CN V, ophthalmic branch.

The decreased sensation in the left nostril could also suggest a CN V lesion (ophthalmic or maxillary branch of CN V).

The temporalis muscle is innervated through the mandibular branch of CN V.

These findings, coupled with the atrophy, suggest that this dog has a trigeminal (CN V) problem involving all branches of this nerve (ophthalmic, maxillary, and mandibular branches). Since there are no other clinical signs, this suggests that the lesion is peripheral in the nerve.

The *differential diagnosis* would include:

- Tumor of the trigeminal nerve
- Inflammation of the trigeminal nerve

The *diagnostic plan* would include:

- Schirmer tear test for KCS
- Check systemic health with CBC, Chem, UA
- MR imaging to assess brain stem and trigeminal nerve
- CFS to rule out encephalitis if other tests are negative

Final Diagnosis. An MR image of the brain showed a lesion in the left trigeminal nerve (fig. A5.9, arrow).

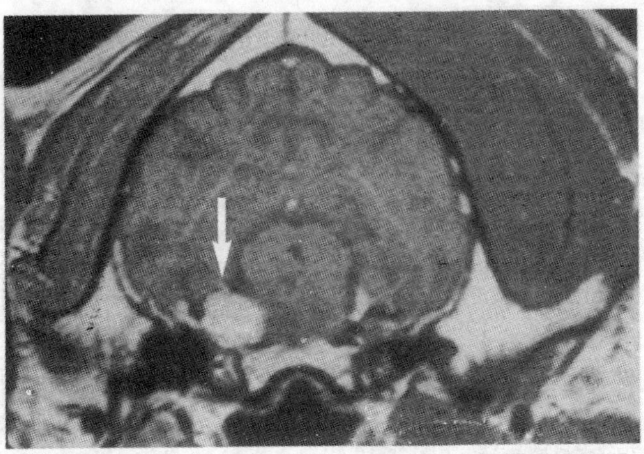

Fig. A5.9.

Case 5.10 Discussion

The hypermetria of the left thoracic limb suggests a neurologic problem, possibly in the cerebellar or vestibular systems, including the spinal cord.

The dog has conscious proprioceptive deficits in the left thoracic and pelvic limbs suggesting a neurologic problem. This is a hemiparesis.

The spinal reflexes are normal, suggesting that the local reflex arcs in the cervical intumescence (C6–T2) and the lumbar intumescence (L4–S1–3) are normal. These findings are consistent with a lesion cranial to the C5 spinal segments.

The dog also has a head tilt. Coupled with the conscious proprioceptive deficits, this suggests vestibular disease. Neuroanatomical localization would be a central vestibular lesion. As the vestibular system is anatomically below the functional crossover, a lesion in the central vestibular area would cause the most deficits on the same side of the lesion. This would suggest a lesion on the left side of the brain stem. The head tilt is usually toward the direction of a peripheral lesion. However, with lesions of the caudal cerebellar peduncle, the head may tilt in the direction opposite to the lesion (i.e., a paradoxical head tilt).

Therefore, the neuroanatomical diagnosis would be a left central vestibular problem.

The *differential diagnosis* would include:

- Brain tumor
- Head trauma
- Acquired hydrocephalus
- Encephalitis
- Cerebrovascular disease
- Metronidazole toxicity (In a dog with vestibular disease, always ask about administration of this drug.)

The *diagnostic plan* would include:

- Advanced intracranial imaging such as MR
- CSF analysis to rule out encephalitis
- Assessment of systemic health with CBC, Chem, UA, blood pressure

Final Diagnosis. An MR image of the brain showed a cystic lesion in the left cerebellopontine area (fig. A5.10, arrow).

Case 5.11 Discussion

The dog has conscious proprioceptive deficits in all limbs suggesting a neurologic problem.

The dog has asymmetric signs and is worse on the left side.

The spinal reflexes are normal in the pelvic limbs suggesting that the local reflex arcs in the lumbar intumescence (L4–S1–3) are normal. The spinal reflexes are decreased in the thoracic limbs suggesting that the local reflex arcs in the cervical intumescence (C6–T2) are involved. These findings are consistent with a lesion in the C6–T2 spinal segments.

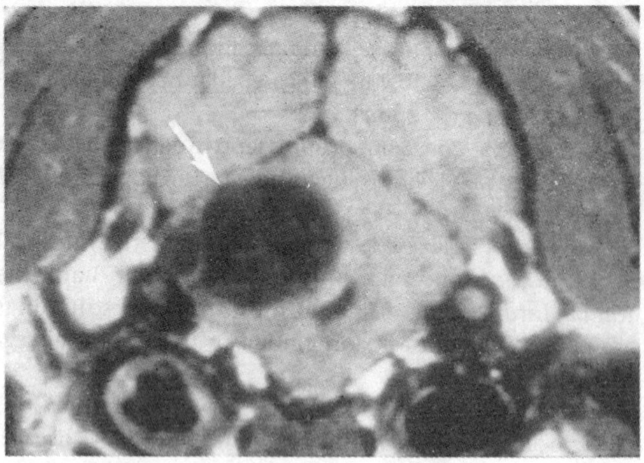

Fig. A5.10.

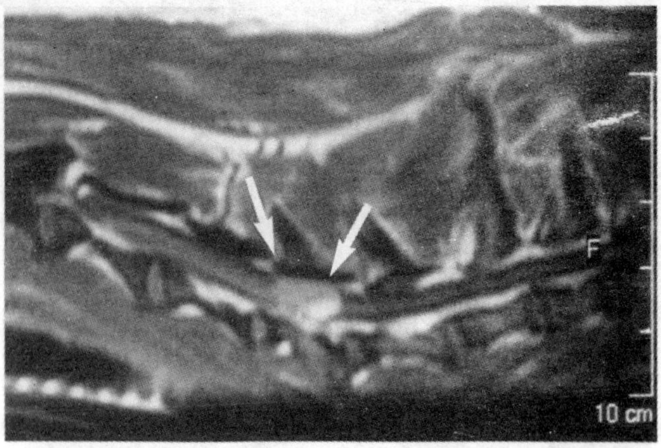

Fig. A5.11.

The cranial nerves are normal, suggesting a problem caudal to the foramen magnum.

Therefore, the neuroanatomical diagnosis is a lesion from *C6 to T2 spinal segments.* The dog is *worse on the left side* suggesting an *asymmetric lesion* more on *the left side.*

The *differential diagnosis* would include:

- Intervertebral disk disease
- Tumor
- Spinal trauma
- Myelitis/meningitis
- Diskospondylitis/osteomyelitis
- Congenital spinal anomaly
- Other spinal defect such as syringomyelia or hydromyelia
- Spinal hemorrhage

The *diagnostic plan* would include:

- Survey spinal radiographs to determine an anatomical spinal cord abnormality, then advanced spinal imaging such as MR, CT, or myelography
- CSF analysis to rule out myelitis

Final Diagnosis. An MR image of the cervical spine showed a lesion in the spinal cord at C5–6 (fig. A5.11, arrows). Diagnosis at surgery was a hematoma.

Case 5.12 Discussion

The cat tends to circle to the left. Circling can indicate a supratentorial or a vestibular problem. Usually, animals will circle in the direction of the lesion.

The cat has conscious proprioceptive deficits in the right thoracic and pelvic limbs suggesting a neurologic problem. This is a right hemiparesis.

The spinal reflexes are normal, suggesting that the local reflex arcs in the cervical intumescence (C6–T2) and the lumbar intumescence (L4–S1–3) are normal. These findings are consistent with a lesion cranial to the C5 spinal segments.

The menace response is abnormal in the right eye. Considering the normal palpebral reflex and the normal pupillary reflex, this suggests a lesion within the opposite (i.e., left) supratentorial area.

We know that the PLR is normal both direct and consensually in the right eye. The lesion must then be caudal to where the fibers leave the right optic tract to result in the PLR. This leaves the right forebrain as abnormal, with this being an example of central blindness.

Considering the circling toward the left side, and the hemiparesis, the neuroanatomical diagnosis is a lesion in the *supratentorial area.* The cat is *worse on the right side* suggesting an *asymmetric lesion* more on *the left side.*

The *differential diagnosis* would include:

- Brain tumor
- Head trauma
- Acquired hydrocephalus
- Encephalitis
- Cerebrovascular disease

The *diagnostic plan* would include:

- Assessment of systemic health with CBC, Chem, UA, blood pressure
- Advanced intracranial imaging such as MR
- CSF analysis to rule out encephalitis

Final Diagnosis. An MR image of the brain showed a tumor in the left supratentorial area (fig. A5.12, arrow; reprinted with permission from R. Bagley, Recognition and localization of intracranial disease [Vet Clin N Am (Small Anim Pract), 1996:667–709, fig. 1]).

Case 5.13 Discussion

A shortened step distance at gait usually indicates a problem with pain or muscle weakness. Muscle weakness can occur as a result of LMN disease.

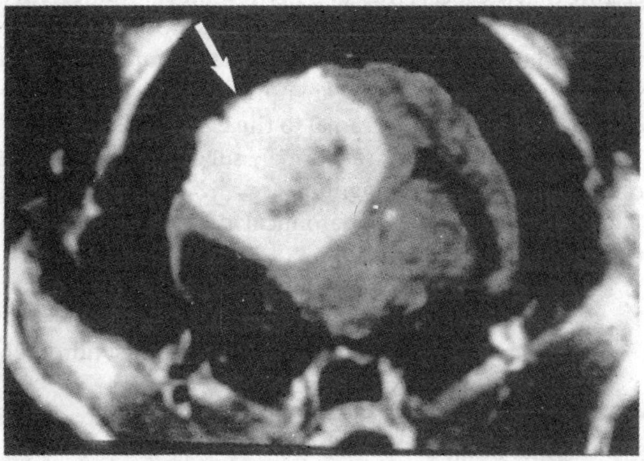

Fig. A5.12.

The dog has conscious proprioceptive deficits when it supports its own body weight, but not when the examiner supports its weight. This suggests a muscle strength problem.

The spinal reflexes are normal, suggesting that the local reflex arcs beginning at the lumbar intumescence (L4–S1–3) are normal.

The menace response and palpebral reflexes are decreased bilaterally suggesting a problem with the facial nerve, or with the orbicularis oculi muscle function or strength.

Therefore, the most likely neuroanatomical diagnosis is a diffuse problem with muscle weakness.

The *differential diagnosis* would include:

- Neuromuscular junction diseases such as myasthenia gravis
- Primary muscle diseases such as myopathy or myositis
- Peripheral nerve disease such as polyneuropathy or polyneuritis (possible but less likely)

The *diagnostic plan* would include:

- Edrophonium (Tensilon) response test
- Serum antiacetylcholine receptor antibody testing for myasthenia gravis
- Serum CK to look for evidence of muscle disease
- Electromyography and nerve conduction studies including decremental responses or single-fiber EMG
- Muscle and nerve biopsies
- If all else is negative, possibly CSF analysis to rule out diffuse myelitis

Final Diagnosis. This dog responded positively to edrophonium administration, and was eventually diagnosed with a positive antiacetylcholine receptor antibody test with myasthenia gravis.

Case 5.14 Discussion

The cat has an abnormal gait wherein the distal pelvic limb drops at the hock or has a plantigrade stance. This suggests poor ability to flex the hock joint. This could indicate a neurologic problem with innervation of the gastrocnemius muscle or the musculoskeletal apparatus necessary to biomechanically flex the hock.

The cat has conscious proprioceptive deficits in the pelvic limbs suggesting a neurologic problem.

The thoracic limbs are normal suggesting a problem caudal to the cervical intumescence (T2).

The spinal reflexes are normal in the thoracic limbs.

The patella reflexes are normal in the pelvic limbs suggesting that the local reflex arcs for the femoral nerve at the lumbar intumescence (L4–L6) are normal. The decreased withdrawal reflex in both pelvic limbs suggests a lesion in the sciatic nerves, either in the cell bodies at the spinal cord (L6–S1–3 spinal segments), in the exiting peripheral nerves, or in the peripheral sciatic nerves distal the spinal canal.

These findings are consistent with a lesion between the *L6 and the S1–3 spinal segments or in the sciatic nerves themselves.*

The *differential diagnosis* for sciatic nerve disease would include:

- Polyneuropathy
- Tumor involving the nerves such as lymphoma
- Diabetic neuropathy
- Myopathies

The *differential diagnosis* for spinal cord disease would include:

- Intervertebral disk disease
- Tumor
- Traumatic injury
- Myelitis/meningitis
- Diskospondylitis/osteomyelitis

The *diagnostic plan* would include:

- Serum CK to assess for evidence of muscle disease
- Electromyography and nerve conduction studies including decremental responses or single-fiber EMG
- Muscle and nerve biopsies
- If all else is negative, possibly CSF to assess for myelitis
- Survey spinal radiographs of LS area
- If radiographs are not definitive, then advanced spinal imaging such as MR, CT, or myelography

Final Diagnosis. This cat had diabetic neuropathy.

Case 5.15 Discussion

This dog has short steps in the thoracic limbs. This suggests pain or LMN weakness. The pelvic limb gait is more characteristic of a problem with UMN influence.

The dog has conscious proprioceptive deficits in all limbs suggesting a neurologic problem.

The spinal reflexes are normal in the pelvic limbs suggesting that the local reflex arcs in the lumbar intumescence (L4–S1–3) are normal. The spinal reflexes are decreased in the thoracic limbs suggesting that the local reflex arcs in the cervical intumescence (C6–T2) are involved. These findings are consistent with a lesion in the C6–T2 spinal segments.

The global gait abnormalities are characteristic of a lesion in the C6–T2 area as well.

Therefore, the neuroanatomical diagnosis is a lesion within the *C6 to T2 spinal segments*.

The *differential diagnosis* would include:

- Intervertebral disk disease
- Tumor
- Spinal trauma
- Myelitis/meningitis
- Diskospondylitis/osteomyelitis
- Congenital spinal anomaly
- Other spinal defect such as syringomyelia or hydromyelia
- Spinal hemorrhage

The *diagnostic plan* would include:

- Survey spinal radiographs to determine an anatomical spinal cord abnormality, then advanced spinal imaging such as MR, CT, or myelography
- CSF analysis to rule out myelitis

Final Diagnosis. The dog has a compressive spinal cord problem consistent with a chronic type II intervertebral disk protrusion at C5–6 and C6–7 intervertebral disk spaces (fig. A5.15, arrows).

Case 5.16 Discussion

This dog shows dragging at gait indicative of a proprioceptive problem in the thoracic limbs.

The dog has conscious proprioceptive deficits in thoracic limbs suggesting a neurologic problem.

The spinal reflexes are normal in the pelvic limbs suggesting that the local reflex arcs in the lumbar intumescence (L4–S1–3) are normal. The spinal reflexes are normal in the thoracic limbs suggesting that the local reflex arcs in the cervical intumescence (C6–T2) are normal. These findings are consistent with a lesion cranial to the C5 spinal segments.

The cranial nerves are normal, suggesting a problem caudal to the foramen magnum.

Therefore, the neuroanatomical diagnosis is a lesion from *C1 to C5 spinal segments*.

The *differential diagnosis* would include:

- Cervical stenosis/malformation (wobbler syndrome)
- Intervertebral disk disease
- Tumor
- Spinal trauma
- Myelitis/meningitis
- Diskospondylitis/osteomyelitis
- Congenital spinal anomaly
- Other spinal defects such as syringomyelia or hydromyelia
- Spinal hemorrhage

The *diagnostic plan* would include:

- Survey spinal radiographs to determine an anatomical spinal cord abnormality, advanced spinal imaging such as MR, CT, or myelography
- CSF analysis to rule out myelitis

Final Diagnosis. The dog has a compressive spinal cord problem consistent with the dorsolateral compression seen with acquired cervical stenosis at C4–5 and C5–6.

A CT image of the cervical spine showed bilateral lateral spinal cord compression due to proliferation of the articular facet joints (fig. A5.16, arrows).

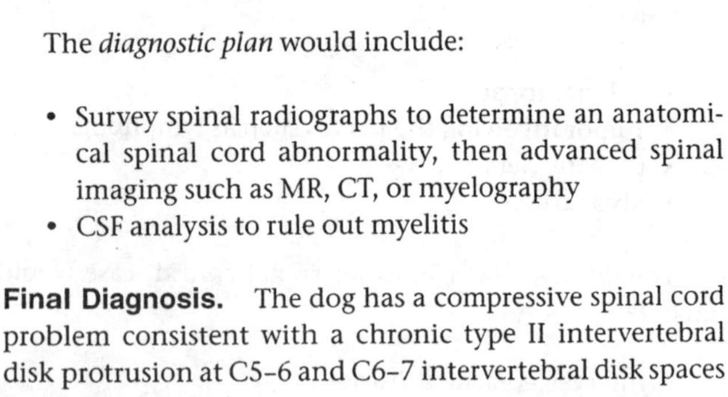

Fig. A5.15.

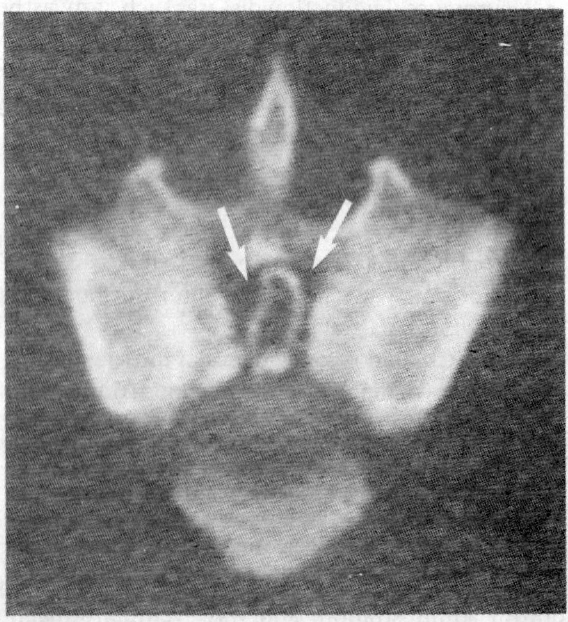

Fig. A5.16.

Case 5.17 Discussion

The dog drags its right pelvic limb suggesting a proprioceptive deficit.

The dog has conscious proprioceptive deficits in the right pelvic limb suggesting a neurologic problem.

The thoracic limbs are normal suggesting a problem caudal to the cervical intumescence (T2).

The spinal reflexes are normal in the thoracic limbs.

The patella and withdrawal reflexes are normal in the left pelvic limbs suggesting that the local reflex arcs for the femoral nerve at the lumbar intumescence (L4–L6) are normal. The patellar reflex is exaggerated in the right pelvic limb, suggesting possible UMN disease. The decreased withdrawal reflex in the right pelvic limbs, however, suggests a lesion in the sciatic nerves, either in the cell bodies at the spinal cord (L6–S1-3 spinal segments), in the exiting peripheral nerves, or in the peripheral sciatic nerves distal the spinal canal on the right side. The L6–S1-3 spinal segments lie over the L4-5 vertebral segments.

When the antagonistic muscles to the patellar reflex (normally innervated by the sciatic nerve) are abnormal, the patellar reflex can appear exaggerated. This may be confused for an associated UMN lesion, however, this *pseudohyperpatellar* reflex can be explained by the sciatic nerve abnormality.

The spinal pain in the caudal lumbar area suggests a lesion in or around these spinal cord segments. These findings are consistent with a lesion between the *L6 and the S1-3 spinal segments or in the sciatic nerve.*

The *differential diagnosis* would include:

- Intervertebral disk disease
- Tumor (spinal or peripheral nerve)
- Traumatic injury
- Myelitis/meningitis/neuritis
- Diskospondylitis/osteomyelitis

The *diagnostic plan* would include:

- Survey spinal radiographs of LS area to evaluate for diskospondylitis, tumor, and fracture
- For definitive diagnosis, advanced spinal imaging such as MR, CT
- EMG helpful in determination of local denervation
- CSF analysis to rule out myelitis

Final Diagnosis. This dog has tumor of the lumbar spine involving the right sciatic nerve and spinal segments (fig. A5.17, arrow).

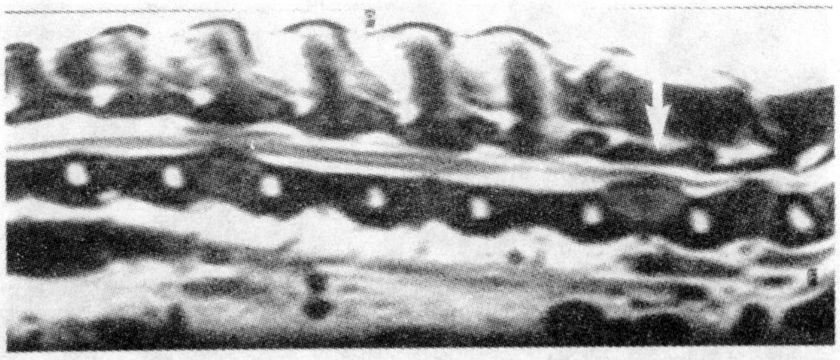

Fig. A5.17.

Case 5.18 Discussion

The dog is lame at gait suggesting pain in the limb. At rest, the dog would sometimes hold the right thoracic limb off of the ground suggesting limb pain or nerve root signature.

The dog has conscious proprioceptive deficits in the right limbs suggesting a neurologic problem. This is a right hemiparesis.

The dog has asymmetric signs and is worse on the right side.

The spinal reflexes are normal in the pelvic limbs suggesting that the local reflex arcs in the lumbar intumescence (L4–S1-3) are normal. The spinal reflexes are decreased in the right thoracic limbs suggesting that the local reflex arcs in the cervical intumescence (C6–T2) are involved. These findings are consistent with a lesion in the C6–T2 spinal segments, on the right side.

The lack of movement of the right cutaneous trunci muscle suggests a problem with the right C8–T1 spinal segments or the associated lateral thoracic nerve.

The cranial nerves are normal, suggesting a problem caudal to the foramen magnum.

The pain in the axillary region suggests a problem in or around this area.

Therefore, the neuroanatomical diagnosis is a lesion from *C6 to T2 spinal segments.* The dog is *worse on the right side* suggesting an *asymmetric lesion* more on *the right side.*

The *differential diagnosis* would include:

- Nerve sheath tumor of the brachial plexus invading the spinal cord
- Intervertebral disk disease
- Spinal trauma
- Myelitis/meningitis
- Diskospondylitis/osteomyelitis
- Other spinal defects, such as syringomyelia or hydromyelia

The *diagnostic plan* would include:

- Survey spinal radiographs
- If radiographs are not definitive, then advanced spinal imaging such as MR, CT, or myelography. MR would provide the advantage of being able to image the soft tissue structures of the brachial plexus area.
- CSF analysis to rule out myelitis
- EMGs of the right thoracic limb to assess innervation of this limb

Final Diagnosis. This dog had tumor of the C7 nerve that was invading and compressing the spinal cord (fig. A5.18).

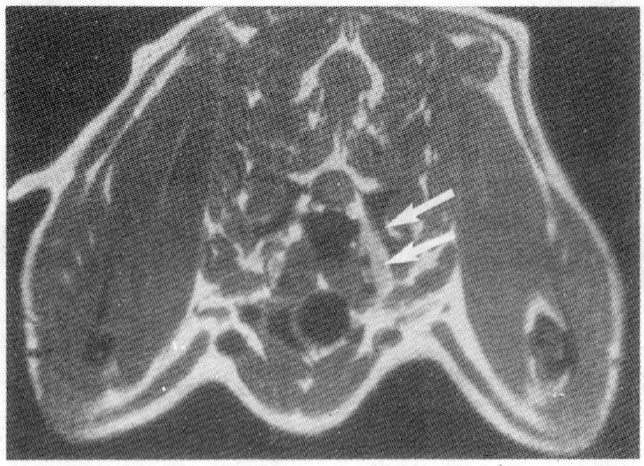

Fig. A5.18.

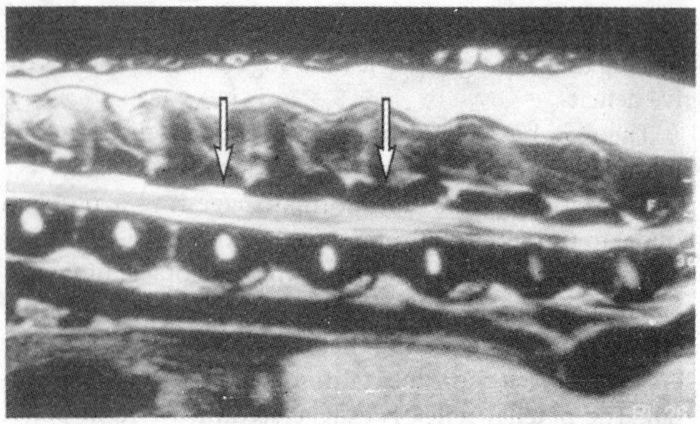

Fig. A5.19.

Case 5.19 Discussion

The dog cannot stand on the pelvic limbs.

The dog has conscious proprioceptive deficits in the both pelvic limbs suggesting a neurologic problem.

The thoracic limbs are normal suggesting a problem caudal to the cervical intumescence (T2).

The spinal reflexes are normal in the thoracic limbs.

The patella and withdrawal reflexes are absent in the left pelvic limbs suggesting the local reflex arcs for the femoral nerve at the lumbar intumescence (L4–S1–3) are abnormal. The patellar reflex and withdrawal reflex are decreased in the right pelvic limbs, suggests a lesion in the femoral and sciatic nerves, either in the cell bodies at the spinal cord (L4–S1–3 spinal segments), in the exiting peripheral nerves, or in the peripheral sciatic nerves distal to the spinal canal on the right side.

The L4–S1–3 spinal segments lie over the L3–5 vertebral segments.

The bladder and bowel signs are suggestive of LMN disease to the S1–3 spinal segments or the pudendal and pelvic nerves.

These signs are indicative of a LMN disease involving the lumbar intumescence spinal segments L4–S1–3, worse on the left, as the deep pain sensation and reflexes are absent on that side.

The *differential diagnosis* would include:

- Intervertebral disk disease
- Tumor
- Spinal trauma
- Myelitis/meningitis
- Diskospondylitis/osteomyelitis
- Spinal cord infarction
- Fibrocartilaginous emboli

The *diagnostic plan* would include:

- Survey spinal radiographs of LS area
- If radiographs are not definitive, then advanced spinal imaging such as MR, CT, or myelography
- CSF analysis to rule out myelitis
- EMGs could be used after 5 days to assess innervation of the pelvic limb muscles

Final Diagnosis. This dog had spinal cord infarcts in the lumbar intumescence (fig. A5.19, arrows).

Case 5.20 discussion

The dog has conscious proprioceptive deficits in all limbs suggesting a neurologic problem.

The dog has asymmetric signs and is worse on the right side.

The spinal reflexes are normal, suggesting that the local reflex arcs in the cervical intumescence (C6–T2) and the lumbar intumescence (L4–S1–3) are normal. These findings are consistent with a lesion cranial to the C5 spinal segments.

The cranial nerves are normal, suggesting a problem caudal to the foramen magnum.

Therefore, the neuroanatomical diagnosis is a lesion from *C1 to C5 spinal segments.* The dog is *worse on the right side* suggesting an *asymmetric lesion* more on *the right side.*

The *differential diagnosis* would include:

- Intervertebral disk disease
- Tumor
- Spinal trauma
- Myelitis/meningitis
- Diskospondylitis/osteomyelitis
- Other spinal defects, such as syringomyelia or hydromyelia

The *diagnostic plan* would include:

- Survey spinal radiographs of cervical area to evaluate for diskospondylitis, tumor, and fracture
- For definitive diagnosis, advanced spinal imaging such as MR, CT
- CSF analysis to rule out myelitis

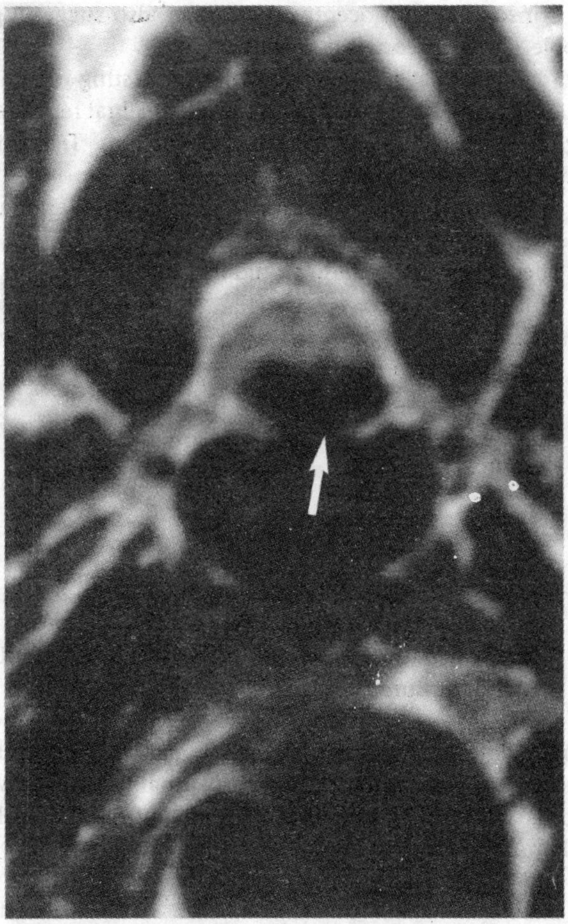

Fig. A5.20.

Final Diagnosis. This dog had a right-sided intervertebral disk extrusion at C2–3 (fig. A5.20). Surgery was performed to remove this disk, and the clinical signs resolved.

Case 5.21 Discussion

The cat has an abnormal head position characterized as a head tilt. Head tilting can indicate vestibular or cerebellar disease. Head tilting is not specific for either central or peripheral disease as it can be seen in both instances. The head tilt is usually in the direction of a peripheral lesion.

The cat has normal conscious proprioceptive in all limbs.

The character of the nystagmus is rotatory, which could be seen with either a central or peripheral vestibular lesion.

As no signs of central vestibular disease are present, a presumptive diagnosis of peripheral vestibular disease would be made.

The *differential diagnosis* peripheral vestibular nerve disease would include:

- Otitis interna/media
- Tumor involving the middle or inner ear
- Trauma
- Toxicity such as aminoglycosides
- Metronidazole toxicity may include other signs such as seizures in cats compared to dogs.
- There is an idiopathic vestibular disease of cats.

The *diagnostic plan* would include:

- Check systemic health with CBC, Chem, UA
- Otoscopic exam of ear
- If middle/inner ear disease suspicious, could perform skull radiographs looking for bulla disease. CT and MR imaging can also assess the bulla.
- Advantage of MR imaging is that it can assess the peripheral structure of the middle/inner ear concurrently with the brain stem and other central nervous system structures.
- CSF to rule out encephalitis if other tests are negative

Final Diagnosis. This cat had a middle ear infection on the right side.

Case 5.22 Discussion

A shortened step distance at gait usually indicates a problem with pain or muscle weakness. Muscle weakness can occur as a result of LMN disease.

The dog has conscious proprioceptive deficits in all limbs suggesting a neurologic problem.

The spinal reflexes are all decreased suggesting that the local reflex arcs are abnormal. This could indicate multiple lesions involving both spinal cord intumescences or, more likely, a diffuse peripheral nerve problem.

The *differential diagnosis* would include:

- Peripheral nerve disease such as polyneuropathy or polyneuritis
- Neuromuscular junction diseases such as myasthenia gravis
- Primary muscle diseases such as myopathy or myositis

The *diagnostic plan* would include:

- Serum CK to look for evidence of muscle disease
- Electromyography and nerve conduction studies including decremental responses or single-fiber EMG
- Muscle and nerve biopsies
- Possibly edrophonium (Tensilon) response test
- Serum antiacetylcholine receptor antibody testing for myasthenia gravis
- If all else is negative, possibly CSF analysis to rule out diffuse myelitis
- Further spinal evaluation with survey radiographs and advanced imaging (MR)

Final Diagnosis. This dog had a peripheral neuropathy common in malamute dogs.

Case 5.23 Discussion

The dog has tetraplegia. The spinal reflexes are absent suggesting a LMN problem.

Diffuse diseases involving the peripheral nerves, NMJ, or muscle should be considered. Possibly diffuse disease of the spinal cord involving nerve roots or both intumescences.

The *differential diagnosis* would include:

- Botulism
- Tick paralysis
- Polyradiculoneuritis (coonhound paralysis)
- Toxicity (OP)
- Diffuse myelitis

The dog is hyperesthetic to minimal stimulation, which would be characteristic of polyradiculoneuritis or coonhound paralysis.

The *diagnostic plan* would include:

- Question regarding toxin exposure
- Blood work including CK and electrolytes
- EMG, NCV studies (Signs may be too early to see EMG changes.)
- CSF analysis to rule out myelitis
- Peripheral nerve/muscle biopsy

Final Diagnosis. This dog had polyradiculoneuritis.

Case 5.24 Discussion

The dog has a wide-based stance suggestive of a proprioceptive problem. The ataxia and hypermetria are suggestive of abnormal unconscious proprioception.

Conscious proprioceptive is normal also suggesting a problem with unconscious proprioception.

The abnormality of menace response testing with normal vision, pupillary light reflex, and palpebral reflex testing suggests a problem with the cerebellum. Tremoring may also be present with cerebellar lesions.

Therefore, the neuroanatomical diagnosis is a lesion diffusely involving the cerebellum.

The *differential diagnosis* would include:

- Encephalitis
- Acquired hydrocephalus
- Cerebrovascular disease
- Head trauma
- Tumor

The *diagnostic plan* would include:

- Advanced intracranial imaging such as MR
- CSF analysis to rule out encephalitis
- Assessment of systemic health with CBC, Chem, UA, blood pressure

Final Diagnosis. Magnetic resonance imaging of the cerebellum was normal. Cerebrospinal fluid analysis showed evidence of inflammation. A diagnosis of cerebellar inflammation was made.

Bibliography

CHAPTERS 1–4: ANATOMY, PHYSIOLOGY, AND CLINICAL ASSESSMENT

Neuroanatomy

Allam, M. W., Lee, D. G., Nulsen, F. E., Fortune, E. A. 1952. The anatomy of the brachial plexus of the dog. Anat Rec 114:173–180.

Anderson, B., McCann, S. M. 1956. The effect of hypothalamic lesions on the water intake of the dog. Acta Physiol Scand 35:312.

Bagley, R. S. 1994. Adipsia and the nervous system. Comp Cont Ed 17:311–318.

Bagley, R. S., Stefanacci, J. D., Hansen, B., Kornegay, J. N., Wheeler, S. J. 1993. Dysphonia in two dogs with cranial cervical intervertebral disc extrusion. JAAHA 29:557–559.

Bailey, C. S., Kitchell, R. L. 1987. Cutaneous sensory testing in the dog. J Vet Intern Med 1:128.

Beitz, A. J., Fletcher, T. F. 1993. The brain. In Miller's Anatomy of the Dog, 3d ed., Evans, H. E., ed. Philadelphia, W. B. Saunders, 894–952.

Braund, KG. 1994. Clinical Syndromes in Veterinary Neurology, 2d ed. St. Louis, Mosby.

Burke, M. J., Colter, S. B. 1990. A practical review of canine and feline spinal cord anatomy. Prog Vet Neurol 1:358–370.

Chrisman, C. L. 1991. Problems in Small Animal Neurology. Philadelphia, Lea & Febiger.

———. 1990. The functional neuroanatomy of the cerebrum and rostral brain stem. Prog Vet Neurol 1:117–122.

Collins, B. K., O'Brien, D. 1990. Autonomic dysfunction of the eye. Seminar Vet Med Surg 5:24.

deLahunta, A. 1983. Veterinary Neuroanatomy and Clinical Neurology, 2d ed. Philadelphia, W. B. Saunders.

———. 1980. Comparative cerebellar disease in domestic animals. The Compendium on Continuing Education 2:8–19.

Dyce, K. M., Sack, W. O., Wensing, C. J. G. 1996a. The neck, back, and vertebral column of the carnivores. In Textbook of Veterinary Anatomy, 2d ed., Dyce, K. M., Sack, W. O., Wensing, C. J. G., eds. Philadelphia, W. B. Saunders, 393–401.

———. 1996b. The nervous system. In Textbook of Veterinary Anatomy, 2d ed., Dyce, K. M., Sack, W. O., Wensing, C. J. G., eds. Philadelphia, W. B. Saunders, 259–324.

Evans, H. E. 1993. The ear. In Miller's Anatomy of the Dog, 3d ed., Evans, H. E., ed. Philadelphia, W. B. Saunders, 988–1008.

Evans, H. E, Kitchell, R. L. 1993. Cranial nerves and cutaneous innervation of the head. In Miller's Anatomy of the Dog, 3d ed., Evans, H. E., ed. Philadelphia, W. B. Saunders, 953–986.

Fletcher, T. F. 1993. Spinal cord and meninges. In Miller's Anatomy of the Dog, 3d ed., Evans HE, ed. Philadelphia, W. B. Saunders, 800–828.

Guyton, A. C., Hall, J. E. 1996. Textbook of Medical Physiology, 9th ed. Philadelphia, W. B. Saunders, 525.

Holliday, T. A. 1979/1980. Clinical signs of acute and chronic experimental lesions of the cerebellum. Veterinary Science Communications 3:259.

Hudson, L. C. 1993. Nervous system. In Atlas of Feline Anatomy for Veterinarians, Hudson, L. C., Hamilton, W. P., eds. Philadelphia, W. B. Saunders, 190–226.

Jenkins, T. W. 1978. Diencephalon. In Functional Mammalian Neuroanatomy, 2d ed., Jenkins, T. W., ed. Philadelphia, Lea & Febiger, 264.

King, A. S. 1987. Physiological and Clinical Anatomy of the Domestic Mammals. Oxford, Oxford University Press.

Kitchell, R. L. 1993. Introduction to the nervous system. In Miller's Anatomy of the Dog, 3d ed., Evans, H. E., ed. Philadelphia, W. B. Saunders, 758–799.

Kitchell, R. L., Evans, H. E. 1993. The spinal nerves. In Miller's Anatomy of the Dog, 3d ed., Evans, H. E., ed. Philadelphia, W. B. Saunders, 829–893.

Kitchell, R. L., Whalen, L. R., Bailey, C. S., Lohse, C. L. 1980. Electrophysiologic studies of cutaneous nerves of the thoracic limb of the dog. Am J Vet Res 41:61.

Kornegay, J. N., Oliver, J. E., Gorgacz, E. J. 1983. Clinicopathologic features of brain herniation in animals. JAVMA 182:1111–1116.

Kot, W., Partlow, G. D., Parent, J. 1994. Anatomical survey of the cat's lumbosacral spinal cord. Prog Vet Neuro 5:162.

Morgan, J. P., Atilola, M., Bailey, C. S. 1987. Vertebral canal and spinal cord mensuration: a comparative study of its effect on lumbosacral myelography in the dachshund and German shepherd dog. JAVMA 191:951–957.

Murphy, C. J., Pollock, R. V. S. 1993. The eye. In Miller's Anatomy of the Dog, 3d ed., Evans, H. E., ed. Philadelphia, W. B. Saunders, 1009–1057.

Oliver, J. E., Hoerlein, B. F., Mayhew, I. G. 1987. Veterinary Neurology. Philadelphia, W. B. Saunders.

Oliver, J. E., Jr., Lorenz, M. D., Kornegay, J. N. 1997. In Handbook of Veterinary Neurology, 3d ed. Philadelphia, W. B. Saunders, 341–402.

Pearson, K., Gordon, J. 2000. Spinal reflexes. In Principles of Neural Science, 4th ed., Kandel, E. R., Schwartz, J. H., Jessell, T. M., eds. New York, McGraw-Hill, 713–736.

Scagliotti, R. H. 1990. Neuro-ophthalmology. Prog Vet Neurol 1:157–170.

Selcer, R. C. 1990. Functional neuroanatomy of the caudal brain stem and cerebellum. Prog Vet Neurol 1:226–231.

Shell, L. G. 1990. The cranial nerves of the brain stem. Prog Vet Neurol 1:233–245.

Yoshitomi, T., Ito, Y. 1986. Double reciprocal innervation in dog iris sphincter and dilator muscles. Investigative Ophthalmology & Visual Science 27:83–91.

Pathophysiology

Allen, R. 1986. Intracranial pressure: a review of clinical problems, measurement techniques and monitoring methods. J Med Eng Tech 10:299–320.

Aucoin, P. J., Rosen Kotilainen, H., Gantz, N. M., Davidson, R., Kellogg, P., Stone, B. 1986. Intracranial pressure monitors, epidemiologic study of risk factors and infections. Am J Med 80:369–376.

Bagley, R. S. 2000. Bleeding in the CNS. Proc 18th ACVIM Forum, Seattle, WA, 334–336.

———. 1996a. Clinical signs and localization of intracranial disease. Vet Clin N Am 26:667–710.

———. 1996b. Intracranial pressure in dogs and cats: physiology and treatment. Comp Cont Ed Pract Vet 18:605–621.

———. 1996c. Pathophysiologic sequelae of intracranial disease. Vet Clin N Am 26:711–733.

———. 1994. Adipsia and the nervous system. Comp Cont Ed 17:311–318.

Bagley, R. S., Baszler, T. V., Harrington, M. L., Pluhar, G. E., Moore, M. P., Keegan, R. D., Greene, S. A. 1995. Clinical effects of longitudinal division of the corpus callosum in dogs. Vet Surg 24:122–127.

Bagley, R. S., Gavin, P. R. 1998. Seizures as a complication of brain tumors. Clin Tech Small Anim Pract 13:178–184.

Bagley, R. S., Gavin, P. R., Moore, M. P., Silver, G. M., Harrington, M. L., Connor, R. 1999. Clinical signs associated with brain tumor in dogs: 97 cases (1992–1997). JAVMA 215:818–819.

Bagley, R. S., Harrington, M. L., Pluhar, G. E., Keegan, R. D., Greene, S. A., Moore, M. P., Gavin, P. R. 1996. Effect of craniectomy/durotomy alone or in combination with hyperventilation, diuretics, and corticosteroids on intracranial pressure in normal dogs. Am J Vet Res 57:116–119.

Bagley, R. S., Keegan, R. D., Greene, S. A., Moore, M. P., Gavin, P. R. 1995. Intraoperative intracranial pressure monitoring in five dogs with space-occupying intracranial lesions. JAVMA 207:588–591.

Barlow, P., Mendelow, A. D, Lawrence, A. E., Barlow, M., Rowan, J. O. 1985. Clinical evaluation of two methods of subdural pressure monitoring. J Neurosurg 63:578–582.

Beitz, A. J., Fletcher, T. F. 1993. The brain. In Miller's Anatomy of the Dog, 3d ed., Evans, H. E., ed. Philadelphia, W. B. Saunders, 894–952.

Berg, R. J., Rucker, N. C. 1985. Pathophysiology and medical management of acute spinal cord injury. Comp Cont Ed 7:646–653.

Bouma, G. J., Muizelaar, J. P., Bandoh, K., Marmarou, A. 1992. Blood pressure and intracranial pressure-volume dynamics in severe head injury: relationship with cerebral blood flow. J Neurosurg 77:15–19.

Braund, K. G., Shores, A., Brawner, W. R. 1990. The etiology, pathology and pathophysiology of acute spinal trauma. Vet Med 85:684–681.

Brinker, T., Seifert, V., Dietz, H. 1992. Cerebral blood flow and intracranial pressure during experimental subarachnoid hemorrhage. Acta Neurochir Wien 115:47–52.

Brock, M., Winkelmüller Pöll, W., Markakis, E., Dietz, H. 1972. Measurement of brain-tissue pressure. Lancet 1:595–596.

Brown, S. A., Hall, E. D. 1992. Role of oxygen-derived free radicals in the pathogenesis of shock and trauma, with focus on central nervous system injuries. JAVMA 200:1849–1859.

Cardoso, E. R., Rowan, J. O., Galbraith, S. 1983. Analysis of the cerebrospinal fluid pulse wave in intracranial pressure. J Neurosurg 59:817–821.

Cornick, J. L. 1992. Anesthetic management of patients with neurologic abnormalities. Comp Cont Ed Pract Vet 14:163–172.

Coulter, D. M., Gooch, W. M. 1993. Falling intracranial pressure: an important element in the genesis of intracranial hemorrhage in the beagle. Biol Neonate 63:316–26.

Crutchfield, J. S., Narayan, R. K., Robertson, C. S., Michael, L. H. 1990. Evaluation of a fiberoptic intracranial pressure monitor. J Neurosurg 72:482–487.

deLahunta, A. 1983. Veterinary Neuroanatomy and Clinical Neurology, 2d ed. Philadelphia, W. B. Saunders.

Enevoldsen, E. M., Jensen, F. T. 1979. Autoregulation and CO_2 responses of cerebral blood flow in patients with acute severe head injury. J Neurosurg 48:689–703.

Feldman, Z., Kanter, M. J., Robertson, C. S., Contant, C. F., et al. 1992. Effect of head elevation on intracranial pressure, cerebral perfusion pressure, and cerebral blood flow in head-injured patients. J Neurosurg 76:207–211.

Fishman, R. A. 1975. Brain Edema. N Eng J Med 293:706–711.

Fletcher, T. F. 1993. Spinal cord and meninges. In Miller's Anatomy of the Dog, 3d ed., Evans, H. E., ed. Philadelphia, W. B. Saunders 800–828.

Foley, P. L., Takenaka, K., Kassell, N. F., Lee, K. S. 1994. Cytotoxic effects of bloody cerebrospinal fluid on cerebral endothelial cells in culture. J Neurosurg 81:87–92.

Germon, K. 1988. Interpretation of ICP pulse waves to determine intracerebral compliance. J Neurosci Nurs 20:344–349.

Graf, C. J., Rossi, N. P. 1978. Catecholamine response to intracranial hypertension. J Neurosurg 49:862–868.

Guyton, A. C., Hall, J. E. 1996. Textbook of Medical Physiology, 9th ed. Philadelphia, W. B. Saunders.

Hariri, R. J., Firlick, A. D., Shepard, S. R., Cohen, D. S., et al. 1993. Traumatic brain injury, hemorrhagic shock, and fluid resuscitation: effects on intracranial pressure and brain compliance. J Neurosurg 79:421–427.

Hassler, W., Steinmetz, H., Gawlowski, J. 1988. Transcranial Doppler ultrasonography in raised intracranial pressure and in intracranial circulatory arrest. J Neurosurg 68:745–751.

Hoerlein, B. F. 1965. Laboratory examinations. In Canine Neurology, Diagnosis and Treatment, Hoerlein, B. F., ed. Philadelphia, W. B. Saunders, 50–54.

Hopkins, A. L., Wheeler, S. J. 1991. Subdural hematoma in a dog. Vet Surg 20:413–417.

Iannotti, F., Hoff, J. T., Schielke, G. P. 1984. Brain tissue pressure: physiological observations in anesthetized cats. J Neurosurg 60:1219–1225.

Janssens, L. A. A. 1991. Mechanical and pathophysiological aspects of acute spinal cord trauma. J Sm An Prac 32:572–578.

Keegan, R. D., Greene, S. A., Bagley, R. S., Moore, M. P., Weil, A. B., Short, C. E. 1995. Effects of medetomidine administration on intracranial pressure and cardiovascular variables of isoflurane anesthetized dogs. Am J Vet Res 56:193–198.

King, A. S. 1987. Physiological and Clinical Anatomy of the Domestic Mammals. Oxford, Oxford University Press.

King, J. M., Roth, L., Haschek, W. M. 1982. Myocardial necrosis secondary to neural lesions in domestic animals. JAVMA 180:144–148.

Kornegay, J. N. 1993. Pathogenesis of diseases of the central nervous system. In Textbook of Small Animal Surgery, 2d ed., Slatter, D., ed. Philadelphia, W. B. Saunders, 1022–1037.

Kornegay, J. N., Oliver, J. E., Gorgacz, E. J. 1983. Clinicopathologic features of brain herniation in animals. JAVMA 182:1111–1116.

Lundberg, N. 1960. Continuous recording and control of ventricular fluid pressure in neurosurgical practice. Acta Psychiatr Neurol Scand 36:1–193.

Lyons, M. K., Meyer, F. B. 1990. Cerebrospinal fluid physiology and the management of increased intracranial pressure. Mayo Clinic Proc 65:684–707.

March, P. A. 1998. Seizures: classification, etiology, and pathophysiology. Clin Tech Small Anim Pract 13:119–131.

Novak, G., Digel, C., Burns, B., James, A. E. 1974. Cerebrospinal fluid pressure measurements and radioisotope cisternography in dogs. Lab Animal 8:85–91.

Olby, N., Jeffery, N. 2003. Pathogenesis of diseases of the central nervous system. In Textbook of Small Animal Surgery, Slatter, D., ed. Philadelphia, W. B. Saunders, 1132–1147.

Ostrup, R. C., Luerssen, T. G., Marshall, L. F., Zornow, M. H. 1987. Continuous monitoring of intracranial pressure with a miniaturized fiberoptic device. J Neurosurg 67:206–209.

Parker, A. J. 1972. The diagnostic uses of cerebro-spinal fluid. J Sm An Prac 13:607–611.

Pender, E. S., Pollack, C. V., Jr. 1993. Neurogenic pulmonary edema: case reports and review. J Emerg Med 10:45–51.

Pluhar, G. E., Bagley, R. S., Keegan, R. D., Bazler, T. V., Moore, M. P. 1996. The effect of acute, unilateral transverse venous sinus occlusion on intracranial pressure in normal dogs. Vet Surg 25:480–486.

Podell, M. 1996. Seizures in dogs. Vet Clin N Am (Small Anim Pract) 26:779–809.

Quencer, R. M., Bunge, R. P. 1996. The injured spinal cord: imaging, histopathologic, clinical correlates, and basic science approaches to enhancing neural function after spinal injury. Spine 21:2064–2066.

Regan, R. F., Panter, S. S. 1993. Neurotoxicity of hemoglobin in cortical cell culture. Neurosci Lett 153:219–222.

Reulen, H. J. 1976.Vasogenic brain oedema: new aspects in its formation, resolution and therapy. Br J Anaesth 48:741–752.

Rosenberg, G. A., Saland, L., Kyner, W. T. 1983. Pathophysiology of periventricular tissue changes with raised CSF pressure. J Neurosurg 59:606–611.

Rosner, M. J., Becker, D. P. 1984. Origin and evolution of plateau waves. J Neurosurg 60:312–324.

Rucker, N. C. 1990. Management of spinal cord trauma. Prog Vet Neurol 1:397–412.

Russo, M. E. 1981. The pathophysiology of epilepsy. Cornell Vet 71:221–247.

Salvati, M., Cosentino, F., Artico, M., Ferrari, M., et al. 1992. Electrocardiographic changes in subarachnoid hemorrhage secondary to cerebral aneurysm. Report of 70 cases. Ital J Neurol Sci 13:409–13.

Schirmer, R. G. 1958. Analysis of the cerebrospinal fluid: its significance in diagnosis. Modern Veterinary Practice 39:38–40.

Shapiro, H. M. 1975. Intracranial hypertension: therapeutic and anesthetic considerations. Anesthesiology 43:445–471.

Shores, A. 1992. Spinal trauma. Vet Clin N Am 22:859–887.

———. 1985. Neuroanesthesia: a review of the effects of anesthetic agents on cerebral blood flow and intracranial pressure in the dog. Vet Surg 14:257–263.

Shores, A., Jevens, D., DeCamp, C. E. May 1991. Intraoperative brain pressure monitoring in the dog. Proc 9th ACVIM Forum, New Orleans, LA, 831–833.

Simpson, S. T. 1987. Manometric values for normal cerebrospinal fluid pressure in dogs. J Am Anim Hosp Assoc 23:629–632.

Simpson, S. T., Reed, R. B. 1987. Cerebrospinal fluid pressure in dogs: technique, normal values and meaning. Proc 5th ACVIM Forum, 275–276.

Summers, B. A., Cummings, J. F., deLahunta, A. 1995. Veterinary Neuropathology. Philadelphia, W. B. Saunders.

Turner, W. D. 1987. Fractures and fracture-luxations of the lumbar spine: a retrospective study in the dog. J Am Anim Hosp Assoc 23:460–464.

van Loon, J., Shivalkar, B., Plets, C., Goffin, J., et al. 1993. Catecholamine response to a gradual increase of intracranial pressure. J Neurosurg 79:705–709.

Weaver, D. D., Winn, H. R., Jane, J. A. 1982. Differential intracranial pressure in patients with unilateral mass lesions. J Neurosurg 56:660–665.

Clinical Neurologic Examination

Adams, R. D., Victor, M. 1993. Principles of Neurology, 5th ed. New York, McGraw-Hill.

Antonini, A., Berlucchi, G., Marzi, C. A., Sprague, J. M. 1979. Behavioral and electrophysiological effects of unilateral optic tract section in ordinary and Siamese cats. J Comp Neur 185:183–202.

Bagley, R. S. 1992 Tremor syndromes in dogs: diagnosis and treatment. J Sm An Prac 33:485–490.

———. 1994. Adipsia and the nervous system. Comp Cont Ed 17:311–318.

———. 2000. Vestibular disease of dogs and cats. In Kirk's Current Veterinary Therapy XII, Bonagura, J., ed. Philadelphia, W. B. Saunders, 966–971.

Bagley, R. S., Gavin, P. G., Silver, G. M., et al. 2000. Syringomyelia and hydromyelia in dogs. Comp Cont Ed 22:471–479.

Bagley, R. S., Pluhar, G. E., Alexander, J. E. 1994. Lateral intervertebral disk extrusion causing lameness in a dog. JAVMA 205:181–183.

Bagley, R. S., Silver, G. M., Seguin, B., Lincoln, J. D., Britt, L. G. 1997. Scoliosis and associated cystic spinal cord abnormality in a dog. JAVMA 211:573–575.

Bagley, R. S., Stefanacci, J. D., Hansen, B., Kornegay, J. N. 1993. Dysphonia in two dogs with cranial cervical intervertebral disk extrusion. J Am Anim Hosp Assoc 29:557–559.

Bailey, C. S., Kitchell, R. L. 1987. Cutaneous sensory testing in the dog. J Vet Intern Med 1:128–135.

Braund, K. G. 1994. Clinical Syndromes in Veterinary Neurology. 2d ed. St. Louis, Mosby.

Breazile, J. E., Blaugh, B. S., Nail, N. 1966. Experimental study of canine distemper myoclonus. Am J Vet Res 27:1375–1379.

Breitschwerdt, E. B., Breazile, J. E., Broadhurst, J. J. 1979. Clinical and electroencephalographic findings associated with ten cases of suspected limbic epilepsy in the dog. J Am Anim Hosp Assoc 15:37–50.

Child, G., Higgins, R. J., Cuddon, P. A. 1986. Acquired scoliosis associated with hydromyelia and syringomyelia in two dogs. JAVMA 189:909–912.

Chrisman, C. L. 1990. Dancing Doberman disease: clinical finding and prognosis. Progress in Veterinary Neurology 1, 83–90.

———. 1991. Problems in Small Animal Neurology. Philadelphia, Lea & Febiger.

Coates, J. R., Dewey, C. W. 1998. Cervical spinal hyperesthesia as a clinical sign of intracranial disease. Compend Cont Ed Pract Vet 20:1025–1037.

Collins, B. K, O'Brien D. 1990. Autonomic dysfunction of the eye. Seminar Vet Med Surg 5:24–36.

Cooper, G., Rodnitzky, R. 2000. The many forms of tremor. Precise classification guides selection of therapy. Postgrad Med 108:57–58, 61–64, 70.

Cummings, J. F., deLahunta, A., Winn, S. S. 1981. Acral mutilation and nociceptive loss in English Pointer dogs. A canine sensory neuropathy. Acta Neuropathol (Berl) 53:119–127.

DeJong, R. N. 1967. The Neurologic Examination, 3d ed. New York, Harper and Row, 6.

deLahunta, A. 1983. In Veterinary Neuroanatomy and Clinical Neurology, 2d ed. Philadelphia, W. B. Saunders.

Fox, J.G., Averill, D. F., Hallett, M., Schunk, K. 1984. Familial reflex myoclonus in Labrador retrievers. Am J Vet Res 45:2367–2376.

Goldfarb, S., Swann, P. G. 1984. Case report—idiopathic tonic pupil or Adie's syndrome in a dog. Aust Vet Pract 14:20.

Griffiths, I. R. 1989. Neurological examination of the limbs and the body. In Manual of Small Animal Neurology, Wheeler, S. J., ed. West Sussex, British Small Animal Veterinary Association.

Guilford, W. G., Shaw, D. P., O'Brien, D. P., Maxwell, V. D. 1990. Fecal incontinence, urinary incontinence, and priapism associated with multifocal distemper encephalomyelitis in a dog. JAVMA 197:90–92.

Guyton, A. C., Hall, J. E. 1996. Textbook of Medical Physiology, 9th ed. Philadelphia, W. B. Saunders, 525.

Hansen, B. May, 1990. Recognition of acute pain and distress in the dog. Proc 8th ACVIM Forum, Washington, DC, 773.

Hendricks, J. C., Morrison, A. R. 1981. Normal and abnormal sleep in mammals. JAVMA 178:121-126.

Herritage, M. E., Palmer, A. C. 1983. Episodic falling in the cavalier King Charles spaniel. Vet Rec 112:458–459.

Holliday, T. A. May 1991. Unilateral neglect (hemi-inattention) syndrome in dogs. Proc 9th ACVIM Forum, New Orleans, LA, 819.

———. 1979/1980. Clinical signs of acute and chronic experimental lesions of the cerebellum. Veterinary Science Communications 3:259–278.

Jacobson, D. M. 1990. Pupillary responses to dilute pilocarpine in preganglionic 3rd nerve disorders. Neurology 40:804–808.

Jenkins, T. W. 1978. Functional Mammalian Neuroanatomy, 2d ed. Philadelphia, Lea & Febiger.

Johnson, B. W. 1991. Congenitally abnormal visual pathways of Siamese cats. Comp Cont Ed Pract Vet 13:374–377.

Joseph, R. J. May 1992. Vestibular eye movement—revisited. Proc 10th ACVIM Forum, San Diego, CA, 762.

Kern, T. J., Aromando, M. C., Erb, H. N. 1989. Horner's syndrome in dogs and cats: 100 cases (1975–1985) JAVMA 195:369–373.

King, A. S. 1987. Physiological and Clinical Anatomy of the Domestic Mammals. Oxford, Oxford University Press.

Kornegay, J. N. 1986. Management of animals with neurologic disease. In Neurologic Disorders—Contemporary Issues in Small Animal Practice, Kornegay, J. N., ed. New York, Churchill Livingstone, 3.

Kornegay, J. N., Oliver, J. E., Gorgacz, E. J. 1983 Clinicopathologic features of brain herniation in animals. JAVMA 182: 1111–1116.

Lewis, D. D. 2000. Gracilis-semitendiosus myopathy. In Kirk's Current Veterinary Therapy XII, Bonagura, J., ed. Philadelphia, W. B. Saunders, 989–992.

Lewis, G. T., Blanchard, G. L., Trapp, A. L., DeCamp, C. E. 1984. Ophthalmoplegia caused by thyroid adenocarcinoma invasion of the cavernous sinuses in the dog. J Am Anim Hosp Assoc 20:805–812.

Malik, R., Church, D. B., Maddison, J. E., Farrow, B. R. 1989. Three cases of local tetanus. J Sm An Prac 30:469–475.

March, P. A., Knowles, K., Thalhammer, J. G. 1993. Reflex myoclonus in two Labrador retriever littermates: a clinical, electrophysiological, and pathological study. Prog Vet Neurol 4:19–24.

McCormick, D. A., Thompson, R. F. 1984. Cerebellum: essential involvement in the classically conditioned eyelid response. Science 223:296–299.

Moore, M. P. 1992. Approach to the patient with spinal disease. Vet Clin N Am 22:750–780.

Moreau, P. M. 1989. Neurological examination of the cranial nerves. In Manual of Small Animal Neurology, Wheeler, S. J., ed. West Sussex, British Small Animal Veterinary Association, 13.

Morgan, R. V., Zanotti, S. W. 1989. Horner's syndrome in dogs and cats: 49 cases (1980–1986). JAVMA 194:1096–1099.

Myers, K. M., Lund, J. E., Padgett, G., Dickson, W. M. 1969. Hyperkinetic episodes in Scottish Terrier dogs. JAVMA 155:129–133.

Myers, L. J. 1990. Dysosmia of the dog in clinical veterinary medicine. Prog Vet Neurol 1:171–179.

Nakahata, K., Uzuka, Y., Matsumoto, H., Gotoh, N., et al. 1992. Hyperkinetic involuntary movements in a young Shetland sheepdog. J Am An Hosp Assoc 28:347–348.

Neer, T. M. 1984. Horner's syndrome: anatomy, diagnosis and causes. Comp Cont Ed Pract Vet 6:740–746.

Neer, T. M., Carter, J. D. 1987. Anisocoria in dogs and cats: ocular and neurologic causes. Comp Cont Ed Pract Vet 9:817–823.

Nelson, R. W., Morrison, W. B., Lurus, A. G., Miller, J. B. 1981. Diencephalic syndrome secondary to intracranial astocytoma in a dog. JAVMA 179:1004–1010.

O'Brien, D. May 1993. Brain damage and behavior. Proc 11th ACVIM Forum, Washington, DC, 542.

O'Brien, D., Longshore, R. C. 2000. Diagnosis and management of dysautonomia in dogs. In Kirk's Current Veterinary Therapy XII, Bonagura, J., ed. Philadelphia, W. B. Saunders, 957–959.

Oliver, J. E., Hoerlein, B. F., Mayhew, I. G. 1987. Veterinary Neurology. Philadelphia, W. B. Saunders.

Oliver, J. E., Jr., Lorenz, M. D., Kornegay, J. N. 1997. In Handbook of Veterinary Neurology, 3d ed. Philadelphia, W. B. Saunders, 341–402.

Palmer, A. C. 1970. Clinical and pathological aspects of cervical disc protrusion and primary tumors of the cervical spinal cord in the dog. J Sm An Prac 11:63–67.

Palmer, A. C., Malinowski, W., Barnet, K. C. 1974. Clinical signs including papilloedema associated with brain tumors in twenty-one dogs. J Sm An Prac 15:359–386.

Parker, A. J. 1990. Behavioral changes of organic neurologic origin. Prog Vet Neurol 1:123–131.

Penderis, J., Franklin, R. J. M. 2001. Dyskinesia in an adult bichon frise. J Sm An Prac 42:24–25.

Prata, R. G., Stoll, S. G. 1973. Ventral decompression and fusion for the treatment of cervical disk disease in the dog. J Am Anim Hosp Assoc 9:462–472.

Ramsey, I. K., Chandler, K. E., Franklin, R. J. M. 1999. A movement disorder in boxer pups. Vet Rec 144:179–180.

Reading, M. J., McKerrell, R. E. 1993. Suspected myokymia in a Yorkshire terrier. Vet Rec 132:587–588.

Roberts, S. R., Vainisi, S. J. 1967. Hemifacial spasm in dogs. JAVMA 150:381–385.

Scagliotti, R. H. 1990. Neuro-ophthalmology. Prog Vet Neurol 1:157–170.

Schwartzman, R. J., McLellan, T. L. 1987. Reflex sympathetic dystrophy, a review. Arch Neurol 44:555–561.

Sharp, N. J. H., Nash, A. S., Griffiths, I. R. 1984. Feline dysautonomia (the Key-Gaskell syndrome): a clinical and pathological study of forty cases. J Sm An Prac 25:599–615.

Shores, A., Vaughn, D. M., Holland, M., Smith, B., Simpson, S. T., Burns J. 1991. Glossopharyngeal neuralgia syndrome in a dog. J Am An Hosp Assoc 27:101–104.

Silver, G. M., Bagley, R. S., Moore, M. P. 1997. Myoclonus of the tongue. Prog Vet Neurol 7:137–140.

Sims, M. H., Brace, J. J., Arthur, D. A., Harvey, R. C. 1991. Otoacoustic emission in a dog. JAVMA 198:1017–1018.

Spaulding, K. S., Sharp, N. J. H. 1990. Ultrasonographic imaging of the lateral cerebral ventricles in the dog. Vet Rad 31:59–64.

Suter, P. F., Watrous B. J. 1980. Oropharyngeal dysphagias in the dog: a cinefluorographic analysis in experimentally induced and spontaneously occurring swallowing disorders. Vet Rad 21:24–39.

Thomas, W. B. 2000. Vestibular dysfunction. Vet Clin N Am (Small Anim Practice) 30:227–250.

Thompson, H. S., Franceschetti, A. T., Thompson, P. M. 1971. Hippus, semantic and historic considerations of the word. Amer J Ophthal 71:1116–1120.

Wheeler, S. J. 1989. Manual of Small Animal Neurology. West Sussex, British Small Animal Veterinary Association.

Wise, L. A., Lappin, M. R. 1991. A syndrome resembling feline dysautonomia (Key-Gaskell syndrome) in a dog. JAVMA 12:2103–2106.

Yoshitomi, T., Ito, Y. 1986. Double reciprocal innervation in dog iris sphincter and dilator muscles. Invest Ophthalmol Visual Sci 27:83–91.

Neuroanatomical Diagnosis

Braund, K. G. 1994. Clinical Syndromes in Veterinary Neurology, 2d ed. St. Louis, Mosby.

Chrisman, C. L. 1991. Problems in Small Animal Neurology. Philadelphia, Lea & Febiger.

deLahunta, A. 1983. Veterinary Neuroanatomy and Clinical Neurology. 2d ed. Philadelphia, W. B. Saunders.

Dewey, C. L. 2003. A Practical Guide to Canine and Feline Neurology, Dewey, C. W., ed. Ames, Iowa State Press.

Holliday, T. A. May, 1991. Unilateral neglect (hemi-inattention) syndrome in dogs. Proc 9th ACVIM Forum, New Orleans, LA, 819–821.

———. 1979/1980. Clinical signs of acute and chronic experimental lesions of the cerebellum. Veterinary Science Communications 3:259–278.

Kot, W., Partlow, G. D., Parent, J. 1994. Anatomical survey of the cat's lumbosacral spinal cord. Prog Vet Neurol 5:162–166.

Morgan, J. P., Atilola, M., Bailey, C. S. 1987. Vertebral canal and spinal cord mensuration: a comparative study of its effect on lumbosacral myelography in the dachshund and German shepherd dog. JAVMA 191:951–957.

O'Brien, D. 1993. Brain damage and behavior. Proc 11th ACVIM Forum, May, Washington, DC, 542.

Oliver, J. E. 1990. Localization of lesions: the anatomic diagnosis. Prog Vet Neurol 1:28–39.

Oliver, J. E., Hoerlein, B. F., Mayhew, I. G. 1987. Veterinary Neurology. Philadelphia, W. B. Saunders.

Oliver, J. E., Jr., Lorenz, M. D., Kornegay, J. N. 1997. Handbook of Veterinary Neurology, 3d ed. Philadelphia, W. B. Saunders, 341–402.

Shelton, G. D., Willard, M. D., Cardinette, G. H., Lindstrom, J. 1990. Acquired myasthenia gravis, selective involvement of esophageal, pharyngeal, and facial muscles. J Vet Intern Med 4:281–284.

Thomas, W. B. 2000. Vestibular dysfunction. Vet Clin N Am (Small Anim Practice) 30:227–250.

CHAPTERS 5–15: DISEASES

General Neurologic Disease References

Bagley, R. S. 2003. Intracranial surgery. In Textbook of Small Animal Surgery, 3d ed., Slatter, D., ed. Philadelphia, W. B. Saunders, 1261–1276.

Braund, K. G. 1994. Clinical Syndromes in Veterinary Neurology, 2d ed. St. Louis, Mosby.

Chrisman, C. L. 1991. Problems in Small Animal Neurology. Philadelphia, Lea & Febiger.

deLahunta, A. 1983. Veterinary Neuroanatomy and Clinical Neurology, 2d ed. Philadelphia, W. B. Saunders.

Dewey, C. L. 2003. In A Practical Guide to Canine and Feline Neurology, Dewey, C. W., ed. Ames, Iowa State Press.

LeCouteur, R. A., Child, G. 1995. Diseases of the spinal cord. In Textbook of Veterinary Internal Medicine: Disease of the Dog and Cat, ed. 4, Ettinger, S. J., Feldman, E. C., eds. Philadelphia, W. B. Saunders, 629–696.

Oliver, J. E., Hoerlein, B. F., Mayhew, I. G. 1987. Veterinary Neurology. Philadelphia, W. B. Saunders.

Oliver, J. E., Jr., Lorenz, M. D., Kornegay, J. N. 1997. In Handbook of Veterinary Neurology, 3d ed. Philadelphia, W. B. Saunders, 341–402.

Shelton, G. D. 2002. Neuromuscular diseases. Vet Clin N Am (Small Animal Pract) 32(1).

———. 1994a. Diseases of the muscle and neuromuscular junction. In The Cat Diseases and Management, R. G. Sherding, ed., 2d ed. New York, Churchill Livingstone, 1569–1576.

———. 1994b. Neuromuscular disorders. In Consultations in Feline Medicine, J. R. August, ed., 2d ed. Philadelphia, W. B. Saunders, 405–412.

Summers, B. A., Cummings, J. F., deLahunta, A. 1995. In Veterinary Neuropathology, St. Louis, Mosby.

Intracranial Disease References

Degenerative Intracranial Diseases

Bagley, R. S. 1997. Common neurologic diseases of older animals. Vet Clin N Am (Small Anim Pract) 27:1451–1486.

Bjerkas, I. 1977. Hereditary "cavitating" leukodystrophy in Dalmation dogs. Acta Neuropathol 40:163–169.

Borrás, D., Ferrer, I., Pumarola, M. 1999. Age-related changes in the brain of the dog. Vet Pathol 36:202–211

Braund, K. G. 1987. Degenerative and developmental diseases. In Veterinary Neurology, Oliver, J. E. J., Hoerlein, B. F., Mayhew, I. B., eds. Philadelphia, W. B. Saunders, 186.

Carmichael, K. P., Howerth, E. W., Oliver, J. R., Jr., Klappenbach, K. 1993. Neuroaxonal dystrophy in a group of related cats. J Vet Diagn Invest 5:585–590.

Celesia, G. C. 2001. Disoders of membrane channels or channelopathies. Clinical neurophysiology 112:2–18.

Chapman, B. L. 1995. Behavioral disorders. In Geriatrics and Gerontology of the Dog and Cat, Goldston, R. T., Hoskins, J. D., eds. Philadelphia, W. B. Saunders, 51.

Coates, J. R., Mine, K. L. 1995. Congenital and inherited neurologic disorders in dogs and cats. In Kirk's Current Veterinary Therapy XII, Bonagura, J. D., ed. Philadelphia, W. B. Saunders, 1111–1120.

Cox, N. R., Kwapien, R. P., Sorjonen, D. C., et al. 1986. Myeloencephalopathy resembling Alexander's disease in a Scottish terrier dog. Acta Neuropathol 71:163–166.

Cummings, B. J., Head, E., Ruehl, W., et al. 1996. The canine as an animal model of human aging and dementia. Neurobiol Aging 17:259–268.

deLahunta, A. 1990. Abiotrophy in domestic animals: a review. Can J Vet Res 54:65–76.

deLahunta, A., Ingram, J. T., Cummings, J. F., Bell, J. S. 1994. Labrador retriever central axonpathy. Prog Vet Neurol 5:117–122.

Eger, C. E., Huxtable, C. R. R., Chester, Z. C., et al. 1998. Progressive tetraparesis and laryngeal paralysis in a young rottweiler with neuronal vacuolation and axonal degeneration: an Australian case. Aust Vet J 76:733–737.

Harkin, K. R., Goggin, I. M., DeBey, B. M., et al. 1999. Magnetic resonance imaging of the brain of a dog with hereditary polioencephalomyelopathy. JAVMA 214;9:1342–1344.

Hart, B. J. 2001. Effect of gonadectomy on subsequent development of age-related cognitive impairment in dogs. JAVMA 219:51–56.

Houpt, K. A. 2001. Cognitive function in geriatric cats. In Consultation in Feline Internal Medicine, 4th ed., August, J. R., ed. Philadelphia, W. B. Saunders, 583–591.

Kortz, G. D., Meier, W. A., Higgins, R. J., et al. 1997. Neuronal vacuolation and spinocerebellar degeneration in young Rottweiler dogs. Vet Pathol 34:296–302.

Kullmann, D. M. 2002. The neuronal channelopathies. Brain 125:1177–1195.

March, P. A. 1996. Degenerative brain disease. Vet Clin N Am (Small Anim Pract) 26:945–971.

Milgram, N. W., Head, E., Weiner, E., et al. 1994. Cognitive functions and aging in the dog: acquisition of non-spatial visual tasks. Behavioral Neuroscience 108;1:57–68.

Milgram, N. W., Ivy, G. O., Head, E., et al. 1993. The effect L-deprenyl on behavior, cognitive function, and biogenic amines in the dog. Neurochem Research 18;12:1211–1219.

Neilson, J. C., Hart, B. J., Cliff, K. D., et al. 2001. Prevalence of behavioral changes associated with age-related cognitive impairment in dogs. JAVMA 218;11:1787–1791.

Palmer, A. C., Cavanagh, J. B. 1995. Encephalomyelopathy in young cats. J Sm Anim Pract 36:57–64.

Palmer, A. C., Payne, J. E., Wallace, M. E. 1973. Hereditary quadriplegia and amblyopia in the Irish setter. J Sm Anim Pract 14:343–352.

Parker, A. J. 1990. Behavioral changes of organic neurologic origin. Prog Vet Neurol 1:123–131.

Richardson, J. A., Tank, K., Burns, D. K. 1991. Myeloencephalopathy with Rosenthal fiber formation in a miniature poodle. Vet Pathol 28:536–538.

Ruehl, W. W., Bruyette, D. S., DePaoli, A., et al. 1995. Canine cognitive dysfunction as a model for human age-related cognitive decline, dementia and Alzheimer's disease: clinical presentation, cognitive testing, pathology and response to l-deprenyl therapy. Prog Brain Research 106:217–225.

Ruehl, W. W., Hart, B. J., Entriken, T. L., et al. 2000. L-deprenyl therapy for canine cognitive dysfunction. In Kirk's Current Veterinary Therapy XIII (Small Animal Practice), Bonagura, J. D., ed. Philadelphia, W. B. Saunders, 53–57.

Sakai, T., Harashima, T., Yamamura, H., et al. 1994. Two cases of hereditary quadriplegia and amblyopia in a litter of Irish setters. J Sm Anim Pract 35:221–223.

Shimada, A., Kuwamura, M., Awakura, T., et al. 1992. An immunohistochemical and ultrastructural study on age-related astrocytic gliosis in the central nervous system of dogs. J Vet Med Sci 54:29–36.

Sorjonen, D. C., Cox, N. R., Kwapien, R. P. 1987. Myeloencephalopathy with eosinophilic refractile bodies (Rosenthal fibers) in a Scottish terrier. JAVMA 190:1004–1006.

Stoffregen, D. A., Huxtable, C. R., Cummings, J. F., deLahunta, A. 1993. Hypomyelination of the central nervous system of two Siamese kitten littermates. Vet Path 30:388–391.

Summers, B. A., Cummings, J. F., deLahunta, A. 1995. In Veterinary Neuropathology. St. Louis, Mosby.

van den Ingh, T. S. G. A. M., Mandigers, P. J., van Nes, J. J. 1998. A neuronal vacuolar disorder in young Rottweiler dogs. Vet Rec 142:245–247.

Wakshlag, J. J., deLahunta, A., Robinson, T., et al. 1999. Subacute necrotising encephalopathy in an Alaskan husky. J Sm Anim Pract 40:585–589.

Yoshino, T., Uchida, K., Tateyama, S., et al. 1996. A retrospective study of canine senile plaques and cerebral amyloid angiopathy. Vet Pathol 33:230–234.

Multineuronal Degeneration

Cummings, J. F., deLahunta, A., Gasteiger, E. L. 1991. Multisystemic chromatolytic neuronal degeneration in Cairn terriers: a case with generalized cataplectic episodes. J Vet Intern Med 5:91–94.

Cummings, J. F., deLahunta, A., Moore, J. J., III. 1988. Multisystemic chromatolytic neuronal degeneration in a Cairn terrier pup. Cornell Vet 78:301–314.

Jaggy, A., Vandevelde, M. 1988. Multisystem neuronal degeneration in cocker spaniels. J Vet Intern Med 2:117–120.

Palmer, A. C., Blakemore, W. F. 1989. A progressive neuronopathy in the young Cairn terrier. J Sm Anim Pract 30:101–106.

Spongiform Encephalopathy and Leukodystrophies

Cachin, M., Vandevelde, M. 1991. Congenital tremor with spongy degeneration of the central nervous system in two puppies. J Vet Intern Med 5:87–90.

Gunn-Moore, D., Harbour, D. A. 2001. Feline spongiform encephalopathies and Borna disease. In Consultatiom in Feline Internal Medicine, 4th ed., August, J. R., ed. Philadelphia, W. B. Saunders, 62–70.

Jones, B. R., Alley, M. R., Shimada, A., Lyon, M. 1992. An encephalomyelopathy in related Birman kittens. NZ Vet J 40:160–16.

Kelly, O. F., Gaskell, C. J. 1976. Spongy degeneration of the central nervous system in kittens. Acta Neuropathol 35:151–158.

Leggett, M. M., Dukes, J., Pirie, H. M. 1990. A spongiform encephalopathy in a cat. Vet Rec 127:586–588.

Mason, R. W., Hartley, W. J., Randall, M. 1979. Spongiform degeneration of the white matter in a Samoyed pup. Aust Vet Pract 9:11–13.

McGrath, J. T., Batt, R. 1975. A leukodystrophy in the dog. J Neuropathol Exp Neurol 34:78.

Morales, C., Bernardini, M., Pumarola, M., et al. 2001. Familial spongy degeneration in Cocker spaniel dogs. J Vet Intern Med 15:72.

Neer, T. M., Kornegay, J. N. 1995. Leucoencephalomalacia and cerebral white matter vacuolar degeneration in two related Labrador retriever puppies. J Vet Intern Med 9:100–104.

O'Brien, D. P., Zachary, J. F. 1985. Clinical features of spongy degeneration of the central nervous system in two Labrador retriever littermates. JAVMA 186:1207–1210.

Richards, R. B., Kakulas, B. A. 1978. Spongiform leukoencephalopathy associated with congenital myoclonia syndrome in the dog. J Comp Pathol 88:317–320.

Wells, G. A. H., McGill, I. S. 1992. Recently described scrapie-like encephalopathies of animals: case definitions. Res Vet Sci 53:1–10.

Wood, S. L., Patterson, J. S. 2001. Shetland sheepdog leukodystrophy. J Vet Intern Med 15:486–493.

Wyatt, J. M., Pearson, G. R., Smerdon, T. N., et al. 1991. Naturally occurring scrapie-like spongiform encephalopathy in five domestic cats. Vet Rec 129:233–236.

Zachary, J. F., O'Brien, D. P. 1985. Spongy degeneration of the central nervous system in two canine littermates. Vet Pathol 22:561–571.

Storage Diseases

Gieselmann, V. 1995. Lysosomal storage diseases. Biochem Biophys Acta 1270:103–136.

Hartley, W. J., Canfield, P. J., Donnelly, T. M. 1982. A suspected new canine storage disease. Acta Neuropathol 56:225–232.

Haskins, M. 1996. Bone marrow transplantation therapy for metabolic disease: animal models as predictors of success and in utero approaches. Bone Marrow Transplant 18 Supp 3:S25–7.

Jolly, R. D., Walkley, S. U. 1997. Lysosomal storage diseases of animals: an essay in comparative pathology. Vet Pathol 34:527–548.

Kaye, E. M. 1995. Therapeutic approaches to lysosomal storage diseases. Curr Opin Pediatr 7:650–654.

March, P. A. 2001. Neuronal storage disorders. In Consultations in Feline Internal Medicine, 4th ed., August, I. R., ed. Philadelphia, W. B. Saunders, 393–404.

Rac, R., Giesecke, P. R. 1975. Lysosomal storage disease in Chihuahuas. Aust Vet J 5:403–404.

Salvetti, A., Heard, J. M., Danos, O. 1995. Gene therapy of lysosomal storage disorders. Br Med Bull 51:106–122.

Ceroid Lipofuscinosis

Appleby, E. C., Longstaffe, J. A., Bell, F. R. 1982. Ceroid lipofuscinosis in two Saluki dogs. J Comp Pathol 92:375–380.

Bichsel, P., Vandevelde, M. 1982. Un cas de lipofuscinose ceroide chez un berger de Yougoslavie. Schweiz Arch Tierheilkd 124:413–418.

Bildfell, R., Matwichuk, C., Mitchell, S., Ward, P. 1995. Neuronal ceroid-lipofuscinosis in a cat. Vet Pathol 32:485–488.

Cantile, C., Buonaccorsi, P. V., Arispici, M. 1996. Juvenile neuronal ceroid-lipofuscinosis (Batten's disease) in a poodle dog. Prog Vet Neurol 7:82–87.

Cho, D. Y., Leipold, H. W., Rudolph, R. 1986. Neuronal ceroidosis (ceroid-lipofuscinosis) in a blue heeler dog. Acta Neuropathol 69:161–164.

Franks, J. N., Dewey, C. W., Walker, M. A., Storts, R. W. 1999. Computed tomographic findings of ceroid lipofuscinosis in a dog. 35:430–435.

Goebel, H. H., Bilzer, T., Dahme, E., Malkusch, F. 1988. Morphological studies in canine (Dalmatian) neuronal ceroid-lipofuscinosis. Am J Med Genet Suppl 5:127–139.

Greene, P. D., Little, P. B. 1974. Neuronal ceroid-lipofuscin storage in Siamese cats. Can J Comp Med 38:207–210.

Hanichen, T., Puschner, H. 1971. Generalized lipofuscinosis with neural complications in a dog. Vet Med Rev 1:27–39.

Hoover, D. M., Little, P. B., Cole, W. D. 1984. Neuronal ceroid-lipofuscinosis in a mature dog. Vet Pathol 21:359–361.

Jolly, R. D., Palmer, D. N., Studdert, V. P., et al. 1994. Canine ceroid-lipofuscinoses: a review and classification. J Sm Anim Pract 35:299–306.

Koppang, N. 1992. English setter model and juvenile ceroid-lipofuscinosis in man. Am J Med Genet 42:599–604.

Minatel, L., Underwood, S. C., Carfagnini, J. C. 2000. Ceroid-lipofuscinosis in a Cocker spaniel dog. Vet Pathol 37:488–490.

Patel, V., Koppang, N., Patelb, Z. W. 1974. Phenylene diamine-mediated peroxidase deficiency in English setters with neuronal ceroid-lipofuscinosis. Lab Invest 30:366–368.

Riis, R. C., Cummings, J. F., Loew, E. R., deLahunta, A. 1992. Tibetan terrier model of canine ceroid lipofuscinosis. Am J Med Genet 42:615–621.

Studdert, V. P., Mitten, R. W. 1991. Clinical features of ceroid lipofuscinosis in border collie dogs. Aust Vet J 68:137–140.

Umemura, T., Sato, H., Goryo, M., Itakura, C. 1985. Generalized lipofuscinosis in a dog. Jpn J Vet Sci 47:673–677.

Vandevelde, M., Fatzer, R. 1980. Neuronal ceroid lipofuscinosis in older dachshunds. Vet Pathol 17:686–692.

Fucosidosis

Barker, C. G., Herrtage, M. E., Shanahan, F., Winchester, B. G. 1988. Fucosidosis in English springer spaniels: results of a trial screening programme. J Sm An Prac 29:623–630.

Keller, C. B., Lamarre, J. 1992. Inherited lysosomal storage disease in an English springer spaniel. JAVMA 200:194–195.

Kelly, W. R., Barnes, R. J., Clague, A. E. 1982. a-L-fucosidase deficiency and storage disease in springer spaniels. Aust Adv Vet Sci 235–236.

Kelly, W. R., Clague, A. E., Barns, R. J., et al. 1983. Canine alpha-L-fucosidosis: a storage disease of Springer spaniels. Acta Neuropathol (Berl) 60:9–13.

Littlewood, J. D., Herttage, M. E., Palmer, A. C. 1983. Neuronal storage disease in English springer spaniels. Vet Rec 112:86–87.

Smith, M. O., Wenger, D. A., Hill, S. L., et al. 1996. Fucosidosis in a family of American-bred English Springer spaniels. JAVMA 209:2088–2090.

Taylor, R. M., Farrow, B. R. H. 1988. Animal models of human disease: fucosidosis. Comp Pathol Bull 20:2–4.

———. 1992. Ceroid lipofuscinosis in the border collie dog: retinal lesions in an animal model of juvenile Batten disease. Am J Med Genet 42:622–627.

Taylor, R. M., Farrow, B. R. H., Healy, P. J. 1987. Canine fucosidosis: clinical findings. J Sm Anim Pract 28:291–300.

Taylor, R. M., Martin, I. C. A., Farrow, B. R. H. 1989. Reproductive abnormalities in canine fucosidosis. J Comp Pathol 100:369–380.

Gangliosidosis

Alroy, J., Orgad, U., Ucci, A. A., Schelling, S. H., et al. 1985. Neurovisceral and skeletal GM1-gangliosidosis in dogs with beta-galactosidase deficiency. Science 229:470–472.

Alroy, J., Orgad, V., DeGasperi, R., Richard, R., et al. 1992. Canine GM1-gangliosidosis: a clinical, morphologic, histochemical, and biochemical comparison of two different models. Am J Pathol 140:675–689.

Baker, H. J., Lindsey, J. R. 1974. Animal model of human disease: human GM1 gangliosidosis. Animal model: feline GM1 gangliosidosis. Am J Pathol 74:649–652.

Baker, H. J., Lindsey, J. R., McKhann, G. M., Farrell, D. F. 1971. Neuronal GM1 gangliosidosis in a Siamese cat with beta-galactosidase deficiency. Science 174:838–839.

Baker, H. J., Reynolds, G. D., Walkley, S. U., Cox, N. R., et al. 1979. The gangliosidoses: comparative features and research applications. Vet Pathol 16:635–649.

Barker, C. G., Blakemore, W. F., Dell, A., Palmer, A. C., et al. 1986. GM1 gangliosidosis (type 1) in a cat. Biochem 235:151–158.

Blakemore, W. F. 1972. GMI Gangliosidosis in a cat. J Comp Pathol 82:179–185.

Blakemore, W. F., Palmer, A. C. 1971. Cerebral lipidoses and leucodystrophies in animals. Vet Ann 12:129–135.

Cork, L. C., Munnell, J. F., Lorenz, M. D. 1978. The pathology of feline GM2 gangliosidosis. Am J Pathol 90:723–734.

Cork, L. C., Munnell, J. F., Lorenz, M. D., Murphy, J. V. 1977. GM2 ganglioside lysosomal storage disease in cats with B-hexosaminidase deficiency. Science 196:1014–1017.

Cummings, J. F., Wood, P. A., Walkley, S. U., deLahunta, A., et al. 1985. GM2 gangliosidosis in a Japanese spaniel. Acta Neuropathol 67:247–253.

Dial, S. M., Mitchell, T. W., LeCouteur, R. A., et al. 1994. GM 1-gangliosidosis (Type II) in three cats. J Am Anim Hosp Assoc 30:355–359.

Eto, Y., Autilio-Gametti, L., McGrath, J. T. 1984. Canine GM2-gangliosiodosis: chemical and enzymatic features. Adv Exp Med Biol 174:431–440.

Eto, Y., Ida, H., Umezawa, F., Ohashi, T., et al. 1987. Partial deficiency of betahexosaminidase activity in canine GM2-gangliosidosis. Tohoku J Exp Med 152:333–338.

Ishikawa, Y., Li, S. C., Wood, P. A., Li, Y. T. 1987. Biochemical basis of type AB GM2 gangliosidosis in a Japanese spaniel. J Neurochem 48:860–864.

Jolly, R. D. 1978. Lysosomal storage diseases. Neuropathol Appl Neurobiol 4:419–427.

Karbe, E. 1973. Animal model of human disease: GM2-gangliosidosis (Amaurotic idiocies) types I, II, and III. Animal model: canine GM2-gangliosidosis. Am J Pathol 71:151–154.

Lange, A. L., Van den Berg, P. B., Baker, M. K. 1977. A suspected lysosomal storage disease in Abyssinian cats. Part II: histopathological and ultrastructural aspects. J S Afr Vet Assoc 48:201–209.

Müller, G., Alldinger, S., Moritz, A., et al. 2001. GM1-gangliosidosis in Alaskan Huskies: clinical and pathological findings. Vet Pathol 38:281–290.

Murray, J. A., Blakemore, W. F., Barnett, K. C. 1977. Ocular lesions in cats with GM1-gangliosidosis with visceral involvement. J Sm An Prac 18:1–10.

Neuwelt, E. A., Johnson, W. G., Blank, N. K., Pagel, M. A., et al. 1985. Characterization of a new model of GM2-gangliosidosis (Sandhoffs disease) in Korat cats. J Clin Invest 76:482–490.

Nowakowski, R. W., Thompson, J. N., Baker, H. J. 1988. Diagnosis of feline GM1 gangliosidosis by enzyme assay of cultured conjunctival cells. Invest Ophthalmol Vis Sci 29:487–490.

Read, D. H., Harrington, D. D., Keenana, T. W., Hinsman, E. J. 1976. Neuronal-visceral GM1 gangliosidosis in a dog with beta-galactosidase deficiency. Science 194:442–445.

Saunders, G. K., Wood, P. A., Myers, R. K., Shell, L. G., Carithers, R. 1988. GM1 gangliosidosis in Portuguese water dogs: pathologic and biochemical findings. Vet Pathol 25:265–269.

Shell, L. G., Potthoff, A. I., Carithers, R., et al. 1989. Neuronal-visceral GM1 gangliosidosis in Portuguese water dogs. J Vet Intern Med 3:1–7.

Singer, H. S., Cork, L. C. 1989. Canine GM2 gangliosidosis: morphological and biochemical analysis. Vet Pathol 26: 114–120.

Van den Berg, P. B., Baker, M. K., Lange, A. L. 1977. A suspected lysosomal storage disease in Abyssinian cats. Part I: genetic clinical and clinical pathological aspects. J S Afr Vet Assoc 48:195–199.

Walkley, S. U. 1987. Further studies on ectopic dendrite growth and other geometrical distortions of neurons in feline GM1 gangliosidosis. Neuroscience 21:313–331.

Walkley, S. U., Pierok, A. L. 1986. Ferric ion-ferrocyanide staining in ganglioside storage disease establishes that meganeurites are of axon hillock origin and distinct from axonal spheroids. Brain Res 382:379–386.

Walkley, S. U., Wurzelmann, S., Purpura, D. P. 1981. Ultrastructure of neurites and meganeurites of cortical pyramidal neurons in feline gangliosidosis as revealed by the combined Golgi-EM technique. Brain Res 211:393–398.

Yamato, O., Ochiai, K., Masuoka, Y., Hayashida, M., et al. 2000. GM1 gangliosidosis in shiba dogs. Vet Rec 146:493–496.

Globoid Cell Leukodystrophy

Boysen, B. G., Tryphonas, L., Harries, N. W. 1974. Globoid cell leukodystrophy in the bluetick hound dog. I. Clinical manifestations. Can Vet J 15:303–308.

Fankhauser, R., Luginbuhl, H., Hartley, W. J. 1965. Leukodystrophie von Typus Krabbe beim Hund. Schweiz Arch Tierheilkd 105:198–207.

Fletcher, T. F., Kurtz, H. J., Low, D. G. 1966. Globoid cell leukodystrophy (Krabbe type) in the dog. JAVMA 149:165–172.

Fletcher, T. F., Kurtz, H. J., Stadlan, E. M. 1971. Experimental wallerian degeneration in peripheral nerves of dogs with globoid cell leukodystrophy. J Neuropathol Exp Neurol 30:593–602.

Fletcher, T. F., Lee, D. G., Hammer, R. F. 1971. Ultrastructural features of globoid-cell leukodystrophy in the dog. Am J Vet Res 32:177–181.

Howell, J. M., Palmer, A. C. 1971. Globoid leukodystrophy in two dogs. J Sm An Prac 12:633–642.

Johnson, G. R., Oliver, J. E, Jr., Selcer, R. 1975. Globoid cell leukodystrophy in a beagle. JAVMA 167:380–384.

Johnson, K. H. 1970. Globoid leukodystrophy in the cat. JAVMA 157:2057–2064.

Kurtz, H. J., Fletcher, T. F. 1970. The peripheral neuropathy of canine globoid-cell leukodystrophy (Krabbe-Type). Acta Neuropath (Berl) 16:226–232.

Luttgen, P. J., Braund, K. G., Storts, R. W. 1983. Globoid leukodystrophy in a bassett hound. J Sm Anim Pract 24:153–160.

McGrath, J. T., et al. 1969. A morphologic and biochemical study of canine globoid cell leukodystrophy. J Neuropathol Exp Neurol 28:171.

Roszel, J. F. 1972. Membrane filtration of canine and feline cerebrospinal fluid for cytologic evaluation. JAVMA 160:720–725.

Selcer, E. S., Selcer, R. R. 1984. Globoid cell leukodystrophy in two West Highland white terriers and one Pomeranian. Compend Contin Educ Pract 6:621–624.

Sigurdson, C. J., Basaraba, R. J., Mazzaferro, E. M., Gould, D. H. 2002. Globoid cell-like leukodystrophy in a domestic longhaired cat. Vet Pathol 39:494–496.

Suzuki, Y., Miyatake, T., Fletcher, T. F., Suzuki, K. 1974. Glycosphingolipid beta-galactosidases: 3. Canine form of globoid cell leukodystrophy; comparison with the human disease. J Biol Chem 249:2109–2112.

Vicini, D. S., Wheaton, L. G., Zachary, J. F., and Parker, A. J. 1988. Peripheral nerve biopsy for diagnosis of globoid cell leukodystrophy in a dog. JAVMA 192:1087–1090.

Zaki, F., Kay, W. J. 1973. Globoid cell leukodystrophy in a miniature poodle. JAVMA 163:248–250.

Glucocerebrosidosis (Gaucher's Disease)

Hartley, W. J., Blakemore, W. F. 1973. Neurovisceral glucocerebroside storage (Gaucher's disease) in a dog. Vet Pathol 10:191–201.

Van De Water, N. S., Jolly, R. D., Farrow, B. R. H. 1979. Canine Gaucher disease—the enzymic defect. Aust J Exp Bio Med Sci 57:551–554.

Glycogenosis

Bardens, J. W. 1966. Glycogen storage disease in puppies. Vet Med Small Anim Clin 61:1174–1176.

Bardens, J. W., Bardens, G. W., Bardens, B. 1961. Clinical observation on a Von Gierke-like syndrome in puppies. Allied Vet 32:4–7.

Ceh, L., et al. 1976. Glycogenesis type III in the dog. Acta Vet Scand 17:210–222.

Coates, J. R., Paxton, R., Cox, N. R., Braund, K. G., et al. 1996. A case presentation and discussion of Type IV glycogen storage disease in a Norwegian Forest Cat. Prog Vet Neurol 7:5–11.

Fyfe, J. C., Giger, U., Van Winkle, T. J., Haskins, M. E., et al. 1992. Glycogen storage disease type IV: inherited deficiency of branching enzyme activity in cats. Pediatr Res 32:719–725.

Harvey, J. W., Calderwood Mays, M. B., Gropp, K. E., Denaro, F. J. 1990. Polysaccharide storage myopathy in canine phosphofructokinase deficiency (type VII glycogen storage disease). Vet Pathol 27:1–8.

Hegreberg, G. A., Norby, D. E. 1973. An inherited storage disease of cats. Fed Prac 32:821.

Rafiquzzaman, M., Svenkerud, R., Strande, A., Hauge, J. G. 1976. Glycogenosis in the dog. Acta Vet Scand 17:196–209.

Walvoort, H. C. 1983. Glyocgen storage diseases in animals and their potential value as models of human disease. J Inherit Metab Dis 6:3–16.

Walvoort, H. C., Nes, J. J. van, Stokhof, A. A., Wolvekamp, W. T. C., et al. 1984. Canine glycogen storage disease type II: a clinical study of four affected Lapland dogs. J Am Anim Hosp Assoc 20:279–286.

Glycoproteinosis (Lafora's Disease)

Cusick, P. K., Cameron, A. M., Parker, A. J. 1976. Canine neuronal glycoproteinosis- Lafora's disease in the dog. J Am Anim Hosp Assoc 12:518–521.

Hall, D. G., Steffens, W. L., Lassiter, L. 1998. Lafora bodies associated with neurologic signs in a cat. Vet Pathol 35:218–220.

Holland, J. M., et al. 1970. Lafora's disease in the dog. Am J Pathol 58:509–529.

Jian, Z., Alley, M. R., Cayzer, J., Swinney, G. R. 1990. Lafora's disease in an epileptic basset hound. NZ Vet J 38:75–79.

Kaiser, E., Krauser, K., Schwartz-Porsche, D. 1991. Lafora-Erkrankung (progressive myoklonus-epilepsie) beim Basset-Hund-Moglichkeiter der Friiherkennung mittels Muskelbiopsie? Tieriirztl Pra 19:290–295.

Montgomery, D. L., Lee, A. C. 1983. Brain damage in the epileptic beagle dog. Vet Pathol 20:160–169.

Moreau, P. M., Warren, C. D., Raghavan, S. S., Daniel, P. F., et al. May 1990. Lafora's disease in basset hounds. Proc 8th ACVIM Forum, Washington, DC, 1045–1049.

Mannosidosis

Alroy, J., et al. 1987. Biochemical, ultrastructural and histochemical studies of cat placentae deficient in activity of lysosomal a-mannosidase. Placenta 8:545–553.

Burditt, U., Chotai, K., Hiran, S., Nugent, PG., et al. 1980. Biochemical studies on a case of feline mannosidosis. Biochem J 189:467–473.

Castagnaro, M. 1990. Lectin histochemistry of the central nervous system in a case of feline a-mannosidosis. Res Vet Sci 49:375–377.

Cummings, J. F., Wood, P. A., deLahunta, A., Walkley, S. U., et al. 1988. The clinical and pathologic heterogeneity of feline alpha mannosidosis. J Vel Intern Med 2:163–170.

Maenhout, T., Kint, J. A., Dacremont, G., Ducatelle, R., et al. 1988. Mannosidosis in a litter of Persian cats. Vel Rec 122: 351–354.

Vandevelde, M., Fankhauser, R., Bichsel, P., Wiesmann, U., Herschkowitz, N. 1982. Hereditary neurovisceral mannosidosis associated with a-mannosidase deficiency in a family of Persian cats. Acta Neuropathol 58:64–68.

Vite, C. H., McGowan, J. C., Braund, K. G., et al. 2001. Histopathology, electrodiagnostic testing, and magnetic resonance imaging show significant peripheral and central nervous system myelin abnormalities in the cat model of alpha-mannosidosis. J Neuropathol Exp Neurol 60:817–828.

Walkley, S. U., Blakemore, W. F., Purpura, D. P. 1981. Alterations in neuron morphology in feline mannosidosis. Acta Neuropalhol 53:75–79.

Walkley, S. U., Siegel, D. A. 1985. Ectopic dendritogenesis occurs on cortical pyramidal neurons in swainsonine-induced feline a-mannosidosis. Dev Brain Res 20:143–148.

Mucopolysaccharidosis

Breider, M. A., Shull, R. M., Constantopoulos, G. 1989. Long-term effects of bone marrow transplantation in dogs with mucopolysaccharidosis I. Am J Pathol 134:677–692.

Breton, L., Guerin, P., Morin, M. 1983. A case of mucopolysaccharidosis VI in a cat. J Am Anim Hosp Assoc 19:891–896.

Crawley, A. C., Muntz, F. H., Haskins, M. E., Jones, B. R., et al. 2003. Prevalence of mucopolysaccharidosis Type VI mutations in Siamese cats. J Vet Intern Med 17:495–498.

Gasper, P. W., Thrall, M. A., Wenger, D. A., Macy, D. W., et al. 1984. Correction of feline arylsulphatase B deficiency (mucopolysaccharidosis VI) by bone marrow transplantation. Nature 312:467–469.

Gitzelmann, R., Bosshard, N. U., Superti-Furga, A., Spycher, M. A., et al. 1994. Feline mucopolysaccharidosis VII due to b-glucuronidase deficiency. Vet Pathol 31:435–443.

Haskins, M. E., Aguirre, G. D., Jezyk, P. F., Patterson, D. F., et al. 1980. The pathology of the feline model of mucopolysaccharidosis VI. Am J Pathol 101:657–674.

Haskins, M. E., Bingel, S. A., Northington, J. W., Newton, C. D., et al. 1983. Spinal cord compression and hindlimb paresis in cats with mucopolysaccharidosis VI. JAVMA 182:983–985.

Haskins, M. E., Jezyk, P. F., Desnick, R. J., McDonough, S. K., et al. 1979. Mucopolysaccharidosis in a domestic short-haired cat-a disease distinct from that seen in the Siamese cat. JAVMA 175:384–387.

Haskins, M. E., McGrath, J. T. 1983. Meningiomas in young cats with mucopolysaccharidosis I. J Neuropathol Exp Neurol 42:664–670.

Hubler, M., Haskins, M. E., Arnold, S., et al. 1996. Mucolipidosis type II in a domestic shorthair cat. J Sm Anim Pract 37:435–441.

Langweiler, M., Haskins, M. E., Jezyk, P. F. 1978. Mucopolysaccharidosis in a litter of cats. J Am Anim Hosp Assoc 14:748–451.

Neer, T. M., Umeda, M., Kamiya, S., Sugiyama, K. May 1992. Mucopolysaccharidosis VI (Marateaux-Lamy syndrome) in a miniature pinscher. Proc 10th ACVIM Forum, San Diego, CA, 807.

Schultheiss, P. C., Gardner, S. A., Owens, J. M., Wenger, D. A., et al. 2000. Mucopolysaccharidosis VII in a cat. Vet Pathol 37:502–505.

Shull, R. M., Hastings, N. E. 1985. Auorometric assay of a-L-iduronidase in serum for detection of affected and carrier animals in a canine model of mucopolysaccharidosis I. Clin Chem 31:826–827.

Spellacy, E., Shull, R. M., Constantopoulos, G., Neufeld, E. F. 1983. A canine model of human a-L-iduronidase deficiency. Prac Natl Acad Sci USA 80:6091–6095.

Walkley, S. U., Haskins, M. E., Shull, R. M. 1988. Alterations in neuron morphology in mucopolysaccharidosis type I. A Golgi study. Acta Neuropathol 75:611–620.

Wilkerson, M. J., Lewis, D. C., Marks, S. L., Prieur, D. J. 1998. Clinical and morphologic features of mucopolysaccharidosis type II in a dog: naturally occurring model of Hunter syndrome. Vet Pathol 35:230–233.

Sphingomyelinosis (Niemann-Pick disease)

Baker, H. J., Wood, P. A., Wenger, D. A., Walkley, S. U., et al. 1987. Sphingomyelin lipidosis in a cat. Vet Pathol 24:386–391.

Bundza, A., Lowden, I. A., Charlton, K. M. 1979. Niemann-Pick disease in a poodle dog. Vet Pathol 16:530–538.

Cuddon, P. A., Higgins, R. J., Duncan, I. D., Miller, S. P., et al. 1989. Polyneuropathy in feline Niemann-Pick disease. Brain 112:1429–1443.

Lowenthal, A. C., Cummings J. F., Wenger, D. A., Thrall, M. A., et al. 1990. Feline sphingolipidosis resembling Niemann-Pick disease type C. Acta Neuropathol 81:189–197.

Muñana, K. R., Luttgen, P. J., Thrall, M. A., Mitchell, T. W., et al. 1994. Neurological manifestations of Niemann-Pick disease Type C in cats. J Vet Intern Med 8:117–121.

Percy, O. H., Iortner, B. S. 1971. Feline lipidosis: light and electron microscopic studies. Arch Pathol 92:136–143.

Snyder, S. P., Kingston, R. S., Wenger, O. A. 1982. Animal model of human disease: Niemann-Pick disease. Sphingomyelinosis of Siamese cats. Am J Pathol 108:252–254.

Walkley, S. U., Baker, H. I. 1984. Sphingomyelin lipidosis in a cat: Golgi studies. Acta Neuropathol 65:138–144.

Yamagami, T., et al. 1989. Neurovisceral sphingomyelinosis in a Siamese cat. Acta Neuropathol 79:330–332.

Anomalous Disease

Barone, G., deLahunta, A., Sandler, J. 2000. An unusual neurological disorder in the Labrador Retriever. J Vet Intern Med 14:315–318.

Coates, J. R., Sullivan, S. A. 2001. Congenital cranial and intracranial malformations. In Consultations in Feline Internal Medicine, 4th ed., August, J. R., ed. Philadelphia, W. B. Saunders, 413–423.

Greene, C. E., Gorgacz, E J., Martin, C. L. 1982. Hydranencephaly associated with feline panleukopenia virus infection. JAVMA 180:767–768.

Jeffery, N. D., Watson, P. J., Abramson, C., Notenboom, A. 2003. Brain malformations associated with primary adipsia identified using magnetic resonance imaging. Vet Rec 152: 436–438.

Milner, R. J., Engela, J., Kirberge, R. M. 1996. Arachnoid cyst in cerebellar pontine area of a cat-diagnosis by magnetic resonance imaging. Vet Radiol Ultrasound 37:34–36.

Rusbridge, C., MacSweeny, J. E., Davies, J. V., et al. 2000. Syringohydromyelia in cavalier King Charles spaniels. J Am Anim Hosp Assoc 36:34–41.

Schmid, V., Lang, J., Wolf, M. 1992. Dandy-Walker-like syndrome in four dogs: cisternography as a diagnostic aid. J Am Anim Hosp Assoc 28:355–360.

Scott, F. W., LaHunta, A., Schultz, R. D., Bistner, S. I., Riis, R. C. 1975. Teratogenesis in cats associated with griseofulvin therapy. Teratology 11:79–86.

Sharp, N. J., Davis, B. J., Guy, J. S., Cullen, J. M., Steingold, S. F., Kornegay, J. N. 1999. Hydranencephaly and cerebellar hypoplasia in two kittens attributed to intrauterine parvovirus infection. J Comp Pathol 21:39–53.

Spondenberg, D. P., Graf-Webster, E. 1986. Hereditary meningoencephalocele in Burmese cats. J Hered 77:60.

Summers, B. A., Cummings, J. F., deLahunta, A. 1995. In Veterinary Neuropathology, Summers, B. A., Cummings, J., deLahunta, A., eds. St. Louis, Mosby, 68–94.

Van Winkle, T. J., Fyfe, J. C., Dayrell-Hart, B., et al. 1994. Blindness due to polymicrogyria and asymmetrical dilation of the lateral ventricles in standard poodles. Prog Vet Neurol 5:66–71.

Vernau, K. M., Kortz, G. D., Koblik, P. D., et al. 1997. Magnetic resonance imaging and computed tomography characteristics of intracranial intraarachnoid cysts in 6 dogs. Vet Radiol Ultrasound 38:171–176.

Regnier, A. M., Ducos de Lahitte, M. J., Delisle, M. B., et al. 1993. Dandy-Walker syndrome in a kitten. J Am Anim Hosp Assoc 29:514–518.

Zook, B. C., Sostaric, B. R., Draper, D. J., Graf-Webster, E. 1983. Encephalocele and other congenital craniofacial anomalies in Bunnese cats. Vet Med Small Anim Clin 78:695–701.

Dermoid Cyst

Howard-Martin, M., Howles, M. H. 1988. Intracranial dermoid cyst in a dog. JAVMA 192:215–216.

Kornegay, J. N., Gorgacz, E. J. 1982. Intracranial epidermoid cysts in three dogs. Vet Pathol 19:646–650.

Mawdesley-Thomas, L. E., Hague, P. H. 1970. An intra-cranial epidermoid cyst in a dog. Vet Rec 87:133–134.

Platt, S. R., Graham, J., Chrisman, C. L., et al. 1999. Canine intracranial epidermoid cyst. Vet Rad Ultrasound 40: 454–458.

Lissencephaly

Dewey, C. L.. 2003. In A Practical Guide to Canine and Feline Neurology, Dewey, C. W., ed. Ames, Iowa State Press.

Greene, C. E., Vandevelde, M., Braund, K. 1976. Lissencephaly in two Lhasa apso dogs. JAVMA 169:405–410.

Zaki, F. A. 1976. Lissencephaly in Lhasa apso dogs. JAVMA 169:1165–1168.

Occipital Dysplasia

Bagley, R. S., Harrington, M. L., Tucker, R. L., Sande, R. D., Root, C. R., Kramer, R. W. 1996. Occipital dysplasia and associated cranial spinal cord abnormalities in two dogs. Vet Rad 37:359–362.

Parker, A. J., Park, R. D. 1974. Occipital dysplasia in the dog. J Am Anim Hosp Assoc 10:520–525.

Simoens, P., Poels, P., Lauwers, H. 1994. Morphometric analysis of the foramen magnum in Pekingese dogs. Am J Vet Res 55:34–39.

Wright, J. A. 1979. A study of the radiographic anatomy of the foramen magnum in dogs. J Sm Anim Pract 20:501–508.

Hydrocephalus

Adams, R. D. Victor, M. 1989. Disturbance of cerebrospinal fluid circulation, including hydrocephalus and meningeal reactions. In Principle of Neurology, 4th ed. New York, McGraw Hill, 501–515.

Baumgärtner, W. K., Krakowka, S., Koestner, A., Everman, J. 1982, Acute encephalitis aNd hydrocephalus in dogs caused by canine parainfluenza virus. Vet Pathol 19:79–92.

Bruinsma, D. L. 1983. Acquired hydrocephalus in an adult cat. Vet Med Small Anim Clin, 1857–1858.

Cantile, C., Arispici, M., Modenato, M., et al. 1997. Hydrocephalus with periventricular encephalitis in the dog. J Vet Med 44:595–60.

Carmichael, S., Griffiths, I. R., Harvey, M. J. A. 1983. Familial cerebellar ataxia with hydrocephalus in bull mastiffs. Vet Rec 112:354–358.

Coates, J. R., Sullivan, S. A. 2001. Congenital cranial and intracranial malformations. In Consultations in Feline Internal Medicine, 4th ed., August, J. R., ed. Philadelphia, W. B. Saunders, 413–423.

Cox, N. R., Shires, A., McCoy, C. P., Burns, J. 1990. Obstructive hydrocephalus due to neoplasia in a Rottweiler puppy. J Am Anim Hosp Assoc 26:335–338.

deLahunta, A. 1983. In Veterinary Neuroanatomy and Clinical Neurology, 2d ed. Philadelphia, W. B. Saunders.

deLahunta, A., Cummings, J. F. 1965. The clinical and electroencephalographic features of hydrocephalus in three dogs. JAVMA 146:954–964.

Dewey, C. W. 2002. External hydrocephalus in a dog with suspected bacterial meningoencephalitis. J Am Anim Hosp Assoc 38:563–567.

Few, A. B. 1966. The diagnosis and surgical treatment of canine hydrocephalus. JAVMA 149:286–293.

Gage, E. D. 1970. Surgical treatment of canine hydrocephalus. JAVMA 157:1729–1740.

Gage, E. D., Hoerlein, B. F. 1968. Surgical treatment of canine hydrocephalus by ventriculoatrial shunting. JAVMA 153:1418–1431.

Greenberg, M. S. 1991. Treatment of Hydrocephalus. In Handbook of Neurosurgery, Lakeland, F. L., Greenberg Graphics, 200–218.

Hale, P. M., McAllister, J. P., II, Katz, S. D., et al. 1992. Improvement of cortical morphology in infantile hydrocephalic animals after ventriculoperitoneal shunt placement. Neurosurgery 31(6):1085–96.

Harrington, M. L., Bagley, R. S., Moore, M. P. 1996. Hydrocephalus. Vet Clin N Am (Small Anim Pract) 26:843–856.

Higgins, R. J., Vandevelde, M., Braund, K. B. 1977. Internal hydrocephalus and associated periventricular encephalitis in young dogs. Vet Pathol 14:236–246.

Hudson, J. A., Cartee, R. E., Simpson, S. T., Buxton, D. F. 1989. Ultrasonographic anatomy of the canine brain. Vet Rad 30:13–21.

Hudson, J. A., Simpson, S. T., Buxton, D. F., Cartee, R. E., et al. 1990. Ultrasonographic diagnosis of canine hydrocephalus. Vet Rad 31:50–58.

Hudson, J. A., Simpson, S. T., Cox, N. R., Buxton, D. F. 1991. Ultrasonographic examination of the normal canine neonatal brain. Vet Rad 32:50–59.

Itoh, T., Nishimura, R., Marsunaga, S., et al. 1996. Syringomyelia and hydrocephalus in a dog. JAVMA 209:934–936.

James, A. E., Burns, B., Flor, W. F., Strecker, E. P., et al. 1975. Pathophysiology of chronic communicating hydrocephalus in dogs (Canis familiaris). J Neurol Sci 24:151–178.

Johnson, L., Rolsma, M., Parker, A. 1992. Syringomyelia, hydromyelia and hydrocephalus in two dogs. Prog Vet Neurol 3:82–86.

Kay, N. D., Holliday, T. A., Hornof, W. J., Gomez, J. 1986. Diagnosis and management of an atypical case of canine hydrocephalus, using computed tomography, ventriculoperitoneal shunting, and nuclear scintigraphy. JAVMA 188:423–426.

Klemm, W. R., Hall, C. L. 1971. Electroencephalograms of anesthetized dogs with hydrocephalus. Am J Vet Res 32:1859–1864.

Kornegay, J. N. 1986. Cerebellar vermian hypoplasia in dogs. Vet Pathol 23:374–379.

Kriebel, R. M., Shah, A. B., McAllister, J. P., et al. 1993. The microstructure of cortical neuropil before and after decompression in experimental infantile hydrocephalus. Exp Neurol 119:89–98.

Krumm, S., Johnson, K., Wilson, J. 1975. Hydrocephalus associated with the noneffusive form of feline infectious peritonitis. JAVMA 167:746–748.

Leggett, M. M., Dukes, J., Pirie, H. M. 1990. A spongiform encephalopathy in a cat. Vet Rec 127:586–588.

Levesque, D. C., Plummer, S. B. 1994. Ventriculoperitoneal shunting as a treatment for hydrocephalus. Proc. 12th ACVIM Forum, 891–893.

McAllister, J. P., II, Cohen, M. I., O'Mara, K. A., et al. 1991. Progression of experimental infantile hydrocephalus and effects of ventriculoperitoneal shunts: an analysis correlating magnetic resonance imaging with gross morphology. Neurosurgery 29(3):329–40.

Oliver, J. E., Hoerlein, B. F. 1987. Cranial Surgery. In Veterinary Neurology, Oliver, J. E., Hoerlein, B. F., Mayhew, I. G., eds. Philadelphia, W. B. Saunders, 486–88.

Piatt, J. H., Jr. 1995. Peritoneal cerebrospinal fluid shunt insertion: a technique for protection of the abdominal catheter. J Neurosurg 82:305–306.

Pumarola, M., van Niel, M. H. F. 1992. Obstructive hydrocephalus produced by parasitic granulomas in a dog. J Vet Med Assoc 39:392–395.

Rivers, W. J., Walter, P. A. 1992. Hydrocephalus in the dog: utility of ultrasonography as an alternate diagnostic imaging technique. JAVMA 28:333–343.

Rosenberg, G. A., Saland, L., Kyner, W. T. 1983 Pathophysiology of periventricular tissue changes with raised CSF pressure. J Neurosurg 59:606–611.

Schmahl, W., Kaiser, E. 1984. Hydrocephalus, syringomyelia, and spinal cord angiodysgenesis in a Lhasa-apso dog. Vet Pathol 21:252–254.

Sahar, A., Hochwald, G. M., Kay, W. J., Ransohoff, J. 1971. Spontaneous canine hydrocephalus: cerebrospinal fluid dynamics. J Neurol Neurosurg Psychiatr 34:308–315.

Selby, L. A., Hayes, H. M. L., Becker, S. V. 1979. Epizootiologic features of canine hydrocephalus. Am J Vet Res 40:411–413.

Silson, M., Robinson, R. 1969. Hereditary hydrocephalus in the cat. Vet Rec 84:477.

Simpson, S. T. 1989. Hydrocephalus. In Current Veterinary Therapy X, Kirk, R. W., ed. Philadelphia, W. B. Saunders, 842–47.

Simpson, S. T., Reed, R. B. 1987. Manometric values for normal cerebrospinal fluid pressure in dogs. J Am Anim Hosp Assoc 23:629–632.

Spaulding, K. A., Sharp, N. J. H. 1990. Ultrasonographic imaging of the lateral cerebral ventricles in the dog. Vet Rad 31:59–64.

Van Winkle, T. J., Fyfe, J. C., Dayrell-Hart, B., Aguire, G. D., et al. 1994. Blindness due to polymicrogyria and asymmetrical dilation of the lateral ventricles in standard poodles. Prog Vet Neurol 5:66–71.

Whittle, I. R, Johnston, I. H., Besser, M. 1985. Intracranial pressure changes in arrested hydrocephalus. J Neurosurg 62:77–82.

Wright, L. C., McAllister, J. P., II, Katz, S. D., et al. 1990–1991. Cytological and cytoarchitectural changes in the feline cerebral cortex during experimental infantile hydrocephalus. Pediatr Neurosurg 16(3):139–55.

Wünschmann, A., Oglesbee, M. 2001. Periventricular changes associated with spontaneous canine hydrocephalus. Vet Pathol 38:67–73.

Yamada, H., Yokota, A., Furuta, A. 1992. Reconstitution of Shunted Mantle in Experimental Hydrocephalus. J Neurosurg 76:856–62.

Metabolic Diseases

Cuddon, P. A. 1996. Metabolic encephalopathies. Vet Clin N Am (Small Anim Pract) 26:893–923.

O'Brien, D. E., Kline, K. L. 1997. Metabolic encephalopathies. In Consultations in Feline Internal Medicine, 3d ed., August, J. R., ed. Philadelphia, W. B. Saunders, 373–379.

O'Brien, D. E., Kroll, R. A. 1992. Metabolic encephalopathies. In Kirk's Current Veterinary Therapy XI, Kirk, R. W., Bonagura, J. D., eds. Philadelphia, W. B. Saunders, 998–1003.

Disorders of Glucose

Bagley, R. S., Levy, J. K., Malarkey, D. E. 1996. Hypoglycemia associated with intra-abdominal leiomyoma and leiomyosarcoma in six dogs. JAVMA 208:69–71.

Beaudry, D., Knapp, D. W., Montgomery, T., et al. 1995. Hypoglycemia in four dogs with smooth muscle tumors. J Vet Intern Med 9:415–418.

Elliott, D. A., Feldman, E. C., Koblik, P. D., et al. 2000. Prevalence of pituitary tumors among diabetic cats with insulin resistance. JAVMA 216:1765–1768.

Howerton, T. L., Shell, L. G. 1992. Neurologic manifestations of altered serum glucose. Prog Vet Neurol 3:57–64.

Kraje, A. C. 2003. Hypoglycemia and irreversible neurologic complications in a cat with insulinoma. JAVMA 223:812–814.

Peterson, M. E., Taylor, R. S., Greco, D. S., Nelson, R. W., et al. 1990. Acromegaly in 14 cats. J Vet Intern Med 4:192–201.

Shimada, A., Morita, T., Ikeda, N., et al. 2000. Hypoglycemic brain lesions in a dog with hypoglycemia. J Comp Pathol 122: 67–71.

Steiner, J. M., Bruyerte, D. S. 1996. Canine insulinoma. Compend Contin Educ Pract Vet 18:13–25.

Whitley, N. T., Drobatz, K. J., Panciera, D. L. 1997. Insulin overdose in dogs and cats: 28 cases (1986–1993). JAVMA 211:326–330.

Disorders of Sodium

Bagley, R. S. 1994. Adipsia and the nervous system. Compend Contin Educ Pract Vet 17:311–319.

Churcher, R. K., Watson, A. D. J., Eaton, A. 1999. Suspected myelinolysis following rapid correction of hyponatremia in a dog. J Am Anim Hosp Assoc 35:493–497.

Fraser, C. L., Arieff, A. I. 1997. Epidemiology, pathophysiology, and management of hyponatremic encephalopathy. Am J Med 102:67–77.

Gregory, C. R., Mathews, K. G., Aronson, L. R., et al. 1997. Central nervous system disorders after renal transplantation in cats. Vet Surg 26:386–392.

Laureno, R., Karp, B. I. 1997. Myelinolysis after correction of hyponatremia. Ann Intern Med 126:57–62.

Mulloy, A. L., Caruana, R. I. 1995. Hyponatremic emergencies. Med Clin North Am 79:155–168.

O'Brien, D. 1992. The CNS effects of sodium imbalances. Proc 10th ACVIM Forum, 741–744.

O'Brien, D. E., Kroll, R. A., Johnson, G. C., et al. 1994. Myelinolysis after correction of hyponatremia in two dogs. J Vet Intern Med 8:40–48.

Disorders of Thyroid

Bichsel, P., Jacobs, G. Oliver, J. E. J. 1988. Neurologic manifestations associated with hypothyroidism in four dogs. JAVMA 192:1745–1747.

Chastain, C. B., Graham, C. L., Riley, M. G. 1982. Myxedema coma in two dogs. Canine Practice 9:20–34.

Coates, I. R. 1997. Neurologic manifestations of hypothyroidism. Canine Practice 22:27–28.

Jaggy, A., Oliver, J. E. 1994. Neurologic manifestations of thyroid disease. Vet Clin N Am (Small Anim Pract) 24:487–494.

Jaggy, A., Oliver, J. E., Ferguson, D. C., Mahaffey, E. A., Glaus, T. J. 1994. Neurological manifestations of hypothyroidism: a retrospective study of 29 dogs. J Vet Intern Med 8:328–336.

Joseph, R. J., Peterson, M. E. 1992. Review and comparison of neuromuscular and central nervous system manifestations of hyperthyroidism in cats and humans. Prog Vet Neurol 3:114–119.

Kelly, M. J., Hill, J. R. 1984. Canine myxedema stupor and coma. Compend Contin Educ Pract Vet 6:1049–1055.

Laureno, R. 1996. Neurologic manifestations of thyroid disease. Endocrinologist 6:467–473.

Liu, S., Tilley, L. P., Tappe, J. P., et al. 1986. Clinical and pathologic findings in dogs with atherosclerosis: 21 cases (1970–1983). J Vet Med Assoc 189:227–232.

Panciera, D. L. 1997. Clinical manifestations of canine hypothyroidism. Veterinary Medicine, 44–49.

Zeiss, C. L., Waddle, G. 1995. Hypothyroidism and atherosclerosis in dogs. Compend Contin Educ Pract Vet 17:1117–1129.

Hepatic Encephalopathy

Allen, L., Stobie, D., Mauldin, G. N., et al. 1999. Clinicopathologic features of dogs with hepatic microvascular dysplasia with and without portosystemic shunts: 42 cases (1991–1996). JAVMA 214:218–220.

Aronson, L. R., Gacad, R. C., Kaminsky-Russ, K., et al. 1997. Endogenous benzodiazepine activity in the peripheral and portal blood of dogs with congenital portosystemic shunts. Vet Surg 26:189–194.

Blaxter, A. C., Holt, P. E., Pearson, G. R., Gibbs, C., Gruffydd-Jones, T. J. 1988. Congenital portosystemic shunts in the cat: a report of nine cases. J Sm An Prac 29:631–645.

Berger, B., et al. 1986. Congenital feline portosystemic shunts. JAVMA 188:517–521.

Bunch, S. E. 1991. Hepatic encephalopathy. Prog Vet Neurol 2:287–296.

Campbell, T. M., Lording, P. M., Wrigley, R. H., Lavelle, R. B. 1980. Portal vein anomaly and hepatic encephalopathy in three dogs. Aust Vet J 56:593–598.

Forster-van Hijfte, M. A., McEvoy, F. J., White, R. N., et al. 1996. Per rectal portal scintigraphy in the diagnosis and management of feline congenital portosystemic shunts. J Sm An Prac 37:7–11.

Hottinger, H. A., Walshaw, R., Hauptman, J. G. 1995. Long-term results of complete and partial ligation of congenital portosystemic shunts in dogs. Vet Surg 24:331–336.

Johnson, C. A., Armstrong, P. J., Hauptman, J. G. 1987. Congenital portosystemic shunts in dogs: 46 cases (1979–1986). JAVMA 191:1478–1483.

Johnson, S. E., Crisp, S. M., Smeak, D. D., Fingeroth, J. M. 1989. Hepatic encephalopathy in two aged dogs secondary to a presumed congenital portalazygous shunt. J Am Anim Hosp Assoc 25:129–137.

Komtebedde, J., Forsyth, S. F., Breznock, E. M., Koblik, P. D. 1991. Intrahepatic portosystemic venous anomaly in the dog: perioperative management and complications. Vet Surg 20:37–42.

Komtebedde, J., Koblik, P. D., Breznock, E. M., et al. 1995. Long-term clinical outcome after partial ligation of single extrahepatic vascular anomalies in 20 dogs. Vet Surg 24:379–383.

Maddison, J. E. 1992. Hepatic encephalopathy. J Vet Intern Med 6:341–353.

———. 1988. Canine congenital portosystemic encephalopathy. Aust Vet J 65:245–249.

Marretta, M., Pask, A. J., Greene, R. W., Liu, S. K. 1981. Urinary calculi associated with portosystemic shunts in six dogs. Am J Vet Res 178:133–137.

Murphy, S. T., Ellison, G. W., Long, M., et al. 2001. A comparison of the ameroid constrictor versus ligation in the surgical management of single extrahepatic portosystemic shunts. J Am Anim Hosp Assoc 37:390–396.

Phillips, L., Tappe, J., Lyman, R. et al. 1996. Hepatic microvascular dysplasia in dogs. Prog Vet Neurol 88–96.

Roy, R. G., Post, G. S., Waters, D. J., Hardy, R. M. 1992. Portal vein thrombosis as a complication of portosystemic shunt ligation in two dogs. J Am Anim Hosp Assoc 28:53–58.

Scavelli, T. D., Hornbuckle, W. E., Roth, L., Rendano, V. T., Jr., et al. 1986. Portosystemic shunts in cats: seven cases (1976–1984). JAVMA 189:317–325.

Schermerhorn, T., Center, S. A., Dykes, N. L., et al. 1996. Characterization of a hepatoportal microvascular dysplasia in a kindred of cairn terriers. J Vet Intern Med 10:219–230.

Schunk, C. M. 1997. Feline portosystemic shunts. Semin Vet Med Surg (Small Anim) 12:45–50.

Swalec, K. M. 1993. Portosystemic shunts. In Disease Mechanismsin Small Animal Surgery, 2d ed., Bojrab, M. J., Smeak, D. D., Bloomberg, M. S., eds. Philadelphia, Lea & Febiger, 298–305.

Taboada, J., Dimski, D. S. 1995. Hepatic encephalopathy: clinical signs, pathogenesis, and treatment. Vet Clin N Am (Small Anim Pract) 25:337–355.

Ware, W. A., Montavon, P., DiBartola, S. P., Couto, C. G. 1986. Atypical portosystemic shunt in a cat. JAVMA 188:187–188.

Wrigley, R. H., Konde, L. J., Park, R. D., Lebel, J. L. 1987. Ultrasonographic diagnosis of portacaval shunts in young dogs. JAVMA 191:421–424.

Vogt, J. C., Krahwinkel, D. J., Bright, R. M., et al. 1996. Gradual occlusion of extrahepatic portosystemic shunts in dogs and cats using the ameroid constrictor. Vet Surg 25:495–502.

Renal Encephalopathy

Fenner, W. R. 1995. Uremic Encephalopathy. In Kirk's Current Veterinary Therapy XII (Small Animal Practice), Bonagura, J. D., ed. Philadelphia, W. B. Saunders, 1158–1161.

Gregory, C. R., Mathews, K. G., Aronson, L. R., Ilkiw, J. E., et al. 1997. Central nervous system disorders after renal transplantation in cats. Vet Surgery 26:386–392

Kyles, A. E., Gregory, C. R., Mathews, K. G., et al. 1998. Management of hypertension controls in postoperative neurologic disorders after renal transplantation in cats. Vet Surg 27:511 (Abstract).

Wolf, A. M. 1980. Canine uremic encephalopathy. J Am Anim Hosp Assoc 16:735–738.

Metabolic Encephalopathies

Brenner, O., deLahunta, A., Cummings, J. F., et al. 2000. A canine encephalomyelopathy with morphological abnormalities in mitochondria. Acta Neuropathol 94:390–397.

Brenner, O., deLahunta, A., Summers, B. A., et al. 1997. Hereditary polioencephalomyelopathy of the Australian Cattle dog. Acta Neuropathol 94:64–66.

Brenner, O., Wakshlag, J. J., Summers, B. A., et al. 2000. Alaskan Husky encephalopathy-a canine neurodegenerative disorder resembling subacute necrotizing encephalomyelopathy (Leigh syndrome). Acta Neuropathol 100:50–62.

Harkin, K. R., Goggin, I. M., DeBey, B. M., et al. 1999. Magnetic resonance imaging of the brain of a dog with hereditary polioencephalomyelopathy. JAVMA 214:1342–1344.

Wakshlag, J., deLahunta, A., Robinson, T., et al. 1999. Subacute necrotizing encephalopathy in the Alaskan Husky. J Sm Anim Pract 40:585–589.

Brain Tumor

Adams, R. D., Victor, M. 1989. In Principles of Neurology, 4th ed. New York, McGraw-Hill.

Axlund, Y. W., McGlasson, M. L., Smith, A. N. 2002. Surgery alone or in combination with radiation therapy for treatment of intracranial meningiomas in dogs: 31 cases (1989–2002). JAVMA 221:1597–1600.

Baarnhart, K. F., Edwards, J. F., Storts, R. W. 2001. Symptomatic granular cell tumor involving the pituitary gland in a dog: a case report and review of the literature. Vet Pathol 38:332–336.

Bagley, R. S., Gavin, P. R., Moore, M. P., Silver, G. M., Harrington, M. L., Connor, R. 1999. Clinical signs associated with brain tumor in dogs: 97 cases (1992–1997). JAVMA 215:818–819.

Bagley, R. S., Kornegay, J. N., Lane, S. B., et al. 1996. Cystic meningiomas in 2 dogs. J Vet Intern Med 10:72–75.

Bagley, R. S., Kornegay, J. N., Page, R. L., et al. 1992. Central nervous system neoplasia. In Textbook of Small Animal Surgery, 3d ed., Slatter, D. H., ed. Philadelphia, W. B. Saunders, 2137.

Bagley, R. S., Wheeler, S. J., Klopp, L., et al. 1998. Clinical features of trigeminal nerve-sheath tumor in 10 dogs. J Am Anim Hosp Assoc 34:19–25.

Bailey, C. S., Higgins, R. J. 1986. Characteristics of cisternal cerebrospinal fluid associated with primary brain tumors in the dog: a retrospective study. JAVMA 4:414–417.

Bindal, R. K., Sawaya, R., Leavens, M., et al. 1993. Surgical treatment of multiple brain metastasis. J Neurosurg 79:210–216.

Braund, K. G. 1984. Neoplasia of the nervous system. Compend Contin Educ Pract Vet 6:717–722.

Braund, K. G., Everett, R. M., Albert, R. A. 1978. Neurologic manifestations of monoclonal IgM gammopathy associated with lymphocytic leukemia in a dog. JAVMA 172:1407–1410.

Braund, K. G., Everett, R. M., Bartels, J. E., DeBuysscher, E. 1979. Neurologic complications of IgA multiple myelomas associated with cryoglobulinemia in a dog. JAVMA 174:1321–1325.

Braund, K. G., Ribas, J. L. 1986. Central nervous system meningiomas. Comp Cont Ed 8:241–248.

Brearly, M. J., Jeffery, N. D., Phillips, S. M., et al. 1999. Hypofractionated radiation therapy of brain masses in dogs: a retrospective analysis of survival of 83 cases (1991–1996). J Vet Intern Med 13:408–412.

Carrillo, J. M., Sarfaty, D., Greenlee, P. 1986. Intracranial neoplasm and associated inflammatory response from the central nervous system. J Am Anim Hosp Assoc 22:367–373.

Cook, J. R. 1990. Chemotherapy for brain tumors. Vet Med Report 2:391–396.

Chamberlain, M. C., Kormanik, P. A. 1998. Practical guidelines for the treatment of malignant gliomas. West J Med 168:114–120.

Couto, C. G., Cullen, J., Pedroia, V., et al. 1984. Central nervous system lymphosarcoma in the dog. JAVMA 184:809–813.

Davidson, M. G., Nasisse, M. P., Breitschwerdt, E. B., et al. 1991. Acute blindness associated with intracranial tumors in dogs and cats: eight cases (1984–1989). JAVMA 199:755–758.

Dernell, W. S., Straw, R. C., Cooper, M. F., et al. 1998. Multilobular osteochondrosarcoma in 39 dogs: 1979–1993. J Am Anim Hosp Assoc 34:11–18.

Dewey, C. W., Coates, J. R., Bahr, A., et al. 2000. How I treat primary brain tumors in dogs and cats. Compend Contin Educ Pract Vet 22:756–762.

Dimiski, D. S., Cook, J. R. 1990. Carmustine-induced partial remission of an astrocytoma in a dog. J Am Anim Hosp Assoc 26:179–182.

Dow, S. W., LeCouteur, R. A., Rosychuk, R. A. W., et al. 1990. Response of dogs with functional pititary macroadenomas and macrocarcinomas to radiation. J Sm An Prac 31:287–294.

Fan, T. M., Kitchell, B. E. 2000. Lomustine. Compend Contin Educ Pract Vet 22:934–936.

Feldman, E. C., Nelson, R. W. 1996. In Canine and Feline Endocrinology and Reproduction. Philadelphia, W. B. Saunders.

Fenner, W. R. 1990. Metastatic neoplasms of the central nervous system. Seminars Vet Med Surg 5:253–261.

Foster, E. S., Carrillo, J. M., Patnaik, A. K. 1988. Clinical signs of tumors affecting the rostral cerebrum in 43 dogs. J Vet Intern Med 2:71–74.

Fulton, L. 1991. The use of lomustine in the treatment of brain masses. In Proc 9th ACVIM Forum, New Orleans, LA, 827.

Gallagher, J. G., Berg, J., Knowles, K. E., et al. 1993. Prognosis after surgical excision of cerebral meningiomas in cats: 17 cases (1986–1992). JAVMA 203:1437–1440.

Gavin, P. R., Fike, J. R., Hoopes, P. J. 1995. Central nervous system tumors. Seminars Vet Med Surg 10:180–189.

Geib, L. W. 1966. Ossifying meningioma with extracranial metastasis in a dog. Pathol Vet 3:247–254.

Glass, E. N., Kapatkin, A., Vite, C., et al. 2000. A modified bilateral transfrontal sinus approach to the canine frontal lobe and olfactory bulb: surgical technique and five cases. J Am Anim Hosp Assoc 36:43–50.

Gordon, L. E., Thacher, C., Matthiesen, D. T., et al. 1994. Results of craniotomy for treatment of cerebral meningioma in 42 cats. Vet Surg 23:94–100.

Hammer, A. S., Weeren, F. R., Weisbrode, S. E., et al. 1995. Prognostic factors in dogs with osteosarcomas of the flat or irregular bones.J Am Anim Hosp Assoc 31:321–326.

Heidner, G. L., Kornegay, J. N., Page, R. L., et al. 1991. Analysis of survival in a retrospective study of 86 dogs with brain tumors. J Vet Intern Med 5:219–226.

Higgins, R. J., Le Couteur, R. A., Vernau, K. M., Sturges, B. K., et al. 2001. Granular cell tumor of the canine central nervous system: two cases. Vet pathol 38:620–627.

Ihle, S. L. 1997. Pituitary corticotroph macrotumors. Diagnosis and treatment. Vet Clin N Am (Small Anim Pract) 27:287–297.

Jeffery, N., Brearley, M. J. 1993. Brain tumours in the dog. Treatment of 10 cases and review of recent literature. J Sm Anim Pract 34:367–372.

Kipperman, B. S., Feldman, E. C., Dybdal, N. O., et al. 1992. Pituitary tumor size, neurologic signs, and relation to endocrine test results in dogs with pituitary-dependent hyperadrenocorticism: 43 cases (1980–1990). JAVMA 201: 762–767.

Koblik, P. D., LeCouteur, R. A., Higgins, R. J., et al. 1999a. CT-guided brain biopsy using a modified Pelorus Mark III stereotactic system: experience with 50 dogs. Vet Rad Ultrasound 40:434–440.

———. 1999b. Modification and application of a Pelorus Mark III Stereo- tactic system for CT-guided brain biopsy in 50 dogs. Vet Rad Ultrasound 40:423–440.

Komarnisky, M. D. 1985. Astrocytoma in a cat. Can Vet J 26:237–240.

Kornegay, J. N. 1990. Imaging brain neoplasms: computed tomography and magnetic resonance imaging. Vet Med Report 2:372–390.

Kostolich, M., Dulisch, M. L. 1987. A surgical approach to the canine olfactory bulb for meningioma removal. Vet Surg 16:273–277.

Kraft, S. L., Gavin, P. R., DeHaan, C., et al. 1997. Retrospective review of canine intracranial tumors evaluated by magnetic resonance imaging. J Vet Intern Med 11:218–225.

Lane, S. B., Kornegay, J. N. 1991. Spinal Lymphosarcoma. Consultations in Feline Internal Medicine, August, J. R., ed. Philadelphia, W. B. Saunders, 487.

Lapointe, J. M., Higgins, R. J., Kortz, G. D., Bailey, C. S., et al. 1997. Intravascular malignant T-cell lymphoma (Malignant angioendotheliomatosis) in a cat. Vet Pathol 34:247–250.

Lawson, D. C., Burk, R. L., Prata, R. G. 1984. Cerebral meningioma in the cat: diagnosis and surgical treatment of ten cases. J Am Anim Hosp Assoc 20:333–342.

LeCouteur, R. A. 2001. Cerebral meningiomas: diagnostic and therapeutic considerations. In Consultations in Feline Internal Medicine, 4th ed., August, J. R., ed. Philadelphia, W. B. Saunders, 385–392.

———. 1996. Tumors of the nervous system. In Small Animal Clinical Oncology, 2d ed., Withrow, S. J., MacEwen, E. G., eds. Philadelphia, W. B. Saunders, 393–419.

———. 1990. Brain tumors of dogs and cats: diagnosis and management. Vet Med Report 2:332–342.

LeCouteur, R. A., Vernau, K. M., Koblik, P. D. 1998. Papillary ependymomas and hydrocephalus in three cats. J Vet Intern Med 12:243.

Lobetti, R. G., Nesbit, J. W., Miller, D. B. 1997. Multiple malignant meningiomas in a young cat. J South Afr Vet Assoc 197, 68:62–65.

Long, S. N., Johnston, P. E. J., Anderson, T. J. 2001. Primary T-cell lymphoma of the central nervous system in a dog. JAVMA 218:719–722.

Lorenzo, V., Pumarola, M., Munoz, A. 1998. Meningioangiomatosis in a dog: magnetic resonance imaging and neuropathological studies. J Sm Anim Pract 39:486–489.

Lu, D., Pockness, A., Lamb, C. R., Targett, M. P. 2003. Concurrent benign and malignant meningiomas in a cat: clinical, MRI and pathological findings. Vet Rec 152:780–782.

McGrath, J. T. 1960. Neurologic Examination of the Dog. 2d ed. Philadelphia, Lea & Febiger, 148–195.

Meij, B. P., Voorhout, G., van den Ingh, T. S., et al. 1998. Results of transsphenoidal hypohysectomy in 52 dogs with pituitary-dependent hyperadrenocorticism. Vet Surg 27:246–261.

Moore, J. A., Taylor, H. W. 1988. Primary pulmonary adenocarcinoma with brain stem metastasis in a dog. JAVMA 192: 219–221.

Moore, M. P., Bagley, R. S., Harrington, M. L., et al. 1996. Intracranial tumors. Vet Clinic North Am 26:759–777.

Moore, M. P., Gavin, P. R., Bagley, R. S., Harrington, M. L. 1994. Cerebrospinal fluid analysis in dogs with intracranial tumors. Proc. 12th ACVIM Forum, 917–921.

Moore, M. P., Gavin, P. R., Kraft, S. L., et al. 1991. MR, CT and clinical features from four dogs with nasal tumors involving the rostral cerebrum. Vet Rad 32:19–25.

Nafe, L. A. Meningiomas in cats. 1979. A retrospective clinical study of 36 cases. JAVMA 174:1224–1227.

———. 1990. The clinical presentation and diagnosis of intracranial neoplasia. Semin Vet and Surg (Small Anim) 5: 223–231.

Niebauer, G. W., Dayrell-Hart, B. L., Speciale, J. 1991. Evaluation of craniotomy in dogs and cats. JAVMA 198:89–95.

Ogilvie, G. K., Moore, A. S. 1995. Clinical briefing: tumors of the nervous system. In Managing the Veterinary Cancer Patient: A Practice Manual, Ogilvie, G. K., Moore, G. E., eds. Trenton, NJ, Veterinary Learning Systems, 291–304.

Palmer, A. C., Malinowski, W., Barnet, K. C. 1974. Clinical signs including papilloedema associated with brain tumors in twenty-one dogs. J Sm Anim Pract 15:359–386.

Patchell, R. A., Tibbs, P. A., Walsh, J. W., et al. 1990. A randomized trial of surgery in the treatment of single brain metastases to the brain. New Engl J Med 322:494–500.

Patnaik, A. K., Kay, W. J., Hurvitz, A. I. 1986. Intracranial meningioma: a comparative pathologic study of 28 dogs. Vet Path 23:369–373.

Pluhar, G. E., Bagley, R. S., Keegan, R. D., Baszler, V., Moore, M. P. 1996. The effect of acute, unilateral transverse venous sinus occlusion on intracranial pressure in normal dogs. Vet Surg 25:480–486.

Porter, B., deLahunta, A., Summers, B. 2003. Gliomatosis cerebri in six dogs. Vet Pathol 40:97–102.

Ribas, J. L., Mena, H., Braund, K. G., et al. 1989. A histologic and immunocytochemical study of choroid plexus tumors in the dog. Vet Path 26:55–64.

Sant' Ana, F. J. F., Serakides, R., Graca, D. L. 2002. Pilocytic astrocytoma in a cat. Vet Path 39:759–761.

Sarfaty, D., Carillo, J. M., Peterson, M. E. 1988. Neurologic, endocrinologic and pathologic findings associated with large pituitary tumors in dogs: eight cases (1976–1984). JAVMA 143:854–856.

Schulman, F. Y., Carpenter, J. L., Ribas, J. L., Brum, D. E. 1992. Cystic papillary meningioma in the sella turcica of a dog. JAVMA 200:67–69.

Schulman, F. Y., Ribas, J. L., Carpenter, J. L., et al. 1992. Intracranial meningioma with pulmonary metastasis in three dogs. Vet Path 29:196–202.

Smith, M. O., Turrel, J. M., Bailey, C. S., et al. 1989. Neurologic abnormalities as the predominant signs of neoplasia of the nasal cavity in dogs and cats: seven cases (1973–1986). JAVMA 195:242–245.

Smith, S. H., Van Winkle, T. 2001. Cerebral vascular hamartomas in five dogs. Vet Path 38:108–112.

Sneed, P. K., McDermort, M. W., Gutin, P. H. 1997. Interstitial brachytherapy procedures for brain tumors. Semin Surg Oncol 13:157–166.

Stacy, B. A., Stevenson, T. L., Lipsitz, D., Higgins, R. J. 2003. Simultaneously occurring oligodendroglioma and meningioma in a dog. J Vet Intern Med 17:357–359.

Straw, R. C., LeCouteur, R. A., Powers, B. A., et al. 1989. Multilobular osteochondrosacroma of the canine skull: 16 cases (1978–1988). JAVMA 195:1764–1769.

Summers, B. A., Cummings, J. F., deLahunta, A. 1995. Tumors of the central nervous system. In Veterinary Neuropathology, Summers, B. A., Cummings, J., deLahunta, A., eds. St. Louis, Mosby, 351–401.

Summers, B. A., Palmer, A. C., Littlewood, J. D., Blakemore, W. F. 1989. Intracranial germ cell tumours in two dogs. J Sm An Prac 30:39–42.

Theon, A. P., Feldman, E. C. 1998. Megavoltage irradiation of pituitary macrotumors in dogs with neurologic signs. JAVMA 213:225–231.

Theon, A. P., LeCouteur, R. A., Carr, E. A. 2000. Influence of tumor cell proliferation and sex hormone receptors on effectiveness of radiation therapy for dogs with incompletely resected meningiomas. JAVMA 216:701–707.

Tucker, R. L., Gavin, P. G. 1996. Brain imaging. Vet Clinic North Am 26:735–758.

Turrel, J. M., Fike, J. R., LeCouteur, R. A., et al. 1986. Computed tomographic characteristics of primary brain tumors in 50 dogs. JAVMA 8:851–856.

Uchida, K., Morozumi, M., Yamaguchi, R., Tateyman, S. 2001. Diffuse leptomeningeal malignant histiocytosis in the brain and spinal cord of a Tibetian terrier. Vet Path 38:219–222.

Valentine, H. A., Summers, B. A., de Lahunta, A., White, C. L., et al. 1988. Suprasellar germ cell tumors in the dog: a report of five cases and review of the literature. Acta Neuropathol 76:94–100.

Vandevelde, M. Sept 1984. Brain tumors in domestic animals: an overview. Abstracts for Conference on Brain Tumors in Man and Animals. Research Triangle Park, NC, National Institute of Environmental Health Sciences.

Vernau, K. M., Higgins, R. J., Bollen, A. W., Jimenez, D. F., et al. 2001. Primary canine and feline nervous system tumors: intraoperative diagnosis using the smear technique. Vet Patholo 38:47–57.

Vernau, K. M., Terio, K. A., LeCouteur, R. A., Berry, W. L., et al. 2000. Acute B-cell lymphoblastic leukemia with meningeal metastasis casuing primary neurology dysfunction in a dog. J Vet Intern Med 14:110–115.

Waters, D. J., Hayden, D. W., Walter, P. A. 1989. Intracranial lesions in dogs with hemangiosarcoma. J Vet Intern Med 3:222–230.

Wolf, M., Pedroia, V., Higgins, R. J., et al. 1995. Intracranial ring enhancing lesions in dogs: a correlative CT scanning and neuropathologic study. Vet Rad Ultrasound 36:16–20.

Zaki, F. A., Nafe, L. A. 1980. Choroid plexus tumors in the dog. JAVMA 176:328–330.

Thiamine Deficiency

Anderson, W. I., Morrow, L. A. 1987. Thiamine deficiency encephalopathy with concurrent mycardial degeneration and polyradiculoneuropathy in a cat. Cornell Vet 77:251–257.

Garosi, L. S., Dennis, R., Platt, S. R., Corletto, F., deLahunta, A., Jakobs, C. 2003. Thiamine deficiency in a dog: clinical, clinicopathologic, and magnetic resonance imaging findings. J Vet Intern Med 17:719–723.

Jubb, K. V., Saunders, L. Z., Coates, H. V. 1956. Thiamine deficiency encephalopathy in cats. J Comp Pathol 66:217–227.

Munday, B. L., King, S. I. 1972 A condition resembling Chastek paralysis in cats. NJ Vet J 20:80–81.

Read, D. H., Harrington, D. D. 1986. Experimentally induced thiamine deficiency in beagle dogs: pathologic changes of the central nervous system. Am J Vet Res 47:2281–2289.

———. 1981. Experimentally induced thiamine deficiency in beagle dogs: clinical observations. Am J Vet Res 42:984–991.

Encephalitis

General

Braund, K. G., Vandevelde, M. 1979. Polioencephalomalacia in the dog. Vet Pathol 16:661–672.

Breitschwerdt, E. B. 2001. Neurologic manifestations of tick-transmitted infectious diseases. Proc 19th ACVIM Forum, Denver, CO, 399–401.

Fenner, W. R. 1998. Central nervous system infections. In Infectious Diseases of the Dog and Cat, 2d ed., Greene, C. E., ed. Philadelphia, W. B. Saunders, 647–657.

Greene, C. E. 1998. Protothecosis. In Infectious Diseaes of the Dog and Cat, 2d ed. Greene, C. E., ed. Philadelphia, W. B. Saunders, 430–435.

Greene, C. E., Appel, M. J., Straubinger, R. K. 1998. Lyme Borreliosis. In Infectious Diseases of the Dog and Cat, 2d ed., Greene, C. E., ed. Philadelphia, W. B. Saunders, 282–293.

Munana, K. R. 1996. Encephalitis and meningitis. Vet Clin N Am (Small Anim Pract) 26:857–874.

Nowotny, N., Weissenböck, H. 1995. Description of feline nonsuppurative meningoencephalomyelitis ("Staggering Disease") and studies of its etiology. J Clin Microbiol 33:1668–1669.

Plummer, S. B., Wheeler, S. J., Thrall, D. E., et al. 1992. Computed tomography of primary inflammatory brain disorders in dogs and cats. Vet Rad Ultrasound 33:307–312.

Summers, B. A., Cummings, J. F., deLahunta, A. 1995. Inflammatory diseases of the central nervous system. In Veterinary Neuropathology, Summers, B. A., Cummings, J., deLahunta, A., eds. St. Louis, Mosby, 95–188.

Tipold, A. 1995. Diagnosis of inflammatory and infectious diseases of the central nervous system in dogs: a retrospective study. J Vet Intern Med 9:304–314.

Thomas, W. B. 1998. Inflammatory diseases of the central nervous system in dogs. Clin Tech Small Anim Pract 13:167–178.

Vandevelde, M. 1998. Neurologic diseases of suspected infectious origin. In Infectious Diseases of the Dog and Cat, 2d ed., Greene, C. E., ed. Philadelphia, W. B. Saunders, 530–539.

Vandevelde, M., Braund, K. G. 1979. Polioencephalomyelitis in cats. Vet Pathol 16:420–427.

Bacterial

Budsberg, S. C. 1998. Musculoskeletal infections. In Infectious Diseases of the Dog and Cat, 2d ed., Greene, C. E., ed. Philadelphia, W. B. Saunders, 555–567.

Mane, M. C., Vives, M. A., Barrera, R., et al. 1992. A putative clostridial myositis in a dog. J Sm Anim Pract 33:345–348.

Poncelet, L. 1991. Polymyositis associated with Leptospira australis infection in a dog. Vet Rec 129:40.

Poonacha, K. B., Donahue, J. M., Nightengale, J. R. 1989. Clostridial myositis in a dog. JAVMA 194:69–70.

Seddon, M. L., Barry, S. J. 1992. Clostridial myositis in dogs. Vet Rec 131; 4:84 (letter).

Thomson, M. J., Eger, C. E. 1997. Management of a femoral fracture complicated by Clostridial myositis. J Sm Anim Pract 38:70–73.

Mycosis

Berthelin, C. F., Bailey, C. S., Kass, P. H., et al. 1994. Cryptococcosis of the nervous system in dogs, Part 1: epidemiologic, clinical, and neuropathologic features. Prog Vet Neurol 5:88–97.

Berthelin, C. F., Legendre, A. M., Bailey, C. S., et al. 1994. Cryptococcosis of the nervous system in dogs, Part 2: diagnosis, treatment, monitoring, and prognosis. Prog Vet Neurol 5:136–146.

Burtch, M. 1998. Granulomatous meningitis caused by Coccidioides immitis in a dog. JAVMA 212:827–829.

Cook, J. R., Evinger, J. V., Wagner, L. A. 1991. Successful combination chemotherapy for canine cryptococcal meningoencephalitis. J Am Anim Hosp Assoc 27:61–64.

Day, M. J. 1998a. Canine disseminated aspergillosis. In Infectious Diseases of the Dog and Cat, 2d ed., Greene, C. E., ed. Philadelphia, W. B. Saunders, 409–412.

———. 1998b. Feline disseminated aspergillosis. In Infectious Diseases of the Dog and Cat, 2d ed., Greene, C. E., ed. Philadelphia, W. B. Saunders, 412–413.

Dillehay, D. L., Ribas, J. L., Newton, J. C., Jr., Kwapien, R. P. 1987. Cerebral phaeohyphomycosis in two dogs and a cat. Vet Pathol 24:192–194.

Foil, C. S. 1998. Miscellaneous fungal infections. In Infectious Diseases of the Dog and Cat, 2d ed., Greene, C. E., ed. Philadelphia, W. B. Saunders, 420–430.

Gerds-Grogan, S., Dayrell-Hart, B. 1997. Feline cryptococcosis: a retrospective evaluation. J Am Anim Hosp Assoc 33:118–122.

Greene, R. T. 1998. Coccidioidomycosis. In Infectious Diseases of the Dog and Cat, 2d ed., Greene, C. E., ed. Philadelphia, W. B. Saunders, 391–398.

Jacobs, G. J., Medleau, L. 1998. Cryptococcosis. In Infectious Diseases of the Dog and Cat, 2d ed., Greene, C. E., ed. Philadelphia, W. B. Saunders, 383–390.

Jasmin, A. M., et al. 1969. Systemic blastomycosis in Siamese cats. Vet Med Small Anim Clin 64:33–37.

Legendre, A. M. 1998. Blastomycosis. In Infectious Diseases of the Dog and Cat, 2d ed., Greene C. E., ed. Philadelphia, W. B. Saunders, 371–377.

Lincoln, S. D., Adcock, I. L. 1968 Disseminated geotrichosis in a dog. Pathol Vet 5:282–289.

Mullaney, T. P., Levin, S., Indrieri, R. J. 1983. Disseminated aspergillosis in a dog. JAVMA 182:516–518.

Nafe, L. A., Turk, J. R., Carter, J. D. 1983. Central nervous system involvement of blastomycosis in the dog. J Am Anim Hosp Assoc 19:933–936.

Newsholme, S. J., Tyrer, M. J. 1980. Cerebral mycosis in a dog caused by Cladosporium trichoides Emmons 1952. Onderstepoort J Vet Res 47:47–49.

O'Toole, T. E., Sata, A. F., Rozanski, E. A. 2003. Cryptococcsis in the central nervous system in a dog. JAVMA 222:1722–1725.

Palmer, A. C., Herrtage, M. E., Kaplan, W. 1981. Cryptococcal infection of the central nervous system of a dog in the United Kingdom. J Sm Anim Pract 22:579–586.

Patterson, I. M., Rosendal, S., Humphrey, J., Teeter, W. G. 1983. A case of disseminated paecilomycosis in the dog. J Am Anim Hosp Assoc 19:569–574.

Pryor, W. H., Huizenga, C. G., Splitter, G. A., Harwell, J. F., Jr. 1972. Coccidioides immitis encephalitis in two dogs. JAVMA 161:1108–1112.

Sims, M. A. 1974. Flavobacterium meningosepticum: a probable cause of meningitis in a cat. Vet Rec 95:567–569.

Sutton, R. H. 1981. Cryptococcosis in dogs: a report on 6 cases. Aust Vet J 57:558–564.

Wilkinson, G. T. 1979. Feline cryptococcosis: a review and seven case reports. J Sm An Prac 20:749–768.

Wolf, A. M. 1998. Histoplasmosis. In Infectious Diseases of the Dog and Cat, Greene, C. E., 2d ed. Philadelphia, W. B. Saunders, 378–383.

Parasitic Migration

Barron, C. N., Saunders, L. Z. 1966. Visceral larva migrans in the dog. Pathol Vet 3:315–330.

Buback, J. L., Schulz, K. S., Walker, M. A., Snowden, K. F. 1996. Magnetic resonance imaging of the brain for diagnosis of neurocysticercosis in a dog. JAVMA 208:1846–1848.

Buick, T. D., Campbell, R. S. F., Hutchinson, G. W. 1977. Spinal nematodiasis of the dog associated with Ancylostoma caninum. Aust Vet J 53:602–603.

Cook, J. R. J., Levesque, D. C., Nuehting, L. P. 1985.Intracranial cuterebral myiasis causing acute lateralizing meningoencephalitis in two cats. J Am Anim Hosp Assoc 21:279–284.

Georgi, J. R., deLahunta, A., Percy, D. H. 1969. Cerebral coenurosis in a cat. Report of a case. Cornell Vet 59:127–134.

Glass, E. N., Cornetta, A. M., deLahunta, A., et al. 1998. Clinical and clinicopathologic features in 11 cats with Cuterebra larvae myiasis of the central nervous system. J Vet Intern Med 12:365–368.

Hatziolos, B. C. 1966. Cuterebra larva in the brain of a cat. JAVMA 148:787–793.

Hayes, M. A., Creighton, S. R. 1978. A coenurus in the brain of a cat. Can Vet J 19:341–343.

Hendrix, C. M., DiPinto, M. N., Cox, N. R., Sartin, E. A., et al. 1989. Aberrant intracranial myiasis caused by larval Cuterebra infection. Compend Contin Educ Pract Vet 550:550–562.

Huss, B. T., Miller, M. A., Corwin, R. M., et al. 1994. Fatal cerebral coenurosis in a cat. JAVMA 205:69–71.

Jauregui, P. H., Marquez-Monter, H. 1977. Cysticercosis of the brain in dogs in Mexico City. Am J Vet Res 38;1641–1642.

Kotani, T., Tomimura, T., Ogura, M., Yoshida, H., et al. 1975. Cerebral infarction caused by Dirofilaria immitis in three dogs. Jpn J Vet Sci 37:379–390.

MacDonald, J. M., deLahunta, A., Georgi, J. 1976. Cuterebra encephalitis in a dog. Cornell Vet 66:372–380.

Mandelke, L., Brutus, R. L. 1971. Feline and canine dirofilaria encephalitis. JAVMA 159:776.

Mason, K. V. 1987. Canine neural angiostrongylosis: the clinical and therapeutic features of 55 natural cases. Aust Vet J 64:201–203.

———. 1989. Haematological and cerebrospinal fluid findings in canine neural angiostrongylosis. Aust Vet J 66:152–154.

Mason, K. V., Prescott, C. W., Kelly, W. R., Waddell, A. H. 1976. Granulomatous encephalomyelitis of puppies due to Angiostrongylus cantonensis. Aust Vet J 52:295.

McKenzie, B. E., Lyles, D. L., Clinkscales, J. A. 1978. Intracerebral migration of Cuterebra larva in a kitten. JAVMA 172: 173–175.

Patton, C. S., Garner, F. M. 1970. Cerebral infarction caused by heartworms (*Dirofilaria immitis*) in a dog. JAVMA 156:600–605.

Pumarola, M., van Niel, M. H. F. 1992. Obstructive hydrocephalus produced by parasitic granulomas in a dog. J Vet Med Assoc 39:392–395.

Richards, M. A., Sloper, J. C. 1964. Hypothalamic involvement by "visceral" larva migrans in a dog suffering from diabetes insipidus. Vet Rec 76:449–451.

Rudmann, D. G., Kazacos, K. R., Storandt, S. T., et al. 1996. Baylisascaris procyonis larva migrans in a puppy: a case report and update for the veterinatian. J Am Anim Hosp Assoc 32:73–76.

Sartin, E. A., Hendrix, C. M., Dillehay, D. L., et al. 1986.Cerebral cuterebrosis in a dog. JAVMA 189:1338–1339.

Slocombe, R. F., Arundel, J. H., Labuc, R., et al. 1989. Cerebral coenuriasis in a domestic cat. Aust Vet J 66:92–93.

Smith, M. C., Bailey, C. S., Baker, N., et al. 1988. Cerebral coenurosis in a cat. JAVMA 192:82–84.

Thomas, J. S., 1988. Encephalomyelitis in a dog caused by Baylisascaris infection. Vet Pathol 25:94–95.

Williams, K. J., Summers, B. A., deLahunta, A. 1998. Cerebrospinal cuterebriasis in cats and its association with feline ischemic encephalopathy. Vet Pathol 35(5):330–43.

Protothecosis

Cook, J. R. J., Tyler, D. E., Coulter, D. B., Chandler, F. W. 1984. Disseminated protothecosis causing acute blindness and deafness in a dog. JAVMA 184:1266–1272.

Gaunt, S. D., McGrath, R. K., Cox, H. U. 1984. Disseminated protothecosis in a dog. JAVMA 185:906–907.

Imes, G. D., Lloyd, J. C., Brightman, M. P. 1977. Disseminated prothothecosis in a dog. Onderstepoort J Vet Res 44:1–6.

Moore, F. M., Schmidt, G. M., Desai, D., et al. 1985. Unsuccessful treatment of disseminated protothecosis in a dog. JAVMA 186:705–708.

Thomas, J. B., Preston, N. 1990. Generalised protothecosis in a collie dog. Aust Vet J 67:25–27, 1990.

Tyler, D. E., Lorenz, M. D., Blue, J. L., Munnell, J. F., et al, 1980. Disseminated protothecosis with central nervous system involvement in a dog. JAVMA 176:987–993.

Protozoal

Averill, D. R. J., deLahunta, A. 1971. Toxoplasmosis of the canine nervous system: clinicopathologic findings in four cases. JAVMA 159:1134–1141.

Barber, J. S., Payne-Johnson, C. E., Trees, A. J. 1996. Distribution of Neospora caninum within the central nervous system and other tissues of six dogs with clinical neosporosis. J Sm Anim Pract 37:568–574.

Basso, W., Venturini, L., Venturini, M. C., et al. 2001. First isolation of Neospora caninum from the feces of a naturally infected dog. J Parasitol 87:612–618.

Coman, B. J., Jones, E. H., Westbury, H. A. 1981. Protozoan and viral infections of feral cats. Aust Vet J 57:319–323.

Cuddon, P., Lin, D. S., Bowman, D. D., et al. 1992. Neospora caninum infection in English Springer Spaniel littermates. Diagnostic evaluation and organism isolation. J Vet Intern Med 6:325–332.

Davidson, M. G. 2000. Toxoplasmosis. Vet Clin N Am (Small Anim Pract) 30:1051–1062.

Dubey, J. P. 1992. Neospora caninum infections. In Kirk's Current Veterinary Therapy XI (Small Animal Practice), Kirk, R. W., Bonagura, J. D., eds. Philadelphia, W. B. Saunders, 263–266.

———. 1990. Neospora caninum: a look at a new toxoplasma-like parasite of dogs and other animals. Compend Contin Educ 12:653–661.

Dubey, J. P., Carpenter, J. L. 1993. Histologically confirmed clinical toxoplasmosis in cats: 100 cases (1952–1990). JAVMA 203:1556–1566.

———. 1993. Unidentified Toxoplasma-like tissue cysts in the brains of three cats. Vet Parasitol 45:319–321.

Dubey, J. P., Carpenter, J. L., Speer, C. A., et al. 1988. Newly recognized fatal protozoan disease of dogs. JAVMA 192:1269–1285.

Dubey, J. P., Higgins, R. J., Barr, B. C., et al. 1994. Sarcocystis-associated meningoencephalomyelitis in a cat. J Vet Diagn Invest 6:118–120.

Dubey, J. P., Lappin, M. R. 1998. Toxoplasmosis and neosporosis. In Infectious Diseases of the Dog and Cat, 2d ed., Greene, C. E., ed. Philadelphia, W. B. Saunders, 493–509.

Dubey, J. P., Lindsay, D. S. 1996. A review of Neospora caninum and neosporosis. Vet. Parasitol. 67:1–59.

———. 1990. Neosporosis in dogs. Vet Parasitol 36:147–151.

Dubey, J. P., Lindsay, O. S., Lipscomb, T. P. 1990. Neosporosis in cats. Vet Pathol 27:335–339.

Dubey, J. P., Slife, L. N. 1990. Fatal encephalitis in a dog associated with an unidentified coccidian parasite. J Vet Diagn Invest 2:233–236.

Greene, C. E., Cook, J. R., Jr., Mahaffey, E. A. 1985. Clindamycin for treatment of toxoplasma polymyositis in a dog. JAVMA 187:631–634.

Hass, J. A., Shell, L., Saunders, G. 1989. Neurological manifestations of Toxoplasmosis: a literature review and case summary. J Am Anim Hosp Assoc 25:253–260.

Knowler, C., Wheeler, S. J. 1995. Neospora caninum infection in three dogs. J ft 36:172–177.

Lappin, M. R. 1989. Feline toxoplasmosis. In Kirk's Current Veterinary Therapy X (Small Animal Practice), Kirk, R. W., ed. Philadelphia, W. B. Saunders, 1112–1115.

Lappin, M. R., Greene, C. E., Prestwood, A. K., Dawe, D. L., Tarleton, R. L. 1989. Diagnosis of recent Toxoplasma gondii infection in cats by use of an enzyme-linked immunosobent assay for immunoglobulin M. Amer J Vet Res 50:1580–1585.

Lindsay, D. S., Blagburn, B. L., Dubey, J. P. 1997. Feline toxoplasmosis and the importance of the toxoplasma gondii oocyst. Compend Contin Educ 19:448–461.

Lindsay, D. S., Dubey, J. P., McAllister, M. 1999. Neospora caninum and the potential for parasite transmission. Compend Contin Educ Pract Vet 21;4:317–321.

Mayhew, I. G., Smith, K. C., Dubey, J. P., et al. 1991. Treatment of encephalomyelitis due to Neospora caninum in a litter of puppies. J Sm An Prac 32:609–612.

Okoh, A. E. J. 1978. A case of cerebral babesiosis in the dog. Bull Anim Health Prod Afr 26:118–119.

Plowright, W. 1952. An encephalitis-nephritis syndrome in the dog probably due to congenital encephalitozoon infection. J Comp Pathol 62:83–92.

Purchase, H. S. 1947. Cerebral babesiosis in dogs. Vet Rec 59:269–270.

Taboada, J., Merchant, S. R. 1991. Babesiosis of companion animals and man. Vet Clin N Am 21:103–123.

Toomey, J. M., Carlisle-Nowak, M. M., Barr, S. C., et al. Concurrent Toxoplasmosis and feline infectious peritonitis in a cat. J Am Anim Hosp Assoc 31:425–428.

Uggla, A., Dubey, J. P., Lundmark, G., et al. 1989. Encephalomyelitis and myositis in a boxer puppy due to a Neospora-like infection. Vet Parasitol 32:255–260.

van Dellen, A. F., et al. 1978. Light and electron microscopic studies on canine encephalitozoonosis: cerebral vasculitis. Onderstepoort J Vet Res 45:165–186.

Rickettsial Meningoencephalitis

Comer, K. M. 1991. Rocky Mountain spotted fever. Vet Clin N Am 21:27–44.

Firneisz, G. D., Cochrane, S. M., Parent, J., Houston, D. M. 1990. Canine ehrlichiosis in Ontario. Canadian Vet J 31:652–653.

Gasser, A. M., Birkenheuer, A. J., Breitschwerdt, E. B. 2001. Canine Rocky Mountain Spotted fever: a retrospective study of 30 cases. J Am Anim Hosp Assoc 37:41–48.

Greene, C. E., Breirschwerdt, E. B. 1998. Rocky mountain spotted fever, Q fever, and Typhus. In Infectious Diseases of the Dog and Cat, 2d ed., Green, C. E., ed. Philadelphia, W. B. Saunders, 155–165.

Greene, C. E., Burgdorfer, W., Cavagnolo, R., Philip, R. N., and Peacock, M. G. 1985. Rocky Mountain spotted fever in dogs and its differentiation from canine ehrlichiosis. JAVMA 186:465–472.

Harvey, J. W. 1998. Canine thrombocytic Ehrlichiosis. In Infectious Diseases of the Dog and Cat, 2d ed., Greene, C. E. Philadelphia, W. B. Saunders, 147–149.

Lappin, M. R. 1998. Feline Ehrlichiosis. In Infectious Diseases of the Dog and Cat, 2d ed., Greene, C. E. Philadelphia, W. B. Saunders, 149–154.

Maretzki, C. H., Fisher, D. J., Greene, C. E. 1994. Granulocytic ehrlichiosis and meningitis in a dog. JAVMA 1554–1556.

Meinkoth, J. H., Ewing, S. A., Cowell, R. L., Dawson, J. E., et al. 1998. Morphologic and molecular evidence of a dural species Ehrlichial infection in a dog presenting with inflammatory central nervous system disease. J Vet Intern Med 12:389–393.

Meinkoth, J. H., Hoover, J. P., Cowell, R. L., Tyler, R. D., Link, J. 1989. Ehrlichiosis in a dog with seizures and nonregenerative anemia. JAVMA 195:1754–1755.

Neer, T. M. 1998. Canine monocytic and granulocytic Ehrlichiosis. In Infectious Diseases of the Dog and Cat, 2d ed., Greene, C. E. Philadelphia, W. B. Saunders, 139–147.

Troy, G. C., Vulgamott, I. C., Tumwald, O. H. 1980. Canine ehrlichiosis: a retrospective study of 30 naturally occurring cases. J Am Anim Hosp Assoc 16:181–187.

Waddle, J. R., Littman, M. P. 1988. A retrospective study of 27 cases of naturally occurring canine ehrlichiosis. J Am Anim Hosp Assoc 24:615–620.

Viral

Baumgärtner, W. K., Krakowka, S., Koestner, A., Everman, J. 1982, Acute encephalitis and hydrocephalus in dogs caused by canine parainfluenza virus. Vet Pathol 19:79–92.

Lundgren, A. L., Ludwig, H. 1993. Clinically diseased cats with nonsuppurative meningoencephalitis have Borna disease virus-specific antibodies. Act Vet Scand 34:101–103.

Quesnel, A. D., Parent, J. M., McDonell, W., et al. 1997. Diagnostic evaluation of cats with seizure disorders: 30 cases (1991–1993). JAVMA 210:65–71.

Rand, J. S., Parent, J., Percy, D., et al. 1994. Clinical, cerebrospinal fluid, and histological data from twenty-seven cats with primary inflammatory disease of the central nervous system. Can Vet J 35:103–110.

Distemper

Adams, J. M. 1975. Old dog encephalitis and demyelinating diseases in man. Vet Pathol 12:220–226.

Alleman, A. R., et al. 1992. Identification of intracytoplasmic inclusion bodies in mononuclear cells from the cerebrospinal fluid of a dog with canine distemper. Vet Pathol 29:84–85.

Braund, K. G., Crawley, R. R., Speakman, C. 1981. Hippocampal necrosis associated with canine distemper virus infection. Vet Rec 109:122–123.

Breazile, J. E., Blaugh, B. S., Nail, N. 1966. Experimental study of canine distemper myoclonus. Am J Vet Res 27:1375–79.

Cornwell, H. J., Thompson, H., McCandlish, I. A., et al. 1988. Encephalitis in dogs associated with a batch of canine distemper (Rockborn) vaccine [published erratum appears in Vet Rec 1988 Feb 20;122(8):187.] Vet Rec 122:54–59.

Fischer, C. A. 1971. Retinal and retinochoroidal lesions in early neuropathic canine distemper. JAVMA 158:740–752.

Greene, C. E., Appel, M. J. 1998. Canine distemper. In Infectious Diseases of the Dog and Cat, 2d ed., Greene, C. E., ed. Philadelphia, W. B. Saunders, 9–22.

Hartley, W. J. 1974. A post-vaccinal inclusion body encephalitis in dogs. Vet Pathol, 301–312

———. 1963. Polioencephalomalacia in dogs. Acta Neuropathol 2:271–281.

Higgins, R. J., Child, G., Vandevelde, M. 1989. Chronic relapsing demyelinating encephalomyelitis associated with persistent spontaneous canine distemper virus infection. Acta Neuropathol 77:441–444.

Lisiak, J. A., Vandevelde, M. 1979. Polioencephalomalacia associated with canine distemper virus infection. Vet Pathol 16:650–660.

McGovern, V. J., et al. 1950. Canine encephalitis causing a syndrome characterized by tremor. Aust J Exp Biol Med Sci 28:433–447.

Sharp, N., Vitek, S., Steingold, S., et al. 2000. A rapid, antemortem diagnostic test for canine distemper virus. J Vet Intern Med 14:342.

Silver, G. M., Bagley, R. S., Moore, M. P. 1997. Myoclonus of the tongue. Prog Vet Neurol 7:137–140.

Sorjonen, D. C., Cox, N. R., Swango, L. J. 1989. Electrophoretic determination of albumin and gamma globulin concentrations in cerebrospinal fluid of dogs with encephalomyelitis attributable to canine distemper virus infection: 13 cases (1980–1987). JAVMA 195:977–980.

Thomas, W. B., Sorjonen, D. C., Steiss, J. E. 1993. A retrospective evaluation of 38 cases of canine distemper encephalomyelitis. J Am Anim Hosp Assoc 29:129–133.

Turnwald, G. H., Barta, O., Taylor, H. W., Kreeger, J., et al. 1988. Cryptosporidiosis associated with immunosuppression attributable to distemper in a pup. JAVMA 192:79–81.

Vandevelde, M., Cachin, M. 1992. The neurologic form of canine distemper. In Kirk's Current Veterinary Therapy XI (Small Animal Practice), Kirk, R. W., Bonagura, J. D., eds. Philadelphia, W. B. Saunders, 1003–1007.

Vandevelde, M., Kristensen, B., Braund, K. G., Greene, C. E., et al. 1980. Chronic distemper virus encephalitis in mature dogs. Vet Pathol 17:17–28.

Vandevelde, M., Zurbriggen, A., Higgins, R. J., et al. 1985. Spread and distribution of viral antigen in nervous canine distemper. Acta Neuropathol (Berl) 67:211–218.

Zurbriggen, A., Vandevelde, M. 1994. The pathogenesis of nervous distemper. Prog Vet Neurol 5:109–116.

Feline Borna Virus

Berg, A-L. 2000. Borna disease in cats. In Kirk's Current Veterinary Therapy XIII (Small Animal Practice), Bonagura, J. D., ed. Philadelphia, W. B. Saunders, 976–978.

Feline Immunodeficiency Virus

Dow, S. W., Poss, M. L., Hoover, E. A. 1990. Feline immunodeficiency virus: a neurotropic lentivirus. J Acquir Immun Disease Syndr 3:658–668.

Gunn-Moore, D. A., Pearson, G. R., Harbour, D. A., Whiting, C. V. 1996. Encephalitis associated with giant cells in a cat with naturally occurring feline immunodeficiency virus infection demonstrated by situ hydridization. Vet Patho 33: 699–703.

Pedersen, N. C., Ho, E. W., Brown, M. L., et al. 1987. Isolation of a T-lymphotropic virus from domestic cats with an immunodeficiency-like syndrome. Science 235:790–793.

Pedersen, N. C., Yamamoto, J. K., Ishida, T., et al. 1989. Feline immunodeficiency virus infection. Vet Immunol Immunopathol 21:111–129.

Podell, M., Oglesbee, M., Mathes, L., et al. 1993. AIDS-associated encephalopathy with experimental feline immunodeficiency virus infection. J Acquir Immune Defic Syndr 6:758–771.

Phillips, T. R., Prospero-Garcia, O., Puaoi, D. L., et al. 1994. Neurological abnormalities associated with feline immunodeficiency virus infection. J Gen Virol 75:979–987.

Sellon, R. K. 1998. Feline immunodeficiency virus infection. In Infectious Diseases of the Dog and Cat, 2d ed., Greene, C. E., ed. Philadelphia, W. B. Saunders, 84–96.

Feline Infectious Peritonitis and Coronavirus

Addie, D. D., Jarrett, A. 1998. Feline coronavirus infection. In Infectious Diseases of the Dog and Cat, 2d ed., Greene, C. E., ed. Philadelphia, W. B. Saunders, 58–69.

Baroni, M, Heinold, Y. 1995. A review of the clinical diagnosis of feline infectious peritonitis viral meningoencephalomyelitis. Prog Vet Neurol 6:88–94.

Evermann, J. F., Henry, C. J., Marks, S. L. 1995. Feline infectious peritonitis. JAVMA 206:1130–1134.

Foley, J. E., Lapointe, J. M., Koblik, P., et al. 1998. Diagnostic features of clinical neurologic feline infectious peritonitis. J Vet Intern Med 12:415–423.

Ingram, P. L. 1971. Feline infectious peritonitis and its differential diagnosis. J Small Anim Pract 12:301–306.

Kline, K. L., Joseph, R. J., Averill, D. R. 1994. Feline infectious peritonitis with neurologic involvement: clinical and pathological findings in 24 cats. J Am Anim Hosp Assoc 30:111–118.

Kornegay, J. N. 1978. Feline infectious peritonitis: the central nervous system form. J Am Anim Hosp Assoc 14:580–584.

Toomey, J. M., Carlisle-Nowak, M. M., Barr, S. C., et al. Concurrent Toxoplasmosis and feline infectious peritonitis in a cat. J Am Anim Hosp Assoc 31:425–428.

Herpes Virus Encephalitis

Burrows, R. 1977. Herpes virus infections of animals—a brief review. J Antimicrob Chemother 3 Suppl A:9–14.

Carmichael, L. E., Greene, C. E. 1998. Canine herpesvirus infection. In Infectious Diseases of the Dog and Cat, 2d ed., Greene, C. E., ed. Philadelphia, W. B. Saunders, 28–32.

Carmichael, L. E., Squire, R. A., Krook, L. 1965. Clinical and pathological features of a fatal virus disease of new-born pups. Am J Vet Res 26:803–814.

Percy, D. H., Carmichael, L. E., Albert, D. M., King, J. M., Jonas, A. M. 1971. Lesions in puppies surviving infection with canine herpesvirus. Vet Pathol 8:37–53.

Percy, D. H., Munnel, J. F., Olander, H. J., Carmichael, L. E. 1970. Pathogenesis of canine herpesvirus encephalitis. Am J Vet Res 31:145–156.

Percy, D. H., Olander, H. J., Carmichael, L. E. 1968. Encephalitis in the newborn pup due to a canine herpesvirus. Pathol Vet 5:135–145.

Parainfluenza

Baumgärtner, W. K., Krakowka, S., Koestner, A., Everman, J. 1982. Acute encephalitis and hydrocephalus in dogs caused by canine parainfluenza virus. Vet Pathol 19:1979–1992.

Parvovirus

Greene, C. E. 1998. Feline panleukopenia. In Infectious Diseases of the Dog and Cat, 2d ed., Greene, C. E., ed. Philadelphia, W. B. Saunders, 52–57.

Johnson, B. J., Castro, A. E. 1984. Isolation of canine parvovirus from a dog brain with severe necrotizing vasculitis and encephalomalacia. JAVMA 184:1398–1399.

Postvaccinal Encephalomyelitis

Bestetti, G., Fatzer, R., Fankhauser, R. 1978. Encephalitis following vaccination against distemper and infectious hepatitis in the dog. An optical and ultrastructural study. Acta Neuropathol 43:69–75.

Cornwell, H. I. C., Thompson, H., McCandlish, I. A. P., Macartney, L., Nash, A. S. 1988. Encephalitis in dogs associated with a batch of canine distemper (Rockborn) vaccine. Vet Rec 112:54–59.

Hartley, W. I. 1974. A post-vaccinal inclusion body encephalitis in dogs. Vet Pathol 11:301–312.

Krakowka, S., Olsen, R. G., Axthelm, M. K., Rice, J., Winters, K. 1982. Canine parvovirus infection potentiates canine distemper encephalitis attributable to modified live-virus vaccine. JAVMA 180:137–139.

McCandlish, I. A. P., Cornwell, H. J. C., Thompson, H., Nash, A. S., Lowe, C. M. 1992. Distemper encephalitis in pups after vacination of the dam. Vet Rec 130:27–30.

Pedersen, N. C., Emmons, R. W., Selcer, R., Woodie, J. D., et al. 1978. Rabies vaccine virus infection in three dogs. JAVMA 172:1092–1096.

Pekadu, M., Baer, G. M. 1980. Recovery from clinical rabies of 2 dogs inoculated with a rabies virus strain from Ethiopia. JAVMA 41:1632–1634.

Wilson, R. B., Holladay, J. A., Cave, J. S. 1986. A neurological syndrome associated with use of a canine coronavirus-parvovirus vaccine in dogs. Compend Contin Educ Pract Vet 8:117–124.

Pseudorabies

Monroe, W. E. 1989. Clinical signs associated with pseudorabies in dogs. JAVMA 195:599–602.

Murdoch, R. S. 1990. Aujeszky's disease in foxhounds. Vet Rec 126:226.

Vandevelde, M. 1998. Pseudorabies. In Infectious Diseases of the Dog and Cat, 2d ed., Greene, C. E., ed. Philadelphia, W. B. Saunders, 126–128.

Rabies

Cran, H. R., 1986. Some clinical observations on rabies. Vet Rec 118:23–24.

Eng, T.R., Fishbein, O. B. 1990. Epidemiologic factors, clinical findings, and vaccination status of rabies in cats and dogs in the United States in 1988. JAVMA 197:201–209.

Fogelman, V., Fischman, H. R., Horman, J. T., et al. 1993. Epidemiologic and clinical characteristics of rabies in cats. JAVMA 202:1829–1833.

Greene, C. E., Dreesen, D. W. 1998. Rabies. In Infectious Diseases of the Dog and Cat, 2d ed., Greene, C. E., ed. Philadelphia, W. B. Saunders, 114–126.

Murphy, F. A. 1977. Rabies pathogenesis. Brief review. Arch Virol 54:279–297.

Noninfectious Diseases

Berrocal, A., Montgomery, D. L., Pumarola, M. 2000. Leukoencephalitis and vasculitis with perivascular demyelination in a Weimaraner dog. Vet Pathol 37:470–472.

Poncelet, L., Balligand, M. 1993. Steroid responsive meningitis in three boxer dogs. Vet Rec 132:361–362.

Eosinophilic Encephalitis

Bennett, P. F., Allan, F. J., Guilford, W. G., et al. 1997. Idiopathic eosinophilic meningoencephalitis in rottweiler dogs: three cases (1992–1997). Aust Vet J 75:786–789.

Schultte, A. E., Cribb, A. E., Tvedten, H. W. 1986. Eosinophilic meningoencephalitis in a cat. J Am Anim Hosp Assoc 22:623–627.

Smith-Maxie, L. L., Parent, J. P., Rand, J., et al.1989. Cerebrospinal fluid analysis and clinical outcome of eight dogs with eosinophilic meningoencephalomyelitis. J Vet Intern Med 3:167–174.

Granulomatous Meningoencephalitis

Alley, M. R., Jones, B. R., Johnstone, A. C. 1983. Granulomatous meningoencephalomyelitis of dogs in New Zealand. NZ Vet J 31:117–119.

Bailey, C. S., Higgins, R. J. 1986. Characteristics of cerebrospinal fluid associated with canine granulomatous meningoencephalomyelitis: a retrospective study. JAVMA 188:418–421.

Bichsel, P., Vandevelde, M., Vandevelde, E., Affolter, U., et al. 1984. Immunoelectrophoretic determination of albumin and IgG in serum and cerebrospinal fluid in dogs with neurological diseases. Res Vet Sci 37:101–107.

Braund, K. G. 1989. Granulomatous meningoencephalomyelitis. In Kirk's Current Veterinary Therapy X (Small Animal Practice), Kirk, R. W., ed. Philadelphia, W. B. Saunders, 854–858.

———. 1985. Granulomatous meningoencephalomyelitis. JAVMA 186:138–141.

Braund, K. G., Vandevelde, M., Walker, T. L., Redding, R. W. 1978. Granulomatous meningoencephalomyelitis in six dogs. JAVMA 172:1195–1200.

Cordy, D. R. 1979. Canine granulomatous meningoencephalomyelitis. Vet Pathol 16:325–333.

Cuddon, P. A., Coates, J. R., Murray, M. 2002. New treatments for granulomatous meningoencephalomyelitis. Proc 20th ACVIM Forum, Dallas, TX, 319–21.

Cuddon, P. A., Smith-Maxie, L. 1984. Reticulosis of the central nervous system in the dog. Compend Contin Educ Pract Vet 6:23–33.

Gearhart, M. A., deLahunta, A., Summers, B. A. 1986. Cerebellar mass in a dog due to granulomatous meningoencephalomyelitis. J Am Anim Hosp Assoc 22:683–686.

Glastonbury, J. R. W., Frauenfelder, A. R. 1981. Granulomatous meningoencephalomyelitis in a dog. Aust Vet J 57:186–189.

Harris, C. W., Didier, P. J., Parker, A. J. 1988. Simultaneous central nervous system reticulosis in two related Afghan hounds. Compend Contin Educ Pract Vet 10:304–310.

Kipar, A., Baumgartner, W., Vogl, C., et al. 1998. Immunohistochemical characterization of inflammatory cells in brains of dogs with granulomatous meningoencephalitis. Vet Pathol 35:43–52.

Munana, K. R., Luttgen, P. J. 1998. Prognostic factors for dogs with granulomatous meningoencephalomyelitis: 42 cases (1982–1996). JAVMA 212:1902–1906.

Murtaugh, R. J., Fenner, W. R., Johnson, G. C. 1985. Focal granulomatous meningoencephalomyelitis in a pup. JAVMA 187: 835–836.

Russo, M. E. 1979. Primary reticulosis of the central nervous system in dogs. JAVMA 174:492–500.

Ryan, K., Marks, S. L., Kerwin, S. C. 2001. Granulomatous meningoencephalomyelitis in dogs. Compend Contin Educ Pract Vet 23;7:644–650.

Sarfaty, D., Carrillo, J. M., Greenlee, P. G. 1986. Differential diagnosis of granulomatous meningoencephalomyelitis, distemper, and suppurative meningoencephalomyelitis in the dog. JAVMA 188:387–392.

Sorjonen, D. C. 1990. Clinical and histopathological features of granulomatous meningoencephalomyelitis in dogs. JAVMA 26:141–147.

Speciale, J., Van Winkle, T. J., Steinberg, S. A., et al. 1992. Computed tomography in the diagnosis of focal granulomatous meningoencephalitis: retrospective evaluation of three cases. J Am Anim Hosp Assoc 28:327–332.

Thomas, J. B., Eger, C. 1989. Granulomatous meningoencephalomyelitis in 21 dogs. J Sm Anim Pract 30:287–293.

Vandevelde, M., Fatzer, R., Fankhauser, R. 1981. Immunohistologic studies in primary reticulosis of the canine brain. Vet Pathol 18:577–588.

Greyhound Encephalitis

Callanan, J. J., Mooney, C. T., Mulcahy, G., Fatzer, R., et al. 2002. A novel nonsuppurative meningoencephalitis in young greyhounds in Ireland. Vet Pathol 39:56–65.

Maltese Encephalitis

Stalis, I. H., Chadwick, B., Dayrell-Hart, B., et al. 1995. Necrotizing meningoencephalitis of Maltese dogs. Vet Pathol 32: 230–235.

Necrotizing Meningoencephalitis in a Pekingese

Cantile, C., Chianini, F., Arispici, M., Fatzer, R. 2001. Necrotizing meningoencephalitis associated with cortical hippocampal hamartia in a pekingese dog. Vet Pathol 38:119–122.

Pug Dog Meningoencephalitis

Bradley, G. A. 1991. Myocardial necrosis in a pug dog with necrotizing meningoencephalitis, Vet Pathol 28:91–93.

Cordy, O. R., Holliday, T. A. 1989. A necrotizing meningoencephalitis of pug dogs. Vet Pathol 26:191–194.

Yorkshire Terrier Encephalitis

Ducote, J. M., Johnson, K. E., Dewey, C. W., et al. 1999. Computed tomography of necrotizing meningoencephalitis in 3 Yorkshire terriers. Vet Rad Ultrasound 40;6:617–621.

Jull, B. A., Merryman, J. I., Thomas, W. B., et al. 1997. Necrotizing encephalitis in a Yorkshire terrier. JAVMA 211:1005–1007.

Kuwamura, M., Adachi, T., Yamate, J., Kotani, T., et al. 2002. Necrotising encephalitis in the Yorkshire terrier: a case report and literature review. J Sm Anim Pract 43:459–463.

Tipold, A., Fatter, R., Zurbriggen, A., et al. 1993. Necrotizing encephalitis in Yorkshire terriers. J Sm Anim Pract 34:623–628.

Spinal Cord Vasculitis

Harcourt, R. A. 1978. Polyarteritis in a colony of beagles. Vet Rec 102:519–522.

Hayes, T. J., Robert, G. K. S., Halliwell, W. H. 1989. An idiopathic febrile necrotizing arteritis syndrome in the beagle dog: beagle pain syndrome. Toxicologic Pathology 17:129–137.

Hoff, E. J., Vandevelde, M. 1981. Case report: necrotizing vasculitis in the central nervous systems of two dogs. Vet Pathol 18:219–223.

Irving, G., Chrisman, C. 1990, Long-term outcome of five cases of corticosteroid-responsive meningomyelitis. J Am Anim Hosp Assoc 26:324–328.

Kelly, D. F., Grunsell, C. S. G., Kenyon, C. J. 1973. Polyarteritis in a dog: a case report. Vet Rec 92:363–366.

Meric, S. M., Child, G., Higgins, R. J. 1986. Necrotizing vasculitis of the spinal pachyleptomeningeal arteries in three Bernese mountain dog littermates. J Am Anim Hosp Assoc 22:459–465.

Meric, S. M., Pennan, V., Hardy, R. M. 1985. Corticosteroid-responsive meningitis in ten dogs. J Am Anim Hosp Assoc 21: 677–684.

Prethus, J. 1991. Aseptic suppurative meningitis in Bernese mountain dogs. Eur J Companion Anim Pract 1:24–28.

Scott-Moncrieff, J. C., Snyder, P. W., Glickman, L. T., et al. 1992. Systemic necrotizing vasculitis in ine young beagles. JAVMA 201:1553–1558.

Snyder, P. W., Kazacos, E. A., Scott-Moncrieff, J. C., et al. 1995. Pathological features of naturally-occuring juvenile polyarteritis in beagle dogs. Vet Pathol 3:337–345.

Tipold, A. 2000. Steroid-responsive meningitis-arteritis in dogs. In Kirk's Current Veterinary Therapy XIII (Small Animal Practice), Bonagura, J. D., ed. Philadelphia, W. B. Saunders, 978–981.

Tipold, A., Jaggy, A. 1994. Steroid-responsive meningitis-arteritis in dogs: long-term study of 32 cases. J Sm An Prac 35:311–316.

Tremor-syndrome Encephalitis

Bagley, R. S. 1992. Tremor syndromes in dogs: diagnosis and treatment. J Sm An Prac 33:485–490.

Bagley, R. S., Kornegay, J. N., Wheeler, S. J., Plummer, S. B., Cauzinille, L. 1993. Generalized tremors in maltese: clinical findings in seven cases. J Am Anim Hosp Assoc 29:141–145.

Farrow, B. R. H. 1986. Generalized tremor syndrome. In Kirk, R. W., ed., Current Veterinary Therapy IX. Philadelphia, W. B. Saunders, 800.

Wagner, S. O., Podell, M., Fenner, W. R. 1997. Generalized tremors in dogs: 24 cases (1984–1995). JAVMA 211:731–735

Idiopathic Diseases

Feline Hyperesthesia

Chrisman, C. L. 1991. Self-mutilation. In Problems in Small Animal Neurology, 2d ed., Chrisman, C. L., ed. Philadelphia, Lea & Febiger, 469–477.

March, P. A., Fischer, J. R., Porthoff, A. 1999. Electromyographic and histologic abnormalities in epaxial muscles of cats with feline hyperesthesia syndrome. J Vet Intern Med 13:238 (abstract).

Quesnel, A. D., Parent, J. M. 1997. Diagnostic approach and medical treatment of seizure disorders. In Consultations in Feline Internal Medicine, August, 3d ed., J. R., ed. Philadelphia, W. B. Saunders, 389–402.

Narcolepsy-cataplexy

Baker, T. L., Mitler, M. M., Foutz, A. .S, et al. 1983. Diagnosis and treatment of narcolepsy in animals. In Current Veterinary Therapy VIII: Small Animal Practice, Kirk, R. W., ed. Philadelphia, W. B. Saunders, 755–759.

Foutz, A. S., Mitler, M. M., Dement, W. C. 1980. Narcolepsy. Vet Clin N Am 10:65–80.

Hendricks, J. C., Hughes, C. 1989. Treatment of cataplexy in a dog with narcolepsy. JAVMA 194:791–792.

Hendricks, J. C., Morrison, A. R., Farnbach, G. L., Steinberg, S. A., et al, 1981. A disorder of rapid cyc movement sleep in a cat. JAVMA 178:55–57.

Katherman, A. E. 1980. A comparative review of canine and human narcolepsy. Compend Contin Educ Pract Vet 11:818–822.

Mignot, E., et al. 1988. Role of central alpha-1 adrenoceptors in canine narcolepsy. J Clin Invest 82:885–894.

Mitler, M. M., Soave, O., Dement, W. C. 1976. Narcolepsy in seven dogs. JAVMA 168:1036–1038.

Shores, A., Redding, R. W. 1987. Narcoleptic hypersomnia syndrome responsive to protriptyline in a Labrador retriever. J Am Anim Hosp Assoc 23:455–458.

Thomas, W. B. 2003. Seizures and narcolepsy. In A Practical Guide to Canine and Feline Neurology, Dewey, C. W., ed. Ames, Iowa State Press, 193–212.

Van Heerden, J., Eckersley, O. N. 1989. Narcolepsy in a long-haired dachshund. J S Afr Vet Assoc 60:151–153.

Seizures

Adusumalli, Y. E., Gilchrist, J. R., Wichmann, J. K., et al. 1992. Pharmacokinetics of felbamate in pediatric and adult beagle dogs. Epilepsia 33:955.

Adusumalli, Y. E., Yang, J. T., Wong, K. K., et al. 1991. Felbamate pharmacokinetics in the rat, rabbit, and dog. Drug Met Disp 19:1116.

Bateman, S. W., Parent, J. M. 1999. Clinical findings, treatment, and outcome of dogs with status epilepticus or cluster seizures: 156 cases (1990–1995). JAVMA 215:1463–1468.

Berendt, M., Gram, L. 1999. Epilepsy and seizure classification in 63 dogs: a reappraisal of veterinary epilepsy terminology. J Vet Intern Med 13:14–20.

Berendt, M., Gredal, H., Pedersen, L. G., Alban, L., Alving, J. 2002. A cross-sectional study of epilepsy in Danish Labrador retrievers: prevalence and selected risk factors. J Vet Intern Med 16:262–268.

Boothe, D. M. 2001. Anticonvulsants and other neurologic therapies. In Small Animal Clinical Pharmacology and Therapeutics, Boothe, D. M., ed. Philadelphia, W. B. Saunders, 431–456.

———. 1998. Anticonvulsant therapy in small animals. Vet Clin N Am (Small Anim Pract) 28:411–448.

Boothe, D. M., George, K., Couch, P., et al. 2002. Disposition and clinical use of bromide in cats. JAVMA 221:1131–1135.

Boothe, D. M., Simpson, G., Foster, T. 1996. Effects of serum separation tubes on serum benzodiazepine and phenobarbital concentrations in clinically normal and epileptic dogs. Am J Vet Res 57:1299–1303.

Breitschwerdt, E. B., Breazile, J. E., Broadhurst, J. J. 1979. Clinical and electroencephalographic findings associated with ten cases of suspected limbic epilepsy in the dog. J Am Anim Hosp Assoc 15:37–50.

Brown, S. A., Forrester, S. D. 1991. Serum disposition of oral clorazepate from regular-release and sustained-delivery tablets in dogs. J Vet Pharmacol Theurap 14:126.

Buckmaster, P. S., Smith, M. O., Buckmaster, C. L., LeCouteur, R. A., Dudek, F. E. 2002. Absence of temporal lobe epilepsy pathology in dogs with medically intractable epilepsy. J Vet Intern Med 16:95–99.

Bunch, S. E., Baldwin, B. H., Hornbuckle, W. E., et al. 1984. Compromised hepatic function in dogs treated with anticonvulsant drugs. JAVMA 184:444–448.

Bunch, S. E., Cascleman, W. L., Baldwin, B. H., et al. 1985. Effects of long-term primidone and phenytoin administration on canine hepatic function and morphology. Am J Vet Res 46:105–115.

Center, S. A., Elston, T. H., Rowland, P. H., et al. 1996. Fulminant hepatic failure associated with oral administration of diazepam in 11 cats. JAVMA 209:618–625.

Chauvet, A. E., Feldman, E. C., Kass, P. H. 1995. Effects of phenobarbital administration on results of serum biochemical analyses and adrenocortical function tests in epileptic dogs. JAVMA 207:1305

Cochrane, S. M., Parent, J. M., Black, W. D., et al. 1990. Pharmacokinetics of phenobarbital in the cat following multiple oral administration. Can J Vet Res 54:309–312.

Crowell-Davis, S. L., Lappin, M. R., Oliver, J. E. 1989. Stimulus-responsive psychomotor epilepsy in a Doberman pinscher. J Am Anim Hosp Assoc 25:57–60.

Cunningham, J. G., Farnbach, G. C. 1988. Inheritance and idiopathic canine epilepsy. J Am Anim Hosp Assoc 24:421–424.

Dayrell-Hart, B., Steinberg, S. A., Van Winkle, T. J., Farnbach, G. C. 1991. Hepatoxicity of phenobarbital in dogs: 18 cases (1985–1989). JAVMA 199:1060–1066.

Dayrell-Hart, B., Tiches, D., Vite, C., et al. 1996. Efficacy and safety of felbamate as an anticonvulsant in dogs with refractory seizures. J Vet Intern Med 10:174.

Dewey, C. W., Ducote, J. M., Coates, J. R., et al. 1999. Intrarectally administered potassium bromide loading in normal dogs. J Vet Intern Med 13:238.

Dichter, M. A., Brodie, M. J. New antiepileptic drugs. N Engl J Med 334;24:1583, 1996.Dodman, N. H., Knowles, K. E., Shuster, L., et al. 1996. Behavioral changes associated with suspected complex partial seizures in Bull terriers. JAVMA 208:688–691.

Dodman, N. H., Miczek, K. A., Knowles, K., et al. 1992. Phenobarbital-responsive episodic dyscontrol (rage) in dogs. JAVMA 201:1580–1583.

Famula, T. R., Oberbauer, A. M. 2000. Segregation analysis of epilepsy in the Belgian Tervuren dog. Vet Rec 147:218–221.

Famula, T. R., Oberbauer, A. M., Brown, K. N. 1997. Heritability of epileptic seizures in the Belgian tervuren. J Sm Anim Pract 38:349–352.

Fatzer, R., Gandini, G., Jaggy, A., Doherr, M., et al. 2000. Necrosis of hippocampus and pyriform lobe in 38 domestic cats with seizures: a retrospective study on clinical and pathologic findings. J Vet Intern Med 14:100–104.

Forrester, S. D., Wilcke, J. R., Jacobson, J. D., Dyer, K. R. 1993. Effects of a 44-day administration of phenobarbital on disposition of clorazepate in dogs. Am J Vet Res 54:1136–1138.

Gaskill, C. L., Cribb, A. E. 2000. Pancreatitis associated with potassium bromide/phenobarbital combination therapy in epileptic dogs. Can Vet J 41:555–558.

Gaskill, C. L., Burton, S. A., Gelens, H. C. J., Ihle, S. L., et al. 1999. Effects of phenobarbital treatment on serum thyroxine and thyroid-stimulated hormone concentration in epileptic dogs. JAVMA 215:489.

Hall, S. J. G., Wallace, R. J.1996. Canine epilepsy: a genetic counseling programme for keeshonds. Vet Rec 138:358–360.

Harden, C. 2001. Safety profile of levetiracetam. Epilepsia 42 (Suppl 4):36.

Heynold, Y., Faissler, D., Steffen, F., Jaggy, A. 1997. Clinical, epidemiological and treatment results of idiopathic epilepsy in 54 Labrador retrievers: a long-term study. J Sm Anim Pract 38:7–14.

Hovinga, C. A. 2001. Levetiracetam: a novel antiepileptic drug. Pharmacotherapy 21;11:1375–1388.

Hughes, D., Moreau, R. E., Overall, K. L., et al. 1996. Acute hepatic necrosis and liver failure associated with benzodiazepine therapy in six cats, 1986–1995. J Vet Emerg Crit Care 6;1:13–20.

Jaggy, A., Bemardini, M. 1998. Idiopathic epilepsy in 125 dogs: a long-term study. Clinical and electroencephalographic findings. J Sm Anim Pract 38:23–29.

Jaggy, A., Faissler, D., Gaillard, C., Srenk, P., Graber, H. 1998. Genetic aspects of idiopathic epilepsy in Labrador retrievers. J Sm Anim Pract 39:275–280.

Kantrowitz, L. B., Peterson, M. E., Trepanier, L. A., Melian, C., et al. 1999. Serum total thyroxine, total triiodothyronine, free thyroxine, and thyrotropin concentrations in epileptic dogs treated with anticonvulsants. JAVMA 214:1804.

Kathmann, I., Jaggy, A., Busato, A., Bartschi, M., et al. 1999. Clinical and genetic investigations of idiopathic epilepsy in the Bernese mountain dog.J Sm Anim Pract 40:319–325.

Knowles, K. 1998. Idiopathic epilepsy. Clin Tech Small Anim Pract 13:144–151.

Krakow, K., Walker, M., Otoul, C., et al.2001. Long-term continuation of levetiracetam in patients with refractory epilepsy. Neurology 56:1772

LeCouteur, R. A., Child, G. 1989. Clinical management of epilepsy in dogs and cats. Prob Vet Med 1:578–595.

Leppik, I. E. 2001. The place of levetiracetam in the treatment of epilepsy. Epilepsia 42 (Suppl 4): 44.

Levitski, R. E., Trepanier, L. A. 2000. Effects of timing of blood collection on serum phenobarbital concentrations in dogs with epilepsy. JAVMA 217:200–204.

Lord, L. K., Podell, M. 1999. Owner perception of the care of long-term phenobarbital-treated epileptic dogs. J Sm Anim Pract 40:11–15.

March, P. A. 1998. Seizures: classification, etiology, and pathophysiology. Clin Tech Small Anim Pract 13:119–131.

Matsumoto, K., Miyazaki, H., Fujii, T., et al. 1983. Absorption, distribution and excretion of 3-(sulfamoyl [^{14}C] methyl)-1,2, benzisoxasole (AD-810) in rats, dogs and monkeys and of AD-810 in men. Drug Res 33:961.

Mellema, L. M., Koblik, P. D., Kortz, G. D., et al. 1999. Reversible magnetic resonance imaging abnormalities in dogs following seizures. Vet Rad Ultrasound 40:588–595.

Müller, P. B., Taboada, J., Hosgood, G., et al. 2000. Effects of long-term phenobarbital treatment on the liver in dogs. J Vet Intern Med 14:165–171.

Müller, P. B., Wolfsheimer, K. J., Taboada, J., Hosgood, G., et al. 2000. Effects of long-term phenobarbital treatment on the thyroid and adrenal axis and adrenal function tests in dogs. J Vet Intern Med 14:157.

Munana, K. R., Vitek, S. M., Tarver, W. B., et al. 2002. Use of vagal nerve stimulation as a treatment for refractory epilepsy in dogs. JAVMA 221:977–983.

Nichols, E. S., Trepanier, L. A., Linn, K. 1996. Bromide toxicosis secondary to renal insufficiency in an epileptic dog. JAVMA 208:23.

Papich, M. G., Alcorn, J. 1995. Absorption of diazepam after its rectal administration in dogs. Am J Vet Res 56:1629–1636.

Penderis, J., Franklin, R. J. M. 2001. Dyskinesia in an adult bichon frise. J Sm Anim Pract 42:24–25.

Platt, S. R., McDonnell, J. J. 2000. Status epilepticus: clinical features and pathophysiology. Compmd Contin Educ Pract Vet 22:660–669.

———. 2000a. Status epilepticus: managing refractory cases and treating out-of-hospital patients. Compend Contin Educ Pract Vet 22:732–741.

———. 2000b. Status epilepticus: patient management and pharmacologic therapy. Compend Contin Educ Pract Vet 22:722–729.

Podell, M. 2004. Seizures. In BSVMA Manual of Canine and Feline Neurology, 3d ed., Platt S. R., Olby, N. J., eds. British Small Animal Veterinary Association, 97–112.

Podell M. 2001. Strategies of antiepileptic drug therapy. In Proc 19th ACVIM Forum, Denver, CO, 430–432.

———. 1998. Antiepileptic drug therapy. Clin Tech Small Anim Pract 13:185–192.

———. 1996. Seizures in dogs. Vet Clin N Am (Small Anim Pract) 26:779–809.

———. 1995. The use of diazepam per rectum at home for the acute management of cluster seizures in dogs. J Vet Intern Med 9:68–74.

Podell, M., Fenner, W. R. 1994. Use of bromide as an antiepileptic drug in dogs. Compend Contin Educ Pract Vet 16:767–774.

———. 1993. Bromide therapy in refractory canine idiopathic epilepsy. J Vet Intern Med 7:318– 327.

Podell, M., Fenner, W. R., Powers, J. D. 1995. Seizure classification in dogs from a nonreferral-based population. JAVMA 206: 1721–1728.

Podell, M., Hadjiconstantinou, M. 1999. Low concentration of cerebrospinal fluid GABA correlate to a reduced response to phenobarbital therapy in primary canine epilepsy J Vet Intern Med 13:89–94.

Podell, M., March, P., Sams, R. 2000. Successful loading by continuous intravenous administration of sodium bromide in the dog. J Vet Intern Med, 14.

Quesnel, A. D., Parent, J. M., McDonell, W., et al. 1997. Clinical management and outcome of cats with seizure disorders: 30 cases (1991–1993). JAVMA 210;1:72–77.

———. 1997. Diagnostic evaluation of cats with seizure disorders: 30 cases (1991–1993). JAVMA 210;1:65–71.Radulovic, L. L., Turck, D., von Hodenberg, A., et al. 1995. Disposition of gabapentin (neurontin) in mice, rats, dogs, and monkeys. Drug Metab Disposition 23;4:441.

Ramsey, I. K., Chandler, K. E., Franklin, R. J. M. 1999. A movement disorder in boxer pups. Vet Rec 144:179–180.

Reading, M. J., McKerrell, R. E. 1993. Suspected myokymia in a Yorkshire terrier. Vet Rec 132:587–588

Ruehlmann, D., Podell, M., March, P. 2001. Treatment of partial seizures and seizure-like activity with felbamate in six dogs. J Sm Anim Pract 42:403.

Russo, M. E. 1981. The pathophysiology of epilepsy. Cornell Vet 71:221–247, 1981.

Saito, M., Munana, K. R., Sharp, N. J., et al. 2001. Risk factors for development of status epilepticus in dogs with idiopathic epilepsy and effects of status epilepticus on outcome and survival time: 32 cases (1990–1996). JAVMA 219:618–623.

Scherkl, R., Kurudi, D., Frey, H. H. 1989. Clorazepate in dogs: tolerance to the anticonvulsant effect and signs of physical dependence. Epilepsy Res 3:144.

Schwartz-Porsche, D., Loscher, W., Frey, H. H. 1985. Therapeutic efficacy of phenobarbital and primidone in canine epilepsy: a comparison. J Vet Pharmacol Therap 8:113–119.

Shell, L. G. 2000. Feline seizure disorders. In Kirk's Current Veterinary Therapy XIII (Small Animal Practice), Bonagura, J. D., ed. Philadelphia, W. B. Saunders, 963–966.

Shorvon, S. D., van Rijckevorsel, K. 2002. A new antiepileptic drug: levetiracetam, a pyrrolidone recently licensed as an epileptic drug (editorial). J Neurol Neurosurg Psychiatry 72:426.

Sorde, A., Pumarola, M., Fondevila, M. D., Anteca, X. 1994. Psychomotor epilepsy associated with metastatic thymoma in a dog. J Am Anim Hop Assoc 35:377–380.

Speciale, J., Dayrell-Hart, B., Steinberg, S. A. 1991. Clinical evaluation of gamma-vinyl-gamma-aminobutyric acid for control of seizures in dogs. JAVMA 198:995.

Srenk P., Jaggy A.1996. Interictal electroencephalographic findings in a family of golden retrievers with idiopathic epilepsy. J Sm Anim Pract 37:317.

Steffen, F., Grasmueck, S. 2000. Propofol for treatment of refractory seizures in dogs and a cat with intracranial disorders. J Sm Anim Pract 41:496–499.

Stonehewer, J., Mackin, A. J., Tasker, S., Simpson, J. W., Mayhew, I. G. 2000. Idiopathic phenobarbital-responsive hypersialosis in the dog: an unusual form of limbic epilepsy. J Sm Anim Pract 41:416–421.

Thomas, W. B. 2003. Seizures and narcolepsy. In A Practical Guide to Canine and Feline Neurology, Dewey, C. W., ed. Ames, Iowa State Press, 193–212.

———. 2000. Idiopathic epilepsy in dogs. Vet Clin N Am (Small Anim Pract) 30;1:183–206.

Trepanier, L. A. 1993. Pharmokinetics and clinical use of bromide. Proc 11th ACVIM Forum, 878–880.

Trepanier, L. A., Schoick, A., Schwark, W. S., et al. 1998. Therapeutic serum drug concentrations in epileptic dogs treated with potassium bromide alone or in combination with other anticonvulsants: 122 cases (1992–1996). JAVMA 213:1449–1453.

Vollmer, K. G., von Hodenberg, A., Kolle, E. U. 1986. Pharmacokinetics and metabolism of gabapentin in rat, dog and man. Drug Res 36;1:830.

Walker, R. M., DiFonzo, C. J., Barsoum, N. J., et al. 1988. Chronic toxicity of the anticonvulsant zonisamide in Beagle dogs. Fundament Appl Toxicology 11:333.

Yohn, S. E., Morrison, W. B., Sharp, P. E. 1992. Bromide toxicosis (bromism) in a dog treated with potassium bromide for refractory seizures. JAVMA 201:468–470.

Anticonvulsants

Boothe, D. M. 2001. Anticonvulsants and other neurologic therapies. In Small Animal Clinical Pharmacology and Therapeutics, Boothe, D. M., ed. Philadelphia, W. B. Saunders, 431–456.

———. 1998. Anticonvulsant therapy in small animals. Vet Clin N Am (Sm Anim Pract} 28:411–448.

Dichter, M. A., Brodie, M. J. 1996. New antiepileptic drugs. N Engl J Med 334;24: 1583–1590.

Knowles, K. 1998. Idiopathic epilepsy. Clin Tech Small Anim Pract 13:144–151.

LeCouteur, R. A., Child, G. 1989. Clinical management of epilepsy in dogs and cats. Prob Vet Med 1:578–595.

Podell, M. 2001. Strategies of antiepileptic drug therapy. In Proc 19th ACVIM Forum, Denver, CO, 430–432.

———. 1998. Antiepileptic drug therapy. Clin Tech Small Anim Pract 13:185–192.

———. 1996. Seizures in dogs. Vet Clin N Am (Small Animal Pract). 26:779–809.

Quesnel, A. D., Parent, J. M., McDonell, W., et al. 1997a. Clinical management and outcome of cats with seizure disorders: 30 cases (1991–1993). JAVMA 210:72–77.

———. 1997b. Diagnostic evaluation of cats with seizure disorders: 30 cases (1991–1993). JAVMA 210:65–71.

Sisson, A. 1997. Current experiences with anticonvulsants in dogs and cats. Proc 15th ACVIM Forum, 596–598.

Thomas, W. B. 2003. Seizures and Narcolepsy. In A Practical Guide to Canine and Feline Neurology, Dewey, C. W., ed. Ames, Iowa State Press, 193–212.

———. 2000. Idiopathic epilepsy in dogs. Vet Clin N Am (Small Anim Pract) 30;1:183–206.

Phenobarbital

Boothe, D. M., Simpson, G., Foster, T. 1996. Effects of serum separation tubes on serum benzodiazepine and phenobarbital concentrations in clinically normal and epileptic dogs. Am J Vet Res 57:1299–1303.

Bunch, S. E., Baldwin, B. H., Hornbuckle, W. E., et al. 1984. Compromised hepatic function in dogs treated with anticonvulsant drugs. JAVMA 184:444–448.

Chauvet, A. E., Feldman, E. C., Kass, P. H. 1995. Effects of phenobarbital administration on results of serum biochemical analyses and adrenocortical function tests in epileptic dogs. JAVMA 207:1305.

Cochrane, S. M., Parent, J. M., Black, W. D., et al. 1990. Pharmacokinetics of phenobarbital in the cat following multiple oral administration. Can J Vet Res 54:309–312.

Dayrell-Hart, B., Steinberg, S. A., Van Winkle, T. J. , Farnbach, G. C. 1991. Hepatoxicity of phenobarbital in dogs: 18 cases (1985–1989). JAVMA 199:1060–1066.

Gaskill, C. L., Burton, S. A., Gelens, H. C. J., Ihle, S. L., et al. 1999. Effects of phenobarbital treatment on serum thyroxine and thyroid-stimulated hormone concentration in epileptic dogs. JAVMA 215:489–496.

Kantrowitz, L. B., Peterson, M. E., Trepanier, L. A., Melian, C., et al. 1999. Serum total thyroxine, total triiodothyronine, free thyroxine, and thyrotropin concentrations in epileptic dogs treated with anticonvulsants. JAVMA 214:1804–1808.

Levitski, R. E., Trepanier, L. A. 2000. Effects of timing of blood collection on serum phenobarbital concentrations in dogs with epilepsy. JAVMA 217:200–204.

Lord, L. K., Podell, M. 1999. Owner perception of the care of long-term phenobarbital-treated epileptic dogs. J Small Anim Pract 40:11–15.

Maguire, P. J., Fettman, M. J., Smith, M. O., Greco, D. S., et al. 2000. Effects of diet on pharmacokinetics of phenobarbital in healthy dogs. JAVMA 217:847–852.

Müller, P. B., Taboada, J., Hosgood, G., et al. 2000. Effects of long-term phenobarbital treatment on the liver in dogs. J Vet Intern Med 14:165–171.

Müller, P. B., Wolfsheimer, K. J., Taboada, J., Hosgood, G., et al. 2000. Effects of long-term phenobarbital treatment on the thyroid and adrenal axis and adrenal function tests in dogs. J Vet Intern Med 14:157–164.

Podell, M., Hadjiconstantinou, M. 1999. Low concentration of cerebrospinal fluid GABA correlate to a reduced response to phenobarbital therapy in primary canine epilepsy. J Vet Intern Med 13:89–94.

Schwartz-Porsche, D., Loscher, W., Frey, H. H. 1985. Therapeutic efficacy of phenobarbital and primidone in canine epilepsy: A comparison. J Vet Pharmacol Therap 8:113–119.

Potassium Bromide

Boothe, D. M., George, K., Couch, P., et al. 2002. Disposition and clinical use of bromide in cats. JAVMA 221:1131–1135.

Gaskill, C. L., Cribb, A. E. 2000. Pancreatitis associated with potassium bromide/phenobarbital combination therapy in epileptic dogs. Can Vet J 41:555–558.

Nichols, E. S. Trepanier, L. A., Linn, K. 1996. Bromide toxicosis secondary to renal insufficiency in an epileptic dog. J Am Vet Med Assoc 208:231–233.

Podell, M., Fenner, W. R. 1994. Use of bromide as an antiepileptic drug in dogs. Compend Cont Ed Pract Vet 16:767–774.

———. 1993. Bromide therapy in refractory canine idiopathic epilepsy. J Vet Intern Med 7:318–327.

Trepanier, L. A. 1993. Pharmokinetics and clinical use of bromide. Proc 11th ACVIM Forum 878–880.

Trepanier, L. A., Schoick, A., Schwark, W. S., et al. 1998. Therapeutic serum drug concentrations in epileptic dogs treated with potassium bromide alone or in combination with other anticonvulsants: 122 cases (1992–1996). JAVMA 213:1449–1453.

Yohn, S. E., Morrison, W. B., Sharp, P. E. 1992. Bromide toxicosis (bromism) in a dog treated with potassium bromide for refractory seizures. JAVMA 201:468–470.

Diazepam

Center, S. A., Elston, T. H., Rowland, P. H., et al. 1996. Fulminant hepatic failure associated with oral administration of diazepam in 11 cats. JAVMA 209:618–625.

Hughes, D., Moreau, R. E., Overall, K. L., et al. 1996. Acute hepatic necrosis and liver failure associated with benzodiazepine therapy in six cats, 1986–1995. J Vet Emerg Crit Care 6;1: 13–20.

Papich, M. G., Alcorn, J. 1995. Absorption of diazepam after its rectal administration in dogs. Am J Vet Res 56:1629–1636.

Primidone

Bunch, S. E., Cascleman, W. L., Baldwin, B. H., et al. 1985. Effects of long-term primidone and phenytoin administration on canine hepatic function and morphology. Am J Vet Res 46:105–115.

Clorazepate

Brown, S. A., Forrester, S. D. 1991. Serum disposition of oral clorazepate from regular-release and sustained-delivery tablets in dogs. J Vet Pharmacol Theurap 14:126–129.

Forrester, S. D., Wilcke, J. R., Jacobson, J. D., Dyer, K. R. 1993. Effects of a 44-day administration of phenobarbital on disposition of clorazepate in dogs. Am J Vet Res 54:1136–1138.

Scherkl, R., Kurudi, D., Frey, H. H. 1989. Clorazepate in dogs: Tolerance to the anticonvulsant effect and signs of physical dependence. Epilepsy Res 3:144–450.

Vigabatrin

Speciale, J., Dayrell-Hart, B., Steinberg, S. A. 1991. Clinical evaluation of gamma-vinyl-gamma-aminobutyric acid for control of seizures in dogs. JAVMA 198:995–1000.

Felbamate

Adusumalli, Y. E., Gilchrist, J. R., Wichmann, J. K., et al. 1992. Pharmacokinetics of felbamate in pediatric and adult beagle dogs. Epilepsia 33:955–960.

Adusumalli, Y. E., Yang, J. T., Wong, K. K., et al. 1991. Felbamate pharmacokinetics in the rat, rabbit, and dog. Drug Met Disp 19:1116–1125.

Dayrell-Hart, B., Tiches, D., Vite, C., et al. 1996. Efficacy and safety of felbamate as an anticonvulsant in dogs with refractory seizures. Proc 14th ACVIM Forum, 756.

Podell, M. 1997. Proc 15th ACVIM Forum, Lake Buena Vista, FL.

Ruehlmann, D., Podell, M., March, P. 2001. Treatment of partial seizures and seizure-like activity with felbamate in six dogs. J Small Anim Pract 42:403–408.

Gabapentin

Podell, M. 2001. Strategies of antiepileptic drug therapy. In Proc. 19th ACVIM Forum, Denver, CO, 430–432.

Radulovic, L. L., Turck, D., von Hodenberg. A, et al. 1995. Disposition of gabapentin (neurontin) in mice, rats, dogs, and monkeys. Drug Metab Disposition 23:441–448.

Vollmer, K. G., von Hodenberg, A., Kolle, E. U. 1986. Pharmacokinetics and metabolism of gabapentin in rat, dog and man. Drug Res 36:830–839.

Zonisamide

Matsumoto, K., Miyazaki, H., Fujii, T., et al. 1983. Absorption, distribution and excretion of 3-(sulfamoyl [^{14}C] methyl)-1,2, benzisoxasole (AD-810) in rats, dogs and monkeys and of AD-810 in men. Drug Res 33:961–968.

Perucca, E. 2000. Is there a role for therapeutic drug monitoring of new anticonvulsants? Clin Pharmacokinet 38;3: 191–204.

Podell, M. 2001. Strategies of antiepileptic drug therapy. In Proc 19th ACVIM Forum, Denver, CO, 430–432.

Walker, R. M., DiFonzo, C. J., Barsoum, N. J., et al. 1988. Chronic toxicity of the anticonvulsant zonisamide in Beagle dogs. Fundamnt Appl Toxicology 11:333–342.

Levetiracetam

Harden, C. 2001. Safety profile of levetiracetam. Epilepsia 42 (Suppl 4):36–39.

Hovinga, C. A. 2001. Levetiracetam: a novel antiepileptic drug. Pharmacotherapy 21;11: 1375–1388.

Krakow, K., Walker, M., Otoul, C., et al. 2001. Long-term continuation of levetiracetam in patients with refractory epilepsy. Neurology 56:1772–1774.

Leppik, I. E. 2001. The place of levetiracetam in the treatment of epilepsy. Epilepsia 42 (Suppl 4): 44–45.

Podell, M. 2001. Strategies of antiepileptic drug therapy. Proc 19th ACVIM Forum, Denver, CO, 430–432.

Shorvon, S. D., van Rijckevorsel, K. 2002 A new antiepileptic drug: Levetiracetam, a pyrrolidone recently licensed as an epileptic drug (Editorial). J Neurol Neurosurg Psychiatry 72: 426–428.

Status Epilepticus

Bateman, S. W., Parent, J. M. 1999. Clinical findings, treatment, and outcome of dogs with status epilepticus or cluster seizures: 156 cases (1990–1995). JAVMA 215:1463–1468.

Dewey, C. W., Ducote, J. M., Coates, J. R., et al. 1999. Intrarectally administered potassium bromide loading in normal dogs. J Vet Intern Med 13:238.

Lowenstein, D. H., Alldredge, B. K. 1998. Status epilepticus. N Engl J Med 338:970–976.

Platt, S. R., McDonnell, J. J. 2000a. Status epilepticus: clinical features and pathophysiology. Compend Cont Ed Pract Vet 22;7:660–669.

———. 2000b. Status epilepticus: managing refractory cases and treating out-of-hospital patients. Compend Cont Ed Pract Vet 22:732–741.

———. 2000c. Status epilepticus: patient management and pharmacologic therapy. Compend Cont Ed Pract Vet 22:722–729.

Podell, M. 1996. Seizures in dogs. Vet Clin N Amer (Sm Anim Pract) 26:779–809.

———. 1995. The use of diazepam per rectum at home for the acute management of cluster seizures in dogs. J Vet Intern Med 9:68–74.

Saito, M., Munana, K. R., Sharp, N. J., et al. 2001. Risk factors for development of status epilepticus in dogs with idiopathic epilepsy and effects of status epilepticus on outcome and survival time: 32 cases (1990–1996). JAVMA 219:618–623.

Steffen, F., Grasmueck, S. 2000. Propofol for treatment of refractory seizures in dogs and a cat with intracranial disorders. J Sm Anim Pract 41:496–499.

Trauma

Braakman, R., Schouten, H. J., Blaauw-van, D. M., Minderhoud, J. M. 1983. Megadose steroids in severe head injury. Results of a prospective double-blind clinical trial. J Neurosurg 58:326–330.

Cooper, P. R., Moody, S., Clark, W. K., et al. 1979. Dexamethasone and severe head injury. A prospective double-blind study. J. Neurosurg. 51:307–316.

Dearden, N. M., Gibson, J. S., McDowall, D. G., Gibson, R. M., Cameron, M. M. 1986. Effect of high-dose dexamethasone on outcome from severe head injury. J. Neurosurg. 64:81–88.

Dewey, C. W. 2000. Emergency management of the head trauma patient: principles and practice. In The Veterinary Clinics of North America: Small Animal Practice, Vassallo, J., ed. Philadelphia, W. B. Saunders, 207–225.

Dewey, C. W., Budsberg, S. C., Oliver, J. E., Jr. 1992. Principles of head trauma management in dogs and cats-part 1. Compend Contin Educ Pract Vet 14:199–206.

Finnie, J. W., Blumbergs, P. C. 2002. Traumatic brain injury. Vet Pathol 39:679–689.

Giannotta, S. L., Weiss, M. H., Apuzzo, M. L., Martin, E. 1984. High dose glucocorticoids in the management of severe head injury. Neurosurgery 15:497–501.

Gudeman, S. K., Miller, J. D., Becker, D. P. 1979. Failure of high-dose steroid therapy to influence intracranial pressure in patients with severe head injury. J Neurosurg 51:301–306.

Hopkins, A. L. 1996. Head Trauma. Vet Clinic North Am 26:875–891.

Procaccio, F., Stocchetti, N., Citero, G., et al. 2000. Guidelines for the treatment of adults with severe head trauma (part II). Criteria for medical treatment. J Neurosurg Sci 44:11–18.

Proulx, J., Dhupa, N. D. 1998. Severe brain injury. Part I. Pathophysiology. Compend Contin Educ Pract Vet 20: 897–905.

———. 1998. Severe brain injury. Part II. Therapy. Compend Contin Educ Pract Vet 20:993–1005.

Saul, T. G., Ducker, T. B., Salcman, M., Carro, E. 1981. Steroids in severe head injury: a prospective randomized clinical trial. J. Neurosurg 54:596–600.

Shores, A. 1989. Craniocerebral trauma. In Current veterinary therapy X, Kirk, R. W., ed. Philadelphia, W. B. Saunders, 847–853.

Syring, R. S., Otto, C. M., Drobatz, K. J. 2001. Hyperglycemia in dogs and cats with head trauma: 122 cases (1997–1999). JAVMA 218:1124–1129.

Toxicity

Dorman, D. C. 1993. Diagnosis and therapy of neurotoxicological syndromes in dogs and cats: selected syndromes induced by pesticides, part 2. Prog Vet Neurol 14:111–120.

———. 2003. Neurotoxicological syndromes. In A Practical Guide to Canine and Feline Neurology, Dewey, C. W., ed. Ames, Iowa State Press, 559–596.

Dorman, D. C., Fikes, J. D. 1993. Diagnosis and therapy of neurotoxicological syndromes in dogs and cats: general concepts, part 1. Prog Vet Neurol 4:95–103.

Edds, G. T., Simpson, C. F. 1974. Hexachlorophene-pHisoHex toxicity in pups. Am J Vet Res 35:1005–1007.

Hadrick, M. K., Bunch, S. E., Kornegay, J. N. 1995. Ivermectin toxicosis in two Australian shepherds. JAVMA 206:1147–1150.

Hanig, J. P., Krop, S., Morrison, Colson, S. H. 1976. Observations on hexachlorophene-induced paralysis in the cat and its antagonism by hypertonic urea (39352). Proc Soc Exp Biol Med 152:165–169.

Hopkins, K. D., Marcella, K. L., Strecker, A. E. 1990. Ivermectin toxicosis in a dog. JAVMA 197:93–94.

Houston, D. M., Parent, J., Matushek, K. J. 1987. Ivermectin toxicosis in a dog. JAVMA 191:78–80.

Levy, J. K. 1991. Ataxia in a kitten treated with griseofulvin. JAVMA 198:105–106.

Lewis, D. T., Merchant, S. R., Neer, T. M. 1994. Ivermectin toxicosis in a kitten. JAVMA 205:584–586.

Osweiler, G. D. 1983. Strychnine poisoning. In Current veterinary therapy, XIII, Kirk, R. W., ed. Philadelphia, W. B. Saunders, 98–100.

Saxon, B., Magne, M. L. 1993. Reversible central nervous system toxicosis associated with metronidazole therapy in three cats. Prog Vet Neurol 4:25–27.

Smith, R. A., Stronski, E. J., Beck, B. E., Wolper, G. G. 1990. Death of a rough collie exposed to an ivermectin-based paste. Can Vet J 31:221.

Thompson, J. P., Senior, D. F., Pinson, D. M., Moriello, K. A. 1987. Neurotoxicosis associated with the use of hexachlorophene in a cat. JAVMA 190:1311–1312.

Ward, B. C., Jones, B. D., Rubin, G. J. 1973. Hexachlorophene toxicity in dogs. J Am Anim Hosp Assoc 9:167–169.

Lead Poisoning

Clarke, E. G. C. 1973. Lead poisoning in small animals. J Sm An Prac 14:183–193.

Hamir, A. N., Sullivan, N. D., Handson, P. D., Barr, S. 1986. A comparison of calcium disodium ethylene diarnine tetra-acetate (CaEDTA) by oral and subcutaneous routes as a treatment of lead poisoning in dogs. J Sm An Prac 27:39–43.

Knecht, C. D., Crabtree, J., Katherman, A. 1979. Clinical, clinicopathologic, and electroencephalographic features of lead poisoning in dogs. JAVMA 175:196–201.

Kowalczyk, D. F. 1983. Lead poisoning. In Current veterinary therapy, VIII, Kirk, R. W., ed. Philadelphia, W. B. Saunders, 107–112.

Maddison, I. E., Allan, G. S. 1990. Megaesophagus attributable to lead toxicosis in a cat. JAVMA 197:1357–1358.

Morgan, R. V., Moore, F. M., Pearce, L. K., Rossi, T. 1991. Clinical and laboratory findings in small companion animals with lead poisoning: 347 cases (1977–1986). JAVMA 199:93–97.

Steiss, I. E., Braund, K. G., Clark, E. G. 1985. Inability to experimentally produce a polyneuropathy in dogs given chronic oral low level lead. Can J Comp Med 49:401–404.

Zook, B. C., Carpenter, J. L., Roberts, R. M. 1972. Lead poisoning in dogs: occurrence source clinical pathology and electroencephalography. Am J Vet Res 33:891–902.

Cerebrovascular Disease

Applewhite, A. A., Wilkens, B. E, McDonald, D. E., Radasche, R. M., Barstad, R. D. 1999. Potential central nervous system complications of Von Willebrand's disease. J Am Anim Hosp Assoc 35:423–429.

Bagley, R. S., Anderson, W. I., deLahunta, A., Kallfelz, F. A., Bowersox, T. S. 1988. Cerebellar infarction caused by arterial thrombosis in a dog. JAVMA 192:785–787.

Cordy, D. R. 1979. Vascular malformations and hemangiomas of the canine spinal cord. Vet Pathol 16:275–282.

Dukes, J. 1992. Hypertension: a review of the mechanisms, manifestations and management. J Sm Anim Pract 33:119–129.

Dunn, K. J., Nicholls, P. K., Dunn, J. K., Herrtage, M. E. 1995. Intracranial haemorrhage in a Doberman puppy with von Willebrand's disease. Vet Rec 136:635–636.

Fankhauser, R., Luginbuhl, H., McGrath, J. T. 1965. Cerebrovascular disease in various animal species. Ann NY Acad Sci 127:817–860.

Hopkins, A. L., Wheeler, S. J. 1991. Subdural hematoma in a dog. Vet Surg 20:413.

Joseph, R. J., Greenlee, P. G., Carrillo, J. M., et al. 1988. Canine cerebrovascular disease: clinical and pathological findings in 17 cases. J Am Anim Hosp Assoc 24:569–576.

Kipar, A., Hetzel, U., Armien, A. G., Baumgärtner, W. 2001. Bilateral focal cerebral angiomatosis associated with nervous signs in a cat. Vet Pathol 38:350–353

Kotani, T., Tomimura, T., Ogura, M., Yoshida, H., et al. 1975. Cerebral infarction caused by *Dirofilaria immitis* in three dogs. Jpn J Vet Sci 37:379–390.

Littman, M. P. 2000. Hypertension. In Textbook of Veterinary Internal Medicine, 2d ed., Ettinger, S. J., Feldman, E. C., eds. Philadelphia, W. B. Saunders, 179–182.

Liu, S. K., Tilley, L. P., Tappe, J. P., et al. 1986. Clinical and pathologic findings in dogs with atherosclerosis: 21 cases (1970–1983). JAVMA 189:227–232.

Norton, F. 1992. Cerebral infarction in a dog. Prog Vet Neurol 3:120–125.

Patterson, S., Rusley, M. S., Zachary, J. F. 1985. Neurologic manifestations of cerebrovascular atherosclerosis associated with primary hypothyroidism in a dog. JAVMA 186:499–503.

Patton, C. S., Garner, F. M. 1970. Cerebral infarction caused by heartworms (Dirofilaria immitis) in a dog. JAVMA 156:600–605.

Platt, S. R., Garosi, L. 2003. Canine cerebrovascular disease: do dogs have strokes. J Am Anim Hosp Assoc 39:337–342.

Smith, S. H., Van Winkle, T. 2001. Cerebral vascular hamartomas in five dogs. 38:108–112.

Snyder, P. W., Cooke, K. L. Management of hypertension. In Textbook of Veterinary Internal Medicine, 6th ed., Ettinger, S. J., Feldman, E. C., eds. St. Louis, Elsevier, 477–79.

Stoffregen, D. A., Kallfelz, F. A., deLahunta, A. 1985. Cerebral hemorrhage in an old dog, J Am Anim Hosp Assoc 21:495–498.

Swanson, J. F., Morgan, S., Green, R. A., Woody, B. J. 1986. Cerebral thrombosis and hemorrhage in association with L-asparaginase administration, J Am Anim Hosp Assoc 22:749–755.

Swayne, D. E., Tyler, D. E., Batker, J. 1988. Cerebral infarction with associated venous thrombosis in a dog, Vet Pathol25:317–320.

Thomas, W. B. 1996. Cerebrovascular disease. Vet Clin N Am (Small Anim Fract) 26:925–943

———. 2001. Vascular disorders. In Consultations in Feline Internal Medicine, August, J. R., ed., 4th ed. Philadelphia, W. B. Saunders, 405–412.

Tidwell, A. S., Mahony, O. M., Moore, R. P., et al. 1994. Computed tomography of an acute hemorrhagic cerebral infarct in a dog. Vet Rad Ultrasound 35:290–296

Zaki, F. A. 1979. Vascular malformation (cavernous angioma) of the spinal cord in a dog. J Sm Anim Pract 20:417–422.

Zeiss, C. L., Waddle, G. 1995. Hypothyroidism and atherosclerosis in dogs. Compend Contin Educ Pract Vet 17:1117–1129.

Feline Ischemic Encephalopathy

Bernstein, N. M., Fiske, R. A. 1986. Feline ischemic encephalopathy in a cat. J Am Anim Hosp Assoc 22:205–206.

deLahunta, A. 1976. Feline neurology. Vet Clin North Am 6:433–452.

King, J. M. 1991. Feline ischemic encephalopathy. Vet Med 86:1062.

Williams, K. J., Summers, B. A., deLahunta, A. 1998. Cerebrospinal cuterebriasis in cats and its association with feline ischemic encephalopathy. Vet Pathol 35:330–343.

Zaki, F. A., Nafe, L. A. 1980. Ischemic encephalopathy and focal granulomatous meningoencephalitis in the cat, J Sm Anim Pract 21:429–438.

Disorders of Blood Viscosity

Evans, L. M., Caylor, K. B. 1995. Polycythemia vera in a cat and management with hydroxyurea. JAAHA 31:434–438.

Cerebellar Disease

General Cerebellar Diseases

Braund, K. G. 1994. Clinical Syndromes in Veterinary Neurology. St. Louis, Mosby.

deLahunta, A. 1990. Abiotrophy in domestic animals: a review. Can J Vet Res 54:65–76.

———. 1980a. Comparative cerebellar disease in domestic animals. The Compendium on Continuing Education 11:8–17.

———. 1980b. Diseases of the cerebellum. Vet. Clin. North Am. Small Anim. Pract. 10:91–101.

Holliday, T. A. 1979/1980 Clinical signs of acute and chronic experimental lesions of the cerebellum. Veterinary Science Communications 1979; 3:259–278.

Kornegay, J. N. 1991. Ataxia, dysmetria, tremor. Cerebellar diseases. Probl. Vet. Med. 3:409–416.

Oliver, J. E., Lorenz, M. D., Kornegay, J. N. 1997. Handbook of Veterinary Neurology. Philadelphia, W. B. Saunders.

Parker, A. J. 1981. Differential diagnosis of brain disease. Part 3. Hypermetria and tremors. Mod Vet Pract 62:919–924.

Sanders, S., Bagley, R. S. 2003. Cerebellar diseases and tremor syndromes. In A Practical Guide to Canine and Feline Neurology, Dewey, C. W., ed. Ames, Iowa State Press, 241–276.

Summers, B. A., Cummings, J. F., deLahunta, A. 1995. Veterinary Neuropathology. St. Louis, Mosby.

Cerebellar Degeneration

Bildfell, R. J., Mitchell, S. K. 1995. Cerebellar cortical degeneration in a Labrador retriever. Can Vet J 36:570–572.

Carmichael, S., Griffiths, I. R., Harvey, M. J. A. 1983. Familial cerebellar ataxia with hydrocephalus in bull mastiffs. Vet Rec 112:354–358.

Chieffo, C., Stalis, I. H., Van Winkle, T. J., et al. 1994. Cerebellar purkinje's cell degeneration and coat color dilution in a family of Rhodesian Ridgeback dogs. J Vet Intern Med 8:112–116.

Coates, J. R., O'Brien, D. P., Kline, K. L., et al. 2002. Neonatal cerebellar ataxia in Coton de Tulear dogs. J Vet Intern Med 16:680–689.

Cordy, D. R., Snelbaker, H. A. 1952. Cerebellar hypoplasia and degeneration in a family of Airdale dogs. J Neuropathol Exp Neurol 11:324–328.

Cummings, J. F., deLahunta, A. 1988. A study of cerebellar and cerebral cortical degeneration in miniature poodle pups with emphasis on the ultrastructure of Purkinje cell changes. Acta Neuropathol 75:261–271.

deLahunta, A. 1990. Abiotrophy in domestic animals: a review. Can J Vet Res 54:65–76.

deLahunta, A., Averill, D. R. 1976. Hereditary cerebellar cortical and extrapyramidal nuclear abiotrophy in Kerry blue terriers JAVMA 168:1119–1124.

deLahunta, A., Fenner, W. R., Indrieri, R. J., et al. 1980. Hereditary cerebellar cortical abiotrophy in the Gordon setter dog. JAVMA 177:538–541.

Franklin, R. J. M., Ramsey, I. K., McKerrell, R. E. 1997. An inherited neurological disorder of the St. Bernard dog characterized by unusual cerebellar cortical dysplasia. Vet Rec 140:656–657.

Gill, J. M., Hewland, M. L. 1980. Cerebellar degeneration in the border collie. NZ Vet J 28:170.

Hartley, W. J., Barker, J. S. F., Wanner, R. A., Farrow, B. R. 1978. Inherited cerebellar degeneration in the rough coated collie. Veterinary Practitioner 8:79–85.

Hartley, W. J., Palmer, A. C. 1973. Ataxia in Jack Russell terriers. Acta Neuropathol (Berl) 26:71–74.

Inada, S., Mochizuki, M., Izumo, S., Kuriyama, M., et al. 1996. Study of hereditary cerebellar degeneration in cats. Am J Vet Res 57:296–301.

Kent, M., Glass, E., deLahunta, A. 2000. Cerebellar cortical abiotrophy in a beagle. J Sm Anim Pract 41:321–323.

Montgomery, D. L., Storts, R. W. 1983a. Herditary striatonigral and cerebelloolivary degeneration of the Kerry Blue terrier: I, gross and light microscopic central nervous system lesions. Vet Pathol 20:143–159.

———. 1983b. Herditary striatonigral and cerebelloolivary degeneration of the Kerry Blue terrier: II, ultrastructural lesions in the caudate nucleus and cerebellar cortex, J Neuropathol Exp Neurol 43:263–275.

Nesbit, J. W., Ueckerman, J. F. 1981. Cerebellar cortical atrophy in a puppy. J S Afr Vet Assoc 52:247–250.

Perille, A. L., Baer, K., Joseph, R. J., Carrillo, J. M. 1991. Postnatal cerebellar cortical degeneration in Labrador retriever puppies. Can Vet J 32:619–621.

Sandy, J. R., Solocombe, R. F., Mitten, R. W., Jedwab, D. 2002. Cerebellar abiotrophy in a family of Border collie dogs. Vet Pathol 39:736–738.

Shamir, M., Perl, S., Sharon, L. 1999. Late onset of cerebellar abiotrophy in a Siamese cat. J Sm Anim Pract 40:343–345.

Steinberg, H. S., Troncoso, J. C., Cork, L. C., Price, D. L. 1981. Clinical features of inherited cerebellar degeneration in Gordon Setters. JAVMA 179:886–890.

Steinberg, H. S., Van Winkle, T., Bell, J. S., et al. 2000. Cerebellar degeneration in Old English sheepdogs. JAVMA 217:1162–1165.

Thomas, J. B., Robertson, D. 1989. Hereditary cerebellar abiotrophy in Australian kelpie dogs. Aust Vet J 66:301–302.

Troncoso, J. C., Cork, L. C., Price, D. L. 1985. Canine inherited ataxia: ultrastructural observations. J Neuropathol Exp Neurol 44:165–175.

Taniyama, H., Takayanagi, S., Izumisawa, Y., et al. 1994. Cerebellar cortical atrophy in a kitten. Vet Pathol 31:710–713.

Van der Merwe, L. L., Lane, E. 2001. Diagnosis of cerebellar cortical degeneration in a Scottish terrier using magnetic resonance imaging. J Sm Anim Pract 42:409–412.

Yasuba, M., Okimoto, K., Iida, M., Itakura, C. 1988. Cerebellar cortical degeneration in beagle dogs. Vet Pathol 25:315–317.

Adult-onset Cerebellar Degneration

Barone, G., Foureman, P., deLahunta, A. 2002. Adult-onset cerebellar corical abiotrophy and retinal degeneration in a domestic shorthair cat. J An Amin Hosp Assoc 38:51–54.

Chrisman, C. L., Spencer, C. P., Crane, S. W., Mayhew, I. G., et al. 1983. Late-onset cerebellar degeneration in a dog. JAVMA 182:717–720.

Higgins, R. J., LeCouteur, R. A., Kornegay, J. N., et al. 1989. Late-onset progressive spinocerebellar degeneration in Brittany Spaniel dogs. Acta Neuropathol 96:97–101.

Shamir, M., Perl, S., Sharon, L. 1999. Late onset cerebellar abiotrophy in a Siamese cat. J Sm Anim Pract 40:343–345.

Tatalick, L. M., Marks, S. L., Baszler, T. V. 1993. Cerebellar abiotrophy characterized by granular cell loss in a Brittany. Vet Pathol 30:385–388.

Cerebellar Hypoplasia

Csiza, C. K. de la, Scott, F. W., Gillespie, J. H. 1972. Spontaneous feline ataxia. Cornell Vet 62:300–322.

Johnson, R. H., Margolis, G., Kilham, L. 1967. Identity of feline ataxia virus on the feline panleukopenia virus. Nature 214:175–177.

Kahn, D. E. 1978. Pathogenesis of feline panleukopenia. JAVMA 173:628–630.

Kay, W. J., Budzelovich, G. N. 1970. Cerebellar hypoplasia and agenesis in the dog. J Neuropathol Exp Neurol 29:156.

Kilham, L., Margolis, G., Colby, E. D. 1971. Cerebellar ataxia and its congenital transmission in cats by feline panleukopenia virus. JAVMA 158:Suppl 2:888+.

Kilham, L., Margolis, G., Colby, E. D. 1967. Congenital infections of cats and ferrets by feline panleukopenia virus manifested by cerebellar hypoplasia. Lab Invest 17:465–480.

Knecht, C. D., Lamar, C. H., Schaible, R, et al. 1979. Cerebellar hypoplasia in Chow Chows. J Am Anim Hosp Assoc 15:51–53.

Kornegay, J. N. 1986. Cerebellar vermian hypoplasia in dogs. Vet Pathol 23:374–379.

Kronevi, T., Ostensson, K., Lesser, J. 1978. A case of partial cerebellar hypoplasia in a cat. Nord Vet Med 30:221–222.

Hypomyelination and Dysmyelination

Comont, P. S. V., Palmer, A. C., Williams, A. E. 1988. Weakness associated with spinal subpial myelopathy in a weimaraner puppy. J Sm Anim Pract 29:367–372.

Cummings, J. F., Summers, B. A., deLahunta, A., Lawson, C., et al. 1986. Tremors in Samoyed pups with oligodendrocyte deficiencies and hypomyelination. Acta Neuropathol 71:267–277.

Duncan, I. D., Hammang, J. P., Jackson, K. F. 1987. Myelin mosaicism in female heterozygotes of the canine shaking pup and myelin-deficient rat mutants. Brain Res 402:168–172.

Greene, C. E., Vandevelde, M., Hoff, E. J. 1977. Congenital cerebrospinal hypomyelinogenesis in a pup. JAVMA 171:534–536.

Griffiths, I. R., Duncan, I. D., McCulloch, M., Harvey, M. J. A. 1981. Shaking pups: a disorder of central myelination in the spaniel dog. Part 1: clinical genetic and light microscopical observations. J Neurol Sci 50:423–433.

Kornegay, J. N., Goodwin, M. A., Spyridakis, L. K. 1987. Hypomyelination in weimaraner dogs. Acta Neuropathol 72:394–401.

Mayhew, I. G., Blakemore, W. F., Palmer, A. C., Clarke, C. J. 1984. Tremor syndrome and hypomyelination in lurcher pups. J Sm Anim Pract 25:551–559.

Nadon, N. L., Duncan, I. D., Hudson, L. D. 1990. A point mutation in the proteolipid protein gene of the "shaking pup" interrupts oligodendrocyte development. Development 110:529–537.

Palmer, A. C., Blakemore, W. F., Wallace, M. E., Wilkes, M. K., et al. 1987. Recognition of "trembler," a hypomyelinating condition in the Bernese mountain dog. Vet Rec 120:609–612.

Stoffregen, D. A., Huxtable, C. R., Cummings, J. F., deLahunta, A. 1993. Hypomyelination of the central nervous system of two Siamese kitten littermates. Vet Path 30:388–391.

Vandevelde, M., Braund, K. G., Luttgen, P. J., Higgins, R. J. 1981. Dysmyelination in chow chow dogs: further studies in older dogs. Acta Neuropathol 55:81–87.

Vandevelde, M., Braund, K. G., Walker, T. L., Kornegay, J. N. 1978. Dysmyelination of the central nervous system in the chow-chow dog. Acta Neuropathol 42:211–215.

Leukoencephalopathy

Chrisman, C. L. 1986. Neuroaxonal dystrophy and Leukoencephalomyelopathy of Rottweiler dogs. In Current Veterinary Therapy, 9th ed., Kirk, R. W., ed. Philadephia, W. B. Saunders, 805–806.

Duncan, I. D. 1987. Abnormalities of myelination of the central nervous system associated with congenital tremor. J Vet Intern Med 1:10–23.

Gamble, D. A., Chrisman, C. L. 1984. A leukoencephalomyelopathy of Rottweiler dogs. Vet Pathol 21:174–180.

Lewis, D. G., Newsholme, S. I. 1987. Pseudo cervical spondylopathy in the Rottweiler. J Sm Anim Pract 28:1178.

Moreau, P. M., Hugon, J., Vallat, J. M. 1989. Leucoencephalomyeloneuropathy in a litter of Birman cats. Proc Eur Soc Vet Neurol 3:75–80.

Moreau, P. M., Vallat, J. M., Hugon, J. 1991. Peripheral and central distal axonopathy of suspected inherited origin in Birman cats. Acta Neuropathol (Berl) 82:143–146.

Slocombe, R. F., Mitten, R., Mason, T. A. 1989. Leucoencephalomyelopathy in Australian Rottweiler dogs. Aust Vet J 66: 147–150.

Wouda, W., van Nes, L. L. 1986. Progressive ataxia due to central demyelination in Rottweiler dogs. Vet Q 8:89–97.

Neuroaxonal Dystrophy

Blakemore, W. F., Palmer, A. C. 1985. Nervous system disease in the Chihuahua characterised by axonal seliings. Vet Rec 117: 498–499.

Carmichael, K. P., Howerth, E. W., Oliver, J. E. J., Klappenbach, K. 1993. Neuroaxonal dystrophy in a group of related cats. J Vet Diagn Invest 5:585–590.

Chrisman, C. L. 1986. Neuroaxonal dystrophy and Leukoencephalomyelopathy of Rottweiler dogs. In Current Veterinary Therapy, 9th ed., Kirk, R. W., ed. Philadephia, W. B. Saunders, 805–806.

Chrisman, C. L., Cork, L. C., Gamble, D. A. 1984. Neuroaxonal dystrophy of Rottweiler dogs. JAVMA 184:464–467.

Clark, R. G., Hartley, W. J., Burgess, G. S., et a1. 1982. Suspected neuroaxonal dystrophy in collie sheep dogs. NZ Vet J 30: 102–103.

Cork, L. C., Troncoso, J. C., Price, D. L. 1981. Canine inherited ataxia. Ann Neurol 9:492–499.

Cork, L. C., Troncoso, J. C., Price, D. L., Stanley, E. F., Griffin, J. W. 1983. Canine neuroaxonal dystrophy. J Neuropathol Exp Neurol 42:286–296.

Evans, M. G., Mullaney, T. P., Lowrie, C. T. 1988. Neuroaxonal dystrophy in a Rottweiler pup. JAVMA 192:1560–1562.

Franklin, R. J., Jeffery, N. D., Ramsey, I. K. 1995. Neuroaxonal dystrophy in a litter of papillon pups. J Sm Anim Pract 36:441–444.

Rodriguez, F., Espinosa de los Monteros, M. M., Herraez, P., Jaber, J. R., Fernandez, A. 1996. Neuroaxonal dystrophy in two Siamese kitten littermates. Vet Rec 138:548–549.

Sacre, B. J., Cummings, J. F., deLahunta, A. 1993. Neuroaxonal dystrophy in a Jack Russell terrier pup resembling human infantile neuroaxonal dystrophy. Cornell Vet 83:133–142.

Walkley, S. U., Baker, H. J., Rattazzi, M. C., Haskins, M. E., Wu, J. Y. 1991. Neuroaxonal dystrophy in neuronal storage disorders: evidence for major GABAergic neuron involvement. J Neurol Sci 104:1–8.

Woodard, J. C., Collins, G. H., Hessler, J. R. 1974. Feline hereditary neuroaxonal dystrophy. Am J Pathol 74:551–566.

Anomalous

Hart, M. N, Malamud, N., Ellis, W. G. 1972. The Dandy-Walker syndrome. A clinicopathological study based on 28 cases. Neurology 22:771–780.

Regnier, A. M., Delisle, M. B. 1993. Dandy-Walker syndrome in a kitten. J Am Anim Hosp Assoc 29:514–518.

Schmid, V. S., Lang, J. L., Wolf, M. 1992. Dandy-walker-like syndrome in four dogs: cisternography as a diagnostic aid. J Am Anim Hosp Assoc 28:355–360.

Cerebellar Neoplasia

Bagley, R. S., Silver, G. M., Gavin, P. R. 2000. Cerebellar cystic meningioma in a dog. J Am Anim Hosp Assoc 36:413–415.

Steinberg, H., Galbreath, E. J. 1998. Cerebellar medulloblastoma with multiple differentiation in a dog. Vet Pathol 5:543–546.

Inflammatory Cerebellar Conditions

Gearhart, M. A., deLahunta, A., Summers, B. A. 1986. Cerebellar mass in a dog due to granulomatous meningoencephalitis. J Am Anim Hosp Assoc 22:683–686.

Lorenzo, V, Pumarola, A, Sisö, S. 2002. Neosporosis with cerebellar involvement in an adult dog. J Sm Anim Pract 43:76–79.

Palmer, A. C., Cavanagh, J. B. 1995. Encephalomyelopathy in young cats. J Sm Anim Pract 36:57–64.

Sorjonen, D. C. 1990. Clinical and histopathological features of granulomatous meningoencephalomyelitis. J Am Anim Hosp Assoc 26:141–147.

Thomas, W. B., Sorjonen, D. C., Steiss, J. E. 1993. A retrospective evaluation of 38 cases of canine distemper encephalomyelitis. J Am Anim Hosp Assoc 29:129–133.

Wyatt, J. M., Pearson, G. R., Smerdon, T. N., et al. 1991. Naturally occurring scrapie-like spongiform encephalopathy in five domestic cats. Vet Rec 129:233–236.

Vascular

Bagley, R. S., Anderson, W. I. de la, Kallfelz, F. A., Bowersox, T. S. 1988. Cerebellar infarction caused by arterial thrombosis in a dog. JAVMA 192:785–787.

Berg, J. M., Joseph, R. J. 2003. Cerebellar infarcts in two dogs diagnosed with magnetic resonance imaging. J Am Anim Hosp Assoc 39:203–207.

Cranial Nerve Disorders

Anosmia

Myers, L. J., Hanrahan, L. A., Swango, L. J., Nusbaum, K. E. 1988. Anosmia associated with canine distemper. Am J Vet Res 49:1295–1297.

Nerves of the Eyes

Antonini, A., Berlucchi, G., Marzi, C. A., Sprague, J. M. 1979. Behavorial and electrophysiological effects of unilateral optic tract section in ordinary and siamese cats. J Comp Neur 185:183–202.

Boydell, P. 2000. Iatrogenic pupillary dilation resembling Pourfour du Petit syndrome in three cats. J Sm An Prac 41:202–203.

———. 1995a. Horner's syndrome following cervical spinal surgery in the dog. J Sm Anim Pract 36:510–512.

———. 1995b. Idiopathic Horner's syndrome in the golden retriever. J Sm Anim Pract 36:382–384.

Boydell, P., Brogan, N. 2000. Horner's syndrome associated with Neospora infection. J Sm Anim Pract 41:571–572.

Dugan, S. J., Schwarz, P. D., Roberts, S. M., Ching, S. V. 1993. Primary optic nerve meningioma and pulmonary metastasis in a dog. J Am Anim Hosp Assoc 29:11–16.

Goldfarb, S., Swann, P. G. 1984. Case report—Idiopathic tonic pupil or Adie's syndrome in a dog. Aust Vet Pract 14:20–23.

Holland, C. T. 1996. Horner's syndrome and ipsilateral hemipelgia in three cats. J Sm Anim Pract 37:442–446.

Melian, C., Morales, M., de los Monteros, A. E., Peterson, M. E. 1996. Horner's syndrome associated with a functional thyroid carcinoma in a dog. J Sm Anim Pract 37:591–593.

Scagliotti, R. H. 1990. Neuro-ophthalmology. Prog Vet Neurol 1:157–170.

Sisó, S., Lorenzo, V., Ferrer, I., Villagrassa, M., et al. 2003. An anaplastic astrocytoma (optic chiasmatic-hypothalamic glioma) in a dog. Vet Path 40:567–569

Optic Neuritis

Nafe, L. A., Carter, I. O. 1981. Canine optic neuritis. Compend Contin Educ Pract Vet 3:978–984.

Optic Nerve Hypoplasia

Barnett, K. C., Grimes, T. O. 1974. Bilateral aplasia of the optic nerve in a cat. Br J Ophthalmol 58:663–667.

Kern, T. I., Riis, R. C. 1981. Optic nerve hypoplasia in three miniature poodles. JAVMA 178:49–54.

Saunders, L. Z. 1952. Congenital optic nerve hypoplasia in collie dogs. Cornell Vet 42:67–80.

Turnquist, S. E., Pace, L. W., Sardinas, I. 1991. Unilateral optic nerve hypoplasia and hydrocephalus in a Pekingese. Cornell Vet 81:305–311.

Cavernous Sinus Syndrome

Lewis, G. T., Blanchard, G. L., Trapp, A. L., DeCamp, C. E. 1984. Ophthalmoplegia caused by thyroid adenocarcinoma invasion of the cavernous sinuses in the dog. J Am Anim Hosp Assoc 20:805–812.

Theisen, S. K., Podell, M., Schneider, T., et al. 1996. A retrospective study of cavernous sinus syndrome in 4 dogs and 8 cats. J Vet Intern Med 10:65–71.

Trigeminal Nerve Disease

Bagley, R. S., Wheeler, S. J., Klopp, L., Sorjonen, D., et al. 1998. Trigeminal nerve sheath tumor in 10 dogs. J Am Anim Hosp Assoc 34:19–25.

Carmichael, S., Griffiths, I. R. 1981. Case of isolated sensory trigeminal neuropathy in a dog. Vet Rec 109:280–282.

Carpenter, J. L., King, N. W., Jr., Abrams, K. L. 1987. Bilateral trigeminal nerve paralysis and Horner's syndrome associated with myelomonocytic neoplasia in a dog. JAVMA 191:1594–1596.

Christopher, M. M., Metz, A. L., Klausner, J., Polzin, D., et al. 1986. Acute myelomonocytic leukemia with neurological manifestations in the dog. Vet Pathol 23:140–147.

Cizinauskas, S., Lang, J., Maier, R., Fatzer, R., Jaggy, A. 2001. Paradoxical vestibular disease with trigeminal nerve-sheath tumor in a dog. Schweiz Arch Tierheilkd 143:419–425.

Pfaff. A. D., March, P. A., Fishman, C. 2000. Acute bilateral trigeminal neuropathy associated with nervous system lymphosarcoma in a dog. J Am Anim Hosp Assoc 36:57–61.

Wheeler, S. J. 1987. Sensory neuropathy in a border collie puppy. J Sm Anim Pract 28:281–289.

Trigeminal Neuritis

Carmichael, S., Griffiths, I. R. 1981. Case of isolated sensory trigeminal neuropathy in a dog. Vet Rec 109:280–282.

Chrisman, C. L., Platt, S. R., Chandra, A. M., et al. 1999. Sensory polyganglioradiculoneuritis in a dog. J Am Anim Hosp Assoc 35:232–235.

Cummings, J. F., deLahunta, A., Mitchell, W. J. L. 1983. Ganglioradiculitis in the dog. A clinical, light- and electron-microscopic study. Acta Neuropathol (Berl) 60:29–39.

deLahunta, A. 1983. Cranial nerve-Lower motor neuron: general somatic efferent system, special visceral efferent system. In Veterinary Neuroanatomy and Clinical Neurology, deLahunta A., ed., 2d ed. Philadelphia, W. B. Saunders, 95–114.

Hoelzle, R. J. 1983. Idiopathic trigeminal neuropathy in a dog. Vet Med Small Anim Clin 78:345.

Humphreys, G. U. 1974. Correspondence: dropped jaw in dogs. Vet Rec 95:222.

Mayhew, P. D., Bush, W. W., Glass, E. N. 2002. Trigeminal neuropathy in dogs: a retrospective study of 29 cases (1991–2000). J Am Anim Hosp Assoc 38:262–270.

Powell, A. K. 1991. Idiopathic trigeminal neuritis in a dog. Can Vet J 32:265.

Facial Nerve Disease

Baringer, J. R. 1996. Herpes simplex virus and Bell palsy (editorial; comment). Ann Intern Med 124:63–65.

Billue, J. S. 1997. Bell's palsy: an update on idiopathic facial paralysis. Nurse Pract 22:88, 97–105.

Jabor, M. A, Gianoli, G. 1996. Management of Bell's palsy. J La State Med Soc 148:279–283.

Jackson, C. G, von Doersten, P. G. 1999. The facial nerve. Current trends in diagnosis, treatment, and rehabilitation. Med Clin North Am 83:179–195.

James, D. G. 1997. Differential diagnosis of facial nerve palsy. Sarcoidosis Vasc Diffise Lung Dis 14:115–120.

Kern, T. J, Erb, H. N. 1987. Facial neuropathy in dogs and cats: 95 cases (1975–1985). JAVMA 191:1604–1609.

Renegar, W. R. 1979. Auriculopalpebral nerve paralysis following prolonged anesthesia in a dog. JAVMA 174:1007–1009.

Roberts, S. R., Vainisi, S. J. 1967. Hemifacial spasm in dogs. JAVMA 150:381–385.

Roob, G., Fazekas, F., Hartung, H. P. 1999. Peripheral facial palsy: etiology, diagnosis and treatment. Eur Neurol 41:3–9.

Selesnick, S. H., Patwardhan, A. 1994. Acute facial paralysis: evaluation and early management. Am J Otolaryngol 15: 387–408.

Wright, J. A. 1988. Ultrastructural findings in idiopathic facial paralysis in the dog. J Comp Pathol 98:111–115.

Vestibular Disease

Bagley, R. S., Silver, G. M., Gavin, P. R. 2000. Cerebellar cystic meningioma in a dog. J Am Anim Hosp Assoc 36:413–415.

Bayens-Simmonds, J., Purcell, T. P., Nation, N. P. 1997. Use of magnetic resonance imaging in the diagnosis of central vestibular disease. Can Vet J 38:38.

Bedford, P. D. C. 1979. Congenital vestibular disease in the English cocker spaniel. Vet Rec 105:530–531.

Burke, E. E., Moise, N. S. de la, Erb, H. N. 1985. Review of idiopathic feline vestibular syndrome in 75 cats. JAVMA 187:941–943.

Busch, D. S., Noxon, J. O., Miller, L. D. 1992. Laryngeal paralysis and peripheral vestibular disease in a cat. J Am Anim Hosp Assoc 28:82–86.

Cizinauskas, S., Lang, J., Maier, R., Fatzer, R., Jaggy, A. 2001. Paradoxical vestibular disease with trigeminal nerve-sheath tumor in a dog. Schweiz Arch Tierheilkd 2001. 143:419–425.

Forbes, S., Cook, J. R., Jr. 1991. Congenital peripheral vestibular disease attributed to lymphocytic labyrinthitis in two related litters of Doberman pinscher pups. JAVMA 198:447–449.

Garosi, L. S., Dennis, R., Penderis, J., et al. 2001. Results of magnetic resonance imaging in dogs with vestibular disorders: 85 cases (1996–1999). JAVMA 218:385–391.

Gasser, A. M., Birkenheuer, A. J., Breitschwerdt, E. B. 2001. Canine Rocky Mountain Spotted fever: a retrospective study of 30 cases. J Am Anim Hosp Assoc 37:41–48.

Ingwersen, W., Groom, S., Parent, J. 1989. Vestibular syndrome associated with an ependymoma in a cat. JAVMA 195:98–100.

Kornegay, J. N. 1991. Ataxia, head tilt, nystagmus. Vestibular diseases. Probl Vet Med 3:417–425.

Lee, M. 1983. Congenital vestibular disease in a German shepherd dog. Vet Rec 113:571.

Morozumi, M., Miyahara, K., Sato, M., Hirose, T. 1997. Computed tomography and magnetic resonance findings in two dogs and a cat with intracranial lesions. J Vet Med Sci 59:807–810.

Quesnel, A. D., Parent, J. M. 1995. Paradoxical vestibular syndrome in a cat with a cerebellar meningioma. Can Vet J 36:230–232.

Sanders, S., Bagley, R. S. 2003. Disorders of hearing and balance: the vestibulocochlear nerve (CN VIII) and associated structures. In A Practical Guide to Canine and Feline Neurology, Dewey, C. W., ed. Ames, Iowa State Press, 213–240.

Schunk, K. L. 1988. Disorders of the vestibular system. Vet Clin N Am (Small Anim Pract) 18:641–665.

Schunk, K. L., Averill, D. R. J. 1983. Peripheral vestibular syndrome in the dog: a review of 83 cases. JAVMA 182:1354–1357.

Skerritt, G. C., Whitbread, T. I. 1985. Two cases of paradoxical vestibular syndrome in rough collies. J Sm Anim Pract 26:603–611.

Sims, M. H., Shull-Selcer, E. 1985. Electrodiagnostic evaluation of deafness in two English setter littermates. JAVMA 187:398–404.

Wilkes, M. K., Palmer, A. C. 1992. Congenital deafness and vestibular deficit in the Dobermann. J Sm Anim Pract 33:218–224.

Otoacoustic Emission

Sims, M. H., Brace, J. J., Arthur, D. A., Harvey, R. C. 1991. Otoacoustic emission in a dog. JAVMA 198:1017–1018.

Ototoxicity

Callaghan, D., Culley, C. D. 1985. Ototoxicity in the dog and cat. Vet Rec 117:291.

Clark, C. H. 1977. Toxicity of aminoglycoside antibiotics. Mod Vet Pract 58:594–598.

Lane, J. G. 1985. Ototoxicity in the dog and cat. Vet Rec 117:94.

Mansfield, P. D. 1990. Ototoxicity in dogs and cats. Compend Contin Educ Pract Vet 12:331–337.

Matz, G. J. 1976. The ototoxic effects of ethacrynic acid in man and animals. Laryngoscope 86:1065–1086.

Merchant, S. R. 1994. Ototoxicity. Vet Clin N Am (Small Anim Pract) 24:971–980.

Pickrell, J. A., Oehme, F. W., Cash, W. C. 1993. Ototoxicity in dogs and cats. Semin Vet Med Surg (Small Anim) 8:42–49.

Metronidazole Toxicity

Caylor, K. B., Cassimatis, M. K. 2001. Metronidazole neurotoxicosis in two cats. J Am Anim Hosp Assoc 37:258–262.

Dow, S. W., LeCouteur, R. A., Poss, M. L., Beadleston, D. 1989. Central nervous system toxicosis associated with metronidazole treatment of dogs: five cases (1984–1987). JAVMA 195:365–368.

Evans, J., Levesque, D., Knowles, K., et al. 2003. Diazepam as a treatment for metronidazole toxicosis in dogs: a retrospective study of 21 cases. J Vet Intern Med 17:304–310.

Saxon, B., Magne, M. L. 1993 Reversible central nervous system toxicosis associated with metronidazole therapy in three cats. Prog Vet Neuro 4:25–27.

Deafness

Adams, E. W. 1956. Hereditary deafness in a family of foxhounds. JAVMA 128:302–303.

Anniko, M., Fabiansson, E., Nilsson, O. 1977. Deafness in an old English sheepdog. A case report. Arch Otorhinolaryngol 218:1–7.

Bergsma, D. R, Brown, K. S. 1971. White fur blue eyes and deafness in the domestic cat. J Hered 62:171–185.

Branis, M., Burda, H. 1985. Inner ear structure in the deaf and normally hearing Dalmatian dog. J Comp Pathol 95:295–299.

Cattanach, B. 1990. The "dalmatian dilemma": white coat colour and deafness. J Sm An Prac 40:193–200.

Erickson, F., Saperstein, G., Leipold, H. W., McKinley, J. 1977. Congenital defects of dogs, part 2. Canine Pract 4:51–61.

Famula, T. R., Oberbauer, A. M., Sousa, C. A. 2000. Complex segregation analysis of deafness in Dalmatians. Am J Vet Res 61:550–553.

Famula, T. R., Oberbauer, A. M., Williams, D. C. 2001. Gender effects in hearing loss in Dalmatians. Prev Vet Med 48:15–24.

Ferrara, M. L., Halnan, C. R. E. 1983. Congenital structural brain defects in the deaf dalmatian. Vet Rec 112:344–346.

Griebrokk, T. 1994. Hereditary Deafness in the Dalmatian: relationship to eye and coat color. J Am Anim Hosp Assoc 30:170–176.

Hayes, H. M., Wilson, G. P., Fenner, W. R., Wyman, M. 1981. Canine congenital deafness: epidemiologic study of 272 cases. J Am Anim Hosp Assoc 17:473–476.

Holliday, T. A., Nelson, H. J., Williams, D. C., Willits, N. 1992. Unilateral and bilateral brainstem auditory-evoked response abnormalities in 900 Dalmatian dogs. J Vet Intern Med 6:166–174.

Johnston, D. E., Cox, B. 1970. The incidence in pure-bred dogs in Australia of abnormalities that may be inherited. Aust Vet J 46:465–474.

Knowles, K., Blauch, B., Leipold, H., Cash, W., et al. 1989. Reduction of spiral ganglion neurons in the aging canine with hearing loss. J Vet Med 36:188–199.

Knowles, K. E., Cash, W. C., Blauch, B. S. 1988. Auditory-evoked responses of dogs with different hearing abilities. Can J Vet Res 52:394–397.

Leipold, H. W. 1978. Nature and causes of congenital defects of dogs. Vet Clin N Am 8:47–77.

Luttgen, P. J. 1994. Deafness in the dog and cat. Vet Clin N Am (Small Anim Pract) 24:981–989.

Mair, I. W. 1976. Hereditary deafness in the dalmatian dog. Arch Otorhinolaryngol 212:1–14.

Munro, K. J., Cox, C. L. 1997. Investigation of hearing impairment in Cavalier King Charles spaniels using auditory brainstem response audiometry. J Sm Anim Pract 38:2–5.

Roberts, S. R. 1967. Color dilution and hereditary defects in collie dogs. Am J Ophthalmol 63:1762–1775.

Sims, M. H. 1989. Hearing loss in small animals: occurrence and diagnosis. In Current Veterinary Therapy X, Kirk, R. W., ed. Philadelphia, W. B. Saunders, 805.

Steinberg, S. A., Klein, E., Killens, R. L., Uhde, T. W. 1994. Inherited deafness among nervous pointer dogs. J Hered 85:56–59.

Strain, G. M. 1999. Congenital deafness and its recognition. Vet Clin N Am (Small Anim Pract) 29:895–907.

——. 1996. Aetiology, prevalence and diagnosis of deafness in dogs and cats. Br Vet J 152:17–36.

——. 1991. Congenital deafness in dogs and cats. Compend Contin Educ Pract Vet 13:245–254.

Strain, G. M., Kearney, M. T., Gignac, I. J., et al. 1992. Brainstem auditory-evoked potential assessment of congenital deafness in Dalmatians: associations with phenotypic markers. J Vet Intern Med 6:175–182.

Strain, G. M., Kearney, M. T., Gignac, I. J., Levesque, D. C., et al. 1992. Brainstem auditory-evoked potential assessment of congenital deafness in Dalmatians: associations with phenotypic markers. J Vet Intern Med 6:175–182.

Townsend, H. G. 1997. 101 Dalmatians—but how many are congenitally deaf? Vet J 154:89–90.

Turner, S. 1994. Deafness in dalmatians and other breeds. Vet Rec 134:200.

Wilkes, M. K., Palmer, A. C. 1992. Congenital deafness and vestibular deficit in the Dobermann. J Sm Anim Pract 33: 218–224.

——. 1987. Deafness in Dobermans. Vet Rec 120:624.

Glossopharyngeal

Shores, A., Vaughn, D. M., Holland, M., Smith, B., Simpson, S. T., Burns, J. 1991. Glossopharyngeal neuralgia syndrome in a dog. J Am Anim Hosp Assoc 27:101–104.

Laryngeal Paralysis

Barr, S., Baker, D., Markovits, J. 1986. Trypanosomiasis and laryngeal paralysis in a dog. JAVMA 188:1307–1309,

Bennett, P. F., Clarke, R. E. 1997. Laryngeal paralysis in a rottweiler with neuroaxonal dystrophy. Aust. Vet. J. 75:784–786.

Bjorling, D. E. 1995. Laryngeal paralysis, In Kirk's Current Veterinary Therapy XII (Small Animal Practice), Bonagura , J. D., ed. Philadelphia, W. B. Saunders, 901–905.

Braund, K. G. 1995. Laryngeal paralysis-polyneuropathy complex in young Dalmatian dogs. In Kirk's Current Veterinary Therapy XII (Small Animal Practice), Bonagura, J. D., ed. Philadelphia, W. B. Saunders, 1136–1140.

Braund, K. G., Shores, A., Cochrane, S., et al. 1994. Laryngeal paralysis-polyneuropathy complex in young Dalmatians. Am J Vet Res 55:534–542.

Braund, K. G., Steinberg, H. S., Shores, A., et al. 1989. Laryngeal paralysis in immature and mature dogs as one sign of a more diffuse polyneuropathy. JAVMA 194:1735–1740.

Burbidge, H. M. 1995. A review of laryngeal paralysis in dogs. Br Vet J 151:71–82.

Gaber, C. E., Amis, T. C., LeCouteur, R. A. 1985. Laryngeal paralysis in dogs: a review of 23 cases. JAVMA 186:377–380.

Hardie, E. M., Kolata, R. I., Stone, E. A., et al. 1981. Laryngeal paralysis in three cats. JAVMA 179:879–882.

Lussier, B., Flanders, J. A., Erb, H. N. 1996. The effect of unilateral arytenoid lateralization on rima glotidis area in canine cadaver larynges. Vet Surg 25:121–126.

MacPhail, C. M., Monnet, E. 2001. Outcome and postoperative complications in dogs undergoing surgical treatment of laryngeal paralysis: 140 cases (1985–1998). JAVMA 218;12: 1949–1956.

Mahony, O. M., Knowles, K. E., Braund, K. G., et al. 1998. Laryngeal paralysis-polyneuropathy complex in young Rottweilers. J Vet Intern Meed 12:330–337.

O'Brien, L. A., Hendriks, L. 1986. Inherited laryngeal paralysis. Analysis in the husky cross. Vet Q 8:301–302.

Ridyard, A. E., Corcoran, B. M., Tasker, S., et al. 2000. Spontaneous laryngeal paralysis in four white-coated German shepherd dogs. J Sm An Prac 41:558–561.

Schacter, S., Norris, C. R. 2000. Laryngeal paralysis in cats: 16 cases (1990–1999). JAVMA 216;7:1100–1103.

Schaer, M., Zaki, F. A., Harvey, H. J., O'Reilly, W. H. 1979. Laryngeal hemiplegia due to neoplasia of the vagus nerve in a cat. JAVMA 174:513–515.

Shelton, G. D., Podell, M., Sullivan, S., et al. 2000. Distal, symmetrical polyneuropathy with laryngeal paralysis in young, related Leonberger dogs. J Vet Intern Med 14;3:339 (abstract).

Venker-van Haagen, A. L. 1992. Diseases of the larynx. Vet Clin N Am (Small Anim Pract) 22:1155–1172.

Venker-van Haagen, A. L., Bouw, L., Hartman, W. 1981. Hereditary transmission of laryngeal paralysis in Bouviers. J Am Anim Hosp Assoc 17:75–76.

Venker-van Haagen, A. L., Hartman, W., Goedegebuure, S. A. 1978. Spontaneous laryngeal paralysis in young Bouviers. J Am Anim Hosp Assoc 14:714–720.

Megaesophagus

Clifford, D. H., Barboza, P. F., Pirschl, G. 1980. The motor nuclei of the vagus nerve in cats with and without congenital achalasia of the oesophagus. Br Vet J 136:74–83.

Cox, V. S., Wallace, L., Anderson, Y. E., et al. 1980. Hereditary esophageal dysfunction in the Miniature Schnauzer dog. Am J Vet Res 41:326–330.

Guilford, W. G. 1990. Megaesophagus in the dog and cat. Semin Vet Med Surg (Small Anim) 5:37–45.

Hoenig, M., Mahaffey, M. B., Parnell, P. G., et al. 1990. Megaesophagus in two cats. JAVMA 196:763–765.

Hoffer, R. E., MacCoy, D. M., Quick, C. B., et al. 1979. Management of acquired achalasia in dogs. JAVMA 175:814–817.

Maddison, J. E., Allan, G. S. 1990. Megaesophagus attributable to lead toxicosis in a cat. JAVMA 197:1357–1358.

McKerrell, R. E., Braund, K. G. 1987. Hereditary myopathy in Labrador retrievers: clinical variations. J Sm Anim Pract 28:479–489.

Moses, L., Harpster, N. K, Beck, K. A., et al. 2000. Esophageal motility dysfunction in cats: a study of 44 cases. J Am Anim Hosp Assoc 36:309–312.

Peeters, M. E., Venker-van Haagen, A. J., Goedegebuure, S. A., Wolvekamp, W. T. 1991. Dysphagia in Bouviers associated with muscular dystrophy; evaluation of 24 cases. Vet Q 13:65–73.

Stickle, R., Sparschu, G., Love, N., et al. 1992. Radiographic evaluation of ésophageal function in Chinese Shar Pei pups. JAVMA 201:81–84.

Strombeck, D. R. 1978. Pathophysiology of esophageal motiltiy disorders in the dog and cat. Application to management and prognosis. Vet Clin N Am (Small Anim Pract) 8:229–244.

Tan, B. J. K., Diamant, N. E. 1987. Assessment of the neural defect in a dog with idiopathic megaesophagus. Dig Dis Sci 32:76–85.

Swallowing

Suter, P. F., Watrous, B. J. 1980. Oropharyngeal dysphagies in the dog: a cineflurographic analysis if experimentally induced and spontaneously occuring swallowing disorders. Vet Rad 21:24–39.

Multiple Cranial Nerve Disease

Carpenter, J. L., King, N. W., Jr., Abrams, K. L. 1987. Bilateral trigeminal nerve paralysis and Horner's syndrome associated with myelomonocytic neoplasia in a dog. JAVMA 191: 1594–1596.

Christopher, M. M., Metz, A. L., Klausner, J., Polzin, D., et al. 1986. Acute myelomonocytic leukemia with neurological manifestations in the dog. Vet Pathol 23:140–147.

Hobbs, S. L., Cobb, M. A. 1990. A cranial neuropathy associated with multicentric lymphosarcoma in a dog. Vet Rec 127: 525–526.

Panciera, R. J., Ritchey, J. W., Baker, J. E., DiGregorio, M. 2002. Trigeminal and polyradiculoneuritis in a dog presenting with masticatory muscle atrophy and Horner's syndrome. Vet Pathol 39:146–149.

Pfaff, A. D., March, P. A., Fishman, C. 2000. Acute bilateral trigeminal neuropathy associated with nervous system lymphosarcoma in a dog. J Am Anim Hosp Assoc 36:57–61.

Zachary, J. F., O'Brien, D. P., Ingles, B. W., Everitt, J. I., Parker, A. J. 1986. Multicentric nerve sheath fibrosarcomas of multiple cranial nerve roots in two dogs. JAVMA 188:723–726.

Spinal Cord Diseases

Degenerative Spinal Diseases

General Degenerative Diseases

Averill, D. R. J., Bronson, R. T. 1977. Inherited necrotizing myelopathy of Afghan hounds. J Neuropathol Exp Neurol 36:734–747.

Bjorck, G., Mair, W., Olsson, S-E., et al. 1962. Hereditary ataxia in fox terriers. Acta Neuropathologica (Suppl I), 45–48.

Chrisman, C. L. 1986. Neuroaxonal dystrophy and leukoencephalomyelopathy of Rottweiler dogs. In Current Veterinary Therapy IX (Small Animal Practice), Kirk, R. W., ed. Philadelphia, W. B. Saunders, 805–806.

Cockrell, B. Y., Herigstad, R. R., Flo, G. L., et al. 1973. Myelomalacia in Afghan hounds. JAVMA 162:362–365.

Cummings, J. F., deLahunta, A. 1978. Hereditary myelopathy of Afghan hounds, a myelinolytic disease. Acta Neuropathol (Berl) 42:173–181.

deLahunta, A., Ingram, J. T., Cummings, J. F., et al. 1994. Labrador retriever central axonopathy. Prog Vet Neurol 5:117–122.

Douglas, S. W., Palmer, A. C. 1961. Idiopathic demyelination of brain-stem and cord in a miniature poodle puppy. J Pathol Bact 82:67–71.

Gamble, D. A., Chrisman, C. L. 1984. A leukoencephalomyelopathy of rottweiler dogs. Vet Path 21:274–280.

Hartley, W. J., Palmer, A. C. 1973. Ataxia in Jack Russell terriers. Acta Neuropathol (Berl) 26:71–74.

Mandigers, P. J., van Nes, J. J., Knol, B. W., et al. 1993. Hereditary necrotising myelopathy in Kooiker dogs. Res Vet Sci 54:118–123.

Matthews, N. S., deLahunta, A. 1985. Degenerative myelopathy in an adult miniature poodle. JAVMA 186:1213–1215.

Palmer, A. C., Cavanagh, J. B. 1995. Encephalomyelopathy in young cats. J Sm Anim Pract 36:57–64.

Richardson, J. A., Tang, K., Burns, O. K. 1991. Myeloencephalopathy with Rosenthal fiber formation in a miniature poodle. Vet Pathol 28:536–538.

Slocombe, R. F., Mitten, R., Mason, T. A. 1989. Leucoencephalomyelopathy in Australian Rottweiler dogs. Aust Vet J 66:147–150.

Vandevelde, M., Braund, K. G. 1979. Polioencephalomyelitis in cats. Vet Pathol 16:420–427.

Wouda, W., van Nes, J. J. 1986. Progressive ataxia due to central demyelination in Rottweiler dogs. Vet Q 8:89–97.

Degenerative Myelopathy

Averill, D. R., Jr. 1973. Degenerative myelopathy in the aging German Shepherd dog: clinical and pathologic findings. JAVMA 162:1045–1051.

Barclay, K. B., Haines, D. M. 1994. Immunohistochemical evidence for immunoglobulin and complement deposition in spinal cord lesions in degenerative myelopathy in German shepherd dogs. Can J Vet Res 58:20–24.

Bichsel, P., Vandevelde, M. 1983. Degenerative myelopathy in a family of Siberian Husky dogs. JAVMA 183:998–1000.

Braund, K. G., Vandevelde, M. 1978. German shepherd dog myelopathy: a morphologic and morphometric study. Am J Vet Res 39:1309–1315.

Clemmons, R. M. 1992. Degenerative myelopathy. Vet Clin N Am (Small Anim Pract) 22:965–971.

———. 1991. Therapeutic considerations for degenerative myelopathy of German shepherds, Proc 9th ACVIM Forum, New Orleans, LA, May, 773–775.

———. 1989. Degenerative myelopathy. In Current Veterinary Therapy, 10th ed. Kirk, R. W., ed. Philadelphia, W. B. Saunders, 830.

Griffiths, I. R., Duncan, I. D. 1975. Chronic degenerative radiculomyelopathy in the dog, J Sm Anim Pract 16:461–471.

Johnston, P. E. J., Barrie, J. A., McCulloch, M. C., Anderson, T. J., et al. 2000. Central nervous system pathology in 25 dogs with chronic degenerative radiculomyelopathy. Vet Rec 146:629–633

Longhofer, S. L., Duncan, I. D., Messing, A. 1990. A degenerative myelopathy in young German shepherd dogs. J Sm An Prac 31:199–203.

Lutgen, P. I. 1990. Common degenerative and vascular neurologic disorders in cats and dogs. Prog Vet Neurol 1:387–395.

Matthews, N. S., deLahunta, A. 1985. Degenerative myelopathy in an adult miniature poodle. JAVMA 186:1213–1215.

Mesfin, G. M., Kusewitt, D., Parker, A. 1980. Degenerative myelopathy in a cat. JAVMA 176:62–64.

Summers, B. A., Cummings, J., deLahunta, A. 1995. Degenerative diseases of the central nervous system. In Veterinary Neuropathology, Summers, B. A., Cummings, J., deLahunta, A., eds. St. Louis, Mosby, 208–350.

Vandevelde, M. 1980. Degenerative diseases of the spinal cord. Vet Clin N Am (Small Anim Pract) 10:147–154.

Waxman, F. J., Clemmons, R. M., Hinrichs, D. J. 1980a. Progressive myelopathy in older German Shepherd dogs II. Presence of circulating suppressor cells. J Immunol 124:1216–1222.

Waxman, F. J., Clemmons, R. M., Johnson, G., et al. 1980b. Progressive myelopathy in older German Shepherd dogs I. Depressed response to thymus-dependent mitogens. J Immunol 124:1209–1215.

Williams, D. A., Batt, R. M., Sharp, N. J. H. 1984. Degenerative myelopathy in German shepherd dogs: an association with mucosal biochemical changes and bacterial overgrowth in the small intestine. Clin Sci 66:25.

Intervertebral Disk Disease

Amsellem, P. M., Toombs, J. P., Laverty, P. H., Breur, G. J. 2003a. Loss of deep pain sensation following thoracolumbar intervertebral disk herniation in dogs: patholophysiology. Compend Contin Ed Pract Vet 25:266–264.

———. 2003b. Loss of deep pain sensation following thoracolumbar intervertebral disk herniation in dogs: treatment and prognosis. Compend Contin Ed Pract Vet 25:266–274.

Atilola, M. A., Bailey, C. S., Morgan, J. P. 1988. Cervical chemonucleolysis in the dog. A surgical technique. Vet Surg 17:135–140.

Atilola, M. A., Cockshutt, J. R., McLaughlin, R., et al. 1993. Collagenase chemonucleolysis—a long term radiographic study in normal dogs. Vet Rad Ultrasound 34:321–324.

Bagley, R. S., Tucker, R., Harrington, M. L. 1996. Lateral and foraminal disk extrusions in dogs. Compend Contin Educ Pract 18:795–804.

Bagley, R. S., Tucker, R. L., Moore, M. P., et al. 1995. Intervertebral disk extrusion in a cat. Vet Rad Ultrasound 36:380–382.

Bailey, C. S. 1992. Chymopapain chemonucleolysis. In Kirk's Current Veterinary Therapy XI (Small Animal Practice), Bonagura, J. D., ed. Philadelphia, W. B. Saunders, 1018–1020.

Ball, M. U., McGuire, J. A., Swaim, S. F., Hoerlein, B. F., et al. 1982. Patterns of occurrence of disk disease among registered dachshunds. JAVMA 180:519–522.

Beal, M. W., Paglia, D. T., Griffin, G. M., et al. 2001. Ventilatory failure, ventilator management, and outcome in dogs with cervical spinal disorders: 14 cases (1991–1999). JAVMA 218:1598–1602.

Bellah, J. R. 1983. Colonic perforation after corticosteroid and surgical treatment of intervertebral disk disease in a dog. JAVMA 183:1002–1003.

Boag, A. K., Otto, C. M., Drobatz, K. J. 2001. Complications of methylprednisolone sodium succinate therapy in Dachshunds with surgically treated intervertebral disc disease. J Vet Emerg Crit Care 11:104–110.

Braund, K. G. 1986. Intervertebral disk disease. In Neurologic disorders: contemporary issues in small animal practice, Kornegay, J. N., ed. New York, Churchill Livingstone, 21–39.

———. 1981. Canine intervertebral disk disease. In Pathophysiology in Small Animal Surgery, Bojrab, M. J., ed. Philadelphia, Lea & Febiger, 739–746.

Braund, K. G., Ghosh, P., Taylor, T. K. F., Larsen, L. H. 1975. Morphological studies on the canine intervertebral disk. The assignment of the beagle to the achondroplastic classification. Res Vet Sci 19:167–172.

———. 1976. The qualitative assessment of glycosaminoglycans in the canine intervertebral disc using a critical electrolyte concentration staining technique. Res Vet Sci 21:314–317.

Bray, J. P., Burbidge, H. M. 1998a. The canine intervertebral disk. Part one: structure and function. J Am Anim Hosp Assoc 34:55–63.

———. 1998b. The canine intervertebral disk. Part two: degenerative changes-nonchondrodystrophoid versus chondrodystrophoid disks. J Am Anim Hosp Assoc 34:135–144.

Butterworth, S. J., Denny, H. R. 1991. Follow-up study of 100 cases with thoracolumbar disc protrusions treated by lateral fenestration. J Sm Anim Pract 32:443–447.

Coates, J. R. 2000. Intervertebral disc disease. Vet Clin N Am (Small Anim Pract) 30 (1):77–110.

Cudia, S. P., Duval, J. M. 1997. Thoracolumbar intervertebral disk disease in large, nonchondrodystrophic dogs: a retrospective study. J Am Anim Hosp Assoc 33:456–460.

Dallman, M. J., Moon, M. L., Giovannirti-Jensen, A. 1991. Comparison of the width of the intervertebral disk space and radiographic changes before and after intervertebral disk fenestration in dogs. Am J Vet Res 52:140–145.

Dallman, M. J., Palettas, P., Bojrab, M. J. 1992. Characteristics of dogs admitted for treatment of cervical intervertebral disk disease: 105 cases (1972–1982). JAVMA 200:2009–2011.

Davis, G. J., Brown, D. C. 2002. Prognostic indicators for time to ambulation following surgical decompression in nonambulatory dogs with acute thoracolumbar disk extrusions: 112 cases. Vet Surg 31;6:513–518.

Dhupa, S, Glickman, NW, Waters, DJ. 1999. Functional outcome in dogs after surgical treatment of caudal lumbar intervertebral disk herniation. J Am Anim Hosp Assoc 35:323–331.

———. 1999. Reoperative neurosurgery in dogs with thoracolumbar disk disease. Vet Surg 28:421–428.

Duval, J., Dewey, C., Roberts, R., et al. 1996. Spinal cord swelling as a myelographic indicator of prognosis: a retrospective study in dogs with intervertebral disc disease and loss of deep pain perception. Vet Surg 25:6–12.

Ghosh, P., Taylor, T. K. F., Braund, K. G. 1977. The variation of the glycosaminoglycans of the canine intervertebral disc with aging. I: chondrodystrophoid breed. Gerontology 23:87–98.

———. 1977. The variation of the glycosaminoglycans of the canine intervertebral disc with aging. II: non-chondrodystrophoid breed. Gerontology 23:99–109.

Ghosh, P., Taylor, T. K., Braund, K. G., Larsen, L. H. 1976a. The collagenous and non-collagenous protein of the canine intervertebral disc and their variation with age, spinal level and breed, Gerontology 22:124–134.

———. 1976b. A comparative chemical and histochemical study of the chondrodystrophoid and non-chondrodystrophoid canine intervertebral disc, Vet Pathol 13:414–427.

Ghosh, P., Taylor, T. K. F., Yarroll, J. M., Braund, K. G., et a1. 1975. Genetic factors in the maturation of the canine intervertebral disk, Res Vet Sci 19:304–311.

Gilmore, D. R. 1983. Extrusion of feline intervertebral disk. Vet Med 207–209.

Griffiths, I. R. 1972a. The extensive myelopathy of intervertebral disc protrusions in dogs ('the ascending syndrome'). J Sm Anim Pract 13:425–437.

———. 1972b. Some aspects of the pathogenesis and diagnosis of lumbar disc protrusion in the dog. J Sm Anim Pract 13:439–447.

———. 1972c. Some aspects of the pathology and pathogenesis of the myelopathy caused by disc protrusions in the dog. J Neurol Neurosurg Psychiatr 35:403–413.

———. 1970. A syndrome produced by dorso-lateral "explosions" of the cervical intervertebral discs. Vet Rec 87:737–741.

Fingeroth, J. M. 1995. Treatment of canine intervertebral disk disease: recommendations and controversies. In Kirk's Current

Veterinary Therapy XII (Small Animal Practice), Bonagura, J. D., ed. Philadelphia, W. B. Saunders 1146–1153.

———. 1989. Fenestration: pros and cons. Prob Vet Med 1:445–466.

Fitch, R. B., Kerwin, Hosgood, G. 2000. Caudal cervical intervertebral disk disease in the small dog: role of distraction and stabilization in ventral slot decompression. J Am Anim Hosp Assoc 36:68–74.

Fourie, S. L., Kirberger, R. M. 1999. Relationship of cervical spinal cord diameter to vertebral dimensions: a radiographic study of normal dogs. Vet Rad Ultrasound 40:137–143.

Fry, T. R., Johnson, A. L. 1991. Chemonucleolysis for treatment of intervertebral disk disease. JAVMA 199:622–627.

Fry, T. R., Johnson, A. L., Hungerford, L., et al. 1991. Surgical treatment of cervical disc herniations in ambulatory dogs. Ventral decompression vs. fenestration, III cases (1980–1988). Prog Vet Neurol 2:165–173.

Gill, P. J., Lippincott, C. L., Anderson, S. M. 1996. Dorsal laminectomy in the treatment of cervical intervertebral disk disease in small dogs: a retrospective study of 30 cases. J Am Anim Hosp Assoc 32:77–80.

Hansen, H. J. 1952. A pathologic-anatomical study on disc degeneration in the dog. Acta Orthop Scand (suppl 11):1–117.

Holmberg, D. L., Palmer, N. C., VanPelt, D., et al. 1990. A comparison of manual and power-assisted thoracolumbar disc fenestration in dogs. Vet Surg 19:323–327.

Hoerlein, B. F., Spano, J. S. 1975. Non-neurological complications following decompressive spinal cord surgery. Arch Am Coli Vet Surg 4:11–16.

Hurlbert, R. J. 2000 Methylprednisolone for acute spinal cord injury: an inappropriate standard of care. J Neurosurg 93 (Suppl 1):1–7.

Janssens, L. A., de Prins, E. M. 1989. Treatment of thoracolumbar disk disease in dogs by means of acupuncture: a comparison of two techniques. J Am Anim Hosp Assoc 25:169–174.

Jerram, R. M., Dewey, C. W. 1999a. Acute thoracolumbar disk extrusion in dogs—part I. Compend Contin Educ Pract Vet 21:922–931.

———. 1999b. Acute thoracolumbar disk extrusion in dogs—part II. Compend Contin Educ Pract Vet 21:1037–1047.

King, A. S., Smith, R. N. 1960a. Disc protrusion in the cat: age incidence of dorsal protrusion. Vet Rec 72:381–383.

———. 1960b. Disc protrusions in the cat: distribution of dorsal protrusions along the vertebral column. Vet Rec 72:335–337.

King, A. S., Smith, R. N., Kon, V. M. 1958. Protrusion of the intervertebral disc in the cat. Vet Rec 70:509–515.

Kirberger, R. M., Roos, C. J., Lubbe, A. M. 1992. The radiological diagnosis of thoracolumbar disc disease in the Dachshund. Vet Rad Ultrasound 33:255–261.

Knapp, D. W., Pope, E. R., Hewett, J. E., Bojrab, M. J. 1990. A retrospective study of thoracolumbar disk fenestration in dogs using a ventral approach: 160 cases (1976 to 1986), J Am Anim Hosp Assoc 26:543–549.

Knipe, M. F., Vernau, K. M., LeCouteur, R. A. 2001. Intervertebral disk extrusion in six cats. J Vet Intern Med 15:318.

Kornegay, J. N. 1992. Intervertebral disk disease: treatment guidelines. In Kirk, R. W., Kirk's Current Veterinary Therapy XI (Small Animal Practice), Bonagura, J. D., eds. Philadelphia, W. B. Saunders, 1013–1018.

Kudo, T., Sumi, A., Hashimoto, A. 1993. Experimental chemonucleolysis with chymopapain in canine intervertebral disks. J Vet Med Sci 55:211–215.

LeCouteur, R. A., Child, G. 1995. Diseases of the spinal cord, in Textbook of Veterinary Internal Medicine. Diseases of the Dog and Cat., Ettinger SJ, Feldman EC, eds, 4th edition, Philadelphia, W.B. Saunders 629–696.

Littlewood, J. D., Herrtage, M. E., Palmer, A. C. 1984. Intervertebral disc protrusion in a cat. J Sm Anim Pract 25:119–127.

Lu, D. S., Shono, Y., Oda, I., et al. 1997. Effects of chondroitinase ABC and chymopapain on spinal motion segment biomechanics. An in vivo biomechanical, radiologic, and histologic canine study. Spine 22:1828–1834.

McKee, W. M. 1992. A comparison of hemilaminectomy (with concomitant disc fenestration) and dorsal laminectomy for the treatment of thoracolumbar disc protrusion in dogs. Vet Rec 130:296–300.

Melrose, J., Taylor, T. K., Ghosh, P., et al. 1996. Intervertebral disc reconstitution after chemonucleolysis with chymopapain is dependent on dosage. Spine 21:9–17.

Miyabayashi, T., Lord, P. F., Dubielzig, R. R., et al. 1992. Chemonucleolysis with collagenase. A radiographic and pathologic study in dogs. Vet Surg 21:189–194.

Moore, R. W., Withrow, S. J. 1982. Gastrointestinal hemorrhage and pancreatitis associated with intervertebral disk disease in the dog. JAVMA 180:1443–1447.

Morgan, P. W., Parent, J., Holmberg, D. L. 1993. Cervical pain secondary to intervertebral disc disease in dogs; radiographic findings and surgical implications. Prog Vet Neurol 4:76–80.

Munana, K. R., Olby, N. J., Sharp, N. J. H., et al. 2000. Intervertebral disk disease in 10 cats. J Am Anim Hosp Assoc 37:384–389.

Muir, P., Johnson, K. A., Manley, P. A., et al. 1995. Comparison of hemilaminectomy and dorsal laminectomy for thoracolumbar intervertebral disc extrusion in dachshunds. J Sm Anim Pract 36:360–367.

Olby, NJ, Dyce, J, Houlton, JE. 1994. Correlation of plain radiographic and lumbar myelographic findings with surgical findings in thoracolumbar disc disease. J Sm An Prac 35:345–350.

Olby, NJ, Munana, KR, Sharp, NJH, et al. 2000. The computed tomographic appearance of acute thoracolumbar intervertebral disc herniations in dogs. Vet Rad Ultrasound 41:396–402.

Prata, RG. 1981. Neurosurgical treatment of thoracolumbar disks: the rationale and value of laminectomy with concomitant disk removal, J Am Anim Hosp Assoc 17:17–26.

Salisbury, S. K., Cook, J. R., Jr. 1988. Recovery of neurological function following focal myelomalacia in a cat. J Am Anim Hosp Assoc 24:227–230.

Sanders, S. G., Bagley, R. S., Gavin, P. R. 2002. Intramedullary spinal cord damage associated with intervertebral disk material in a dog. JAVMA 221:1594–1596.

Schulz, K. S., Walker, M., Moon, M., et al. 1998. Correlation of clinical, radiographic, and surgical localization of intervertebral disc extrusion in small-breed dogs: a prospective study of 50 cases. Vet Surg 27:105–111.

Schwarz, T., Owen, M. R., Long, S., Sullivan, M. 2000. Vacuum disk and facet phenomenon in a dog with cauda equina syndrome. JAVMA 217:862–864.

Scott, H. W. 1997. Hemilaminectomy for the treatment of thoracolumbar disc disease in the dog: a follow-up study of 40 cases. J Sm Anim Pract 38:488–494.

Scott, H. W., McKee, W. M. 1999. Laminectomy for 34 dogs with thoracolumbar intervertebral disc disease and loss of deep pain perception. J Sm Anim Pract 40:417–422.

Seim, H. B. 1996. Conditions of the thoracolumbar spine. Semin Vet Med Surg (Small Anim Pract) 11:235–253.

Seim, H. B., III, Nafe, L. A. 1981. Spontaneous intervertebral disk extrusion with associated myelopathy in a cat. J Am Anim Hosp Assoc 17:201–204.

Shires, P. K., Waldron, D. R., Hedlund, C. S., Blass, C. E., Massoudi, L. 1991. A biochemical study of rotational instability in unrelated and surgically altered canine thoracolumbar vertebral motion units. Prog Vet Neurol 2:6–14.

Simpson, S. T. 1992. Intervertebral disc disease. Vet Clin N Am (Small Anim Pract) 22:889–897.

Smith, J. D., Newell, S. M., Budsberg, S. C., Bennett, R. A. 1997. Incidence of contralateral versus ipsilateral neurological signs associated with lateralised Hansen type I disc extrusion. J Sm Anim Pract 38:495–497.

Sparkes, A. H., Skerry, T. M. 1990. Successful management of a prolapsed intervertebral disc in a Siamese cat. Feline Pract 18:7–9.

Stigen, O. 1996. Calcification of intervertebral discs in the dachshund: a radiographic study of 115 dogs at 1 and 5 yr of age. Acta Vet Scand 37:229–237.

———. 1991. Calcification of intervertebral discs in the dachshund. A radiographic study of 327 young dogs. Acta Vet Scand 32:197–203.

Stigen, O., Christensen, K. 1993. Calcification of intervertebral discs in the dachshund: an estimation of heritability. Acta Vet Scand 34:357–361.

Still, J. 1989. Analgesic effects of acupuncture in thoracolumbar disc disease in dogs. J Sm Anim Pract 30:298–301.

Sukhiani, H. R., Parent, J. M., Atilola, M. A., et al. 1996. Intervertebral disk disease in dogs with signs of back pain alone: 25 cases (1986–1993). JAVMA 209:1275–1279.

Thomson, C. E., Kornegay, J. N., Stevens, J. B. 1989. Canine intervertebral disc disease: changes in the cerebrospinal fluid. J Sm Anim Pract 30:685–688.

Tomlinson, J. 1996. Surgical conditions of the cervical spine. Semin Vet Med Surg (Small Anim) 11:225–234.

Toombs, J. P. 1992. Cervical intervertebral disk disease in dogs. Compend Contin Educ Pract Vet 14:1477–1489.

Toombs, J. P., Caywood, D. D., Lipowitz, A. J., Stevens, J. B. 1980. Colonic perforation following neurosurgical procedures and corticosteroid therapy in four dogs, JAVMA 177:68–72.

Toombs, J. P., Collins, L. G., Graves, G. M., et al. 1986. Colonic perforation in corticosteroid-treated dogs. J Vet Med Assoc 188:145–150.

Trevor, P. B., Martin, R. A., Saunders, G. K., et al. 1991. Healing characteristics of free and pedicle fat grafts after dorsal laminectomy and durotomy in dogs. Vet Surg 20:282–290.

Waldron, D. R., Shires, P. K., McCain, W., Hedlund, C., Blass, C. E. 1991. The rotational stabilizing effect of spinal fixation techniques in an unstable vertebral model. Prog Vet Neurol 2:105–110.

Wright, F., Palmer, A. C. 1969. Morphological changes caused by pressure on the spinal cord, Pathol Vet 6:355–368.

Wobbler Syndrome

Adamo, P. F., Cherubini, G. B., Mocavero, A., et al. 2001. Short and long term results in eight cases of caudal cervical spondylomyelopathy by using an interbody methylmethacrylate plug. J Vet Internal Med 15:75 (abstract).

Al-Mefty, O., Harkey, H. L., Marawi, I., et al. 1993. Experimental chronic compressive cervical myelopathy. J Neurosurg 79:550.

Baum, F., III, deLahunta, A., Trotter, E. J. 1992. Cervical fibrotic stenosis in a young Rottweiler. JAVMA 2001:1222–1224.

Bruecker, K. A., Seim, H. B., III, Blass, C. E. 1989. Caudal cervical spondylomyelopathy: decompression by linear traction and stabilization with Steinmann pins and polymethyl methacrylate. J Am Anim Hosp Assoc 25:677–683.

Bruecker, K. A., Seim, H. B., Withrow, S. I. 1989. Clinical evaluation of three surgical methods for treatment of caudal cervical spondylomyelopathy of dogs. Vet Surg 18:197–203.

Chambers, J. N., Oliver, J. E., Jr., Bjorling, D. E. 1986. Update on ventral decompression for caudal cervical disk herniation in Doberman pinschers. J Am Anim Hosp Assoc 22:775–778.

deLahunta, A. 1983. In Veterinary Neuroanatomy and Clinical Neurology, 2d ed. Philadelphia, W. B. Saunders.

Denny, H. R., Gibbs, C., Gaskell, C. J. 1977. Cervical spondylopathy in the dog: a review of thirty-five cases. J Small Animl Pract 18:117–132.

DeRisio, L., Munana, K., Murray, M., et al. 2002. Dorsal laminectomy for caudal cervical spondylomyelopathy: postoperative recovery and long-term follow-up in 20 dogs. Vet Surg 31:418–427.

Dickinson, P. I., LeCouteur, R. A., Sturges, B. K., et al. 1999. Extradural spinal synovial cysts in two dogs: clinical and pathological features. J Vet Intern Med 13:241 (Abstract).

Dixon, B. C., Tomblinson, J. L., Kraus, K. H. 1995. A modified distraction-stabilization technique for canine caudal cervical spondylomyelopathy using an interbody polymethyl methacrylate plug. Vet Surg 24:425

Dixon, B. C., Tomlinson, I. L., Kraus, K. H. 1996. Modified distraction-stabilization technique using an interbody polymethyl methacrylate plug in dogs with caudal cervical spondylomyelopathy. JAVMA 208:61–68.

Ellison, G. W., Seim, H. B., Clemmons, R. M. 1988. Distracted cervical spinal fusion for management of caudal cervical spondylomyelopathy in large-breed dogs. JAVMA 193:447–453

Goring, R. L., Beale, B. S., Faulkner, R. F. 1991. The inverted cone decompression technique: a surgical treatment for cervical vertebral instability "wobbler syndrome" in Doberman pinschers. Part 1, J Am Anim Hosp Asso 27:403–409.

Hurov, L. 1979. Dorsal decompressive cervical laminectomy in the dog: surgical considerations and clinical cases. J Am Anim Hosp Assoc 15:301–309.

Jaggy, A., Gaillard, C., Lang, J., Vandevelde, M. 1988. Hereditary cervical spondylopathy (wobbler syndrome) in the Borzoi dog, J Am Anim Hosp Assoc 24:453–460.

LeMarie, R. J., Kerwin, S. C., Partington, B. P., et al. 2000. Vertebral subluxation following ventral cervical decompression in the dog. J Am Anim Hosp Assoc 36:348–358.

Levitski, R. E., Chauvet, A. E., Lipsitz, D. 1999. Cervical myelopathy associated with extradural synovial cysts in 4 dogs. J Vet Intern Med 13:181–186.

Lewis, D. G. 1991. Radiological assessment of the cervical spine of the doberman with reference to cervical spondylo-myelopathy. J Sm Anim Pract 32:75–82.

———. 1989. Cervical spondylo-myelopathy ('wobbler' syndrome) in the dog: a study based on 224 cases. J Sm Anim Pract 30:657–665.

Lipsitz, D., Levitski, R. E., Chauvet, A. E., et al. 2001. Magnetic resonance imaging features of cervical stenotic myelopathy in 21 dogs. Vet Rad Ultrasound 42:20–27.

Lyman, R. 1991. Continuous dorsal laminectomy is the procedure of choice. Prog Vet Neurol 2:143–146.

McKee, W. M., Lavelle, R. B., Mason, T. A. 1989. Vertebral stabilisation for cervical spondylopathy using a screw and washer technique. J Sm An Prac 30:337–342.

Pitch, R. B., Kerwin, S. C., Hosgood, G. 2000. Caudal cervical intervertebral disk disease in the small dog: role of distraction and stabilization in ventral slot decompression. J Am Anim Hosp Assoc 36:68–74.

Read, R. A., Robins, G. M., Carlisle, C. H. 1983. Caudal cervical spondylo-myelopathy (wobbler syndrome) in the dog: a review of thirty cases. J Sm Anim Pract 24:605–621.

Rusbridge, C., Wheeler, S. I., Torrington, A. M., et al. 1998. Comparison of two surgical techniques for the management of cervical spondylomyelopathy in dobermanns. J Sm Anim Pract 39:425–431.

Seim, H. B., III. 1989. Wobbler syndrome in the Doberman pinscher. In Kirk, R. W., ed., Current Veterinary Therapy X (Small Animal Practice). Philadelphia, W. B. Saunders, 858–862.

Seim, H. B., III, Withrow, S. J. 1982. Pathophysiology and diagnosis of caudal cervical spondylo-myelopathy with emphasis on the Doberman Pinscher. J Am Anim Hosp Assoc 18: 241–251.

Sharp, N. J., Cofone, M., Robertson, I. D., et al. 1995. Computed tomography in the evaluation of caudal cervical spondylomyelopathy of the Doberman pinscher. Vet Rad Ultrasound 36:100–108.

Sharp, N. J., Wheeler, S. J., Cofone, M. 1992. Radiological evaluation of 'Wobbler' syndrome-caudal cervical spondylomyelopathy. Journal of Small Animal Practice 33, 491–499.

Trotter, E. J., deLahunta, A., Geary, J. C., et al. 1976. Caudal cervical vertebral malformation-malarticulation in Great danes and Doberman pinshcers. JAVMA 168:917–930.

VanGundy, T. E. 1989a. Canine wobbler syndrome. Part 1: pathophysiology and diagnosis. Compend Contin Educ Pract Vet 11:144–158.

———. 1989b. Canine wobbler syndrome part II. Treatment. Compend Contin Educ Pract Vet 11:269–284.

———. 1988. Disc-associated wobbler syndrome in the Doberman pinscher. Vet Clin N Am (Small Anim Pract) 18:667–696.

Wilson, E. R., Aron, D. N., Roberts, R. E. 1994. Observation of a secondary compressive lesion after treatment of caudal cervical spondylomyelopathy in a dog. JAVMA 205:1297–1299.

Lumbosacral Disease

Adams, W. H., Daniel, G. B., Pardo, A. D., Selcer, R. R. 1995. Magnetic resonance imaging of the caudal lumbar and lumbosacral spine in 13 dogs (1990–1993). Vet Radiol Ultrasound 36:3–13.

Bagley, R. S. 2003. Surgical Stabilization of the lumbosacral joint. In Textbook of Small Animal Surgery, 3d ed., Slatter, D., ed. Philadelphia, W. B. Saunders, 1238–1243.

———. 1992. Tremor syndromes in dogs: diagnosis and treatment. J Sm Anim Pract 33:485–490.

Bodner, D. R., Delamarter, R. B., Bohlman, H. H., et al. 1990. Urologic changes after cauda equina compression in dogs. J Urol 143:186–190.

Chambers, J. N. 1989a. Degenerative lumbosacral stenosis in dogs. Vet Med Rep 1:166–189.

———. 1989b. Optimal treatment for degenerative lumbosacral stenosis: surgical exploration and excision of tissue. Vet Med Report 1:248–252.

Chambers, J. N., Barbara, A., Selcer, B. A., et al. 1988. Results of treatment of degenerative lumbosacral stenosis in dogs by exploration and excision. Vet Comp Orthop Trauma 3:130–133.

Chambers, J. N., Selcer, B. A., Butler, T. W., et al. 1994. A comparison of computed tomography to epidurography for the diagnosis of suspected compressive lesions at the lumbosacral junction in dogs. Prog Vet Neurol 5:30–34.

Danielsson, F., Sjöström, L. 1999. Surgical treatment of degenerative lumbosacral stenosis in dogs. Vet Surg 28:91–98.

deHaan, J. J., Shelton, S. B., Ackerman, N. 1993. Magnetic resonance imaging in the diagnosis of degenerative lumbosacral stenosis in four dogs. Vet Surg 22:1–4.

Denny, H. R., Gibbs, C., Holt, P. R. 1982. The diagnosis and treatment of cauda equina lesions in the dog. J Sm An Prac 23:425–443.

Gilmore, D. R. 1987. Lumbosacral diskospondylitis in 21 dogs. J Am Anim Hosp Assoc 23:57–61.

Griffiths, I. R., Carmichael, S., Mayer, S. J., Sharp, N. J. H. 1983. Polyradiculoneuritis in two dogs presenting as neuritis of the cauda equina. Vet Rec 112:360–361.

Hathcock, J. T., Pechman, R. D., Dillon, A. R., et al. 1988. Comparison of three radiographic contrast procedures in the evaluation of the canine lumbosacral vertebral canal. Vet Radiol 29:4–15.

Hurov, L. 1985. Laminectomy for treatment of cauda equina syndrome in a cat. JAVMA 186:504–505.

Indrieri, R. J. 1988. Lumbosacral stenosis and injury of the cauda equina. Vet Clin N Am (Small Anim Pract) 18:697–710.

Jones, J. C., Hudson, J. A., Sorjonen, D. C., Hoffman, C. E., et al. 1996. Effects of experimental nerve root compression on arterial blood flow velocity in the seventh lumbar spinal ganglion of the dog: measurement using intraoperative doppler ultrasonography. Vet Rad Ultrasound 37:133–140.

Jones, J. C., Inzana, K. D. 2000. Subclinical CT abnormalities in the lumbosacral spine of older large-breed dogs. Vet Rad Ultrasound 41:19–26.

Jones, J. C., Shires, P. K., Inzana, K. D., Sponenberg, D. P., et al. 1999. Evaluation of canine lumbosacral stenosis using intravenous contrast-enhanced computed tomography. Vet Rad US 40:108–114.

Jones, J. C., Wright, J. C., Bartels, J. E. 1995. Computed tomographic morphometry of the lumbosacral spine of dogs. Am J Vet Res 56:1125–1132.

Lang, J. 1988. Flexion-extension myelography of the canine cauda equina. Vet Radiol 1988, 29:242–257.

Lenehan, T. M. 1983. Canine cauda equina syndrome. Compend Contin Educ Pract Vet 5:941–951.

Linn, L. L., Bartels, K. E., Rochat, M. C., Payton, M. E., et al. 2003. Lumbosacral stenosis in 29 military working dogs: epidemiologic findings and outcome after surgical intervention (1990–1999). 32:21–29.

Mattoon, J. S., Koblik, P. D. 1993. Quantitative survery radiographic evaluation of the lumbosacral spine of normal dogs and dogs with degenerative lumbosacral stenosis. Vet Rad Ultasound 34:194–206.

McKee, W. M., Mitten, R. W., Labuc, R. H. 1990. Surgical treatment of lumbosacral discospondylitis by a distraction-fusion technique. J Sm Anim Pract 31:15–20.

Morgan, J. P., Bailey, C. S. 1990. Cauda equina syndrome in the dog: radiographic evaluation. J Sm Anim Pract 31:69–77.

Morgan, J. P., Bahr, A., Franti, C. E., Bailey, C. S. 1993. Lumbosacral transitional vertebrae as a predisposing cause of cauda equine syndrome in German Shepherd dogs: 161 cases (1987–1990). JAVMA 202:1877–1882.

Ness, M. G. 1994. Degenerative lumbosacral stenosis in the dog: a review of 30 cases. J Sm Anim Pract 35:185–190.

Oliver, J. E., Selcer, R. R., Simpson, S. 1978. Cauda equina compression from lumbosacral malarticulation and malformation in the dog. JAVMA 1978, 173:207–214.

Palmer, R. H., Chambers, J. N. 1991a. Canine lumbosacral diseases. Part I. Anatomy, pathophysiology, and clinical presentation. Comp Cont Ed 13:61–68.

———. 1991b. Canine lumbosacral diseases. Part II. Diagnosis, treatment, and prognosis. Comp Cont Ed 13:213–221.

Prata, R. G. 1992. Cauda equina syndrome. In Textbook of Small Animal Surgery, 2d ed., Slatter, D. H., ed. Philadelphia, W. B. Saunders, 1094.

Schmid, V., Lang, J. 1993. Measurements of the lumbosacral junction in normal dogs and those with cauda equina compression. J Sm Anim Pract 34:437–442.

Schulman, A. L., Lippincott, C. L. 1988. Canine cauda equina syndrome. Comp Contin Educ Pract Vet 10:835–844.

Sisson, A. F., LeCouteur, R. A., Ingram, J. T., et al. 1992. Diagnosis of cauda equina abnormalities by using electromyography, discography, and epidurography in dogs. J Vet Intern Med 6:253–263.

Slocum, B., Devine, T. 1989. Optimal treatment for degenerative lumbosacral stenosis: traction, internal fixation, and fusion. Vet Med Report 1:249–257.

———. 1986. L7-S1 fixation-fusion for treatment of cauda equina compression in the dog. JAVMA 188:31–35.

Slocum, B., Slocum, T. D. 1992. L7-S1 fixation-fusion for cauda equina compression-An alternative view. In Textbook of Small Animal Surgery, 2d ed., Slatter, D. H., ed. Philadelphia, W. B. Saunders, 1105–1110.

Sjöström, L. 2003. Lumbosacral disorders. In Textbook of Small Animal Surgery, 3d ed., Slatter, D., ed. Philadelphia, W. B. Saunders, 1227–137

Summers, B. A., Cummings, J. F., deLahunta, A. 1995. In Veterinary Neuropathology. St. Louis, Mosby.

Tarvin, G., Prata, R. G. 1980. Lumbosacral stenosis is dogs. JAVMA 177:154–159.

Watt, P. R. 1991. Degenerative lumbosacral stenosis in 18 dogs. J Sm Anim Pract 32:125–134.

Spondylosis

Bagley, R. S., Tucker, R. L. 1996. Specialty board review, neuroradiology. Prog Vet Neuro 7:62

Goldman, A. L. 1992. Hypervitaminosis A in a cat. JAVMA 200:1970–1972.

Langeland, M., Lingaas, F. 1995. Spondylosis deformans in the boxer: estimates of heritability. J Sm Anim Pract 36:166–169.

Larsen, JS, Selby, LA. 1981. Spondylosis deforma in large dogs-relative risk by breed and sex, J Am Anim Hosp Assoc 17: 623–62.

Morgan, J. P., Biery, D. N. 1985. Spondylosis deformans. In Textbook of Small Animal Orthopaedics. Newton, C. D., Nunamaker, D. M., eds. Philadelphia, J. P. Lippincott, 733.

Morgan, J. P., Hansson, K., Miyabayashi, T. 1989. Spondylosis deformans in the female beagle dog: a radiographic study. J Sm An Prac 30:457–460.

Morgan, J. P., Ljunggren, G., Read, R. 1967. Spondyosis deformans (vertebral osteophytosis) in the dog. J Sm Anim Pract 8:57–66.

Morgan, J. P., Stavenborn, M. 1991. Disseminated idiopathic skeletal hyperostosis (DISH) in a dog. Vet Radiology 32:65–70.

Woodard, J. C., Poulos, P. W. J., Parker, R. B., et al. 1985. Canine diffuse idiopathic skeletal hyperostosis. Vet Pathol 22:317–326.

Dural Ossification

Morgan, J. P. 1969. Spinal dural ossification in the dog: incidence and distribution based on a radiographic study. J Am Vet Radiol Soc 10:43–48.

Wilson, J. W., Greene, H. J., Leipold, H. W. 1975. Osseous metaplasia of the spinal dura mater in a Great Dane. JAVMA 167:75–77.

Anomalous Spinal Diseases

Sacrococcygeal Dysgenesis

Deforest, M. E., Basrur, P. K. 1979. Malformations and the Manx syndrome in cats. Can Vet J 20:304–314.

James, C. C., Lassman, L. P., Tomlinson, B. E. 1968. Congenital anomalies of the lower spine and spinal cord in Manx cats. J Pathol 97:269–276.

Leipold, H. W., et al. 1974. Congenital defects of the caudal vertebral column and spinal cord in Manx cats. JAVMA 164: 520–523.

Vertebral Anomalies

Bailey, C. S. 1975. An embryological approach to the clinical significance of congenital vertebral and spinal cord abnormalities. J Am Anim Hosp Assoc 11:426–434.

Done, S. H., Drew, R. A., Robins, G. M., Lane, J. G. 1975. Hemivertebra in the dog: clinical and pathological observations. Vet Rec 96:313–317.

Drew, R. A. 1974. Possible association between abnormal vertebral development and neonatal mortality in bulldogs. Vet Rec 94:480–481.

Kramer, J. W., Schiffer, S. P., Sande, R. D., Rantanen, N. W., et al. 1982. Characterization of heritable thoracic hemivertebra of the German shorthaired pointer. JAVMA 181:814–815.

Morgan, J. P. 1968. Congenital anomalies of the vertebral column of the dog: a study of the incidence and significance based on a radiographic and morphometric study. J Am Vet Radiol Soc 9:21–29.

Spina Bifida

Chesney, C. J. 1973. A case of spina bifida in a Chihuahua. Vet Rec 93:120–121.

Clarke, L., Carlisle, C. H. 1975. Spina bifida with syringomyelia and meningocoele in a short-tailed cat. Aust Vet J 51:392–394.

Fingeroth, J. M,. et al. 1989. Neuroradiographic diagnosis and surgical repair of tethered cord syndrome in an English bulldog with spina bifida and myeloschisis. JAVMA 194:1300–1302.

Frye, F. L., McFarland, L. Z. 1965. Spina bifida with rachischisis in a kitten. JAVMA 146:481–482.

Fumeaux, R. W., Doige, C. E., Kaye, M. M. 1973. Syringomyelia and spina bifida occulta in a Samoyed dog, Can Vet J 14:317–321.

Parker, A. J., Byerly, C. S. 1973. Meningomyelocoele in a dog, Vet Pathol 10:266–273.

Plummer, S. B., Bunch, S. E., Khoo, L. H., Spaulding, K. A., Kornegay, J. N. 1993. Tethered spinal cord and an intradural lipoma associated with a meningocele in a Manx-type cat. JAVMA 203:1159–1161.

McGrath, J. T. 1965. Spinal dysraphism in the dog, Pathol Vet [Suppl] 2:1–36.

Oieb, L. W., Bistner, S. I. 1967. Spinal cord dysraphism in a dog. JAVMA 150:618–620.

Neufeld, I. L., Little, P. B. 1974. Spinal dysraphism in a dalmation dog, Can Vet J 15:335–336.

Shell, L. G., Carrig, C. B., Sponenberg, D. P., Jortner, B. S. 1988. Spinal dysraphism, hemivertebra, and stenosis of the spinal canal in a Rottweiler puppy. J Am Anim Hosp Assoc 24:341–344.

Wilson, J. W., Kurtz, H. J., Leipold, H. W., Lees, G. E. 1979. Spina bifida in the dog, Vet Pathol 16:165–179.

Myelodysplasia

Confer, A. W., Ward, B. C. 1972. Spinal dysraphism: a congenital myelodysplasia in the Weimaraner. JAVMA 160:1423–1426.

Engel, H. N., Draper, D. D. 1982. Comparative prenatal development of the spinal cord in normal and dysraphic dogs: embryonic stage. Am J Vet Res 43:1729–1734.

———. 1982. Comparative prenatal development of the spinal cord in normal and dysraphic dogs: fetal stage. Am J Vet Res 43:1735–1743.

Geib, L. W., Bistner, S. I. 1967. Spinal cord dysraphism in a dog. JAVMA 150:618–620.

McGrath, J. T. 1965. Spinal dysraphism in the dog. With comments on syringomyelia. Pathol Vet 2:Suppl:1– 36.

Rishniw, M., Wilkerson, M. J., deLahunta, A. 1994. Myelodysplasia in an Alaskan Malamute dog with adult onset of clinical signs. Prog Vet Neurol 5:35–38.

Summers, B. A., Cummings, J. F., deLahunta, A. 1995. Malformations of the central nervous system. In Veterinary Neuropathology, Summers, B. A., Cummings, J. F., deLahunta, A., eds. St. Louis, Mosby, 68–94.

Till, K. 1969. Spinal dysraphism. A study of congenital malformations of the lower back. J Bone Joint Surg 51:415–422.

Tomlinson, J., Higgins, R. J., LeCouteur, R. A., Knapp, D. 1988. Intraspinal epidermoid cyst in a dog, JAVMA 193:1435–1436.

Dermoid Sinus

Antin, I. P. 1970. Dermoid sinus in a Rhodesian ridgeback dog. JAVMA 157:961–962.

Fatone, G., Brunetti, A., Lamagna, F., Potena, A. 1995. Dermoid sinus and spinal malformations in a Yorkshire terrier: diagnosis and follow-up. J Sm Anim Pract 36:178–180.

Gammie, J. S. 1986. Dermoid sinus removal in a Rhodesian ridgeback dog. Can Vet J 27:250–251.

Henderson, J. P., Pearson, G. R., Smerdon, T. N. 1993. Dermoid cyst of the spinal cord associated with ataxia in a cat. J Sm Anim Pract 34:402–404.

Hofmeyr, C. F. B. 1963. Dermoid sinus in the ridgeback dog. J Sm Anim Pract 4(suppl):5–8.

Marks, S. M., Harari, J., Dernell, W. S. 1993. Dermoid sinus in a Rhodesian ridgeback. J Sm Anim Pract 34:356–358.

Pratt, J. N., Knottenbelt, C. M., Welsh, E. M. 2000. Dermoid sinus at the lumbosacral junction in an English springer spaniel. J Sm Anim Pract 41:24–26.

Selcer, E. A., Helman, R. G., Selcer, R. R. 1984. Dermoid sinus in a Shih Tzu and a Boxer. J Am Anim Hosp Assoc 20:634–636.

Tshamala, M., Moens, Y. 2000. True dermoid cyst in a Rhodesian ridgeback. J Sm Anim Pract 41:352–353.

Atlantoaxial Subluxation

Bailey, C. S., Morgan, J. P. 1992. Congenital spinal malformations. Vet Clin N Am (Small Anim Pract) 22:985–1015.

Beaver, O. P., Ellison, G. W., Lewis, D. D. 2000. Risk factors affecting the outcome of surgery for atlantoaxial subluxation in dogs: 46 cases (1978–1998). JAVMA 216:1104–1109.

Chambers, J. N., Betts, C. W., Oliver, J. E. 1977. The use of nonmetallic suture material for stabilization of atlantoaxial subluxation. J Am Anim Hosp Assoc 13:602–604.

Cook, J. R., Jr., Oliver, J. E., Jr. 1981. Atlantoaxial luxation in the dog. Compend Contin Educ Pract Vet 3:242–252.

DeCamp, C. E., Schirmer, R. G., Stickle, R. L. 1991. Traumatic atlantooccipital subluxation in a dog. J Am Anim Hosp Assoc 27:415–418.

Denny, H. R., Gibbs, C., Waterman, A. 1988. Atlanto-axial subluxation in the dog: a review of thirty cases and an evaluation of treatment by lag screw fixation. J Sm Anim Pract 29:37–47.

Gage, E. D. 1975. Atlanto-axial subluxation. In Current techniques in small animal surgery, Bojrab, M. J., ed. Philadelphia, Lea & Febiger, 376–383.

Gage, E. D., Hoerlein, B. F. 1973. Surgical repair of cervical subluxation and spondylolisthesis in the dog. J Am Anim Hosp Assoc 9:385–390.

Geary, J. C. 1969. Canine spinal lesions not involving disks. JAVMA 155:2038–2044.

Geary, J. C., Oliver, J. E., Hoerlein, B. F. 1967. Atlanto axial subluxation in the canine. J Sm An Prac 8:577–582.

Gilmore, D. R. 1984. Nonsurgical management of four cases of atlantoaxial subluxation in the dog. J Am Anim Hosp Assoc 20:93–96.

Greenwood, K. M., Oliver, J. E., Jr. 1978. Traumatic atlanto-occipital dislocation in two dogs. JAVMA 173:1324–1327.

Hosgood, G., Toombs, J., Blevins, W. 1989. Traumatic atlantooccipital instability in a dog. Aust Vet Pract 19:88–91.

Jaggy, A., Hutto, V. L., Roberts, R. S., Oliver, J. E. 1991. Occipitoatlantoaxial malformation with atlantoaxial subluxation in a cat. J Sm Anim Pract 32:366–372.

Jeffery, N. D. 1996. Dorsal cross pinning of the atlantoaxial joint: new surgical technique for atlantoaxial subluxation. J Sm An Prac 37:26–9.

Kishigami, M. 1982. Application of an atlantoaxial retractor for atlantoaxial subluxation in the cat and dog. J Am Anim Hosp Assoc 20:413–419.

Ladds, P., Guffy, M., Blauch, B., Splitter, G. 1971. Congenital odontoid process separation in two dogs. J Sm An Prac 12:463–471.

Lappin, M. R., Dow, S. 1983. Traumatic atlanto-occipital luxation in a cat. Vet Surg 12:30–32.

LeCouteur, R. A., McKeown, D., Johnson, J., et al. 1980. Stabilization of atlantoaxial subluxation in the dog, using the nuchal ligament. JAVMA 177:1011–7.

McCarthy, R. J., Lewis, D. D., Hosgood, G. 1995. Atlantoaxial subluxation in dogs. Compend Contin Educ Pract Vet 17:215–227.

Oliver, J. E., Jr., Lewis, P. E. 1973. Lesions of the atlas and axis in dogs, J Am Anim Hosp Assoc 9:304–313.

Parker, A. J., Park, R.D. Atlanto-axial subluxation in small breeds of dogs: diagnosis and pathogenesis. Vet Med Small Anim Clin 68:1133–1137.

Richter, K., Lorenzana, R., Ettinger, S. J. 1983. Traumatic displacement of the dens in a cat: case report. J Am Anim Hosp Assoc 19:751–753.

Read, R. 1987. Instability of the occipito-atlanto-axial joint complex. Aust Vet Pract 17:179–182.

Read, R., Brett, S., Cahill, J. 1987. Surgical treatment of occipito-atlanto-axial malformation in the dog, Aust Vet Pract 17:184–189.

Renegar, W. R., Stoll, S. G. 1979. The use of methylmethacrylate bone cement in the repair of atlantoaxial subluxation stabilization failures—case report and discussion. J Amer An Hospl Assoc 15:313–318.

Sanders, S. G., Bagley, R. S., Silver, G. M. 2000. Complications associated with ventral screws, pins, and polymethylmethacrylate for the treatment of atlantoaxial instability: 8 dogs. J Vet Intern Med 14:339

Schulz, K. S., Waldron, O. R., Fahie, M. 1997. Application of ventral pins and polymethylmethacrylate for the management of atlantoaxial instability: results in nine dogs. Vet Surg 26: 317–325.

Shelton, S. B., Bellah, J. Chrisman, C., McMullen, D. 1991. Hypoplasia of the odontoid process and secondary atlantoaxial luxation in a Siamese cat. Prog Vet Neurol 2:209–211.

Sorjonen, D. C., Shires, P. K. 1981. Atlantoaxial instability: a ventral surgical technique for decompression, fixation, and fusion. Vet Surg 1:22–29.

Thomas, W. B., Sorjonen, D. C., Simpson, S. T. 1991. Surgical management of atlantoaxial subluxation in 23 dogs. Vet Surg 20:409–412.

van Ee, R. T., Pechman, R., van Ee, R. M. 1989. Failure of the atlantoaxial tension band in two dogs. J Am Anim Hosp Assoc 25:707–712.

Watson, A. G. 1979. Congenital occipitoatlantoaxial malformation (OAM) in a dog. Anat Histol Embryol 8:187.

Watson, A. G., deLahunta, A. 1989. Atlantoaxial subluxation and absence of transverse ligament of the atlas in a dog. JAVMA 195:235–237.

Watson, A. G., Hall, M. A., deLahunta, A. 1985. Congenital occipitoatlantoaxial malformation in a cat. Compend Contin Educ Pract Vet 7:245–254.

Watson, A. G., Stewart, J. S. 1990. Postnatal ossification centers of the atlas and axis in miniature schnauzers. Am J Vet Res 51:264–268.

Wheeler, S. J. 1992. Atlantoaxial subluxation with absence of the dens in a Rottweiler. J Sm An Prac 33:90–93.

Wheeler, S. J., Sharp, N. J. H. 1994. Small animal spinal disorders: diagnosis and surgery. London, Mosby-Wolfe, 71–75.

Syringomyelia

Bagley, R. S., Gavin, P. G., Silver, G. M., Moore, M. P., Kippenes, H., Connors, R. 2000. Syringomyelia and Hydromyelia in dogs. Comp Cont Ed 22:471–479.

Bagley, R. S., Harrington, M. L., Tucker, R. L., Sande, R. D., Root, C. R., Kramer, R. W. 1996. Occipital dysplasia and associated cranial spinal cord abnormalities in two dogs. Vet Rad 37:359–362.

Bagley, R. S., Silver, G. M., Seguin, B., Lincoln, J. D., Britt, L. G. 1997. Scoliosis and associated cystic spinal cord abnormality in a dog. JAVMA 211:573–575.

Bone, D. L., Wilson, R. B. 1982. Primary syringomyelia in a kitten. JAVMA 181:928–929.

Cauzinille, L., Kornegay, J. N. 1992. Acquired syringomyelia in a dog. JAVMA 201:1225–1228.

Chauvet, A. E., Darien, D. L., Steinberg, H. 1996. What is your neurological diagnosis? J Vet Med Assoc 208:1387–1389.

Child, G., Higgins, R. J., Cuddon, P. A. 1986. Acquired scoliosis associated with hydromyelia and syringomyelia in two dogs. JAVMA 189:909–912.

Chuma, A., Kitahara, H., Minami S., et al. 1997. Structural scoliosis model in dogs with experimentally induced syringomyelia Spine 22:589–594.

Fumeaux, R. W., Doige, C. E., Kaye, M. M. 1973. Syringomyelia and spina bifida occulta in a Samoyed dog. Can Vet J 14:317–321.

Hida, K., Iwasaki, Y., Koyanagi, I., et al. 1995. Surgical indication and results of foramen magnum decompression versus syringosubarachnoid shunting for syringomyelia associated with Chiari I malformation. Neurosurgery 37:673–678.

Itoh, T., Nishimura, R., Matsunaga, S., et al. 1996. Syringomyelia and hydrocephalus in a dog. JAVMA 209:934–936.

Itoh, T., Nishimura, R., Matsunaga, S., Kadosawa, T., et al. 1996 Syringomyelia and hydrocephalus in a dog. JAVMA 209: 934–936.

Johnson, L., Rolsma, M., Parker, A. 1992. Syringomyelia, hydromyelia and hydrocephalus in two dogs. Prog Vet Neurol 3:82–86.

Kirberger, R. M., Jacobson, L. S., Davies, J. V., Engela, J. Hydromyelia in the dog. 1997. Vet Rad and Ultrasound 38:30–38.

Levy, E. I., Heiss, J. D., Kent, M. S., et al. 2000. Spinal cord swelling preceding syrinx development. J Neurosurg 92:93–97.

Lu, D., Lab, Pfeiffer, D. U., Targett, M. P. 2003. Neurological signs and results of magnetic resonance imaging in 40 cavalier King Charles spaniels with Chiari type1-like malformations. Vet Rec 153:260–263.

Mariani, C., Cislaghi, M. G., Barbieri, S., et al. 1991. The natural history and results of surgery in 50 cases of syringomyelia. J Neurol 238:433–438.

Milhorat, T. H., Capocelli, A. L., Anzil, A. P., Kotsen, R. M., et al. 1995. Pathological basis of spinal cord cavitation in syringomyelia: analysis of 105 autopsy cases. J Neurosurg 82:802–812.

Oldfield, E. H., Muraszko, K., Shawker, T. H., Patronas, N. J. 1994. Pathophysiology of syringomyelia associated with Chiari I malformation of the cerebellar tonsils. J Neurosurg 80:3–15.

Rusbridge, C., Knowler, S. P. 2003. Hereitary aspects of occipital bone hypoplasia and syringomyelia (Chiari type I malformation) in Cavalier King Charles spaniels. Vet Rec 153:107–112.

Rusbridge, C., MacSweeny, J. E., Davies, J. V., et al. 2000. Syringohydromyelia in Cavalier King Charles Spaniels. J Am Anim Hosp Assoc 36:34–41.

Schmahl, W., Kaiser, E. 1984. Hydrocephalus, syringomyelia, and spinal cord angiodysgenesis in a Lhasa-apso dog. Vet Pathol 21:252–254.

Tage, A., Taura, Y., Nakaichi, M., et al. 2000 Magnetic resonance imaging of syringomyelia in five dogs. J Sm An Prac 41:362–365.

Williams B. 1993. Pathogenesis of syringomyelia. Acta Neurochir (Wim) 123:159–165.

———. 1990. Syringomyelia. Neurosurg Clin N Am 1:653–685.

———. 1986. Progress in syringomyelia. Neurol Res 8:130–145.

Scoliosis

Bagley, R. S., Silver, G. M., Seguin, B., Lincoln, J. D., Britt, L. G. 1997. Scoliosis and associated cystic spinal cord abnormality in a dog. JAVMA 211:573–575.

Child, G., Higgins, R. J., Cuddon, P. A. 1986. Acquired scoliosis associated with hydromyelia and syringomyelia in two dogs. JAVMA 189:909–912.

Arachnoid Cysts

Bentley, J. F., Simpson, S. T., Hathcock, J. T. 1991. Spinal arachnoid cyst in a dog. J Am Anim Hosp Assoc 27:549–551.

Cambridge, A. J., Bagley, R. S., Britt, L. G., et al. 1997. Radiographic diagnosis: arachnoid cyst in a dog. Vet Rad Ultrasound 38:434–436.

Dyce, J., Herrtage, M. E., Houlton, J. E. F., Palmer, A. C. 1991. Canine spinal arachnoid cysts. J Sm An Prac 32:433–437.

English, P. B., Seawright, A. A. 1964. Deforming cervical spondylosis of the cat. Aust Vet J 40:376– 381.

Frykman, O. F. 1999. Spinal arachnoid cyst in four dogs: diagnosis, surgical treatment and follow-up results. J Sm Anim Pract 40:544–549.

Gage, E. D., Hoerlein, B. F., Bartels, J. E. 1968. Spinal cord compression resulting from a leptomeningeal cyst in a dog. JAVMA 152:1664–1670.

Galloway, A. M., Curtis, N. C., Sommerlad, S. F., et al. 1999 Correlative imaging findings in seven dogs and one cat with spinal arachnoid cysts. Vet Rad Ultrasound 40:445–452.

Hardie, R. J., Linn, K. A, Rendano, V. T. 1996. Spinal meningeal cyst in a dog: a case report and literature review. J Am Anim Hosp Assoc 32:477–480.

McKee, W. M., Renwick, P. W. 1994. Marsupialisation of an arachnoid cysts in a dog. J Sm An Prac 35:108–11.

Ness, M. G. 1998. Spinal arachnoid cysts in two shih tzu littermates. Vet Rec 142:515–516.

Parker, A. J., Adams, W. M., Zachary, J. F. 1983. Spinal arachnoid cysts in the dog. J Am Anim Hosp Assoc 19:1001–1008.

Parker, A. J., Smith, C. W. 1974. Meningeal cysts in a dog. J Am Anim Hosp Assoc 10:595–597.

Rylander, H., Lipsitz, D., Berry, W. L., Sturges, B. K., et al. 2002. Retrospective analysis of spinal arachnoid cysts in 14 dogs. J Vet Intern Med 16:690–696.

Shamir, M. H., Shahar, R., Aizenberg, I. 1997. Subarchnoid cyst in a cat. J Am Anim Hosp 33:123–125.

Vignoli, M., Rossi, F., Sarli, G. 1999. Spinal subarchnoid cyst in a cat. Vet Rad Ultrasound 40:116–119.

Spinal Tumor

Bagley, R. S., Tucker, R. L. 1996. Specialty Board Review, Neuroradiology. Prog Vet Neurol 7:62

Bailey, C. S. 1990. Long-term survival after surgical excision of a schwannoma of the sixth cervical spinal nerve in a dog. JAVMA 196:754–756.

Bell, F. W., Fenney, D. A., O'Brien, T. J., Caywood, D. D., et al. 1992. External beam radiation therapy for recurrent intraspinal meningioma in a dog. J Am Anim Hosp Assoc 28:318–322.

Bentley, J. F., Simpson, S. T., Hathcock, J. T., Brawner, W. R., Jr., et al. 1990. Metastatic thyroid solid-follicular carcinoma of the cervical portion of the spine of a dog. JAVMA 197:1498–1500.

Blass, C. E., Kirby, B. M., Kreeger, J. M., Gossett, K. A., 1988. Teratomatous medulloepithelioma in the spinal cord of a dog. J Am Anim Hosp Assoc 24:51–54.

Bradley, R. L., Withrow, S. J., Snyder, S. P. 1982. Nerve sheath tumors in the dog. J Am Anim Hosp Assoc 18:915–921.

Brehm, D. M., Vite, C. H., Steinberg, H. S., et al. 1995. A retrospective evaluation of 51 cases of peripheral nerve sheath tumors in the dog. J Am Anim Hosp Assoc 31:349–359.

Byrne, T. N. 1992. Spinal cord compression from epidural metastasis. New Engl J Med 327:614

Clemmons, R. M., Gorman, N. T., Calderwood Mays, M. B. 1983. Lumbar epidural chondrosarcoma in a dog treated by excision and chemotherapy. JAVMA 183:1006–1007.

Cooley, D. M., Waters, D. J. 1998. Skeletal metastasis as the initial clinical manifestation of metastatic carcinoma in 19 dogs. J Vet Intern Med 12:288–93.

Cooley, O. M., Waters, D. L. 1997. Skeletal neoplasms of small dogs: a retrospective study and literature review. J Am Anim Hosp Assoc 33:11–23.

Couto, C. G., Cullen, J., Pedroia, V., et al. 1984. Central nervous system lymphosarcoma in the dog. J Vet Med Assoc 184:809–813.

Dallman, M. I., Saunders, G. K. 1986. Primary spinal cord lymphosarcoma in a dog. JAVMA 189:1348–1349.

deLahunta, A. 1983. Veterinary Neuroanatomy and Clinical Neurology, 2d ed. Philadelphia, W. B. Saunders.

Dernell, W. S., Van Vechten, B. J., Straw, R. C., LaRue, S. M., et al. 2000. Outcome following treatment of vertebral tumors in 20 dogs (1986–1995). J Am Anim Hosp Assoc 36:245–251.

De Vries-Chalmers Hoynk van Paperdrecht, H. R., Vos, J. H., van Nes, J. J. 1988. Spinal cord ependymoma in two young dogs. Vet Quarterly 10:205–210.

Doige, C. E., Pharr, J. W., Withrow, S. J. 1978. Chondrosarcoma arising in multiple cartilagenous exostoses in a dog. J Am Anim Hosp Assoc 14:605–611.

Drost, W. R., Love, N. E., Berry, C. R. 1996. Comparison of radiography, myelography and computed tomography for the evaluation of canine vertebral and spinal cord tumors in sixteen dogs. Vet Rad Ultrasound 37:28–33.

Durán, M. E., Ezquerra, J., Roncero, V., et al. 1992. Acute necrotizing myelopathy associated with a hepatocarcinoma. Prog Vet Neurol 3:35–38.

Ferretti, A., Scanziani, E., Colombo, S. 1993. Surgical treatment of a spinal cord tumor resembling nephroblastoma in a young dog. Prog Vet Neurol 4:84–87.

Fingeroth, J. M., Prata, R. G., Patnaik, A. K. 1987. Spinal meningiomas in dogs: 13 cases (1972–1987). JAVMA 191:720–726.

Gilmore, D. R. 1983. Intraspinal tumors in the dog. Comp Cont Ed 5:55–64.

———. 1983. Neoplasia of the cervical spinal cord and vertebrae in the dog. J Am Anim Hosp Assoc 19:1009–1014.

Irving, G., McMillan, M. C. 1990. Fluoroscopically guided percutaneous fine-needle aspiration biopsy of thoracolumbar spinal lesions in cats. Prog Vet Neurol 1:473–475.

Jeffery, N. D. 1991. Treatment of epidural haemangiosarcoma in a dog. J Sm An Prac 32:359–362.

Jeffery, N. D., Phillips, S. M. 1995. Surgical treatment of intramedullary spinal cord neoplasia in two dogs. J Smal Animal Pract 36:553–557.

Kippenes, H., Gavin, P. R., Bagley, R. S., Silver, G. M., et al. 1999. Magnetic resonance imaging features of tumors of the spine and spinal cord. Vet Rad Ultrasound 40:627–633.

Lane, S. B., Kornegay, J. N. 1991. Spinal Lymphosarcoma. In Consultations in Feline Internal Medicine, August, J. R., ed. Philadelphia, W. B. Saunders, 487.

LeCouteur, R. A. 2001. Tumors of the Nervous System, in Withrow, S. J., MacEwen, E. G., eds., Small Animal Clinical Oncology, 3d ed. Philadelphia, W. B. Saunders, 500–531.

LeCouteur, R. A., Child, G. 1995. Diseases of the spinal cord, In Textbook of Veterinary Internal Medicine: Disease of the Dog and Cat, Ettinger, S. J., Feldman, E. C., eds., 4. Philadelphia, W. B. Saunders, 629–696.

Levy, M. S., Kapatkin, A. S., Patnaik, A. K., et al. 1997. Spinal tumors in 37 dogs: clinical outcome and long-term survival (1987–1994). J Am Anim Hosp Assoc 33:307–312.

Levy, M. S., Mauldin, G., Kapatkin, A. S., et al. 1997. Nonlymphoid vertebral canal tumors in cats: 11 cases (1987–1995). J Am Anim Hosp Assoc 210:663–664.

Lewis, D. D., Kim, D. Y., Paulsen, D. B., Kerwin, S. C. 1991. Extradural spinal liposarcoma in a dog, JAVMA 199: 1606–1607.

Lipsitz, D., Bailey, C. S. 1992. Lateral approach for cervical spinal cord decompression. Prog Vet Neurol 3:39–44.

Long, S. N., Johnston, P. E. J., Anderson, T. J. 2001. Primary T-cell lymphoma of the central nervous system in a dog. JAVMA 218:719–722.

Luttgen, P. J. 1992. Neoplasms of the spine. Vet Clin N Am (Small Anim Pract) 22:973–984.

———. 1990. Spinal neoplasia: diagnosis and treatment. Semin Vet Med Surg (Small Anim) 5:246–252.

Luttgen, P. J., Braund, K. G., Brawner, W. R., Jr., Vandevelde, M. 1980. A retrospective study of twenty-nine spinal tumours in the dogs and cat. J Sm An Prac 21:213–226.

Macpherson, G. C., Chadwick, B. J., Robbins, P. D. 1993. Intramedullary spinal cord metastasis of a primary lung tumour in a dog. J Sm An Prac 34:242–246.

Macri, N. P., Van Alstine, W., Coolman, R. A. 1997. Canine spinal nephroblastoma. J Am Anim Hosp Assoc 33:302–306.

Marks, S. L., Bellah, J. R., Wells, M. 1991. Resolution of quadriparesis caused by cervical tumoral calcinosis in a dog. J Am Anim Hosp Assoc 27:72–76.

McCarthy, R. J., Feeney, D. A., Lipowitz, A. J. 1993. Preoperative diagnosis of tumors of the brachial plexus by use of computed tomography in three dogs. JAVMA 202:291–294.

McEntee, M. C. 1997. Radiation therapy in the management of bone tumors. Vet Clin N Am (Small Anim Pract) 27:131–138.

Moissonnier, P., Abbott, D. P. 1993. Canine neuroepithelioma: case report and literature review. J Am Anim Hosp Assoc 29: 397–401.

Monon, O. 1985. Chondrosarcoma arising in a multilobular chondroma in a cat. JAVMA 186:804–806.

Morgan, J. P., Ackerman, N., Bailey, C. S., et al. 1980. Vertebral tumors in the dog: a clinical, radiologic, and pathologic study of 61 primary and secondary lesions. Vet Radiology 21:197–212.

Morgan, J. P., Ackerman, N., Bailey, C. S., Pool, R. R. 1980. Vertebral tumors in the dog: a clinical radiologic and pathologic study of 61 primary and secondary lesions. Vet Rad Ultrasound 21:197–212.

Ogilvie, G. K., Moore, A. S. 1995. Clinical briefing: tumors of the nervous system. In Managing the Veterinary Cancer Patient: A Practice Manual, Ogilvie, G. K., Moore, G. E., eds. Trenton, NJ, Veterinary Learning Systems, 291–304.

Parker, A. J., Park, R. D. 1974. Successful removal of a spinal cord tumor. Canine Pract 1:35–37.

Platt, S. R., Sheppard, B. J., Graham, J., Uhl, E. W., et al. 1998. Pheochromocytoma in the vertebral canal of two dogs. J Am Anim Hosp Assoc 34:365–371.

Powers, B. E., Beck, E. R., Gillette, E. L., Gould, D. H., et al. 1992. Pathology of radiation injury to the canine spinal cord. Int J Radiation Oncol Biol Phys 23:539–549.

Prata, R. G. 1977. Diagnosis of spinal cord tumors in the dog. Vet Clin N Am (Small Anim Pract) 7:165–185.

Raskin, R. E. 1984. An atypical spinal meningioma in a dog. Vet Pathol 27:538–540.

Reif, U., Lowrie, C. T., Fitzgerald, S. D. 1998. Extradural spinal angiolipoma associated with bone lysis in a dog. J Am Anim Hosp Assoc 34:373–376.

Rosin, A. 1982. Neurologic diseases associated with lymphosarcoma in ten dogs. JAVMA 181:50–53.

Rusbridge, C., Wheeler, S. J., Lamb, C. R., et al. 1999. Vertebral plasma cell tumors in 8 dogs. J Vet Intern Med 13:126–133.

Schueler, R. O., Roush, J. K., Oyster, R. A. 1993. Spinal ganglioneuroma in a dog. J Am Vet Med Assoc 203:539–541.

Schulz, K., Chickering, W. R., Shell, L., et al. 1994. Fluoroscopic-guided and direct spinal cord aspiration in the normal dog. Prog Vet Neurol 5:46–48.

Seigel, S., Kornegay, J. N., Thrall, D. E. 1996. Postoperative irradiation of spinal cord tumors in 9 dogs. Vet Rad Ultrasound 37:150–153.

Seppälä, M. T., Haltia, M. J. J., Sankila, R. J., et al. 1995. Long-term outcome after removal of spinal schwannoma: a clinicopathological study of 187 cases. J Neurosurg 83:621–626.

Shamir, M. H., Lichovsky, D., Aizenberg, I., Chrisman, C. L. 1999. Partial surgical removal of an intramedullary epidermoid cyst from the spinal cord of a dog. J Sm An Practice 40:439–442.

Sharp, N. J. H. 1988. Craniolateral approach to the canine brachial plexus. Vet Surg 17:18–21.

Shell, L, Dallman, M, Sponenburg, P. 1987. Chondrosacroma in a cat presenting with forelimb monoparalysis. Comp Cont Ed 9:391–397.

Spodnick, G. J., Berg, J., Moore, F. M., Cotter, S. M. 1992. Spinal lymphoma in cats: 21 cases (1976–1989). JAVMA 200:373–376.

Steinberg, H. S. 1988. Brachial plexus injuries and dysfunction. Vet Clinic N Amer 18:565–580.

Stoica, G., Tasca, S. I., Kim, H. T. 2001. Point mutation of *neu* oncogen in animal peripheral nerve sheath tumors. Vet Pathol 38:679–688.

Suess, R. P., Jr., Martin, R. A., Shell, L. G., Carrig, C. B., et al. 1990. Vertebral lymphosacroma in a cat. J Am V et Med Assoc 197:101–103.

Summers, B. A., Cummings, J. F., deLahunta, A. 1995. Veterinary Neuropathology, St. Louis:Mosby.

Summers, B. A., deLahunta, A., McEntee, M., Kuhajda, F. P. 1988. A novel intradural extramedullary spinal cord tumor in young dogs. Act Neuropath 75:402–410.

Targett, M. P., Dyce, J., Houlton, J. E. F. 1993. Tumours involving the nerve sheaths of the forelimb in dogs. J Sm An Prac 34:221–225.

Tomlinson, J., Higgins, R. J., LeCouteur, R. A., Knapp, D. 1988. Intraspinal epidermoid cyst in a dog, JAVMA 193:1435–1436.

Turner, J. L., Luttgen, P. J., VanGundy, T. E., et al. 1992. Multicentric osseous lymphoma with spinal extradural involvement in a dog. JAVMA 200:196–198.

Uchida, K., Morozumi, M., Yamaguchi, R., Tateyama, S. 2001. Diffuse leptomeningeal malignant histocytosis in the brain and spinal cord of a Tibetian Terrier. Vet Path 38:219–222.

Umphlet, R. C., Vicini, O. S., Godshalk, C. P. 1989. Intradural-extramedullary lipoma in a dog, Compend Contin Educ Pract Vet 11:1192–1196.

Van Ham, L., van Bree, H., Maenhout, T., Tshamala, M., et al. 1991. Metastatic pilomatrixoma presenting as paraplegia in a dog. J Sm Anim Pract 32:27–30.

Waters, D. J., Hayden, D. W. 1990. Intramedullary spinal cord metastasis in the dog. J Vet Intern Med 4:207–215.

Wright, J. A. 1985. The pathological features associated with spinal tumours in 29 dogs. J Comp Path 95:549–557.

Wright, J. A., Bell, D. A., Clayton-Jones, D. G. 1979. The clinical and radiological features associated with spinal tumours in thirty dogs. J Sm Anim Pract 20:461–472.

Wells, M. Y., Weisbrode, S. E. 1987. Vascular malformations in the thoracic vertebrae of three cats. Vet Pathol 24:360–361.

Yoshioka, M. M. 1987. Meningioma of the spinal cord in a cat. Comp Cont Ed 9:34–38.

Yturraspe, D. J., Lumb, W. V., Young, S., Gorman, H. A. 1975. Neurologic and pathologial effects of second lumbar spondylectomy and spinal column shortening in the dog. J Neurosurg 42:47–58.

Zaki, F. A., Prata, R. G., Hurvitz, A. I., Kay, W. J. 1975. Primary tumors of the spinal cord and meninges in six dogs. JAVMA 166:511–517.

Multiple Cartilaginous Exostoses

Acton, C. E. 1987. Spinal cord compression in young dogs due to cartilaginous exostosis. Calif Vet 41:7–8, 26.

Alexander, J. W. 1983. Selected skeletal dysplasias: craniomandibular osteopathy, multiple cartilaginous exostoses, and hypertrophic osteodystrophy. Vet Clin N Am (Small Anim Pract) 13:55–70.

Banks, W. C., Bridges, C. H. 1956. Multiple cartilaginous exostoses in a dog. JAVMA 129:131–135.

Bhatti, S., Van Ham, L., Putcuyps, De Bosschere, H., et al. 2001. Atlantoaxial cartilaginous exostosis causing spinal cord compression in a mature Bernese mountain dog. J Sm An Prac 42:79–81.

Bichsel, P., Lang, J., Vandevelde, M., Haeni, H. J., et al. 1985. Solitary cartilaginous exostoses associated with spinal cord compression in three large-breed dogs. J Am Anim Hosp Assoc 21:619–622.

Caporn, T. M., Read, R. A. 1996. Osteochondromatosis of the cervical spine causing compressive myelopathy in a dog. J Sm An Prac 37:133–137.

Chester, D. K. 1971. Multiple catilaginous exostoses in two generations of dogs. JAVMA 159:895–897.

Gambardella, P. C., Osborne, C. A., Stevens, J. B. 1975. Multiple cartilaginous exostoses in the dog, J Am Vet Med Assoc 166:761–768.

Gee, B. R., Ooige, C. E. 1970. Multiple cartilaginous exostoses in a litter of dogs. J Vet Med Assoc 156:53–59.

Jacobson, L. S., Kirberger, R. M. 1996. Canine multiple cartilaginous exostoses: unusual manifestations and a review of the literature. J Am Anim Hosp Assoc 32:45–51.

Liu, S. K., Thacher, C. 1990. Case report 622. Multiple cartilaginous exostoses. Skeletal Radial 19:383–385.

Monon, O. 1985. Chondrosarcoma arising in a multilobular chondroma in a cat. JAVMA 186:804–806.

Ooige, C. E. 1987. Multiple cartilaginous exostoses in dogs. Vet Pathol 24:276–278.

Owen, L. N., Bostock, D. E. 1971. Multiple catilaginous exostoses with development of a metastasizing osteosarcoma in a shetland sheepdog. J Sm Aim Pract 12:507–512.

Pool, R. R., Carrig, C. B. 1972. Multiple cartilaginous exostoses in a cat. Vet Path 9:350–359.

Prata, R. A., Stoll, S. O., Zaki, F. A. 1975. Spinal cord compression caused by osteocartilaginous exostoses of the spine in two dogs. JAVMA 166:371–375.

Nutrition

Clark, L. O., Seawright, A. A., Hrdlicka, J. 1970 Exostoses in hypervitaminotic A cats with optimal calcium-phosphorus intakes. J Sm An Prac 11:553–561.

Goldman, A. L. 1992. Hypervitaminosis A in a cat. JAVMA 200:1970–1972.

Lucke, V. M., Baskerville, A., Bardgett, P. L., Mann, P. G. H., et al. 1968. Deforming cervical spondylosis in the cat associated with hypervitaminosis A, Vet Rec 82:141–142.

Palmer, A. C. 1988. Hound ataxia. Vet Rec 122:263.

Palmer, A. C., Medd, R. K., Wilkinson, G. T. 1984. Spinal cord degeneration in hound ataxia. J Sm Anim Pract 25:139–148.

Sheahan, B. J., Caffrey, J. F., Gunn, H. M., et al. 1991. Structural and biochemical changes in a spinal myelinopathy in twelve English foxhounds and two harriers. Vet Pathol 28:117–124.

Idiopathic Spinal Conditions

Calcinosis Circumscripta

Berrocal, A., Tjalsma, E. J., Koeman, J. P. 1992. Calcinosis circumscripta in two cats, Feline Pract 20:9–12.

Bichsel, P., Lang, J., Vandevelde, M., Haeni, H. J., et al. 1985. Solitary cartilaginous exostoses associated with spinal cord compression in three large-breed dogs, J Am Anim Hosp Assoc 21:619–622.

DeRisio, L., Olby, N. May, 2000. Tumoral calcinosis of the thoracic spine: a case report and literature review. Vet Neurol Neurosurg (http://www.neurovet.org/tumoral calcinosis).

Dukes McEwan, J., Thomson, C., Sullivan, M., et al. 1992. Thoracic spinal calcinosis circumscripta causing cord compression in two German shepherd dog littermates. Vet Rec 130:575–578.

Lewis, D. G., Kelly, D. F. 1990. Calcinosis circumscripta in dogs as a cause of spinal ataxia, J Sm An Prac 31:36–38.

Marks, S. L., Bellah, J. R., Wells, M. 1991. Resolution of quadriparesis caused by cervical tumoral calcinosis in a dog. J Am Anim Hosp Assoc 27:72–76

McEwan, J. D., Thomson, C., Sullivan, M., Callanan, S., et al. 1992. Thoracic spinal calcinosis circumscripta causing cord compression in two German shepherd dog littermates, Vet Rec 130:575–578.

Roudebush, P., Maslin, W. R., Cooper, R. C. 1988. Canine tumoral calcinosis, Comp Small Anim 10:1162–1164.

Inflammatory Spinal Conditions

Myelitis

Addie, D. D., Jarrett, A. 1998. Feline coronavirus infection. In Infectious Diseases of the Dog and Cat, 2d ed., Greene, C. E., ed. Philadelphia, W. B. Saunders, 58–69.

Averill, D. R. J., DeLahunta, A. 1971. Toxoplasmosis of the canine nervous system: clinicopathologic findings in four cases. JAVMA 159:1134–1141.

Azuma, Y., Kawamura, K., Isogai, H., et al. 1993. Neurologic abnormalities in two dogs with suspected Lyme disease. Microbiol Immunol 37:325–329.

Bailey, C. S., Higgins, R. J. 1986. Characteristics of cerebrospinal fluid associated with canine granulomatous meningoencephalomyelitis: a retrospective study.JAVMA 188:418–421.

Baroni, M., Heinold, Y. 1995. A review of the clinical diagnosis of feline infectious peritonitis viral meningoencephalomyelitis. Prog Vet Neurol 6:88–94.

Basso, W., Venturini, L., Venturini, M. C., et al. 2001. First isolation of Neospora caninum from the feces of a naturally infected dog. J Parasitol 87:612–618.

Bennett, P. F., Allan, F. J., Guilford, W. G., et al. 1997. Idiopathic eosinophilic meningoencephalitis in rottweiler dogs: three cases (1992–1997). Aust Vet J 75:786–789.

Berg, A-L. 2000. Borna disease in cats. In Kirk's Current Veterinary Therapy XIII (Small Animal Practice), Bonagura, J. D., ed. Philadelphia, W. B. Saunders, 976–978.

Berthelin, C. F., Bailey, C. S., Kass, P. H., et al. 1994. Cryptococcosis of the nervous system in dogs, Part 1: epidemiologic, clinical, and neuropathologic features. Prog Vet Neurol 5:88–97.

Berthelin, C. F., Legendre, A. M., Bailey, C. S., et al. 1994. Cryptococcosis of the nervous system in dogs, Part 2: diagnosis, treatment, monitoring, and prognosis. Prog Vet Neurol 5:136–146.

Bestetti, G., Buhlmann, V., Nicolet, J., Fankhauser, R. 1977. Paraplegia due to Actinomyces viscosus infection in a cat. Acta Neuropathol 39:231–235.

Braund, K. G. 1980. Encephalitis and meningitis. Vet Clin N Am (Small Anim Pract) 10:31–56.

———. 1989. Granulomatous meningoencephalomyelitis. In Kirk's Current Veterinary Therapy X (Small Animal Practice), Kirk, R. W., ed. Philadelphia, W. B. Saunders, 854–858.

Braund, K. G., Vandevelde, M., Walker, T. L., Redding, R. W. 1978. Granulomatous meningoencephalomyelitis in six dogs. JAVMA 172:1195–1200.

Carmichael, K. P., Bienzle, D., McDonnell, J. J. 2002. Feline leukemia virus-associated myelopathy in cats. Vet Pathol 39:536–545.

Cherrone, K. L., Eich, C. S., Bonzynski, J. J. 2002. Suspected paraspinal abscess and spinal epidural empyema in a dog. J Am Anim Hosp Assoc 38:149–151.

Coman, B. J., Jones, E. H., Westbury, H. A. 1981. Protozoan and viral infections of feral cats. Aust. Vet. J. 57:319–323.

Cook, J. R. J., Evinger, J. V., Wagner, L. A. 1991. Successful combination chemotherapy for canine cryptococcal meningoencephalitis. J Am Anim Hosp Assoc 27:61–64.

Cook, J. R. J., Tyler, D. E., Coulter, D. B., Chandler, F. W. 1984. Disseminated protothecosis causing acute blindness and deafness in a dog. JAVMA 184:1266–1272.

Cuddon, P., Lin, D. S., Bowman, D. D., et al. 1992. Neospora caninum infection in English Springer Spaniel littermates. Diagnostic evaluation and organism isolation. J Vet. Intern. Med. 6:325–332.

Cummings, J. F., deLahunta, A., Suter, M. M., Jacobson, R. H. 1988. Canine protozoan polyradiculoneuritis, Acta Neuropathol 76:46–54.

Davidson, M. G. 2000. Toxoplasmosis. Vet Clin N Am (Small Anim Pract) 30:1051–1062.

Day, M. J. 1998a. Canine disseminated aspergillosis. In Infectious Diseases of the Dog and Cat, 2d ed., Greene, C. E., ed. Philadelphia, W. B. Saunders. 409–412.

———. 1998b. Feline disseminated aspergillosis. In Infectious Diseases of the Dog and Cat, 2d ed., Greene, C. E., ed. Philadelphia, W. B. Saunders, 412–413.

Dewey, C. W., Kortz, G. D., Bailey, C. S. 1998. Spinal empyema in two dogs. J Am Anim Hosp 34:305–308.

Dougherry, S. A., Center, S. A., Shaw, E. E. et al. 1991. Juvenile-onset polyarthritis syndrome in Akitas. JAVMA 198:849–856.

Dow, S. W., Poss, M. L., Hoover, E. A. 1990. Feline immunodeficiency virus: a neurotropic lentivirus. J Acquir Immun Disease Syndr 3:658–668.

Dubey, J. P. 1992. *Neospora caninum* infections. In Current Veterinary Therapy XI (Small Animal Practice), Kirk, R. W., Bonagura, J. D., eds. Philadelphia, W. B. Saunders, 263–266.

———. 1990. *Neospora caninum:* a look at a new toxoplasma-like parasite of dogs and other animals. Compend Contin Educ 12:653–661.

Dubey, J. P., Carpenter, J. L. 1993. Histologically confirmed clinical toxoplasmosis in cats: 100 cases (1952–1990). JAVMA 203:1556–1566.

———. 1993. Unidentified Toxoplasma-like tissue cysts in the brains of three cats. Vet Parasitol 45:319–321.

Dubey, J. P., Carpenter, J. L., Speer, C. A., et al. 1988. Newly recognized fatal protozoan disease of dogs. JAVMA 192:1269–1285.

Dubey, J. P., Fenner, W. R. 1992. Clinical segmental myelitis associated with an unidentified Toxoplasma-like parasite in a cat. J Vet Diagn Invest 5:472–480.

Dubey, J. P., Higgins, R. J., Barr, B. C., et al. 1994. Sarcocystis-associated meningoencephalomyelitis in a cat. J Vet Diagn Invest 6:118–120.

Dubey, J. P., Lappin, M. R. 1998. Toxoplasmosis and neosporosis. In Infectious Diseases of the Dog and Cat, 2d ed., Greene, C. E., ed. Philadelphia, W. B. Saunders, 493–509.

Dubey, J. P., Lindsay, D. S. 1996. A review of Neospora caninum and neosporosis. Vet. Parasitol 67:1–59.

———. 1990. Neosporosis in dogs. Vet Parasitol 36:147–151.

Dubey, J. P., Lindsay, O. S., Lipscomb ,T. P. 1990. Neosporosis in cats. Vet Pathol 27:335–339

Edwards, D. F., Nyland, T. G., Weigel, J. P. 1988. Thoracic, abdominal, and vertebral actinomycosis, J Vet Intern Med 2:184–191.

Fenner, W. R. 1998. Central nervous system infections. In Infectious Diseases of the Dog and Cat, 2d ed., Greene, C. E., ed. Philadelphia, W. B. Saunders, 647–657.

Foil, C. S. 1998. Miscellaneous fungal infections. In Infectious Diseases of the Dog and Cat, 2d ed., Greene, C. E., ed. Philadelphia, W. B. Saunders, 420–430.

Foley, J. E., Lapointe, J. M., Koblik, P., et al. 1998. Diagnostic features of clinical neurologic feline infectious peritonitis.J Vet Intern Med 12:415–423.

Gerds-Grogan, S., Dayrell-Hart, B. 1997. Feline cryptococcosis: a retrospective evaluation. J Am Anim Hosp Assoc 33:118–122.

Glass, E. N., Cornetta, A. M., DeLahunta, A., et al. 1998. Clinical and clinicopathologic features in 11 cats with Cuterebra larvae myiasis of the central nervous system. J Vet Intern Med 12:365–368.

Greene, R. T. 1998. Coccidioidomycosis. In Infectious Diseases of the Dog and Cat. 2d ed, Greene, C. E., ed. Philadelphia, W. B. Saunders, 391–398.

Greene, C. E. 1998a. Feline panleukopenia. In Infectious Diseases of the Dog and Cat, 2d ed., Greene, C. E., ed. Philadelphia, W. B. Saunders, 52–57.

———. 1998b. Protothecosis. In Infectious Diseases of the Dog and Cat, 2d ed., Greene, C. E., ed. Philadelphia, W. B. Saunders, 430–435.

Greene, C. E., Appel, M. J. 1998. Canine distemper. In Infectious Diseases of the Dog and Cat, 2d ed., Greene, C. E., ed. Philadelphia, W. B. Saunders, 9–22.

Greene, C. E., Appel, M. J., Straubinger, R. K. 1998. Lyme Borreliosis. In Infectious Diseases of the Dog and Cat, 2d ed. Greene, C. E ed. Philadelphia, W. B. Saunders, 282–293.

Greene, C. E., Burgdorfer, W., Cavagnolo, R., Philip, R. N., Peacock, M. G. 1985. Rocky Mountain spotted fever in dogs and its differentiation from canine ehrlichiosis. JAVMA 186:465–472.

Greene, C. E., Cook, J. R.. Jr., Mahaffey, E. A. 1985. Clindamycin for treatment of toxoplasma polymyositis in a dog. JAVMA 187:631–634.

Gunn-Moore, D., Harbour, D. A. 2001. Feline spongiform encephalopathies and Borna disease. In Consultatiom in Feline Internal Medicine, 4th ed., August, J. R., ed. Philadelphia, W. B. Saunders, 62–70.

Harvey, J. W. 1998. Canine thrombocytic Ehrlichiosis. In Infectious Diseases of the Dog and Cat, 2d ed., Greene, C. E., ed. Philadelphia, W. B. Saunders, 147–149.

Hass, J. A., Shell, L., Saunders, G. 1989. Neurological manifestations of Toxoplasmosis: a literature review and case summary. J Am Anim Hosp Assoc 25:253–260.

Heidel, J. R., Dubey, J. P., Blythe, L. L., Walker, L. L., et al. 1990. Myelitis in a cat infected with Toxoplasma gondii and feline immunodeficiency virus. JAVMA 196:316–318.

Hess, P. R., Sellon, R. K. 1997. Steroid-responsive, cervical pyogranulomatous pachymeningitis in a dog. J Am Anim Hosp Assoc 33:461–468.

Imes, G. D., Lloyd, J. C., Brightman, M. P. 1977. Disseminated protothecosis in a dog. Onderstepoort. J Vet Res. 44:1–6.

Irwin, P. J., Parry, B. W. 1999. Streptococcal meningoencephalitis in a dog. J Am Anim Hosp Assoc 35:417–422.

Jacobs, G. J., Medleau, L. 1998. Cryptococcosis. In Infectious Diseases of the Dog and Cat, 2d ed., Greene, C. E., ed. Philadelphia, W. B. Saunders, 383–390.

Jerram, R. M., Dewey, C. W. 1998. Suspected spinal epidural empyema and associated vertebral osteomyelitis (physitis) in a dog. J Vet Emerg Crit Care 8:216–221.

Kerwin, S. C., McCarthy, R. J., VanSteenhouse, J. L., et al. 1998. Cervical spinal cord compression caused by cryptococcosis in a dog: successful treatment with surgery and fluconazole. J Am Anim Hosp Assoc 34:523–526.

Kipar, A., Baumgartner, W., Vogl, C., et al. 1998. Immunohistochemical characterization of inflammatory cells in brains of dogs with granulomatous meningoencephalitis. Vet Pathol 35:43–52.

Kline, K. L., Joseph, R. J., Averill, D. R. 1994. Feline infectious peritonitis with neurologic involvement: clinical and pathological findings in 24 cats. J Am Anim Hosp Assoc 30:111–118.

Lappin, M. R. 1989. Feline Toxoplasmosis. In Kirk's Current Veterinary Therapy X (Small Animal Practice), Kirk, R. W., ed. Philadelphia, W. B. Saunders, 1112–1115.

Lappin, M. R., Greene, C. E., Prestwood, A. K., Dawe, D. L., Tarleton, R. L. 1989. Diagnosis of recent Toxoplasma gondii infection in cats by use of an enzyme-linked immunosobent assay for immunoglobulin M. Am J Vet Res 50:580–1585.

Legendre, A. M. 1998. Blastomycosis. In Infectious Diseases of the Dog and Cat, 2d ed., Greene, C. E., ed. Philadelphia, W. B. Saunders, 371–377.

Legendre, A. M., Whitenack, D. L. 1975. Feline infectious peritonitis with spinal cord involvement in two cats, JAVMA 167:931–932.

Lindsay, D. S., Dubey, J. P., McAllister, M. 1999. Neospora caninum and the potential for parasite transmission. Compend Contin Educ Pract Vet 21:317–321.

Lundgren, A. L., Ludwig, H. 1993. Clinically diseased cats with nonsuppurative meningoencephalitis have Borna disease virus-specific antibodies. Act Vet Scand 34:101–103.

Luttgen, P. J., Crawley, R. R. 1981. Posterior paralysis caused by epidural dirofilariasis in a dog. J Am Anim Hosp Assoc 17:57–59.

Mandel, N. S., Senker, E. G., Schneider, E. M., et al. 1993. Intrathecal production of Borrelia burgdorferi- Specific antibodies in a dog with central nervous system Lyme Boreliosis. Compend Contin Educ Pract Vet 15:581–586.

Maretzki, C. H., Fisher, D. J., Greene, C. E. 1994. Granulocytic ehrlichiosis and meningitis in a dog. JAVMA :1554–1556.

Mayhew, I. G., Smith, K. C., Dubey, J. P., et al. 1991. Treatment of encephalomyelitis due to Neospora caninum in a litter of puppies. J Sm An Prac 32:609–612.

Meric, S. M. 1992. Breed-specific meningitis in dogs. In Current Veterinary Therapy XI (Small Animal Practice), Kirk, R. W., ed. Philadelphia, W. B. Saunders, 1007–1009.

———. 1988. Canine meningitis. A changing emphasis. J Vet Intern Med 2:26–35.

Moore, F. M., Schmidt, G. M., Desai, D., et al. 1985. Unsuccessful treatment of disseminated protothecosis in a dog. JAVMA 186:705–708.

Munana, K. R. 1996. Encephalitis and meningitis. Vet Clin N Am (Small Anim Pract) 26:857–874.

Munana, K. R., Luttgen, P. J. 1998. Prognostic factors for dogs with granulomatous meningoencephalomyelitis: 42 cases (1982–1996). JAVMA 212:1902–1906.

Ndikuwera, J., Knottenbelt, D. C., Lawrence, J., Hill, F. W. G. 1987. Spinal abscess in a dog, Vet Rec 120:554–555.

Nesbit, J. W., Lourens, D. C., Williams, M. C. 1981. Spastic paresis in two littermate pups caused by Toxoplasma gondii. J S Afr Vet Assoc 52:243–246.

O'Toole, T. E., Sata, A. F., Rozanski, E. A. 2003. Cryptococcsis in the central nervous system in a dog. JAVMA 222:1722–1725.

Pedersen, N. C., Ho, E. W., Brown, M. L., et al. 1987. Isolation of a T-lymphotropic virus from domestic cats with an immunodeficiency-like syndrome. Science 235:790–793.

Pedersen, N. C., Yamamoto, J. K., Ishida, T., et al. 1989. Feline immunodeficiency virus infection. Vet Immunol Immunopathol 21:111–129.

Phillips, T. R., Prospero-Garcia, O., Puaoi, D. L., et al. 1994. Neurological abnormalities associated with feline immunodeficiency virus infection. J Gen Viro 175:979–987.

Poncelet, L. O., Balligand, M. 1993. Steroid responsive meningitis in three boxer dogs. Vet Rec 132:361–362.

Radaelli, S. T., Platt, S. R. 2002. Bacterial meningoencephalitis in dogs: a retrospective study of 23 cases (1990–1999). J Vet Intern Med 16:159–163.

Rand, J. S., Parent, J., Percy, D., et al. 1994. Clinical, cerebrospinal fluid, and histological data from twenty-seven cats with primary inflammatory disease of the central nervous system. Can Vet J 35:103–110.

Ryan, K., Marks, S. L., Kerwin, S. C. 2001. Granulomatous meningoencephalomyelitis in dogs. Compend Contin Educ Pract Vet 23:644–650.

Schultte, A. E., Cribb, A. E., Tvedten, H. W. 1986.Eosinophilic meningoencephalitis in a cat. J Am Anim Hosp Assoc 22:623–627.

Scott-Moncrieff, J. C., Snyder, P. W., Glickman, L. T., et al. 1992. Systemic necrotizing vasculitis in nine young beagles. JAVMA 201:1553–1558.

Sellon, R. K. 1998. Feline immunodeficiency virus infection. In Infectious Diseases of the Dog and Cat, 2d ed., Greene, C. E., ed. Philadelphia, W. B. Saunders, 84–96.

Sharp, N., Vitek, S., Steingold, S., et al. 2000. A rapid, antemortem diagnostic test for canine distemper virus. J Vet Intern Med 14:342.

Smith-Maxie, L. L., Parent, J. P., Rand, J., et al. 1989. Cerebrospinal fluid analysis and clinical outcome of eight dogs with eosinophilic meningoencephalomyelitis. J Vet Intern Med 3:167–174.

Sorjonen, D.C., Cox, N.R., Swango, L.J. 1989. Electrophoretic determination of albumin and gamma globulin concentrations in cerebrospinal fluid of dogs with encephalomyelitis attributable to canine distemper virus infection: 13 cases (1980–1987). JAVMA 195:977–980.

Stowater, J. L., Codner, E. C., McCoy, J. C. 1978. Actinomycosis in the spinal canal of a cat. Feline Pract 8:26–27.

Thomas, J. B., Eger, C. 1989. Granulomatous meningoencephalomyelitis in 21 dogs. J Sm Anim Pract 30:287–293.

Thomas, J. B., Preston, N. 1990. Generalised protothecosis in a collie dog. Aust Vet J 67:25–27.

Thomas, J. S. 1988. Encephalomyelitis in a dog caused by Baylisascaris infection. Vet Pathol 25:94–95.

Thomas, W. B., Sorjonen, D. C., Steiss, J. E. 1993. A retrospective evaluation of 38 cases of canine distemper encephalomyelitis. J Am Anim Hosp Assoc 29:129–133.

Tipold, A. 1995. Diagnosis of inflammatory and infectious diseases of the central nervous system in dogs: a retrospective study. J Vet Intern Med 9:304–314.

Tipold, A., Jaggy, A. 1994. Steroid responsive meningitis-arteritis in dogs: long-term study of 32 cases. J Sm Anim Pract 35:311–316.

Tipold, A., Vandevelde, M., Zurbriggen, A. 1995. Neuroimmunological studies in steroid-responsive meningitis arteritis in dogs. Res Vet Sci 58:103–108.

Uggla, A., Dubey, J. P., Lundmark, G., et al. 1989. Encephalomyelitis and myositis in a boxer puppy due to a Neospora-like infection. Vet Parasitol 32:255–260.

Vandevelde, M. 1998. Neurologic diseases of suspected infectious origin. In Infectious Diseases of the Dog and Cat, 2d ed., Greene, C. E., ed. Philadelphia, W. B. Saunders, 530–539.

Vandevelde. M., Braund, K. G. 1979. Polioencephalomyelitis in cats. Vet Pathol 16:420–427.

Vandevelde, M., Cachin, M. 1992. The neurologic form of canine distemper. In Kirk's Current Veterinary Therapy XI (Small Animal Practice), Kirk, R. W., Bonagura, J. D., ed. Philadelphia, W. B. Saunders, 1003–1007.

Vandevelde, M., Zurbriggen, A., Higgins, R. J., et al. 1985. Spread and distribution of viral antigen in nervous canine distemper. Acta Neuropathol (Berl) 67:211–218.

Wolf, A. M. 1998. Histoplasmosis. In Infectious Diseases of the Dog and Cat, 2d ed., Greene, C. E., ed. Philadelphia, W. B. Saunders, 378–383.

Zurbriggen, A., Vandevelde, M. 1994. The pathogenesis of nervous distemper. Prog Vet Neurol 5:109–116.

Diskospondylitis

Bennett, D., Carmichael, S., Griffiths, I. R. 1981. Discospondylitis in the dog, J Sm Anim Pract 22:539–547.

Carpenter, J. L., Myers, A. M., Conner, M. W., Schelling, S. H., et al. 1988. Tuberculosis in five basset hounds, JAVMA 192:1563–1568.

Dallman, M. J., Dew, T. L., Tobias, L., Doss, R., et al. 1992. Disseminated aspergillosis in a dog with diskospondylitis and neurological deficits. JAVMA 200:511–513.

Davis, M. J., Dewey, C. W., Walker, M. A., et al. 2000. Contrast radiographic findings in canine bacterial discospondylitis: a multicenter, retrospective study of 27 cases. J Am Anim Hosp Assoc 36:82–85.

Gilmore, D. R. 1987. Lumbosacral diskospondylitis in 21 dogs. J Am Anim Hosp Assoc 23:57– 61.

Henderson, R. A., Hoerlein, B. F., Kramer, T. T., Meyer, M. E. 1974. Discospondylitis in three dogs infected with Brucella canis. JAVMA 165:451–455.

Hurov, L., Troy, G., Turnwald, G. 1978. Diskospondylitis in the dog: 27 cases. JAVMA 173:275–281.

Johnson, D. E., Summers, B. A. 1971. Osteomyelitis of the lumbar vertebrae in dogs caused by grass-seed foreign bodies. Aust Vet J 47:289–294.

Johnson, K. A. 1995. Treatment of osteomyelitis, discospondylitis, and septic arthritis. In Kirk's Current Veterinary Therapy XII (Small Animal Practice), Kirk, R. W., Bonagura J. D., eds. Philadelphia, W. B. Saunders, 1200–1204.

Johnson, R. G., Prata, R. G. 1983. Intradiskalosteomyelitis: a conservative approach, J Am Anim Hosp Assoc 19:743–750.

Kerwin, S. C., Lewis, D. D., Hribernik, T. N., Partington, B., et al. 1992. Diskospondylitis associated with Brucella canis infection in dogs: 14 cases (1980–1991). J Am Vet Med Asso 201:1253–1257.

Kornegay, J. N. 1992. Discospondylitis. In Textbook of Small Animal Surgery, 2d ed., Slatter, D., ed. Philadelphia, W. B. Saunders, 1087.

Kornegay, J. N., Barber, D. L. 1980. Diskospondylitis in dogs. JAVMA 177:337–341.

LaCroix, J. A. 1973. Vertebral body osteomyelitis: a case report, Am Vet Radiol J 14:17–21.

Lobetti, R. G. 1994. Subarachnoid abscess as a complication of discospondylitis in a dog. J Sm Anim Pract 35:480–483.

Malik, R., Latter, M., Love, D. N. 1990. Bacterial discospondylitis in a cat. J Sm An Prac 31:404–406.

Norsworthy, G. D. 1979. Discospondylitis as a cause of posterior paresis. Feline Pract 9:39–40.

Patnaik, A. K., Liu, S. K., Wilkins, R. J., Johnson, G. F. 1972. Paecilomycosis in a dog. JAVMA 161:806–813.

Turnwald, G. H., Shires, P. K., Turk, M. A., Cox, H. U. 1986. Diskospondylitis in a kennel of dogs: clinicopathologic findings. JAVMA 188:178–183.

Watson, E., Roberts, R. E. 1993. Discospondylitis in a cat. Vet Rad 34:397–398.

Wood, G. L., Hirsh, D. C., Selcer, R. R., Rinaldi, M. G. 1978. Disseminated aspergillosis in a dog. JAVMA 172:704–707.

Trauma

Bagley, R. S. 2000a. Exogenous spinal trauma: surgical therapy and aftercare. Comp Cont Ed 22:218–230.

———. 2000b. Spinal fracture or luxation. Vet Clinic North America 30:133–153.

———. 1999. Exogenous spinal trauma. Clinical assessment and clinical management. Comp Cont Ed 21:1138–1144.

Basinger, R. R., Bjorling, D. E., Chambers, J. N. 1986. Cervical spinal luxation in two dogs with entrapment of the cranial articular process of C6 over the caudal articular process of C5. JAVMA 188:865–867.

Berg, R. J., Rucker, N. C. 1985. Pathophysiology and medical management of acute spinal cord injury. Comp Cont Ed 7:646–653.

Bergman, R., Lanz, O., Shell, L. 2000. A review of experimental and clinical treatments for acute spinal cord injury. Vet Med (November):855–866.

Blass, C. E., Waldron, D. R., van Ee, R. T. 1988. Cervical stabilization in three dogs using Steinmann pins and methylmethacrylate. J Am Anim Hosp Assoc 24:61–68.

Bracken, M. B., Shepard, M. J., Collins, W. F., Holford, T. R., et al. 1990. A randomized controlled study of methylprednisolone or naloxone in the treatment of acute spinal-cord injury. New Eng J Med 322:1405–1411.

Bracken, M. B., Shepard, M. J., Collins, W. F., Jr., Holford, T. R., et al. 1992. Methylprednisolone or naloxone treatment after acute spinal cord injury: 1-year follow-up data. J Neurosurg 76:23–31.

Braund, K. G., Shores, A., Brawner, W. R. 1990. The etiology, pathology and pathophysiology of acute spinal trauma. Vet Med 85:684–681.

Chiles, B. W., Cooper, P. R. 1996. Acute spinal injury. N Engl J Med 334:514–520.

Coughlan, A. R. 1993. Secondary injury mechanisms in acute spinal cord trauma. J Sm Anim Pract 34:117–122.

Harrington, M. L., Bagley, R. S. 1998. Realignment of lumbosacral fracture/luxations in two dogs using a Senn retractor. J Am Anim Hosp Assoc 34:377–380.

Hawthorne, J. C., Blevins, W. E., Wallace, L. J., et al. 1999. Cervical vertebral fractures in 56 dogs: a retrospective study. J Am Anim Hosp Assoc 35:135–146.

Hoerlein, B. F., Redding, R. W., Hoff, E. J., McGuire, J. A. 1985. Evaluation of Naloxone, Crocetin, Thyrotropin releasing hormone, methylprednisolone, partial myelotomy, and hemilaminectomy in the treatment of acute spinal cord trauma. J Am Anim Hosp Assoc. 21:67–77.

Janssens, L. A. A. 1991. Mechanical and pathophysiological aspects of acute spinal cord trauma. J Sm Anim Pract 32:572–578.

Kraus, K. H. 1996. The pathophysiology of spinal cord injury and its clinical implications. Semin Vet Med Surg (Small Anim) 11:201–207.

Matthiesen, D. T. 1983. Thoracolumbar spinal fractures/luxations: surgical management. Compend Contin Educ Pract Vet 5:867–878.

McKee, W. M. 1990. Spinal trauma in dogs and cats: a review of 51 cases. Vet Rec 126:285–289.

Meintjes, E., Hosgood, G., Daniloff, J. 1996. Pharmaceutic treatment of acute spinal cord trauma. Compend Contin Educ Pract Vet 18:625–636.

Olby, N. 1999. Current concepts in the management of acute spinal cord injury. J Vet Intern Med 13:399–407.

Quencer, R. M., Bunge, R. P. 1996. The injured spinal cord: imaging, histopathologic, clinical correlates, and basic science approaches to enhancing neural function after spinal injury. Spine 21:2064–2066.

Rucker, N. C. 1990. Management of spinal cord trauma. Prog Vet Neurol 1:397–412.

Selcer, R. R., Bubb, W. J., Walker, T. L. 1991. Management of vertebral column fractures in dogs and cats: 211 cases (1977–1985). JAVMA 198:1965–1968.

Siemering, G. B. 1992. High dose methylprednisolone sodium succinate: an adjunct to surgery for canine intervertebral disc herniation. Scientific meeting abstracts, ACVS, 406.

Shires, P. K., Waldron, D. R., Hedlund, C. S., et al. 1991. A biomechanical study of rotational instability in unaltered and surgically altered canine thoracolumbar vertebral motion units. Prog Vet Neurol 2:6–14.

Shores, A. 1992. Spinal trauma. Pathophysiology and management of traumatic spinal injuries. Vet Clin N Am (Small Anim Pract) 22:859–888.

Shores, A., Braund, K. G., Brawner, W. R., Jr. 1990. Management of acute spinal cord trauma. Vet Med 85:724–739.

Turner, W. D. 1987. Fractures and fracture-luxations of the lumbar spine: a retrospective study in the dog. J Am Anim Hosp Assoc 23:460–464.

Waldron, D. R., Shires, P. K., McCain, W., Hedlund, C., Blass, C. E. 1991. The rotational stabilizing effect of spinal fixation techniques in an unstable vertebral model. Prog Vet Neurol 2:105–110.

Vascular Spinal Conditions

Fibrocartilagenous Emboli

Cauzinille, L., Kornegay, J. N. 1996. Fibrocartilaginous embolism of the spinal cord in dogs: review of 36 histologically confirmed cases and retrospective study of 26 suspected cases. J Vet Intern Med 10:241

Cook, J. R. J. 1988. Fibrocartilaginous embolism. Vet Clin N Am (Small Anim Pract) 18:581–592.

Doige, C. E., Parent, J. M. 1983. Fibrocartilaginous embolism and ischemic myelopathy in a four month old German shepherd dog, Can J Comp Med 47:499–500.

Dyce, J., Houlton, J. E. F. 1993. Fibrocartilaginous embolism in the dog. J Sm Anim Pract 34:332–336.

Gandini, G., Cizinauskas, S., Lang, J., et al. 2003. Fibrocartilaginous embolism in 75 dogs: clinical findings and factors influencing the recovery rate. J Sm Anim Pract 44:76–80.

Gaschen, L., Lang, J., Haeni, H. 1995. Intravertebral disc herniation (Schmorl's Node) in five dogs. Vet Rad Ultrasound 36:509–516.

Gilmore, D. R., deLahunta, A. 1987. Necrotizing myelopathy secondary to presumed or confirmed fibrocartilaginous embolism in 24 dogs, J Am Anim Hosp Assoc 23:373–376.

Greene, C. E., Higgins, R. J. 1976. Fibrocartilaginous emboli as the cause of ischemic myelopathy in a dog. Cornell Vet 66:131–142.

Griffiths, I. R. 1973. Spinal cord infarction due to emboli arising from the intervertebral discs in the dog. J Comp Pathol 83:225–232.

Hawthorne, J. C., Wallace, L. J., Fenner, R. W., et al. 2001. Fibrocartilaginous embolic myelopathy in Miniature Schnauzers. J Am Anim Hosp Assoc 37:374–383.

Hay, C. W., Muir, P. 2000. Tearing of the dura mater in three dogs. Vet Rec 146:279–282.

Hayes. M. A. 1978. Acute necrotizing myelopathy from nucleus pulposus embolism in dogs with intervertebral disk degeneration, JAVMA 169:289–295.

Neer, T. M. 1992. Fibrocartilaginous emboli. Vet Clin N Am (Small Anim Pract) 22:1017–1026.

Sanders, S., Bagley, R. S., Tucker, R. L., Nelson, N. 1999. Focal spinal cord malacia in a cat. Vet Rad 40:122–125.

Scott, H. W., O'Leary, M. T. 1996. Fibrocartilaginous embolism in a cat. J Sm Anim Pract 37:228–231.

Yarrow, T. G., Jeffery, N. D. 2000. Dura mater laceration associated with acute paraplegia in three dogs. Vet Rec 146:138–139.

Zaki, F. A., Prata, R. G. 1976. Necrotizing myelopathy secondary to embolization of herniated intervertebral disk material in the dog. JAVMA 169:222–228.

Zaki, F. A., Prata, R. G., Kay, W. J. 1974. Necrotizing myelopathy in five great Danes. JAVMA 165:1080–1084.

Zaki, F. A., Prata, R. G., Werner, L. L. 1976. Necrotizing myelopathy in a cat. JAVMA 169:228–229.

Spinal Hemorrhage

Applewhite, A. A., Wilkens, B. E., McDonald, D. E., Radasche, R. M., Barstad, R. D. 1999. Potential central nervous system complications of Von Willebrand's disease. J Am Anim Hosp Assoc 35, 423–429.

Martin, R. A., Shell, L. G., Dodds, W. J. 1986. Spinal cord hematoma. J Am Anim Hosp Assoc 22:545–550.

Stokol, T., Parry, B. W., Mansell, P. D., Richardson, J. L. 1994. Hematorrhachis associated with hemophilia A in three German Shepherd dogs. J Am Anim Hosp Assoc 30:239–243.

Withrow, S. J., Doige, C. E. 1979. Subperiosteal vertebral hematoma as a cause of acute paraplegia in two dogs. J Am Anim Hosp Assoc 15:295–299.

Diseases of the Peripheral Nerves, Neuromuscular Junction, and Muscle

Nerve and Muscle Biopsy

Braund, K. G. 1991. Nerve and muscle biopsy techniques. Prog Vet Neurol 2:35.

Degenerative Diseases

Degenerative Neuropathies

Blakemore, W. F., Mitten, R. W., Palmer, A. C., et al. 1974. Value of a nerve biopsy in diagnosis of globoid cell leucodystrophy in the dog. Vet Rec 94:70–71.

Braund, K. G. 1996a. Degenerative causes of neuropathies in dogs and cats. Vet Med 91:722–739.

———. 1996b. Endogenous causes of neuropathies in dogs and cats. Vet Med 91:740–754.

———. 1996c. Idiopathic and exogenous causes of neuropathies in dogs and cats. Vet Med 91:755–769.

———. 1995a. Laryngeal paralysis-polyneuropathy complex in young Dalmatian dogs. In Kirk's Current Veterinary Therapy XII (Small Animal Practice), Bonagura, J. D., ed. Philadelphia, W. B. Saunders, 1136–1140.

———. 1995b. Peripheral nerve disorders, In Textbook of Veterinary Internal Medicine. Diseases of the Dog and Cat, 4th ed., Ettinger, S. J., Feldman, E. C., eds. Philadelphia, W. B. Saunders, 701–726.

———. 1987. Degenerative and developmental diseases. In Veterinary Neurology, Oliver, J.E., Jr., Hoerlein, B.F., and Mayhew, I.B., eds. Philadephia, W. B. Saunders, 186.

Braund, K. G., Luttgen, P. J., Redding, R. W., et al. 1980. Distal symmetrical polyneuropathy in a dog. Vet Pathol 17:422–435.

Braund, K. G., Luttgen, P. J., Sorjonen, D. C., et al. 1979. Idiopathic facial paralysis in the dog. Vet Rec 105:297–299.

Braund, K. G., Mehta, J. R., Toivio-Kinnucan, M., et al. 1989. Congenital hypomyelinating polyneuropathy in two golden retriever littermates. Vet Pathol 26:202–208.

Braund, K. G., Shores, A., Cochrane, S., et al. 1994. Laryngeal paralysis-polyneuropathy complex in young Dalmatians. Am J Vet Res 55:534–542.

Braund, K. G., Shores, A., Lowrie, C. R., et al. 1997. Idiopathic polyneuropathy in Alaskan malamutes. J Vet Intern Me-d 11:243–249.

Braund, K. G., Simpson, S. T., Steiss, J. E., Cox, N. R., et al. 1995. Idiopathic neuromyopathy in a young American cocker spaniel. J Vet Intern Med 9:370.

Braund, K. G., Steinberg, H. S., Mehta, J. R., Amling, K. A. 1990. Investigating a degenerative polymyopathy in four related Bouvier des Flandres dogs. Vet Med 85:558–570.

Braund, K. G., Steinberg, H. S., Shores, A., et al. 1989. Laryngeal paralysis in immature and mature dogs as one sign of a more diffuse polyneuropathy. JAVMA 194:1735–1740.

Braund, K. G., Toivio-Kinnucan, M., Vallat, J. M., et al. 1994. Distal sensorimotor polyneuropathy in mature Rottweiler dogs. Vet Pathol 31:316–326.

Burbidge, H. M. 1995. A review of laryngeal paralysis in dogs. Br Vet J 151:71–82.

Chrisman, C. L. 2000. Polyneuropathies of cats. Small Anim Pract 41:384–389.

———. 1990. Dancing Doberman disease: clinical findings and prognosis. Prog Vet Neurol 1:83–90.

Cooper, B. J., deLahunta, A., Cummings, J. F., et al. 1984. Canine inherited hypertrophic neuropathy: clinical and electrodiagnostic studies. Am J Vet Res 45:1172–1177.

Cooper, B. J., Duncan, I., Cummings, J., deLahunta, A. 1984. Defective Schwann cell function in canine inherited hypertrophic neuropathy, Acta Neuropathol 63:51–56.

Cuddon, P. A., Higgins, R. J., Duncan, I. D., Miller, S. P. 1989. Polyneuropathy in feline Niemann-Pick disease. Brain 112:1429–1443.

Cummings, J. F., Cooper, B. J., deLahunta, A., et al. 1981. Canine inherited hypertrophic neuropathy. Acta Neuropathol (Berl) 53:137–143.

Duncan, I. D. 1990. Peripheral neuropathy in the dog and cat. Prog Vet Neurol 2:111–128.

Duncan, I. D., Griffiths, I. R. 1977. Canine giant axonal neuropathy. Vet Rec 101:438–441.

Duncan, I. D., Griffiths, I. R., Carmichael, S., et al. 1981. Inherited canine giant axonal neuropathy. Muscle Nerve 4:223–227.

Furuoka, H., Amanai, H., Taniyama, H., et al. 1992. Peripheral neuropathy in German shepherd dogs. J Comp Pathol 107:169–177.

Gerritsen, R. J., van Nes, J. J., van Niel, M. H. F., van den Ingh, T. S. G. A. M, et al. 1996. Acute idiopathic polyneuropathy in nine cats. Vet Quart 18:63–65.

Griffiths, I. R. 1989. Progressive axonopathy of Boxer dogs. In Current Veterinary Therapy X (Small Animal Practice) Kirk, R. W., ed. Philadelphia, W. B. Saunders, 828–830.

———. 1985. Progressive axonopathy: an inherited neuropathy of Boxer dogs. I. Further studies of the clinical and electrophysiological features. J Sm An Prac 26:381–392.

Griffiths, I. R., Duncan, I. 1979a. Distal denervating disease: a degenerative neuropathy of the distal motor axon in dogs.J Sm An Prac 20:579–592.

Griffiths, I. R., Duncan, I. D., Barker, J. 1980. A progressive axonopathy of Boxer dogs affecting the central and peripheral nervous systems. J Sm An Prac 21:29–43.

Hardie, E. M., Kolata, R. L., Stone, E. A., et al. 1981. Laryngeal paralysis in three cats. JAVMA 179:879–882.

Henricks, P. M., Steiss, J., Petterson, J. R. 1987. Distal peripheral polyneuropathy in a Great Dane. Can Vet J 28:165–167.

LaHue, T. R. 1995. Laryngeal paralysis. Semin Vet Med Surg (Small Anim) 10:94–100.

Mahony, O. M., Knowles, K. E., Braund, K. G., et al. 1998. Laryngeal paralysis-polyneuropathy complex in young Rottweilers. J Vet Intern Med 12:330–337.

Matz, M. E., Shell, L., Braund, K. 1990. Peripheral hypomyelinization in two golden retriever littermates. JAVMA 197:228–230.

Moe L. 1992. Hereditary polyneuropathy of Alaskan Malamutes. In Current Veterinary Therapy XI (Small Animal Practice), Kirk, R. W., Bonagura, J. D., eds. Philadelphia, W. B. Saunders, 1038–1039.

Moreau, P. M., Vallat, J. M., Hugon, J., et al. 1991. Peripheral and central distal axonopathy of suspected inherited origin in Birman cats. Acta Neuropathol (Berl) 82:143–146.

O'Brien, L. A., Hendriks, L. 1986. Inherited laryngeal paralysis. Analysis in the husky cross. Vet Q 8:301–302.

Peeters, M. E., Venker-van Haagen, A. J., Goedegebuure, S. A., et al. 1991. Dysphagia in Bouviers associated with muscular dystrophy; evaluation of 24 cases. Vet Q 13:65–73.

Reisner, I. 1991. The pathophysiologic basis of behavior problems. Vet Clin N Am (Small Anim Pract) 21:207–224.

Ridyard, A. E., Corcoran, B. M., Tasker, S., et al. 2000. Spontaneous laryngeal paralysis in four white-coated German shepherd dogs. J Sm An Prac 41:558–561.

Schacter, S., Norris, C. R. 2000. Laryngeal paralysis in cats: 16 cases (1990–1999) JAVMA 216:1100–1103.

Shelton, G. D., Podell, M., Sullivan, S., et al. 2000. Distal, symmetrical polyneuropathy with laryngeal paralysis in young, related Leonberger dogs. J Vet Intern Med 14:339 (abstract).

Sponenberg, D. P., DeLahunta, A. 1981. Hereditary hypertrophic neuropathy in Tibetan Mastiff dogs. J Hered 72:287.

Venker-van Haagen, A. L. 1992. Diseases of the larynx. Vet Clin N Am (Small Anim Pract) 22:1155–1172.

Venker-van Haagen, A. L, Bouw, L., Hartman, W. 1981. Hereditary transmission of laryngeal paralysis in Bouviers. J Am Anim Hosp Assoc 17:75–76.

Venker-van Haagen, A. L., Hartman, W., Goedegebuure, S. A. 1978. Spontaneous laryngeal paralysis in young Bouviers. J Am Anim Hosp Assoc 14:714–720.

Vicini, D. S., Wheaton, L. G., Zachary, J. F., Parker, A.J. 1988. Peripheral nerve biopsy for diagnosis of globoid cell leukodystrophy in a dog. JAVMA 192, 1087–1090.

Motor Neuron Disease

Cork, L. C. 1991. Hereditary canine spinal muscular atrophy: an animal model of motor neuron disease. Can J Neurol Sci 18:432–434.

Cork, L. C., Green, S. L., Pinter, M. J. 1997. Hereditary canine spinal muscular atrophy: genetics, neurophysiology, and pathology. J Neurol Sci 152 Suppl 1:S74.

Cork, L. C., Kin, C. A., Struble, R. G., et al. 1987. Animal models of degenerative neurological disease. Prog Clin Biol Res 229:241–269.

Cork, L. C., Price, D. L., Griffin, J. W., et al. 1990. Hereditary canine spinal muscular atrophy: canine motor neuron disease. Can J Vet Res54:77–82.

Cork, L. C., Struble, R. G., Gold, B. G., et al. 1989. Changes in size of motor axons in hereditary canine spinal muscular atrophy. Lab Invest 61:333–342.

Cummings, J. F., deLahunta, A. 1995. Canine neurodegenerative diseases involving motor neurons. In Kirk's Current Veterinary Therapy XII (Small Animal Practice), Bonagura, J. D., ed. Philadelphia, W. B. Saunders, 1132–1136.

Cummings, J. F., deLahunta, A., Gasteiger, E. L. 1991. Multisystemic chromatolytic neuronal degeneration in Cairn terriers: a case with generalized cataplectic episodes, J Vet Intern Med 5:91–94.

Cummings, J. F., deLahunta, A., Moore, J. J., III. 1988. Multisystemic chromatolytic neuronal degeneration in a Cairn terrier pup. Cornell Vet 78:301–314.

Cummings, J. F., George, C., deLahunta, A., et al. 1989. Focal spinal muscular atrophy in two German shepherd pups. Acta Neuropathol (Em) 79:113–116.

deLahunta, A., Shively, G. N. 1975. Neurofibrillary accumulation in a puppy. Cornell Vet 65:240–247.

Hartley, W. J. 1963. Lower motor neuron disease in dogs. Acta Neuropathol 2:334–342.

Izumo, S., Ikuta, F., Igata, A., Osame, M., et al. 1983. Morphological study on the hereditary neurogenic amyotrophic dogs: accumulation of lipid compound-like structures in the lower motor neuron, Acta Neuropathol 61:270–276.

Kent, M., Knowles, K., Glass, E., et al. 1999. Motor neuron abiotrophy in a saluki. J Am Anim Hosp Assoc 35:436–439.

Lorenz, M. D., Cork, L. C., Griffin, J. W., et al. 1979. Hereditary spinal muscular atrophy in Brittany Spaniels: clinical manifestations. JAVMA 175:833–839.

Mandara, M. T., Di Meo, A. 1998. Lower motor neuron disease in the Griffon Briquet Vendeen dog. Vet Pathol 35:412–414.

Muma, N. A., Cork, L. C. 1993. Alterations in neurofilament mRNA in hereditary canine spinal muscular atrophy. Lab Invest 69:436–442.

Palmer, A. C., Blakemore, W. F. 1989. A progressive neuronopathy in the young Cairn terrier, J Sm An Prac 30:101–106.

Pinter, M. J., Waldeck, R. F., Cope, T. C., et al. 1997. Effects of 4-aminopyridine on muscle and motor unit force in canine motor neuron disease. J Neurosci 17:4500–4507.

Pinter, M. J., Waldeck, R. F., Wallace, N., et al. 1995. Motor unit behavior in canine motor neuron disease. J Neurosci 15:3447–3457.

Pioro, E. P., Mitsumoto, H. 1995. Animal models of ALS. Clin Neurosci 3:375–385.

Presthus, J. 1988. Spinal muscular atrophy in Rottweilers. Nor Veterinaertidssk 100:821.

Sack, G. H. J., Cork, L. C., Morris, J. M. et al. 1984. Autosomal dominant inheritance of hereditary canine spinal muscular atrophy. Ann Neurol 15:369–373.

Sandefeldt, E., Cummings, J. F., deLahunta, A., et al. 1976. Animal model of human disease. Infantile spinal mus- cular atrophy, Werdnig-Hoffman disease. Animal model: hereditary neuronal abiotrophy in Swedish Lapland dogs. Am J Pathol 82:649–652.

Shell, L. G., Jorner, B. S., Leib, M. S. 1987. Familial motor neuron disease in Rottweiler dogs: neuropathologic studies. Vet Pathol 24:135–139.

———. 1987. Spinal muscular atrophy in two Rottweiler littermates. JAVMA 190:878–880.

Shelton, G. D., Hopkins, A. L., Ginn, P. E., et al. 1998. Adult-onset motor neuron disease in three cats. JAVMA 212:1271–1275.

Stockard, C. R. 1936. An hereditary lethal factor for localized motor and preganglionic neurons. Am J Anat 59:1–53.

Tsai, G., Cork, L. C., Slusher, B. S., et al. 1993. Abnormal acidic amino acids and N-acetylaspartylglutamate in hereditary canine motoneuron disease. Brain Res 629:305–309.

Vandevelde, M., Greene, C. E., Hoff, E. J. 1976. Lower motor neuron disease with accumulation of neurofilaments in a cat. Vet Pathol 13:428–435.

Degenerative Myopathies

Amann, J. F., Laughlin, M. H., Kotthuis, R. J. 1988. Muscle hemodynamics in hereditary myopathy of Labrador retrievers. Am J Vet Res 49:1127–1130.

Averill, D. R. 1980. Diseases of the muscle. Vet Clin N Am (Small Anim Pract) 10;1:223–234.

Braund, K. G. 1994. Pediatric myopathies. Semin Vet Med Surg (Sm Anim) 9;2:99–107.

———. 1991. Nerve and muscle biopsy techniques. Prog Vet Neurol 2:35–56.

———. 1986. Identifying degenerative and developmental myopathies. Vet Med August: 713–718.

Braund, K. G., Amling, K. A., Mehta, J. R., et al. 1995. Histochemical and morphometric study of fiber types in ten skeletal muscles of healthy young adult cats. Am J Vet Res 56:349–357.

Braund, K. G., Hoff, E. J., Richardson, K. E. Y. 1978. Histochemical identification of fiber types in canine skeletal muscle. Am J Vet Res 39:561–565.

Braund, K. G., Steinberg, H. S. 1989 (May). Degenerative myopathy of Bouvier des Flandres. Proc 7th ACVIM Forum, San Diego, CA, 995.

Cardinet, G. H., Holliday, T. A. 1979. Neuromuscular diseases of domestic animals: a summary of muscle biopsies from 159 cases. Ann NY Acad Sci 317:290–313.

Carpenter, J. L., Hoffman, E. P., Romanul, F. C. A., et al. 1989. Feline muscular dystrophy with dystrophin deficiency. Am J Pathol 135:909–919.

Frackowiak, A. 1987. Generalized muscle weakness in Labradors. Vet Rec 120;19:466.

Gaschen, F., Gaschen, L., Seiler, G., et al. 1998. Lethal peracute rhabdomyolysis associated with stress and general anesthesia in three dystrophin-deficient cats. Vet Pathol 35:117–123.

Gaschen, F. P., Hoffman, E. P., Gorospe, J. R. F., et al. 1992. Dystrophin deficiency causes lethal muscle hypertrophy in cats. J Neurol Sci 110:149–159.

Goedegebuure, S. A. 1987. Spontaneous primary myopathies in domestic animals: a review. Vet Quarterly 9:155–171.

Gottel, K., Houston, D. M., Kuiken, T., et al. 1996. Inherited myopathy in a litter of Labrador retrievers. Can Vet J 37:108–110.

Hanson, S. M., Smith, M. O., Walker, T. L., et al. 1998. Juvenile-onset distal myopathy in RottWeiler dogs. J Vet Intern Med 12:103–108.

Holland, C. T., Canfield, P. J., Watson, A. D. J., et al. 1991. Dyserythropoiesis. polymyopathy. and cardiac disease in three related English Springer spaniels. J Vet Intern Med 5:151–159.

Howell, J. M., Fletcher, S., Kakulas, B. A., et al. 1997. Use of the dog model for Duchenne muscular dystrophy in gene therapy trials. Neuromusc Disord 7:325–328.

Huxtable, C. R., Chadwick, B., Eger, C., Shaw, S. 1994. Severe subacute progressive myopathy in a young silky terrier. Prog Vet Neurol 5:21–27.

Jones, B. R., Callanan, J. J., Mooney, C. F., et al. 2001. Muscular dystrophy in Japanese Spitz dogs. J Vet Intern Med, 15:290.

Karpati, G., Gilbett, R., Petrof, B. J., et al. 1997. Gene therapy research for Duchenne and Becker muscular dystrophies. Curr Opin Neurol 10; 5; 430–435.

Klopp, L. S., Smith, B. F. 2000. Autosomal recessive muscular dystrophy in Labrador retrievers. Compend Contin Educ Pract Vet 22:121–130.

Kornegay, J. N. 1995. Disorders of the skeletal muscles. In Textbook of Veterinary Internal Medicine, 4th ed. Ettinger, S. J., Feldman, E. C., eds. Philadelphia, W. B. Saunders, 727–736.

———. 1992. The X-linked muscular dystrophies. In Current Veterinary Therapy X: Small Animal Practice, Kirk, R. W., Bonagura, J. D., eds. Philadelphia, W. B. Saunders, 1042–1047.

Kramer, J. W., Hegreberg, G. A., Bryan, G. M., et al. 1976. A muscle disorder of Labrador retrievers characterized by deficiency of Type II muscle fibers. JAVMA 169:817–820.

Luttgen, P. J. 1989. Miscellaneous myopathies. Semin Vet Med Surg (Sm Anim) 4:168–176.

Malik, R., Mepstead, K., Yang, F., Harper, C. 1993. Hereditary myopathy of Devon rex cats. J Sm An Prac 34:539–546.

McGavin, M. D. 1983. Muscle biopsy in veterinary practice. Vet Clin N Am (Small Anim Pract) 13:135–144.

McKerrell, R. E., Braund, K. G. 1989. Hereditary myopathy of Labrador retrievers. In Current Veterinary Therapy. Small Animal Practice, Kirk, R. W., ed. Philadelphia, W. B. Saunders, 820–822.

———. 1987. Hereditary myopathy in Labrador retrievers: clinical variations. J Sm An Prac 28:479–489.

———. 1986. Hereditary myopathy in Labrador retrievers; a morphologic study. Vet Pathol 23:411–417.

Newsholme, S. J., Gaskell, C. J. 1987. Myopathy with core-like structures in a dog. J Comp Path 97:597–600.

Niederhauser, U. B., Holliday, T. A. 1989. Electrodiagnostic studies in diseases of muscles and neuromuscular junctions. Semin Vet Med Surg (Sm Animal)4:116–125.

O'Brien, D. P., Johnson, G. C., Liu, L., et al. 2000. Laminin alpha 2 deficient muscular dystrophy in two cats. J Vet Intern Med 14; 386.

Ozawa, E., Hagiwara, Y., Yoshida, M. 1999. Creatine kinase, cell membrane, and Duchenne muscular dystrophy., Mol Cell Biochem 190:143–151.

Paola, J. P., Podell, M., Shelton, G. D. 1993. Muscular dystrophy in a miniature Schnauzer. Prog Vet Neurol 4:14–18.

Peeters, M. E., Venker-van Haagen, A. J., Goedegebuure, S. A., et al. 1991. Dysphagia in Bouviers associated with muscular dystrophy: evaluation of 24 cases. Vet Quarterly 13:65–73.

Presthus, J., Nordstoga, K. 1993. Congenital myopathy in a litter of Samoyed dogs. Prog Vet Neurol 4:37–40.

Schatzberg, S. J., Olby, N. J., Breen, M., et al. 1999. Molecular analysis of a spontaneous dystrophin "knockout" dog. Neuromuscul Disord 9:289–295.

Sharp, N. J. H., Kornegay, J. N., Lane, S. B. 1989. The muscular dystrophies. Semin Vet Med Surg (Sm Animal) 4:133–140.

Shelton, G. D. 1991. Differential diagnosis of muscle diseases in companion animals. Prog Vet Neurol 2:27–33.

Shelton, G. D., Cardinet, G. H. 1987. Pathophysiologic basis of canine muscle disorders. J Vet Intern Med I:36–44.

Shelton, G. D., Liu, A., Guo, L. T., et al. 2001. Muscular dystrophy in female dogs. J Vet Intern Med 15:240–244.

Sirns, M. H. 1983. Electrodiagnostic techniques in the evaluation of diseases affecting skeletal muscle. Vet Clin N Am (Small Anim Pract) 13:145–162.

Taylor, S. M. 2000.Selected disorders of the muscle and neuromuscular junction. Vet Clin N Am (Small Anim Pract) 30:59–75.

Valentine, B. A., Blue, J. T., Shelley, S. M., et al. 1990. Increased serum alanine aminotransferase activity associated with muscle necrosis in the dog. J Vet Intern Med 4:140–143.

Valentine, B. A., Cooper, B. J., deLahunta, A., et al. 1988. Canine X-linked muscular dystrophy. J Neurol Sci 88:69–91.

Van Ham, L. M. L., Desmidt, M., Tshamala, M., et al. 1993. Canine X-linked muscular dystrophy in Belgian Groenendaeler Shepherds. J Am Anim Hosp Assoc 29:570–574.

Van Ham, L. M. L., Roels, S., Hoorens, J. K. 1995. Congenital dystrophy-like myopathy in a Brittany Spaniel puppy. Prog Vet Neurol 6:135–138.

Vos, J. H., Van Der Linde-Sipman, J. S., Goedegebuure, S. A. 1986. Dystrophy-like myopathy in the cat. J Comp Path 96:335–341.

Watson, A. D. J., Farrow, B. R. H., Middleton, D. J., et al. 1998. Myopathy in a Labrador retriever. Austr Vet J 65:226–227.

Wentink, G. H., Van Der Linde-Sipman, J. S., Meijer, A. E. F. H., et al. 1972. Myopathy with a possible recessive X-linked inheritance in a litter of Irish terriers. Vet Path 9:328–349.

Wetterman, C. A., Harkin, K. R., Cash, W. C., et al. 2000. Hypertrophic muscular dystrophy in a young dog. JAVMA 216:878–881.

Ytterberg, S. R. 1991. Animal models of myopathy. Curr Opin Rheum 3:934–940.

Muscular Dystrophy

Carpenter, J. L., Hoffman, E. P., Romanul, F. C., Kunkel, L. M., et al. 1989. Feline muscular dystrophy with dystrophin deficiency, Am J Pathol 135:909–919.

Cooper, B. J., Valentine, B. A., Wilson, S., Patterson, D. F., et al. 1988. Canine muscular dystrophy: confirmation of X-linked inheritance. J Hered 79:405–408.

Gaschen, F., Gaschen, L., Seiler, G., Welle, M., Jaunin, V. B., Jmaa, D. G., Neiger-Aeschbacher, G., Ade-Damilano, M. 1998. Lethal peracute rhabdomyolysis associated with stress and general anesthesia in three dystrophin-deficient cats. Vet Pathol 35:117–123.

Gaschen, F. P., Hoffman, E. P., Gorospe, J. R., Uhl, E. W., Senior, D. F., Cardinet, G. H., III, Pearce, L. K. 1992. Dystrophin deficiency causes lethal muscle hypertrophy in cats. J Neurol Sci 110:149–159.

Kornegay, J. N., Tuler, S. M., Miller, D. M., Levesque, D. C. 1988. Muscular dystrophy in a litter of golden retriever dogs. Muscle Nerve 11:1056–1064.

Obrien, D. P., Johnson, G. C., Liu, L., et al. 2000. Laminin alpha 2 deficient muscular dystrophy in two cats. J Vet Intern Med 14:386.

Paola, J. P., Podell, M., Shelton, G. D. 1993. Muscular dystrophy in a minature schnauzer. Prog Vet Neurol 4:14.

Peeters, M. E., Ubbink, G. J. 1994. Dysphagia-associated muscular dystrophy: a familial trait in the Bouvier des Flandres. Vet Rec 134:444–446.

Schatzberg, S., Whittemore, J., Morgan, E., et al. 2003. Sarcoglyanpathy in 3 dogs. Proc 21st ACVIM Forum, Charlotte, NC, 956.

Sharp, N. J., Kornegay, J. N., Lane, S. B. 1989. The muscular dystrophies. Semin Vet Med Surg (Small Anim) 4:133–140.

Shelton, G. D., Liu, L. A., Guo, L. T., et al. 2001. Muscular dystrophy in female dogs. J Vet Intern Med 15:240–244.

Shimatsu, Y., Katagiri, K., Furuta, T., Nakura, M., Tanioka, Y., Yuasa, K., Tomohiro, M., Kornegay, J. N., Nonaka, I., Takeda, S. 2003. Canine X-linked muscular dystrophy in Japan (CXMDJ). Exp Anim 52:93–97.

Valentine, B. A., Blue, J. T., Cooper, B. J. 1989. The effect of exercise on canine muscular dystrophy. Ann Neurol 26:588.

Valentine, B. A., Cooper, B. J., Cummings, J. F., deLahunta, A. 1990. Canine X-linked muscular dystrophy: morphologic lesions. J Neurol Sci 97:1–23.

Valentine, B. A., Cooper, B. J., deLahunta, A., O'Quinn, R. 1988. Canine X-linked muscular dystrophy. An animal model of Duchenne muscular dystrophy: clinical studies. J Neurol Sci 88:69–81.

Valentine, B. A., Winand, N. J., Pradhan, D., Moise, N. S., deLahunta, A., Kornegay, J. N., Cooper, B. J. 1992. Canine X-linked muscular dystrophy as an animal model of Duchenne muscular dystrophy: a review. Am J Med Genet 42:352–356.

Vos, J. H., van der Linde-Sipman, J. S., Goedegebuure, S. A. 1986. Dystrophy-like myopathy in the cat. J Comp Pathol 96:335–341.

Wetterman, C. A., Harkin, K. R., Cash, W. C., et al. 2000. Hypertrophic muscular dystrophy in a young dog. JAVMA 216:878.

Labrador Retriever Hereditary Myopathy

Amann, I. F., Laughlin, M. H., Korthuis, R. J. 1988. Muscle hemodynamics in hereditary myopathy of Labrador retrievers. Am J Vet Res 49:1127–1130.

Braund, K. G. et al. 1989. Animal models: muscular dystrophy. Comp Pathol Bull 21:2–4.

Kramer, J. W., Hegreberg, G. A., Bryan, G. M., et al. 1976. A muscle disorder of Labrador retrievers characterized by deficiency of type II muscle fibers, JAVMA 169:817–820

Kramer, J. W., Hegreberg, G. A., Hamilton, M. J. 1981. Inheritance of a neuromuscular disorder of Labrador retriever dogs. JAVMA 179:380–381.

McKerrell, R. E., Braund, K. G. 1987. Hereditary myopathy in Labrador retrievers: clinical variations. J Sm An Prac 28:479–489.

———. 1986. Hereditary myopathy in Labrador retrievers: a morphologic study. Vet Pathol 23:411–417.

McKerrell, R. E., et al. 1984. Generalized muscle weakness in the Labrador retriever. Vet Rec 115:276

Mehta, J. R., Braund, K. G., Hegreberg, G. A., Thukral, V. 1991. Lipid fluidity and composition of the erythrocyte membrane from healthy dogs and Labrador retrievers with hereditary muscular dystrophy, Neurochem Res 16:129–135.

Mehta, J. R., Braund, K. G., McKerrell, R. E., Toivio-Kinnucan, M. 1989a. Analysis of muscle elements, water, and total lipids from healthy dogs and Labrador retrievers with hereditary muscular dystrophy. Am J Vet Res 50:640–644.

———. 1989b. Isoelectric focusing under dissociating conditions for analysis of muscle protein from clinically normal dogs and Labrador retrievers with hereditary myopathy. Am J Vet Res 50:633–639.

Hereditary Myopathy of Devon Rex Cats

Malik, R., Mepstead, K., Yang, F., Harper, C. 1993. Hereditary myopathy of Devon rex cats. J Sm An Prac 34:539–546.

Nemaline Rod Myopathy

Cooper, B. J., deLahunta, A., Gallagher, E. A., et al. 1986. Nemaline myopathy of cats. Muscle Nerve 9:618–625.

Delauche, A. J., Cuddon, P. A., Podell, M., et al. 1998. Nemaline rods in canine myopathies: 4 case reports and literature review. J Vet Intern Med 12:424–430.

Newsholme, S. J., Gaskell, C. J. 1987. Myopathy with core-like structures in a dog. J Comp Path 97:597–600.

Targett, M. P., Franklin, R. J. M., Olby, N. J., et al. 1994. Central core myopathy in a great dane. J Sm Anim Pract 35:100–103.

Metabolic Neuropathies

Diabetic Neuropathy

Anderson, P. G., Braund, K. G., Dillon, A. R., Sartin, J. L. 1986. Polyneuropathy and hormone profiles in a chow puppy with hypoplasia of the Islets of Langerhans, Vet Pathol 23:528–531.

Braund, K. G., Steiss, J. E. 1982. Distal neuropathy in spontaneous diabetes mellitus in the dog. Acta Neuropathol (Berl) 57:263–269.

Ghani, M., Malik, R. A., Walker, D., et al. 1999. Perineural abnormalities in the spontaneously diabetic dog. Acta Neuropathol (Berl) 97:98–102.

Johnson, C. A., Kittleson, M. D., Indrieri, R. J. 1983. Peripheral neuropathy and hypotension in a diabetic dog, JAVMA 183:1007–1009.

Katherman, A. E., Braund, K. G. 1983. Polyneuropathy associated with diabetes mellitus in a dog. JAVMA 182:522–524.

Kramek, B. A., Moise, N. S., Cooper, B., et al. 1984. Neuropathy associated with diabetes mellitus in the cat. JAVMA 184:42–45.

Mizisin, A. P., Shelton, G. D., Wagner, S., et al. 1998. Myelin splitting, Schwann cell injury and demyelination in feline diabetic neuropathy. Acta Neuropathol (Berl) 95:171–174.

Munana, K. R. 1995. Long-term complications of diabetes mellitus, part 1: retinopathy, nephropathy, neuropathy. Vet Clin North Am (Small Anim Pract) 25:715–730.

Steiss, J. E., Orsher, A. N., Bowen, J. M. 1981. Electrodiagnostic analysis of peripheral neuropathy in dogs with diabetes mellitus. Am J Vet Res 42:2061–2064.

Insulinoma Neuropathy

Braund, K. G., Steiss, J. E., Amling, K. A., et al. 1987. Insulinoma and subclinical peripheral neuropathy in two dogs. J Vet Intern Med 1:86–90.

Bergman, P. J., Bruyette, D. S., Coyne, B. E., et al. 1994. Canine clinical peripheral neuropathy associated with pancreatic islet cell carcinoma. Prog Vet Neurol 5:57–62.

Dyer, K. R., Duncan, I. D., Hammang, J. P., Dubielzig, R. R. 1986. Peripheral neuropathy in two dogs: correlation between clinical, electro- physiological and pathological findings, J Sm An Prac 27:133–146.

Dyer, K. R., Messing, A. 1989. Peripheral neuropathy associated with functional islet cell adenomas in SV40 transgenic mice. J Neuropath Exp Neurol 48:399.

Schrauwen, E., Van Ham, L., Hoorens, J. 1996. Peripheral polyneuropathy associated with insulinoma in the dog: clinical, pathological, and electrodiagnostic features. Prog Vet Neurol 7:16–19.

Shahar, R., Rousseaux, C., Steiss, J. 1985. Peripheral polyneuropathy in a dog with functional islet B-cell tumor and widespread metastasis. JAVMA 187:175–177.

Van Ham, L., Braund, K. G., Roels, S., Putcuyps, I. 1997. Treatment of a dog with an insulinoma-related peripheral polyneuropathy with corticosteroids. Vet Rec 141:98–100.

Hypocalcemia

Forbes, S., Nelson, R. W., Guptill, L. 1990. Primary hypoparathyroidism in a cat. JAVMA 196:1285–1287.

Kornegay, J. N., Greene, C. E., Martin, C., Gorgacz, E. J., et al. 1980. Idiopathic hypocalcemia in four dogs, J Am Anim Hosp Assoc 16:723–734.

Peterson, M. E., James, K. M., Wallace, M., Timothy, S. D., et al. 1991. Idiopathic hypoparathyroidism in five cats. J Vet Intern Med 5:47–51.

Hypothyroidism

Bichsel, P., Jacobs, G., Oliver, J. E. J. 1988. Neurologic manifestations associated with hypothyroidism in four dogs. JAVMA 192:1745–1747.

Budsberg, S. C., Moore, G. E., Klappenbach, K. 1993. Thyroxine-responsive unilateral forelimb lameness and generalize neuromuscular disease in four hypothyroid dogs. JAVMA 202:1859–1860.

Coates, J. R. 1997. Neurologic manifestations of hypothyroidism. Canine Practice 22:27–28.

Dewey, C. W., Shelton, G. D., Bailey, C. S., et al. 1995. Neuromuscular dysfunction in five dogs with acquired myasthenia gravis and presumptive hypothyroidism. Prog Vet Neurol 6:117–123.

Indrieri, R. J., Whalen, L. R., Cardinet, G. H., Holliday, T. A. 1987. Neuromuscular abnormalities associated with hypothyroidism and lymphocytic thyroiditis in three dogs, JAVMA 190:544–548.

Jaggy, A., Oliver, J. E. 1994. Neurologic manifestations of thyroid disease. Vet Clin N Am (Small Anim Pract) 24:487–494.

Jaggy, A., Oliver, J. E., Ferguson, D. C., et al. 1994. Neurological manifestations of hypothyroidism: a retrospective study of 29 dogs. J Vet Intern Med 8:328–336.

Kemppainen, R. J., Behrend, E. N. 2000. CVT update: interpretation of endocrine diagnostic test results for adrenal and thyroid disease. In Kirk's Current Veterinary Therapy XIII (Small Animal Practice), Bonagura, J. D., ed. Philadelphia, W. B. Saunders, 321–324.

Hyperchylomicronemia

Johnstone, A. C., Jones, B. R., Thompson, J. C., et al. 1990. The pathology of an inherited hyperlipoproteinaemia of cats. J Comp Pathol 102:125–137.

Jones, B. R., Johnstone, A. C., Cahill, J. I., Hancock, W. S. 1986. Peripheral neuropathy in cats with inherited primary hyperchylocomicronaemia. Vet Rec119:268–272.

Watson, T. D. G., Gaffney, D., Mooney, C. T., et al. 1992. Inherited hyperchylomicronaemia in the cat: lipoprotein lipase function and gene structure. J Sm An Prac 33:207–212.

Hyperoxaluria

McKerrell, R. E., Blakemore, W. F., Heath, M. F., et al. 1989. Primary hyperoxaluria (L-glyceric aciduria) in the cat: a newly recognised inherited disease. Vet Rec 125:31–34.

Metabolic Myopathies

Breitschwerdt, E. B., Kornegay, I. N., Wheeler, S. I., et al. 1992. Episodic weakness associated with exertional lactic acidosis and myopathy in Old English sheepdog littermates. JAVMA 201; 5:731–736.

Coates, I. R., Paxton, R., Cox, N. R. 1996. A case presentation and discussion of Type IV glycogen storage disease in a Norwegian forest cat. Prog Vet Neurol 7:5–11.

Duran, M., Loof, N. E., Ketting, D., et al. 1990. Secondary camitine deficiency. J Clin Chem Clin Biochem 28 359–363.

Forbes, S., Nelson, R. W., Guptill, L. 1990. Primary hypoparathyroidism in a cat. JAVMA 196:1285–1287.

Giger, U., Argov, Z., Schnall, M., et al. 1988. Metabolic myopathy in canine muscle-type phosphofructokinase deficiency. Muscle Nerve 11:1260–1265.

Giger, U., Smith, B. F., Woods, C. B., et al. 1992. Inherited phosphofructokinase deficiency in an American Cocker spaniel. JAVMA 201:1569–1571.

Griffiths, I. R., Duncan, I. D. 1979b. Collapsing Clumber spaniels. Vet Rec Oct:405 (letter).

Harding, A. E., Holt, II. 1989. Mitochondrial myopathies. Br Med Bull 45:760–771.

Harvey, J. W., Calderwood Mays, M. B., Gropp, K. E. et al. 1990. Polysaccharide storage myopathy in canine phosphofructokinase deficiency (Type VII glycogen storage disease). Vet Pathol 27:1–8.

Herrtage, M. E., Houlton, J. E. F. 1979. Collapsing clumber spaniels. Vet Rec 105:334.

Houlton, J. E. F., Herrtage, M. E. 1980. Mitochondrial myopathy in the Sussex spaniel. Vet Rec 106:206.

Olby, N. I., Chan, K. K., Targett, M. P., et al. 1997. Suspected mitochondrial myopathy in a Jack Russell terrier. J Sm Anim Pract 38:213–216.

Peterson, M. E., James, K. M., Wallace, M., Timothy, S. D., et al. 1991. Idiopathic hypoparathyroidism in five cats. J Vet Intern Med 5:47–51.

Platt, S. R., Chrisman, C. L., Shelton, G. D. 1999. Lipid storage myopathy in a cocker spaniel. J Sm Anim Pract 40:31–34.

Scholte, H. R., Pereira, R. R., Delonge, P. C., et al. 1990. Primary carnitine deficiency. J Clin Chem Clin Biochem 28:351–357.

Shelton, G. D. 1995. Canine lipid storage myopathies. In Kirk's Current Veterinary Therapy XII (Small Animal Practice), Bonagura, J. D., ed. Philadelphia, W. B. Saunders, 1161–1163.

Shelton, G. D., Nyhan, W. L., Kass, P. H., et al. 1998. Analysis of organic acids, amino acids, and carnitine in dogs with lipid storage myopathy. Muscle Nerve 21:1202–1205.

Smith, M. O. 1989. Idiopathic myositides in dogs. Semin Vet Med Surg (Sm Anim) 4:156–160.

Walvoort, H. C., van Ness, I. I., Stokhof, A. A., et al. 1984. Canine glycogen storage disease type II: a clinical study of four affected Lapland dogs. J Am Anim Hosp Assoc 20:279–286.

Endocrine Myopathies

Kendall-Taylor, P., Turnbull, D. M. 1983. Endocrine myopathies. Br Med J 287:705–708.

LeCouteur, R. A., Dow, S. W., Sisson, A. F. 1989. Metabolic and endocrine myopathies of dogs and cats. Semin Vet Med Surg (Sm Anim) 4;2:146–155.

Hypokalemic Myopathy

Blaxter, A. C., Lievesley, P., Gruffydd-Jones, T., et al. 1986. Periodic muscle weakness in Burmese kittens. Vet Rec 118:619–620, (letter).

Dow, S. W., Fettman, M. J., Curtis, C. R., LeCouteur, R. A. 1989. Hypokalemia in cats: 186 cases (1984–1987). JAVMA 194: 1604–1608.

Dow, S. W., LeCouteur, R. A. 1989. Hypokalemic polymyopathy of cats. InCurrent Veterinary Therapy X. Small Animal Practice, Kirk, R. W., ed. Philadelphia, W. B. Saunders, 812–815.

Dow, S. W., LeCouteur, R. A., Fettman, M. J. et al. 1987. Potassium depletion in cats: hypokalemic polymyopathy. JAVMA 191; 12:1563–1567.

Fettman, M. J. 1989. Feline kaliopenic polymyopathy/nephropathy syndrome. Vet Clin North Am 19:415–432.

Hopkins, A. L. 1989. Sporadic feline hypokalemic polymyopathy. Vet Rec 125; 17:830.

Jones, B. R. 2000. Hypokalemic myopathy in cats. In Kirk's Current Veterinary Therapy XIII (Small Animal Practice), Bonagura, J. D., ed. Philadelphia, W. B. Saunders, 985–987.

Jones, B. R., Gruffydd-Jones, T. J. 1990. Hypokalemia in the cat. Cornell Vet 8:13–16.

Jones, B. R., Swinney, G. W., Alley, M. R. 1988. Hypokalaemic myopathy in Burmese kittens. NZ Vet J 36:150–151.

Leon, A., Bain, S., Levick, W. R. 1992. Hypokalemic episodic polymyopathy in cats fed a vegetarian diet. Austr Vet J 69; 10:249–254.

Nemzek, J. A., Kruger, J. M., Walshaw, R. W., et al. 1994. Acute onset of hypokalemia and muscular weakness in four hyperthyroid cats. JAVMA 205:65–68.

Hyperkalemic Myopathy

Jezyk, P. F. 1982. Hyperkalemic periodic paralysis in a dog. J Am Anim Hosp Assoc 18:977–980.

Hypernatremic Myopathy

Dow, S. W., Fettman, M. J., LeCouteur, R. A., Allen, T. A. 1987. Hypodipsic hypernatremia and associated myopathy in a hydrocephalic cat with transient hypopituitarism, JAVMA 191:217–221.

Hyperadrenocorticism Myopathy

Braund, K. G., Dillon, A. R., Mikeal, R. L. 1980. Experimental investigation of glucocorticoid-induced myopathy in the dog, Exp Neurol 68:50–71.

Braund, K. G., Dillon, A. R., Mikeal, R. L., et al. 1980. Subclinical myopathy associated with hyperadrenocorticism in the dog. Vet Pathol 17:134–148.

Duncan, I. D., Griffiths, I. R., Nash, A. S. 1977. Myotonia in canine Cushing's disease, Vet Rec 100:30–31.

Greene, C. E., Lorenz, M. D., Munnell, J. F., et al. 1979. Myopathy associated with hyperadrenocorticism in the dog. JAVMA 174:1310–1315.

Hoskins, J. D., Nafe, L. A., Cho, D. Y. 1982. Myopathy associated with hyperadrenocorticism in a dog: a case report. Vet Med Small Anim Clin 77:760–764.

Reusch, C. E., Feldman, E. C. 1991. Canine hyperadrenocorticism due to adrenocortical neoplasia. J Vet Intern Med 5:3–10.

Hypothyroid Myopathy

Braund, K. G., Dillon, A. R., August, J. R., et al. 1981. Hypothyroid myopathy in two dogs. Vet Pathol 18:589–598.

Chastain, C. B. 1982. Canine hypothyroidism. JAVMA 181; 4:349–353.

Indrieri, R. J., Whalen, L. R., Cardinet, G. H., et al. 1987. Neuromuscular abnormalities associated with hypothyroidism and lymphocytic thyroiditis in three dogs. JAVMA 190; 5:544–548.

Neoplasia

Bailey, C. S. 1990. Long-term survival after surgical excision of a schwannoma of the sixth cervical spinal nerve in a dog. JAVMA 196:754–756.

Bradley, R. L., Withrow, S. J., Snyder, S. P. 1982. Nerve sheath tumors in the dog. J Am Anim Hosp Assoc 18:915–921.

Brehm, D. M., Vite, C. H., Steinberg, H. S., et al. 1995. A retrospective evaluation of 51 cases of peripheral nerve sheath tumors in the dog. J Am Anim Hosp Assoc 31:349–359.

LeCouteur, R. A. 2001. Tumors of the Nervous System, in Withrow, S. J., MacEwen, E. G., eds., Small Animal Clinical Oncology, 3d ed. Philadelphia, W. B. Saunders, 500–531.

McCarthy, R. J., Feeney, D. A., Lipowitz, A. J. 1993. Preoperative diagnosis of tumors of the brachial plexus by use of computed tomography in three dogs. JAVMA 202:291–294.

Seppälä, M. T., Haltia, M. J. J., Sankila, R. J., et al. 1995. Long-term outcome after removal of spinal schwannoma: a clinicopathological study of 187 cases. J Neurosurg 83:621–626.

Steinberg, H. S. 1988. Brachial plexus injuries and dysfunction. Vet Clinic N Amer 18:565–580.

Summers, B. A., Cummings, J. F., deLahunta, A. 1995. In Veterinary Neuropathology, St. Louis:Mosby.

Targett, M. P., Dyce, J., Houlton, J. E. F. 1993. Tumours involving the nerve sheaths of the forelimb in dogs. J Sm An Prac 34:221–225.

Muscle

Harkin, K. R., Kennedy, G. A., Moore, W. E., Schoning, P. 2000. Skeletal muscle lymphoma in a bullmastiff. J Am Anim Hosp Assoc 36:63–66.

Paraneoplasic Neuropathy

Braund, K. G. 1990. Remote effects of cancer on the nervous system. Semin Vet Med Surg 5:262–270.

Braund, K. G., McGuire, J. A., Amling, K. A., Henderson, R. A. 1987. Peripheral neuropathy associated with malignant neoplasms in dogs. Veterinary Pathology 24: 16–21.

Mariani C. L., Shelton, S. B., Alsup, J. C. 1999. Paraneoplastic polyneuropathy and subsequent recovery following tumor removal in a dog. J Am Anim Hosp Assoc 35: 302–305.

Sorjonen, D. C., Braund, K. G., Hoff, P. J. 1982. Paraplegia and subclinical neuromyopathy associated with a primary lung tumor in a dog. JAVMA 180:1209–1211.

Villiers, E., Dobson, J. 1998. Multiple myeloma with associated polyneuropathy in a German shepherd dog. J Sm Anim Pract 39:249–251.

Nutritional Myopathy

Dennis, I. M., Alexander, R. W. 1982. Nutritional myopathy in a cat. Vet Rec 111:195–196.

Kaspar, L. V., Lombard, L. S. 1963. Nutritional myodegeneration in a litter of beagles. JAVMA 143:284–288.

Manktelow, B. W. 1963. Myopathy of dogs resembling white muscle disease of sheep. NZ Vet J 11:52–55.

Polyneuritis/ Polyradiculoneuritis

Brachial Plexus Neuritis

Alexander, J. W., deLahunta, A., Scott, D. W. 1974. A case of brachial plexus neuropathy in a dog. J Am Anim Hosp Assoc 10:515–517.

Bright, R. M., Crabtree, B. J., Knecht, C. D. 1978. Brachial plexus neuropathy in the cat: a case report. J Am Anim Hosp Assoc 14:612–615.

Cummings, J. F., Lorenz, M. D., deLahunta, A., et al. 1973. Canine brachial plexus neuritis: a syndrome resembling serum neuritis in man. Cornell Vet 63:589–617.

deLahunta, A. 1983. Veterinary Neuroanatomy and Clinical Neurology, 2d ed. Philadelphia, W. B. Saunders.

Sharp, N. J. H. 1988. Craniolateral approach to the canine brachial plexus. Vet Surg 17:18–21.

Steinberg, H. S. 1988. Brachial plexus injuries and dysfunctions. Vet Clin North Am 18:565–580.

Protozoal Neuritis

Barber, J. S., Trees, A. J. 1996. Clinical aspects of 27 cases of neosporosis in dogs. Vet Rec 139:439–443.

Braund, K. G., Blagburn, B. L., Toivio-Kinnucan, M., et al. 1988. Toxoplasma polymyositis/polyneuropathy-a new clinical variant in two mature dogs. J Am Anim Hosp Assoc 24:93–97.

Core, O. M., Hoff, E. J., and Milton, J. L. 1983. Hindlimb hyperextension as a result of Toxoplasma gondii polyradiculitis. J Am Anim Hosp Assoc 19:713–716.

Cuddon, P., Lin, D. S., Bowman, D. D., et al. 1992. Neospora caninum infection in English Springer Spaniel litter-mates. Diagnostic evaluation and organism isolation. J Vet Intern Med 6:325–332

Cummings, J. F., deLahunta, A., Suter, M. M., et al. 1988. Canine protozoan polyradiculoneuritis. Acta Neuropathol (Berl) 76:46–54.

Dubey, J. P., Carpenter, J. L., Speer, C. A., et al. 1988. Newly recognized fatal protozoan disease of dogs. JAVMA 192:1269–1285.

Knowler, C., Skerritt, G. 1994. Canine neosporosis and toxoplasmosis. Prog Vet Neurol 5:167–169.

Trigeminal Neuritis

Carmichael, S., Griffiths, I. R. 1981. Case of isolated sensory trigeminal neuropathy in a dog. Vet Rec 109:280–282.

Chrisman, C. L., Platt, S. R., Chandra, A. M., et al. 1999. Sensory polyganglioradiculoneuritis in a dog. J Am Anim Hosp Assoc 35:232–235.

Cummings, J. F., deLahunta, A., Mitchell, W. J. L. 1983. Ganglioradiculitis in the dog. A clinical, light- and electron-microscopic study. Acta Neuropathol (Berl) 60:29–39.

deLahunta, A. 1983. Veterinary Neuroanatomy and Clinical Neurology, 2d ed. Philadelphia, W. B. Saunders, 95–114.

Hoelzle, R. J. 1983. Idiopathic trigeminal neuropathy in a dog. Vet Med Small Anim Clin 78:345.

Humphreys, G. U. 1974. Correspondence: dropped jaw in dogs. Vet Rec 95:222.

Powell, A. K. 1991. Idiopathic trigeminal neuritis in a dog. Can Vet J 32:265.

Myositis

Bacterial Myositis

Budsberg, S. C. 1998. Musculoskeletal infections. In Infectious Diseases of the Dog and Cat, 2d ed., Greene, C. E., ed. Philadelphia, W. B. Saunders, 555–567.

Mane, M. C., Vives, M. A., Barrera, R., et al. 1992. A putative clostridial myositis in a dog. J Sm Anim Pract 33:345–348.

Poncelet, L. 1991. Polymyositis associated with *Leptospira australis* infection in a dog, Vet Rec 129:40.

Poonacha, K. B., Donahue, J. M., Nightengale, J. R. 1989. Clostridial myositis in a dog. JAVMA 194:69–70.

Seddon, M. L., Barry, S. J. 1992. Clostridial myositis in dogs. Vet Rec 131; 4:84 (letter).

Thomson, M. J., Eger, C. E. 1997. Management of a femoral fracture complicated by Clostridial myositis. J Sm Anim Pract 38:70–73.

Dermatomyositis

Hargis, A. M., Haupt, K. H. 1990. Review of familial canine dematomyositis. Vet Annual 30:277–282.

Hargis, A. M., Haupt, K. H., Prieur, D. J., et al. 1985. A skin disorder in three Shetland sheepdogs: comparison with familial canine dermatomyositis of collies. Compend Contin Educ Pract Vet 7:306–315.

Hargis, A. M., Mundell, A. C. 1992. Familial canine dermatomyositis. Compend Contin Educ Pract Vet 14:855–864.

Haupt, K. H., Hargis, A. M. 1989. Familial canine dermatomyositis. In Current Veterinary Therapy X. Small Animal Practice, Kirk, R. W., ed. Philadelphia, W. B. Saunders, 606–609.

Haupt, K. H., Prieur, D. J., Hargis, A. M., et al. 1985. Familial canine dermatomyositis: clinicopathologic, immunologic, and serologic studies. Am J Vet Res 46:1870–1875.

Haupt, K. H., Prieur, D. J., Moore, M. P., et al. 1985. Familial canine dermatomyositis: clinical, electrodiagnostic, and genetic studies. Am J Vet Res 46:1861–1869.

Kasper, C. S., White, C. L., Freeman, R. G. 1988. Pathology and immunopathology of polymyositis/dermatomyositis. Clin Dermatol 6:64–75.

Kunkle, G. A., Gross, T. L., Fadok, V., et al. 1985. Dermatomyositis in Collie dogs. Compend Contin Educ Pract Vet 7; 3:185–192.

Plamondon, S., Dent, P. B., Reed, A. M. 1999. Familial dermatomyositis. J Rheumatol 26:2691–2692.

White, S. D., Shelton, G. D., Sisson, A., et al. 1992. Dermatomyositis in an adult Pembroke Welsh Corgi. J Am Anim Hosp Assoc 28:398–401.

Extraocular Polymyositis

Boydell, P. 2001. Ultrasonographic appearance of extraocular myositis in the dog. J Vet Intern Med 15:80(abstract).

Carpenter, J. L., Schmidt, G. M., Moore, F. M., et al. 1989. Canine bilateral extraocular polymyositis. Vet Pathol 26:510–512.

Glauberg, A., Beaumont, P. R. 1979. Sudden blindess as the presenting sign of eosinophilic myositis: a case report. J Am Anim Hosp Assoc 15:609–611.

Hepatozoonosis

Baker, J. L., Craig, T. M., Barton, C. C. L., Scott, D. W. 1988. Hepatozoon canis in a dog with oral pyogranulomas and neurological disease. Cornell Vet 78:179–183.

Craig, T. M., Jones, L. P., Nordgren, R. M. 1984. Diagnosis of Hepatazoon canis by muscle biopsy. J Am Anim Hosp Assoc 20:301–303.

Murata, T., Shiramizu, K., Hara, Y., Inoue, M., et al. 1991. First case of Hepatozoon canis infection of a dog in Japan. J Vet Med Sci 53:1097–1099.

Masticatory Myopathy

Anderson, I. G., Harvey, C. E. 1993. Masticatory muscle myositis. J Vet Dent 10:6–8.

Gilmour, M. A., Morgan, R. V., Moore, F. M. 1992. Masticatory myopathy in the dog: a retrospective study of 18 cases. J Am Anim Hosp Assoc 28:300–306.

Lantz, G. C., Cantwell, H. D. 1986. Intermittent open-mouth lower jaw locking in five dogs. JAVMA 188:1403–1405.

Orvis, I. S., Cardinet, G. H. 1981. Canine muscle fiber types and susceptibility of masticatory muscles to myositis. Muscle Nerve 4:354–359.

Roberts, K. E., Hanson, P. O., Zaslow, I. M. 1975. Masticator myopathy in the dog (A review of two cases). Vet Med (Sm Anim Clin) 70:840–843.

Shelton, G. D., Bandman, E., Cardinet, G. H. 1985. Electrophoretic comparison of myosins from masticatory muscles and selected limb muscles in the dog. Am J Vet Res 46:493–498.

Shelton, G. D., Cardinet, G. H. 1989. Canine masticatory muscle disorders. In Current Veterinary Therapy X: Small Animal Practice, Kirk, R. W., ed. Philadelphia, W. B. Saunders, 816–819.

Shelton, G. D., Cardinet, G. H., Bandman, E. 1987. Canine masticatory muscle disorders: a study of 29 cases. Muscle Nerve 10:753–766.

Vamvakidis, C. D., Koutinas, A. F., Kanakoudis, G., Georgiadis, G., et al. 2000. Masticatory and skeletal muscle myositis in canine leishmaniasis (Leishmania infantum). Vet Rec 146:698–703.

Vilafranca, M., Wohlsein, P., Borras, D, et al. 1995. Muscle fiber expression of transforming growth factor-Bl and latent transforming growth factor-B binding protein in canine masticatory muscle myositis. J Comp Path 112:299–306.

Polymyositis

Buoro, I. B. J., Kanui, T. I., Atwell, R. B., Njenga, K. M., Gathumbi, P. K. 1990, Polymyositis associated with Ehrlichia canis infection in two dogs. J Sm Anim Pract 31:624–627.

Cuddon, P. A., Shelton, G. D. 1999. Breed associated polymyositis of young Newfoundlands. J Vet Intern Med 13:239

Evans, J., Levesque, D., Shelton, G. D. 2003. Canine inflammatory myopathies: a review of 200 cases. Proc 21st ACVIM Forum, Charlotte, NC, 955.

Giger, U., Werner, L. L., Millichamp, N. J., et al. 1985. Sulfadiazine-induced allergy in six Doberman pinschers. JAVMA 186:479–484.

Gorman, N. T., Werner, L. L. 1986. Immune mediated-diseases of the dogs and cat. II. Immune-mediated diseases of the hemolymphatic and musculoskeletal system. Br Vet J 142:403–410.

Kornegay, I. N., Gorgacz, E. J., Dawe, D. L., et al. 1980. Polymyositis in dogs. JAVMA 176:431–438.

Lewis, R. M. 1994. Immune-mediated muscle disease. Vet Clin N Am (Small Anim Pract) 24:703–711.

Morozurni, M., Oyama, Y., Kurosu, Y., Nakayama, H., et al. 1991. Immune-mediated polymyositis in a dog. J Vet Med Sci 53:511–512.

Presthus, J., Lindboe, C. F. 1988. Polymyositis in two German wirehaired pointer littermates. J Small Anim Pract 29:239–248.

Tiches, D., Shelton, S., Shelton, G. D. 1996. Vasculitic neuromyopathy in a dog. Prog Vet Neurol 7:77–81.

Werner, L. L., Gorman, N. T. 1988. Immune-mediated disorders of cats. Vet Clin N Am (Small Anim Pract) 14:1039–1064.

Whitney, I. C. 1955. Eosinophilic myositis in dogs. Vet Rec 67:1140–1143.

Protozoal Myositis

Baneth, G., Harmelin, A., Presentey, B. Z. 1995. Hepatozoon canis infection in two dogs. JAVMA 206:1891–1894.

Braund, K. G., Blagburn, B. L., Toivio-Kinnucan, M., et al. 1988. Toxoplasma polymyositis/polyneuropathy-A new clinical variant in two mature dogs. J Am Anim Hosp Assoc 24:93–97.

Cuddon, P., Lin, D. S., Bowman, D. D., et al. 1992. Neospora caninum infection in English Springer spaniel littermates: diagnostic evaluation and organism isolation. J Vet Intern Med 6:325–332.

Greene, C. E., Cook, J. R., Mahaffey, E. A. 1985. Clindamycin for treatment of Toxoplasma polymyositis in a dog. JAVMA 187:631–634.

Jacobson, L. S., Jardine, J. E. 1993. Neospora caninum infection in three Labrador littermates. J S Afr Vet Assoc 64:47–51.

Macintire, D. K., Vincent-Johnson, N., Dillon, A. R., et al. 1997. Hepatozoonosis in dogs: 22 cases (1989–1994). JAVMA 210:916–922.

Macintire, D. K., Vincent-Johnson, N. A., Kane, C. W., et al. 2001. Treatment of dogs infected with Hepatozoon americanum: 53 cases (1989–1998). JAVMA 218:77–81.

Viral Myopathy

Podell, M., Chen, E., Shelton, G. D. 1998. Feline immunodeficiency virus associated myopathy in the adult cat. Muscle Nerve 21:1680–1685.

Myasthenia Gravis

Atwater, S. W., Powers, B. E., Park, R. D., et al. 1994. Thymoma in dogs: 23 cases (1980–1991). JAVMA 205:1007–1013.

Bartges, J. W., Klausner, J. S., BostWick, E. F., et al. 1990. Clinical remission following plasmapheresis and corticosteroid treatment in a dog with acquired myasthenia gravis. JAVMA 196:1276–1278.

Cuddon, P. A. 1989. Acquired immune-mediated myasthenia gravis in a cat. J Sm Anim Pract 30:511–516.

Dewey, C. W. 1998. Acquired myasthenia gravis in dogs, part 2. Compend Contin Educ Pract Vet 20:47–57.

———. 1997. Acquired myasthenia gravis in dogs, part 1. Compend Contin Educ Pract Vet 19:1340–1353.

Dewey, C. W., Bailey, C. S., Shelton, G. D., et al. 1997. Clinical forms of acquired myasthenia gravis in dogs: 25 cases (1988–1995). J Vet Intern Med 11:50–57.

Dewey, C. W., Boothe, D. M., Rjnn, K. L., et al. 2000. Treatment of a myasthenic dog with mycophenolate mofetil. J Vet Emerg Crit Care 10:177–187.

Dewey, C. W., Coates, J. R., Ducote, J. M., et al. 1999. Azathioprine therapy for acquired myasthenia gravis in five dogs. J Am Anim Hosp Assoc 35:396–402.

Dewey, C. W., Shelton, G. D., Bailey, C. S., et al. 1995. Neuromuscular dysfunction in five dogs with acquired myasthenis gravis and presumptive hypothyroidism. Prog Vet Neurol 6(4):117–123.

Ducote, J. M., Dewey, C. W. 2001. Acquired myasthenia gravis and other disorders of the neuromuscular junction. In Consultations in Feline Internal Medicine, 4th ed., August, J. R., ed. Philadelphia, W. B. Saunders, 200:374–80.

Ducote, J. M., Dewey, C. W., Coates, J. R. 1999. Clinical forms of acquired myasthenia gravis in cats. Compend Contin Educ Pract Vet 21:440–448.

Flagstad, A. 1993. Development of the electrophysiological pattern in congenital myasthenic syndrome. Prog Vet Neurol 4;4:126–134.

Flagstad, A., Trojaborg, W., Garnmeltoft, S. 1989. Congenital myasthenic syndrome in the dog breed Gammel Dansk Honsehund: clinical, electrophysiological, pharmacological and immunological comparison with acquired myasthenia gravis. Acta Vet Scand 30:89–102.

Hackett, T. B., Van Pelt, D. R., Willard, M. D., et al. 1995. Third degree atrioventricular block and acquired myasthenia gravis in four dogs. JAVMA 206:1173–1176, 1995.

Hitt, M. E., Shaw, D. P., Hogan, P. M., et al. 1987. Radiation treatment for thymoma in a dog. JAVMA 190:1187–1190.

Hopkins, A. L., Howard, J. F., Wheeler, S. J., et al. 1993. Stimulated single fibre electromyography in normal dogs. J Sm An Prac 34:271–276.

Indrieri, R. J., Creighton, S. R., Lambert, E. H., Lennon, V. A. 1983. Myasthenia gravis in two cats, JAVMA 182:57–60.

Johnson, R. P., Ho, S., Church, D. B. 1975. Myasthenia in springer spaniel littermates: J Small Anim Prac 16:641–647.

Joseph, R. J., Carrillo, J. M., Lennon, V. A. 1988. Myasthenia gravis in the cat. J Vet Internal Med 2:75–79.

King, L. G., Vite, C. H. 1998. Acute fuminating myasthenia gravis in five dogs. JAVMA 212:830–834.

Klebanow, E. R. 1992. Thymoma and acquired myasthenia gravis in the dog: a case report and review of 13 additional cases. J Am Anim Hosp Assoc 28:63–70.

Krotje, L. J., Fix, A. S., Porrhoff, A. D. 1990. Acquired myasthenia gravis and cholangiocellular carcinoma in a dog. JAVMA 197:488–490.

Lainesse, M. F., Taylor, S. M., Myers, S. L., et al 1996. Focal myasthenia gravis as aparaneoplastic syndrome of canine thymoma: improvement following thymectomy. J Am Anim Hosp Assoc 32:111–117.

Lipsitz, D., Berry, J. L., Shelton, D. 1999. Inherited predisposition to myasthenia gravis in Newfoundlands. JAVMA 215;7:956.

Malik, R., Gabor, L., Hunt, G. B., et al. 1997. Benign cranial mediastinal lesions in three cats. Aust Vet J 75:183–187.

Malik, R., Ho, S., Church, D. B. 1989. The normal response to repetitive motor nerve stimulation in dogs. J Sm An Prac 30:20.

Mason, K. V. 1976. A case of myasthenia gravis in a cat. J Sm An Prac 17:467–472,

Miller, L. M., Hegreberg, G. A., Prieur, D. J., et al. 1984. Inheritance of congenital myasthenia gravis in Smooth Fox terriers. J Hered 75:163–166.

Miller, L. M., Lennon, V. A., Lambert, E. H., Reed, S. M., et al. 1983. Congenital myasthenia gravis in 13 smooth fox terriers. JAVMA 182:694–697.

Moore, A. S., Madewell, B. R., Cardinet, G. H., III, et al. 1990. Osteogenic sarcoma and myasthenia gravis in a dog. JAVMA 197:226–227.

O'Dair, H. A., Holt, P. E., Pearson, G. R., Gruffydd-Jones, T. J. 1991. Acquired immune-mediated myasthenia gravis in a cat associated with a cystic thymus. J Sm Anim Pract 32:198–202.

Palmer, A. C., Goodyear, J. V. 1978. Congenital myasthenia in the Jack Russell terrier. Vet Rec 103:433–434.

Pflugfelder, C. M., Cardinet, G. H., Lutz, H., et al. 1981. Acquired canine myasthenia gravis: immunocytochemical localization of immune complexes at neuromuscular junctions. Muscle Nerve 4:289–295.

Ridyard, A. E., Rhind, S. M., French, A. T., et al. 2000. Myasthenia gravis associated with cutaneous lymphoma in a dog. J Sm An Prac 41:348–351.

Rusbtidge, C., White, R. N., Elwood, C. M., et al. 1996. Treatment of acquired myasthenia gravis associated with thymoma in two dogs. J Sm Anim Pract 37:376–380.

Scott-Moncrieff, J. C., Cook, J. R. J., Lantz, G. C. 1990. Acquired myasthenia gravis in a cat with thymoma. JAVMA 196:1291–1293.

Shelton, G. D. 1998. Myasthenia gravis: lessons from the past 10 years. J Sm An Prac 39:368–372.

———. 1998. Neuromuscular disease. Proc 41st BSAVA Congress. Birmingham, Br Sm Anim Vet Assoc., 4–6.

———. 1996. Myasthenia gravis: 1000 cases later. Proc 14th ACVIM Forum, 658.

———. 1992a. Canine myasthenia gravis. In Current Veterinary Therapy XI. Kirk, R. W., Bonagura, J. D., eds. Philadelphia, W. B. Saunders, 1039–1042.

———. 1992b. Megaesophagus secondary to acquired myasthenia gravis. In Current Veterinary Therapy XI (Small Animal Practice), Kirk, R. W., Bonagura, J. D., eds. Philadelphia, W. B. Saunders, 580–583.

———. 1989a. Canine seronegative acquired myasthenia gravis. Proc 11th ACVIM Forum, 999–1002

———. 1989b. Disorders of neuromuscular transmission. Semin Vet Med Surg (Small Anim) 4:126–132.

Shelton, G. D., Cardinet, G. H., III, Lindstrom, J. M. 1988. Canine and human myasthenia gravis autoantibodies recognize similar regions on the acetylcholine receptor. Neurology 38:1417–1423.

Shelton, G. D., Ho, M., Kass, P. H. 2000. Risk factors for acquired myasthenia gravis in cats: 105 cases (1986–1998). JAVMA 216:55–57.

Shelton, G. D., Schule, A., Kass, P. H. 1997. Rick factors for acquired myasthenia gravis in dogs: 1,154 cases (1991–1995) J Am Vet Med Assos 211 1428–1431.

Shelton, G. D., Willard, M. D., Cardinette, G. H., Lindstrom, J. 1990. Acquired myasthenia gravis, selective involvement of esophageal, pharyngeal, and facial muscles. J Vet Intern Med 4, 281–284.

Sirns, M. H., McLean, R. A. 1990. Use of repetitive nerve stimulation to assess neuromuscular function in dogs: a test protocol for suspected myasthenia gravis. Prog Vet Neurol 1:311–319, 1990.

Van Ham, L. M. L. 1993. A myasthenic-like syndrome in young related mongrel dogs. Prog Vet Neurol 3:135.

Wallace, M. E., Palmer, A. C. 1984. Recessive mode of inheritance in myasthenia gravis in the Jack Russell terrier. Vet Rec 114:350.

Wheeler, S. J. 1990 Disorders of the neuromuscular junction. Prog Vet Neurol 2:129–135, 1990.

Wilkes, M. K., McKerrell, R. E., Patterson, R. C., Palmer, A. C. 1987. Ultrastructure of motor endplates in canine congenital myasthenia gravis, J Comp Pathol 97:247–256.

Yam, P. S., Shelton, G. D., Simpson, J. W. 1996. Megaoesophagus secondary to acquired myasthenia gravis. J Sm An Prac 37:179–183.

Neuropathies and Myopathies Without a Known Cause

Blakemore, W. F., Mitten, R. W., Palmer, A. C., et al. 1974. Value of a nerve biopsy in diagnosis of globoid cell leucodystrophy in the dog. Vet Rec 94:70–71.

Braund, K. G. 1996a. Degenerative causes of neuropathies in dogs and cats. Vet Med 722–739.

———. 1996b. Endogenous causes of neuropathies in dogs and cats. Vet Med, 740–754.

———. 1996c. Idiopathic and exogenous causes of neuropathies in dogs and cats. Vet Med 755–769.

———. 1995a. Laryngeal paralysis-polyneuropathy complex in young Dalmatian dogs. In Kirk's Current Veterinary Therapy XII (Small Animal Practice), Bonagura, J. D., ed. Philadelphia, W. B. Saunders, 1136–1140.

———. 1995b. Peripheral nerve disorders. In Textbook of Veterinary Internal Medicine, Diseases of the Dog and Cat, 4th ed., Ettinger, S. J., Feldman, E. C., eds. Philadelphia, W. B. Saunders, 701–726.

———. 1987. Degenerative and developmental diseases. In Veterinary Neurology, Oliver, J. E., Jr., Hoerlein, B. F., Mayhew, I. B., eds. Philadelphia, W. B. Saunders, 186.

Braund, K. G., Luttgen, P. J., Redding, R. W., et al. 1980. Distal symmetrical polyneuropathy in a dog. Vet Pathol 17:422–435.

Braund, K. G., Luttgen, P. J., Sorjonen, D. C., et al. 1979. Idiopathic facial paralysis in the dog. Vet Rec 105:297–299.

Braund, K. G., Mehta, L. R., Toivio-Kinnucan, M., et al. 1989. Congenital hypomyelinating polyneuropathy in two golden retriever littermates. Vet Pathol 26:202–208.

Braund, K. G., Shores, A., Cochrane, S., et al. 1994. Laryngeal paralysis-polyneuropathy complex in young Dalmatians. Am J Vet Res 55:534–542.

Braund, K. G., Shores, A., Lowrie, C. R., et al. 1997. Idiopathic polyneuropathy in Alaskan malamutes. J Vet Intern Med 11:243–249.

Braund, K. G., Steinberg, H. S., Shores, A., et al. 1989. Laryngeal paralysis in immature and mature dogs as one sign of a more diffuse polyneuropathy. JAVMA 194:1735–1740.

Braund, K. G., Toivio-Kinnucan, M., Vallat, J. M., et al. 1994. Distal sensorimotor polyneuropathy in mature Rottweiler dogs. Vet Pathol 31:316–326.

Braund, K. G., et al. 1991. Distal polyneuropathy in mature Rottweiler dogs. J Vet Intern Med 5:147.

Chrisman, C. L. 2000. Polyneuropathies of cats. Small Anim Pract 41:384–389.

———. 1990. Dancing Doberman disease: clinical findings and prognosis. Prog Vet Neurol 1:83–90.

Cooper, B. L., DeLahunta, A., Cummings, I. F., et al. 1984. Canine inherited hypertrophic neuropathy: clinical and electrodiagnostic studies. Am J Vet Res 45:1172–1177

Cummings, I. F., Cooper, B. L., deLahunta, A., et al. 1981. Canine inherited hypertrophic neuropathy. Acta Neuropathol (Berl) 53:137–143.

Duncan, I. D. 1990. Peripheral neuropathy in the dog and cat. Prog Vet Neurol 2(2):111–128

Duncan, I. D., Griffiths, I. R. 1977. Canine giant axonal neuropathy. Vet Rec 101:438–441

Duncan, I. D., Griffiths, I. R., Carmichael, S., et al. 1981. Inherited canine giant axonal neuropathy. Muscle Nerve 4:223–227.

Furuoka, H., Amanai, H., Taniyama, H., et al. 1992. Peripheral neuropathy in German shepherd dogs. J Comp Pathol 107: 169–177.

Griffiths, I. R. 1989. Progressive axonopathy of Boxer dogs. In Current Veterinary Therapy X (Small Animal Practice), Kirk, R. W., ed. Philadelphia, W. B. Saunders Co 828–830.

———. 1985. Progressive axonopathy: an inherited neuropathy of boxer dogs. I: Further studies of the clinical and electrophysiological features. J Sm Anim Pract 26:381–392.

Griffiths, I. R., Duncan, I. 1979. Distal denervating disease: a degenerative neuropathy of the distal motor axon in dogs. J Sm An Prac 20:579–592.

Griffiths, I. R., Duncan, I. D., Barker, J. 1980. A progressive axonopathy of Boxer dogs affecting the central and peripheral nervous systems.J Sm An Prac 21:29–43.

Henricks, P. M., Steiss, J., Petterson, J. R. 1987. Distal peripheral polyneuropathy in a Great Dane. Can Vet J 28;4:165–167.

LaHue, T. R. 1995. Laryngeal paralysis. Semin Vet Med Surg (Small Anim) 10:94–100

Matz, M. E., Shell, L., Braund, K. 1990. Peripheral hypomyelinization in two golden retriever littermates. JAVMA 197:228–230.

Moe, L. 1992. Hereditary polyneuropathy of Alaskan Malamutes. In Current Veterinary Therapy XI (Small Animal Practice), Kirk, R. W., Bonagura, J. D., eds. Philadelphia, W. B. Saunders, 1038–1039.

Moreau, P. M., Vallat, J. M., Hugon, J., et al. 1991. Peripheral and central distal axonopathy of suspected inherited origin in Birman cats. Acta Neuropathol (Berl) 82:143–146.

Newsholme, S. J., Gaskell, C. J. 1987. Myopathy with core-like structures in a dog. J Comp Pathol 97:597–600.

Reisner, I. 1991. The pathophysiologic basis of behavior problems. Vet Clin N Am (SmallAnim Pract) 21:207–224.

Robinson, R. 1992. "Spasticity" in the Devon rex cat. Vet Rec 130:302.

Sponenberg, D. P., deLahunta, A. 1981. Hereditary hypertrophic neuropathy in Tibetan Mastiff dogs. J Hered 72:287.

Wheeler, S. J., Jaggy, A., Van Nes, J., et al. 1997. Outbreak of polyneuropathy in cats related to food contaminated by salinoymycin. Proc 15th ACVIM Forum, 667.

Sensory Neuropathy

Carmichael, S., Griffiths, I. R. 1981. Case of isolated sensory trigeminal neuropathy in a dog. Vet Rec 109:280–282.

Chrisman, C. L., Platt, S. R., Chandra, A. M. S., deLahunta, A., Shelton, G. D. 1999. Sensory polyganglioradiculoneuritis in a dog. 35, 232–235.

Cummings, J. F., deLahunta, A., Braund, K. G., et al. 1983. Hereditary sensory neuropathy. Nociceptive loss andacral mutilation in pointer dogs: canine hereditary sensory neuropathy. Am J Pathol 112:136–138.

Cummings, J. F., deLahunta, A., Braund, K. G., Mitchell, W. J. 1983 Animal model of human disease: hereditary sensory neuropathy. Am J Pathol 112:136–138.

Cummings, J. F., deLahunta, A., Simpson, S. T., et al. 1984. Reduced substance P-like immunoreactivity in hereditary sensory neuropathy of pointer dogs. Acta Neuropathol (Berl) 63:33–40.

Cummings, J. F., deLahunta, A., Winn, S. S. 1981. Acral mutilation and nociceptive loss in English pointer dogs. A canine sensory neuropathy. Acta Neuropathol (Berl) 53:119–127.

Duncan, I. D., Cuddon, P. A. 1989. Sensory neuropathy. In Current Veterinary Therapy (Small Animal Practice), Kirk, R. W., ed. Philadelphia, W. B. Saunders, 822–827.

Duncan, I. D., Griffiths, I. R., Munz, M. 1982. The pathology of a sensory neuropathy affecting long haired Dachshund dogs. Acta Neuropathol (Berl) 58:141–151.

Franklin, R. J. M., Olby, N. J., Targett, M. P., Houlton, J. E. F. 1992. Sensory neuropathy in a Jack Russell terrier. J Sm An Prac 33:402–404.

Goldberger, E., Rapopory, J. L. 1991. Canine acral lick dermatitis: response to the antiobsessional drug clomipramine. J Am Anim Hosp Assoc 27:179–182.

Porter, B., Schatzberg, S., McDonough, S., Mertens, D., et al. 2002. Ganglioradiculitis (sensory neuronopathy) in a dog: clinical, morphologic, and immunohistochemical findings. Vet Pathol 39:598–602.

Steiss, J. E., Pook, H. A., Clark, E. G., Braund, K. G. 1987. Sensory neuronopathy in a dog. JAVMA 190:205–208.

van Nes, J. J. 1986. Electrophysiological evidence of sensory nerve dysfunction in 10 dogs with acral lick dermatitis. J Am Anim Hosp Assoc 22:157–160.

Wouda, W., et al. 1983. Sensory neuropathy in dogs: a study of four cases. J Comp Pathol 93:437–350.

Wheeler, S. J. 1987. Sensory neuropathy in a border colliẹ puppy. J Sm An Prac 28:281–289

Wright, J. A., Brownlie, S. 1985. Progressive ataxia in a Pyrenean mountain dog. Vet Rec 116:410–411.

Laryngeal Paralysis

Barr, S., Baker, D., Markovits, J. 1986. Trypanosomiasis and laryngeal paralysis in a dog. JAVMA 188:1307–1309.

Bennett, P. F., Clarke, R. E. 1997. Laryngeal paralysis in a rottweiler with neuroaxonal dystrophy. Aust Vet J 75:784–786.

Bjorling, D. E. 1995. Laryngeal paralysis. In Kirk's Current Veterinary Therapy XII (Small Animal Practice), Bonagura, L. D., ed. Philadelphia, W. B. Saunders, 901–905.

Braund, K. G. 1995. Laryngeal paralysis-polyneuropathy complex in young Dalmatian dogs. In Kirk's Current Veterinary Therapy XII (Small Animal Practice), Bonagura, J. D., ed. Philadelphia, W. B. Saunders, 1136–1140.

Braund, K. G., Shores, A., Cochrane, S., et al. 1994. Laryngeal paralysis-polyneuropathy complex in young Dalmatians. Am J Vet Res 55:534–542.

Braund, K. G., Steinberg, H. S., Shores, A., et al. 1989. Laryngeal paralysis in immature and mature dogs as one sign of a more diffuse polyneuropathy. JAVMA 194:1735–1740.

Burbidge, H. M. 1995. A review of laryngeal paralysis in dogs. Br Vet J 151:71–82.

Busch, D. S., Noxon, J. O., Miller, L. D. 1992. Laryngeal paralysis and peripheral vestibular disease in a cat. J Am Anim Hosp Assoc 28:82–86.

Gaber, C. E., Amis, T. C., LeCouteur, R. A. 1985. Laryngeal paralysis in dogs: a review of 23 cases. JAVMA 186:377–380.

Hardie, E. M., Kolata, R. L., Stone, E. A., et al. 1981. Laryngeal paralysis in three cats. JAVMA 179:879–882.

Lussier, B., Flanders, J. A., Erb, H. N. 1996. The effect of unilateral arytenoid lateralization on rima glortidis area in canine cadaver larynges. Vet Surg 25:121–126.

MacPhail, C. M., Monnet, E. 2001. Outcome and postoperative complications in dogs undergoing surgical treatment of laryngeal paralysis: 140 cases (1985–1998). JAVMA 218:1949–1956.

Mahony, O. M., Knowles, K. E., Braund, K. G., et al. 1998. Laryngeal paralysis-polyneuropathy complex in young Rottweilers. J Vet Intern Med 12:330–337.

O'Brien, L. A., Hendriks, L. 1986. Inherited laryngeal paralysis. Analysis in the husky cross. Vet Q 8:301–302.

Ridyard, A. E., Corcoran, B. M., Tasker, S., et al. 2000. Spontaneous laryngeal paralysis in four white-coated German shepherd dogs. J Sm An Prac 41:558–561.

Schacter, S., Norris, C. R. 2000. Laryngeal paralysis in cats: 16 cases (1990–1999). JAVMA 216:1100–1103.

Schaer, M., Zaki, F. A., Harvey, H. J., O'Reilly, W. H. 1979. Laryngeal hemiplegia due to neoplasia of the vagus nerve in a cat. JAVMA 174:513–515.

Shelton, G. D., Podell, M., Sullivan, S., et al. 2000. Distal, symmetrical polyneuropathy with laryngeal paralysis in young, related Leonberger dogs. J Vet Intern Med 14:339 (abstract).

Venker-van Haagen, A. L. 1992. Diseases of the larynx. Vet Clin N Am (Small Anim Pract) 22:1155–1172.

Venker-van Haagen, A. L., Bouw, L., Hartman, W. 1981. Hereditary transmission of laryngeal paralysis in Bouviers. J Am Anim Hosp Assoc 17:75–76.

Venker-van Haagen, A. L., Hartman, W., and Goedegebuure, S. A. 1978. Spontaneous laryngeal paralysis in young Bouviers. J Am Anim Hosp Assoc 14:714–720.

Cricopharyngeal Achalasia

Goring, R. L., Kagan, K. G. 1982. Cricopharyngeal achalasia in the dog: radiographic evaluation and surgical management. Compend Contin Educ Pract Vet 4;5:438–444.

Ladlow, J., Hardie, R. J. 2000. Cricopharyngeal achalasia in dogs. Compend Contin Educ Pract Vet 22;4:750–755.

Mattson, A. 1994. Pharyngeal disorders. Vet Clin N Am (Small Anim Pract) 24;5:825–855.

Niles, J. D., Williams, J. M., Sullivan, M., et al. 2001. Resolution of dysphagia following cricopharyngeal myectomy in six young dogs. J Sm Anim Pract 42:32–35.

Rosin, E., Hanlon, G. F. 1972. Canine cricopharyngeal achalasia. JAVMA 160;11:1496–1499.

Ryer, K. A., Ryer, J. 1980. Acquired achalasia: a case report. Vet Med November, 1703–1704.

Shelton, G. D. 1982. Swallowing disorders in the dog. Compend Contin Educ Pract Vet 4;7:607–613.

Weaver, A. D. 1983. Cricopharyngeal achalasia in Cocker spaniels. J Sm An Prac 24:209–214.

Megaesophagus

Clifford, D. H., Barboza, P. F., Pirsch, L. G. 1980. The motor nuclei of the vagus nerve in cats with and without congenital achalasia of the oesophagus. Br Vet J 136:74–83.

Cox, V. S., Wallace, L., Anderson, Y. E., et al. 1980. Hereditary esophageal dysfunction in the Miniature Schnauzer dog. Am J Vet Res 41:326–330.

Guilford, W. G. 1990. Megaesophagus in the dog and cat. Semin Vet Med Surg (Small Anim) 5:37–45

Hoenig, M., Mahaffey, M. B., Parnell, P. G., et al. 1990. Megaesophagus in two cats. JAVMA 196:763–765.

Hoffer, R. E., MacCoy, D. M., Quick, C. B., et al. 1979 Management of acquired achalasia in dogs. JAVMA 175:814–817.

Maddison, J. E., Allan, G. S. 1990. Megaesophagus attributable to lead toxicosis in a cat, J Am Vet MedAssoc 197:1357–1358.

McKerrell, R. E., Braund, K. G. 1987. Hereditary myopathy in Labrador retrievers: clinical variations, J Sm An Prac 28: 479–489.

Moses, L., Harpster, N. K., Beck, K. A., et al. 2000. Esophageal motility dysfunction in cats: a study of 44 cases. J Am Anim Hosp Assoc 36:309–312.

Peeters, M. E., et al. 1991. Dysphagia in Bouviers associated with muscular dystrophy; evaluation of 24 cases, Vet Q 13:65–73.

Stickle, R., Sparschu, G., Love, N., et al. 1992. Radiographic evaluation of esophageal function in Chinese Shar Pei pups. J Am Vet MedAssoc 201:81–84.

Strombeck, D. R. 1978. Pathophysiology of esophageal motilitiy disorders in the dog and cat. Application to management and prognosis. Vet Clin N Am (Small Anim Pract) 8:229–244.

Tan, B. J. K., Diamant, N. E. 1987. Assessment of the neural defect in a dog with idiopathic megaesophagus. Dig Dis Sci 32:76–85.

Dysautonomia

Beban, H. J., Beban, R. L. G., Lindsay, R. G., Bentall, H. P. 1987. A suspected case of feline dysautonomia, NZ Vet J 35:58.

Berghaus, R. D., O'Brien, D. R., Johnson, G. C., et al. 2001. Risk factors for development of dysautonomia in dogs. JAVMA 218;8:1285–1290.

Bjerkas, E., Skancke, E. 1994. Feline dysautonomia in Norway [letter]. Vet Rec 135:463

Bromberg, N. M., Cabaniss, L. D. 1986. Feline dysautonomia: a case report, J Am Anim Hosp Assoc 24:106–108.

Canton, D. D., Sharp, N. J., Aguirre, G. D. 1988. Dysautonomia in a cat. J Am Vet MedAssoc 192:1293–1296

Detweiler, D. A., Biller, D. S., Hoskinson, J. J., Harkin, K. R. 2001. Radiographic findings of canine dysautonomia in twenty-four dogs. Vet Radiol Ultrasound 42:108–112.

Griffiths, I. R., Nash, A. S., Sharp, N. J. H. 1982. The Key-Gaskell syndrome: the current situation, Vet Rec 111:532–533.

Griffiths, I. R., Sharp, N. J. H., McCulloch, M. C. 1985. Feline dysautonomia (the Key-Gaskell syndrome): an ultra structural study of autonomic ganglia and nerves, Neuropathol Appl Neurobiol 11:17–29.

Harkin, K. R., Andrews, G. A., Nietfeld, J. C. 2002. Dysautonomia in dogs: 65 cases (1993–2000). JAVMA 220:633–630.

Harkin, K. R., Nietfeld, J., Fischer, J. R. 2002. Dysautonomia in a family of German shorthaired pointers. J Am Anim Hosp Assoc 38:55–59.

Goodman, M. M., Clark, M. I., Warner, K. 1998. Key-Gaskell syndrome in three cats [letter]. Vet Rec 143:428.

Guilford, W. G., O'Brien, D. R., Allert, A., et al. 1988. Diagnosis of dysautonomia in a cat by autonomic nervous system function testing. JAVMA 193:823–828.

Key, T. J. A. , Gaskell, C. J. 1982. Puzzling syndrome in cats associated with pupillary dilation, Vet Rec 110:160.

Levy, J. K., James, K. M., Cowgill, L. D., et al. 1994. Decreased urinary catecholamines in a cat with dysautonomia. JAVMA 205:842–844.

Longshore, R. C., O'Brien, D. R., Johnson, G. C., et al. 1996. Dysautonomia in dogs: a retrospective study. J Vet Intern Med10:103–109.

Nash, A. S., Griffiths, I. R., Sharp, N. J. H. 1982. The Key-Gaskell syndrome: an autonomic polyganglionopathy. Vet Rec 111:307–308.

Pollin, M., Sullivan, M. 1986. A canine dysautonomia resembling the Key-Gaskell syndrome. Vet Rec 118:402–403.

Presthus, J., Bjerkas, I. 1987. Canine dysautonomia in Norway. Vet Rec 120:463–464.

Rochlitz, L., Bennett, A. M. 1983. Key-Gaskell syndrome in a bitch. Vet Rec 112:614–615.

Schrauwen, E., Van Ham Lo Maenhout, T., et al. 1991. Canine dysautonomia: a case report. Vet Rec 128:524–525.

Sharp, N. J. 1990. Feline dysautonomia. Semin Vet Med Surg (Small Anim) 5:67–71.

Sharp, N. J., Nash, A. S., Griffiths, I. R. 1984. Feline dysautonomia (the Key-Gaskell syndrome): a clinical and pathological study of forty cases. J Sm An Prac 25:599–615.

Schoen, A. M. 1991. Decision-making concerning pets with loss of autonomic function. Probl Vet Med 3;1:61–72.

Symonds, H. W., McWilliams, R., Thompson, H., et al. 1995. A cluster of cases of feline dysautonomia (Key-Gaskell syndrome) in a closed colony of cats. Vet Rec 136:353–355.

Wise, L. A., Lappin, M. R. 1991. A syndrome resembling feline dysautonomia (Key-Gaskell syndrome) in a dog. Am Vet Med Assoc 198:2103–2106.

———. 1990. Canine dysautonomia. Semin Vet Med Surg (Small Anim) 5:72–74.

Exercise Induced Collapse in Labrador Retrievers

Shelton, G. D., Taylor, S. M. 2002. The syndrome of exercise induced collapse in Labrador retrievers. Proc 20th ACVIM Forum, Dallas, TX, 317–318.

Taylor, S. M., Shelton, G. D. 2002. The syndrome of exercise induced collapse in Labrador retrievers. Proc 20th ACVIM Forum, Dallas, TX, 315–316.

Exertional Rhabdomyolysis

Gannon, J. R. 1980. Exertional rhabdomyolysis (myoglobinuria) in the racing greyhound. In Current Veterinary Therapy VII: Small Animal Practice, Kirk, R. W., ed. Philadelphia, W. B. Saunders, 783–787.

Porzio, P., Render, J. A., Baptiste, K. E. 1997. Exertional rhabdomyolysis in an adult Siberian husky. J Vet Med Emerg Crit Care 7; 1:43–48.

Spangler, W. L., Muggli, F. M. 1978. Seizure-induced rhabdomyolysis accompanied by acute renal failure in a dog, JAVMA 172:1190–1194.

Malignant Hyperthermia

Bagshaw, R. J., Cox, R. H., Knight, D. H., et al. 1978. Malignant hyperthermia in a greyhound. Am Vet Med Assoc 170:61–62.

Bellah, J. R., Robertson, S. A., Buergelt, C. D., et al. 1989. Suspected malignant hyperthermia after halothane anesthesia in a cat. Vet Surg 18; 6:483–488.

DeJong, R. H., Heavner, J. E., Amory, D. W. 1974. Malignant hyperpyrexia in the cat. Anesth 41; 6:608–9.

Drobatz, K. J., Macintire, D. K. 1996. Heat-induced illness in dogs: 42 cases (1976–1993). JAVMA 209;11:1894–1899.

Duncan, K. L., Hare, W. R., Buck, W. B. 1997. Malignant hyperthermia-like reaction secondary to ingestion of hops in five dogs. JAVMA 210; 1:51–54.

Kirmayer, A. H., Klide, A. M., Purvance, J. E. 1984. Malignant hyperthermia in a dog: case report and review of the syndrome. JAVMA 185; 9:978–982.

Leary, S. L., Anderson, L. C., Manning, P. J. 1983. Recurrent malignant hyperthermia in a Greyhound. JAVMA 182; 5:521–522.

Nelson, T. E. 1991. Malignant hyperthermia in dogs. JAVMA 198; 6:989–994.

O'Brien, P. J., Cribb, P. H., White, R. J., et al. 1983. Canine malignant hyperthermia: diagnosis of susceptibility in a breeding colony. Can Vet J 24:172–177.

Rand, J. S., O'Brien, P. J. 1987. Exercise-induced malignant hyperthermia in an English Springer spaniel. JAVMA 190;8:1013–1014.

Fibrotic Myopathy

Clarke, R. E. 1989. Fibrosis and contracture of the semitendinosus muscle in a dog. Austr Vet J 66;8:259–261.

Lewis, D. D. 2000. Gracilis-semitendinosus myopathy. In Kirk's Current Veterinary Therapy XIII (Small Animal Practice), Bonagura, J. D., ed. Philadelphia, W. B. Saunders, 989–992.

———. 1988. Fibrotic myopathy of the semitendinosus muscle in a cat. JAVMA 193;2:240–241.

Lewis, D. D., Shelton, G. D., Picas, A. 1997. Gracilis or semitendinosus myopathy in 18 dogs. J Am Anim Hosp Assoc 33:177–188.

Lobetti, R. G., Hill, T. P. 1994. Sartorius muscle contracture in a dog. J S Afr Vet Assoc 65; 1:28–30.

Montgomery, R., Fitch, R. 2003. Tendon and muscle disorders. In Textbook of Small Animal Surgery, 3d ed., Slatter, D., ed. Philadelphia, W. B. Saunders, 2264–2272.

Moore, R. W., Rouse, G. P., Piermattei, D. L., Ferguson, H. R. 1981. Fibrotic myopathy of the semitendinosus muscle in four dogs. Vet Surg 10:169–174.

Norris, A. M., Pallett, L., Wilcock, H. 1980. Generalized myositis ossificans in a cat, J Am Anim Hosp Assoc 16:659–663.

Valentine, H. A., George, C., Randolph, J. F., Center, S. A., et al. 1992. Fibrodysplasia ossificans progressiva in the cat. A case report. J Vet Intern Med 6:335–340.

Vaughan, L. C. 1979. Muscle and tendon injuries in dogs. J Sm An Prac 20:711–736.

Cramping Syndromes

Andersson, B., Andersson, M. 1982. On the etiology of "Scotty cramp" and "splay"-two motoring disorders common in the Scottish terrier breed. Acta Vet Scand 23:550–558.

Furber, R. M. 1984. Cramp in Notwich terriers. Vet Rec 115:46 (letter).

Herrtage, M. E., Palmer, A. C. 1983. Episodic falling in the cavalier King Charles spaniel. Vet Rec 112:,458–459.

Joshua, J. O. 1956. Scottie cramp. Vet Rec 68:411–412.

Meyers, K. M., Dickson, W. M., Lund, J. E., et al. 1971. Muscular hypertonicity: episodes in Scottish terrier dogs. Arch Neurol 25:61–68.

Meyers, K. M., Lund, J. E., Padgett, G., et al. 1969. Hyperkinetic episodes in Scottish terrier dogs. JAVMA 155;2:129–133.

Meyers, K. M., Padgen, G. A., Dickson, W. M. 1970. The genetic basis of a kinetic disorder of Scottish terrier dogs. J Heter 61:189–192.

Meyers, K. M., Schaub, R. G. 1974. The relationship of serotonin to a motor disorder of Scottish terrier dogs. Life Sci 14:1895–1906.

Peeters, R. I., Meyers, K. M. 1977. Precursor regulation of serotonergic neuronal function in Scottish terrier dogs. J Neurochem 29:753–755.

Smythe, R. H. 1945. Recurrent tetany in the dog. Vet Rec 32;57:380.

Woods, C. B. 1977. Hyperkinetic episodes in two Dalmatian dogs. J Am Anim Hosp Assoc 13:255–257.

Wright, J. A., Brownlie, S. E., Smyth, J. B. A., et al. 1986. Muscle hypertonicity in the cavalier King Charles spaniel—myopathic features. Vet Rec 118:511–512.

Wright, J. A., Smyth, J. B. A., Brownlie, S. E., et al. 1987. A myopathy associated with muscle hypertonicity in the cavalierKing Charles spaniel. J Comp Path 97:559–565.

Myotonia

Amann, J. F.,Tomlinson, J., Hankison, J. K. 1985. Myotonia in a Chow Chow. JAVMA 187;4:415–417.

Berardinelli, A., Gorni, K., Orcesi, S. 2000 Response to carbamazepine of recessive-type myotonia congenita. Muscle Nerve January: 138–139.

Duncan, I. D., Griffiths, I. R. 1975. A myopathy associated with myotonia in the dog. Acta Neuropath (Berl) 31:297–303.

Farrow, B. R., Malik, R. 1981. Hereditary myotonia in the chow chow, J Sm An Prac 22:451–465.

Griffiths, I. R., Duncan, I. D. 1973. Myotonia in the dog: a report of four cases. Vet Rec 93:184–188.

Harrington, M. L., Moore, M. P., Talcott, P. A., Bagley, R. S., Sandmeier, P. 1996. Suspected herbicide toxicosis in a dog. JAVMA 209:2085–2087.

Hickford, F. H., Jones, B. R. 2000. Congenital myotonia in the cat. In Kirk's Current Veterinary Therapy XIII (Small Animal Practice), Bonagura, J. D., ed. Philadelphia, W. B. Saunders, 987–989.

Hickford, F. H., Jones, B. R., Gething, M. A., et al. 1998. Congenital myotonia in related kittens. J Sm Anim Pract 39:281–285.

Hill, S. L., Shelton, G. D., Lenehan, T. M. 1995. Myotonia in a Cocker Spaniel. J Am Anim Hosp Assoc 31:506–509.

Honhold, N., Smith, D. A. 1986. Myotonia in the Great Dane. Vet Rec 119; 7:162.

Jones, H. R., et al. 1977 Myotonia in related chow chow dogs. N Z Vet J 25:217–220.

Koch, M. C., Steinmeyer, K., Lorenz, C. 1992. The skeletal muscle chloride channel in dominant and recessive human myotonia. Science 257;7:797–800.

Kortz, G. 1989. Canine myotonia. Sem Vet Med Surg (Sm Anim) 4;2:141–145.

Rhodes, T. H., Vite, C. H., Giger, U., et al. 1999. A missense mutation in canine CIC-1 causes recessive myotonia congenita in the dog. FEBS letters 456:54–58.

Sasaki, R., Ichiyasu, H., Ito, N., et al. 1999. Novel chloride channel gene mutations in two unrelated Japanese families with Becker's autosomal recessive generalized myotonia. Neuromusc Disord 9:587–592.

Shires, P. K., Nafe, L. A., Hulse, D. A. 1983. Myotonia in a Staffordshire terrier. JAVMA 183:229–232.

Shores, A., Redding, R. W., Braund, K. G., et al. 1986. Myotonia congenita in a Chow Chow pup. JAVMA 188;5:532–533.

Simpson, S. T., Braund, K. G. 1985. Myotonic dystrophy-like disease in a dog. JAVMA 186;5:495–498.

Steiss, J. E., Braund, K. G., Clark, E. A. 1987. Neuromuscular effects of acute 2,4 dichlorophenoxyacetic acid (2,4-D) exposure in dogs. J Neurol Sci 78:295–301.

Toll, J., Cooper, B., Altschul, M. 1998. Congenital myotonia in 2 domestic cats. J Vet Intern Med 12:116–119.

Vite, C. H., Cozzi, F., Rich, M., et al. 1998. Myotonic myopathy in a Miniature Schnauzer: case report and data suggesting abnormal chloride conductance across the muscle membrane. J Vet Intern Med 12:394–397.

Vite, C. H., Melniczek, J., Patterson, D., et al. 1999. Congenital myotonic myopathy in the Miniature Schnauzer:An autosomal recessive trait. J Hered 90;5:578–580.

Zhang, J., Bendahhou, S., Sanguinetti, M. C., et al. 2000. Functional consequences of chloride channel gene (CICN1) mutations causing myotonia congenita. Neurology 54:937–942.

Zhang, J., Sanguinetti, M. C., Kwiecinski, H., et al. 2000. Mechanism of inverted activation of CIC-1 channels caused by a novel myotonia congenira mutation. J Bio Chem 275; 4:2999–3005.

Feline Hyperesthesia

Chrisman, C. L. 1991. Self-mutilation. In Problems in Small Animal Neurology, 2d ed., Chrisman, C. L., ed. Philadelphia, Lea & Febiger, 469–477.

March, P. A., Fischer, J. R., Porthoff, A. 1999. Electromyographic and histologic abnormalities in epaxial muscles of cats with feline hyperesthesia syndrome. J Vet Intern Med 13:238 (abstract).

Quesnel, A. D., Parent, J. M. 1997. Diagnostic approach and medical treatment of seizure disorders. In Consultations in Feline Internal Medicine, August, 3d ed., J. R., ed. Philadelphia, W. B. Saunders, 389–402.

Reflex Sympathetic Dystrophy

Kasdan, M. L., Johnson, A. L. 1998. Reflex sympathetic dystrophy. Occup Med 13:521–531.

LaBarre, A., Coyne, B. E. 1999. Reflex sympathetic dystrophy in a dog. J Am Anim Hosp Assoc 35:229–231.

Parrillo, S. J. 1998. Reflex sympathetic dystrophy in children. Pediatr Emerg Care 14:217–220.

Schwartzman, R. J., McLellan, T. L. 1987. Reflex sympathetic dystrophy, a review. Arch Neurol 44:555.

Peripheral Nerve Trauma

Basinger, R. R., Aron, O. N., Crowe, D. T., et al. 1987. Osteofascial compartment syndrome in the dog. Vet Surg 1 16:427–434.

Chambers, I. N., Hardie, E. M. 1986. Localization and management of sciatic nerve injury due to ischial or acetabular fracture. J Am Anim Hosp Assoc 22:539–544.

DeHaan, J., Beale, B. S. 1993. Compartment syndrome in the dog: case report and literature review. J Am Anim Hosp Assoc 29:134–140.

Fanton, J. W., Blass, C. E., Withrow, S. J. 1983. Sciatic nerve injury as a complication of intramedullary pin fixation of femoral fractures. J Am Anim Hosp Assoc 19:687–694.

Gilmore, D. R. 1984. Sciatic nerve injury in twenty-nine dogs. J Am Anim Hosp Assoc 20:403–407.

Sorjonen, O. C., Milton, J. L., Steiss, J. E., et al. 1990. Hip dysplasia with bilateral ischiatic nerve entrapment in a dog. JAVMA 197:495–497.

Tollens, T., Lanzing, H., Broos, P. 1998. The pathophysiology of the acute compartment syndrome. Acta Chirurg 98:171–175.

Brachial Plexus Trauma

Bailey, C. S. 1984. Patterns of cutaneous anesthesia associated with brachial plexus avulsions in the dog. JAVMA 185:889–899.

Baiiey, C. S., Kitchen, R. L. 1987. Cutaneous sensory testing in the dog. J Vet Intern Med 1:128–135

Bailey, C. S., Kitchen, R. L., Johnson, R. D. 1982. Spinal nerve root origins of the cutaneous nerves arising from the canine brachial plexus. Am J Vet Res 43:820–825.

Casaus, J. U., Ezquerra, L. J., Vives, M. A., et al. 1991. Treatment of distal radial paralysis by implantation of the palmar branch of the ulnar nerve; Compared to transposition of the humeral head of the flexor carpi ulnaris muscle. Prog Vet Neurol 2:269–278.

Dewey, C. W. 2000. Peripheral nerve surgery. In Veterinary Surgical Secrets, Harari, J., ed. Philadelphia, Hanley & Belfus, Inc., 324–325.

Griffiths, I. R. 1977. Avulsion of the brachial plexus in the dog. In Current Veterinary Therapy VI (Small Animal Practice). Kirk, R. W., ed. Philadelphia, W. B. Saunders, 828–831.

Griffiths, I. R. 1974a. Avulsion of the brachial plexus: 1. Neuropathology of the spinal cord and peripheral nerves. J Sm An Prac 15:165–176.

———. 1974b. Avulsion of the brachial plexus: 2. Clinical aspects. J Sm An Prac 15:177–182.

Kitchen, R. L., Canton, D. D., Johnson, R. D., et al. 1982. Electrophysiologic studies of cutaneous nerves of the forelimb of the cat. Comp Neurol 210:400–410.

Rodkey, W. G. 1993. Peripheral nerve surgery. In Textbook of Small Animal Surgery, 2d ed. Slatter, D., ed. Philadelphia, W. B. Saunders, 1135–1141.

Sharp, N. J. H. 1998. Disorders of the peripheral nervous system. ACVS Veterinary Symposium (26th Annual Surgical Forum, 33rd Annual Scientific Meeting), 84–86.

Shores, A. 1998. Nervous system, In Current Techniques in Small Animal Surgery, 4th ed. Bojrab, M. J., Ellison, G. W., Slocum, B., eds. Baltimore, Williams & Wilkins, 73–82.

Steinberg, H. S. 1979. The use of electrodiagnostic techniques in evaluating traumatic brachial plexus root injuries. J Am Anim Hosp Assoc 15:621–626.

———. 1988. Brachial plexus injuries and dysfunctions. Vet Clin N Am (Small Anim Pract) 18:565–580.

Wheeler, S. J., Clayton-Jones, D. G., Wright, J. A. 1986. The diagnosis of brachial plexus disorders in dogs: a review of twenty-two cases. J Sm Anim Pract 27:147–157.

Muscle Trauma

Bennett, R. A. 1986. Contracture of the infraspinatus muscle in dogs: a review of 12 cases. J Am Anim Hosp Assoc 22:481–487.

Bonneau, N. H., Olivieri, M., Breton, L. 1983. Avulsion of the gastrcnemius tendon in the dog causing flexion of the hock and digits. J Am Anim Hosp Assoc 19:717–722.

Braund, K. G., Shires, P. K., Mikeal, R. L. 1980. Type I fiber atrophy in the vastus lateralis muscle in dogs with femoral fractures treated by hyperextension. Vet Pathol 17:164–176.

Breur, G. J., Blevins, W. E. 1997. Traumatic injury of the iliopsoas muscle in three dogs. JAVMA 210; 11:1631–1634.

Bruce, W. J., Spence, S., Miller, A. 1977. Teres minor myopathy as a cause of lameness in a dog. J Sm Anim Pract 38:74–77.

Carberry, C. A., Gilmore, D. R. 1986. Infraspinatus muscle contracture associated with trauma in a dog. JAVMA 188; 5:533–534

Mughannam, A. J., Reinke, J. D. 1994. Avulsion of the gastrocnemius tendon in three cats. J Am Anim Hosp Assoc 30:550–556.

Reinke, J. D., Mughannam, A. J., Owens, J. M. 1993. Avulsion of the gastrocnemius tendon in 11 dogs. J Am Anim Hosp Assoc 29:410–418.

Rewerts, J. M., Grooters, A. M., Payne, J. T., et al. 1997. Atraumatic rupture of the gastrocnemius muscle after corticosteroid administration in a dog. JAVMA 210; 5:655–657.

Robinson, A. 1999. Atraumatic bilateral avulsion of the origins of the gastrocnemius muscle. J Sm Animal Pract 40:498–500.

Siems, L. L., Breur, G. J., Blevins, W. E., et al. 1998. Use of two-dimensional real-time ultrasonography for diagnosing contracture and strain of the infraspinatus muscle in a dog. JAVMA 212; 1:77–80.

Watt, P. R. 1992. Posttraumatic myositis ossificans and fibrotic myopathy in the rectus gemoris muscle in a dog: a case report and literature review. J Am Anim Hosp Assoc 28:560–564.

Tail Injury

Steiss, J., Braund, K., Wright, J., et al. 1999. Coccygeal muscle injury in English pointers (limber tail). J Vet Intern Med 13:540–548.

Steiss, J. E., Braund, K. G. 1997. Frozen tail or limber tail in working dogs. Vet Rec 141; 7:179 (letter).

Toxic Neuropathies and Myopathies

Gunn, G. J., Rafferty, A. G., Rafferty, G. C., et al. 1992. Fatal canine neurotoxicosis attributed to blue-green algae (cyanobacteria). Vet Rec 130:301–302.

Maddison, J. E., Allan, G. S. 1990. Megaesophagus attributable to lead toxicosis in a cat. JAVMA 197:1357–1358.

Botulism

Barsanti, JA. 1998. Botulism. In Infectious Diseases of the Dog and Cat, 2d ed. Greene, C. E., ed. Philadelphia, W. B. Saunders, 263–267.

Barsanti, J. A., Walser, M., Hatheway, C. L., et al. 1978. Type C botulism in American Foxhounds. JAVMA 172:809–813.

Blakemore, W. F., Rees-Evans, E. T., Wheeler, P. E. G. 1977. Botulism in foxhounds. Vet Rec 100:57–58.

Coleman, E. S. 1998. Clostridial neurotoxins: tetanus and botulism. Comp Cont Ed Pract Vet 20;10:1089–1096.

Comelissen, J. M., Haagsma, J., van Nes, J. J. 1985. Type C botulism in five dogs. J Am Anim Hosp Assoc 21:401–404.

Darke, P. G. G., Roberts, T. A., Smart, J. L., Bradshaw, P. R. 1976. Suspected botulism in foxhounds. Vet Rec 99:98–99.

Kao, I., Drachman, D. B., Price, D. L. 1976. Botulinum toxin: mechanism of presynaptic blockade. Science 193:1256–1258.

van Nes, J. J., van der Most van Spijk, D. 1986. Electrophysiologic evidence of peripheral nerve dysfunction in six dogs with botulism type C. Res Vet Sci 40:372–276.

Tick Paralysis

Atwell, R. B., Campbell, F. E. 2001. Reactions to tick antitoxin serum and the role of atropine in treatment of dogs and cats with tick paralysis caused by *Ixodes holocyclus*; a pilot survey. Aust Vet J 79:394–397.

Atwell, R. B., Campbell, F. E., Evans, E. A. 2001. Prospective survey of tick paralysis in dogs. Aust Vet J 79; 6:412–418.

Ilkiw, J. E., Turner, D. M. 1987a. Infestation in the dog by the paralysis tick Ixodes holocyclus. 2: blood-gas and pH, haematological and biochemical findings. Aust Vet J 64:139–142

———. 1987b. Infestation in the dog by the paralysis tick Ixodes holocyclus. 3: respiratory effects. Aust Vet J 64:142–144.

Ilkiw, J. E., Turner, D. M., Howlett, C. R. 1987. Infestation in the dog by the paralysis tick Ixodes holocyclus. I: clinical and histological findings. Aust Vet J 64:137–139

Kocan, A. A. 1988. Tick paralysis. JAVMA 192;11:1498–1500.

Malik, R., Farrow, B. R. 1991. Tick paralysis in North America and Australia. Vet Clin N Am (Small Anim Pract) 21:157–171.

Malik, R., King, J., Allan, O. S. 1988. Mega oesophagus associated with tick paralysis in three dogs, Aust Vet Pract 18:156–159.

Nafe, L. A. 1988. Selected neurotoxins. Vet Clin N Am (Small Anim Pract) 18; 3:593–604.

Viljoen, G. I., Bezuidenhout, I. D., Oberem, P. T., et al. 1986. Isolation of a neurotoxin from the salivary glands of female Rhipicephalus evertsi evertsi. J Parasitol 72:865–874.

NMJ Toxins

Andonopoulos, A. P., Terzis, E., Tsibri, E., et al. 1994. D-penicillamine induced myasthenia gravis in rheumatoid arthritis: an unpredictable common occurrence? Clin Rheumatol 13:586–588.

Clemmons, R. M., Meyer, D. J., Sundlof, S. F., Rappaport, J. J., et al. 1984. Correction of organophosphate-induced neuromuscular blockade by diphenhydramine. Am J Vet Res 45:2167–2169.

Coleman, E. S. 1998. Clostridial neurotoxins: tetanus and botulism. Compend Contin Educ Pract Vet 20;10:1089–1096.

Fiekers, J. F. 1983a. Effects of the aminoglycoside antibiotics, streptomycin and neomycin, on neuromuscular transmission. I. Presynaptic considerations. J Pharmacol Exp Ther 225:487–495.

———. 1983b. Effects of the aminoglycoside antibiotics, streptomycin and neomycin, on neuromuscular transmission. II. Postsynaptic considerations. J Pharmacol Exp Ther 225:496–502.

Fowler, M. E. 1993. Veterinary Zootoxicology. Boca Raton, Florida, CRC Press.

Mahmood, N. A., Carmichael, W. W., Pfahler, D. 1988. Anticholinesterase poisonings in dogs from a cyanobacterial (blue-green algae) bloom dominated by Anabaena flos-aquae. Am J Vet Res 49:500–503.

Osweiler, G. D. 1996. Arachnids. In Toxicology. Philadelphia, Williams and Wilkins, 438–439.

Peterson, M. E., Meerdink, G. L. 1989. Bites and stings of venomous animals. In Current Veterinary Therapy X (Small Animal Practice), Kirk, R. W., ed. Philadelphia, W. B. Saunders, 177–186.

Pritchard, C. W. 1940 Black widow spider and snake venom in small animals. JAVMA 96:356 358.

Twedt, D. C., Cuddon, P. A., Horn, T. W. 1999. Black widow spider envenomation in a cat. J Vet Intern Med 13:613–616.

Toxic Neuropathies

Gunn, G. J., Rafferty, A. G., Rafferty, G. C., et al. 1992. Fatal canine neurotoxicosis attributed to blue-green algae (cyanobacteria). Vet Rec 130:301–302.

Maddison, J. E., Allan, G. S. 1990. Megaesophagus attributable to lead toxicosis in a cat. JAVMA 197:1357–1358.

Snake Envenomenation

Chrisman, C. L., Hopkins, A. L., Ford, S. L., et al. 1996. Acute, flaccid quadriplegia in three cats with suspected coral snake envenomation. J Am Anim Hosp Assoc 32:343–349.

Kremer, K. A., Schaer, M. 1995. Coral snake (Micrurus fulvius fulvius) envenomation in five dogs: present and earlier findings. J Vet Emerg Crit Care 5;1:9–15.

Marks, S. L., Mannella, C., Schaer, M. 1990. Coral snake envenomation in the dog: report of four cases and review of the literature. J Am Anim Hosp Assoc 26:629–634.

Minschin, P. J., Masci, P., Paton, D. C., et al. 1998. Snake bites recorded by veterinary practices in Australia. Aust Vet J 76:195–198.

Tetanus

Bagley, R. S., Dougherty, S. A., Randolph, J. F. 1994. Tetanus subsequent to ovariohysterectomy in a dog. Prog Vet Neur 5;2:63–65.

Baker, J. L., Waters, D. J., deLahunta, A. 1988. Tetanus in two cats. J Amer An Hospital Assoc 24:159–164.

Coleman, E. S. 1998. Clostridial neurotoxins: tetanus and botulism. Comp Cont Ed Pract Vet 20;10:1089–1096.

Dieringer, T. M., Wolf, A. M. 1991 Esophageal hiatal hernia and megaesophagus complicating tetanus in two dogs. J Vet Med Assoc 199:87–89.

Godwin, R. L. G. 1985. Tetanus in a cat. Vet Rec 116; 21:574 (letter).

Greene, CE. 1998. Tetanus. In Infectious Diseases of the Dog and Cat, 2d ed. Greene, C. E. Philadelphia, W. B. Saunders, 267–273.

Hanson, C. J. 1982. Tetanus in a dog: a case report. Vet Rec 110:336–337.

Kazakos, G., Georgiadis, G., Sabasias, N. 2001. Local tetanus in the cat: a report of two cases. J Vet Intern Med 15; 1:81.

Malik, R., Church, D. B., Maddison, J. E., Farrow, B. R. 1989. Three cases of local tetanus. J Sm An Prac 30:469–473.

Matthews, B. R., Forbes, D. C. 1985. Tetanus in a dog. Can Vet J 26:159–161.

Panciera, D. L., Baldwin, C. J., Keene, B. W. 1988. Electrocardiographic abnormalities associated with tetanus in two dogs. JAVMA 192:225–227.

Ratcliffe I. 1989. Tetanus in a dog. Vet Rec 124:666.

Robinson, L. R. 1985. Tetanus in a cat. Vet Rec 116; 26:699 (letter).

Ryer, K. A. 1979. Tetanus in a dog. Vet Med June: 830–832

Stogdale, L. 1976. Canine tetanus. S Afr Vet Assoc 47;4:299–302.

Saranta, J. T. 1977. Tetanus in a cat. Am Vet Med Assoc 170;1:3 (letter).

Van Ham, L., van Bree, H. 1992. Conservative treatment of tetanus associated with hiatus hernia and gastro-oesophageal reflux, J Sm An Prac 33:289–294.

Zontine, W. J., Uno, T. 1968. Tetanus in a dog: a case report. Vet Med 63; 4:341–344.

Vascular Neuropathies and Myopathies

Atkins, C. E., Gallo, A. M., Kurzman, I. D., Cowen, P. 1992. Risk factors, clinical signs, and survival in cats with a clinical diagnosis of idiopathic hypertrophic cardiomyopathy: 74 cases (1985–1989). JAVMA 201:613–618.

Dillon, A. R., Braund, K. G. 1982. Distal polyneuropathy after canine heartworm disease therapy complicated by disseminated intravascular coagulation. JAVMA 181:239–242.

Flanders, J. A. 1986. Feline aortic thromboembolism. Compend Contin Educ Pract Vet 8:473–484.

Griffiths, I. R., Duncan, I. D. 1979d. Ischaemic neuromyopathy in cats. Vet Rec 104:518–522.

Langelier, R. M. 1982. Ischemic neuromyopathy associated with steel pellet BB shot: aortic obstruction in a cat. Can Vet J 23:187–189.

Tilley, L. P., Liu, S-K. 1975. Cardiomyopathy and thromboembolism in the cat. Feline Pract 5:32–41. .

Muscle Hemorrhage

Dueland, R. T., Wagner, S. D., Parker, R. B. 1990. Von Willebrand heterotopic osteochondrofibrosis in Doberman pinschers: five cases (1980–1987). JAVMA 197:383–388.

Diagnostic Testing

Adams, R. D., Victor, M. 1993. In Principles of Neurology, 5th ed., Adams, R. D., and Victor, M., eds. New York, McGraw-Hill, 10–15.

Bagley, R. S. 2003a. How to obtain a CSF sample in dogs and cats. Vet Med, June, 475–486.

———. 2003b. Interpreting the result of CSF analysis in dogs and cats. Vet Med, June, 499–506.

———. 2003c. Intracranial surgery. In Textbook of Small Animal Surgery, 3d ed., Slatter, D., ed. Philadelphia, W. B. Saunders, 1261–1276.

Bagley, R. S., Baszler, T. V., Harrington, M. L., et al. 1995a. Clinical effects of longitudinal division of the corpus callosum in dogs. Vet Surg 24:122–127.

Bagley, R. S., Harrington, M. L., Pluhar, G. E., Gavin, P. R., Moore, M. P. 1997. Acute, unilateral transverse sinus occlusion during craniectomy in 7 dogs with space-occupying intracranial disease. Vet Surg, 26:195–201.

Bagley, R. S., Harrington, M. L., Pluhar, G. E., Keegan, R. D., Greene, S. A., Moore, M. P., Gavin, P. R.. 1996a. Effect of craniectomy/durotomy alone or in combination with hyperventilation, diuretics, and corticosteroids on intracranial pressure in normal dogs. Am J Vet Res 57:116–119.

Bagley, R. S., Keegan, R. D., Greene, S. A., et al. 1995b. Intraoperative intracranial pressure monitoring in five dogs with structural brain disease. JAVMA 207:588–591.

Bagley, R. S., Keegan, R. D., Greene, S. A., Harrington M. L., Moore, M. P. 1995c. Pathologic effects in brain following intracranial pressure monitoring in normal dogs using a fiberoptic monitoring system. Am J Vet Res 56:1475–1478.

Bagley, R. S., Kornegay, J. N., Wheeler, S. J., Plummer, S. B., Cauzinille, L. 1993. Generalized tremor in Maltese terriers: a retrospective study of 7 cases (1984–1990). JAAHA 29:141–145.

Bagley, R. S., Tucker, R. T., Gavin, P. R., Keegan, R. D., Greene, S. A. 1997. Transcranial Doppler measurements of intracranial blood flow during increasing intracranial pressure in dogs: preliminary results of waveform analysis. J Vet Intern Med 11:119.

Bagley, R. S., Tucker, R., Harrington, M. L. 1996. Lateral and foraminal disk extrusions in dogs. Compend Contin Educ Pract 18:795–804.

Bailey, C. S., Higgins, R. J. 1986. Characteristics of cisternal cerebrospinal fluid associated with primary brain tumors in the dog: a retrospective study. JAVMA 4:414.

Baroni, M., Heinold Y. 1995. A review of the clinical diagnosis of feline infectious peritonitis viral meningoencephalomyelitis. Prog Vet Neurol 6:88–94.

Bennett, P. F., Allan, F. J., Guilford, W. G., Julian, A. F., et al. 1997. Idiopathic eosinophilic meningoencephalitis in Rottweiler dogs: three cases. Aust Vet J 75:786–789.

Berry, C. R. 2002. Physical principles of computed tomography and magnetic resonance imaging. In Text of Veterinary Diagnostic Radiology, 4th ed., Thrall, D. E., ed., Philadelphia, W. B. Saunders, 28–35

Bichsel, P., Vandevelde, M., Vandevelde, E., Affolter, U., Pfister, H. 1984. Immunoelectrophoretic determination of albumin and IgG in serum and cerebrospinal fluid in dogs with neurological diseases. Res Vet Sci 37:101–7.

Bienzle, D., McDonnell, J. J., Stanton, J. B. 2000 Analysis of cerebrospinal fluid from dogs and cats after 24 and 48 hours of storage. JAVMA 216:1761–4.

Bohn, A. A., Bagley, R. S., Bohn, A. A. 2003. CSF sample handling and examination. Vet Med, June, 488–498.

Braund, K. G. 1994. Clinical Syndromes in Veterinary Neurology. 2d ed. St. Louis, Mosby.

———. 1991. Nerve and muscle biopsy techniques. Prog Vet Neurol 2:35.

Bush, W. W., Barr, C. S., Darrin, E. W., Shofer, F. S., Vite, C. H., Steinburg, S. A. 2002. Results of cerebrospinal fluid analysis, neurologic examination findings, and age of onset of seizures as predictors for results of magnetic resonance imaging of the brain in dogs examined. JAVMA 220:781–783.

Cardoso, E. R., Rowan, J. O., Galbraith, S. 1983. Analysis of the cerebrospinal fluid pulse wave in intracranial pressure. J Neurosurg 59:817–821.

Carrillo, J. M., Sarfaty, D., Greenlee, P. 1986. Intracranial neoplasm and associated inflammatory response from the central nervous system. J Am Anim Hosp Assoc 22:367.

Chrisman, C. L. 1992. Cerebrospinal fluid analysis. Vet Clin N Am 22:781–810.

———. 1991. Problems in Small Animal Neurology. Philadelphia, Lea & Febiger.

———. 1983. Cerebrospinal fluid evaluation. In Kirk, R. W., ed. Current Veterinary Therapy. Philadelphia, W. B. Saunders, 676–681.

Christopher, M. M., Perman, V., Hardy, R. M. 1988. Reassessment of cytologic values in canine cerebrospinal fluid by use of cytocentrifugation. JAVMA 171:1726–1729.

Cook, J. R., Jr., DeNicola, D. B. 1988. Cerebrospinal fluid. Vet Clin N Am (Small Anim Pract) 18:475–99.

Cuddon, P. A. 1998. Electrophysiologic assessment of acute polyradiculoneuropathy in dogs: comparison with Guillain-Barrá syndrome in people. J Vet Intern Med 12:294–303.

Daniel, G. B., Twardoock, A. R., Tucker, R. L., et al. 1992. Brain scintigraphy. Prog Vet Neurol 3:25–34.

deLahunta, A. 1983. Veterinary Neuroanatomy and Clinical Neurology, 2d ed. Philadelphia, W. B. Saunders.

Dewey, C. L. 2003. In A Practical Guide to Canine and Feline Neurology, Dewey, C. W., ed. Ames, Iowa State Press.

Dykes, N. L., Warnick, L. D., Summers, B. A., et al. 1994. Retrospective analysis of brain scintigraphy in 116 dogs and cats. Vet Rad Ultrasound 35:59–65.

Fischer, A., Obermaier, G. 1994. Brainstem auditory-evoked potentials and neuropathologic correlates in 26 dogs with brain tumor. J Vet Intern Med 8:363.

Forrest, L. J. 2002 The cranial and nasal cavities—canine and feline. In Text of Veterinary Diagnostic Radiology, 4th ed., Thrall, D. E., ed. Philadelphia, W. B. Saunders, 71–86.

Gallagher, J. G., Penninck, D., Boudrieau, R. J., Schelling, S. H., et al. Ultrasonography of the brain and vertebral canal in dogs and cats: 15 cases (1988–1993). JAVMA 207:1320.

Germon, K. 1988. Interpretation of ICP pulse waves to determine intracerebral compliance. J Neurosci Nurs 20:344–349.

Harrington, M. L., Bagley, R. S., Moore, M. P., Tyler, J. W. 1996. Effect of craniectomy, durotomy and wound closure on intracranial pressure in healthy cats. AJVR 57:1659–1661.

Hassler, W., Steinmetz, H., Gawlowski, J. 1988. Transcranial Doppler ultrasonography in raised intracranial pressure and in intracranial circulatory arrest. J Neurosurg 68:745–751.

Hoerlein, B. F. 1978. Canine Neurology Diagnosis and Treatment, 3d ed. Philadelphia, W. B. Saunders, 143–145.

———. 1965.Laboratory examinations. In Canine Neurology, Diagnosis and Treatment, Hoerlein, B. F., ed. Philadelphia, W. B. Saunders, 50–54.

Holliday, T. A. 1992. Electrodiagnostic evaluation, Somatosensory evoked potentials and electromyography. Vet Clin N Am 22:833.

Holliday, T. A., Nelson, H. J., Williams, D. C., Willits, N. 1992. Unilateral and bilateral brainstem auditory-evoked response abnormalities in 900 Dalmatian dogs. J Vet Intern Med 6:166–174.

Hopkins, A. L., Howard, J. F., Wheeler, S. J., Kornegay, J. N. 1993. Stimulated single fibre electromyography in normal dogs. J Sm An Prac 34:271.

Hurtt, A. E., Smith, M. O. 1997. Effects of iatrogenic blood contamination or results of cerebrospinal fluid analysis in clinically normal dogs and dogs with neurologic disease. JAVMA 211:866–867.

Iannotti, F., Hoff, J. T., Schielke, G. P. 1984. Brain tissue pressure: physiological observations in anesthetized cats. J Neurosurg 60:1219–1225.

Irving, G., McMillan, M. C. 1990. Fluoroscopically guided percutaneous fine-needle aspiration biopsy of thoracolumbar spinal lesions in cats. Prog Vet Neurol 1:473–475.

Jamison, E. M., Lumsden, J. H. 1988. Cerebrospinal fluid analysis in the dog: methodology and interpretation. Semin Vet Med Surg (Small Anim) 3:122–32.

Johnston, I. H., Johnston, J. A., Jennett, B. Intracranial-pressure changes following head injury. Lancet 2:433–436, 1970.

Keegan, R. D., Greene, S. A., Bagley, R. S., et al. 1995. Effects of medetomidine administration on intracranial pressure and cardiovascular variables of isoflurane anesthetized dogs. Am J Vet Res 56:193–98.

Knecht, C. D., Redding, R. W., Wilson, S. 1985. Characteristics of F and H waves of ulnar and tibial nerves in cats: reference values. Am J Vet Res 46:977.

Kornegay, J. N. 1981. Cerebrospinal fluid collection, examination and interpretation in dogs and cats. Comp Cont 3:85–90.

Lavely, J. A., Lipsitz, D., Williams, D. C., et al. 2003. Evaluation of jitter by stimulated single fiber electromyography in normal cats. Proc 21st ACVIM Forum, Charlotte, NC, 955.

LeCouteur, R. A., Child, G. 1995. Diseases of the spinal cord. In Ettinger, S. J., Feldman, E. C. eds. Textbook of Veterinary Internal Medicine: Disease of the Dog and Cat, ed. 4. Philadelphia, W. B. Saunders, 629–696.

Lundberg, N. 1960. Continuous recording and control of ventricular fluid pressure in neurosurgical practice. Acta Psychiatr Neurol Scand 36:1–193.

Lyons, M. K., Meyer, F. B. 1990. Cerebrospinal fluid physiology and the management of increased intracranial pressure. Mayo Clinic Proc 65:684–707.

Mayhew, I. G., Beal, C. R. 1980. Techniques of analysis of cerebrospinal fluid. Vet Clin N Am (Small Anim Pract) 10:155–76.

Meric, S. M. 1988. Canine Meningitis. Vet Int Med 2:26–35.

Meric, S. M., Perman, V., Hardy, R. M. 1985. Corticosteroid-responsive meningitis in ten dogs. JAAHA, 21:677–684.

Novak, G., Digel, C., Burns, B., James, A. E. 1974. Cerebrospinal fluid pressure measurements and radioisotope cisternography in dogs. Lab Animal 8:85–91.

Obrist, W. D., Langfitt, T. W., Jaggi, J. L., et al. 1984. Cerebral blood flow and metabolism in comatose patients with acute head injury. J Neurosurg 61:241–253.

Olby, N. J., Dyce, J., Houlton, J. E. 1994. Correlation of plain radiographic and lumbar myelographic findings with surgical findings in thoracolumbar disc disease. J Sm An Prac 35:345–350.

Oliver, J. E. 1969. Cranial sinus venography in the dog. Am J Vet Res 10:66.

Oliver, J. E., Hoerlein, B. F., Mayhew, I. G. 1987. Veterinary Neurology, Philadelphia, W. B. Saunders.

Oliver, J. E., Jr., Lorenz, M. D., Kornegay, J. N. 1997. Handbook of Veterinary Neurology, 3d ed. Philadelphia, W. B. Saunders, 341–402.

Parker, A. J. 1972. The diagnostic uses of cerebrospinal fluid. J Sm An Prac 13:607–611.

Pluhar, G. E., Bagley, R. S., Keegan, R. D., Moore, M. P. 1994. The effect of acute, unilateral transverse venous sinus occlusion on intracranial pressure in normal beagles. Vet Surg 23:425.

Rand, J. S., Parent, J., Jacobs, R., Percy, D. 1990. Reference intervals for feline cerebrospinal fluid: cell counts and cytologic features. Am J Vet Res, 51:1044–1048.

Rand, J. S., Parent, J., Percy, D., Jocobs, R. 1994. Clinical, cerebrospinal fluid, and histologic data from twenty-seven cats with primary inflammatory disease of the central nervous system. Can Vet J 35:103–109.

Redding, R. W. 1990. Electroencephalography. Prog Vet Neurol 1:181–188.

Roberts, R. E., Selcer, B. A. 1993. Myelography and epidurography. Vet Clin N Am (Small Anim Pract) 23:307–329.

Rosner, M. J., Becker, D. P. 1984. Origin and evolution of plateau waves. J Neurosurg 60:312–324.

Schirmer, R. G. 1958. Analysis of the cerebrospinal fluid: its significance in diagnosis. Mod Vet Pract 39:38–40.

Schultze, A. E., Cribb, A. E., Tvedten, H. W. 1986. Eosinophilic meningoencephalitis in a cat. J Am Anim Hosp Assoc 22:623–627.

Schulz, K., Chickering, W. R., Shell, L., et al. 1994. Fluoroscopic-guided and direct spinal cord aspiration in the normal dog. Prog Vet Neurol 5:46–48.

Shapiro, H. M. 1975. Intracranial hypertension: therapeutic and anesthetic considerations. Anesthesiology 43:445–471.

Shelton, G. D., Willard, M. D., Cardinette, G. H., and Lindstrom, J. 1990. Acquired myasthenia gravis, selective involvement of esophageal, pharyngeal, and facial muscles. J Vet Intern Med 4:281–284.

Shores, A., Jevens, D., DeCamp, C. E. 1991. Intraoperative brain pressure monitoring in the dog. Proc ACVIM Forum 9:831–83.

Simpson, S. T., Reed, R. B. 1987. Manometric values for normal cerebrospinal fluid pressure in dogs. J Am Anim Hosp Assoc 23:629–632.

Sims, M. H., Selcer, R. R. 1981. Occurrence and evaluation of a reflex-evoked muscle potential (H reflex) in the normal dog. Am J Vet Res 42:975.

Smith-Maxie, L. L., Parent, J. P., Rand, J., Wilcock, B. P., et al. 1989. Cerebrospinal fluid analysis and clinical outcome of eight dogs with eosinophilis meningoencephalomyelitis. J Vet Intern Med 3:167–174.

Sorjonen, D. C. 1987. Total protein, albumin quota, and electrophoretic patterns in cerebrospinal fluid of dogs with central nervous system disorders. Am J Vet Res 48:301.

Sorjonen, D. C., Cox, N. R., Swango, L. J. 1989. Electrophoretic determination of albumin and gamma globulin concentrations in the cerebrospinal fluid of dogs with encephalomyelitis attributable to canine distemper virus infection: 13 cases (1980–1987). JAVMA 195:977.

Sorjonen, D. C., Warren, J. N., Schultz R. D. 1981. Qualitative and quantitative determination of albumin, IgG, IgM, and IgA in normal cerebrospinal fluid of dogs. J Am Anim Hosp Assoc 17:833.

Speciale J., Steinberg, S. A., Van Winkle, T. 1995. Morbidity and mortality related to cerebellomedullary spinal tap in dogs and cats. J Vet Intern Med 9:208.

Steiss, J. E. 1984. Linear regression to determine the relationship between F-wave latency and limb length in control dogs. Am J Vet Res45:2649.

Steiss, J. E., Cox, N. R, Hathcock, J. T. 1994. Brain stem auditory-evoked response abnormalities in 14 dogs with confirmed central nervous system lesions. J Vet Intern Med8:293.

Steiss, J. E., Cox, N. R., Kneckt, C. D. 1990. Electroencephalographic and histopathologic correlations in eight dogs with intracranial meass lesions. Am J Vet Res 51:1286–1291.

Strain, G. M., Kearney, M. T., Gignac, I. J., Levesque, D. C., et al. 1992. Brainstem auditory-evoked potential assessment of congenital deafness in Dalmatians: associations with phenotypic markers, J Vet Intern Med 6:175–182.

Summers, B. A., Cummings, J. F., deLahunta, A. 1995. In Veterinary Neuropathology. St. Louis, Mosby.

Thomas, W. B., Sorjonen, D. C., Hudson, J. A., Cox, N. R. 1993a. Ultrasound-guided brain biopsy in dogs. Am J Vet Res 54:1942–1947.

Thomas, W. B., Sorjonen, D. C., Steiss, J. E. 1993b. A retrospective of 38 cases of canine distemper encephalomyelitis. JAAHA 29:129–133.

Thomson, C. E., Kornegay, J. N., Stevens, J. B. 1990. Analysis of cerebrospinal fluid from the cerebellomedullary and lumbar cisterns of dogs with focal neurologic disease: 145 cases (1985–1987). JAVMA 196:1841–1844.

Tipold, A. 1995. Diagnosis of inflammatory and infectious diseases of the central nervous system in dogs: a retrospective study. J Vet Intern Med 9:304–314.

Tipold, A., Pfister, H., Zurbriggen, A., Vandevelde, M. 1994. Intrathecal synthesis of major immunoglobulin classes in inflammatory diseases of the canine CNS. Vet Immunol Immunopathol 42:149–59.

Tucker, R. L., Bagley, R. S., Gavin, P. R., Greene, S. A., Keegan, R. D. 1997. Technical considerations in transcranial Doppler ultrasound. J Vet Intern Med 11:119.

Tyler, D. E., Lorenz, M. D., Blue, J. L., et al. 1980. Disseminated protothecosis with central nervous system involvement in a dog. JAVMA 176:987–992.

Vandevelde, M., Spano, J. S. 1977. Cerebrospinal fluid cytology in canine neurologic disease. Am J Vet Res 38:1827–1832.

van Loon, J., Shivalkar, B., Plets, C., et al. 1993. Catecholamine response to a gradual increase of intracranial pressure. J Neurosurg 79:705–709.

Vaughn, D. M., Coleman, E., Simpson, S. T., Satjawatcharaphong, C. 1988. Analysis of neurotransmitter metabolite concentrations in canine cerebrospinal fluid. Am J Vet Res 49:1302–6.

Vaughn, D. M., Coleman, E., Simpson, S. T., Whitmer, B., Satjawatcharaphong, C. 1988. A rostrocaudal gradient for neurotransmitter metabolites and a caudorostral gradient for protein in canine cerebrospinal fluid. Am J Vet Res 49:2134–37.

Walker, M. A. 2002. The vertebrae—canine and feline. In Text of Veterinary Diagnostic Radiology, 4th ed., Thrall, D. E., ed. Philadelphia, W. B. Saunders, 98–109.

Weaver, D. D., Winn, H. R., Jane, J. A. 1982. Differential intracranial pressure in patients with unilateral mass lesions. J Neurosurg 56:660–665.

Widmer, W. R., Thrall, D. E. 2002. Canine and feline intervertebral disc disease, myelography, and spinal disease. In Text of Veterinary Diagnostic Radiology, 4th ed., Thrall, D. E., ed. Philadelphia, W. B. Saunders, 28–35.

Wilson, J. W., Stevens, J. B. 1977. Effects of blood contamination on cerebrospinal fluid analysis. JAVMA 171(3):256–258.

APPENDIXES

Appendix 3 Anticonvulsants

Phenobarbital

Boothe, D. M., Simpson, G., Foster, T. 1996. Effects of serum separation tubes on serum benzodiazepine and phenobarbital concentrations in clinically normal and epileptic dogs. Am J Vet Res 57:1299–1303.

Bunch, S. E., Baldwin, B. H., Hornbuckle, W. E., et al. 1984. Compromised hepatic function in dogs treated with anticonvulsant drugs. JAVMA 184:444–448.

Chauvet, A. E., Feldman, E. C., Kass, P. H. 1995. Effects of phenobarbital administration on results of serum biochemical analyses and adrenocortical function tests in epileptic dogs. JAVMA 207:1305.

Cochrane, S. M., Parent, J. M., Black, W. D., et al. 1990. Pharmacokinetics of phenobarbital in the cat following multiple oral administration. Can J Vet Res 54:309–312.

Dayrell-Hart, B., Steinberg, S. A., Van Winkle, T. J., Farnbach, G. C. 1991. Hepatoxicity of phenobarbital in dogs: 18 cases (1985–1989). JAVMA 199:1060–1066.

Gaskill, C. L., Burton, S. A., Gelens, H. C. J., Ihle, S. L., et al. 1999. Effects of phenobarbital treatment on serum thyroxine and thyroid-stimulated hormone concentration in epileptic dogs. JAVMA 215:489–496.

Kantrowitz, L. B., Peterson, M. E., Trepanier, L. A., Melian, C., et al. 1999. Serum total thyroxine, total triiodothyronine, free thyroxine, and thyrotropin concentrations in epileptic dogs treated with anticonvulsants. JAVMA 214:1804–1808.

Levitski, R. E., Trepanier, L. A. 2000. Effects of timing of blood collection on serum phenobarbital concentrations in dogs with epilepsy. JAVMA 217:200–204.

Lord, L. K., Podell, M. 1999. Owner perception of the care of long-term phenobarbital-treated epileptic dogs. J Small Anim Pract 40:11–15.

Maguire, P. J., Fettman, M. J., Smith, M. O., Greco, D. S., et al. 2000. Effects of diet on pharmacokinetics of phenobarbital in healthy dogs. JAVMA 217:847–852.

Müller, P. B., Taboada, J., Hosgood, G., et al. 2000. Effects of long-term phenobarbital treatment on the liver in dogs. J Vet Intern Med 14:165–171.

Müller, P. B., Wolfsheimer, K. J., Taboada, J., Hosgood, G., et al. 2000. Effects of long-term phenobarbital treatment on the thyroid and adrenal axis and adrenal function tests in dogs. J Vet Intern Med 14:157–164.

Podell, M., Hadjiconstantinou, M. 1999. Low concentration of cerebrospinal fluid GABA correlate to a reduced response to phenobarbital therapy in primary canine epilepsy. J Vet Intern Med 13:89–94.

Schwartz-Porsche, D., Loscher, W., Frey, H. H. 1985. Therapeutic efficacy of phenobarbital and primidone in canine epilepsy: A comparison. J Vet Pharmacol Therap 8:113–119.

Potassium Bromide

Boothe, D. M., George, K., Couch, P., et al. 2002. Disposition and clinical use of bromide in cats. JAVMA 221:1131–1135.

Gaskill, C. L., Cribb, A. E. 2000. Pancreatitis associated with potassium bromide/phenobarbital combination therapy in epileptic dogs. Can Vet J 41:555–558.

Nichols, E. S. Trepanier, L. A., Linn, K. 1996. Bromide toxicosis secondary to renal insufficiency in an epileptic dog. J Am Vet Med Assoc 208:231–233.

Podell, M., Fenner, W. R. 1994. Use of bromide as an antiepileptic drug in dogs. Compend Cont Ed Pract Vet 16:767–774.

———. 1993. Bromide therapy in refractory canine idiopathic epilepsy. J Vet Intern Med 7:318–327.

Trepanier, L. A. 1993. Pharmokinetics and clinical use of bromide. Proc 11th ACVIM Forum 878–880.

Trepanier, L. A., Schoick, A., Schwark, W. S., et al. 1998. Therapeutic serum drug concentrations in epileptic dogs treated with potassium bromide alone or in combination with other anticonvulsants: 122 cases (1992– 1996). JAVMA 213: 1449–1453.

ohn, S. E., Morrison, W. B., Sharp, P. E. 1992. Bromide toxicosis (bromism) in a dog treated with potassium bromide for refractory seizures. JAVMA 201:468–470.

Diazepam

Center, S. A., Elston, T. H., Rowland, P. H., et al. 1996. Fulminant hepatic failure associated with oral administration of diazepam in 11 cats. JAVMA 209:618–625.

Hughes, D., Moreau, R. E., Overall, K. L., et al. 1996. Acute hepatic necrosis and liver failure associated with benzodiazepine therapy in six cats, 1986–1995. J Vet Emerg Crit Care 6;1:13–20.

Papich, M. G., Alcorn, J. 1995. Absorption of diazepam after its rectal administration in dogs. Am J Vet Res 56:1629–1636.

Primidone

Bunch, S. E., Cascleman, W. L., Baldwin, B. H., et al. 1985. Effects of long-term primidone and phenytoin administration on canine hepatic function and morphology. Am J Vet Res 46:105–115.

Clorazepate

Brown, S. A., Forrester, S. D. 1991. Serum disposition of oral clorazepate from regular-release and sustained-delivery tablets in dogs. J Vet Pharmacol Theurap 14:126–129.

Forrester, S. D., Wilcke, J. R., Jacobson, J. D., Dyer, K. R. 1993. Effects of a 44-day administration of phenobarbital on disposition of clorazepate in dogs. Am J Vet Res 54:1136–1138.

Scherkl, R., Kurudi, D., Frey, H. H. 1989. Clorazepate in dogs: Tolerance to the anticonvulsant effect and signs of physical dependence. Epilepsy Res 3:144–450.

Vigabatrin

Speciale, J., Dayrell-Hart, B., Steinberg, S. A. 1991. Clinical evaluation of gamma-vinyl-gamma-aminobutyric acid for control of seizures in dogs. JAVMA 198:995–1000.

Felbamate

Adusumalli, Y. E., Gilchrist, J. R., Wichmann, J. K., et al. 1992. Pharmacokinetics of felbamate in pediatric and adult beagle dogs. Epilepsia 33:955–960.

Adusumalli, Y. E., Yang, J. T., Wong, K. K., et al. 1991. Felbamate pharmacokinetics in the rat, rabbit, and dog. Drug Met Disp 19:1116–1125.

Dayrell-Hart, B., Tiches, D., Vite, C., et al. 1996. Efficacy and safety of felbamate as an anticonvulsant in dogs with refractory seizures. Proc 14th ACVIM Forum, 756.

Podell, M. 1997. Proc 15th ACVIM Forum, Lake Buena Vista, FL.

Ruehlmann, D., Podell, M., March, P. 2001. Treatment of partial seizures and seizure-like activity with felbamate in six dogs. J Small Anim Pract 42:403–408.

Gabapentin

Podell, M. 2001. Strategies of antiepileptic drug therapy. In Proc. 19th ACVIM Forum, Denver, CO, 430–432.

Radulovic, L. L., Turck, D., von Hodenberg. A, et al. 1995. Disposition of gabapentin (neurontin) in mice, rats, dogs, and monkeys. Drug Metab Disposition 23:441–448.

Vollmer, K. G., von Hodenberg, A., Kolle, E. U. 1986. Pharmacokinetics and metabolism of gabapentin in rat, dog and man. Drug Res 36:830–839.

Zonisamide

Matsumoto, K., Miyazaki, H., Fujii, T., et al. 1983. Absorption, distribution and excretion of 3-(sulfamoyl [^{14}C] methyl)-1,2, benzisoxasole (AD-810) in rats, dogs and monkeys and of AD-810 in men. Drug Res 33:961–968.

Perucca, E. 2000. Is there a role for therapeutic drug monitoring of new anticonvulsants? Clin Pharmacokinet 38;3: 191–204.

Podell, M. 2001. Strategies of antiepileptic drug therapy. In Proc 19th ACVIM Forum, Denver, CO, 430–432.

Walker, R. M., DiFonzo, C. J., Barsoum, N. J., et al. 1988. Chronic toxicity of the anticonvulsant zonisamide in Beagle dogs. Fundamnt Appl Toxicology 11:333–342.

Levetiracetam

Harden, C. 2001. Safety profile of levetiracetam. Epilepsia 42 (Suppl 4):36–39.

Hovinga, C. A. 2001. Levetiracetam: a novel antiepileptic drug. Pharmacotherapy 21;11: 1375–1388.

Krakow, K., Walker, M., Otoul, C., et al. 2001. Long-term continuation of levetiracetam in patients with refractory epilepsy. Neurology 56:1772–1774.

Leppik, I. E. 2001. The place of levetiracetam in the treatment of epilepsy. Epilepsia 42 (Suppl 4): 44–45.

Podell, M. 2001. Strategies of antiepileptic drug therapy. Proc 19th ACVIM Forum, Denver, CO, 430–432.

Shorvon, S. D., van Rijckevorsel, K. 2002 A new antiepileptic drug: Levetiracetam, a pyrrolidone recently licensed as an epileptic drug (Editorial). J Neurol Neurosurg Psychiatry 72: 426–428.

Status Epilepticus

Bateman, S. W., Parent, J. M. 1999. Clinical findings, treatment, and outcome of dogs with status epilepticus or cluster seizures: 156 cases (1990–1995). JAVMA 215:1463–1468.

Dewey, C. W., Ducote, J. M., Coates, J. R., et al. 1999. Intrarectally administered potassium bromide loading in normal dogs. J Vet Intern Med 13:238.

Lowenstein, D. H., Alldredge, B. K. 1998. Status epilepticus. N Engl J Med 338:970–976.

Platt, S. R., McDonnell, J. J. 2000a. Status epilepticus: clinical features and pathophysiology. Compend Cont Ed Pract Vet 22;7:660–669.

———. 2000b. Status epilepticus: managing refractory cases and treating out-of-hospital patients. Compend Cont Ed Pract Vet 22:732–741.

———. 2000c. Status epilepticus: patient management and pharmacologic therapy. Compend Cont Ed Pract Vet 22:722–729.

Podell, M. 1996. Seizures in dogs. Vet Clin N Amer (Sm Anim Pract) 26:779–809.

———. 1995. The use of diazepam per rectum at home for the acute management of cluster seizures in dogs. J Vet Intern Med 9:68–74.

Saito, M., Munana, K. R., Sharp, N. J., et al. 2001. Risk factors for development of status epilepticus in dogs with idiopathic epilepsy and effects of status epilepticus on outcome and survival time: 32 cases (1990–1996). JAVMA 219:618–623.

Steffen, F., Grasmueck, S. 2000. Propofol for treatment of refractory seizures in dogs and a cat with intracranial disorders. J Sm Anim Pract 41:496–499.

Index

Page references in *italics* denote figures.